VASCULAR DISEASES

SURGICAL & INTERVENTIONAL THERAPY

Volume 1

VASCULAR DISEASES

SURGICAL & INTERVENTIONAL THERAPY

Edited by

D. Eugene Strandness, Jr., M.D.
Professor
Department of Surgery
University of Washington School of Medicine
Chief, Division of Vascular Surgery
Department of Surgery
University of Washington Medical Center
Seattle, Washington

Arina van Breda, M.D.
Clinical Professor
Department of Radiology
George Washington University School of Medicine
Washington, D.C.
Director
Cardiovascular and Interventional Radiology
Alexandria Hospital
Alexandria, Virginia

Churchill Livingstone
New York, Edinburgh, London, Madrid, Melbourne, Tokyo

Library of Congress Cataloging-in-Publication Data

Vascular diseases : surgical and interventional therapy / edited by D.
   Eugene Strandness Jr., Arina van Breda.
       p.   cm.
   Includes bibliographical references and index.
   ISBN 0-443-08841-1
    1. Blood-vessels—Surgery. 2. Blood-vessels—Endoscopic surgery.
   3. Blood-vessels—Diseases.   I. Strandness, D. E. (Donald Eugene),
   Date.   II. Van Breda, Arina.
    [DNLM: 1. Vascular Diseases—therapy. 2. Vascular Surgery—
   methods.   WG 500 V33145 1994]
   RD598.5V3445 1994
   617.4'13—dc20
   DNLM/DLC
   for Library of Congress   93-6033
                                    CIP

© Churchill Livingstone Inc. 1994

Distributed in the United Kingdom by Churchill Livingstone, Robert Stevenson House, 1–3
Baxter's Place, Leith Walk, Edinburgh EH1 3AF, and by associated companies, branches, and
representatives throughout the world.

Accurate indications, adverse reactions, and dosage schedules for drugs are provided in this
book, but it is possible that they may change. The reader is urged to review the package information data of the manufacturers of the medications mentioned.

The Publishers have made every effort to trace the copyright holders for borrowed material. If
they have inadvertently overlooked any, they will be pleased to make the necessary arrange-
ments at the first opportunity.

Acquisitions Editor: *Nancy Mullins*
Assistant Editor: *Ann Ruzycka*
Copy Editor: *Paul Bernstein*
Production Supervisor: *Sharon Tuder*
Cover Design: *Jeannette Jacobs*

Printed in the United States of America

First published in 1994   7 6 5 4 3 2 1

To our patients,
who will benefit from continued cooperation
among those physicians involved in the care
of patients with vascular disease.

Contributors

Arthur B. Abt, M.D.
Professor, Department of Pathology, The Pennsylvania State University College of Medicine; Chief, Division of Anatomic Pathology, Department of Pathology, The Milton S. Hershey Medical Center, Hershey, Pennsylvania

Samuel S. Ahn, M.D.
Associate Professor, Department of Surgery, University of California, Los Angeles, UCLA School of Medicine, Los Angeles, California; Chief, Vascular Surgery, Olive View Medical Center, Sylmar, California

Enrico Ascer, M.D.
Professor, Department of Surgery, State University of New York Health Science Center at Brooklyn College of Medicine; Chief, Vascular Surgery Services, Maimonides Medical Center, Brooklyn, New York

Robert G. Atnip, M.D.
Associate Professor, Department of Surgery, Pennsylvania State University College of Medicine; Attending Vascular Surgeon, Milton S. Hershey Medical Center, Hershey, Pennsylvania

David J. Ballard, M.D., Ph.D.
Associate Professor, Departments of Health Evaluation Sciences and Internal Medicine, University of Virginia School of Medicine; Director, Thomas Jefferson Health Policy Institute, Charlottesville, Virginia

Dennis F. Bandyk, M.D.
Professor, Department of Surgery, University of South Florida College of Medicine; Director, Division of Surgery, Tampa, Florida

Robert E. Barton, M.D.
Fellow, Department of Radiologic Imaging, University of Texas Southwestern Medical Center at Dallas, Dallas, Texas

B. Timothy Baxter, M.D.
Assistant Professor, Department of Surgery, University of Nebraska College of Medicine, Omaha, Nebraska

Fritz R. Bech, M.D.
Fellow, Division of Vascular Surgery, Department of Surgery, University of Chicago Division of the Biological Sciences Pritzker School of Medicine, Chicago, Illinois

Hugh G. Beebe, M.D.
Associate Professor, Department of Surgery, Medical College of Ohio, Toledo, Ohio; Clinical Professor, Department of Surgery, Uniformed Services University of the Health Sciences F. Edward Hébert School of Medicine, Bethesda, Maryland; Adjunct Professor, Department of Surgery, University of Michigan School of Medicine, Ann Arbor, Michigan; Director and Chief, Division of Vascular Surgery, Jobst Vascular Center, Toledo, Ohio

Michael Belkin, M.D.
Associate Professor, Department of Surgery, Tufts University School of Medicine; Attending Surgeon, Department of Surgery, New England Medical Center, Boston, Massachusetts

William R. Bell, M.D.
Professor, Departments of Radiology, Nuclear Medicine; Edythe Harris Lucas-Clara Lucas Lynn Professor, Division of Hematology, Department of Medicine, The Johns Hopkins University School of Medicine; Director, Special Coagulation Laboratory, The Johns Hopkins Hospital, Baltimore, Maryland

Robert S. Bennion, M.D.
Associate Professor, Department of Surgery, University of California, Los Angeles, UCLA School of Medicine, Los Angeles, California; Physician Specialist, Department of Surgery, Olive View Medical Center, Sylmar, California

Thomas M. Bergamini, M.D.
Assistant Professor, Department of Surgery, University of Louisville School of Medicine, Louisville, Kentucky

Joseph Bonn, M.S.
Assistant Professor, Department of Radiology, Jefferson Medical School of Thomas Jefferson University; Attending Radiologist, Department of Radiology, Thomas Jefferson University Hospital, Philadelphia, Pennsylvania

Joseph J. Bookstein, M.D.
Professor, Department of Radiology, University of California, San Diego, School of Medicine; Chief, Cardiovascular Radiology, UCSD Medical Center, San Diego, California

Thomas C. Bower, M.D.
Assistant Professor, Department of Surgery, Mayo Graduate School of Medicine; Consultant, Division of Surgery, Mayo Clinic and Mayo Foundation, Rochester, Minnesota

David C. Brewster, M.D.
Associate Clinical Professor, Department of Surgery, Harvard Medical School; Senior Attending Surgeon, Division of Vascular Surgery, Massachusetts General Hospital, Boston, Massachusetts

W. R. Castaneda-Zuniga, M.D.
Professor and Chairman, Department of Radiology, Louisiana State University School of Medicine; Director, Department of Radiology, Medical Center of Louisiana at New Orleans, New Orleans, Louisiana

Timothy R. Cheatle, M.Ch., F.R.C.S.I.
Surgical Registrar, Vascular Surgery Unit, University College Hospital, London, England

Arun Chervu, M.D.
Assistant Professor, Division of Vascular Surgery, Department of General Surgery, University of Texas Southwestern Medical Center at Dallas Southwestern Medical School; Attending Surgeon, Parkland Memorial Hospital and Zale Lipshy University Hospital; Staff Physician, Dallas Department of Veterans Affairs Medical Center, Dallas, Texas

J. K. Chin, M.D.
Instructor, Department of Radiology, Harvard Medical School; Assistant, Division of Neuroradiology, Massachusetts General Hospital, Boston, Massachusetts

Richard W. Chitwood, M.D.
Research Fellow, Division of Vascular Surgery, Department of Surgery, Oregon Health Sciences University School of Medicine, Portland, Oregon; Resident, Department of General Surgery, St. Joseph Mercy Hospital, Ann Arbor, Michigan

Alexander W. Clowes, M.D.
Professor, Department of Surgery, University of Washington School of Medicine, Seattle, Washington

Douglas Coe, M.D.
Research Fellow, Section of Vascular Surgery, Department of General Surgery, University of Florida College of Medicine; Resident, Department of Surgery, Shands Hospital, Gainesville, Florida

Jon R. Cohen, M.D.
Associate Professor, Department of Surgery, Albert Einstein College of Medicine of Yeshiva University, Bronx, New York; Acting Chairman, Department of Surgery, Long Island Jewish Medical Center, New Hyde Park, New York

P. Macke Consigny, M.D.
Associate Professor, Department of Radiology, Jefferson Medical School of Thomas Jefferson University; Director, Physiologic Research, Thomas Jefferson Hospital, Philadelphia, Pennsylvania

Andrew H. Cragg, M.D.
Instructor, Department of Radiology, University of Minnesota Medical School—Minneapolis, Minneapolis, Minnesota

John J. Cronan, M.D.
Clinical Associate Professor, Department of Radiation Medicine, Brown University School of Medicine; Associate Director, Department of Diagnostic Imaging, Rhode Island Hospital, Providence, Rhode Island

Jack L. Cronenwett, M.D.
Professor, Department of Surgery, Dartmouth Medical School; Surgeon, Section of Vascular Surgery, Dartmouth-Hitchcock Medical Center, Lebanon, New Hampshire

Michael D. Darcy, M.D.
Associate Professor, Department of Radiology, Mallinckrodt Institute of Radiology, Washington University School of Medicine, Saint Louis, Missouri

David L. Dawson, M.D.
Assistant Professor, Department of Surgery, Uniformed Services University of the Health Sciences F. Edward Hébert School of Medicine, Bethesda, Maryland; Director, Vascular Laboratory, Wiford Hall USAF Medical Center, Lackland Air Force Base, Texas

Larry-Stuart Deutsch, M.D.
Associate Professor, Department of Radiology, University of California, Irvine, School of Medicine; Chief of Service, Cardiac/Vascular/Interventional Radiology, University of California, Irvine, Medical Center, Orange, California

Gary S. Dorfman, M.D.
Associate Clinical Professor, Department of Radiation Medicine, Brown University School of Medicine; Director, Vascular and Interventional Radiology, Department of Diagnostic Imaging, Rhode Island Hospital, Providence, Rhode Island

Janette D. Durham, M.D.
Assistant Professor, Department of Radiology, University of Colorado School of Medicine, Denver, Colorado

Joseph R. Durham, M.D.
Associate Professor, Division of Vascular Surgery, Department of Surgery, Northwestern University Medical School; Attending Surgeon and Chief, Section of Vascular Surgery, Columbus Hospital, Chicago, Illinois

John F. Eidt, M.D.
Associate Professor, Department of Surgery, University of Arkansas College of Medicine; Staff Surgeon, Department of Surgery, John L. McClellan Memorial Veterans Hospital, Little Rock, Arkansas

Bo Eklof, M.D., Ph.D.
Visiting Professor, Department of Surgery, University of Hawaii John A. Burns School of Medicine; Consultant, Department of Vascular Surgery, Straub Clinic and Hospital, Honolulu, Hawaii

Frederick S. Ey, M.D.
Assistant Professor, Division of Hematology and Medical Oncology, Department of Medicine, Oregon Health Sciences University School of Medicine, Portland, Oregon

William R. Flinn, M.D.
Associate Professor, Department of Surgery, Northwestern University Medical School; Director, Center for Vascular Research, Columbia Hospital, Chicago, Illinois

Julie A. Freischlag, M.D.
Associate Professor, Department of Vascular Surgery, Medical College of Wisconsin; Chief, Vascular Surgery, Zablocki VA Medical Center, Milwaukee, Wisconsin

Geoffrey A. Gardiner, Jr., M.D.
Associate Professor, Department of Radiology, Jefferson Medical College of Thomas Jefferson University; Director, Division of Cardiovascular Interventional Radiology, Thomas Jefferson University Hospital, Philadelphia, Pennsylvania

Stuart C. Geller, M.D.
Assistant Professor, Department of Radiology, Harvard Medical School; Associate Radiologist, Department of Radiology, Massachusetts General Hospital, Boston, Massachusetts

Mark Gennaro, M.D.
Clinical Vascular Fellow, Department of Surgery, Maimonides Medical Center, Brooklyn, New York

Bruce L. Gewertz, M.D.
Dallas B. Phemister Professor and Chairman, Department of Surgery, University of Chicago Division of the Biological Sciences Pritzker School of Medicine, Chicago, Illinois

Mark C. Goldberg, M.D.
Assistant Professor, Division of Vascular Surgery, Department of Surgery, Tufts University School of Medicine, Boston, Massachusetts

Samuel Z. Goldhaber, M.D.
Associate Professor, Department of Medicine, Harvard Medical School; Staff Cardiologist, Cardiovascular Division, Brigham and Women's Hospital, Boston, Massachusetts

Linda M. Graham, M.D.
Professor, Department of Surgery, Case Western Reserve University School of Medicine; Chief, Vascular Surgery Service, Veterans Administration Medical Center, Cleveland, Ohio

John W. Hallett, Jr., M.D.
Associate Professor, Department of Surgery, Mayo Medical School; Director of Education, Department of Surgery, and Program Director, Vascular Surgery Fellowship, Mayo Clinic, Rochester, Minnesota

Timothy R. S. Harward, M.D.
Assistant Professor, Section of Vascular Surgery, Department of Surgery, University of Florida College of Medicine; Resident, Vascular Surgery Research Fellow, Section of Vascular Surgery, Department of General Surgery, Gainesville, Florida

Thomas S. Hatsukami, M.D.
Assistant Professor, Department of Surgery, University of Washington School of Medicine; Staff Surgeon, Peripheral Vascular Service, Veterans Administration Medical Center, Seattle, Washington

Marshall E. Hicks, M.D.
Associate Professor, Section of Vascular and Interventional Radiology, Mallinckrodt Institute of Radiology, Washington University School of Medicine, Saint Louis, Missouri

Randall T. Higashida, M.D.
Associate Professor, Departments of Radiology and Neurological Surgery, University of California, San Francisco, School of Medicine, San Francisco, California

John D. Horowitz, M.D.
Fellow, Department of Surgery, Ohio State University School of Medicine; Ohio State University Hospital, Columbus, Ohio

Jill V. Hunter, M.D.
Instructor, Department of Radiology, Harvard Medical School; Staff Neuroradiologist, Department of Radiology, Massachusetts General Hospital, Boston, Massachusetts

Danna E. Johnson, M.D.
Assistant Professor, Department of Pathology, Virginia Commonwealth University Medical College of Virginia School of Medicine; Staff Pathologist, Department of Surgical Pathology, Johnston-Willis Hospital, Richmond, Virginia

John W. Joyce, M.D.
Associate Professor, Department of Cardiovascular Disease and Internal Medicine, Mayo Medical School, Rochester, Minnesota

Louis I. Juravsky, M.D.
Assistant Professor, Department of Radiology, Dartmouth Medical School; Radiologist, Department of Radiology, Dartmouth-Hitchcock Medical Center, Lebanon, New Hampshire

John A. Kaufman, M.D.
Instructor, Department of Radiology, Harvard Medical School; Assistant Radiologist, Department of Radiology, Massachusetts General Hospital, Boston, Massachusetts

Frederick S. Keller, M.D.
Professor, Department of Radiology, University of Alabama School of Medicine, University of Alabama at Birmingham; Chief, Vascular and Interventional Radiology, University of Alabama Hospital, Birmingham, Alabama

Robert L. Kistner M.D.
Clinical Professor, Department of Surgery, University of Hawaii John A. Burns School of Medicine; Consultant, Department of Vascular Surgery, Straub Clinic and Hospital, Honolulu, Hawaii

David W. Knutson, M.D.
Professor and Associate Chairman, Department of Medicine, The Pennsylvania State University College of Medicine, Hershey, Pennsylvania; Chief, Medical Service, Lebanon Veterans Affairs Medical Center, Lebanon, Pennsylvania

Ted R. Kohler, M.D.
Associate Professor, Department of Surgery, University of Washington School of Medicine; Acting Chief, Surgical Service, Veterans Administration Medical Center, Seattle, Washington

David N. Ku, M.D., Ph.D.
Associate Professor, Department of Mechanical Engineering, Georgia Institute of Technology; Associate Professor, Department of Surgery, Emory University School of Medicine, Atlanta, Georgia

David A. Kumpe, M.D.
Professor, Departments of Radiology and Surgery, University of Colorado School of Medicine; Chief, Interventional Radiology, University Hospital, Denver, Colorado

Stephen G. Lalka, M.D.
Associate Professor, Department of Surgery, Indiana University School of Medicine; Attending Vascular Surgeon, Indiana University Medical Center, Wishard Memorial Hospital, Richard L. Roudebush Veterans Affairs Medical Center, Indianapolis, Indiana

Michael P. Lilly, M.D.
Assistant Professor, Department of Surgery, University of Maryland School of Medicine; Director, Noninvasive Vascular Laboratory, University of Maryland Hospital, Baltimore, Maryland

Alan Lumsden, M.D.
Assistant Professor, Department of Surgery, Emory University School of Medicine, Atlanta, Georgia; Staff Surgeon, Veterans Administration Medical Center, Decatur, Georgia

William C. Mackey, M.D.
Associate Professor, Department of Surgery, Tufts University School of Medicine; Attending Surgeon, Department of Surgery, New England Medical Center, Boston, Massachusetts

Louis G. Martin, M.D.
Associate Professor, Department of Radiology, Emory University School of Medicine; Vascular Interventional Radiologist, Department of Radiology, Emory University Hospital, Atlanta, Georgia

Gordon K. McLean, M.D.
Director, Vascular and Interventional Radiology, Department of Radiology, Western Pennsylvania Hospital, Pittsburgh, Pennsylvania

Thomas O. McNamara, M.D.
Professor, Department of Radiological Sciences, University of California, Los Angeles, UCLA School of Medicine; Chief, Cardiovascular Radiology, and Co-Director, Endovascular Therapy, UCLA Medical Center, Los Angeles, California

Mark W. Mewissen, M.D.
Associate Professor, Department of Radiology, Medical College of Wisconsin; Director, Angio-Interventional Radiology, Milwaukee County Medical Complex, Milwaukee, Wisconsin

Joseph L. Mills, M.D.
Associate Professor, Department of Surgery, University of South Florida College of Medicine; Chief, Vascular Surgery, James A. Haley Veterans Administration Hospital, Tampa, Florida

Gregory L. Moneta, M.D.
Associate Professor, Department of Surgery, Oregon Health Sciences University School of Medicine; Attending Physician, Department of Surgery, Veterans Administration Hospital, Portland, Oregon

Timothy V. Myers, M.D.
Instructor, Department of Radiology, University of Missouri—Kansas City School of Medicine, Kansas City, Missouri

Stephen H. Nantel, M.D.
Clinical Instructor, Division of Hematology, Department of Medicine, University of British Columbia Faculty of Medicine; Staff Hematologist, Department of Hematology, Vancouver General Hospital, Vancouver, British Columbia, Canada

Albert A. Nemcek, Jr., M.D.
Assistant Professor, Department of Radiology, Northwestern University Medical School; Chief, Section of Ultrasonography, Associate, Vascular and Interventional Radiology, Department of Radiology, Northwestern Memorial Hospital, Chicago, Illinois

Glenn E. Newman, M.D.
Assistant Professor, Department of Radiology, Duke University School of Medicine; Chief, Vascular Interventional Radiology, Duke University Medical Center, Durham, North Carolina

Timothy O'Bryant, M.D.
Vascular and Interventional Radiologist, Department of Radiology, Medical City Dallas Hospital, Dallas, Texas

Thomas F. O'Donnell, Jr., M.D.
Professor, Department of Vascular Surgery, Tufts University School of Medicine; Chief, Vascular Surgery, New England Medical Center, Boston, Massachusetts

B. Clay Parker, M.D.
Assistant Professor, Department of Radiology, George Washington University School of Medicine, Washington, D.C.; Section of Cardiovascular and Interventional Radiology, Alexandria Hospital, Alexandria, Virginia

William H. Pearce, M.D.
Associate Professor, Department of Surgery, Northwestern University Medical School, Chicago, Illinois

Daniel Picus, M.D.
Assocate Professor, Department of Radiology, Mallinckrodt Institute of Radiology, Washington University School of Medicine, Saint Louis, Missouri

John M. Porter, M.D.
Professor, Department of Surgery, Head, Division of Vascular Surgery, Oregon Health Sciences University School of Medicine, Portland, Oregon

Chet R. Rees, M.D.
Associate Attending Physician, Vascular and Interventional Radiology, Department of Radiology, Baylor University Medical Center, Dallas, Texas

Kenneth S. Rholl, M.D.
Assistant Professor, Department of Radiology, George Washington University Schoool of Medicine, Washington, D.C.; Section of Cardiovascular and Interventional Radiology, Alexandria Hospital, Alexandria, Virginia

Thomas S. Riles, M.D.
Professor, Department of Surgery, New York University School of Medicine; Director, Division of Vascular Surgery, Department of Surgery, New York University Medical Center, New York, New York

Anne C. Roberts, M.D.
Associate Professor, Department of Surgery, University of California, San Diego, School of Medicine; Chief, Vascular Radiology, Department of Radiology, Veterans Affairs Medical Center, San Diego, California

Josef Rösch, M.D.
Professor, Departments of Radiology and Surgery, Oregon Health Sciences University School of Medicine; Director, Charles Dotter Institute, Portland, Oregon

Robert J. Rosen, M.D.
Associate Professor, Department of Radiology, New York University School of Medicine; Director, Division of Interventional Radiology, Department of Radiology, New York University Medical Center, New York, New York

Jeffrey R. Rubin, M.D.
Professor, Department of Surgery, Northwestern Ohio Universities College of Medicine; Chairman, Department of Surgery, Western Reserve Care System, Youngstown, Ohio

Donald E. Schwarten, M.D.
Chief, Cardiovascular Laboratory, St. Vincent's Hospital, Indianapolis, Indiana

Kenneth W. Sniderman, M.D., F.R.C.P.(C)
Associate Professor, Department of Radiology, University of Toronto Faculty of Medicine; Director, Angiography Section, The Toronto Hospital, Toronto, Ontario, Canada

Maurice M. Solis, M.D.
Associate Professor and Director of Vascular Laboratory, Department of Surgery, Mercer University School of Medicine, Macon, Georgia

H. Dirk Sostman, M.D.
Professor, Department of Radiology, Duke University School of Medicine; Director of Academics, Duke University Medical Center, Durham, North Carolina

Michael C. Soulen, M.D.
Assistant Professor, Department of Radiology, University of Pennsylvania School of Medicine; Staff Interventional Radiologist, Department of Radiology, Hospital of the University of Pennsylvania, Philadelphia, Pennsylvania

James C. Stanley, M.D.
Professor and Associate Chairman, Department of Surgery, University of Michigan Medical School; Chief, Section of Vascular Surgery, Department of Surgery, University of Michigan Medical Center, Ann Arbor, Michigan

Anthony W. Stanson, M.D.
Associate Professor, Department of Radiology, Mayo Medical School; Consultant, Diagnostic Radiology, Mayo Clinic, Rochester, Minnesota

D. Eugene Strandness, Jr., M.D.
Professor, Department of Surgery, University of Washington School of Medicine; Chief, Division of Vascular Surgery, Department of Surgery, University of Washington Medical Center, Seattle, Washington

Michael Streiff, M.D.
Post-Doctoral Fellow, Division of Hematology, Department of Medicine, The Johns Hopkins University School of Medicine; Attending Physician, Hematology/Oncology, The Johns Hopkins Hospital, Baltimore, Maryland

Kevin L. Sullivan, M.D.
Associate Professor, Department of Radiology, Jefferson Medical College of Thomas Jefferson University; Attending Physician, Division of Cardiovascular Interventional Radiology, Department of Radiology, Thomas Jefferson University Hospital, Philadelphia, Pennsylvania

David C. Taylor, M.D.
Clinical Assistant Professor, Division of Vascular Surgery, Department of Surgery, University of British Columbia Faculty of Medicine, Vancouver, British Columbia, Canada

Lloyd M. Taylor, Jr., M.D.
Professor, Division of Vascular Surgery, Department of Surgery, Oregon Health Sciences University School of Medicine, Portland, Oregon

Brian L. Thiele, M.D.
Professor, Department of Surgery, Pennsylvania State University College of Medicine; Chief, Vascular Surgery, Milton S. Hershey Medical Center, Hershey, Pennsylvania

Bernard W. Thompson, M.D.
Professor, Department of Surgery, University of Arkansas College of Medicine; Assistant Chief, Surgical Service, John L. McClellan Memorial Veterans Hospital, Little Rock, Arkansas

Fong Y. Tsai, M.D.
Professor, Department of Radiology, University of Missouri—Kansas City School of Medicine; Chairman, Department of Radiology, Truman Medical Center, Kansas City, Missouri

Barry T. Uchida, M.D.
Assistant Professor, Department of Radiology, Oregon Health Sciences University School of Medicine; Technical Research Director, Charles Dotter Institute, Portland, Oregon

Renan Uflacker, M.D.
Chief, Department of Vascular and Interventional Radiology, MED-IMAGEM, Hospital Beneficencia Portuguesa, São Paulo, Brazil

Joseph L. Unthank, Ph.D.
Associate Professor, Department of Physiology and Biophysics, Indiana University School of Medicine, Indianapolis, Indiana

Karim Valji, M.D.
Assistant Professor, Department of Radiology, University of California, San Diego, School of Medicine, San Diego, California

Paul S. van Bemmelen, M.D.
Fellow, Section of Peripheral Vascular Surgery, Department of Surgery, Southern Illinois University School of Medicine, Springfield, Illinois

Arina van Breda, M.D.
Clinical Professor, Department of Radiology, George Washington University School of Medicine, Washington, D.C.; Director, Cardiovascular and Interventional Radiology, Alexandria Hospital, Alexandria, Virginia

Robert L. Vogelzang, M.D.
Associate Professor, Department of Radiology, Northwestern University Medical School; Chief, Section of Vascular and Interventional Radiology, Department of Radiology, Northwestern Memorial Hospital, Chicago, Illinois

Bruce F. Waller, M.D.
Clinical Professor, Departments of Pathology and Medicine, Indiana University School of Medicine; Director, Cardiovascular Pathology Registry, St. Vincent Hospital; Cardiologist, Nasser, Smith, Pinkerton Cardiology, Inc., and Indiana Heart Institute, Indianapolis, Indiana

Daniel B. Walsh, M.D.
Associate Professor, Department of Surgery, Dartmouth Medical School; Surgeon, Section of Vascular Surgery, Department of Surgery, Dartmouth-Hitchcock Medical Center, Lebanon, New Hampshire

Arthur Waltman, M.D.
Associate Professor, Department of Radiology, Harvard Medical School; Director, Interventional Radiology, Massachusetts General Hospital, Boston, Massachusetts

Harold J. Welch, M.D.
Clinical Assistant Professor, Department of Surgery, Uniformed Services University of the Health Services F. Edward Hébert School of Medicine, Bethesda, Maryland; Head, Division of Vascular Surgery, Department of Surgery, U.S. Naval Hospital, Portsmouth, Virginia

E. Kent Yucel, M.D.
Associate Professor, Department of Radiology, Boston University Medical School; Director of MRI, Boston University Medical Center, Boston, Massachusetts

Gerald Zemel, M.D.
Clinical Assistant Professor, Department of Radiology, University of Miami School of Medicine; Radiologist, Miami Vascular Institute, Baptist Hospital of Miami, Miami, Florida

R. Eugene Zierler, M.D.
Associate Professor, Division of Vascular Surgery, Department of Surgery, University of Washington School of Medicine, Seattle, Washington

Robert M. Zwolak, M.D.
Assistant Professor, Department of Surgery, Dartmouth Medical School; Surgeon, Section of Vascular Surgery, Dartmouth-Hitchcock Medical Center, Lebanon, New Hampshire

Preface

For centuries, surgical treatment of vascular diseases was limited to simple ligature for trauma or amputation. The advent of modern vascular surgery was dependent on both the development of appropriate instrumentation and materials, and the improved diagnosis allowed by arteriography. The disciplines of vascular surgery and vascular radiology have thus been closely intertwined since their early stages, with vascular surgeons traditionally providing clinical diagnosis and management and radiologists the requisite imaging. Both fields have seen quantum improvements over the last three decades, in many instances, as a result of their close cooperative relationship.

Within a decade of the advent of successful vascular bypass techniques, the pioneering efforts of interventional radiologist Charles Dotter established the feasibility of endovascular treatment of vascular disorders. These efforts were met with great skepticism by vascular surgeons, as they seemed to violate many "time-tested" principles. (How could a diseased artery be expected to remain patent after a tear had been made?) Despite these concerns, interventional techniques continued to improve and proliferate, stimulated by the introduction of the balloon catheter by Andreas Grüntzig, to the point that endovascular techniques are now established as an important and permanent addition to the available options for patient care. With this recognition has come an even closer relationship between the disciplines of vascular surgery and interventional radiology, far exceeding any that previously existed. Whereas interactions in the past may have been limited to discussions of a diagnostic approach or procedure, now the dialogue is likely to include a decision regarding which therapeutic technique—surgery, endovascular intervention, or a combination of the two—is likely to yield the best short- and long-term benefit to the patient.

While some physicians consider surgery and endovascular intervention to be competitive methods, in many circulatory beds this is not the case. Few vascular surgeons would disagree that balloon angioplasty is the procedure of choice in short segment stenotic aortoiliac disease. Endovascular treatment in this area has greatly improved the care of these patients with less morbidity and discomfort, shorter hospitalizations and recuperative periods, and significantly lower cost. In other areas of the vascular system, the appropriate therapy may be less certain or even controversial, but continuing clinical experience should eventually allow an understanding of the relative role of each approach. However, many of the specific advantages of endovascular therapy are being sought by an increasingly educated and cognizant patient population and potentially, in the future, by the payors of health care. It is thus important that all physicians involved in the treatment of patients with vascular disease be aware of the options available, an awareness that we hope will be furthered by this text.

The last few decades have seen an explosion in our knowledge of vascular disease. Our understanding of vascular pathology and physiology has been significantly advanced, allowing improved pharmacologic and structural approaches in the treatment of vascular disease. New diagnostic modalities including ultrasound, computed tomography, magnetic resonance imaging, and magnetic resonance angiography already allow unprecedented and unparalleled noninvasive means of evaluating our patients. Vascular ultrasound is well established as an excellent diagnostic tool in many circulatory beds, with technical improvements allowing an ever-increasing application of this tool. Further improvements in all these diagnostic techniques may eventually obviate the need for diagnostic angiography and limit the need for invasive procedures to purely therapeutic ends.

Yet even with an improved understanding of how the vascular system works and enhanced diagnostic abilities, vascular therapy remains limited by our inability to moderate the response of the vessel wall to injury. A review of the contributions herein highlights the extent to which myointimal hyperplasia compromises the results of all vascular intervention. A further frustration is the variability of patient response: why do some vascular grafts function flawlessly for years while others fail within weeks or months of placement? Why are some patients "cured" after a single angioplasty while others develop rapidly progressive worsening of occlusive disease? Clearly our challenge for the future will be to definitively address the underlying pathologic response to vascular injury. It is likely that future breakthroughs in the treatment of vascular disease will be at a cellular or pharmacologic level rather than a purely structural or anatomic one.

We hope that this major effort on the part of so many authors will fill a real need in our approaches to the treatment of vascular disease. This is a dynamic field that is rapidly changing, but these contributions reflect the standards of practice in the United States today. We believe that this effort should allow all practitioners caring for vascular patients to have the benefit of a comprehensive overview of treatment options. It is our hope that this text will lead to a further mutual respect between our two disciplines that will be the framework for the exciting advances to come. Our disciplines will continue to overlap and grow together; a dialogue between them, as represented by this text, will allow this relationship to be most productive. There is much that our specialties, working together, have brought to the treatment of vascular disease, and there is no field in medicine where cooperation between two specialties is likely to bring greater benefit to our patients.

D. Eugene Strandness, M.D.
Arina van Breda, M.D.

Contents

Color plates follow pages 164 and 872.

Section I

Pathology of Arterial Injury and Repair

Over the last 50 years, a number of approaches have been developed to restore circulation to the limbs of patients with arterial occlusive disease. Because diseased arteries readily delaminate, endarterectomy was applied at first as a means for removing the obstructing lesion. Endarterectomy cleanly removes the plaque and several layers of media and leaves behind a smooth surface. It also results in massive injury to the vessel and induces a reparative response that causes wall thickening and luminal narrowing within months of the surgery. For this reason, endarterectomy has largely been abandoned in favor of bypass grafting, except in selected circumstances. It is unfortunate that bypass grafts can also develop stenosis. Less invasive techniques for the treatment of occlusive disease, including angioplasty and atherectomy, have provided the physician and the patient with less morbid alternatives to open arterial reconstruction. However, these forms of treatment also injure arteries and, particularly in small vessels, are associated with a high restenosis rate. It is important to bear in mind that the types of injury differ substantially even though the vessel response is often the same. Endarterectomy removes all the intima and two-thirds of the media, angioplasty does not remove arterial tissue, and atherectomy removes only a portion of the diseased wall. In addition, the starting point differs depending on the circumstance. In most situations, the vessel has a history of disease, while in others the vessel is normal (vein grafts, arteries subjected to balloon embolectomy).

We have come to recognize the hard truth that *all forms of vascular reconstruction cause injury* and that injury increases the risk of intimal hyperplasia, restenosis, and thrombosis. For this reason there has been a resurgence of interest in arterial wound healing and the factors that regulate wall mass and luminal diameter. In this section, we attempt to define the role of injury in the reparative process after vascular reconstruction and to describe new approaches to controlling restenosis.

Anatomic Aspects of Vascular Disease

Danna E. Johnson

The past decade has witnessed the emergence of a variety of new techniques and devices for the treatment of atherosclerotic vascular disease. An appreciation of the morphology of normal and diseased vessels is useful for greater understanding of the mechanisms of action and potential short-term and long-term complications of these new therapies. This chapter reviews the structure of normal arteries, the important pathologic features of atherosclerosis, and the pathologic changes that occur in biologic and synthetic bypass grafts.

NORMAL ARTERIAL STRUCTURE

Three types of arteries exist, differing with regard to size and function.[1] Large elastic arteries, such as the aorta and common iliac arteries, serve as conduits for blood flow and, because of their abundant elastic fibers, recoil during diastole, thereby assisting in maintenance of hydrostatic blood pressure (Fig. 1-1). Medium and small muscular arteries, such as the coronary and superficial femoral arteries, regulate blood flow distribution, while the small arterioles modulate vascular tone.

Regardless of size, all arteries are composed of three layers, or tunics: tunica intima, tunica media, and tunica adventitia[1] (Fig. 1-1). The intima consists of a single layer of endothelial cells overlying a basement membrane, subendothelial connective tissue, and the internal elastic lamina. Normally, the intima is very thin, but it does become thickened with advancing age or secondary to disease such as atherosclerosis. Endothelial cells are spindle-shaped mesenchymal cells whose characteristic ultrastructural features include a basal lamina surrounding the cell, pinocytotic vesicles, and small intracytoplasmic structures known as Weibel-Palade bodies.[2] Weibel-Palade bodies are electron-dense, rod-shaped structures associated with von Willebrand factor secretion. The endothelium has a crucial role in angiogenesis, hemostasis, inflammation, and regulation of vascular tone.[3] Through a system of pinocytotic vesicles, the endothelium permits transcellular transport of molecules between the blood and vessel wall. Many vital substances are produced and secreted by endothelial cells, a partial list of which is presented in Table 1-1.[3]

The arterial media is composed of smooth muscle cells surrounded by a connective tissue matrix, arranged as a helix that wraps around the vessel wall. This layer is normally thicker than the intima or adventitia, particularly in muscular arteries (Fig. 1-2). The smooth muscle cells contain actin and myosin filaments whose contraction and relaxation allow these cells to regulate vessel size. Smooth muscle cells also produce much of the connective tissue of the vessel. Migration and proliferation of medial smooth muscle cells play an important role in the pathogenesis of inti-

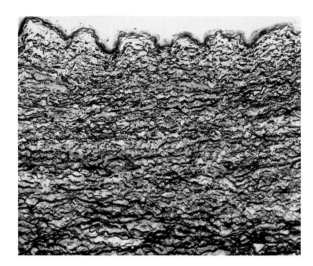

Figure 1-1 Normal aorta has abundant elastic fibers. (VVG, ×330.)

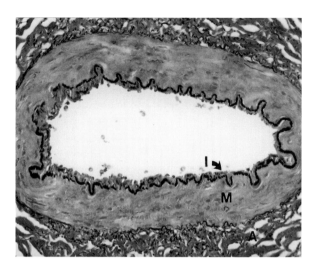

Figure 1-2 Normal small muscular artery. I, intima; M, media; A, adventitia. (VVG, ×650.)

mal thickening and atherosclerosis.[4,5] The adventitia is an ill-defined layer that lies external to the external elastic lamina. Loose connective tissue, elastic fibers, nerves, lymphatic channels, and nutrient vessels known as the vasa vasorum, comprise the adventitia of normal arteries.

Table 1-1 Products of Endothelial Cells

Platelet function
 von Willebrand factor
 Prostacyclin (PGI$_2$)

Procoagulation
 Factor V
 Tissue factor

Anticoagulation
 Tissue plasminogen activator
 Heparan sulfate
 Thrombomodulin

Vascular tone
 Endothelium-derived growth factor
 Endothelin
 Angiotensin converting enzyme

Growth factors
 Endothelium-derived growth factor
 Platelet-derived growth factor-like factor
 Colony stimulating activity

Connective tissue
 Collagens
 Elastin
 Laminin
 Fibronectin
 Thrombospondin

Immunologic
 ABO blood group antigens
 Histocompatibility antigens
 Leukocyte adhesion molecules

PATHOLOGY OF ATHEROSCLEROSIS

Potential Precursor Lesions

Identification of possible precursors to atherosclerotic plaques has been an area of much investigation and some controversy. One candidate lesion is the fatty streak. Fatty streaks are flat to slightly raised yellow intimal lesions that occur in all human populations, regardless of race or genetic predisposition to atherosclerosis.[6] Histologically, fatty streaks are small intimal collections of large cells with clear slightly vacuolated cytoplasm—the so-called foam cell (Fig. 1-3A). Foam cells have been shown to be lipid-rich macrophages and smooth muscle cells by ultrastructural and immunohistochemical methods.[7-9] Fatty streaks are found in the aorta as early as the first decade of life and in the proximal coronary arteries in early adulthood.[6] The prevailing view is that a few fatty streaks, particularly those in the proximal coronary arteries, may evolve into atherosclerotic plaques over time. Hemodynamic stresses may encourage the progression of lesions situated in areas of altered blood flow.[10] However, most fatty streaks, especially those of the ascending aorta, probably coalesce to form larger streaks, regress, or remain unchanged.[11]

Branch pads and intimal thickenings have also been proposed as possible precursors to the atherosclerotic plaque.[12] Seen first in early childhood, these lesions are slightly thickened fibrotic areas that contain smooth muscle cells located at branch points or elsewhere within the proximal to mid-regions of the coronary and other muscular arteries[7,8] (Fig. 1-3B). These are the

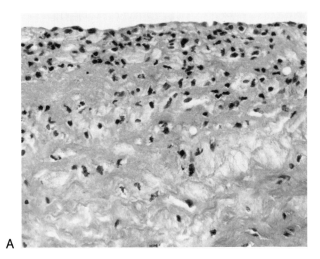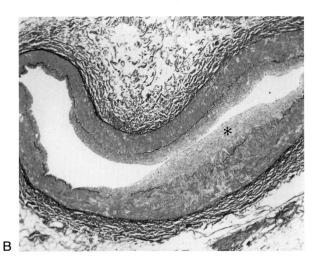

Figure 1-3 (**A**) Aortic fatty streak, from a 17-year-old boy. (H&E, orig mag ×1020.) (**B**) Proximal coronary artery fibrous intimal thickening *(asterisk).* (VVG, ×160.)

same sites favored by atherosclerotic plaques; in one study, histologic evidence for progression of these lesions to early plaques was demonstrated.[12]

Simple Atherosclerotic Plaques

The basic lesion of atherosclerosis is the atherosclerotic plaque. Plaques are heterogeneous structures that vary significantly from person to person in their number, size, distribution, and composition. As a general rule, atherosclerotic plaques most commonly involve the abdominal aorta, proximal coronary arteries, popliteal arteries, internal carotid arteries, and arteries of the circle of Willis.[13] However, virtually any artery may be affected by atherosclerosis.

Fibrous Plaques

The simplest lesions are predominantly fibrous plaques. These lesions are concentric or eccentric white-tan intimal thickenings composed largely of connective tissue elements and smooth muscle cells, with very little lipid. Collagen accounts for up to 60 percent of the dry weight of fibrous plaques, most of which is type I collagen, with smaller amounts of type III, IV, and V collagen.[14] Proteoglycans and fibronectin are also present, but their concentrations relative to collagen diminish as lesions grow older and larger.[15,16]

The extracellular matrix of plaques is produced and secreted by smooth muscle cells that have migrated into the lesion from the deep intima or the media.[17] However, some of these smooth muscle cells differ significantly from those of the normal media in that they have increased numbers of synthetic organelles, such as rough endoplasmic reticulum, Golgi apparatus, and mitochondria, as well as decreased concentrations of actin and myosin filaments.[18] These modified smooth muscle cells have been called synthetic type smooth muscle cells, in contrast to the contractile smooth muscle cells that populate the normal arterial media.[19,20] Generally, synthetic smooth muscle cells are most numerous in the superficial regions of relatively young atherosclerotic lesions.

Atheromatous Plaques

In contrast to the fibrous plaque, the atheromatous plaque has a cap of fibrous tissue that overlies a central necrotic lipid core (Fig. 1-4A). Plasma-derived lipids insudate into the plaque, bind to collagen and elastin fibers, and eventually coalesce to form large pools.[21,22] Most of the lipids are free cholesterol or cholesterol esters that can crystallize to form cholesterol clefts[21] (Fig. 1-4B). Present in smaller quantities are apolipoprotein B, a constituent of low-density lipoproteins and very-low-density lipoproteins; apolipoprotein (a); and apolipoprotein E, which is important in reverse cholesterol transport.[23-26] Lipid-laden foam cells, most of which are macrophages and a few of which are smooth muscle cells, frequently infiltrate the center or periphery of the plaque lipid core[27-29] (Fig. 1-4C). Elongated or stellate-shaped smooth muscle cells are also often seen in the fibrous caps of atheromas, along with scattered T lymphocytes.[27,30-32] Other features commonly observed are vascularization of plaques caused by ingrowth of the vasa vasorum and thinning and fibrosis of the underlying media due to pressure atrophy[33,34] (Fig. 1-4D).

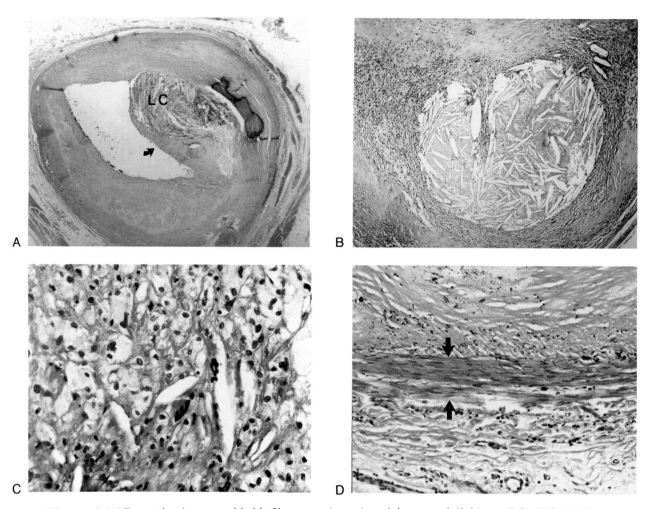

Figure 1-4 (A) Eccentric atheroma, with thin fibrous cap *(arrow)* overlying necrotic lipid core (LC). (H&E, ×50.) (B) Needle-shaped cholesterol clefts occupy the central lipid core. (H&E, ×160.) (C) Lipid-laden foam cells and cholesterol clefts. (H&E, ×820.) (D) Media *(between arrows)* is thinned and partially fibrotic. (H&E, ×510.)

Complicated Atherosclerotic Plaques

While the simple fibrous and atheromatous plaques can give rise to ischemic symptoms, many clinically significant lesions are advanced complicated plaques. Features of complex plaques may include (1) calcification, (2) plaque surface erosion or frank ulceration, (3) thrombosis, (4) intraplaque bleeding, and (5) aneurysm formation.

Dystrophic Calcification

Dystrophic calcification of atherosclerotic plaques occurs by means of a vesicle matrix mechanism; calcium carbonate apatites, sodium, and magnesium are the principal minerals deposited in vascular lesions.[35] Initiating factors may include changes in the acidity and collagen and proteoglycan structure of the plaque.[36] Calcium deposition occurs along collagen and elastic fibers and within the lipid core, but tends to be most pronounced within the connective tissue near the base of a plaque[37] (Fig. 1-5). The severity of plaque calcification may increase in parallel with patient age.[37,38]

Erosions

Erosions of the plaque surface may occur secondary to acute focal injury caused by hemodynamic stress, vasospasm, changes in blood pressure, or vessel wall bending, as with motion or cardiac contraction.[39] Softening of the lipid core, thinning of the fibrous cap, and infiltration by macrophages may be predisposing factors for acute plaque fissuring[40,41] (Fig. 1-6A). Small superficial erosions often heal spontaneously. However, some may progress to deep ulcers of the plaque.

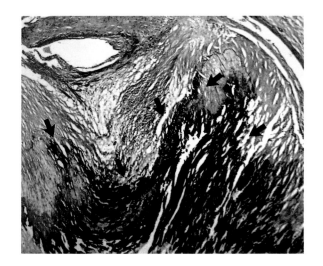

Figure 1-5 Extensive calcification of plaque collagen *(arrows)*. (H&E, ×160.)

Ulceration of atheromas can have dire consequences, including thrombosis, plaque hemorrhage, and athero-embolization.

Thrombosis

Most patients with chronic ischemic syndromes, such as stable angina and intermittent claudication, have fixed stenoses that are not complicated by thrombus. By contrast, most patients with acute ischemic syndromes, such as myocardial infarction, unstable angina, limb-threatening ischemia, and strokes, are found by angiography or at autopsy to have recent thrombosis superimposed on a high-grade athero-sclerotic stenosis (Fig. 1-6B). Distal embolization of thrombus fragments may also cause clinical symptoms such as transient ischemic attacks and the "blue toe syndrome."[42,43] Careful pathologic studies have shown

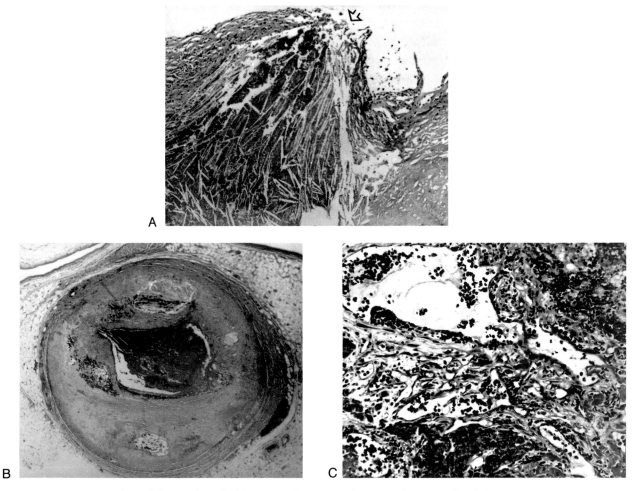

Figure 1-6 **(A)** Superficial erosion of a fibrous cap *(open arrow)* exposes the underlying lipid core. (H&E, ×820.) **(B)** Acute thrombotic occlusion in a case of fatal myocardial infarction. (H&E, ×50.) **(C)** Neovascularization of a thrombus undergoing organization. (H&E, ×820.)

that acute plaque surface disruption is the most common precipitating factor leading to coronary artery thrombosis.[39,40,44,45] Total thrombotic occlusion is most likely to occur at very high-grade stenoses (>90 percent area stenosis).[46,47] Also, atheromas with a high lipid content are more likely to be complicated by ulceration and thrombosis than are fibrous plaques.[39,40]

Injury to the plaque surface initiates thrombosis through denudation of the endothelium, exposure of the underlying collagen and lipid to the bloodstream, and subsequent platelet adhesion, aggregation, and degranulation. The composition of early thrombi is greatly influenced by hemodynamic factors. High shear stress at stenotic sites induces platelet activation, while the lower shear stress and vortices distal to stenoses favor fibrin polymerization.[48] As such, early thrombi have platelet-rich heads directly overlying the ulcerated lesion, while the distal tail consists of fibrin with entrapped erythrocytes.[49,50] Frequently, cholesterol clefts, foam cells, and other debris from the necrotic lipid core are also embedded within the developing thrombus.

Thrombi are ever-changing structures, with new thrombus formation occurring simultaneously with thrombus dissolution through fibrinolysis and embolization of small thrombus fragments. The ultimate fate of a thrombus is dependent on a number of variables, including blood flow, severity of the pre-existing stenosis, whether a thrombus is totally or only partially occlusive, the coagulation status of the patient, and whether thrombolytic therapy is administered. Many young thrombi lyse completely, although reocclusion is common. Thrombi that do not lyse undergo a process known as *organization.* Substances released from

acute and chronic inflammatory cells that have infiltrated a thrombus promote enzymatic degradation of the thrombus, encourage capillary ingrowth (neovascularization), and recruit fibroblasts and myofibroblasts into the lesion (Fig. 1-6C). The fibroblasts and myofibroblasts produce the collagen matrix that eventually replaces the thrombus. Neovascularization can sometimes recanalize a thrombus, but the degree of luminal reconstitution is usually insufficient to permit adequate blood flow.[49] The organization of a thrombus follows a variable time course, is often incomplete, and may be complicated by fresh thrombus deposition. It is not uncommon, for example, to see a layer of recent thrombus coating the surface of older, nearly organized, thrombus.

Intraplaque Hemorrhage

Intraplaque hemorrhage can occur by two mechanisms: (1) rupture of small branches of the vasa vasorum at the base of a plaque, and (2) leakage of blood into a lesion through a disrupted plaque surface (Fig. 1-7). Bleeding from the vasa vasorum is usually minor and of little consequence. Hemorrhage through an eroded plaque surface, however, causes intraplaque pressure to rise with consequent plaque rupture.[46,51] Hemorrhage into high-grade atheromas frequently is accompanied by thrombosis of the vessel lumen.[46]

ANEURYSMS

Aneurysms are localized dilatations of arteries that may result from a number of diseases but are seen most frequently in the setting of severe atherosclerosis.[52] Any artery may be affected, but the abdominal aorta below

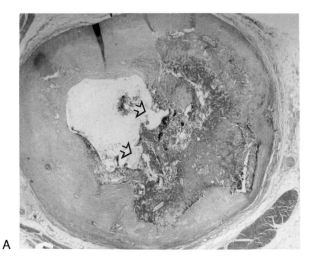

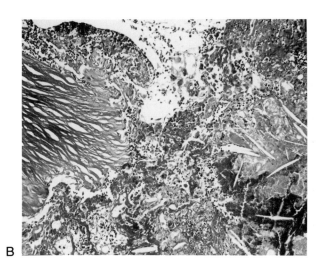

A   B

Figure 1-7 (A) Acute plaque ulceration *(arrows)* complicated by hemorrhage into the lipid core. (H&E, ×50.)
(B) Higher power magnification of the disrupted lesion shown in Fig. A. (H&E, ×650.)

the renal arteries and the iliac arteries are favored sites of aneurysm formation. Some patients have multiple aneurysms at various locations. Aneurysms develop through progressive atrophy and fibrosis of the arterial media underlying intimal atherosclerotic plaques. The weakened arterial wall may then bulge outward, producing fusiform or, less often, saccular aneurysms. Microscopic sections through aneurysms demonstrate marked attenuation of the vessel wall, an atherosclerotic plaque overlying a media obliterated by fibrous tissue, and surface thrombus. This thrombus often appears to have been laid down in layers, producing the characteristic lines of Zahn, and may completely fill the aneurysm cavity. Some aneurysms show a marked periaortic chronic inflammatory reaction, the so-called inflammatory aneurysm.[53] Complications of aneurysms include thromboembolization, compression of adjacent vessels or other structures, secondary infection, perianeurysmal hematoma, and rupture. The risk of rupture is particularly high for those abdominal aortic aneurysms measuring 5 cm or more in diameter.[54]

NATURAL HISTORY OF ATHEROSCLEROSIS

The traditional view is that atherosclerosis is a chronic and progressive disorder, characterized by increasing numbers and severity of atherosclerotic lesions over time.[55-57] Indeed, this is the pattern the disease follows in most patients; certain cardiovascular risk factors, such as diabetes mellitus, hypertension, and dyslipidemia, may accelerate the progression of atherosclerosis. However, recent experimental and clinical evidence shows that some atherosclerotic lesions may partially regress.[58,59]

As discussed previously, mature atherosclerotic plaques have complex compositions and contain variable quantities of collagen, proteoglycans, free cholesterol, esterified cholesterol, phospholipids, calcium, and magnesium salts. Crystalline and bound cholesterol, collagen, and mineral deposits are probably resistant to significant removal from atherosclerotic lesions. However, much of the unbound cholesterol exchanges freely with the plasma through reverse cholesterol transport pathways, suggesting a potential for net efflux of free cholesterol from plaques if serum lipid levels are lowered. Reversal of fatty lesions has been documented in several animal models of diet-induced atherosclerosis when the afflicted animals are placed on low cholesterol diets or are treated with lipid-lowering drugs.[58]

There is also recent evidence that dietary and pharmacologic therapies directed at control of risk factors may retard plaque growth and cause plaque regression in humans. For example, the Cholesterol Lowering Atherosclerosis Study (CLAS) demonstrated a decreased incidence of coronary artery and saphenous vein bypass graft atherosclerotic plaque progression and new lesion formation in patients treated with colestipol and niacin, as compared with a placebo-treated control group.[60] Overall, lesion regression occurred in 16.2 percent of treated versus 2.4 percent of control patients. In the more recent Familial Atherosclerosis Treatment Study (FATS) conducted at the University of Washington, patients treated with lovastatin and colestipol, niacin and colestipol, and placebo were compared after a $2\frac{1}{2}$-year period.[61] Forty-six percent of patients in the placebo-treated group showed lesion progression as the only change, compared with only 21 percent of patients treated with lovastatin/colestipol and 25 percent of those treated with niacin/colestipol. Also, only 11 percent of control patients had lesion regression as the only change, while 32 percent of patients treated with lovastatin/colestipol and 39 percent of those treated with niacin/colestipol had lesion regression. The treated groups also had lower incidences of death, myocardial infarction, and bypass graft surgery. These studies confirm the dynamic nature of atherosclerosis and provide an impetus for further study of the natural history and response to dietary or pharmacologic therapies for this vascular disease.

PATHOLOGY OF AUTOLOGOUS SAPHENOUS VEIN BYPASS GRAFTS

The autologous saphenous vein has been used successfully for many years as a conduit for revascularization of ischemic organs and limbs. Unfortunately, a significant impediment to long-term patency is the development of obstructive vascular lesions in femoropopliteal and aortocoronary saphenous vein bypass grafts that in many ways resemble arterial atherosclerotic plaques.[62-69]

Early Vein Bypass Graft Morphology

Acute thrombotic occlusion has been found in 10 to 35 percent of aortocoronary saphenous vein bypass grafts from patients who died 1 to 30 days after surgery.[63,64,69,70] Thrombosis most often occurs at the distal anastomosis but is sometimes observed at the ostial anastomosis or along the entire length of the graft. Poor distal runoff due to severe distal artery atherosclerosis and concurrent endarterectomy of the diseased artery

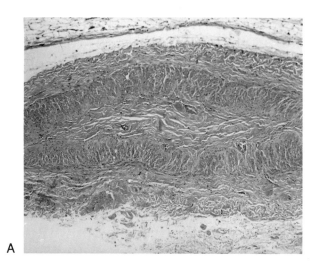
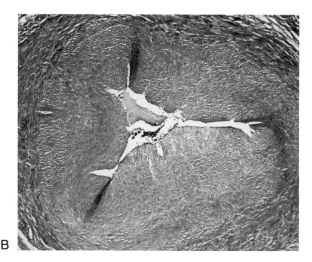

Figure 1-8 (A) Fibrous luminal obliteration of a thrombosed saphenous vein bypass graft. (H&E, ×220.)
(B) Concentric fibrous intimal thickening of a 26-month-old vein graft. (H&E, ×130.)

have been implicated as factors contributing to acute thrombosis of grafts.[63,70] If the patient survives, the thrombus will eventually organize, with conversion of these grafts, into thin fibrous cords with completely obliterated lumens[66] (Fig. 1-8A).

Patent aortocoronary saphenous vein grafts from patients who die during surgery show signs of surgical trauma, including edema, acute hemorrhage, and loss of endothelium. By 12 hours postoperatively, nearly three-quarters of grafts possess scattered platelet-fibrin microthrombi, most conspicuous near the venous valves.[63] These microthrombi persist for about 3 months after surgery, after which time they gradually disappear due to fibrous organization.[63,69]

Fibrous intimal thickening is a change found in all grafts that remain patent for more than a few weeks. Intimal proliferation is first seen at about 2 weeks post-operatively and involves virtually 100 percent of grafts studied at 1 or more months after surgery.[63,64,71,72] The mitogenic effects of growth factors, a reparative response to ischemia or elevated blood pressure, poor distal runoff, and organization of thrombus have all been proposed as mechanisms for fibrous intimal thickening of vein grafts.[63,69,73–75] This process is usually concentric about the lumen and affects the entire length of the graft, but it is often most severe at the graft anastomosis[63,66,71,72] (Fig. 1-8B). Microscopically, fibrous intimal thickening appears as proliferation of modified smooth muscle cells within a variably collagenous stroma containing an abundance of proteoglycans.[63,64,71,76] With time, the smooth muscle cell density decreases and the amount of collagen increases, so that these lesions come to closely resemble fibrous atherosclerotic plaques.[64,73,77] But unlike arteries, the diseased

vein graft never develops well-formed elastic laminae, evidence against true "arterialization" of the vein graft. The severity of luminal narrowing increases in proportion to the elapsed time from surgery and is also affected by hyperlipidemia, hypertension, and a greatly narrowed artery distal to the distal anastomosis.[63,66,67,71,77,78]

Late Vein Bypass Graft Morphology

Early manifestations of "atherosclerosis" are seen in some grafts beginning at about 1 year after surgery. The first change is infiltration of the thickened intima by lipid-laden foam cells.[71,72] By 2 to 3 years, some grafts have lesions that resemble atheromatous plaques with extracellular lipid and cholesterol clefts.[64,66,68,72] Aortocoronary saphenous vein bypass grafts examined 6 to 12 years postoperatively often have advanced high-grade atheromatous lesions that can lead to recurrence of ischemic signs and symptoms. Atheromas develop more frequently in grafts from patients with hyperlipidemia, and the quantity of lipid within individual lesions increases as a function of graft age.[67,68,71]

Although the late vascular lesions of vein bypass grafts resemble those of native coronary arteries, there are some significant differences. Atherosclerosis tends to involve the implanted graft diffusely, rather than occurring as discrete focal stenoses.[68,72] Graft lesions are usually concentric, while about two-thirds of coronary artery plaques are eccentric.[37,70,72] Plaques from saphenous vein bypass grafts are less likely to be heavily calcified than are those of coronary arteries.[68,77] Lipid-rich foam cells are more numerous in diseased vein grafts than in native arteries; frequently, these cells replace and erode the fibrous cap of a plaque.[66,72] This may make vein graft lesions extremely susceptible to ulceration and consequent thrombosis (Fig. 1-9). Indeed, thrombosis is the most common cause of late graft failure; in one study of long-term vein grafts surgically excised during repeat bypass operation, 51 percent of grafts were completely occluded by recent thrombus, usually overlying ruptured or ulcerated atheromas.[77] Finally, a marked chronic inflammatory cell infiltrate is more frequently encountered in vein bypass graft lesions than in atherosclerotic plaques from coronary arteries.[72]

PATHOLOGY OF SYNTHETIC VASCULAR GRAFTS

A variety of synthetic prosthetic graft materials has been used for vascular reconstruction, mainly for aortic and peripheral vascular disease.[78] The ideal substance for vascular grafts should be nontoxic, nonallergenic, porous, and resistant to thrombosis, degradation, kinking, and infection. Knitted Dacron grafts have shown good results when used for aortic or aortoiliac reconstruction but have high rates of thrombosis when used as femoropopliteal grafts. Expanded polytetrafluorethylene (ePTFE) has been a successful material for femoropopliteal grafts and hemodialysis shunts.[79]

The morphologic changes that occur when synthetic grafts are placed into animals have been reported in detail. Soon after surgery, a thin layer of platelets, fibrin, and white blood cells coats the luminal surface of the graft. Experimental studies in baboons show that,

by 1 month postoperatively, smooth muscle cells and endothelial cells from the adjacent artery have proliferated and migrated onto the blood-contacting surface of the graft.[80] These cells form an endothelialized neointima that grows at a rate of about 0.2 mm/d, may completely cover the graft's luminal border, and provides a thromboresistant surface. Eventually, cellular proliferation declines, although patchy areas of endothelial cell replication persist, probably in response to ongoing endothelial cell injury. Smooth muscle cell division at anastomotic sites also continues and can eventually lead to intimal fibrosis and even late stenosis.

In synthetic grafts placed into humans, an intact neointima lined by a continuous layer of endothelium does not develop. Endothelium will grow over the graft anastomoses and may extend for roughly 1 cm onto the graft surface but usually does not proliferate further.[81-83] The remaining graft surface is covered by a compact layer of platelets, fibrin, and leukocytes that has been called a pseudointima or inner capsule (Fig. 1-10A). Healing also produces an outer capsule that surrounds the graft. This outer capsule is initially composed of granulation tissue, but is eventually converted to a sheath of fibrous scar (Fig. 1-10B). In grafts with large pores, the histiocytes, fibroblasts, capillaries, and collagen grow from the outer capsule through the pores and into the basal region of the inner capsule. These bridges anchor the pseudointima to the graft and help prevent sloughing and distal embolization of the inner capsule. Ingrowth of smooth muscle cells from the adjacent native vessel and of fibroblasts and capillaries through the graft pores converts the thrombus of the inner capsule to fibrous tissue.

The pseudointima of synthetic grafts is less throm-

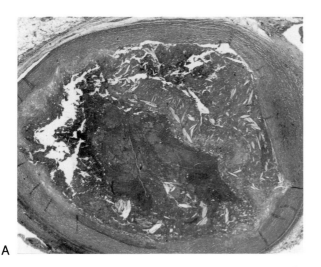
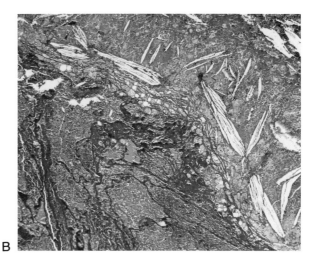

Figure 1-9 (A) Ulceration and acute thrombosis of atherosclerotic vein graft, age 107 months. (H&E, ×50.) **(B)** Higher power magnification of the lesion shown in Fig. A. (H&E, ×330.)

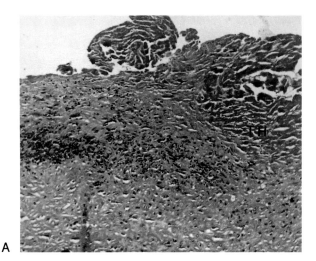
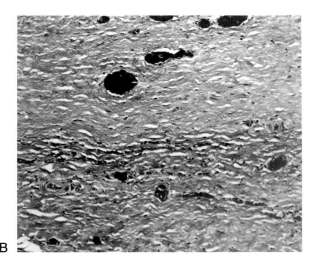

Figure 1-10 (A) Compact pseudointima of synthetic graft with thrombus (TH). (H&E, ×330.) (B) Fibrotic outer capsule has numerous vascular channels. (H&E, ×330.)

boresistant than endothelialized autologous vein grafts. As such, platelets adherent to synthetic graft surfaces can be found for years after surgery.[83,84] These platelet deposits may promote early or late thrombotic occlusion. Early thrombosis often can be linked to technical surgical problems. Late thrombosis occurs most often in small grafts and is related to progressive distal atherosclerotic narrowing and poor distal runoff.[85] Another cause of late patency loss, especially in smaller conduits, is a marked fibroproliferative reaction at the anastomoses, leading to focal severe stenoses.[85-87] Ongoing vascular injury, release of platelet-derived growth factors from platelets deposited upstream to the distal anastomosis, marked discrepancies in the compliance of native artery and graft materials, and turbulent blood flow with increased wall tension at anastomoses promote this intimal hyperplasia.[88-91] Accumulation of lipids and organization of surface thrombus cause further enlargement of stenotic lesions.[87] Other possible complications of synthetic vascular grafts include disintegration of sutures, kinking, perigraft hematoma and seroma, aortoenteric fistula, infection, false aneurysm formation, and degeneration of the graft at anastomotic sites.[92]

REFERENCES

1. Simionescu N, Simionescu M: The cardiovascular system. p. 372. In Weiss L (ed): Histology, Cell and Tissue Biology. Elsevier Biomedical, New York, 1983
2. Palade GE: Blood capillaries of the heart and other organs. Circulation 24:368, 1961
3. Fajardo LF: The complexity of endothelial cells. A review. Am J Clin Pathol 92:241, 1989
4. Ross R: The pathogenesis of atherosclerosis—an update. N Engl J Med 314:488, 1986
5. Schwartz SM, Reidy MA: Common mechanisms of proliferation of smooth muscle in atherosclerosis and hypertension. Hum Pathol 18:240, 1987
6. McGill HC, Jr: Fatty streaks in the coronary arteries and aorta. Lab Invest 18:560, 1968
7. Haust MD: The morphogenesis and fate of potential and early atherosclerotic lesions in man. Hum Pathol 2:1, 1971
8. Geer JC: Fine structure of human aortic intimal thickening and fatty streaks. Lab Invest 14:1764, 1965
9. Munro JM, van der Walt JD, Munro CS et al: An immunohistochemical analysis of human aortic fatty streaks. Hum Pathol 18:375, 1987
10. Stary HC: Evolution and progression of atherosclerotic lesions in coronary arteries of children and young adults. Arteriosclerosis, suppl. 1. 9:1, 1989
11. McGill HC, Jr: Persistent problems in the pathogenesis of atherosclerosis. Arteriosclerosis 4:443, 1984
12. Velican C, Velican D: The precursors of coronary atherosclerotic plaques in subjects up to 40 years old. Atherosclerosis 37:33, 1980
13. Cotran RS: Blood vessels. p. 563. In Cotran RS, Kumar V, Robbins SL (eds): Robbins Pathologic Basis of Disease. 4th Ed. WB Saunders, Philadelphia, 1989
14. Barnes MJ: Collagens in atherosclerosis. Coll Relat Res 5:65, 1985
15. Berenson GS, Radhakrishnamurthy B, Srinivasan SR et al: Arterial wall injury and proteoglycan changes in atherosclerosis. Arch Pathol Lab Med 112:1002, 1988
16. Shekhonin BV, Domogatsky SP, Idelson GL et al: Relative distribution of fibronectin and type I, III, IV, V collagens in normal and atherosclerotic intima of human arteries. Atherosclerosis 67:9, 1987

17. Burke JM, Ross R: Synthesis of connective tissue macromolecules by smooth muscle. Int Rev Connect Tissue Res 8:119, 1979

18. Mosse PRL, Campbell GR, Wang ZL, Campbell JH: Smooth muscle phenotypic expression in human carotid arteries. I. Comparison of cells from diffuse intimal thickenings adjacent to atheromatous plaques with those of the media. Lab Invest 53:556, 1985

19. Chamley-Campbell JH, Campbell GR, Ross R: Phenotype-dependent response of cultured aortic smooth muscle to serum mitogens. J Cell Biol 89:379, 1981

20. Campbell GR, Campbell JH: Smooth muscle phenotypic changes in arterial wall homeostasis: implications for the pathogenesis of atherosclerosis. Exp Mol Pathol 42:139, 1985

21. Smith EP: The relationship between plasma and tissue lipids in human atherosclerosis. Adv Lipid Res 12:1, 1974

22. Bocan TMA, Schifani TA, Guyton JR: Ultrastructure of the human aortic fibrolipid lesion. Formation of the atherosclerotic lipid-rich core. Am J Pathol 123:413, 1986

23. Bedossa P, Poynard T, Abella A et al: Localization of apolipoprotein A-I and apolipoprotein A-II in human atherosclerotic arteries. Arch Pathol Lab Med 113:777, 1989

24. Yomantas S, Elner VM, Schaffner T, Wissler RW: Immunohistochemical localization of apolipoprotein B in human atherosclerotic lesions. Arch Pathol Lab Med 108:374, 1984

25. Rath M, Niendorf A, Reblin T et al: Detection and quantification of lipoprotein (a) in the arterial wall of 107 coronary bypass patients. Arteriosclerosis 9:579, 1989

26. Vollmer E, Roessner A, Bosse A et al: Immunohistochemical double labeling of macrophages, smooth muscle cells, and apolipoprotein E in the atherosclerotic plaque. Pathol Res Pract 187:184, 1991

27. Gown AM, Tsukada T, Ross R: Human atherosclerosis. II. Immunocytochemical analysis of the cellular composition of human atherosclerotic lesions. Am J Pathol 125:191, 1986

28. Aqel NM, Ball RY, Waldmann H, Mitchinson MJ: Identification of macrophages and smooth muscle cells in human atherosclerosis using monoclonal antibodies. J Pathol 146:197, 1985

29. Klurfeld DM: Identification of foam cells in human atherosclerotic lesions as macrophages using monoclonal antibodies. Arch Pathol Lab Med 109:445, 1985

30. Emeson EE, Robertson AL, Jr: T lymphocytes in aortic and coronary intimas. Am J Pathol 130:369, 1988

31. van der Wal AC: Atherosclerotic lesions in human. In situ immunophenotypic analysis suggesting an immune mediated response. Lab Invest 61:166, 1989

32. Hansson GK, Holm J, Jonasson L: Detection of activated T lymphocytes in the human atherosclerotic plaque. Am J Pathol 135:169, 1989

33. Zamir M, Silver MD: Vasculature in the walls of human coronary arteries. Arch Pathol Lab Med 109:659, 1985

34. Isner JM, Donaldson RF, Fortin AH et al: Attenuation of the media of coronary arteries in advanced atherosclerosis. Am J Cardiol 58:937, 1986

35. Tomazic BB, Brown WE, Queral LA, Sadovnik M: Physicochemical characterization of cardiovascular calcified deposits. I. Isolation, purification, and instrumental analysis. Atherosclerosis 69:5, 1988

36. Glimcher MJ: Mechanism of calcification: Role of collagen fibrils—phosphoprotein complexes in vitro and in vivo. Anat Rec 224:139, 1989

37. Vlodaver Z, Edwards JE: Pathology of coronary atherosclerosis. Prog Cardiovasc Dis 14:256, 1971

38. Dollar AL, Kragel AH, Fernicola DJ et al: Composition of atherosclerotic plaques in coronary arteries in women <40 years of age with fatal coronary artery disease and implications for plaque reversibility. Am J Cardiol 67:1223, 1991

39. Falk E: Morphologic features of unstable atherothrombotic plaques underlying acute coronary syndromes. Am J Cardiol 63:114E, 1989

40. Tracy RE, Devaney K, Kissling G: Characteristics of the plaque under a coronary thrombus. Virchows Arch [A] 405:411, 1985

41. Sato T, Takebayashi S, Kohchi K: Increased subendothelial infiltration of the coronary arteries with monocytes/macrophages in patients with unstable angina. Histological data on 14 autopsied patients. Atherosclerosis 68:191, 1987

42. Moore WS, Hall AD: Importance of emboli from carotid bifurcation in pathogenesis of cerebral ischemic attacks. Arch Surg 101:708, 1970

43. Karmody AM, Powers SR, Monaco VJ, Leather RP: "Blue toe" syndrome: An indication for limb salvage surgery. Arch Surg 111:1263, 1976

44. Ridolfi RL, Hutchins GM: The relationship between coronary artery lesions and myocardial infarcts: ulceration of atherosclerotic plaques precipitating coronary thrombosis. Am Heart J 93:468, 1977

45. Davies MJ, Thomas AC: Plaque fissuring—the cause of acute myocardial infarction, sudden ischaemic death and crescendo angina. Br Heart J 53:363, 1985

46. Falk E: Plaque rupture with severe pre-existing stenosis precipitating coronary thrombosis. Characteristics of coronary atherosclerotic plaques underlying fatal occlusive thrombi. Br Heart J 50:127, 1983

47. Qiao J-H, Fishbein MC: The severity of coronary atherosclerosis at sites of plaque rupture with occlusive thrombosis. J Am Coll Cardiol 17:1138, 1991

48. Fuster V, Badimon L, Cohen M et al: Insights into the pathogenesis of acute ischemic syndromes. Circulation 77:1213, 1988

49. Friedman M: The coronary thrombus: its origin and fate. Hum Pathol 2:81, 1971

50. Davies MJ, Fulton WFM, Robertson WB: The relation of coronary thrombosis to ischaemic myocardial necrosis. J Pathol 127:99, 1979

51. Buja LM, Willerson JT: The role of coronary artery lesions in ischemic heart disease: insights from recent clin-

icopathologic, coronary arteriographic, and experimental studies. Hum Pathol 18:451, 1987

52. d'Amati G, Silver MD: Atherosclerosis of the aorta and its complications. p. 284. In Silver MD (ed): Cardiovascular Pathology. 2nd Ed. Churchill Livingstone, New York, 1991

53. Walker DI, Bloor K, Williams G, Gillie I: Inflammatory aneurysms of the abdominal aorta. Br J Surg 59:609, 1972

54. Crawford ES, Hess KR: Abdominal aortic aneurysm. N Engl J Med 321:1040, 1989

55. Velican C, Velican D: Progression of coronary atherosclerosis from adolescents to mature adults. Atherosclerosis 47:131, 1983

56. Bruschke AVG, Wijers TS, Kolsters W, Landmann J: The anatomic evolution of coronary artery disease demonstrated by coronary arteriography in 256 nonoperated patients. Circulation 63:527, 1981

57. Hertzer NR: The natural history of peripheral vascular disease. Implications for its management. Circulation, suppl I. 83:I-12, 1991

58. Wissler RW, Vesselinovitch D: Can atherosclerotic plaques regress? Anatomic and biochemical evidence from nonhuman animal models. Am J Cardiol 65:33F, 1990

59. Blankenhorn DH, Kramsch DM: Reversal of atherosis and sclerosis. The two components of atherosclerosis. Circulation 79:1, 1989

60. Blankenhorn DH, Nession SA, Johnson RL et al: Beneficial effects of combined colestipol-niacin therapy on coronary atherosclerosis and coronary venous bypass grafts. J Am Med Assoc 257:3233, 1987

61. Brown G, Albers JJ, Fisher LD et al: Regression of coronary artery disease as a result of intensive lipid-lowering therapy in men with high levels of apolipoprotein B. N Engl J Med 323:1289, 1990

62. Szilagyi DE, Elliott JP, Hageman JH et al: Biologic fate of autogenous vein implants as arterial substitutes. Clinical, angiographic and histopathologic observations in femoro-popliteal operations for atherosclerosis. Ann Surg 178:232, 1973

63. Bulkley BH, Hutchins GM: Accelerated "atherosclerosis." A morphologic study of 97 saphenous vein coronary artery bypass grafts. Circulation 55:163, 1977

64. Batayias GE, Barboriak JJ, Korns ME, Pintar K: The spectrum of pathologic changes in aortocoronary saphenous vein grafts. Circulation, suppl 2. 56:II-18, 1977

65. Kern WH, Wells WJ, Meyer BW: The pathology of surgically excised aortocoronary saphenous vein bypass grafts. Am J Surg Pathol 5:491, 1981

66. Smith SH, Geer JC: Morphology of saphenous vein-coronary artery bypass grafts. Seven to 116 months after surgery. Arch Pathol Lab Med 107:13, 1983

67. Atkinson JB, Forman MB, Vaughn WK et al: Morphologic changes in long-term saphenous vein bypass grafts. Chest 88:341, 1985

68. Kalan JM, Roberts WC: Morphologic findings in saphenous veins used as coronary arterial bypass conduits for longer than 1 year: necropsy analysis of 53 patients, 123 saphenous veins, and 1865 five-millimeter segments of veins. Am Heart J 119:1164, 1990

69. Yutani C, Imakita M, Ishibashii Veda H: Histopathological study of aorto-coronary bypass grafts with special reference to fibrin deposits on grafted saphenous veins. Acta Pathol Jpn 39:425, 1989

70. Vlodaver Z, Edwards JE: Pathologic analysis in fatal cases following saphenous vein coronary arterial bypass. Chest 64:555, 1973

71. Lie JT, Lawrie GM, Morris GC, Jr: Aortocoronary bypass saphenous vein graft atherosclerosis. Anatomic study of 99 vein grafts from normal and hyperlipoproteinemic patients up to 75 months postoperatively. Am J Cardiol 40:906, 1977

72. Ratliff NB, Myles JL: Rapidly progressive atherosclerosis in aortocoronary saphenous vein grafts. Possible immune-mediated disease. Arch Pathol Lab Med 113:772, 1989

73. Spray TL, Roberts WC: Changes in saphenous veins used as aortocoronary bypass grafts. Am Heart J 94:500, 1977

74. Unni KK, Kottke BA, Titus JL et al: Pathologic changes in aortocoronary saphenous vein grafts. Am J Cardiol 34:526, 1974

75. Brody WR, Kosek JC, Angell WW, Shumway NE: Changes in vein grafts following aorto-coronary bypass induced by pressure and ischemia. J Thorac Cardiovasc Surg 64:847, 1972

76. Kern WH, Dermer GB, Lindesmith GG: The intimal proliferation in aortic-coronary saphenous vein grafts. Light and electron microscopic studies. Am Heart J 84:771, 1972

77. Neitzel GF, Barboriak JJ, Pintar K, Qureshi I: Atherosclerosis in aortocoronary bypass grafts. Morphologic study and risk factor analysis 6 to 12 years after surgery. Arteriosclerosis 6:594, 1986

78. Guidoin R, Couture J, Assayed F, Gosselin C: New frontiers of vascular grafting. Int Surg 73:241, 1988

79. Jarrell BE, Williams SK, Hoch JR, Carabasi RA: Perspectives in vascular surgery. Biocompatible surfaces: the past and future role of endothelial cells. Bull NY Acad Med 63:156, 1987

80. Clowes AW, Gown AM, Hanson SR, Reidy MA: Mechanisms of arterial graft failure. I. Role of cellular proliferation in early healing of PTFE prostheses. Am J Pathol 118:43, 1985

81. Sauvage LR, Berger KE, Wood SJ et al: Interspecies healing of porous arterial prostheses. Arch Surg 109:698, 1974

82. Camilleri JP, Phat VN, Bruneval P et al: Surface healing and histologic maturation of patent polytetrafluoroethylene grafts implanted in patients for up to 60 months. Arch Pathol Lab Med 109:833, 1985

83. Stratton JR, Thiele BL, Ritchie JL: Natural history of platelet deposition on Dacron aortic bifurcation grafts in the first year after implantation. Am J Cardiol 52:371, 1983

84. Goldman M, Norcott HC, Hawker RJ et al: Platelet accumulation on mature Dacron grafts in man. Br J Surg, suppl. 69:S38, 1982

85. Echave V, Koornick AR, Haimov M, Jacobseon JH: Intimal hyperplasia as a complication of the use of the polytetrafluoroethylene graft for femoro-popliteal bypass. Surgery 86:791, 1986

86. Orekhova NM, Andreeva ER, Shekhonin BV et al: Spontaneous atherosclerotic plaque and obstruction of distal anastomosis in femoral artery. Comparative morphologic study. Arch Pathol Lab Med 111:1163, 1987

87. Walton KW, Slaney G, Ashton F: Atherosclerosis in vascular grafts for peripheral vascular disease. Part 2. Synthetic arterial prostheses. Atherosclerosis 61:155, 1986

88. Swedberg S, Brown BG, Sigley R et al: Intimal fibromuscular hyperplasia at the venous anastomosis of PTFE grafts in hemodialysis patients. Clinical, immunocyto-chemical, light and electron microscopic assessment. Circulation 80:1726, 1989

89. Abbott WM, Megerman J, Hasson JE et al: Effect of compliance mismatch on vascular graft patency. J Vasc Surg 5:376, 1987

90. Leung DYM, Glagov S, Matthews MB: Cyclic stretching stimulates synthesis of matrix components by arterial smooth muscle cells in vitro. Science 191:475, 1976

91. Walden R, L'Italien GJ, Megerman J, Abbott WM: Matched elastic properties and successful arterial grafting. Arch Surg 115:1166, 1980

92. Silver MD, Wilson GJ: Pathology of mechanical heart valve prostheses and vascular grafts made of artificial materials. p. 1534. In Silver MD (ed): Cardiovascular Pathology. 2nd Ed. Churchill Livingstone, New York, 1991

2

Response of the Artery to Injury: The Role of Intimal Hyperplasia in the Failure of Vascular Reconstruction

Ted R. Kohler
Alexander W. Clowes

Intimal hyperplasia is a universal response of the arterial wall to all types of injury, including surgical endarterectomy, balloon catheter dilatation, hydrostatic stretch, and exposure to toxins. Rates of restenosis due to intimal hyperplasia are remarkably constant and independent of the type of inciting injury. While great technologic strides have been made in vascular reconstruction over the past two decades, all methods are still subject to late failure due to this process. Intimal hyperplasia is caused by proliferation of medial smooth muscle cells (SMCs) and production by these cells of matrix components (collagen, elastin, and proteoglycans). The result is wall thickening and lumen narrowing, which may lead to pressure and flow reduction and eventual thrombosis. This chapter reviews the pathophysiology of intimal hyperplasia and explores possible methods of controlling it.

CLINICAL PRESENTATION

The clinical presentation of intimal hyperplasia has been best described following percutaneous transluminal coronary angioplasty (PTCA), carotid endarterectomy, atherectomy, and vein bypass grafting. In the coronary circulation, the problem is well defined because restenosis is frequently symptomatic and follow-up angiograms have been obtained in large numbers of patients. Restenosis rates are typically within the range of 30 percent following PTCA.[1-5] The lesions of restenosis tend to occur within the first 6 months of angioplasty[3] and have not been prevented by antiplatelet therapy, steroids, calcium channel blockers, or a 24-hour administration of heparin.[4-6] Specimens obtained by atherectomy confirm that these lesions differ from the primary coronary atherosclerotic plaques and

17

are caused principally by SMC proliferation.[7-9] Restenosis rates of 50 percent have been reported after atherectomy.[9]

Reported rates of restenosis after carotid endarterectomy are similar to those following PTCA ranging from 9 to 36 percent, with most lesions occurring in the first 12 months.[10-13] Pathologic examination of specimens from reoperations demonstrates that early lesions tend to be composed of SMC and matrix components, while later-appearing lesions develop the features of atherosclerosis (calcium, collagen, foam cells).[14,15] Regression occurs in approximately 10 percent of cases.[10,12] Unlike restenosis in the coronary circulation, which frequently causes clinically important flow reduction, carotid narrowing due to restenosis is generally asymptomatic.[12,13] This is in part due to the rich supply of collateral circulation. In addition, these lesions rarely progress to total occlusion and, unlike atherosclerotic plaques, they do not undergo ulceration and embolization.

Approximately 30 percent of vein grafts used as arterial substitutes in both the coronary and lower extremity circulation fail within 5 years of operation.[16-22] Intimal hyperplasia is responsible for up to one-third of the failures that occur during the first 2 postoperative years.[16,23,24] These lesions are similar to those described above, consisting of SMC proliferation and matrix deposition forming a fibrous thickening.[1,7,19,25-29] They most commonly occur at sites of anastomoses, at venous valves, and in association with clamp injuries.

INVESTIGATION IN ANIMAL MODELS

Intimal hyperplasia begins as a response of the vascular wall to injury caused by surgical or angiographic manipulation. The extent of the resulting wall thickening depends on the severity of the injury, the composition of the wall, local hemodynamic factors, and the presence or absence of systemic risk factors. The cellular biology of the injury response has been studied extensively in animal models. While human arteries may respond slightly differently than those of rodents or subhuman primates, the basic cellular responses are likely to be the same. Indeed, specimens of human restenotic lesions obtained by atherectomy closely resemble those seen in laboratory animals.

The best characterized animal model uses balloon injury of the rat common carotid artery.[30] This artery is particularly useful because it has few branches; therefore, denuding injuries are not rapidly repaired by ingrowth of endothelium from branch orifices. A defined and reproducible injury to the common carotid artery is produced by passing a distended 2 French balloon catheter into the common carotid artery either retrograde through the external carotid artery or antegrade through the femoral vessels. This technique produces complete endothelial denudation as well as loss of approximately 20 percent of medial SMCs (as assessed by DNA measurements). Thus, the model combines a denudation injury with vessel distension and medial SMC damage. Similar injuries are likely to result from endarterectomy or angioplasty of human vessels.

Within minutes, the denuded surface of the rat carotid artery is covered with a sheet of platelets, which adhere, spread, and degranulate, releasing SMC mitogens and chemoattractants such as transforming growth factor β, platelet-derived growth factor (PDGF), and an epidermal growth factor-like protein. Interestingly, after 1 day, the surface is no longer thrombogenic, perhaps because it becomes coated with plasma proteins that may prevent platelet adhesion. Studies using ornithine decarboxylase as an early cell cycle marker demonstrate that SMCs synchronously enter the cell cycle within hours of the injury.[31] Studies using continuous labeling of cells with tritiated thymidine have demonstrated that the number of nondividing cells remains constant, suggesting that SMCs either proliferate within the first 48 hours after injury or not at all. Both proliferating and nonproliferating cells may migrate across the internal elastic lamina onto the luminal surface where proliferation continues. Rates of cell division reach a peak by 48 hours, at which time 40 percent have entered the cell cycle as indicated by their incorporation of radiolabeled thymidine. Proliferation rates drop to 20 percent by 1 week and reach quiescent levels (0.05 percent) by 4 weeks. During this early phase, the arterial wall thickens due to both SMC proliferation and matrix production by these cells (collagen, elastin, and proteoglycans). Wall thickening continues for up to 3 months, well after proliferation has ceased, due to continued matrix production (Fig. 2-1).

This hyperplastic process consists of two distinct SMC responses: proliferation and migration from the media across the internal elastic lamina into the intima. Recent studies suggest that proliferation is stimulated primarily by SMC damage at the time of the balloon injury, while migration is caused by the release of platelet products. The work of Ross and Glomset suggested that PDGFs released from degranulating platelets could stimulate SMC proliferation in early atherogenesis.[32,33] Platelets were assumed to play an important role in the development of intimal hyperplasia as well. This concept was supported by the early work of Friedman et al.,[34] who demonstrated reduced intimal hyperplasia following balloon injury in rabbits rendered thrombocytopenic with antiplatelet antibod-

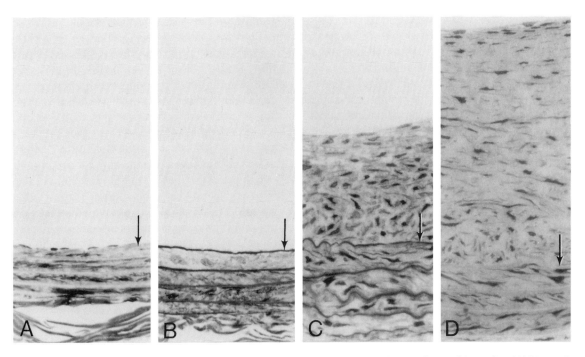

Figure 2-1 Histologic cross sections of the region lacking endothelium of injured left carotid arteries. **(A)** Normal vessel. Note single layer of endothelium in intima. **(B)** Denuded vessel at 2 days. Note loss of endothelium. **(C)** Denuded vessel at 2 weeks. Intima is now markedly thickened because of smooth muscle proliferation. **(D)** Denuded vessel at 12 weeks. Further intimal thickening has occurred. Internal elastic lamina indicated by arrow. Lumen is at the top. (×260.) (From Clowes et al.,[127] with permission.)

ies. Subsequent work by Fingerle et al.,[35] using thrombocytopenic rats, suggested that the primary role of platelets may be stimulation of migration rather than proliferation. They, like Friedman, found reduced intimal thickening in these animals, but they also found that rates of SMC proliferation were not affected. They explained this inhibition of intimal thickening in the presence of significant SMC proliferation by postulating that the primary role of platelets is to stimulate SMC migration from the media into the intima.[35]

Other studies using the rat model suggest that one of the principal mitogens contained in platelets, PDGF, stimulates migration of SMC, rather than their proliferation. Jawien et al.[36] infused recombinant PDGF-BB (the primary isoform found in platelets) intravenously following balloon injury and found a significant increase in SMC migration with only a slight increase of SMC proliferation. The work of Ferns et al.,[37] using a polyclonal antibody to PDGF, further supports the role of PDGF in stimulating migration in vivo. These investigators used athymic nude rats, since these animals do not mount an immune response capable of neutralizing foreign proteins such as the anti-PDGF antibody. They found that an infusion of a polyclonal antibody to PDGF caused a marked inhibition of intimal lesion

formation following balloon injury of the carotid artery, even though SMC proliferation was unaltered. These data again suggest that the primary role of PDGF is to stimulate SMC migration, rather than proliferation.

If platelets are not responsible for the marked increase in SMC proliferation following arterial injury, what is? Recent work suggests that the release of mitogens from injured SMCs may play a key role. Studies in which arteries were hydrostatically distended without balloon catheter injury demonstrated medial SMC proliferation in the absence of significant endothelial injury.[38] Also, very little SMC migration was observed, perhaps due to the absence of platelet factors.[38] Conversely, very little SMC proliferation takes place when the endothelium is gently denuded using a fine nylon loop that does not injure the media.[39,40] The mitogenic effect of SMC injury may be due to the release of growth factors such as PDGF or basic fibroblast growth factor (bFGF) from the injured SMCs. SMCs are capable of synthesizing many growth factors and may secrete them at an increased rate after injury, stimulating proliferation in a paracrine fashion. When grown in culture SMCs derived from injured media produce up to five times more PDGF than do cells from uninjured arteries.[41] SMCs from ballooned carotid arteries also express mRNA for insulin-like growth factor[42] and transforming growth factor β (unpublished data), which are mitogenic for SMCs in culture.

bFGF is synthesized by the arterial wall and may be released when SMCs cells are injured.[43] Infusion of bFGF following gentle denudation of the rat carotid artery markedly increases SMC proliferation.[43] Conversely, systemic injection of a neutralizing antibody against bFGF before balloon catheterization decreases the induced SMC proliferation by approximately 80 percent.[44] These data suggest that endogenous bFGF is the major mitogen controlling the growth of vascular smooth muscle cells following injury. The factors influencing SMC proliferation, migration, and matrix deposition are summarized in Fig. 2-2.

In the balloon injury model, SMCs stop proliferating after several weeks. This may occur because mitogens such as bFGF that are released after injury become depleted, or it may result from an active inhibition of proliferation. Cytokines released from lymphocytes in the vessel wall may inhibit SMC growth. Hansson et al.[45] demonstrated that γ-interferon, a secretory product of activated T lymphocytes, inhibits SMC proliferation in vitro and induces the expression of class II major histocompatibility complex antigens (Ia). These workers found a strong negative correlation in vivo between Ia expression and thymidine incorporation in intimal SMCs following balloon injury, suggesting that γ-interferon regulates SMC growth after injury. The endothelium may also produce factors that inhibit SMC growth. In the rat balloon injury model, SMCs

stop proliferating much sooner in regions in which the endothelium has regrown. This may be because luminal SMCs, unlike endothelial cells, form loose junctions that allow nutrients and mitogens to enter the wall. Alternatively, the endothelium may secrete molecules that inhibit SMC growth, such as heparan sulfate. The endothelium is capable of producing both growth promoters (transforming growth factor β, PDGF, fibroblast growth factor, and interleukin-1) and growth inhibitors (heparan sulfate and endothelium-derived relaxing factor [EDRF]).[46-50] Heparan sulfate, when released from its proteoglycan, can inhibit SMC growth. The drug heparin is a related molecule and is a potent inhibitor of neointimal growth in the rat injury model.

After injury, endothelial cells proliferate and migrate onto the denuded surface. However this process is limited. In the rat model, the endothelium advances approximately 0.2 mm/d and stops after 8 to 12 weeks. Large segments of artery remain denuded for up to 1 year.[51] It is not known why the endothelium stops growing before a complete monolayer is formed. Cell senescence is not a factor, since the endothelium can be stimulated to replicate if it is reinjured.[52] Regenerating endothelial cells produce bFGF, while quiescent cells do not.[53] This growth factor may play a critical role in modulating endothelial regrowth. Addition of bFGF to balloon injured rats stimulates endothelial proliferation in both normal and injured arteries and results in complete endothelialization of denuded carotid arteries within 10 weeks.[54] There are distinct species differences in the extent to which endothelium can regrow. There are no good data regarding endothelial regrowth in humans, as this is very difficult to assess either noninvasively or by standard pathologic evaluation. However, endothelial growth is probably limited in humans, since outgrowth onto the surface of prosthetic grafts is limited to 1 to 2 cm.

While injury causes lesion formation, the ultimate extent of the intimal thickening may be dependent on local hemodynamic factors. It is well known that wall structure is modified by pressure and flow. More than a century ago, the German anatomist Thoma noted that the diameter of developing chick arteries changes in proportion to the velocity of blood flowing through them.[55] In this way, nutrient arteries adjust their caliber to maintain constant shear at the wall. The same phenomenon is observed in mature arteries when flow is increased by creation of an arteriovenous fistula.[56-59] The feeding artery gradually dilates until wall shear is normalized. Conversely, when flow is decreased (e.g., by ligation of outflow vessels), arterial diameter is reduced.[60] While flow rate affects arterial caliber in a way that maintains constant shear, pressure affects wall

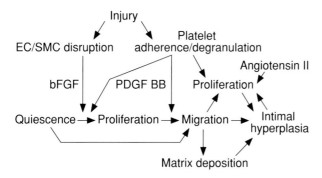

Figure 2-2 Diagram illustrating how injury to the artery might cause endothelial (EC) and smooth muscle cell (SMC) disruption and release of intracellular mitogens such as basic fibroblast growth factor (bFGF). bFGF then stimulates medial smooth muscle proliferation. Factors from platelets (PDGF) regulate movement of the smooth muscle cells from the media to the intima. Angiotensin II also affects the intimal thickening process. (From Clowes,[85] with permission.)

thickness in a manner that maintains constant wall tension. The wall thickens when pressure is increased. Thus, the pulmonary artery and the aorta have the same caliber, as they carry the same blood flow. Yet the aorta is much thicker, since its intraluminal pressure is much greater.

Hemodynamic factors are also important determinants of artery wall structure in diseased states. For example, the arterial wall thickening has been demonstrated in animal models of hypertension.[61] Furthermore, the type of wall thickening can be quite different, depending on the cause of hypertension. Thus, increased SMC proliferation and hyperplasia occurs in rats made hypertensive by aortic coarctation, while aortic medial hypertrophy due to SMC hypertrophy and hyperploidy without hyperplasia occurs in Goldblatt or spontaneously hypertensive rats.[62] The vessel wall response to injury is also influenced by hypertension. Intimal hyperplasia in balloon-injured arteries of spontaneously hypertensive rats is markedly enhanced compared with animals whose blood pressure is lowered by drug treatment.[63]

Intimal hyperplasia occurs in vein grafts placed in the arterial circulation. This was described when Carrel and Guthrie reported the first use of veins as arterial substitutes.[64,65] These investigators correctly interpreted this thickening as adaptation to the arterial circulation. The vein wall is thinner than that of arteries and does not have the lamellar structure that enables arterial wall to withstand systemic pressure. As a result,

wall tension is extremely high when veins are placed in the arterial circulation. Wall thickening due to intimal hyperplasia reduces wall stress to relatively normal levels.[66] In support of this concept, we found that intimal hyperplasia was reduced when wall stress was diminished by supporting the vein graft with a rigid external wrap in a rabbit model of vein graft hyperplasia.[67]

Shear is an important determinant of wall thickening in atherosclerosis, vein graft hyperplasia, and following arterial injury. Atherosclerosis tends to occur in areas of reduced or oscillating shear, such as the lateral carotid bulb.[68-70] Atherosclerotic vessels also appear to adjust their diameter in response to blood flow. Glagov et al.[71] found that when human coronary arteries are moderately constricted by atherosclerotic plaque the vessels dilate in a manner that maintains normal shear. Several studies have demonstrated increased wall thickening in vein grafts when shear is decreased.[72-75] We found that increased flow caused by creation of a distal arteriovenous fistula was associated with reduced intimal thickening in porous polytetrafluoroethylene (PTFE) grafts placed in baboons[76] (Fig. 2-3). The endothelium might play an important role in this response, since these grafts have a complete endothelial lining.[77] Flow rate also affects intimal hyperplasia in ballooned arteries in which endothelium is absent. Studies using the rat carotid injury model demonstrated increased wall thickening when flow was reduced by ligation of outflow vessels.[78]

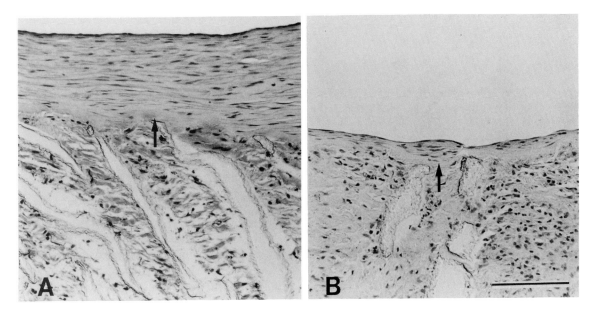

Figure 2-3 Cross sections of PTFE grafts 3 months after placement in baboons. **(A)** Control side. **(B)** Side with a distal arteriovenous fistula causing increased flow. Arrows indicate the junction of the graft and neointima. Bar = 100 μm. (From Kohler et al.,[76] with permission.)

METHODS OF CONTROL

There are several potential strategies for controlling intimal hyperplasia. These include using various drugs to prevent SMC proliferation or to promote endothelial regrowth, using mechanical methods to reduce injury at the time of vessel manipulation or to stent the vessel to prevent narrowing, and introducing specific inhibitor genes by seeding injured segments with genetically altered cells or by injecting genes directly into the vessel wall.

Pharmacologic Methods

Pharmacologic intervention for the prevention of intimal hyperplasia may be directed at any of the relevant cellular processes, including platelet aggregation, SMC proliferation, SMC migration, endothelial regrowth, and matrix deposition. Several classes of drugs are of potential benefit, such as inhibitors of platelet adherence, aggregation, and degranulation, and agents that inhibit SMC mitogenesis or migration.

Antiplatelet Agents

Several clinical trials have been conducted using antiplatelet agents, primarily aspirin with or without dipyridamole, to prevent intimal hyperplasia in vein grafts. Several large studies of coronary artery bypass vein graft failure suggest that aspirin and perhaps ticlopidine, when given during the immediate perioperative period, can improve short-term patency rates, probably by reducing early thrombosis.[79-81] Dipyridamole does not appear to add substantially to the effects of aspirin.[82] Similar studies of lower-extremity bypass grafts have had mixed results. Some have shown a slight improvement in the patency of synthetic femoropopliteal grafts and vein grafts to tibial vessels, but others have not.[83-85] Although some experimental work has suggested that aspirin and dipyridamole can decrease intimal hyperplasia in vein grafts,[86,87] these agents appear to have little effect on the long-term problem of intimal hyperplasia. This is consistent with the previously described animal data demonstrating that platelets are not necessary for SMC proliferation, although they are important in stimulating migration into the intima. Alternatively, antiplatelet agents may not affect intimal hyperplasia because they do not prevent the single layer of platelet deposition that occurs after vein grafting (a complete blockage of platelet adherence would lead to exsanguination).[88]

Fuster and Chesebro[88,89] have summarized the experimental and clinical data regarding the role of aspirin in preventing aortocoronary artery bypass graft failure. They describe four distinct phases of vein graft occlusive disease. The role of antiplatelet therapy is different in each phase. Graft occlusion in the early phase is caused by thrombosis and is significantly reduced by platelet inhibitors. Because platelet deposition occurs immediately after blood flow is restored to the graft, antiplatelet agents must be present at the time of surgery to be effective. The second, intermediate phase extends from the first postoperative month to 1 year after surgery. During this time, intimal hyperplasia is the primary cause of graft narrowing. Platelets may be important during this phase, perhaps mostly as stimulants for SMC migration into the intima. However, platelet inhibitors such as aspirin are not effective in controlling intimal hyperplasia, possibly because they do not prevent platelet adhesion to injured surfaces.[90,91] Although aspirin with or without dipyridamole is not effective in preventing restenosis after PTCA, there is some suggestion that these drugs may reduce the severity of this recurrent lesion.[92] Newer and more potent agents that interfere with platelet adherence, such as monoclonal antibodies to the glycoprotein IIb/IIIa integrin complex and von Willebrand factor, may be more effective in preventing intimal hyperplasia. However, these may not be practical because of their greater effects on hemostasis.[91] In the third phase of late occlusion, vein grafts fail due to thrombosis of critically narrowed segments. Here the data of Chesebro and others suggest that antiplatelet agents may have some benefit, although not as great as in the early phase. Finally, beyond 1 year, vein grafts begin to develop atherosclerotic changes. The possible role of antiplatelet agents in preventing this process is not known, although there are suggestive experimental data.[93] While there is some suggestion that aspirin may help prevent progression of atherosclerosis in arteries and in vein grafts,[94,95] most studies are unconvincing.[83] Lipid-lowering drugs may be more effective in this regard. Recent evidence suggests that increased levels of low-density lipoproteins (LDLs) and apolipoprotein B (apoB) are major risk factors for atherosclerosis in vein grafts.

Calcium Channel Blockers

Calcium channel blockers, when begun early, have been effective in reducing intimal hyperplasia in animal models of vein graft hyperplasia, atherosclerosis induced by fat feeding, and intimal thickening after balloon injury.[96-101] It is not known how they act on the cellular level, but it has been suggested that they may reduce atherosclerosis by protecting arterial cells from calcium overload by inhibiting calcium flux.[102] They may also influence SMC migration and matrix synthesis and the cellular handling of lipoproteins and intracellular cholesterol ester stores.[102] As yet, no clinical trials have demonstrated benefit of these agents in reducing intimal hyperplasia, although there is a suggestion that nifedipine can reduce the incidence of new atherosclerotic lesions in coronary vessels[103] and may improve success rates following PTCA in patients who have coronary artery spasm.[104]

Heparin

Heparin reduces intimal hyperplasia after arterial injury and vein graft hyperplasia in some animal models.[31,105,106] Its principal effect is inhibition of SMC proliferation,[31,107-110] although it also limits migration.[107,111] Studies with cell cycle markers reveal that heparin exerts its effect early in the cell cycle (late G_0 or early G_1). It has to be present only 24 to 72 hours after the injury to be effective.[31] It also causes reduced production of elastin and collagen and increased proteoglycan accumulation.[112] It does not adversely affect endothelial regrowth,[109] and may enhance it.[108] The mechanism of action is not fully understood. It is possible that this agent acts by binding basic FGF and releasing it from the matrix. Work in our laboratory suggests that heparin decreases the expression of tissue-type plasminogen activator and displaces urokinase from the cell layer.[113,114] These effects may interfere with the ability of SMCs to degrade their surrounding matrix, which is a necessary step for their migration and proliferation.[115]

The effects of heparin are not related to its anticoagulant properties since some nonanticoagulant fractions that do not bind antithrombin III are equally effective.[116] Nonanticoagulant fractions of heparin are particularly promising for clinical use; clinical trials with these agents are currently under way. On the basis of experimental data from animal models, heparin administration for prevention of intimal hyperplasia should be started within 24 hours of injury and continued throughout the period of maximal proliferation. This period is approximately 7 days in rats after a single injury to a previously healthy vessel. In this model, 7 days of heparin therapy is as effective as 28 days of treatment.[107]

Angiotensin Converting Enzyme Inhibitors

The angiotensin system, which is an important regulator of systemic blood pressure, may also play an important role in local control of vascular wall structure. This enzyme may affect the local metabolism of angiotensin I in the vessel wall. Angiotensin converting enzyme (ACE) inhibitor activity is present in vascular endothelium and has recently been found in other types of vascular cells.[117] Control of the conversion of angiotensin I may be important since angiotensin II can stimulate SMC proliferation. ACE inhibitors and the specific angiotensin II receptor antagonist, Dup 753, have been shown to reduce intimal hyperplasia following balloon catheter injury in animal models.[101,118] Preliminary data from our laboratory suggest that ACE inhibitors and heparin act by way of different mechanisms since the combination of these two drugs is more effective than either agent alone in reducing intimal hyperplasia after balloon injury.

Other Drugs

Various other growth inhibitors have been used in an attempt to control the SMC proliferation of intimal hyperplasia. Among these are cytotoxic agents used for chemotherapy or for prevention of rejection after transplantation. Unless local delivery systems become available for these agents, their systemic effects will limit their usefulness. Part of the vascular injury response is inflammatory with the invasion of macrophages into the vessel wall. The role of these cells is not well defined, but there is a suggestion that inhibitors of inflammation, such as steroids, can limit the hyperplastic response. There is a suggestion that steroids can limit intimal hyperplasia following balloon catheter injury in an animal model[119] and may act synergistically with heparin, but they have failed to reduce restenosis following coronary angioplasty.[120] Fish oil has also been tested in animal models; it has been found to reduce intimal hyperplasia, perhaps by reducing platelet aggregation and cellular production of PDGF.[121-123] There are as yet no prospective clinical trials using fish oils as antithrombotic or antiatherogenic agents.[122]

Mechanical Factors

Because intimal hyperplasia is a response to vessel injury, reduction of trauma to the arterial wall should result in reduced wall thickening. This is the reason that vascular surgeons have sought methods to minimize damage to veins during preparation for bypass grafting. It has been shown that venous segments that are handled roughly or that are overvigorously distended lose a significant amount of endothelium and have more wall thickening than do veins that are handled more gently.[23] Indeed, reduction of injury is one of the main reasons that in situ saphenous vein bypass grafting has regained popularity for lower-extremity revascularization. Reduction of injury is also a concern for balloon catheter angioplasty techniques. Proponents of atherectomy and laser angioplasty suggest that their devices remove plaque without producing as much damage to the underlying structures as occurs with balloon dilatation, although this is not proven. The extent of injury caused by these devices does appear to have an effect on outcome. For example, the degree of intimal hyperplasia following atherectomy for vein graft stenosis or for restenosis after balloon angioplasty appears to be related to the depth of tissue resection, with higher restenosis rates following deeper injury.[9] It may be possible to alter catheter design to reduce wall trauma. For example, linear extrusion devices for angioplasty may reduce endothelial damage by eliminating shear forces. Finally, mechanical stents are being used to maintain patency after angioplasty. The clinical value of these devices has not been established. It is unlikely that they can prevent intimal hyperplasia.[124]

As mentioned earlier, atherosclerosis, vein graft thickening, and intimal hyperplasia after arterial injury all seem to be increased when flow is reduced. For this reason, flow through arterial bypass grafts or segments that have been dilated should be maximized. Therefore, it is important to achieve the maximum possible lumen diameter when performing angioplasty. Flow may be increased also by greater attention to distal occlusive disease or even by creation of a distal arteriovenous fistula. Some workers have advocated the use of arteriovenous fistulae to maintain the patency of tenuous bypasses to tibial vessels.[125] Although animal research suggests that this technique may reduce injury-induced intimal hyperplasia or neointimal thickening in synthetic bypass grafts, extending this concept to revascularizations in humans remains premature.

Cell Seeding

Cell seeding techniques can be used to provide an endothelial surface for prosthetic grafts, denuded vessels, and stents. The main goal of cell seeding is to prevent thrombosis. However, denuded arterial surfaces can become nonthrombogenic in less time than it takes for seeded cells to regenerate an intact endothelium. Antiplatelet therapy may be a more practical approach to prevent thrombosis. The clinical efficacy of cell seeding has not been proved. Preliminary studies suggest that cell seeding of PTFE arterial grafts results in a less thrombogenic surface,[126] but the long-term durability of the endothelium and its effect on patency have not been fully evaluated. There are other possible benefits of an intact endothelium in addition to reduction of thrombogenicity. As previously mentioned, endothelial cells produce a heparin-like factor that inhib-

its SMC proliferation; in animal models, SMCs cease proliferating in reendothelialized regions, while in chronically denuded regions, SMCs near the lumen continue to proliferate.[46,127] Bush et al.[128] found that intimal hyperplasia following endarterectomy in dogs was significantly less in segments that were seeded with endothelial cells. However, endothelial cells that grow onto denuded segments may not function like normal endothelium and could even produce factors that stimulate rather than inhibit wall thickening. Endothelium on the surface of artificial vascular grafts has a much higher than normal rate of proliferation, suggesting chronic injury.[127,129] Injured endothelium can produce factors, such as bFGF, that are mitogenic for SMC and therefore may stimulate intimal thickening. It may also produce reduced amounts of EDRF.[130] Therefore, the long-term value of this technique in clinical practice remains to be established.

While most workers have concentrated on cell seeding to provide an endothelial surface for synthetic grafts, an alternative approach is to make the graft sufficiently porous to permit ingrowth of capillaries. Animal studies indicate that when capillaries reach the lumen of the graft, they change from a tubular morphology, spread across the luminal surface, coalesce, and form an intact endothelial lining. SMCs then grow in under the endothelium and proliferate, forming a neointima. This has been observed in baboon models using both Dacron and highly porous (60-μm internodal distance) PTFE grafts.[76,131-133] However, angiogenesis in humans may be more limited. Neither Dacron nor highly porous PTFE grafts appears to endothelialize by capillary ingrowth in humans.[134-137]

Genetic Manipulation

Perhaps the most dramatic method of controlling intimal hyperplasia is to introduce genes with specific growth promoters or inhibitors directly into the cells of the vessel wall. Several investigators have been able to implant genes into endothelial cells or SMCs and then demonstrate function of these genes in viable cells that have been seeded onto PTFE grafts or onto denuded arterial segments.[138-142] One mechanism for reducing intimal hyperplasia is the introduction of mutant receptors for mitogens. For example, Williams et al.[143,144] suggested that mutant PDGF receptors that bind PDGF but that do not promote SMC growth could inhibit PDGF-stimulated proliferation. An alternative approach is to use mutant mitogens to occupy receptor sites. Altered forms of bFGF may be particularly useful in view of their probable role in promoting SMC proliferation after arterial injury. Mutated acidic FGF (aFGF) molecules lacking a heparin binding region or nuclear translocation sequence have been produced. These molecules do not stimulate mesenchymal cell growth but do bind to the aFGF receptor blocking the action of authentic aFGF.[145-147] Genetic manipulation may also be useful in blocking thrombogenesis. Dichek and others have used endothelial cells with an added plasminogen activator gene to coat a fibronectin-coated metal stent to make the prosthesis less thrombogenic.[148]

While genes introduced into cells in the vascular wall or on synthetic grafts have great potential for manipulating local intimal hyperplasia, they may also provide a mechanism to treat systemic illnesses caused by acquired (e.g., diabetes mellitus) or inherited (e.g., adenosine deaminase deficiency) gene deficiencies. The possible therapeutic use of genetically altered SMCs was suggested by the recent work of Lynch et al.[142] These investigators demonstrated that SMC retrovirally infected with genes expressing human adenosine deaminase yielded potentially therapeutic levels of the enzyme 6 months after these cells were seeded into injured rat arteries.

SUMMARY

Intimal hyperplasia is a universal response to vessel injury that consists primarily of SMC proliferation and migration into the intima and production by these cells of matrix components. The result is a thickened wall that may cause flow reduction or vessel occlusion. This process is responsible for most failures of revascularization that occur 1 month to 2 years after the procedure. While the controlling mechanisms of this process are still under investigation, recent work suggests that migration of SMCs into the intima is stimulated by the release of PDGF from platelets that adhere to the injured surface and that medial SMC proliferation is largely due to release of bFGF from injured SMCs and endothelial cells. After the acute injury, cellular events may be influenced by the paracrine and autocrine release of various mitogens and growth inhibitors from endothelial cells, macrophages in the vessel wall, and SMCs. Hemodynamic forces are also important, with increased wall thickening occurring in areas of reduced flow. Potential mechanisms for controlling this process include the use of antiplatelet or antiproliferative drugs, the introduction of genes for growth inhibitors or promoters into cells in the vessel wall, and the use of improved methods of revascularization that minimize trauma to the vessel wall.

REFERENCES

1. Liu MW, Roubin GS, King SB: Restenosis after coronary angioplasty, potential biologic determinants and role of intimal hyperplasia. Circulation 79:1374, 1989
2. Macdonald RG, Henderson MA, Hirshfeld JW, Jr et al: Patient-related variables and restenosis after percutaneous transluminal coronary angioplasty—a report from the M-HEART group. Am J Cardiol 66:926, 1990
3. Holmes DR, Jr, Vlietstra RE, Smith HC: Restenosis after percutaneous transluminal coronary angioplasty (PTCA): a report from the PTCA registry of the National Heart, Lung and Blood Institute. Am J Cardiol 53:77C, 1984
4. Meier B: Restenosis after coronary angioplasty: review of the literature. Eur Heart J, suppl. C. 9:1, 1988
5. Pepine CJ, Hirshfeld JW, Macdonald RG et al: A controlled trial of corticosteroids to prevent restenosis after coronary angioplasty. Circulation 81:1753, 1990
6. Meier B: Prevention of restenosis after coronary angioplasty: a pharmacological approach. Eur Heart J 10:64, 1989
7. Garratt KN, Edwards WD, Kaufmann UP et al: Differential histopathology of primary atherosclerotic and restenotic lesions in coronary arteries and saphenous vein bypass grafts: analysis of tissue obtained from 73 patients by directional atherectomy. J Am Coll Cardiol 17:442, 1991
8. Safian RD, Gelbfish JS, Erny RE et al: Coronary atherectomy. Clinical, angiographic, and histological findings and observations. Circulation 82:69, 1990
9. Garratt KN, Holmes DR, Jr, Bell MR et al: Restenosis after directional coronary atherectomy: differences between primary atheromatous and restenosis lesions and influence of subintimal tissue resection. J Am Coll Cardiol 16:1665, 1990
10. Zierler RE, Bandyk DF, Thiele BL, Strandness DE, Jr: Carotid artery stenosis following endarterectomy. Arch Surg 117:1408, 1982
11. Thomas M, Otis SM, Rush M et al: Recurrent carotid artery stenosis following endarterectomy. Ann Surg 200:74, 1984
12. Healy DA, Zierler RE, Nicholls SC et al: Long-term follow-up and clinical outcome of carotid restenosis. J Vasc Surg 10:662, 1989
13. Bernstein EF, Torem S, Dilley RB: Does carotid restenosis predict an increased risk of late symptoms, stroke, or death? Ann Surg 212:629, 1990
14. Clagett CP, Robinowitz M, Youkey JR et al: Morphogenesis and clinicopathologic characteristics of recurrent carotid disease. J Vasc Surg 3:10, 1986
15. Sterpetti AV, Schultz RD, Feldhaus RJ et al: Natural history of recurrent carotid artery disease. Surg Gynecol Obstet 168:217, 1989
16. Szilagyi DE, Elliott JP, Hageman JH et al: Biologic fate of autogenous vein implants as arterial substitutes. Ann Surg 178:232, 1973

17. Whittemore AD, Clowes AW, Couch NP, Mannick JA: Secondary femoropopliteal reconstruction. Ann Surg 193:35, 1981

18. Lie JT, Lawrie GM, Morris GC: Aortocoronary bypass saphenous vein graft atherosclerosis. Anatomic study of 99 vein grafts from normal and hyperlipoproteinemic patients up to 75 months postoperatively. Am J Cardiol 40:906, 1977

19. Lawrie GM, Lie JT, Morris GC, Beazley HL: Vein graft patency and intimal proliferation after aortocoronary bypass. Early and long-term angiopathologic correlations. Am J Cardiol 38:856, 1976

20. Grondin CM, Campeau L, Lesperance J, Solymoss BC: Atherosclerotic changes in coronary vein grafts six years after operation: angiographic aspect in 110 patients. J Thorac Cardiovasc Surg 77:24, 1979

21. Campeau L, Enjalbert M, Lesperance J, Bourassa MG: The relation of risk factors to the development of atherosclerosis in saphenous-vein bypass grafts and the progression of disease in the native circulation. N Engl J Med 311:1329, 1984

22. Bourassa MG, Fisher LD, Campeau L et al: Long-term fate of bypass grafts: the Coronary Artery Surgery Study (CASS) and Montreal Heart Institute experiences. Circulation, suppl. V. 72:V-71, 1985

23. LoGerfo FW, Quist WC, Cantelmo NL, Haudenschild CC: Integrity of vein grafts as a function of initial intimal and medial preservation. Circulation, suppl. II. 68:II-117, 1983

24. Imparato AM, Bracco A, Kim GE, Zeff R: Intimal and neointimal fibrous proliferation causing failure of arterial reconstructions. Surgery 72:1007, 1972

25. Barboriak JJ, Pintar K, Van Horn DK et al: Pathologic findings in the aortocoronary vein grafts. A scanning electron microscope study. Atherosclerosis 29:69, 1978

26. Marti MC, Bouchardy B, Cox JN: Aorto-coronary bypass with autogenous saphenous vein grafts: histopathological aspects. Virchows Arch [A] 352:255, 1971

27. Unni KK, Kottke BA, Titus JL et al: Pathologic changes in aortocoronary saphenous vein grafts. Am J Cardiol 34:526, 1974

28. Vlodaver Z, Edwards JE: Pathologic changes in aortic-coronary arterial saphenous vein grafts. Circulation 44:719, 1971

29. Jones M, Conkle DM, Ferrans VJ et al: Lesions observed in arterial autogenous vein grafts. Light and electron microscopic evaluation. Circulation 47:198, 1973

30. Clowes AW, Reidy MA, Clowes MM: Mechanisms of stenosis after arterial injury. Lab Invest 49:208, 1983

31. Majesky MW, Schwartz SM, Clowes MM, Clowes AW: Heparin regulates smooth muscle S phase entry in the injured rat carotid artery. Circ Res 61:296, 1987

32. Ross R, Glomset JA: The pathogenesis of atherosclerosis (second of two parts). N Engl J Med 295:420, 1976

33. Ross R, Glomset JA: The pathogenesis of atherosclerosis (first of two parts). N Engl J Med 295:369, 1976

34. Friedman RJ, Stemerman MB, Wenz B et al: The effect of thrombocytopenia on experimental arteriosclerotic lesion formation in rabbits. Smooth muscle cell proliferation and re-endothelialization. J Clin Invest 60:1191, 1977

35. Fingerle J, Johnson R, Clowes AW et al: Role of platelets in smooth muscle cell proliferation and migration after vascular injury in rat carotid artery. Proc Natl Acad Sci USA 86:8412, 1989

36. Jawien A, Bowen-Pope DF, Clowes AW: Platelet-derived growth factor promotes smooth muscle migration and intimal thickening in a rat model of balloon angioplasty. J Clin Invest 89:507, 1992

37. Ferns GAA, Raines EW, Sprugel KH et al: Inhibition of neointimal smooth muscle accumulation after angioplasty by an antibody to PDGF. Science 253:1129, 1991

38. Clowes AW, Clowes MM, Fingerle S, Reidy MA: Kinetics of cellular proliferation after arterial injury. V. Role of acute distension in the induction of smooth muscle proliferation. Lab Invest. 60:360, 1989

39. Tada T, Reidy MA: Endothelial regeneration. IX. Arterial injury followed by rapid endothelial repair induces smooth-muscle-cell proliferation but not intimal thickening. Am J Pathol 129:429, 1987

40. Fingerle J, Au YPT, Clowes AW, Reidy MA: Intimal lesion formation in rat carotid arteries after endothelial denudation in absence of medial injury. Arteriosclerosis 10:1082, 1990

41. Walker LN, Bowen-Pope DF, Reidy MA: Production of platelet-derived growth factor-like molecules by cultured arterial smooth muscle cells accompanies proliferation after arterial injury. Proc Natl Acad Sci 83:7311, 1986

42. Cercek B, Fishbein MC, Forrester JS et al: Induction of insulin-like growth factor I messenger RNA in rat aorta after balloon denudation. Circ Res 66:1755, 1990

43. Lindner V, Lappi DA, Baird A et al: Role of basic fibroblast growth factor in vascular lesion formation. Circ Res 68:106, 1991

44. Lindner V, Reidy MA: Proliferation of smooth muscle cells after vascular injury is inhibited by an antibody against basic fibroblast growth factor. Proc Natl Acad Sci USA 88:3739, 1991

45. Hansson GK, Jonasson L, Holm J et al: Gamma-interferon regulates vascular smooth muscle proliferation and Ia antigen expression in vivo and in vitro. Circ Res 63:712, 1988

46. Castellot JJ Jr, Addonizio ML, Rosenberg R, Karnovsky MJ: Cultured endothelial cells produce a heparin-like inhibitor of smooth muscle cell growth. J Cell Biol 90:372, 1981

47. Cooke JP, Stamler J, Andon N et al: Flow stimulates endothelial cells to release a nitrovasodilator that is potentiated by reduced thiol. Am J Physiol Heart Circ Physiol 259:H804, 1990

48. Buga GM, Gold ME, Fukuto JM, Ignarro LJ: Shear stress-induced release of nitric oxide from endothelial cells grown on beads. Hypertension 17:187, 1991

49. Ralevic V, Milner P, Hudlicka O et al: Substance P is

released from the endothelium of normal and capsaicin-treated rat hindlimb vasculature, in vivo, by increased flow. Circ Res 66:1178, 1990

50. Hsieh H-J, Li N-Q, Frangos JA: Shear stress increases endothelial platelet-derived growth factor mRNA levels. Am J Physiol Heart Circ Physiol 260:H642, 1991

51. Clowes AW, Clowes MM, Reidy MA: Kinetics of cellular proliferation after arterial injury. III. Endothelial and smooth muscle growth in chronically denuded vessels. Lab Invest 54:295, 1986

52. Reidy MA, Clowes AW, Schwartz SM: Endothelial regeneration. V. Inhibition of endothelial regrowth in arteries of rat and rabbit. Lab Invest 49:569, 1983

53. Lindner V, Reidy MA, Fingerle J: Regrowth of arterial endothelium: Denudation with minimal trauma leads to complete endothelial cell regrowth. Lab Invest 61:556, 1989

54. Lindner V, Majack RA, Reidy MA: Basic fibroblast factor stimulates endothelial regrowth and proliferation in denuded arteries. J Clin Invest 85:2004, 1990

55. Thoma R: Untersuchungen uber die Histogenese und Histomechanik des Gefassystems. Enke, Stuttgart, 1893

56. Holman E: The anatomic and physiologic effects of an arteriovenous fistula. Surgery 8:362, 1940

57. Hull SS, Romig GD, Sparks HV, Jaffe MD: Flow induced vasodilation of large arteries is dependant on endothelium. Fed Proc 43:900, 1984

58. Kamiya A, Togawa T: Adaptive regulation of wall shear stress to flow change in the canine carotid artery. Am J Physiol 239:14, 1980

59. Zarins CK, Zatina MA, Giddens DP et al: Shear stress regulation of artery lumen diameter in experimental atherogenesis. J Vasc Surg 5:413, 1987

60. Langille BL, O'Donnell F: Reductions in arterial diameter produced by chronic decreases in blood flow are endothelium-dependent. Science 231:405, 1986

61. Wolinsky H: Effects of hypertension and its reversal on the thoracic aorta of male and female rats. Circ Res 28:622, 1971

62. Owens GK, Reidy MA: Hyperplastic growth response of vascular smooth muscle cells following induction of acute hypertension in rats by aortic coarctation. Circ Res 57:695, 1985

63. Clowes AW, Clowes MM: Influence of chronic hypertension on injured and uninjured arteries in spontaneously hypertensive rats. Lab Invest 6:535, 1980

64. Carrel A, Guthrie CC: Results of the biterminal transplantation of veins. Am J Med Sci 132:415, 1906

65. Carrel A, Guthrie CC: Uniterminal and biterminal venous transplantations. Surg Gynecol Obstet 2:266, 1906

66. Zwolak RM, Adams MC, Clowes AW: Kinetics of vein graft hyperplasia. Association with tangential stress. J Vasc Surg 5:126, 1987

67. Kohler TR, Kirkman TR, Clowes AW: The effect of rigid external support on vein graft adaptation to the arterial circulation. J Vasc Surg 9:277, 1989

68. Ku DN, Giddens DP, Zarins C, Glagov S: Pulsatile flow and atherosclerosis in the human carotid bifurcation. Arteriosclerosis 5:293, 1985

69. Zarins CK, Giddens DP, Bharadvaj BK et al: Carotid bifurcation atherosclerosis: quantitative correlation of plaque localization with flow velocity profiles and wall shear stress. Circ Res 53:502, 1983

70. Friedman MH, Hutchins GM, Bargeron CB et al: Correlation between intimal thickness and fluid shear in human arteries. Atherosclerosis 39:425, 1981

71. Glagov S, Weisenberg E, Zarins CK, Stankunavicius R: Compensatory enlargement of human atherosclerotic coronary arteries. N Engl J Med 316:1371, 1987

72. Berguer R, Higgins RF, Reddy DJ: Intimal hyperplasia. Arch Surg 115:332, 1980

73. Rittgers SE, Karayannacos PE, Guy JF: Velocity distribution and intimal proliferation in autologous vein grafts in dogs. Circ Res 42:792, 1978

74. Morinaga K, Okadome K, Kuroki M et al: Effect of wall shear stress on intimal thickening of arterially transplanted autogenous veins in dogs. J Vasc Surg 2:430, 1985

75. Mii S, Okadome K, Onohara T et al: Intimal thickening and permeability of arterial autogenous vein graft in a canine poor-runoff model: transmission electron microscopic evidence. Surgery 108:81, 1990

76. Kohler TR, Kirkman TR, Kraiss LW et al: Increased blood flow inhibits neointimal hyperplasia in endothelialized vascular grafts. Circ Res 69:1557, 1991

77. Clowes AW, Kirkman TR, Reidy MA: Mechanisms of arterial graft healing. III. Rapid transmural capillary ingrowth provides a source of intimal endothelium and smooth muscle in porous PTFE prostheses. Am J Pathol 123:220, 1986

78. Kohler TR, Jawien A: Flow affects development of intimal hyperplasia following arterial injury in rats. Arterioscles. Thromb. 12:963, 1992

79. Goldman S, Copeland J, Moritz T et al: Improvement in early saphenous vein graft patency after coronary artery bypass surgery with antiplatelet therapy: results of a Veterans Administration Cooperative Study. Circulation 77:1324, 1988

80. Chevigné M, David J-L, Rigo P, Limet R: Effect of ticlopidine on saphenous vein bypass patency rates: a double-blind study. Ann Thorac Surg 37:371, 1984

81. Goldman S, Copeland J, Moritz T et al: Saphenous vein graft patency 1 year after coronary artery bypass surgery and effects of antiplatelet therapy: results of a Veterans Administration Cooperative Study. Circulation 80:1190, 1989

82. Fitzgerald GA: Dipyridamole. N Engl J Med 316:1247, 1987

83. Clagett GP, Genton E, Salzman EW: Antithrombotic therapy in peripheral vascular disease. Chest 95:128S, 1989

84. Clowes AW: The role of aspirin in enhancing arterial graft patency. J Vasc Surg 3:381, 1986

85. Clowes AW, Reidy MA: Prevention of stenosis after

vascular reconstruction: pharmacologic control of intimal hyperplasia—a review. J Vasc Surg 13:885, 1991

86. McCann RL, Hagen PO, Fuchs JCA: Aspirin and dipyridamole decrease intimal hyperplasia in experimental vein grafts. Ann Surg 191:238, 1980

87. Satiani B: A prospective randomized trial of aspirin in femoral popiteal and tibial bypass grafts. Angiology 36:608, 1985

88. Fuster V, Chesebro JH: Aortocoronary artery vein-graft disease: experimental and clinical approach for the understanding of the role of platelets and platelet inhibitors. Circulation, suppl. V. 72:V-65, 1985

89. Fluster V, Chesebro JH: Role of platelets and platelet inhibitors in aortocoronary artery vein-graft disease. Circulation 73:227, 1986

90. de Gaetano G, Cerletti C, Dejana E: Current issues in thrombosis prevention with antiplatelet drugs. Drugs 31:517, 1986

91. Gershlick AH, De Bono DP: Restenosis after angioplasty. Br Heart J 64:351, 1990

92. Schwartz L, Lesperance J, Bourassa MG: The role of antiplatelet agents in modifying the extent of restenosis following percutaneous transluminal coronary angioplasty. Am Heart J 119:232, 1990

93. Landymore RW, Karmazyn M, MacAulay MA et al: Correlation between the effects of aspirin and dipyridamole on platelet function and prevention of intimal hyperplasia in autologous vein grafts. Can J Cardiol 4:56, 1988

94. Bonchek LI, Boerboom LE, Olinger GN: Prevention of lipid accumulation in experimental vein bypass grafts by antiplatelet therapy. Circulation 66:338, 1982

95. Hess H, Mietaschk A, Deichsel G: Drug-induced inhibition of platelet function delays progression of peripheral occlusive arterial disease. Lancet 1:415, 1985

96. El-Sanadiki MN, Cross KS, Murray JJ et al: Reduction of intimal hyperplasia and enhanced reactivity of experimental vein bypass grafts with verapamil treatment. Ann Surg 212:87, 1990

97. Atkinson JB, Swift LL: Nifedipine reduces atherogenesis in cholesterol-fed heterozygous WHHL rabbits. Atherosclerosis 84:195, 1990

98. Paniszyn CC: Reduction of intimal hyperplasia and enhanced reactivity of experimental vein bypass grafts with verapamil treatment. Ann Surg 213:374, 1991

99. Jackson CL, Bush RC, Bowyer DE: Mechanism of antiatherogenic action of calcium antagonists. Atherosclerosis 80:17, 1989

100. Jackson CL, Bush RC, Bowyer DE: Inhibitory effect of calcium antagonists on balloon catheter-induced arterial smooth muscle cell proliferation and lesion size. Atherosclerosis 69:115, 1988

101. Powell JS, Müller RKM, Rouge M et al: The proliferative response to vascular injury is suppressed by angiotensin-converting enzyme inhibition. J Cardiovasc Pharmacol, suppl. 4. 16:S42, 1990

102. Sowers JR: Calcium channel blockers and atherosclerosis. Am J Kidney Dis, suppl. 1. 16:3, 1990

103. Lichtlen PR, Hugenholtz PG, Rafflenbeul W et al: Nifedipine trial. Lancet 335:1109, 1990

104. Schlant RC, King SB, III: Usefulness of calcium entry blockers during and after percutaneous transluminal coronary artery angioplasty. Circulation, suppl. 80:IV88, 1989

105. Hirsch GM, Karnovsky MJ: Inhibition of vein graft intimal proliferative lesions in the rat by heparin. Am J Pathol 139:581, 1991

106. Kohler TR, Kirkman TR, Clowes AW: Effect of heparin on adaptation of vein grafts to arterial circulation. Arteriosclerosis 9:523, 1989

107. Clowes AW, Clowes MM: Kinetics of cellular proliferation after arterial injury. IV. Heparin inhibits rat smooth muscle mitogenesis and migration. Circ Res 58:839, 1986

108. Hoover RL, Rosenberg R, Haering W, Karnovsky MJ: Inhibition of rat arterial smooth muscle cell proliferation by heparin. II. In vitro studies. Circ Res 47:578, 1980

109. Clowes AW, Clowes MM: Kinetics of cellular proliferation after arterial injury. II. Inhibition of smooth muscle growth by heparin. Lab Invest 52:611, 1985

110. Clowes AW, Karnovsky MJ: Suppression by heparin of smooth muscle cell proliferation in injured arteries. Nature 265:625, 1977

111. Majack RA, Clowes AW: Inhibition of vascular smooth muscle cell migration by heparin-like glycosaminoglycans. J Cell Physiol 118:253, 1984

112. Snow AD, Bolender RP, Wight TN, Clowes AW: Heparin modulates the composition of the extracellular matrix domain surrounding arterial smooth muscle cells. Am J Pathol 137:313, 1990

113. Au YPT, Kenagy RD, Clowes AW: Heparin selectively inhibits the transcription of tissue-type plasminogen activator in primate arterial smooth muscle cells during mitogenesis. J Biol Chem 267:3438, 1992

114. Kenagy RD, Welgus HG, Clowes AW: Heparin inhibits the expression of matrix metalloproteases by smooth muscle cells, abstracted. J Cell Biol 115:138a, 1991

115. Clowes AW, Clowes MM, Au YPT et al: Smooth muscle cells express urokinase during mitogenesis and tissue-type plasminogen activator during migration in injured rat carotid artery. Circ Res 67:61, 1990

116. Guyton JR, Rosenberg RD, Clowes AW, Karnovsky MJ: Inhibition of rat arterial smooth muscle cell proliferation by heparin. I. In vivo studies with anticoagulant and non-anticoagulant heparin. Circ Res 46:625, 1980

117. Pipili E, Manolopoulos VG, Catravas JD, Maragoudakis ME: Angiotensin converting enzyme activity is present in the endothelium-denuded aorta. Br J Pharmacol 98:333, 1989

118. Powell JS, Clozel JP, Muler RKM et al: Inhibitors of angiotensin-converting enzyme prevent myointimal proliferation after vascular injury. Science 245:186, 1989

119. Chervu A, Moore WS, Quiñones-Baldrich WJ, Henderson T: Efficacy of corticosteroids in suppression of intimal hyperplasia. J Vasc Surg 10:129, 1989

3

Pathophysiology of Vascular Intervention

P. Macke Consigny
Andrew H. Cragg
Bruce F. Waller

The introduction of transluminal balloon angioplasty by Andreas Gruentzig in 1978[1] dramatically changed the way in which peripheral and coronary arterial stenoses and occlusions are treated. However, the limitations of balloon angioplasty have fostered the development of a multitude of alternative interventional techniques, including stents, laser angioplasty, atherectomy, and atheroablation. This chapter describes the pathologic changes that occur in the arterial wall as a result of balloon angioplasty and alternative interventions.

PATHOPHYSIOLOGY OF ARTERIAL REPAIR

Although each of the interventions discussed in this chapter injures the artery in slightly different ways, the pathologic changes that occur are all remarkably similar. The most commonly observed change is restenosis, due primarily to intimal smooth muscle hyperplasia. The mechanisms responsible for this hyperplasia are not clearly understood but, on the basis of current

knowledge, the artery's response to interventions that ultimately lead to restenosis can be divided into five stages.

Thrombosis Secondary to Arterial Injury

The luminal surfaces of arteries are normally covered with a monolayer of endothelial cells. These cells maintain a normal patent lumen by secreting factors that (1) inhibit platelet adhesion and aggregation (prostacyclin, endothelium-derived relaxing factor [EDRF]); (2) promote thrombolysis (tissue-type plasminogen activator [tPA]); (3) relax vascular smooth muscle [EDRF]; and (4) inhibit smooth muscle cell proliferation (heparan sulfate, EDRF, prostanoids).[2-7] All of the interventions discussed below destroy the endothelium and thereby diminish the production of these factors. Furthermore, endothelial denudation and stretching or cutting of plaque expose thrombogenic surfaces to blood. These changes immediately activate the coagulation cascade, producing changes that range from the formation of platelet aggregates on the denuded luminal surface over the first 24 hours after injury[8,9] to the formation of totally occlusive thrombi that can remain indefinitely.

Medial Smooth Muscle Cell Proliferation Secondary to Medial Injury

Balloon angioplasty and many other interventions injure or destroy the smooth muscle cells of the media.[10-12] Within 2 days of this injury, medial smooth muscle cell proliferation is initiated. This proliferation replaces the destroyed cells but does not increase medial thickness.[10,13,14] Although the cause of this proliferative response is unknown, recent studies suggest that basic fibroblast growth factor (bFGF) is intimately involved.[15] Experimental observations that support the role of bFGF in this proliferative process include the following: (1) smooth muscle cells express mRNA for bFGF and proliferate in response to bFGF[16]; (2) bFGF may be released from smooth muscle cells after injury, as bFGF content within the smooth muscle cells of normal artery is reduced after balloon injury[17]; (3) high-affinity bFGF receptors are expressed on smooth muscle cells in the blood vessel after injury[18]; (4) injections of bFGF promote medial smooth muscle cell proliferation after injury[19]; and (5) antibodies against bFGF partially inhibit medial smooth muscle cell proliferation after angioplasty.[15] Experimental findings that indicate that PDGF of platelet origin is not involved include (1) injury-induced medial smooth muscle cell proliferation occurs in thrombocytopenia[20] and in the absence of endothelial denudation,[21] (2) medial smooth muscle cell proliferation does not occur after gentle endothelial denudation if there is no medial injury,[22] and (3) injection of PDGF immediately after balloon injury does not enhance medial smooth muscle cell proliferation.[23]

Smooth Muscle Cell Migration and Intimal Proliferation

The process of intimal smooth muscle cell migration and proliferation that results in restenosis begins approximately 4 days after angioplasty. The 4-day delay in appearance of the smooth muscle cells in the intima is attributed to the fact that the smooth muscle cells in the media must convert from a contractile to a noncontractile phenotype and then free themselves from their surrounding matrix. This later step of matrix deg-

radation most likely involves the release by smooth muscle cells[24] of the plasminogen activators tPA and urokinase plasminogen activator (uPA) that convert plasminogen to plasmin. The resultant plasmin is capable of degrading extracellular matrix either directly or by converting procollagenase to an active enzyme. Upon matrix degradation, the smooth muscle cells are free to respond to chemoattractants present in the intima, including PDGF[20] and fibrin.[25]

Upon arriving in the intima, smooth muscle cells begin to proliferate. Several observations support the role of PDGF in this migratory and proliferative response: (1) intimal proliferation is retarded by thrombocytopenia,[20] (2) infusion of PDGF increases intimal thickening,[23] and (3) the injection of an antibody to PDGF reduces intimal thickening.[26] The source of the PDGF responsible for intimal proliferation is uncertain but may include platelets,[20] smooth muscle cells,[27-29] macrophages,[30] and endothelial cells.[31]

A second factor that may be involved in this proliferative response is insulin growth factor-I (IGF-I), since (1) IGF-1 is a progression factor that acts synergistically with PDGF to stimulate SMC proliferation,[32] and (2) IGF-1 gene expression is increased by arterial injury and remains elevated during the period of intimal proliferation and endothelial regeneration.[33,34]

Thrombin is a third factor that may be involved. There are several pieces of evidence implicating thrombin: (1) thrombin is produced in high concentrations on the luminal surface of injured arteries artery, where it binds to fibrin and is thereby protected from inactivation[35]; (2) restenotic lesions in man often contain thrombi undergoing cellular reorganization[36]; (3) thrombin receptors are present on proliferating smooth muscle cells, and thrombin increases the rate of proliferation of serum-treated smooth muscle cells[37,38]; (4) thrombin induces the release of PDGF from endothelial cells that could further promote proliferation[39,40]; and (5) hirudin, a specific thrombin inhibitor, reduced intimal proliferation in balloon-dilated atherosclerotic rabbit femoral arteries.[41] One factor that does not appear to be involved in intimal hyperplasia is bFGF, since the injection of antibodies to bFGF has no effect on intimal proliferation after balloon injury.[15,17]

Production of Extracellular Matrix Within the Neointima

In the latter stages of neointimal formation, there is an increase in extracellular matrix deposition. One factor that appears to be involved in this phase of neointimal formation is transforming growth factor beta

(TGF-β).[42] TGF-β is a growth factor secreted as a latent molecule by both endothelial cells and smooth muscle cells that is converted to an active molecule by the action of plasmin and other proteases.[43] TGF-β promotes matrix formation by (1) stimulating endothelial cells and smooth muscle cells to secrete matrix proteins including collagen and glycosaminoglycans; (2) inhibiting the synthesis of matrix degrading proteases; and (3) stimulating the synthesis of protease inhibitors, including plasminogen activator inhibitor-1 and the tissue inhibitor of metalloproteinases TIMP-1.[44-47]

Re-endothelialization

In the case of small focal injuries, endothelial cell regrowth is an early event in repair, occurring over the surface of a mural thrombus before there is a cellular infiltrate. However, in cases in which large areas of luminal surface are denuded of endothelium, re-endothelialization is often the final event in repair, occurring over a fully formed neointima. In either case, re-endothelialization is the result of the migration and proliferation of endothelial cells originating from the proximal and distal ends of the injured artery and from arterial side branches present at the site of injury. In animal studies, the sites of arterial injury that re-endothelialize first typically have least amount of intimal proliferation, suggesting that the endothelium may inhibit smooth muscle hyperplasia.[14,22,48,49] Factors released by the endothelium that may mediate this inhibition include heparan sulfate,[5] prostanoids,[6] and EDRF.[7]

BALLOON ANGIOPLASTY

Balloon angioplasty has become the mainstay of percutaneous intervention in vascular disease and plays a major role in the care of the vascular patient. Understanding of the mechanism of angioplasty has increased over the last 15 years due to the pioneering work of Castaneda-Zuniga et al.[50] and others,[51,52] who elucidated the morphologic effects of balloon dilatation, and to later work by many investigators who defined the significance of physiologic changes in the vessel wall after angioplasty.[53-57] This work has served as a standard for evaluating the effects of new revascularization techniques described in this chapter and, even more importantly, has directed us toward what may be the most significant area of future research: reduction of restenosis by modification of the process of arterial injury and repair.

Morphologic Vessel Wall Changes After Angioplasty

It is not uncommon for a highly stenotic atherosclerotic vessel to appear angiographically to be "almost normal" after successful balloon angioplasty (Fig. 3-1). Just as common, however, is the irregular angiographic appearance, generally labeled "a therapeutic angioplasty-induced dissection" (Fig. 3-2).

Early speculation that angioplasty worked by compression and remodeling of plaque soon gave way under the scrutiny of histologic examination to the notion that the major mechanism of balloon angioplasty was splitting or cracking of the intimal plaque and stretching of the underlying media[50,51] (Fig. 3-3). This makes intuitive sense, since most atherosclerotic stenoses are at least partially calcified, and they would be expected to yield to the mechanical stress of a relatively rigid balloon by tearing or cracking.

Early work in this area demonstrated that large areas of intimal-medial dehiscence were produced by angioplasty in humans.[58-60] These dissections, which commonly arise at the junction of plaque with disease-free wall in cases of eccentric stenosis, may be well tolerated, even though they extend in a large arc around the

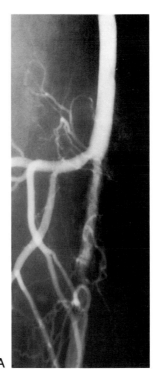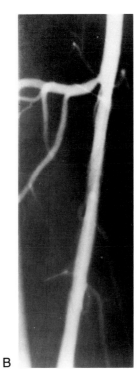

A   B

Figure 3-1 Atherosclerotic superficial femoral artery stenosis before (**A**) and after (**B**) angioplasty. Occasionally, in such cases, angiographic evidence of dissection is minimal, and the dilated vessel appears "almost normal."

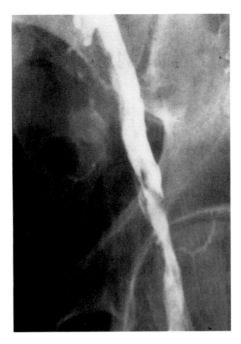

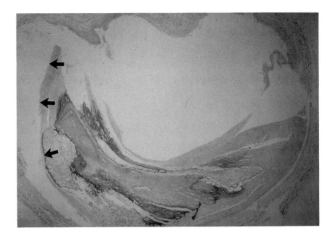

Figure 3-4 Histologic specimen of previously dilated artery demonstrates a large intimal cleft extending around a portion of the circumference of the vessel *(arrows)*. Plaque fracture and intimal-medial dehiscence are typical features of most successful angioplasty procedures.

Figure 3-2 External iliac artery after angioplasty demonstrates a typical angiographic picture of intimal-medial dissection. The size of the dissection in this case limits flow and produces a suboptimal result.

circumference of the vessel (Fig. 3-4). It has been our experience that angiography significantly underestimates the extent of "intimal flap" formation after angioplasty. This impression has now been substantiated by angioscopy, which can demonstrate large mobile intimal flaps in the presence of a very satisfactory angiographic result.[61]

Certainly, flaplike abrupt closure of the dilated vessel is one mechanism of failure; however, this is a very uncommon event in the peripheral circulation,[62] and in most cases the vessel heals by permanent enlargement of the new vessel channel.

In addition to plaque fracture, it now seems clear that stretching of the exposed media is an important mechanism of angioplasty. Waller and others[63-65] have elegantly shown that eccentric atherosclerotic stenoses are common and that stretching of the disease-free wall can produce permanent vessel dilation. Exceeding the elastic limit of the media by overstretching has been shown experimentally to produce prolonged vessel dilatation.[50] Failure to do so clinically may result in another important mechanism of early angioplasty failure: elastic recoil. Although acute elastic recoil shortly after balloon angioplasty is a generally well-recognized mechanism of abrupt narrowing, chronic elastic recoil as a mechanism of late luminal narrowing is not well understood. Possible explanations for chronic recoil of overstretched eccentric segments involve recovery from temporary or permanent injury to medial smooth muscle cells. Temporary dysfunction ("stunned smooth muscle cells") over a period of weeks to months may eventually regain their function, thereby setting

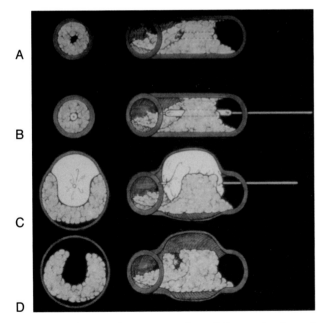

Figure 3-3 Schematic representation of the mechanism of angioplasty. **(A–C)** During balloon inflation, **(D)** separation of plaque and stretching of the disease-free wall occur, resulting in enlargement of the vascular lumen.

the stage for late recoil. By contrast, acute injury of the smooth muscle cells during dilatation may result eventually in replacement rather than repair of these cells. Replacement with normal functioning smooth muscle cells over a period of weeks to months permits the possibility of recoil on a late basis.

Late morphologic changes that occur after angioplasty are clearly the most important and interesting in terms of understanding both why angioplasty fails and how to improve it. Pathologic specimens obtained at autopsy and after atherectomy of previous angioplasty lesions show that the major mechanism of restenosis after angioplasty is intimal hyperplasia[64,66] (Fig. 3-5). Biologic variability may result in more exuberant intimal hyperplasia formation in some patients than in others. Modifying the response to injury is an exciting area of research, which, it is hoped, will ultimately benefit this group of patients.

Physiologic Vessel Wall Changes After Angioplasty

Early research experience with transluminal angioplasty suggested that the profound morphologic changes produced by the technique could also result in local physiologic changes as well, which could have a significant effect on vessel healing. Complex local alterations in vessel physiology could be responsible for early angioplasty failure due to spasm or for late failure due to intimal hyperplasia.

Vascular tone is regulated by a complex interaction of neurohumoral mechanisms. Important among these are arachidonic acid pathways via prostaglandins, thromboxanes, and hydroperoxy acids.[67,68]

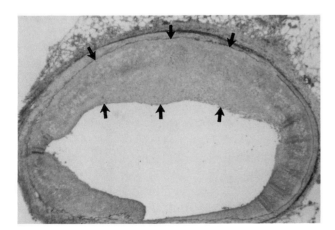

Figure 3-5 Intimal proliferation *(arrows)* is seen as part of the healing process after all types of endovascular injury. Exuberant intimal hyperplasia formation is responsible for most restenosis cases after successful angioplasty.

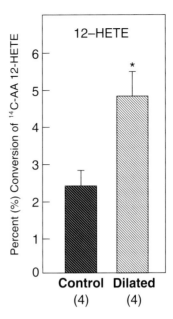

Figure 3-6 Production of vascular hydroxyeicosatetraenoic acid (HETE) is significantly elevated after angioplasty. HETE is a potent vasoconstricting substance that could mediate spasm after angioplasty. *, $p < 0.05$ (control versus dilated).

Angioplasty significantly stimulates the production of hydroperoxy acids, which are known to mediate vessel spasm and inflammation[55] (Fig. 3-6). At the same time, endothelial denudation results in loss of prostaglandin I_2 production a potent angioaggretory vasodilating agent. An imbalance between these and other related metabolites could mediate spasm in the acute phase after angioplasty and facilitate platelet deposition and activation with its attendant consequences. Acute coronary occlusion after angioplasty has been linked to elevated thromboxane levels in blood taken from the coronary sinus in humans.[69]

In addition, angioplasty produces profound vessel wall hyperemia.[52] This increased flow occurs in the vasa vasorum supplying the dilated mural segment. The significance of this finding is not clear. It may be a nonspecific response to the injury process or perhaps may be related again to altered arachidonic acid metabolism. Interestingly, this phenomenon is almost completely suppressed by aspirin, which is known to act in part by inhibiting the cyclooxygenase pathway of arachidonic acid[53] (Fig. 3-7). Aspirin clearly has a significant effect on vessel wall physiology after angioplasty. Aspirin has been widely prescribed and is still used with the hope that it will favorably affect restenosis; disappointingly, however, this has not been the case.[70]

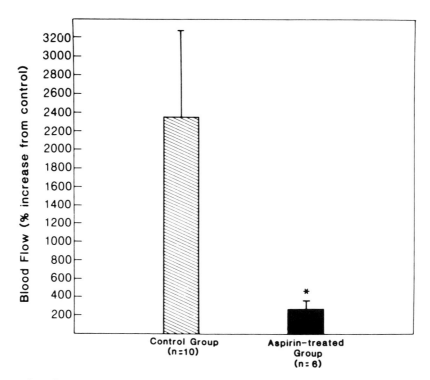

Figure 3-7 Stretching of the vessel wall during angioplasty results in local hyperemia due to increased blood flow through mural vasa vasorum. Aspirin attenuates this hyperemia, suggesting that the process is mediated by arachidonic acid pathways. *, $p < 0.05$ (control versus aspirin). (From Cragg et al.,[54] with permission.)

Numerous other drugs have been investigated with the hope of preventing intimal hyperplasia and restenosis. Agents that have been tried, among others, include heparin,[71] warfarin,[72] and calcium channel blockers.[73] To date none has been successful; however, it seems likely that some medication, perhaps locally delivered, can be found to "derail" the sequence of events leading to intimal hyperplasia.

Most recently, the effect of antineoplastic agents on smooth muscle proliferation has been investigated with interesting results. In culture, 5-fluorouracil produced a significant dose-dependent reduction in smooth muscle proliferation (unpublished data) (Fig. 3-8). While few would consider systemic infusion of cytotoxic agents to prevent restenosis, it is entirely possible that novel local drug delivery systems (e.g., biodegradable stents) could make this approach feasible.

Cragg has also investigated local hyperthermia during angioplasty as a means of modifying the pathophysiologic vessel response in both the short and long term.[74,75] In this system, the saline-contrast solution in a conventional angioplasty balloon is heated during inflation to conduct heat to the vessel wall. Preliminary work has shown that heat application during angioplasty reduces elastic recoil in the acute period compared with conventional angioplasty.[74] Other investigators have shown that plaque softening and remodelling can occur at balloon temperatures of 60 to 70°C.[76] Medial collagen may also soften at these temperatures, promoting greater vessel expansion.

Histologically, the technique results in ablation of medial smooth muscle at the site of balloon inflation.[74] While adverse long-term sequelae (e.g., aneurysms, thrombosis) have not been seen as a result of the technique,[75] it remains to be seen whether intimal proliferation can be reduced by ablation of the cellular substrate (smooth muscle) responsible for its formation. Initial clinical testing of this hypothesis is under way (Fig. 3-8).

Successful treatment strategies for balloon angioplasty restenosis will depend primarily on the morphologic-histologic response at the angioplasty site. If the lesion consists of intimal proliferation tissue, various mechanical, pharmacologic, and/or immunologic approaches may be undertaken (Table 3-1; Figs. 3-9 and 3-10). If, alternatively, the restenosis lesion represents recoil of an overstretched arc of disease-free wall, other treatment strategies, including thermal dilatation ("pyroplasty") and "antirecoil" pharmacologic therapy, may be useful.

Conventional techniques do not allow reliable differentiation of the cause of restenosis in a specific case.

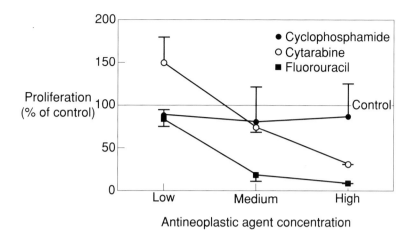

Figure 3-8 Effect of three antineoplastic agents on smooth muscle proliferation in vitro. Two-hour preincubation of porcine pulmonary smooth muscle cells with various concentrations of antiproliferative agents resulted in a significant reduction of cellular proliferation. This effect was most pronounced with fluorouracil. Local drug delivery by stents or other means could allow successful use of relatively potent agents such as cytoxic agents to limit intimal hyperplasia after angioplasty.

Appropriate use of any strategem to reduce restenosis awaits improved diagnostic capabilities. New technologies, including angioscopy and intravascular ultrasound, have not yet met this challenge.

OTHER VASCULAR INTERVENTIONS

Stents

Although the first intravascular stents were developed by Dotter in 1969,[77] it was not until the mid 1980s that stent development and testing really began. Stent

Table 3-1 Possible Solutions to Late Balloon Angioplasty: Angioplasty Restenosis

---

Intimal fibrous proliferation
  Specific smooth muscle cell monoclonal antibodies to block cellular response, delivered by balloons ("rubbing off"), stents ("secreting"), and other methods
  Destruction/reduction of medial smooth muscle cells at site of balloon angioplasty, accomplished by thermal balloons, "heated" stents, and other techniques
Elastic recoil
  Clinical recognition of eccentric plaque by intravascular ultrasound
  Cautious overdilatation of disease-free wall to delay/prevent elastic recoil
  Use of thermal balloons to eliminate/reduce elastic recoil of eccentric lesion
  Stents

---

development accelerated at this time in part because of the success of balloon angioplasty and in part as an attempt to alleviate or avoid some of the problems associated with angioplasty; these problems include abrupt closures and restenoses, which occur in approximately 5 percent and 30 percent of all cases, respectively. The stents that have thus far been developed can be divided into two categories, the balloon expandable stents (Palmaz, Palmaz-Schatz, Gianturco-Roubin, Strecker) and the self-expandable stents (nitinol, Wallstent, Gianturco, zigzag stent). Although these stents have individual differences and behave somewhat differently in vivo, the following discussion will provide a generalized description of the pathologic changes that occur in the artery subsequent to intra-arterial stent placement.

Acute Increases in Lumen Diameter

The luminal diameter of arteries that have undergone balloon angioplasty is usually less than the diameter of the balloon used to perform the dilatation. This smaller diameter after angioplasty suggests that the dilated artery recoils after being stretched by the balloon. One of the principal advantages of stents is that they eliminate or reduce this recoil, and as a result, the diameter of the lumen is greater after stent placement than after balloon dilatation.[78] Furthermore, with the self-expandable Wallstent, lumen diameter may increase over the initial 24 hours after stent placement.[79]

One beneficial effect of the greater increase in lumen diameter after stent placement is that both Poiseuille and turbulent resistance are reduced.[80] These reduc-

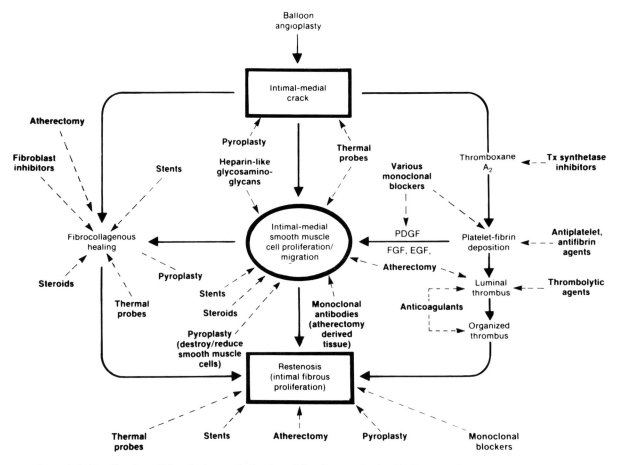

Figure 3-9 Details of possible solutions to intimal proliferation as a basis of balloon angioplasty restenosis. (From Waller and Pinkerton,[162] with permission.)

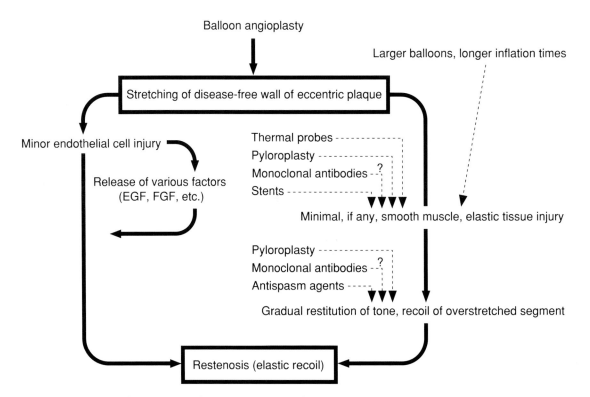

Figure 3-10 Details of possible solutions to "stretch-recoil" as a basis of balloon angioplasty restenosis. (From Waller and Pinkerton,[162] with permission.)

tions in resistance are observed clinically as a greater decrease in the pressure gradient across the residual stenosis after stent placement than after balloon angioplasty.[80,81] Additional studies have suggested that the decrease in residual stenosis and pressure gradient after stent placement could possibly reduce the incidence of thromboses and restenoses.[82,83]

Platelet/Fibrin Deposition

Subsequent to the initial increase in lumen diameter, a series of pathologic events occur that result in the incorporation of the stent into the arterial wall. These changes have been documented in animal studies for several stents including the Palmaz,[84-86] Palmaz-Schatz,[87] Gianturco-Roubin,[88-90] Wallstent,[91-94] Strecker,[95,96] and Gianturco,[97,98] among others.[99-101]

The first event that occurs after stent placement is the interaction of the stent with the circulating blood. Within 30 minutes of placement, stents are covered with adherent platelets, platelet aggregates, erythrocytes, and leukocytes encased in a fibrin matrix[84,86,89] (Fig. 3-11). The reasons for this thrombosis are many, including the surface charge of the metal used for the stent, the surface area of the stent (a function of the diameter of the stent after deployment and the length and thickness of the stent material), and blood flow through the vessel.[84,95,102] Thrombosis generally extends to include the surfaces of the artery between the struts of the stent where the endothelium was destroyed during stent placement.[89] In addition, thrombosis can continue until the artery is completely occluded, particularly if no anticoagulant is used.[84,88] However, with adequate anticoagulation, thrombosis can be confined to the surface of the stent (Fig. 3-12).[103]

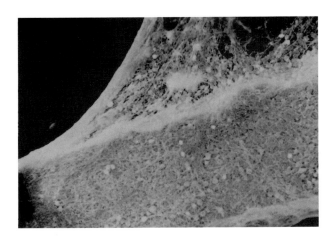

Figure 3-11 Scanning electron micrograph of a thrombus that has developed around a Palmaz stent shortly after its placement in a balloon-dilated rabbit infrarenal abdominal aorta. (×640.) (From Miller et al.,[86] with permission.)

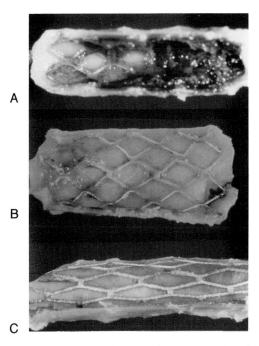

Figure 3-12 Effects of anticoagulation on thrombus formation 3 hours after Palmaz stent placement in the hind legs of dogs. Prior to stent placement, the dogs received (**A**) no anticoagulation; (**B**) heparin, aspirin, and dipyridamole; (**C**) heparin, aspirin, dipyridamole, and dextran. (From Schatz,[103] with permission.)

Re-endothelialization

The endothelium is a monolayer of cells that covers the surface of blood vessels and serves as a nonthrombogenic surface. Invariably, some endothelial cells are destroyed during the deployment of stents and, until the artery and the stent are covered with endothelium, the stented area remains thrombogenic. Consequently, in some applications, anticoagulants must be used until re-endothelialization is complete.[104]

One response of the artery to the intra-arterial placement of a stent is to cover the injured segment with endothelium. This re-endothelialization involves both the migration and the proliferation of endothelial cells. The endothelial cells originate and migrate from side branches and from areas proximal and distal to the stented area; this migration requires that the stent be covered with fibrin, since endothelial cells cannot migrate over bare metal surfaces.[87,89] In animal studies, re-endothelialization has been observed to have begun 72 hours after stent placement.[105] By 1 week, partial coverage of the stent and lumen surface has been observed, and by 3 weeks complete re-endothelialization has been observed. Initially, the new endothelial monolayer has an immature appearance (Fig. 3-13A), characterized by ovoid-appearing cells that have loose in-

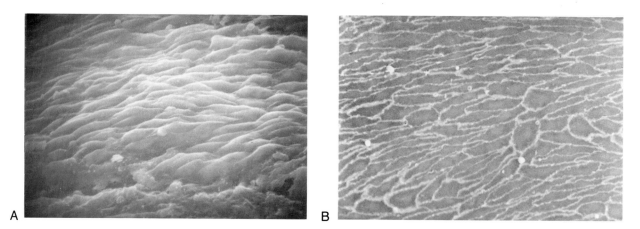

Figure 3-13 Re-endothelialization of Palmaz-Schatz stents placed in normal coronary arteries of dogs treated with aspirin and dipyridamole. **(A)** Monolayer of immature endothelial cells observed 3 weeks after stent placement. **(B)** Monolayer of mature endothelial cells observed 32 weeks after stent placement. (From Schatz et al.,[87] with permission.)

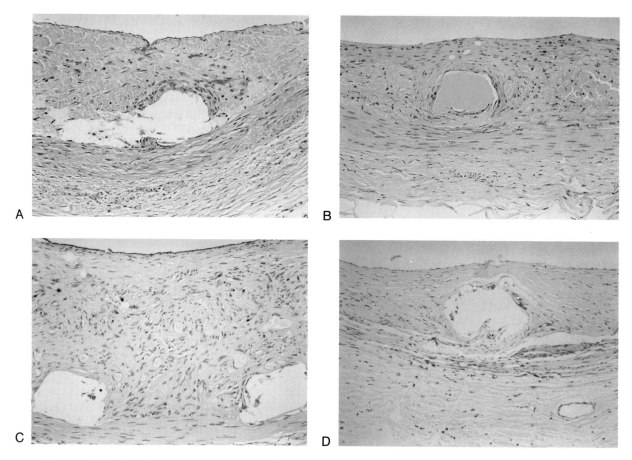

Figure 3-14 Light microscopic cross sections of canine coronary arteries removed at different times after deployment of a Palmaz-Schatz stent. Dogs were treated with aspirin and dipyridamole for the first 3 months of the study. **(A)** One week after stent placement, the luminal surface is covered with thrombus and fibrin. **(B)** Three weeks after stent placement, the thrombus is infiltrated with proliferating smooth muscle cells (myofibroblasts). There is medial thinning beneath the strut. **(C)** Eight weeks after stent placement, the neointima reaches its maximal thickness. The neointima consists predominantly of smooth muscle cells. There is further medial thinning. **(D)** Thirty-two weeks after stent placement, there is thinning of the neointima and further atrophy of the media. (From Schatz et al.,[87] with permission.)

tercellular connections and no orientation relative to the direction of blood flow. However, over the next several months, the endothelial cells take on a mature appearance (Fig. 3-13B), characterized by cells tightly joined together and elongated in the direction of blood flow.[87,88,104-106]

Formation of Neointima and Restenosis

As re-endothelialization is occurring over the luminal surface of the artery, beneath the endothelium a new intima or neointima is being formed. Neointimal formation involves the infiltration of the thrombus that formed over the stent and artery with cells, particularly leukocytes and smooth muscle cells (Fig. 3-14A and B). As the neointima matures, smooth muscle cells become the predominant cell type[89,107,108] (Fig. 3-14C). The end result of this neointimal formation is the incorporation of the stent into the arterial wall.

In animal studies, peak neointimal thickness has been observed from 8 weeks[87,96,98] (Fig. 3-14D) to 6 months[89,106] (Fig. 3-15) after stent placement. At these times, the thickness of the intima has ranged from less than 0.1 mm[85] to 0.4 mm.[89] However, in several studies, after intimal thickness reached a peak, intimal thickness began to decrease with time[89,96,106] (Figs. 3-14D and 3-15).

In clinical studies, intimal thickening and restenosis have been observed 3 to 6 months after stenting. In general, the magnitude of intimal thickening observed in clinical studies has been greater than that observed in animal studies; intimal thicknesses measurements have ranged from an average of .45 mm for Palmaz stents placed in iliac arteries of four patients[109] to an average of 1.45 mm for Palmaz-Schatz stents placed in the coronary arteries of seven patients that developed restenosis.[110] Thinning of the neointima has not been reported in man.

Medial Thinning

Immediately after stent placement, there is a thinning of the media which is the direct effect of arterial stretching[98,106] (Fig. 3-15). This stretching can also fracture the internal elastic lamina, which may provide a pathway for smooth muscle cells to migrate from the media to the intima, where they can proliferate and form the neointima.[84,96,98] Several weeks after stent placement, there is a further thinning of the media beneath the struts of the stent (Fig. 3-14C); this thinning has been attributed to reductions in pulsatile pressure and circumferential wall stress placed on the medial smooth muscle cells.[87] Several months after stent placement, there is further thinning and atrophy of the

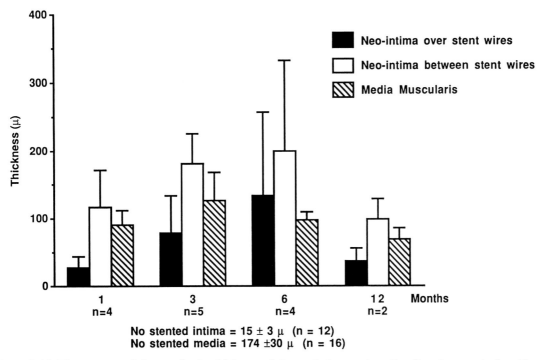

Figure 3-15 Time course of changes in the thickness of the neointima and media after placement of a self-expanding metallic zigzag stent in the coronary artery of dogs treated with aspirin. (From Bonan et al.,[106] with permission.)

media (Fig. 3-14D). Despite these later changes, there is no evidence of stent-induced aneurysm formation, presumably because the circumferential wall force is distributed over the thickened neointima.[87]

In summary, the findings of animal and clinical studies suggest that the deployment of stents in arteries has two principal pathologic effects: acute thrombosis leading to vessel closure and intimal proliferation leading to restenosis. Acute thrombosis can be reduced by aggressive use of anticoagulants and antiplatelet agents. However, there is no way to prevent the restenosis that occurs.

Lasers

In recent years, lasers have received much attention as a means of treating atherosclerosis. This attention arose because of potential advantages that laser angioplasty offered over balloon angioplasty. One such advantage was that lasers might reduce the incidence of restenosis, since lasers recanalize arteries by tissue ablation (debulking), rather than by stretching. A second advantage was that lasers could be used to treat arteries that were so severely stenotic or occluded that they could not be treated by balloon angioplasty.

Laser Systems

Three types of laser system are available: direct, indirect, and hybrid. In direct systems, laser energy is applied directly to the tissue through a fiberoptic. In indirect systems, the laser energy is directed at a metal cap at the end of the fiberoptic (laser probe or hot-tip) where the energy is converted into heat. This heat is then transferred to the arterial wall by direct contact. Hybrid systems, such as sapphire probes and laser hot balloons, are a combination of direct and indirect systems; a portion of the laser energy is applied directly to the tissue, while the remainder is converted to heat, which is then applied to the tissue by direct contact.[111]

In direct systems, the interaction of the laser emissions with the tissue are dependent, in part, on the optical properties of the tissue; these properties include transmittance, reflectance, scattering, and absorption. Laser-tissue interactions are also dependent upon the wavelength of the emission. Furthermore, once the laser emissions are absorbed by the tissue, the effects of that emission are dependent on the energy delivered; measures of such delivery include irradiance (power/area), fluence (energy/area), and exposure time (continuous or pulsed).[111]

Mechanisms of Tissue Ablation

In direct systems the mechanism of tissue ablation is dependent upon the wavelength of the laser emission that is absorbed. The absorption of short wavelength, ultraviolet excimer laser emissions can ablate tissue by breaking intramolecular bonds, a photochemical process. By contrast, the absorption of argon, Nd:YAG, CO_2, and possibly excimer emissions can ablate tissue by heating the tissue, a photothermal process.

In indirect systems, tissue ablation is due solely to the transfer of heat to tissue. As summarized in Table 3-2, the tissue effects of heat are dependent upon the temperature attained. For example, the temperature needed to ablate plaque with a hot-tip laser probe was reported to be approximately 180°C.[112] Important determinants of tissue temperature include the thermal conductivity of the tissue (calcified plaque > normal artery ≥ fibrotic plaque > fatty plaque) and the thermal conductivity of the environment (water > blood > air). Thus, a fatty plaque heated in air will reach a higher temperature and be ablated more readily than a fibrotic plaque heated in water.[113]

The events that occur during the photoablation of atheromatous tissue by argon and Nd:YAG lasers have been documented using high-speed photography.[114,115] The first change observed was blanching of the tissue as the laser energy was absorbed by chromophores within the tissue. Thereafter, the tissue began to melt, forming a pool of molten tissue. As the molten material began to boil, both steam and particulate debris were released. Finally, ablation of tissue resulted in the formation of a crater lined with carbonized material. The gases typically released during such lasing include water vapor, carbon dioxide, nitrogen, hydrogen, and light hydrocarbons.[116,117] The debris formed by argon laser ablation of atherosclerotic plaque ranged from 10 to 50 μM in diameter.[118]

Table 3-2   Effects of Temperature on the Arterial Wall

Temperature (°C)	Biologic Effect
43–48	Cell injury, inflamation, repair
42–65	Protein denaturation
>60	Type I collagen denaturation; cell death
95–140	Optimal temperatures for vascular welding
>100	Boiling of cell water producing vacuoles in tissue
136	Temperature required for radiofrequency hot tip to pass through muscle
>180	Ablation of tissue by laser probe
>500	Ablation of calcified plaque

(Modified from Gardiner and Consigny,[121] with permission.)

Effects of Laser Ablation on the Arterial Wall

Three zones of injury have been identified in histologic sections of arteries treated with lasers[112] (Fig. 3-16). The first and most superficial zone is a layer of carbonization formed by the oxidation of tissue. The second zone is a more peripheral layer of protein coagulation necrosis; this zone contains denatured proteins that readily bind eosin and appear red when tissue sections are stained with hematoxylin and eosin (H&E). The third, and most peripheral, zone is a layer of vacuoles created by explosive expansion of water vapor and other gases formed during the boiling of the tissue.

The nature of the craters and zones of thermal injury surrounding the crater differ depending on the type of laser and laser system used. For example, in a comparative study performed by Lammer et al.,[119] direct irradiation of atheromatous tissue with an Nd:YAG laser (535 J/cm^2 s for 2 seconds) through a fiberoptic resulted in the formation of a crater 1.8 mm deep and 1 mm wide (Fig. 3-17). This crater was surrounded by a 100- to 200-μM zone of thermal necrosis with minimal carbonization or vacuolization. By contrast, indirect treatment of atheromatous tissue with a laser probe heated with 30 J of laser energy produced a crater 0.2 mm deep and 2.4 mm wide (Fig. 3-18). Adjacent to the crater, a 400- to 600-μM layer of thermal necrosis was present which covered an even thicker layer of tissue vacuolization. Treatment of atheromatous tissue with a hybrid sapphire probe (30 J of Nd:YAG energy with 90 percent transmittance) produced an irregular crater 1.5 mm deep and 2.8 mm wide (Fig. 3-19). The deep inner crater was created by the laser light trans-

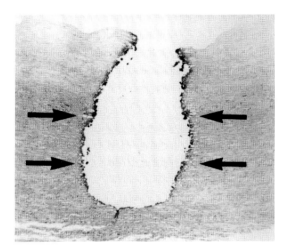

Figure 3-17 Photomicrograph of crater formed in an atherosclerotic aorta by direct Nd:YAG irradiation (30 J) through a 600-μM fiberoptic. (From Lammer et al.,[119] with permission.)

mitted through the focused tip of the sapphire lense; the outer crater was created by heat transmitted by direct contact between the heated sapphire probe and the tissue. In a separate study, treatment of atheromatous tissue with excimer irradiation (308-nM wavelength, 102 pulses, 35 mJ/10-ns pulse) produced a crater which had a shape similar to the laser beam[129] (Fig. 3-20). There were no zones of thermal necrosis or vacuolization surrounding the crater. This absence of thermal injury with excimer laser treatment is attributed to the fact that the laser is pulsed at a rate that allows the tissue

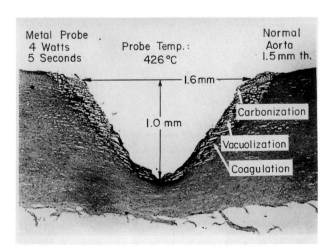

Figure 3-16 Photomicrograph of crater formed in atherosclerotic aorta by a hot-tip laser probe heated with an argon laser (4 W for 5 seconds). (From Welch et al.,[112] with permission.)

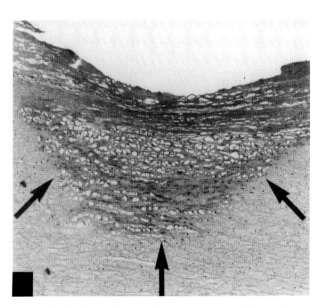

Figure 3-18 Photomicrograph of crater created in an atherosclerotic aorta by hot-tip laser probe heated with an Nd:YAG laser (30 J). (From Lammer et al.,[119] with permission.)

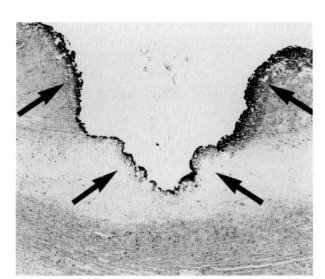

Figure 3-19 Photomicrograph of crater created in an atherosclerotic aorta by a sapphire probe irradiated with an Nd:YAG laser (30 J). (From Lammer et al.,[119] with permission.)

to cool between pulses. As a result of this pulsing, tissue temperature does not exceed 63.5°C before vaporization.

In addition to ablating plaque, both direct and indirect laser irradiation affect vascular function.[121] For example, platelet adhesion studies have demonstrated

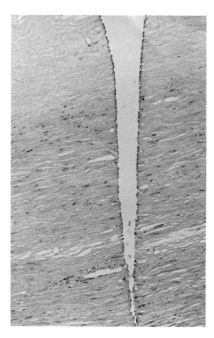

Figure 3-20 Photomicrograph of crater created in an atheromatous aorta by direct excimer irradiation (308 nM, 102 pulses, 35 mJ/10-ns pulse). (From Forrester et al.,[120] with permission.)

that excimer lasing of atherosclerotic plaque increased platelet adhesion slightly (24 percent), whereas hot-tip laser probe ablation (325°C) reduced platelet adhesion by 74 percent.[122] This effect was most likely thermal, since heating subendothelial matrix formed in tissue culture to 55°C, a temperature similar to that produced by the excimer laser, increased platelet adhesion 35 percent, whereas heating the matrix to 100°C, a temperature lower than that produced by the hot-tip, decreased platelet adhesion by 83 percent.[123]

Vascular smooth muscle function is also affected by laser irradiation. For example, exposure of arteries to argon irradiation that raised arterial temperatures to 57 to 75°C elicited reversible arterial contractions.[124] However, temperatures in excess of 75°C can elicit irreversible contractions.[125] By contrast, exposure of arteries to excimer ultraviolet light elicited endothelium-independent relaxations of arterial rings in vitro.[126]

After laser irradiation, arterial repair begins. The repair process has been characterized after CO_2 irradiation of the aortic intima of normal and atherosclerotic swine.[127] Two days after irradiation, the craters created by the laser were filled with platelet-fibrin thrombi and adherent leukocytes. By 2 weeks, the craters were re-endothelialized. Beneath the endothelium, residual thrombus was present and contained numerous macrophages. By 8 weeks, a fibrotic cap of smooth muscle cells was present beneath the endothelium. Beneath this cap, a necrotic core was still present.

The repair process was somewhat similar after argon laser irradiation of normal canine and atherosclerotic primate arteries.[128] Within 1 hour, the craters created by the laser were filled with coagulum of blood and cellular debris. Platelets were present but few in number. Perforations created by the laser were filled with thrombus at this time. By 1 week, the surface of the crater was partially re-endothelialized. Beneath, the thrombus within the crater was partially infiltrated with smooth muscle cells and undifferentiated mesenchymal cells (possibly fibroblasts). However, few mononuclear, and no polymorphonuclear, leukocytes were present. By 30 to 60 days, cellular infiltration and re-endothelialization were complete, but there was no sign of accelerated atherosclerosis.

A somewhat similar scenario was observed after excimer laser irradiation of normal canine arteries.[129] Two hours after irradiation, the craters were filled with thrombus composed of fibrin, red blood cells, and platelets. Two days after irradiation, the thrombus was still coated with platelets and polymorphonuclear leukocytes, and endothelial cells were present at the rim of the crater. Ten days after irradiation, the surface of the thrombus within the crater was almost completely re-endothelialized, and the thrombus beneath was infiltrated with macrophages and fibroblasts. At 42 days, re-endothelialization and fibrocellular infiltration were complete without any signs of intimal hyperplasia.

Although no signs of enhanced proliferation were observed in these three studies, significant proliferation and restenosis have been observed in clinical studies.[130-134] Until this problem can be resolved, it is difficult to justify the added cost associated with lasers except to recanalize arterial occlusions that are resistant to recanalization by other mechanical methods.

Atherectomy Devices

A number of mechanical devices have been designed to remove atheroma physically from within the artery. These devices can be divided into two groups, the atherectomy devices and the atheroablation devices.[135] Atherectomy devices, such as the Simpson AtheroCath (directional atherectomy catheter)[136] and the pullback atherectomy catheter,[137] cut and remove the plaque.[138] The effects of these devices on artery wall pathology have been best documented in experimental and clinical studies using the Simpson AtheroCath. These studies have demonstrated that the acute effects of atherectomy differ from those of balloon angioplasty in two respects. First, angiographic studies have documented that atherectomy produces fewer dissections than are achieved with PTCA (0 to 5 percent versus 50 percent or more).[136,138,139] Second, residual stenoses are less after atherectomy than after balloon angioplasty (5 percent versus 32 to 43 percent in one study[139] and 22 percent versus 44 percent in a second[140]).

There are several mechanisms by which atherectomy may increase lumen diameter. The first and most obvious mechanism is by removing plaque (Fig. 3-21). However, at least two studies have found that the increases in lumen diameter after Simpson atherectomy exceeded the increases in diameter predicted by the mass of plaque removed.[139,141] These findings suggest that other mechanisms must be involved. An additional mechanism by which these devices may increase lumen diameter is by producing a "Dotter" effect; this effect refers to the increase in lumen diameter that occurs when a catheter is passed through a vessel that has a lumen diameter smaller than the outer diameter of the catheter.[142-144] The Simpson AtheroCath may also increase lumen diameter by balloon dilatation of the artery, since positioning of the cutting chamber of this device against the arterial wall requires the inflation of a balloon to pressures up to 35 PSI (2.4 atm).[136,144] Finally, atherectomy devices may increase lumen diameter by cutting the internal and external

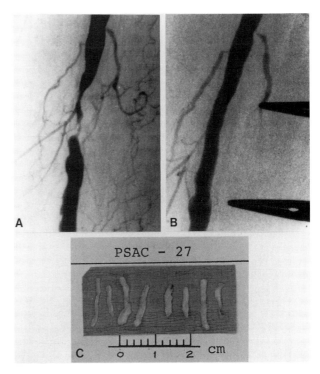

Figure 3-21 Treatment of a superficial femoral artery stenosis with a Simpson AtheroCath. **(A)** Angiogram before atherectomy showing 95 percent stenosis. **(B)** Angiogram after atherectomy showing a 10 percent residual stenosis. **(C)** Gross morphology of eight tissue specimens removed by the atherectomy device. (From Simpson et al.,[136] with permission.)

elastic laminae (Fig. 3-22), structures within the artery which restrict arterial expansion circumferentially. Histologic analyses of Simpson AtheroCath specimens have documented that the internal elastic lamina and media are present in up to 67 percent of samples collected, and the external elastic lamina and adventitia are present in up to 27 percent of samples collected.[139,143,145-147]

The pathologic changes that occur in the artery after atherectomy appear to be similar to those observed after balloon angioplasty. For example, within hours after atherectomy, thrombus forms on the surface of the resected plaque (Fig. 3-23). This thrombosis is initiated by thrombogenic factors, such as collagen and tissue factor, within the plaque that are exposed after resection.[144,147] In the months thereafter, the troughs created by atherectomy device become filled with smooth muscle cells and myofibroblasts (Fig. 3-24). In some cases, this proliferation is so exuberant that restenosis occurs (Fig. 3-25). The rates of restenosis appear to be related to the artery being treated[144] (30 to 36 percent for coronary arteries[136,139]; 51 percent for su-

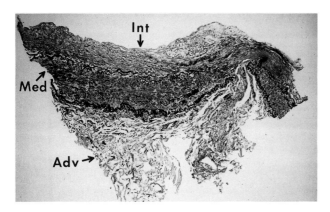

Figure 3-22 Photomicrograph of tissue resected from a coronary artery by a Simpson AtheroCath. Luminal and abluminal borders of media are demarcated by the internal and external elastic laminae, respectively. (Elastic-van Gieson stain.) (Courtesy of Kirk N. Garratt, M.D.)

perficial femoral arteries; 80 percent for tibial peroneal arteries[148]). Restenoses after atherectomy may also be directly related to the severity of the residual stenosis after treatment[136] and to resection through the internal elastic lamina[146] (Fig. 3-25).

In addition to being used as a clinical tool, the Simpson AtheroCath has been used as a research tool to provide valuable information regarding the pathology and cell biology of primary atherosclerotic and secondary restenotic lesions.[149-152]

Atheroablation Devices

In contrast to atherectomy devices, atheroablation devices pulverize the plaque and then either permit the debris to pass through the circulation (Kensey catheter,[153] Auth Rotoblator[154]) or remove the debris

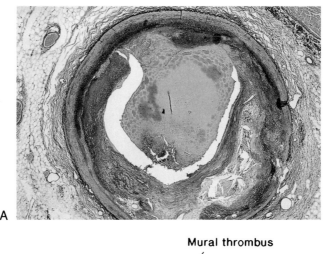

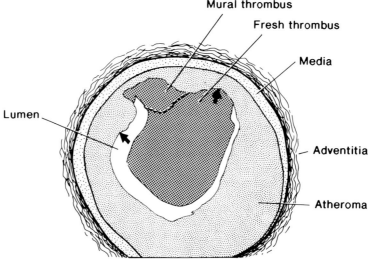

Figure 3-23 **(A)** Histologic cross section and **(B)** corresponding diagram of an atherectomy site in the left anterior descending coronary artery of a patient who died 12 hours after atherectomy. The trough created by the Simpson AtheroCath is filled with partially organized thrombus. The lumen is partially filled with fresh thrombus that presumably developed on the mural thrombus after the patient's heparinization was reversed. (Verhoeff-van Gieson stain.) (From Garratt et al.,[144] with permission.)

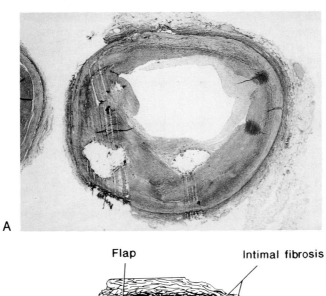

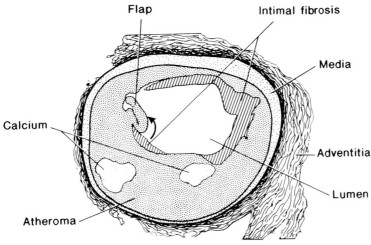

Figure 3-24 (A) Histologic cross section and (B) corresponding diagram of a left anterior descending coronary artery obtained 28 days after atherectomy. The troughs created by the Simpson AtheroCath are filled with smooth muscle cells and myofibroblasts. The residual plaque has an intimal flap but no fissures are present. (Verhoeff-van Gieson stain.) (From Garratt et al.,[144] with permission.)

(transluminal extraction catheter).[155] The Kensey catheter was the first mechanical atheroablation device to be developed.[153] This device and the Auth Rotoblator were both designed to pulverize plaque into pieces too small to affect the distal circulation. Nevertheless, the potential for distal embolization has been a primary concern. Coleman et al.[156] have evaluated the effluent from human cadaver legs after recanalization with a Kensey catheter and found that plaque composition determined the nature of the debris formed. Ablation of soft atherosclerotic lesions produced a mixture of fibrin particles as small as 10 μM and intimal strips as large as 2000 μM. By contrast, ablation of complicated, calcified lesions produced particles as small as 50 μM and intimal strips as long as 800 μM.

The debris generated by the Auth Rotoblator have been measured and found to be smaller than the debris generated by the Kensey catheter. For example, in one study,[157] 90 percent of the debris produced by ablation of atheromatous lesions in human limbs was less than 8 μM in diameter, 5 percent were 7 to 41 μM in diameter, and 5 percent were 41 to 250 μM in diameter. Similarly, only 2 percent of the particles created by ablation of atherosclerotic lesions in rabbit iliac arteries were greater than 10 μM.[158]

The debris produced by atheroablation devices have had somewhat varied effects on the physiology and pathology of the distal circulation. When human atheromatous debris produced by the Kensey catheter were injected into either the coronary or renal circulations of dogs, infarcts developed.[156] By contrast, when human atheromatous debris produced by Auth Rotoblator were collected, labeled with technetium 99m, and then injected into the femoral artery of dogs, most of the radioactivity passed through the microcirculation and lodged in the liver and lungs. There was no

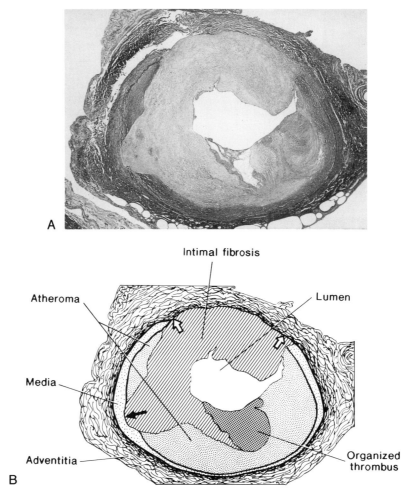

Figure 3-25 (A) Histologic cross section and **(B)** corresponding diagram of a saphenous vein graft obtained 85 days after atherectomy. The troughs created by the Simpson AtheroCath are filled with intimal hyperplasia and organized thrombus. The areas of greatest hyperplasia correspond to the areas where the atherectomy device cut through the internal elastic lamina *(arrow).* (Verhoeff-van Gieson stain.) (From Garratt et al.,[144] with permission.)

evidence of ischemia or infarction up to 28 days post-injection.[154] Similar results were noted when human atheromatous debris were injected into the left circumflex artery of pigs.[157] However, Prevosti et al.[159] observed that the injection of debris from calcified human lesions into the coronary artery of dogs reduced coronary blood flow and subsequently produced severe left ventricular failure; debris from uncalcified lesions had no such effect. Other adverse effects observed after atheroablation include destruction of red blood cells, hemoglobinuria, and vasospasm.[160] In addition, the use of suction to remove debris created by the transluminal extraction catheter may result in a significant loss of blood volume.

The acute effects of atheroablation on the arterial wall pathology appear to be device dependent. Use of the Kensey catheter produces irregular lumen surfaces,

arterial dissections, and perforations.[156] By contrast, use of the Auth Rotoblator produces intimal surfaces that appear smooth and polished but does not routinely penetrate the arterial wall beyond the internal elastic lamina and inner media.[154,158,161] However, evidence of thermal injury to the arterial wall has been observed.[160] The long-term effects of atheroablation on arterial wall pathology have not been reported.

REFERENCES

1. Gruentzig AR: Transluminal dilatation of coronary artery stenoses. Lancet 1:263, 1978
2. Cohen RA, Shepherd JT, Vanhoutte PM: Inhibitory role of the endothelium in the response of isolated coronary arteries to platelets. Science 221:273, 1983

3. Furlong B, Henderson AH, Lewis MJ, Smith JA: Endothelium-derived relaxing factor inhibits in vitro platelet aggregation. Br J Pharmacol 90:687, 1987

4. Furchgott RF, Zawadzki JV: The obligatory role of endothelial cells in the relaxation of arterial smooth muscle by acetylcholine. Nature 299:373, 1980

5. Castellot JJ, Addonizio ML, Rosenberg R, Karnovsky MJ: Cultured endothelial cells produce a heparinlike inhibitor of smooth muscle cell growth. J Cell Biol 90:372, 1981

6. Libby P: Interleukin 1: a mitogen for human vascular smooth muscle cells that induces the release of growth-inhibitory prostanoids. J Clin Invest 81:487, 1988

7. Garg U, Hassid A: Nitric-oxide generating vasodilators and 8-bromo-cyclic guanosine monophosphate inhibit mitogenesis and proliferation of cultured rat vascular smooth muscle cells. J Clin Invest 83:1774, 1989

8. Steele PM, Chesebro JH, Stanson AW et al: Balloon angioplasty: natural history of the pathophysiologic response to injury in a pig model. Circ Res 57:105, 1985

9. Wilentz JR, Sanborn TA, Haudenschild C et al: Platelet accumulation in experimental angioplasty: time course and relation to vascular injury. Circulation 75:636, 1987

10. Consigny PM, Tulenko TN, Nicosia RF: Immediate and long-term effects of angioplasty-balloon dilation on normal rabbit iliac artery. Arteriosclerosis 6:265, 1986

11. Consigny PM, LeVeen RF: Effects of angioplasty balloon inflation time on arterial contractions and mechanics. Invest Radiol 23:271, 1988

12. Consigny PM, Teitelbaum GP, Gardiner GA, Jr, Kerns WD: Effects of laser thermal angioplasty on arterial contractions and mechanics. Cardiovasc Intervent Radiol 12:83, 1989

13. Consigny PM, Gardiner GA, Jr: Comparison of balloon angioplasty and laser-assisted balloon angioplasty on atherosclerotic rabbit iliac arteries. J Vasc Intervent Radiol 2:253, 1991

14. Bjornsson TD, Dryjski M, Tluczek J et al: Acidic fibroblast growth factor promotes vascular repair. Proc Natl Acad Sci USA 88:8651, 1991

15. Lindner V, Reidy MA: Proliferation of smooth muscle cells after vascular injury is inhibited by an antibody against basic fibroblast growth factor. Proc Natl Acad Sci USA 88:3739, 1991

16. Winkles JA, Friesel R, Burgess WH et al: Human vascular smooth muscle cells both express and respond to heparin-binding growth factor I (endothelial cell growth factor). Proc Natl Acad Sci USA 84:7124, 1987

17. Olson NE, Chao S, Lindner V, Reidy MA: Intimal smooth muscle cell proliferation after balloon catheter injury. The role of basic fibroblast growth factor. Am J Pathol 140:1017, 1992

18. Lindner V, Lappi DA, Baird A et al: Role of basic fibroblast growth factor in vascular lesion formation. Circ Res 68:106, 1991

19. Lindner V, Majack RA, Reidy MA: Basic fibroblast growth factor stimulates endothelial regrowth and proliferation in denuded arteries. J Clin Invest 85:2004, 1990

20. Fingerle J, Johnson R, Clowes AW et al: Role of platelets in smooth muscle cell proliferation and migration after vascular injury in rat carotid artery. Proc Natl Acad Sci USA 86:8412, 1989

21. Reidy MA, Schwartz SM: Endothelial regeneration. III. Time course of intimal changes after small defined injury to rat aortic endothelium. Lab Invest 44:310, 1981

22. Fingerle J, Au YP, Clowes AW, Reidy MA: Intimal lesion formation in rat carotid arteries after endothelial denudation in absence of medial injury. Arteriosclerosis 10:1082, 1990

23. Jawien AD, Bowen-Pope DF, Lindner V et al: Platelet-derived growth factor promotes smooth muscle migration and intimal thickening in a rat model of balloon angioplasty. J Clin Invest 89:507, 1992

24. Clowes AW, Clowes MM, Au YPT et al: Smooth muscle cells express urokinase during mitogenesis and tissue-type plasminogen activator during migration in injured rat carotid artery. Circ Res 67:61, 1990

25. Naito M, Hayashi T, Kuzuya M et al: Effects of fibrinogen and fibrin on the migration of vascular smooth muscle cells in vitro. Atherosclerosis 83:9, 1990

26. Ferns GAA, Raines EW, Sprugel KH et al: Inhibition of neointimal smooth muscle accumulation after angioplasty by an antibody to PDGF. Science 253:1129, 1991

27. Nilsson J, Sjolund M, Palmberg I et al: Arterial smooth muscle cells in primary culture produce a platelet-derived growth factor-like protein. Proc Natl Acad Sci USA 82:4418, 1985

28. Libby P, Warner SJC, Salomon RN, Birinyi LK: Production of platelet-derived growth factor like mitogen by smooth muscle cells from human atheroma. N Engl J Med 318:1493, 1988

29. Majesky MW, Reidy MA, Bowen-Pope DF et al: PDGF ligand and receptor gene expression during repair of arterial injury. J Cell Biol 111:2149, 1990

30. Ross R, Masuda J, Raines EW et al: Localization of PDGF-B protein in macrophages in all phases of atherogenesis. Science 248:1009, 1990

31. DiCorletto PE, Bowen-Pope DF: Cultured endothelial cells produce a platelet-derived growth factor-like protein. Proc Natl Acad Sci USA 80:1919, 1983

32. Clemmons DR, Van Wyk J: Evidence for a functional role of endogenously produced somatomedin-like peptides in the regulation of DNA synthesis in cultured human fibroblasts and porcine smooth muscle cells. J Clin Invest 75:1914, 1985

33. Cercek B, Fishbein MC, Forrester JS et al: Induction of insulin-like growth factor I messenger RNA in rat aorta after balloon denudation. Circ Res 66:1755, 1990

34. Hansson HA, Jennische E, Skottner A: Regenerating endothelial cells express insulin-like growth factor I immunoreactivity after arterial injury. Cell Tissue Res 250:499, 1987

35. Weitz JI, Hudoba M, Massel D et al: Clot-bound thrombin is protected from inhibition by heparin-antithrombin III but is susceptible to inactivation by antithrombin III-independent inhibitors. J Clin Invest 86:385, 1990

36. Johnson DE, Hinohara T, Selmon MR et al: Primary peripheral arterial stenoses and restenoses excised by transluminal atherectomy: a histopathologic study. J Am Coll Cardiol 15:419, 1990

37. Graham DJ, Alexander JJ: The effects of thrombin on bovine aortic endothelial cells and smooth muscle cells. J Vasc Surg 11:307, 1990

38. Bar-Shavit R, Benezra M, Eldor A et al: Thrombin immobilized to extracellular matrix is a potent mitogen for vascular smooth muscle cells: nonenzymatic mode of action. Cell Regul 1:453, 1990

39. Harlan JM, Thompson PJ, Ross RR, Bowen-Pope DF: α-Thrombin induces release of platelet-derived growth factor-like molecules by cultured human endothelial cells. J Cell Biol 103:1129, 1986

40. Daniel TO, Gibbs VC, Milfay DF et al: Thrombin stimulates c-sis gene expression in microvascular endothelial cells. J Biol Chem 261:9679, 1986

41. Sarembock IJ, Gertz SD, Gimple LW et al: Effectiveness of recombinant desulphatohirudin in reducing restenosis after balloon angioplasty of atherosclerotic femoral arteries in rabbits. Circulation 84:232, 1991

42. Majesky MW, Lindner V, Twardzik DR et al: Production of transforming growth factor beta 1 during repair of arterial injury. J Clin Invest 88:904, 1991

43. Lyons RM, Keski-Oja J, Moses HL: Proteolytic activation of latent transforming growth factor-β from fibroblast conditioned medium. J Cell Biol 106:1659, 1988

44. Roberts AB, Sporn MB, Assoian RK et al: Transforming growth factor type-beta: rapid induction of fibrosis and angiogenesis in vivo and stimulation of collagen formation in vitro. Proc Natl Acad Sci USA 83:4167, 1986

45. Sporn MB, Roberts AB, Wakefield LM, de Crombrugghe B: Some recent advances in the chemistry and biology of transforming growth factor-β. J Cell Biol 105:1039, 1987

46. Chiang CP, Nilsen-Hamilton M: Opposite and selective effects of epidermal growth factor and human platelet transforming growth factor-β on the production of secreted proteins by murine 3T3 cells and human fibroblasts. J Biol Chem 261:10478, 1986

47. Sporn MB, Roberts AB: Transforming growth factor-β. Multiple actions and potential clinical applications. JAMA 262:938, 1989

48. Fishman JA, Ryan GB, Karnovsky MJ: Endothelial regeneration in the rat carotid artery and the significance of endothelial denudation in the pathogenesis of myointimal thickening. Lab Invest 32:339, 1975

49. Stemerman MB, Spaet TH, Pitlick F et al: Intimal healing. The pattern of reendothelialization and intimal thickening. Am J Pathol 87:125, 1977

50. Castaneda-Zuniga WR, Formanek A, Tadavarthy M et al: The mechanism of angioplasty. Radiology 135:565, 1980

51. Block PC, Baughman KL, Pasternak RC, Fallon JT: Transluminal angioplasty: correlation of morphologic and angiographic findings in an experimental model. Circulation 61:778, 1980

52. Saffitz JE, Totty WG, McClennan BL, Gilula LA: Percutaneous transluminal angioplasty. Radiological-pathological correlation. Radiology 141:651, 1981

53. Cragg AH, Einzig S, Rysavy JA et al: The vasa vasorum and angioplasty. Radiology 148:75, 1983

54. Cragg A, Einzig S, Rysavy J et al: Effect of aspirin on angioplasty-induced vessel wall hyperemia. AJR 140:1233, 1983

55. Cragg A, Einzig S, Castaneda-Zuniga W et al: Vessel wall arachidonate metabolism after angioplasty: possible mediators of postangioplasty vasospasm. Am J Cardiol 51:1441, 1983

56. Steele PM, Cheseboro JH, Stanson AW et al: Balloon angioplasty: natural history of the pathophysiological response to injury in a pig model. Circ Res 57:105, 1985

57. Zollikofer CL, Cragg AH, Einzig S et al: Prostaglandins and angioplasty: an experimental study in canine arteries. Radiology 149:681, 1983

58. Block PC, Myler RK, Stertzer S, Fallon JT: Morphology after transluminal angioplasty in human beings. N Engl J Med 305:382, 1981

59. Waller BF: Early and late morphologic changes in human coronary arteries after percutaneous transluminal coronary angioplasty. Clin Cardiol 6:363, 1983

60. Mizuno K, Kurita A, Imazeki N: Pathological findings after percutaneous transluminal coronary angioplasty. Br Heart J 52:588, 1984

61. Uchida Y, Hasegawa K, Kawamura K, Shibuya I: Angioscopic observation of the coronary luminal changes induced by percutaneous transluminal coronary angioplasty. Am Heart J 117:769, 1989

62. Weibull H, Bergquist D, Jonsson K et al: Complications after percutaneous transluminal angioplasty in the iliac, femoral, and popliteal arteries. J Vasc Surg 5:681, 1987

63. Waller BF: Pathology of transluminal balloon angioplasty used in the treatment of coronary heart disease. Hum Pathol 18:476, 1987

64. Waller BF: Early and late morphologic changes in human coronary arteries after precutaneous transluminal coronary angioplasty. A review. Clin Cardiol 6:363, 1983

65. Waller BF: The eccentric coronary atherosclerotic plaque: morphologic observations and clinical relevance. Clin Cardiol 12:14, 1988

66. Johnson DE, Hinohara T, Selmon MR et al: Primary peripheral arterial stenoses and restenoses excised by transluminal atherectomy: a histopathologic study. J Am Coll Cardiol 15:419, 1990

67. Kalsner S: Endogenous prostaglandin release contributes directly to coronary artery tone. Can J Physiol Pharmacol 53:560, 1975

68. Greenwald JE, Bianchine JR, Wong LK: The production of the arachidonate metabolite HETE in vascular tissue. Nature 281:588, 1979

69. Peterson MB, Machaj V, Block PC et al: Thromboxane release during percutaneous transluminal coronary angioplasty. Am Heart J 111:1, 1986

70. Schwartz L, Bourassa MG, Lesperance J et al: Failure of

antiplatelet agents to reduce restenosis after PTCA in a double blind placebo controlled trial. J Am Coll Cardiol 11:236A, 1988

71. Ellis SG, Roubin GS, Wilenz J et al: Results of a randomized trial of heparin and aspirin vs. aspirin alone for prevention of acute closure and restenosis after angioplasty (PTCA), abstracted. Circulation, suppl. 76:213, 1987

72. Thornton MA, Gruentzig AR, Hollman J et al: Coumadin and aspirin in prevention of recurrence after transluminal coronary angioplasty: a randomized study. Circulation 69:721, 1984

73. Whitworth HB, Roubin GS, Hollman J et al: Effect of nifedipine on recurrent stenosis after percutaneous coronary angioplasty. J Am Coll Cardiol 8:1271, 1986

74. Gleason T, Cragg AH, Smith TP et al: Preliminary results of thermal balloon angioplasty in a canine model. J Vasc Intervent Radiol 1:121, 1990

75. Cragg AH, Smith TP, Landas SK et al: Six month follow-up after thermal balloon angioplasty in canine iliac arteries. Cardiovasc Intervent Radiol 14:230, 1991

76. Deutsch E, Martin JL, Budjak R et al: Low stress angioplasty at 60°Celsius: attenuated arterial barotrauma. Circulation, suppl. III. 82:72, 1990

77. Dotter CT: Transluminally placed coil spring endarterial tube grafts—long term patency in canine popliteal artery. Invest Radiol 4:329, 1969

78. Muller DWM, Ellis SG, Debowey DL, Topol EJ: Quantitative angiographic comparison of the immediate success of coronary angioplasty, coronary atherectomy and endoluminal stenting. Am J Cardiol 66:938, 1990

79. Serruys PW, Juilliere Y, Bertrand ME et al: Additional improvement of stenosis geometry in human coronary arteries by stenting after balloon dilatation. Am J Cardiol 61:71G, 1988

80. Puel J, Juilliere Y, Bertrand ME et al: Early and late assessment of stenosis geometry after coronary arterial stenting. Am J Cardiol 61:546, 1988

81. Bonn J, Gardiner GA Jr, Shapiro MJ et al: Palmaz vascular stent: initial clinical experience. Radiology 174:741, 1990

82. Leimgruber PP, Roubin GS, Hollman J et al: Restenosis after successful coronary angioplasty in patients with single vessel disease. Circulation 73:710, 1986

83. Liu MW, Roubin GS, King SB III: Restenosis after coronary angioplasty. Potential biologic determinants and role of intimal hyperplasia. Circulation 79:1374, 1989

84. Palmaz JC, Sibbitt RR, Tio FO et al: Expandable intraluminal vascular graft: a feasibility study. Surgery 99:199, 1986

85. Palmaz JC, Windeler SA, Garcia F et al: Atherosclerotic rabbit aortas: Expandable intraluminal grafting. Radiology 160:723, 1986

86. Miller D, Boulet AJ, Tio FO et al: In vivo technitium-99m S12 antibody imaging of platelet α-granules in rabbit endothelial neointimal proliferation after angioplasty. Circulation 83:224, 1991

87. Schatz RA, Palmaz JC, Tio FO et al: Balloon-expandable intracoronary stents in the adult dog. Circulation 76:450, 1987

88. Roubin GS, Robinson KA, Sing SB III et al: Early and late results of intracoronary arterial stenting after coronary angioplasty in dogs. Circulation 76:891, 1987

89. Robinson KA, Roubin G, King S et al: Correlated microscopic observations of arterial responses to intravascular stenting. Scann Microsc 3:665, 1989

90. Rodgers GP, Minor ST, Robinson K et al: Adjuvant therapy for intracoronary stents. Investigations in atherosclerotic swine. Circulation 82:560, 1990

91. Sigwart U, Puel J, Mirkovitch V et al: Intravascular stents to prevent occlusion and restenosis after transluminal angioplasty. N Engl J Med 316:701, 1987

92. Rousseau H, Puel J, Joffre F et al: Self expanding endovascular prosthesis: an experimental study. Radiology 164:709, 1987

93. Rousseau H, Joffre F, Raillat C et al: Self-expanding endovascular stent in experimental atherosclerosis. Radiology 170:773, 1989

94. van der Giessen WJ, Serruys PW, Visser WJ et al: Endothelialization of intravascular stents. J Intervent Cardiol 1:109, 1988

95. Strecker EP, Liermann D, Barth KH et al: Expandable tubular stents for treatment of arterial occlusive diseases: experimental and clinical results. Radiology 175:97, 1990

96. Barth KH, Virmani R, Strecker EP et al: Flexible tantalum stents implanted in aortas and iliac arteries: effects in normal canines. Radiology 175:91, 1990

97. Wright KC, Wallace S, Charnsangavej C et al: Percutaneous endovascular stents: an experimental evaluation. Radiology 156:69, 1985

98. Rollins N, Wright KC, Charnasangavej C et al: Self-expanding metallic stents: preliminary evaluation in an atherosclerotic model. Radiology 163:739, 1987

99. Bonan R, Bhat K, Lefevre T et al: Coronary artery stenting after angioplasty with self-expanding parallel wire metallic stents. Am Heart J 121:1522, 1991

100. van der Giessen WJ, Serruys PW, van Beusekom HMM et al: Coronary stenting with a new, radiopaque, balloon-expandable endoprosthesis in pigs. Circulation 83:1788, 1991

101. Sutton CS, Tominaga R, Harasaki H et al: Vascular stenting in normal and atherosclerotic rabbits. Studies of the intravascular endoprosthesis of titanium-nickel-alloy. Circulation 81:667, 1990

102. Lembo NJ, Roubin GS: Intravascular stents. Cardiol Clin 7:877, 1989

103. Schatz RA: A view of vascular stents. Circulation 79:445, 1989

104. Bucx JJJ, de Scheerder I, Beatt K et al: The importance of adequate anticoagulation to prevent early thrombosis after stenting of stenosed venous bypass grafts. Am Heart J 121:1389, 1991

105. Palmaz JC: Balloon expandable intravascular stent. AJR 150:1263, 1988

106. Bonan R, Bhat K, Lefevre T et al: Coronary artery

stenting after angioplasty with self-expanding parallel wire metallic stents. Am Heart J 121:1522, 1991

107. Vorwerk D and Guenther RW: Removal of intimal hyperplasia in vascular endoprostheses by atherectomy and balloon dilatation. AJR 154:617, 1990

108. Gunther RW, Vorwerk D, Bohndorf K et al: Iliac and femoral artery stenoses and occlusions: treatment with intravascular stents. Radiology 172:725, 1989

109. Rees CR, Palmaz JC, Garcia O et al: Angioplasty and stenting of completely occluded arteries. Radiology 172:953, 1989

110. Levine MJ, Leonard BM, Burke JA et al: Clinical and angiographic results of balloon-expandable intracoronary stents in right coronary artery stenoses. J Am Coll Cardiol 16:332, 1990

111. Cragg AH, Gardiner GA, Jr, Smith TP: Vascular applications of laser. Radiology 172:925, 1989

112. Welch AJ, Bradley AB, Torres JH et al: Laser probe ablation of normal and atherosclerotic human aorta in vitro: a first thermographic and histologic analysis. Circulation 76:1353, 1987

113. Welch AJ, Valvano JW, Pearce JA et al: Effect of laser radiation on tissue during laser angioplasty. Lasers Surg Med 5:251, 1985

114. Grundfest WS, Litvack FI, Doyle DL, Forrester JS: Laser-tissue interactions: considerations for cardiovascular applications. p. 32. In White RA, Grundfest WSI (eds): Lasers in Cardiovascular Disease: Clinical Applications, Alternative Angioplasty Devices, and Guidance Systems. 2nd Ed. Year Book Medical Publishers, Chicago, 1989

115. Litvack F, Grundfest WS, Papaioannou T et al: Role of laser and thermal ablation devices in the treatment of vascular diseases. Am J Cardiol 61:81G, 1988

116. Choy DSJ: Laser applications in cardiovascular disease. Semin Intervent Radiol 3:1, 1986

117. Clark RH, Donaldson RF, Isner JM: Identification of photoproducts liberated by in vitro laser irradiation of atherosclerotic plaque, calcified valves, and myocardium. Lasers Surg Med 3:358, 1984

118. Grewe DD, Castaneda-Zuniga WR, Nordstrom LA et al: Debris analysis after laser photorecanalization of atherosclerotic plaque. Semin Intervent Radiol 3:53, 1986

119. Lammer J, Kleinert R, Pilger E et al: Contact probes for intravascular laser recanalization: experimental evaluation. Invest Radiol 24:190, 1989

120. Forrester JS, Litvack F, Grundfest WS: Laser angioplasty and cardiovascular disease. Am J Cardiol 57:990, 1986

121. Gardiner GA, Jr, Consigny PM: Effects of thermal energy on the arterial wall. Semin Intervent Radiol 8:94, 1991

122. Prevosti LG, Lawrence JB, Leon MB et al: Surface thrombogencity after excimer laser and hot-tip thermal ablation of plaque: morphometric studies using an annular perfusion chamber. Surg For 38:330, 1988

123. Borst C, Bos AN, Zwaginga JJ et al: Loss of blood platelet adhesion after heating native and cultured human subendothelium to 100°Celsius. Cardiovasc Res 24:665, 1990

124. Steg PG, Gal D, Rongionne AJ et al: Effect of argon laser irradiation on rabbit aortic smooth muscle: evidence for endothelium dependent contraction and relaxation. Cardiovasc Res 22:747, 1988

125. Gorisch W, Boergen KP: Heat-induced contraction of blood vessels. Lasers Surg Med 2:1, 1982

126. Steg PG, Kongtione AJ, Gal D et al: Pulsed ultraviolet laser irradiation produces endothelium-independent relaxation of vascular smooth muscle. Circulation 79:189, 1989

127. Gerrity RG, Loop FD, Golding LAR et al: Arterial response to laser operation for removal of atherosclerotic plaques. J Thorac Cardiovasc Surg 85:409, 1983

128. Abela GS, Crea F, Seeger JM et al: The healing process in normal canine arteries and in atherosclerotic monkey arteries after transluminal laser irradiation. Am J Cardiol 56:983, 1985

129. Prevosti LG, Leon MB, Smith PD et al: Early and late healing responses of normal canine artery to excimer laser irradiation. J Thorac Cardiovasc Surg 96:150, 1988

130. Bonn J: Clinical utility of laser recanalization in occluded peripheral arteries. Radiology 178:323, 1991

131. Perler BA, Osterman FA, White RI, Jr, Williams GM: Percutaneous laser probe femoropopliteal angioplasty: a preliminary experience. J Vasc Surg 10:351, 1989

132. Werner G, Buchwald A, Unterberg C et al: Excimer laser angioplasty in coronary artery disease. Eur Heart J 12:24, 1991

133. Lammer J, Pilger E, Karnel F et al: Laser angioplasty: results of a prospective multicenter study at 3-year follow-up. Radiology 178:335, 1991

134. Geschwind HJ, Aptecar E, Boussignac G et al: Results and follow-up after percutaneous pulsed laser-assisted balloon angioplasty guided by spectroscopy. Circulation 83:787, 1991

135. Fischell TA, Stadium ML: New technologies for the treatment of obstructive arterial disease. Cathet Cardiovasc Diagn 22:205, 1991

136. Simpson JB, Selmon MR, Robertson GC et al: Transluminal atherectomy for occlusive peripheral vascular disease. Am J Cardiol 61:96, 1988

137. Fischell TA, Fischell RE, White RI, Jr, Chapolini R: Ex-vivo results using a new pullback atherectomy catheter (PAC). Cathet Cardiovasc Diagn 21:287, 1990

138. Hinohara T, Selmon MR, Robertson GC et al: Directional atherectomy. New approaches for treatment of obstructive coronary and peripheral vascular disease. Circulation, suppl. IV. 81:IV-79, 1990

139. Safian RD, Gelbfish JS, Erny RE et al: Coronary atherectomy. Clinical, angiographic and histological findings and observations regarding potential mechanisms. Circulation 82:69, 1990

140. Muller DWM, Ellis SG, Debowey DL, Topol EJ: Quantitative angiographic comparison of the immediate success of coronary angioplasty, coronary atherec-

tomy and endoluminal stenting. Am J Cardiol 66:938, 1990

141. Penny WF, Schmidt DA, Safian RD et al: Insights into the mechanism of luminal improvement after directional coronary atherectomy. Am J Cardiol 67:435, 1991

142. Dotter CT, Judkins MP: Transluminal treatment of arteriosclerotic obstruction: description of a new technique and a preliminary report of its application. Circulation 30:654, 1964

143. Johnson DE, Braden L, Simpson JB: Mechanism of directed transluminal atherectomy. Am J Cardiol 65:389, 1990

144. Garratt KN, Edwards WD, Vlietstra RE et al: Coronary morphology after percutaneous directional coronary atherectomy in humans: autopsy analysis of three patients. J Am Coll Cardiol 16:1432, 1990

145. Dorros G, Lewin RF, Sachdev N, Mathiak L: Percutaneous atherectomy of occlusive peripheral vascular disease: Stenoses and/or occlusions. Cathet Cardiovasc Diagn 18:1, 1989

146. Garratt KN, Kaufmann UP, Edwards WD et al: Safety of percutaneous coronary atherectomy with deep arterial resection. Am J Cardiol 64:538, 1989

146. Garratt KN, Holmes DR, Jr, Bell MR et al: Restenosis after directional coronary atherectomy: differences between primary atheromatous and restenosis lesions and influence of subintimal tissue resection. J Am Coll Cardiol 16:1665, 1990

147. Wilcox JN, Smith KM, Williams LT et al: Platelet-derived growth factor mRNA detection in human atherosclerotic plaques by in situ hybridization. J Clin Invest 82:1134, 1988

148. Dorros G, Iyer S, Lewin R et al: Angiographic follow-up and clinical outcome of 126 patients after percutaneous directional atherectomy (Simpson AtheroCath) for occlusive peripheral vascular disease. Cathet Cardiovasc Diagn 22:79, 1991

149. Barbano EF, Newman GE, McCann RL et al: Correlation of clinical history with quantitative histology of lower extremity atheroma biopsies obtained with the Simpson atherectomy catheter. Atherosclerosis 78:183, 1989

150. Dartsch PC, Bauriedel G, Schinko I et al: Cell constitution and characteristics of human atherosclerotic plaques selectively removed by percutaneous atherectomy. Atherosclerosis 80:149, 1989

151. Dartsch PC, Voisard R, Bauriedel G et al: Growth characteristics and cytoskeletal organization of cultured smooth muscle cells from human primary stenosing and restenosing lesions. Arteriosclerosis 10:62, 1990

152. Garratt KN, Edwards WD, Kaufmann UP et al: Differential histopathology of primary atherosclerotic and restenotic lesions in coronary arteries and saphenous vein bypass grafts: analysis of tissue obtained from 73 patients by directional atherectomy. J Am Coll Cardiol 17:442, 1991

153. Kensey KR, Nash JE, Abrahams C, Zarins CK: Recanalization of obstructed arteries with a flexible, rotating tip catheter. Radiology 163:387, 1987

154. Ahn SS, Auth D, Marcus DR, Moore WS: Removal of focal atheromatous lesions by angioscopically guided high-speed rotary atherectomy. J Vasc Surg 7:292, 1988

155. Wholey MH, Jarmolowski CR: New reperfusion devices: the Kensey catheter, the atherolytic reperfusion wire device, and the transluminal extraction catheter. Radiology 172:947, 1989

156. Coleman CC, Posalaky IP, Robinson JD et al: Atheroablation with the Kensey catheter: a pathologic study. Radiology 170:391, 1989

157. Zacca NM, Raizner AE, Noon GP et al: Treatment of symptomatic peripheral atherosclerotic disease with a rotational atherectomy device. Am J Cardiol 63:77, 1989

158. Hansen DD, Auth DC, Vracko R, Ritchie JL: Rotational atherectomy in atherosclerotic rabbit iliac arteries. Am Heart J 115:160, 1988

159. Prevosti LG, Cook JA, Unger EF et al: Particulate debris from rotational atherectomy: Size distribution and physiologic effects. Circulation, suppl. II. 78:II-83, 1988

160. Dorros G, Iyer S, Zaitoun R et al: Acute angiographic and clinical outcome of high speed percutaneous rotational atherectomy (Rotoblator) Cathet Cardiovasc Diagn 22:157, 1991

161. Fourier JL, Stankowiak C, LaBlanche J et al: Histopathology after rotational angioplasty of peripheral arteries in human beings. J Am Coll Cardiol 11:109A, 1988

162. Waller BF, Pinkerton CA: Coronary balloon angioplasty restenosis: pathogenesis and treatment strategies from a morphologic perspective. J Int Cardiol 3:167, 1989

Section II

Physiology of Arterial Narrowing and Occlusion

A working knowledge of the physiologic principles that govern blood flow in the arterial system is essential in the management of patients with vascular disease. The chapters in this section are intended to provide a theoretical foundation for subsequent discussions of specific diagnostic and therapeutic techniques. Since an appreciation of normal physiology is a logical prerequisite to understanding the effects of disease, the section begins with Chapter 4, on the hemodynamic and mechanical properties that result in normal arterial flow patterns. Although blood pressure is a concept that is familiar to all physicians, it is important to recognize that there are other forms of fluid energy that drive the circulation. These additional potential and kinetic energy components contribute to the total fluid energy. Gradual changes in size and wall properties provide favorable hemodynamic conditions as blood flows from the large elastic arteries of the thorax to the small muscular arterioles. Thus, arteries are remarkably efficient conduits for blood, and relatively little energy is lost as blood flows through the normal arterial system.

If blood flow through normal arteries is regarded as a response to differences in total fluid energy, then the effects of arterial disease can be understood as manifestations of energy loss. The hemodynamic consequences of arterial stenoses are discussed in Chapter 5. Energy losses related to arterial lesions are associated with turbulent flow patterns and pressure gradients, both of which can be objectively documented by various noninvasive and invasive vascular tests. Criti-

cal arterial stenosis and the significance of stenosis diameter are important concepts for explaining the hemodynamic effects of arterial disease. The collateral circulation plays a crucial role in compensating for arterial occlusive lesions, although this ability to provide distal flow is limited by the anatomic and physiologic characteristics of the collateral vessels.

A specific example of normal and abnormal arterial hemodynamics is covered in Chapter 6. The predominant feature of the normal carotid artery bifurcation is a bulb that typically occupies the distal common and proximal internal carotid arteries. This unique diverging and converging geometry gives rise to complex flow patterns that include areas of reversed flow and flow separation. These flow patterns can be identified by noninvasive testing and must be recognized in order to distinguish them from the flow patterns related to arterial disease. The hemodynamics of the carotid bifurcation are of interest not only because of the unusual flow patterns found there, but also because of the association between atherosclerosis of the carotid bulb and stroke. Evaluation of patients with carotid artery disease has provided an opportunity to study the relationship between hemodynamic patterns, arterial pathology, and clinical outcome. Since the cerebral circulation also depends on the vertebrobasilar system, it is appropriate to review subclavian steal syndromes and the cerebral collateral circulation.

The final chapter in this section, Chapter 7 discusses the application of hemodynamic principles to arterial reconstruction. If the goal of an arterial operation is to restore normal physiologic conditions, then the hemodynamic principles reviewed in the previous chapters must be observed. Within the technical limitations that exist, a procedure should be designed to provide blood flow with minimal energy losses. This requires selecting graft materials of proper size and performing anastomoses that produce the least amount of flow disturbance. However, even the most adept arterial reconstruction is rarely as hemodynamically efficient as a normal arterial segment. With this observation in mind, the study of arterial physiology provides useful models for further improvements in techniques for arterial reconstruction.

4

Normal Arterial Physiology

R. Eugene Zierler

The flow of blood through the arterial system is governed by a set of hemodynamic principles that describe the relationships among parameters such as fluid energy, pressure, velocity, and resistance. These principles, together with the mechanical characteristics of the arterial wall, arterial geometry, and certain properties of the blood, influence arterial flow patterns. While some energy loss occurs as blood flows through normal arteries, the arterial system is a remarkably efficient conduit for blood, and pressure gradients are minimal. However, arterial occlusive disease can produce marked flow disturbances that reduce distal pressure and flow. Since the effects of arterial disease are best understood and analyzed as derangements of normal arterial physiology, this chapter provides the necessary background for more detailed discussions of arterial disease.

FLUID ENERGY

Blood Pressure

Fluid pressure is defined as force per area, given in standard units of dynes per square centimeter (dyn/cm^2). Conversion to the more commonly used millimeters of mercury depends on the density of mercury, making 1 mmHg equivalent to 1330 dyn/cm^2. The intravascular arterial pressure (P) has three major components: (1) the dynamic pressure resulting from cardiac contraction, (2) hydrostatic pressure, and (3) static filling pressure. Hydrostatic pressure is determined by the density of blood (ρ), the acceleration due to gravity (g), and the height (h) of the point of measurement relative to a specific reference level. This can be expressed as

$$P \text{ (hydrostatic)} = -\rho gh$$

where ρ is 1.056 g/cm^3, g is 980 cm/s^2, and h is the distance in centimeters (cm) above or below the right atrium. In a man 5 feet 8 inches tall standing erect, the hydrostatic pressure component at ankle level is approximately 89 mmHg.[1]

Static filling pressure is the pressure that would be present in the arterial system without cardiac contractions. This pressure component, typically in the range of 5 to 10 mmHg, is determined by blood volume and the elastic properties of the arterial wall.

Energy Losses in Blood Flow

Bernoulli's Principle

Although pressure gradients are the most obvious forces that drive the circulation, blood flows through the arterial system in response to differences in total fluid energy. The total fluid energy (E) is the sum of potential energy (E$_p$) and kinetic energy (E$_k$). Potential energy consists of the intravascular pressure (P) and gravitational potential energy. The formula for gravitational potential energy is the same as that for hydrostatic pressure, but with the opposite sign, $+\rho gh$. This form of potential energy represents the ability of blood to do work because of its height above a specific reference level. Because static filling pressure is relatively low, and hydrostatic pressure and gravitational potential energy usually cancel each other out, the predominant component of potential energy is the dynamic pressure of cardiac contraction. Thus, potential energy can be expressed as

$$E_p = P + (\rho gh)$$

Kinetic energy is related to the motion of the blood and is proportional to the density of blood and the square of blood velocity (v) in centimeters per second:

$$E_k = \tfrac{1}{2}\rho v^2$$

Combining these two equations provides an expression for total fluid energy per unit volume of blood, with E in units of ergs (dyn · cm) per cubic centimeter:

$$E = P + (\rho gh) + (\tfrac{1}{2}\rho v^2)$$

Bernoulli's principle states that when fluid flows from one point to another, its total energy remains constant, provided that flow is steady and there are no frictional losses. In the horizontal diverging tube shown in Figure 4-1, steady flow between points 1 and 2 is accompanied by an increase in cross-sectional area and by a decrease in flow velocity. Although the fluid gains potential energy and appears to move against a pressure gradient of 2.5 mmHg, the total fluid energy is unchanged due to a decrease in velocity and a proportional loss of kinetic energy. Thus, widening of the tube results in the conversion of kinetic energy to potential energy. This situation is not found in the arterial system because the idealized flow conditions specified by Ber-

noulli's principle do not exist. The energy lost in the movement of blood is dissipated mainly in the form of heat.

Viscosity

The energy losses that occur as blood flows through the arterial system can be described as either viscous or inertial. Viscous losses are the result of frictional forces, while inertial losses are related to changes in the velocity or direction of flow. Viscosity describes the resistance of a fluid to flow that arises from intermolecular attractions. For a moving fluid, the coefficient of viscosity (η) can be defined as the ratio of shear stress (τ) to shear rate (D):

$$\eta = \frac{\tau}{D}$$

where shear stress represents energy loss due to friction between adjacent fluid layers, and shear rate refers to the relative velocity of the fluid layers. Fluids with strong intermolecular attractions offer a high resistance to flow and have high coefficients of viscosity. The unit of viscosity is the poise, which is equivalent to 1 dyn · s/cm². Relative viscosity is a convenient way of expressing viscous properties by comparing the viscosity of a fluid to that of water. The relative viscosity of whole blood is in the range of 3 to 4; the relative viscosity of plasma is approximately 1.8.

The concentration of red blood cells, or hematocrit, is the most important determinant of blood viscosity. Plasma viscosity depends primarily on the concentration of plasma proteins. The cellular and molecular components of blood are responsible for its non-Newtonian characteristics. In a Newtonian fluid, viscosity is independent of shear rate or flow velocity. However, because blood is a heterogeneous suspension of cells and large protein molecules its viscosity varies with the shear rate. As shown in Figure 4-2, blood viscosity increases rapidly at low shear rates and approaches a constant value at higher shear rates.[2] Because the normal shear rates in large and medium-sized arteries place the viscosity on the asymptotic segment of this curve, arterial blood generally resembles a Newtonian fluid.

Poiseuille's Law

The viscous energy losses in an idealized fluid system can be estimated using the relationship of pressure, flow, and resistance. When this is expressed as

$$\text{Pressure} = \text{flow} \times \text{resistance}$$

it is analogous to Ohm's law of electrical circuits.

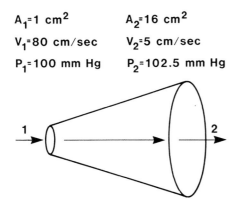

$$A_1 = 1 \text{ cm}^2 \qquad A_2 = 16 \text{ cm}^2$$
$$V_1 = 80 \text{ cm/sec} \qquad V_2 = 5 \text{ cm/sec}$$
$$P_1 = 100 \text{ mm Hg} \qquad P_2 = 102.5 \text{ mm Hg}$$

Figure 4-1 Effect of increasing cross-sectional area on pressure and velocity in a frictionless fluid system. Although pressure increases, total fluid energy remains constant due to a decrease in velocity. (Modified from Sumner,[1] with permission.)

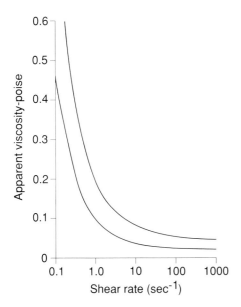

Figure 4-2 Viscosity of human blood as a function of shear rate. Values range between the two curves. (Adapted from Whitmore,[17] with permission.)

Poiseuille's law states that the pressure gradient along a tube $(P_1 - P_2)$ is directly proportional to the mean flow velocity (V) or volume flow (Q), the tube length (L), and the fluid viscosity (η), and inversely proportional to the tube radius (r):

$$P_1 - P_2 = V \frac{8L\eta}{r^2} = Q \frac{8L\eta}{\pi r^4}$$

The application of Poiseuille's law is based on the steady laminar flow of a Newtonian fluid through a straight, rigid, cylindrical tube. Since these conditions rarely exist in the arterial system, Poiseuille's law can only be used to predict the minimum pressure gradient produced by arterial flow. These viscous energy losses are often much less than the energy losses due to inertial effects, particularly when arterial occlusive disease is present.

Vascular Resistance

Hemodynamic resistance (R) can be defined as the ratio of energy drop between two points along a vessel $(E_1 - E_2)$ and volume flow:

$$R = \frac{E_1 - E_2}{Q}$$

If the artery is assumed to be horizontal, so the gravitational potential energy term $(+\rho gh)$ is not significant,

and the kinetic energy term ($\frac{1}{2}\rho v^2$) is considered a relatively small component of the total energy, resistance can be expressed as the ratio of pressure gradient $(P_1 - P_2)$ to volume flow:

$$R \cong \frac{P_1 - P_2}{Q}$$

This formula for resistance is a rearranged version of Poiseuille's law, and the resistance term is

$$R = \frac{8L\eta}{\pi r^4}$$

The standard units of hemodynamic resistance are dyne seconds per centimeter to the fifth power (dyn $\cdot$ s/cm^5). A more useful way of expressing resistance is the peripheral resistance unit (PRU), where one PRU is approximately 8×10^4 dyn $\cdot$ s/cm^5.

For an artery of a particular lumen size, hemodynamic resistance increases as flow velocity increases. These energy losses are related to inertial effects and are proportional to $\frac{1}{2}\rho v^2$ (Fig. 4-3). Inertial energy losses (ΔE) result from the changes in blood flow velocity caused by cardiac contractions, variations in lumen diameter, and arterial branching. Since inertial energy losses are proportional to kinetic energy, they can be expressed as

$$\Delta E = K \tfrac{1}{2}\rho v^2$$

where K is a constant. Figure 4-4 illustrates the combined effects of viscous and inertial energy losses across an arterial segment. The relationship between pressure drop and flow rate is depicted by a curved line that has both linear (viscous) and squared (inertial) terms.

The factor that has the greatest effect on hemodynamic resistance is the vessel radius, which is raised to the fourth power in the denominator of the resistance term. Figure 4-5 shows the relationship between radius and pressure drop for various flow rates. Pressure drop is minimal until the radius is approximately 0.3 cm but increases rapidly with further reductions in lumen size. These observations help explain the frequent failure of autogenous vein femoropopliteal bypass grafts less than 4 mm in diameter[3] and the marked hemodynamic effects of profunda femoris artery stenosis in the presence of superficial artery occlusion.[4]

About 10 percent of the total hemodynamic resistance in the human circulation results from venous flow, arterioles and capillaries are responsible for approximately 70 percent, and the large and medium-size arteries account for only about 20 percent.[5] Thus, the arteries most commonly affected by atherosclerosis normally offer relatively little resistance to arterial flow.

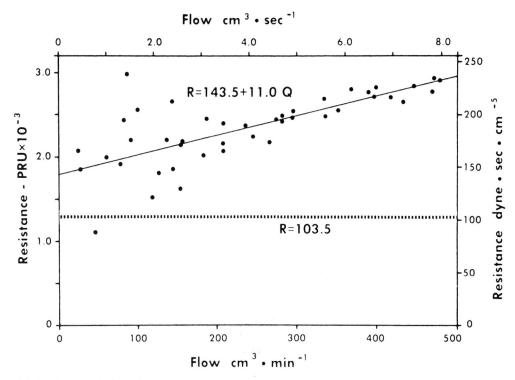

Figure 4-3 Resistance derived from the pressure-flow curve in Figure 4-4. The increase in resistance with increasing flow is due to inertial effects. Constant resistance predicted by Poiseuille's law is indicated by the dotted line. PRU, peripheral resistance unit; R, resistance. (From Sumner,[1] with permission.)

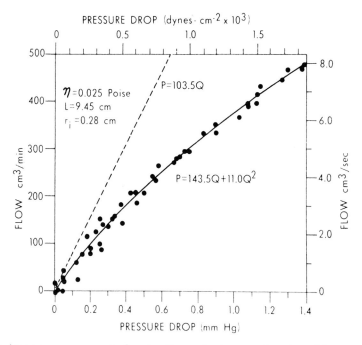

Figure 4-4 Pressure drop across a segment of canine femoral artery as a function of flow rate. Measured values *(solid line)* lie along a curve with both linear and squared terms, corresponding to viscous and inertial energy losses. The pressure-flow relationship predicted by Poiseuille's law *(dashed line)* indicates lower energy losses than those observed. (From Sumner,[1] with permission.)

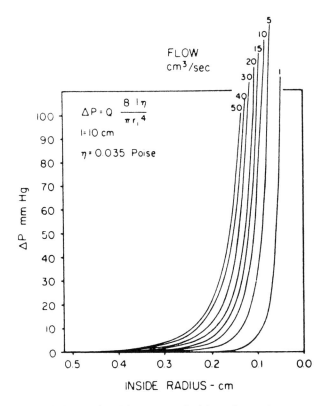

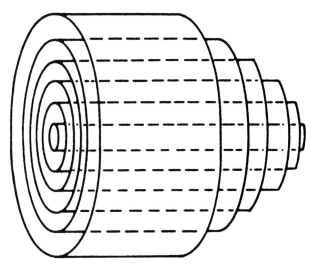

Figure 4-6 Laminar flow from left to right in a cylindrical tube. Central laminae move more rapidly than those near the periphery of the tube. (From Strandness and Sumner,[2] with permission.)

Figure 4-5 Relationship between inside radius and pressure drop for various rates of steady laminar flow through a cylindrical tube 10 cm in length. Flow rates are comparable to those found in the human iliac artery. (From Strandness and Sumner,[2] with permission.)

ARTERIAL FLOW PATTERNS

Laminar Flow

When the motion of the blood is parallel to the walls of the vessel and the blood is arranged in concentric layers or laminae, a laminar flow pattern is present (Fig. 4-6). This is the flow state specified by Poiseuille's law, in which the velocity within each lamina remains constant. The velocities are lowest adjacent to the vessel wall and highest in the center of the lumen, resulting in a parabolic flow profile.

Turbulent Flow

Turbulence is a flow pattern in which velocity varies at random with respect to both space and time. This disorderly flow state can result in considerable energy loss. The transition between laminar and turbulent flow depends primarily on the vessel diameter (d) and the mean flow velocity. The Reynolds number (Re),

which describes the ratio of inertial forces to viscous forces acting on the blood, is expressed as

$$Re = \frac{dV\rho}{\eta}$$

At an Re of less than 2000, minor flow disturbances are damped out by viscous forces and turbulence does not occur. When the Re is greater than 2000, inertial forces tend to disrupt laminar flow and produce turbulent flow. In normal arteries, the Re is usually less than 2000, and true turbulence is rare. However, small areas of turbulence may be found in the normal ascending aorta where the Re exceeds the critical value.[2] A disturbed flow state is a transient disruption of the laminar streamlines that disappears a short distance downstream. Disturbed flow can be considered as an intermediate pattern between stable laminar flow and fully developed turbulence. Areas of disturbed arterial flow may occur at points of curvature or branching.

Boundary Layer Separation

The boundary layer is the portion of flowing blood adjacent to the vessel wall. At certain branch points and areas at which the lumen size changes abruptly, small pressure gradients are created that cause the boundary layer to slow down or change direction. This results in a complex localized flow pattern called boundary layer separation or flow separation.[6] Regions of boundary layer separation have been observed in model studies of arterial bifurcations and anastomoses.[7,8]

The unique geometry of the normal human carotid bifurcation produces an area of flow separation along the outer wall of the carotid bulb, which includes complex vortices and reversed flow.[9,10] This separation zone is limited to the bulb, and a more laminar flow pattern is present in the distal internal carotid artery. Along the inner wall of the bulb, adjacent to the flow divider, the flow pattern is also more laminar. These flow patterns have been documented by pulsed Doppler studies.[9,11] In Figure 4-7, the spectral waveform taken near the outer wall of the bulb shows low velocities with periods of both forward and reverse flow during each cardiac cycle. These features are consistent with flow separation and are considered normal, particularly in young individuals.[11] Increased wall thickness and changes in arterial wall distensibility make this area of flow separation less prominent in older individuals.[12] Spectral waveforms obtained near the inner wall of the bulb along the flow divider depict a forward, quasi-steady flow pattern typical of the internal carotid artery. A more detailed discussion of the flow patterns in the carotid bifurcation is given in Chapter 6.

Regions of boundary layer separation with reversed or stagnant flow components often coincide with areas where atherosclerotic plaques tend to develop.[10,13] For example, intimal thickening and atherosclerosis are found primarily along the outer wall of the carotid bulb, while the inner wall is relatively spared.[8] These

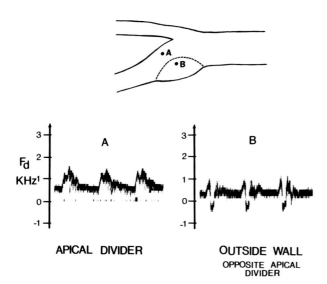

Figure 4-7 Flow separation in the normal carotid bulb, as demonstrated by pulsed Doppler spectral analysis. The flow pattern near the flow divider (**A**) is forward throughout the cardiac cycle but, near the outer wall of the bulb (**B**), the spectral waveform contains both forward and reversed flow components, indicating an area of flow separation. (From Zierler and Strandness,[18] with permission.)

observations suggest that atherosclerotic plaques form in segments of the arterial wall that are subject to low shear stresses.

Pulsatile Flow and Velocity Waveforms

When flow is pulsatile, pressure and velocity vary continuously with time. The hemodynamic principles presented in this chapter are based on steady flow and do not permit a precise description of the arterial system. As previously stated, the resistance term of Poiseuille's law estimates the viscous energy losses in steady flow; however, it does not account for the inertial effects, arterial wall properties, and wave reflections that influence pulsatile flow. The term *vascular impedance* is used to describe the resistance of a peripheral vascular bed to pulsatile flow.

The peak systolic pressure is amplified as blood moves away from the heart and down the limbs. This results from a progressive reduction in arterial compliance and reflections originating from the relatively high peripheral resistance. In order to keep blood moving in the proper direction, the diastolic and mean pressures gradually decrease. The fall in mean arterial pressure between the heart and the ankle is normally less than 10 mmHg. Thus, as the pressure pulse moves distally, systolic pressure rises, diastolic pressure falls, and the pulse pressure widens. This explains why the systolic pressure at the ankle is higher than that in the upper arm and the ankle-arm pressure ratio (ankle-arm index) is greater than one. The normal resting ankle-arm index has a mean value of 1.11 ± 0.10.[14] Lower limb exercise in normal individuals produces little or no drop in ankle systolic pressure.

The velocity pattern in the peripheral arteries is normally triphasic. As shown in Figure 4-8, the initial large forward velocity phase resulting from cardiac systole is followed by a brief phase of reversed flow in early diastole and a smaller phase of forward flow in late diastole. This triphasic pattern is modified by changes in peripheral arterial resistance and the presence of proximal arterial lesions. The reversed flow phase is particularly sensitive to changes in peripheral resistance. Body heating, which causes vasodilatation and decreased resistance, will diminish or eliminate the reversed flow phase; exposure to cold increases resistance and makes the reversed flow phase more prominent.

Bifurcations and Branches

While the branching geometry of the arterial system can produce dramatic changes in flow patterns, the effects of branching on energy loss or pressure drop in

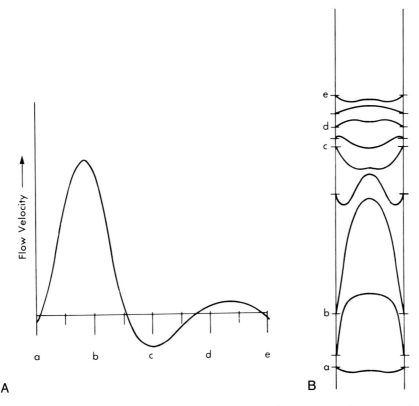

Figure 4-8 Velocity waveform (**A**) and velocity profiles (**B**) representing normal peripheral arterial flow. Lower-case letters indicate corresponding points in the cardiac cycle. Maximum forward velocity occurs near point b, where the flow profile is parabolic. Reversed flow is most prominent at point c. (From Sumner,[1] with permission.)

normal arterial flow are relatively small. The flow pattern across a bifurcation is determined mainly by its area ratio and branch angle, where the area ratio is defined as the combined area of the secondary branches divided by the area of the primary artery. According to Poiseuille's law, an area ratio of 1.41 allows the pressure gradient to remain constant across a bifurcation. An area ratio of 1.0 produces a bifurcation with no change in flow velocity. The most efficient transmission of pulsatile energy occurs when the impedance of the primary artery equals that of the secondary branches. This situation exists when the area ratio is 1.15 for larger arteries and 1.35 for smaller arteries.[15] Human infants have a favorable area ratio of 1.11 at the aortic bifurcation. However, this area ratio decreases with age, dropping to less than 1.0 in the second decade of life and to less than 0.8 by the fifth decade.[16] This fall in the area ratio at the aortic bifurcation leads to an increase in both the iliac artery flow velocity and the amount of reflected pulsatile energy. With an area ratio of 0.8, approximately 22 percent of the incident pulsatile energy is reflected back up the infrarenal aorta.

Curvature and angulation also contribute to the development of flow disturbances at arterial bifurcations.

Centrifugal forces acting on blood flowing around a curve can result in complex helical flow patterns such as those found in the carotid bulb.[9] The tendency to develop disturbed or turbulent flow increases as the angle between the secondary branches of a bifurcation widens. While the average angle between the iliac arteries is 54 degrees, this angle can approach 180 degrees when the arteries are diseased or tortuous.[2]

THE ARTERIAL WALL

Composition

Although blood flow patterns are determined primarily by arterial geometry, the physical characteristics of the arterial wall also have hemodynamic importance. The viscoelastic properties of the arteries depend on the ratio of elastin to collagen in their walls. Elastin, which is the main component of the thoracic aorta, allows energy to be stored during cardiac systole and returned to the circulation in diastole. Collagen is much less extensible than elastin and provides the arterial wall with strength and stiffness. As blood moves from the large central arteries of the thorax and abdomen to the medium-size arteries of the extremities, the relative amount of elastin in the vessel wall decreases and the amount of collagen increases. Thus, the more distal arteries, such as the superficial femoral and popliteal, do not store energy but serve mainly as conduits for blood. Arterioles are specialized vessels with walls that consist almost entirely of smooth muscle. The arterioles control blood pressure and distribute flow to various vascular beds by actively altering their lumen diameter.

Tangential Stress and Tension

Laplace's law defines the tangential tension (T) of a curved surface as the product of pressure and radius:

$$T = Pr$$

where tension is given in units of force per tube length (dyn/cm). Although Laplace's law can be used to characterize thin-walled structures, it is not suitable for describing the stresses in arterial walls. Tangential stress (τ) within the wall of a blood vessel can be expressed as

$$\tau = P \frac{r}{\delta}$$

where r is the internal radius, and δ is the thickness of the vessel wall. Stress is given in units of force per area of tube wall (dyn/cm^2). Thus, tangential stress is directly proportional to pressure and radius but inversely proportional to wall thickness.

The tendency of arterial aneurysms to expand and rupture is readily explained by the effects of increasing radius and decreasing wall thickness on tangential stress. Rupture is likely to occur when the tangential stress within the arterial wall becomes greater than the tensile strength of its components. The relationship between blood pressure and tangential stress emphasizes the importance of hypertension as a risk factor for aneurysm rupture.

REFERENCES

1. Sumner DS: Essential hemodynamic principles. p. 18. In Rutherford RB (ed): Vascular Surgery. 3rd Ed. WB Saunders, Philadelphia, 1989
2. Strandness DE, Jr, Sumner DS: Hemodynamics for Surgeons. Grune & Stratton, Orlando, FL, 1975
3. Barnes RW: Hemodynamics for the vascular surgeon. Arch Surg 115:216, 1980
4. Berguer R, Higgens RF, Cotton LT: Geometry, blood flow, and reconstruction of the deep femoral artery. Am J Surg 130:68, 1975
5. Burns PN: Hemodynamics. p. 46. In Taylor KJW, Burns PN, Wells PNT (eds): Clinical Applications of Doppler Ultrasound. Raven Press, New York, 1988
6. Gutstein WH, Schneck DJ, Marks JO: In vitro studies of local blood flow disturbances in a region of separation. J Atherosclerosis Res 8:381, 1968
7. Logerfo FW, Soncrant T, Teel T, Dewey F: Boundary layer separation in models of side-to-end arterial anastomoses. Arch Surg 114:1364, 1979
8. Zarins CK, Giddens DP, Glagov S: Atherosclerotic plaque distribution and flow velocity profiles in the carotid bifurcation. p. 19. In Bergan JJ, Yao JST (eds): Cerebrovascular Insufficiency. Grune & Stratton, Orlando, FL, 1983
9. Ku DN, Giddens DP, Phillips DJ et al: Hemodynamics of the normal human carotid bifurcation — in vitro and in vivo studies. Ultrasound Med Biol 11:13, 1985
10. Wong PKC, Eng B, Johnston KW et al: Computer simulation of blood flow patterns in arteries of various geometries. J Vasc Surg 14:658, 1991
11. Phillips DJ, Greene FM, Jr, Langlois Y et al: Flow velocity patterns in the carotid bifurcations of young, presumed normal subjects. Ultrasound Med Biol 1:39, 1983
12. Reneman RS, van Merode T, Hick P et al: Flow velocity patterns in and distensibility of the carotid artery bulb in subjects of various ages. Circulation 71:500, 1985
13. Fox JA, Hugh AE: Localization of atheroma: a theory based on boundary layer separation. Br Heart J 28:388, 1966
14. Yao JST: Hemodynamic studies in peripheral arterial disease. Br J Surg 57:761, 1970
15. McDonald DA: Blood Flow in Arteries. 2nd Ed. Edward Arnold, London, 1974
16. Gosling RG, Newman DL, Bowden NLR et al: The area ratio of normal aortic junctions — aortic configuration and pulse wave reflection. Br J Radiol 44:850, 1971
17. Whitmore RL: Rheology of the Circulation. p. 11. Pergamon Press, New York, 1968
18. Zierler RE, Strandness DE, Jr: Hemodynamics for the vascular surgeon. p. 170. In Moore WS (ed): Vascular Surgery: A Comprehensive Review. 2nd Ed. Grune & Stratton, Orlando, FL, 1986

5

Hemodynamics of Arterial Occlusive Disease

Ted R. Kohler

The basic principles of normal arterial hemodynamics are outlined in Chapter 4. This chapter discusses how arterial stenoses cause pressure and flow reduction and how these lesions should be evaluated clinically. The hemodynamics of the collateral circulation are described as well. A complete understanding of these principles is necessary for the proper diagnosis and treatment of arterial occlusive disease.

ENERGY LOSSES DUE TO STENOSIS

The primary function of the arterial circulation is to provide adequate blood flow for maintenance of healthy tissue. Because there is no simple method for determining blood flow at the bedside, clinicians have generally relied on pressure measurement as an indirect assessment of the adequacy of arterial flow. Changes in pressure reflect similar changes in flow, since arterial lesions reduce both flow and pressure at approximately the same level of stenosis, and further reductions in diameter affect pressure and flow equally (Fig. 5-1). Reductions in flow and pressure occur in parallel because both are manifestations of energy loss at sites of stenosis. Energy losses occur as a result of either viscous effects, described by Poiseuille's law or inertial forces (see Ch. 4). Viscous energy losses are important at the level of arterioles and capillaries but

are generally inconsequential in normal arteries. Inertial effects are responsible for most of the energy loss at stenoses. These can be understood by examining the total fluid energy along the artery.

As blood travels through a stenosis, the velocity of flow must increase to maintain the same flow volume in the narrowed segment as in the vessel just proximal to it. This increased velocity produces greater kinetic energy in the stenosis. Since no energy is added to the system, this increase in kinetic energy must correspond exactly to a decrease in potential energy (i.e., pressure). This relationship is described by the Bernoulli equation (see Ch. 4). As long as flow remains ordered and laminar at the entrance and exit to the stenosis, energy is efficiently converted between pressure (potential energy) and velocity (kinetic energy). However, when turbulence develops, energy is lost, resulting in reduced flow and pressure. The extent of turbulence depends on the severity of the stenosis and on the geometry of the lesion. A smoothly tapered inlet and exit from a stenosis can greatly reduce, or even eliminate, turbulence. Abrupt changes in diameter or rough irregular narrowings increase turbulence. In high-grade arterial lesions, most of the kinetic energy within the stenosis is dissipated in turbulence.[1] These relationships are depicted in Figure 5-2, which shows the energy losses due to a 1-cm-long stenosis. Viscous energy losses are small and occur mainly in the region of the stenosis. Most of the

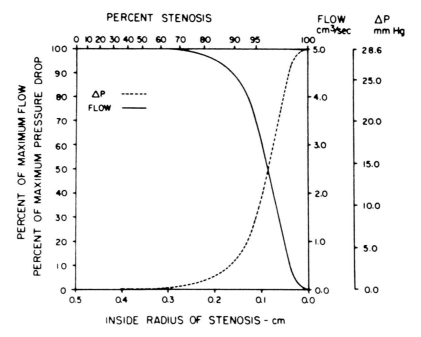

Figure 5-1 Effect of increasing stenosis on blood flow and pressure drop across the stenotic segment. Collateral and peripheral resistances are considered to be fixed. The stenosis is 1 cm long; the 10-cm-long artery has a radius of 0.5 cm. Flow = 5 cm³/s. (From Strandness and Sumner,[10] with permission.)

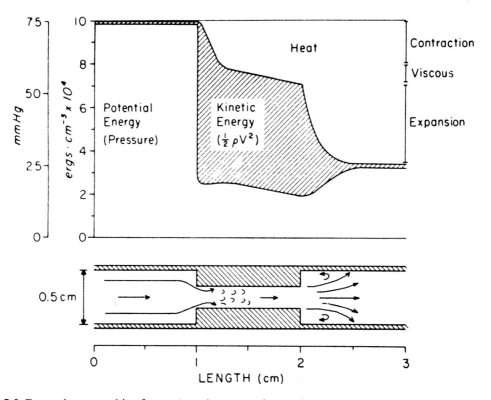

Figure 5-2 Energy losses resulting from a 1-cm-long stenosis. Inertial losses at the entrance and exit are much greater than the viscous losses. (From Sumner,[1] with permission.)

energy loss results from inertial effects related to turbulence at the entrance (contraction) and exit (expansion) of the stenosis. Ultimately, the energy loss is in the form of heat generated by the turbulent flow, although the increased temperature is not significant enough to be measurable.

The Bernoulli equation, which describes the relationship among total energy, pressure, and kinetic energy, has been used quite successfully to calculate pressure gradients across stenotic cardiac valves from velocities measured with Doppler ultrasound.[2] Similar attempts to calculate energy losses across peripheral arterial lesions using this equation, along with velocity measurements, have not been as successful.[3] Significant differences between valvular stenoses and peripheral arterial lesions account for this failure.

While valvular lesions act as a simple outlet stenosis from a reservoir of nonmoving blood, peripheral lesions have significant length and irregularity, and the proximal and distal blood flow has considerable kinetic energy. In addition, most of the kinetic energy of the jet flow across a stenotic valve is lost as turbulence beyond the orifice, while in peripheral lesions a significant amount of the kinetic energy may be recovered as increased pressure beyond the stenosis. Finally, accurate measurement of velocity is often more difficult for peripheral arteries than it is for cardiac valves.

CRITICAL STENOSES

The extent of the energy loss and of the resulting reduction in pressure and flow due to stenosis is exquisitely sensitive to stenosis diameter. This is because the magnitude of energy loss attributable to both inertial and viscous forces varies inversely with the fourth power of the radius of the stenosis lumen. For viscous losses, this follows from Poiseuille's law (see Ch. 4). In the case of inertial losses, this is because the kinetic energy of blood in the stenosis is proportional to the square of the velocity, which in turn varies with the square of the radius.

Arterial lesions are considered critical if they cause reduction in blood flow. This generally occurs at a level of stenosis that also results in reduced systolic pressure. Because energy loss due to both viscous and inertial forces is inversely proportional to the fourth power of the radius of the stenosis, the relationship between the pressure drop and radius is exponential.[4] The extent of pressure loss at a given radius is also dependent on the velocity of flow across the segment. Inertial energy losses increase with velocity as a result of greater kinetic energy in the stenosis and an associated increase in turbulence. The effects of lumen reduction at various flow rates are shown in Figure 5-3. The curves have a sharp bend at the point at which small changes in radius

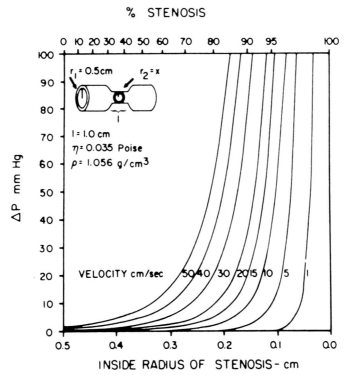

Figure 5-3 Relationship of pressure drop across a stenosis to the radius of the stenotic segment and the flow velocity. (From Strandness and Sumner,[10] with permission.)

result in large reductions in pressure—and flow. This is the point of the critical stenosis, which occurs at a diameter reduction of approximately 50 percent.

Because both viscous and inertial energy losses increase with increased flow velocity, flow rate is an important determinant of energy loss. Pressure loss across a stenosis increases with increased blood flow. Flow is augmented when peripheral resistance is lowered either by exercise, reactive hyperemia, or administration of vasodilators.[5] Any of these factors will therefore cause an accentuation of energy losses across a stenosis and may cause pressure reduction across lesions that are not critical under conditions of resting flow. The exquisite sensitivity of pressure and flow to peripheral resistance is the basis of the exercise test in the noninvasive laboratory and of administration of peripheral dilating agents at the time of pressure measurements during arteriography. This principle is particularly important because it is often difficult to determine the hemodynamic significance of atherosclerotic lesions on the basis of their angiographic appearance alone.

The relationship of pressure and flow outlined above does not take into account the variability of peripheral arterial resistance. Distal arterial beds can compensate for diminished perfusion pressure to some extent by decreasing arterial resistance. This phenomenon of autoregulation permits maintenance of flow despite diminished pressure. Autoregulation makes normal perfusion of skeletal muscle possible down to pressures as low as 20 mmHg and of cerebral perfusion down to pressures of 50 mmHg.[1] Beyond these levels, peripheral vessels are maximally dilated, and further decreases in pressure are mirrored by reductions in flow.

Atherosclerotic lesions are frequently multiple and occur in series. Viscous energy losses are small in comparison to inertial energy losses. Because viscous energy losses are proportional to the length of the lesion, the energy loss due to viscous forces across a single lesion is approximately the same as that of two tandem lesions of the same diameter and total length. This is not the case for the more significant inertial energy losses, caused by turbulence at the entrance and exit to the stenosis. When lesions occur in tandem, the inertial energy losses are additive, much as when two resistors are placed in series in an electric circuit, due to the additional entrance and exit effects. Therefore, multiple noncritical lesions in series may act as a single critical stenosis, causing pressure and flow reduction. In practical terms, when there are two lesions of equal diameter in tandem, both should be repaired, if possible. When tandem lesions are of unequal diameter, repair of the tighter lesion should take precedence, regardless of its location. This is because energy loss is very sensitive to radius and the primary source of pressure and flow reduction of tandem lesions is caused by the narrower lesion, regardless of whether it is the more proximal or distal.

It should be emphasized that this principle applies only to unbranched arteries. A hemodynamically significant proximal stenosis that occurs in an artery that supplies significant collateral blood flow should always be repaired, even if there is a significant stenosis or occlusion in a distal vessel. A classic example is the case of an iliac stenosis proximal to a superficial femoral artery occlusion. Repair of the iliac lesion can greatly increase blood flow to the lower extremity by supplying the profunda-geniculate collateral system. While improving inflow in this situation may not provide adequate flow to heal ulceration of the foot, it is usually sufficient to relieve rest pain or to improve claudication.

COLLATERAL CIRCULATION

The collateral circulation provides a parallel pathway for blood flow when major branches become occluded or significantly narrowed. This system consists proximally of large branches that serve as stem arteries, a network of smaller midzone intramuscular channels, and vessels that enter the major artery distal to the occlusion (Fig. 5-4). This network develops as a result of enlargement of pre-existing arteries, rather than development of new vessels. The stimulus for these arteries to increase their diameter is an increase in blood flow and velocity due to reduced peripheral resistance. It has long been known that, during development, arteries enlarge if flow through them increases; if flow decreases, they atrophy.[6] Similarly, mature arteries increase in diameter if flow is chronically increased, such as occurs with an arteriovenous fistula,[7] and decrease in diameter if flow is reduced.[8]

Changes in arterial diameter and wall structure in response to changes in flow are probably mediated by the endothelium.[8] Endothelial cells alter many of their functions in response to flow and are capable of producing many factors that can influence the function of underlying smooth muscle cells.[9] Many of the arterial responses to flow that have been observed in vitro and in vivo are dependent on an intact endothelium. Dilatation of arteries supplying collateral blood flow is largely responsible for the improvement in symptoms experienced by many patients with lower-extremity arterial occlusive disease.

The efficiency of collateral blood flow varies greatly with anatomic location, since it is dependent on enlargement of pre-existing vessels. This is why occlusion of the brachial artery above the profunda takeoff is

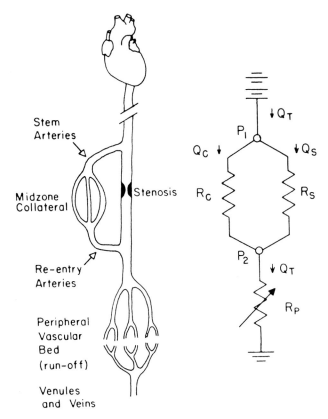

Figure 5-4 Components of the collateral circulation with the analogous electrical circuit. Resistance of the stenosis (Rs) and collateral circulation (Rc) is fixed, while that of the peripheral resistance (Rp) is variable. When the stenosis is severe, peripheral resistance may be fixed at its minimum value. (From Sumner,[1] with permission.)

poorly tolerated while occlusion below results in very little impairment. The collateral network around the most common sites of lower extremity arterial occlusions, the iliac and superficial femoral arteries, is fairly extensive and occlusion at these levels is relatively well tolerated. Dilatation of collateral vessels occurs gradually over a period of weeks to months; therefore, slowly progressive chronic occlusions are much better tolerated than are acute occlusions of previously normal vessels. Even total occlusion of the infrarenal aorta can be tolerated with minimal symptoms if it occurs gradually due to collateral flow through lumbar and mesenteric branches (Fig. 5-5).

No matter how well developed the collateral network, collateral resistance is always greater than that of the normal unobstructed artery. In addition, peripheral resistance vessels beyond major occlusions are usually maximally dilated, even under resting conditions. Therefore, flow through collateral channels cannot be increased significantly with exercise, resulting in clau-

dication. Furthermore, while collateral channels can generally compensate adequately for single level occlusions, they cannot compensate for multiple level occlusions. Thus, iliac or femoral artery occlusions may be well tolerated when they occur singly, but may result in severe ischemia when they occur in tandem.

ABNORMAL PULSES AND WAVEFORMS

Arterial stenosis results in reduction of pressure due to loss of energy. This reduction is first manifested by a decrease in the peak systolic pressure and only later is reflected in a decrease in mean pressure. Therefore, peak pressure is a much more sensitive indicator of the presence or absence of significant stenosis, and it is this parameter, rather than the mean pressure, that should be measured at angiography or surgery. In addition, stenoses will result in a damping of both the pressure and flow waveform. The flow velocity waveform pattern in normal arteries of resting extremities is triphasic, with a reverse flow component in early diastole (see Ch. 11). This pattern changes to one of forward flow throughout the cardiac cycle if peripheral resistance is lowered by exercise, dilating agents, or postischemic hyperemia. The waveforms are also damped by proximal stenoses and change from triphasic, to biphasic, to monophasic, and finally become absent[10] (Fig. 5-6). These changes can be appreciated by listening to Doppler signals from peripheral vessels. The presence of a monophasic signal at the ankle level indicates significant proximal occlusive disease.

CLINICAL APPLICATIONS OF HEMODYNAMIC PRINCIPLES TO THE DIAGNOSIS OF VASCULAR DISEASE

History and physical examination are usually sufficient to determine whether a patient has lower-extremity arterial occlusive disease requiring intervention. Further testing is required to quantitate and locate areas of stenosis. The simplest bedside method is measurement of the systolic blood pressure at the ankle level, using continuous wave Doppler. Reductions in blood pressure are generally accompanied by decreased flow; therefore, abnormal ankle pressures indicate significant arterial occlusive disease. However, ankle pressures can be normal in the presence of clinically significant disease. The extent of energy loss across a stenosis is dependent on the rate of flow, and some lesions that are not significant at resting flow rates be-

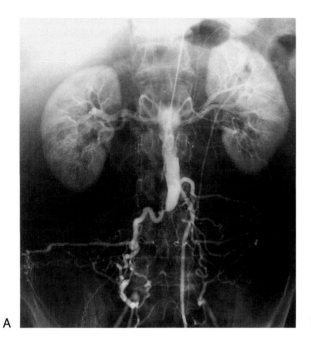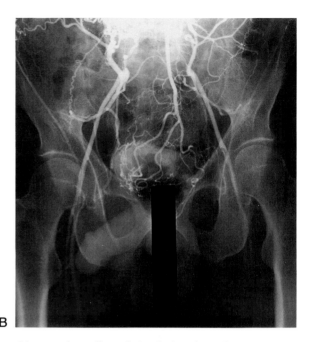

Figure 5-5 (A & B) Arteriograms showing aortic occlusion with extensive collateral circulation through mesenteric and lumbar branches. (Courtesy of David Glickerman, M.D.)

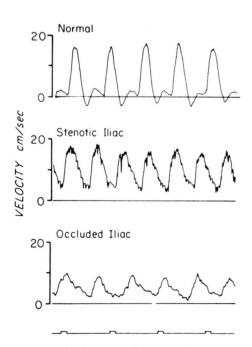

Figure 5-6 Velocity flow waveforms obtained with a directional Doppler velocity detector from the femoral artery of a normal subject, a patient with external iliac stenosis, and a patient with common iliac occlusion. (From Strandness and Sumner,[10] with permission.)

come pressure reducing if flow is increased. In general, clinically important lesions produce a systolic pressure drop of at least 15 mmHg at rest or 10 mmHg with vasodilatation. Conversely, arterial insufficiency can be ruled out as a cause of claudication if no pressure drop occurs when symptoms develop during a treadmill exercise test.

Indirect tests such as ankle or segmental pressure measurement or analysis of flow velocity waveforms at sites distant from diseased arterial segments lack sensitivity, specificity, and anatomic detail. These limitations are overcome by the use of duplex scanning.[11,12] With this technique, velocity waveforms can be obtained from above, below, and within sites of arterial narrowing. Increased velocity due to reduction in lumen diameter is reliably detected. Turbulence associated with arterial narrowing is manifested as spectral broadening, which is a widening of the velocity waveform and indicates nonuniform flow. Moderate stenoses that are not clinically important are associated with spectral broadening, only modest increases in velocity, and no change in waveform morphology. Lesions that are flow reducing are associated with a greater than 100 percent increase in peak systolic velocity within the lesion (compared with the normal proximal segment) and marked spectral broadening. The waveform pattern is also changed; the reverse flow component normally seen in diastole disappears as a result of a significant pressure gradient across the narrowed segment throughout the cardiac cycle. The waveforms proximal and distal to the stenosis are also markedly changed with diminished velocities and a blunted monophasic pattern. These patterns are used to classify degrees of stenosis in diseased arteries; similar parameters can be used to document the natural history of atherosclerotic disease or to follow the results of intervention. Because duplex scanning can identify increased velocity due to narrowing that is not severe enough to cause a pressure drop, it is a more sensitive technique than ankle pressure measurement for detecting restenosis.

Noninvasive studies can supplement and enhance arteriography. Duplex scanning can identify lesions that may be amenable to angioplasty and can direct the examination to specific sites of probable disease, thereby increasing the sensitivity of arteriography. Pressure measurements at arteriography with or without vasodilators help determine the clinical significance of lesions and can be used to document the hemodynamic results of intervention.

The proper application of the basic hemodynamic principles outlined in this chapter greatly enhances our ability to diagnose and treat arterial occlusive disease effectively and to follow the results of our interventions. Their importance for the rational planning of intervention is discussed in Chapters 11 and 12.

REFERENCES

1. Sumner DS: Essential hemodynamic principles. p. 18. In Rutherford RB (ed): Vascular Surgery. 3rd Ed. WB Saunders, Philadelphia, 1989

2. Hatle L, Angelsen BA, Tromsdal A: Non-invasive assessment of aortic stenosis by Doppler ultrasound. Br Heart J 43:284, 1980

3. Kohler TR, Nicholls SC, Zierler RE et al: Assessment of pressure gradient by Doppler ultrasound: experimental and clinical observations. J Vasc Surg 6:460, 1987

4. Kohler TR, Strandness DE, Jr: Use of the Bernoulli principle in the peripheral circulation. p. 275. In Salmasi AM, Nicolaides AN (eds): Cardiovascular Applications of Doppler Ultrasound. Churchill Livingstone, London, 1989

5. Strandness DE, Jr, Bell JW: Hemodynamic response of the claudicating extremity to exercise. Surg Gynecol Obstet 119:1237, 1964

6. Hughes AFW: Studies on the area vasculosa of the embryo chick. II. The influence of the circulation on the diameter of the vessels. J Anat 72:1, 1937

7. Zarins CK, Zatina MA, Giddens DP et al: Shear stress regulation of artery lumen diameter in experimental atherogenesis. J Vasc Surg 5:413, 1987

8. Langille BL, O'Donnell F: Reductions in arterial diameter produced by chronic decreases in blood flow are endothelium-dependent. Science 231:405, 1986

9. Davies PF, Dull RO: How does the arterial endothelium sense flow? Hemodynamic forces and signal transduction. Adv Exp Med Biol 273:281, 1990

10. Strandness DE, Jr, Sumner DS: Hemodynamics for Surgeons. Grune & Stratton, New York, 1975

11. Jager KA, Phillips DJ, Martin RL et al: Noninvasive mapping of lower limb arterial lesions. Ultrasound Med Biol 11:515, 1985

12. Kohler TR, Nance DR, Cramer MM et al: Duplex scanning for diagnosis of aortoiliac and femoropopliteal disease: a prospective study. Circulation 76:1074, 1987

6

Blood Flow Patterns in Cerebrovascular Disease

David N. Ku
Alan Lumsden

HEMODYNAMICS OF THE CAROTID BIFURCATION

Atherosclerotic disease at the carotid artery bifurcation has important clinical significance in the development of transient ischemic attacks and stroke. The detection of disease at this location depends on a detailed knowledge of the complex fluid mechanics at this bifurcation. Because of pulsatile hemodynamics and the formation of transient vortex structures, the complex flow field must be examined through the use of laboratory models. Several investigators have used the geometry defined by Bharadvaj et al. to simulate the flow in glass models.[1-4] By combining flow visualization and studies with quantitative laser Doppler anemometer studies, a comprehensive picture of carotid bifurcation hemodynamics can be formed.

Normal Carotid Flow

Dye injection and hydrogen bubble visualization are useful in pictorially representing the physical trajectories of the fluid at this bifurcation.[5] A quantitative picture of the velocity flow field can be obtained through laser Doppler anemometry studies.[6,7] The complicated flow field near the carotid sinus is illustrated in Figure 6-1. Flow can be divided into (1) the primary flow, which follows the direction of a tube or branch, and (2) secondary flows, which move in a more complicated manner that is different from the primary flow. In the carotid sinus, the primary flow hits the apex of the bifurcation and then continues directly up the internal and external carotid branches. A secondary flow vortex pair develops along the posterior wall of the internal carotid in the shape of corkscrew helices. These helices move retrograde back toward the heart and are separate from the mainstream, hence the term *flow separation.* The formation of a separated flow region near the posterior outer wall produces a reverse flow in the velocity in this region (Fig. 6-2A), but velocity near the flow divider continues in a forward direction throughout the cardiac cycle (Fig. 6-2B). The velocity and shear stress at the flow divider reach their maximum value when flow actually reverses at the outer wall. The secondary helices arise from centripetal forces due to the curvature of the sinus and can convect downstream. Flow separation occurs because the linear momentum of the mainstream cannot follow the sharp curve of the carotid sinus expansion. In arterial bifurcations that have a smaller branch angle, less secondary flow would be

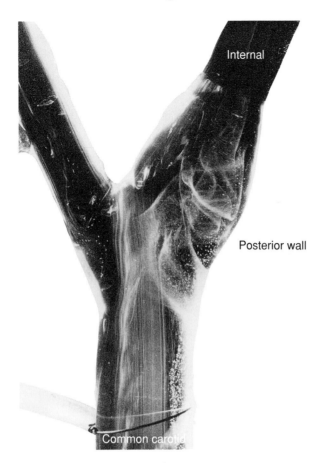

Figure 6-1 Visualization of the complex helical secondary flows in the carotid sinus during systole.

expected. Smaller sinuses would also generate less separation.

The pulsatile nature of the flow further complicates the hemodynamics at the carotid bifurcation. During early systole, the upstream pressure is so high that little separation or secondary flow can develop. All velocity is axial and forward throughout the sinus, with no reverse flow. Near peak systole, large circumferential helices form along the side walls. However, during late systole, the blood decelerates, producing separation and secondary flow. At other times during the cardiac cycle, flow is much more uniform and laminar.

The deceleration of total flow during late systole results in an enlarged separation region with moderate retrograde velocities. Reverse flow velocities, combined with the unstable nature of deceleration, can cause small amounts of turbulent-like vortex formation. These vortices are located predominantly at the outer wall of the proximal internal carotid and can appear in pulsed Doppler spectral waveforms as spectral broadening. Thus, spectral broadening can occur

in the normal carotid bifurcation, independent of any local stenosis. However, flow separation at the outer wall is dependent on a relatively disease-free carotid sinus. Thus, a more specific indication of normal carotid artery anatomy would be a large transient area of flow separation at the posterior wall, not the absence of any spectral broadening.[7]

The pulsatile flow waveform generated by the heart and influenced by the distal resistance can also affect the local hemodynamics at the carotid bifurcation. Reverse flow at the walls can be augmented by rapidly decelerating flow waveforms. These waveform shapes can also affect the onset of turbulence. While it is difficult to extrapolate exactly which waveform shapes will cause augmented reverse flow and turbulence in the three-dimensional carotid bifurcation, it is important to note that in some cases pulsatility can exert a stronger influence than local anatomy or flow divisions between the branches.

Stenotic Carotid Flow

The local hemodynamics in the normal carotid bifurcation have been shown to correlate strongly with the location of atherosclerotic plaque. However, it is unclear whether hemodynamics affects the progression of disease or the intimal hyperplasia that follows balloon angioplasty or direct arterial surgery. Nonetheless, the carotid hemodynamics are strongly altered with severe stenosis.

As the origin of the internal carotid artery becomes stenotic, the velocity patterns change. Downstream from the stenosis, a jet of high velocity develops with a surrounding region of separated reverse velocities. The jet may often be skewed to one side. Because the velocity gradient is so high in the jet region, a wide range of velocities will be measured by Doppler ultrasound. This wide range of velocities appears as spectral broadening (Fig. 6-3). Measurements made by LeGouguec indicate that most of the broadening stems from the large sample volume, as opposed to high levels of turbulence.[8] Because of the relatively large size of the pulsed Doppler sample volume, the peak velocities are averaged to a lower value.

With stenoses greater than 75 percent by diameter, the pressure within the stenosis falls and can go below the external tissue pressure. Bernoulli's equation for pressure within a stenosis indicates that

$$P_{stenosis} \simeq P_{upstream} - \tfrac{1}{2}\rho \overline{V}^2_{upstream} \, (\% \text{ stenosis})^4$$

Thus, with a stenosis greater than 75 percent by diameter, the pressure within the narrower part of the stenosis (throat) can fall below the tissue pressure.[9,10] When this

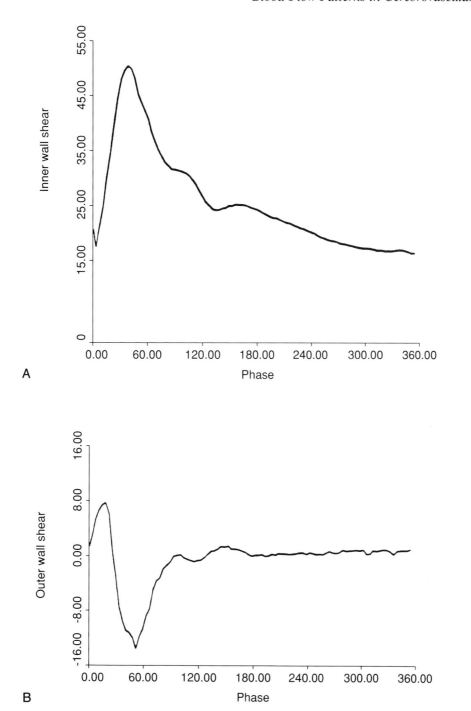

Figure 6-2 Velocity trace at the **(A)** inner wall and **(B)** outer wall at the origin of the internal carotid artery sinus obtained by laser Doppler anemometry studies of a model bifurcation.

occurs, the stenosis will no longer be pressurized and a more severe stenosis may result. Thus, the hemodynamics within this stenosis can decrease the size of the lumen, causing a more severe constriction.

These resistance changes have been detected in the coronary circulation and in biologic preparations by Santamore, Schwartz, Gould, and their co-workers.[11-13] Passive narrowing from decreases in lateral pressure can increase the viscous pressure losses in the stenosis and decrease cerebral blood flow (Fig. 6-4). The lower pressure within the throat also results in a lower transmural pressure and can augment any basal

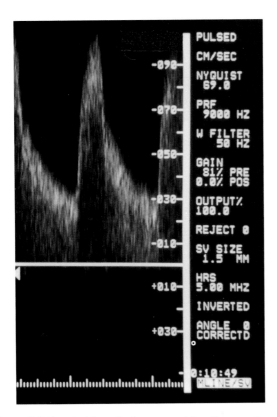

PULSED
CM/SEC
NYQUIST
69.0
PRF
9000 HZ
W FILTER
50 HZ
GAIN
81% PRE
0.0% POS
OUTPUT%
100.0
REJECT 0
SV SIZE
1.5 MM
HRS
5.00 MHZ
INVERTED
ANGLE 0
CORRECTD

Figure 6-3 Spectral broadening present in ultrasound measurements of normal arteries using a commercial duplex scanner.

constriction by the medial smooth muscle cells. Finally, the flexible wall of the artery may actually collapse with the negative pressures within the throat. All the above factors can contribute to large dynamic resistance changes within the stenosis. Stenotic resistance changes are dependent on the downstream resistance in the brain, presence of collateral flow, velocity in the throat of the stenosis, and compliance of the plaque. Significant clinical reductions in the flow to the brain will be governed by the balance of these factors. This mechanism may contribute to the formation of transient ischemic attacks in the absence of either total thrombotic occlusion or distal embolization.

The collapse of a compliant stenosis may also contribute to the instability of the fibrous cap overlaying an atheroma. Cyclic mechanical tests of biologic material, such as porcine heart valves and human arteries, have indicated that compression can lead to mechanical fatigue of these collagenous structures.[14,15] It is therefore possible that the local hemodynamics may accelerate fatigue of the plaque cap, inducing plaque rupture with subsequent distal embolization.

Some comments should be made regarding the va-

lidity of detailed hemodynamic measurements in models as compared with the in vivo physiologic situation. Primary fluid mechanic parameters governing the detailed flow field include the anatomy of the bifurcation, the flow divisions between the branches, and the pulsatile flow waveform. Secondary considerations include the elasticity of the vessel and the non-Newtonian viscosity of the blood. Ultrasound studies of wall motion at the carotid bifurcation indicate that the elasticity at the carotid bulb decreases significantly with age, becoming very rigid during the sixth decade of life.[16] Detailed laser Doppler anemometry studies of a carotid bifurcation with elastic properties have shown that the flow field does not change significantly.[17] Finally, investigators have included the non-Newtonian viscosity in calculated solutions of flow through the carotid bifurcation.[18] Although detectable, these viscosity changes clearly do not strongly affect the flow field characteristics by comparison with the variations seen in the primary factors.

In summary, the fluid mechanics at the human carotid bifurcation are complicated and pulsatile in nature. Flow at the posterior wall of the internal carotid sinus shows transient separation that is more prominent during the end of systole than at the beginning. Flow vortices form within the separated region and can contribute to spectral broadening, even in normal carotid arteries with no stenosis. Flow waveforms and placement of the Doppler sample volume are critical to the measurement of spectral broadening and peak velocities in normal and stenotic arteries. Lastly, the hemodynamics associated with a compliant high-grade stenosis may influence the local resistance and eventual rupture of the plaque cap.

SUBCLAVIAN STEAL SYNDROMES

Contorni, in 1960, demonstrated retrograde flow in the vertebral artery of an asymptomatic patient with an ipsilateral subclavian stenosis.[19] Reivich, in 1961, first recognized an association between this phenomenon and neurologic symptoms.[20] Fisher dubbed this the "subclavian steal syndrome," suggesting that blood is stolen by the ipsilateral vertebral artery from the contralateral vertebral by way of the basilar artery.[21] Because a subclavian stenosis results in a lower pressure in the distal subclavian artery, blood flows in a retrograde direction down the ipsilateral vertebral artery away from the brain stem. Whether this "steal" actually produces clinical signs of brain stem ischemia has been a source of considerable controversy. Undoubtedly, a few patients have symptomatic disease; however, in the

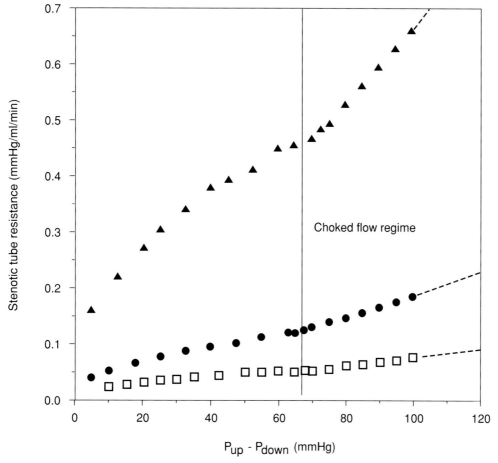

Figure 6-4 Hemodynamic resistance increases as a function of stenosis severity during the collapse of a compliant stenosis. □, 70 percent stenosis data; ●, 80 percent stenosis data; ▲, 90 percent stenosis data. P_{up}, 70 mmHg; P_{ext}, 0 mmHg.

majority, the finding of "angiographic steal" appears to be clinically insignificant and is not associated with an increased risk of vertebrobasilar ischemia.[22]

Symptoms and Signs

Most patients with angiographic subclavian steal are asymptomatic. In a minority, vertebrobasilar symptoms develop, including dizziness, diplopia, nystagmus, ataxia, vertigo, or visual disturbances, such as bilateral blurred vision. Arm claudication, parasthesias, or numbness of the extremity occur in one-third of patients, but trophic changes are rare. Arm exercise increases blood flow to the arm and, by decreasing arm arterial resistance, can precipitate symptoms. On examination, the patient may have a decreased pulse and blood pressure in the affected limb (> 20 mmHg differential in 66 percent), and a supraclavicular bruit may be audible. Steal is much more common on the left

side, perhaps due to a more acute origin of the subclavian artery, resulting in accelerated atherosclerosis from increased turbulence.[23]

Asymptomatic Patient With Steal

In a retrospective angiographic study of patients with symptomatic cerebrovascular disease, Lord et al[24] noted severe proximal subclavian stenosis in 23 percent of patients. This was associated with reversed flow in the ipsilateral vertebral in 6 percent. Similarly, the Joint Study of Extracranial Arterial Occlusion reported a 17 percent incidence of subclavian or innominate stenosis, but angiographic steal occurred in only 2.5 percent.[25] Thus, steal as defined by angiography occurs in only a minority of patients with subclavian stenosis. Vertebral steal, as determined by continuous wave (CW) Doppler is apparent in 6.4 percent of patients with asymptomatic neck bruits.[26] In this group, no vertebrobasilar symptoms developed during a 2-year follow-up period. Indeed, from such Doppler evaluations, there is evidence that even when reversed flow occurs in the vertebral artery, prograde basilar arterial flow persists and may even be increased.[26]

Recently, considerable doubt has been expressed regarding whether an angiographic steal is ever the principal cause of cerebral ischemic symptoms. This is based on a number of observations: (1) re-establishment of prograde flow may not relieve symptoms; (2) rarely are cerebral symptoms provoked by arm exercise; (3) concurrent disease in the other extracranial vessels is very common and may be the principal source of symptoms; and (4) recent reports using the transcranial Doppler have demonstrated that reversed flow in the vertebral arteries is even more common than had been suspected from angiographic data.

Collateral Arterial Flow

Quality of collateral blood supply and the capacity to increase collateral flow may be the principal determinants as to which patients become symptomatic. The most important collateral route is through the circle of Willis, particularly the posterior communicating artery from the internal carotid artery (ICA). This short artery arises close to the bifurcation of the ICA into the anterior and middle cerebral arteries. It then runs posteriorly, communicating with the posterior cerebral artery, a branch of the basilar artery. The posterior communicating artery varies in size from being so large that the posterior cerebral artery appears to arise from the ICA (embryonic variant), to being extremely small or absent. When the principal supply to the posterior communicating artery is from the ICA, the segment arising from the basilar artery may be hypoplastic or atretic.[27] Only 20 percent of patients have the classically described complete circle of Willis. Hypoplasia or absence of one or both posterior communicating arteries occurs in 25 to 30 percent of patients.[28] Such an arrangement may effectively separate the carotid system from the vertebrobasilar system. Anomalies of the circle of Willis occur with increased frequency in patients with symptomatic subclavian steal.[24]

Another potential collateral pathway connecting the carotid, vertebral, and subclavian arteries is through the occipital artery. Arising from the external carotid artery (ECA), the descending branch of the occipital artery courses inferiorly in the posterior neck, where it forms anastomotic connections with the vertebral artery and the deep cervical artery, the latter being a branch of the costocervical trunk of the subclavian artery. Anastomoses between the superior and inferior thyroid arteries form yet another potential collateral pathway between the ECA and the subclavian.[24]

Other rare communications between the carotid and vertebrobasilar system occur with persistence of fetal vessels: hypoglossal, otic, trigeminal, and proatlantal intersegmental arteries.[29]

Doppler Studies of the Vertebrobasilar System

Although anatomic collateral pathways are well defined and may be demonstrated angiographically, the development of the transcranial Doppler and CW Doppler has enabled the dynamics of this complex system to be functionally evaluated. Noninvasive tests further lend themselves to longitudinal follow-up evaluation of patients with asymptomatic steal phenomena. Severe stenosis (>80 percent narrowing) of the proximal subclavian artery is associated with permanent flow reversal in the ipsilateral vertebral artery in 65 percent of cases and with intermittent reversal in 30 percent. In 5 percent of these patients, systolic flow deceleration alone was identified.[29] Patients with moderate stenosis (about 50 percent narrowing) showed permanent flow reversal in the vertebral artery in 56 percent, intermittent in 36 percent, and systolic deceleration alone in 8 percent. In a three-year follow-up study of 41 patients with severe subclavian stenosis, 33 of whom had reversed vertebral flow, no neurologic symptoms developed. None of these patients had reversed or bidirectional basilar arterial flow either at rest or following the subclavian steal test of inflating a blood pressure cuff on the ipsilateral arm to greater than systolic pressure for 3 minutes.[26] Antegrade blood flow, with normal flow velocity in the basilar artery, is present in most patients regardless of the flow pattern in the vertebral artery. Systolic deceleration in the basilar artery occurred in 7 of 47 patients studied, including two patients with bilateral vertebral steal. By contrast, Bornstein et al. reported increased basilar artery flow associated with unilateral reversed vertebral flow.[22] This increased basilar velocity was attributed to either increased flow in the normal vertebral or constriction of the vertebral causing increased velocity despite reduced basilar flow.

Bilateral vertebral flow reversal may be associated with an increased risk of nonlateralizing cerebral ischemia. Brain stem dysfunction from arm exercise was seen only in patients with bilateral reversed flow.[29] However, persistent retrograde flow in the basilar artery, with collateral blood supply from the internal carotid arteries, has been reported in a patient without any neurologic or upper-extremity symptoms.[30] The situation is further complicated by the observation of vertebral compression by head movement (usually rotation of the face towards the opposite side). This may cause vertebral artery compression, further compromising flow intermittently.[31]

Clearly, many patients have clinically insignificant "steal." What, then, precipitates vertebrobasilar symptoms in a few patients? One likely possibility is that symptoms occur only in the presence of hemodynamically significant stenoses elsewhere in the cerebral system, that compromise the collateral circulation. Prospective studies of patients with documented steal show that such patients have a very low incidence of nonhemispheric (posterior circulation) ischemic events. By contrast, they are more likely to develop hemispheric ischemia due to concurrent progressive carotid disease. Identification of subclavian steal is therefore a risk factor for generalized atherosclerosis. These patients have compromised collateral pathways, which places them at risk, principally from carotid territory cerebrovascular events.

INTERNAL CAROTID TO EXTERNAL CAROTID ANASTOMOSES

Anatomic Considerations

The ECA is usually smaller than the ICA and has numerous branches that supply the face, scalp, oropharynx, skull, and meninges (Table 6-1). Under normal circumstances, it makes no significant contribution to the cerebral circulation; however, in the presence of ICA occlusive disease, the external to internal carotid anastomoses (Table 6-2) may provide crucial collateral blood supply (Fig. 6-5). The ICA supplies most of the anterior circulation to the cerebrum. No branches arise in the cervical portion of the ICA. The intracranial ICA may be conveniently divided into three parts: petrous, cavernous, and cerebral[32] (Table 6-3). Those branches that communicate with the ECA

Table 6-1 Branches of the External Carotid Artery

Superior thyroid
Ascending pharyngeal
Lingual
Facial
Occipital
Posterior auricular
Superficial temporal
Maxillary

Table 6-2 Branches of the External Carotid Artery That Participate in Anastomoses With the Internal Carotid Artery

Facial artery
Angular branch
Lateral nasal branch
Posterior auricular artery
Stylomastoid branch
Superfical temporal artery
Transverse facial branch
Zygomatico-orbital branch
Frontal branch
Maxillary
Deep temporal branch
Sphenopalatine branch
Anterior tympanic branch
Middle meningeal branch

arise from the petrous and cavernous segments and are considered in detail (Table 6-4). Within the dura mater, 8 mm beyond the clinoid process, the ICA gives rise to the posterior communicating artery, which runs to the posterior cerebral artery, effectively linking the anterior and posterior cerebral circulations.[33]

Caroticotympanic Artery

The caroticotympanic artery is a small branch arising from the petrous portion of the ICA. It reaches the tympanic cavity through a small foramen in the carotid canal. In the tympanic cavity, it joins with the anterior tympanic branch of the maxillary artery and, with the stylomastoid artery, a branch of the posterior auricular artery.

Artery of the Pterygoid Canal

The artery of the pterygoid canal is a small, occasionally absent, branch that passes into the pterygoid canal (a foramen in the sphenoid, medial to the foramen rotundum). There it anastomoses with branches from the maxillary artery.

Cavernous Branches

The cavernous branches arise from the ICA in the cavernous sinus; these numerous small branches supply the pituitary gland, the trigeminal ganglion, and the walls of the cavernous and inferior petrosal sinus. Some of these branches communicate with the middle meningeal artery, a large branch of the maxillary artery.

Anterior Meningeal Artery

The anterior meningeal artery is a small branch that crosses the lesser wing of the sphenoid bone to supply the dura mater in the anterior cranial fossa. There it

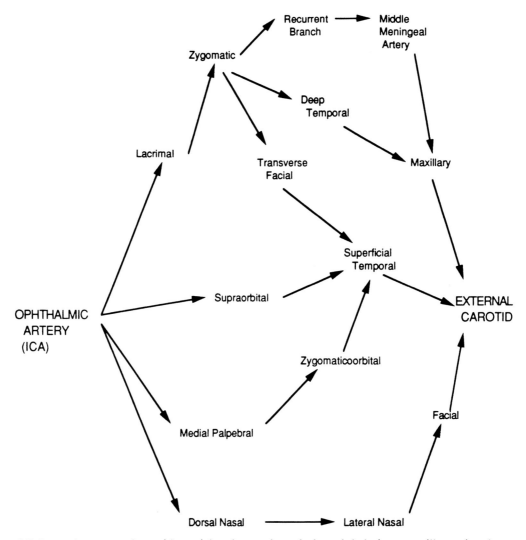

Figure 6-5 Internal to external carotid arterial pathways through the ophthalmic artery, illustrating the many anastomotic connections between the two systems.

Table 6-3 Branches of the Internal Carotid Artery

Petrous portion
   Caroticotympanic
   Artery of the pterygoid canal
   Cavernous
   Hypophyseal
Cavernous portion
   Ganglionic
   Anterior meningeal
   Ophthalmic
   Anterior cerebral
   Middle cerebral
Cerebral portion
   Posterior communicating
   Anterior choroidal

communicates with the meningeal branches of the posterior ethmoidal artery (a branch of the ophthalmic artery), which in turn communicates with the spheno-palatine artery, a branch of the maxillary artery from the ECA.

Table 6-4 Branches of the Internal Carotid Artery That Anastomose With the External Carotid Artery

Caroticotympanic
Artery of the pterygoid canal
Cavernous branches
Anterior meningeal
Ophthalmic

Ophthalmic Artery

The ophthalmic artery is a large artery with numerous branches dispersed to the nasal sinuses, forehead, and contents of the orbit. It represents a principal collateral pathway between the internal and external carotid system and is the anastomosis most intensively studied (see Fig. 6-5).

The ophthalmic artery arises from the ICA just as that artery is emerging from the cavernous sinus. It passes anteriorly, entering the orbit through the optic canal. Initially inferior and lateral to the optic nerve, it crosses to the medial wall of the orbit, coursing along the inferior border of the superior oblique muscle, where it divides into two terminal branches: the supratrochlear and dorsal nasal arteries. The branches of the ophthalmic artery may be divided into an orbital and an ocular group. The latter supply the globe and its contents but do not form significant anastomoses with the external carotid circulation.

The lacrimal artery (orbital group) arises close to the optic foramen and supplies the lacrimal gland, the eyelids, and conjunctiva. It gives off zygomatic branches that reach the temporal fossa, where they anastomose with the deep temporal arteries (maxillary artery), through the zygomaticofacial foramen, they also anastomose with the transverse facial artery (superficial temporal artery). A recurrent branch passes back through the superior orbital fissure to anastomose with a branch of the middle meningeal artery (maxillary artery).

The supraorbital artery (orbital group) exits the orbit at the supraorbital foramen, where it divides into a superficial and a deep branch. These arteries supply the muscles and pericranium of the forehead, anastomosing with the supratrochlear artery, the frontal branch of the superficial temporal artery, and the supraorbital artery of the contralateral side.

The posterior ethmoidal artery supplies the posterior ethmoidal air cells and enters the cranium, where it supplies meningeal branches to the dura of the anterior cranial fossa. There it gives off nasal branches that descend through the cribriform plate, anastomosing with branches of the sphenopalatine artery (maxillary artery). The medial palpebral arteries leave the orbit medially, encircle the eyelids, and anastomose laterally with the zygomaticoorbital branch of the temporal artery. The dorsal nasal artery leaves the orbit above the medial palpebral ligament. It courses inferiorly along the dorsum of the nose and anastomoses with the lateral nasal branch of the facial artery.

In addition to these collateral pathways, additional collaterals may form from the dural or meningeal vessels (external carotid system) to the cerebral vessels.

These collaterals take considerable time to develop and are seen predominantly in slowly progressive cerebral ischemia, as in Moyamoya disease.[34]

Vertebral to External Carotid Anastomoses

The occipital artery arises from the posterior part of the ECA opposite the facial branch, close to the inferior border of the posterior belly of the digastric muscle. Its largest branch is the descending branch, which runs inferiorly in the posterior neck, where it divides into a superficial and a deep portion. The latter branch runs inferiorly between the semispinalis capitis and cervicis, anastomosing with the vertebral artery and the deep cervical artery, a branch of the costocervical trunk.[32] This provides a potential collateral pathway among the carotid, vertebral, and subclavian systems.[33]

Functional Considerations

The anatomy of these collateral pathways is well documented, but their practical importance is supported by the occurrence of new neurologic deficits following ICA occlusion and the therapeutic benefit of ECA endarterectomy.

The Joint Study of Extracranial Arterial Disease[35] reported that 78 percent of patients with angiographically demonstrated unilateral ICA occlusion and 67 percent with bilateral occlusion have neurologic deficits. However, a considerable number of patients sustain complete occlusion of the ICA and are asymptomatic, testimony to the presence of adequate collaterals. Nevertheless, 25 percent of patients with ICA occlusion sustained new strokes during a 44-month follow-up period.[35] Indeed, the follow-up stroke rate after ICA occlusion ranges from 3 to 20 percent per year.[35,36] Several mechanisms for these strokes may be postulated: (1) global low flow, (2) embolization from the distal occluded ICA, and (3) embolization from an ICA stump through collateral vessels. The ECA-ICA collaterals may be up to 3 mm in size, which is more than adequate to permit atheroembolization.[37] Clearly, collateral pathways may be protective in the face of ICA occlusion, but they may also become conduits for cerebral embolization. Such collaterals have been demonstrated both radiologically and anatomically. However, Fogelholm and Vuolio[38] showed that only 41 percent of those patients with ICA occlusion had angiographic evidence of collateral filling of the ipsilateral ophthalmic artery-carotid siphon system. Angiography does not reliably demonstrate collaterals, nor is it a reliable predictor of benefit from ECA endarterectomy.[39]

Several observations support the importance of ECA-ICA collaterals: (1) it has been demonstrated that with an occluded internal carotid, the external system may provide up to 30 percent of the ipsilateral cerebral blood flow[40]; (2) internal carotid stump pressure is increased by 21 percent (mean, 10.1 mmHg) after flow has been re-established through the ECA[41] following internal carotid endarterectomy; and (3) reversed flow in the ophthalmic artery distal to an ICA occlusion may be demonstrated using periorbital and transorbital Doppler ultrasound.[42]

The importance of ECA-ICA collaterals is further supported by the beneficial effects of ECA endarterectomy in patients with a totally occluded ICA.[43] A significant increase in ophthalmic artery pressure (mean, 16.1 mmHg) occurs after ipsilateral ECA endarterectomy.[44] Zarins et al.[45] reported a 15 to 39 percent increase in ipsilateral cerebral perfusion following external carotid endarterectomy, using a Xenon inhalation technique. Similarly, subclavian to external carotid bypass in patients with an occluded ICA and ECA stenosis resulted in a 21.6 mmHg increase in oculoplethysmographic pressure.[46]

ACKNOWLEDGMENTS

This work was supported in part by grant R29 HL 39437 from the National Institutes of Health.

REFERENCES

1. Bhradvaj BK, Mabon RF, Giddens DP: Steady flow in a model of a human carotid bifurcation. Part 1. Flow visualization. J Biomech 15:363, 1982
2. Ku DN, Giddens DP, Zarins CK, Glagov S: Pulsatile flow and atherosclerosis in the human carotid bifurcation. Positive correlation between plaque location and oscillating shear stress. Arteriosclerosis 5:293, 1985
3. Perktold K, Resch M, Reinfried OP: Three-dimensional numerical analysis of pulsatile flow and wall shear stress in the carotid artery bifurcation. J Biomech 24:409, 1991
4. Rindt CCM, Steenhoven AA van, Janssen JD et al: A numerical analysis of steady flow in a three-dimensional model of the carotid artery bifurcation. J Biomech 23:461, 1990
5. Ku DN, Giddens DP: Pulsatile flow in a model carotid bifurcation. Arteriosclerosis 5:31, 1983
6. Ku DN, Giddens DP: Laser doppler anamometer measurements of pulsatile flow in a model carotid bifurcation. J Biomech 20:407, 1987
7. Ku DN, Phillips DJ, Giddens DP, Strandness DE: He-modynamics of the normal human carotid bifurcation —in vitro and in vivo studies. Ultrasound Med Biol 11:13, 1985
8. LeGouguec HA: Velocity measurements with a 2 MHz pulsed doppler ultrasound probe in normal and stenosed models of the carotid bifurcation. MS thesis. Georgia Institute of Technology, Atlanta, 1991
9. Binns RL, Ku DN: Effect of stenosis on wall motion—a possible mechanism of stroke and transient ischemic attack. Arteriosclerosis 9:842, 1989
10. Ku DN, Zeigler MN, Downing JM: One-dimensional steady inviscid flow through a stenotic collapsible tube. J Biomech Eng 112:444, 1990
11. Santamore WP, Bove AA: A theoretical model of a compliant arterial stenosis. Am J Physiol 248:274, 1985
12. Schwartz JS, Carlyle PF, Cohn JN: Effect of dilation of the distal coronary bed on flow and resistance in severely stenotic coronary arteries in the dog. Am J Cardiol 43:219, 1979
13. Gould KL: Dynamic coronary stenosis. Am J Cardiol 45:286, 1980
14. Broom ND: The stress/strain and fatigue behavior of glutaraldehyde preserved heart-valve tissue. J Biomech 10:707, 1977
15. McKinsey J, McCord BN, Aoki T, Ku DN: Can mechanical stress cause fatigue of the atherosclerotic plaque? Surg Forum 42:318, 1991
16. Reneman RS, VanMerode T, Hick P, Hoeks APG: Flow velocity patterns in and distensibility of the carotid bulb in subjects of various ages. Circulation 71:500, 1985
17. Anayiotos A: Fluid dynamics at a compliant bifurcation model. PhD thesis. Georgia Institute of Technology, Atlanta, 1990
18. Reuderink P: Analysis of the flow in a 3d distensible model of the carotid artery bifurcation. PhD thesis. Eindhoven University, Eindhoven, the Netherlands, 1991
19. Contorni L: Il circolo collaterale vertebro-vertebrale nelle obliterazione dell'arteria succlavia alla sua origine. Minerva Chir 15:268, 1960
20. Reivich M, Holling HE, Roberts B, Toole JF: Reversal of blood flow through the vertebral artery and its effect on cerebral circulation. N Engl J Med 265:878, 1961
21. Fisher CM: A new vascular syndrome: "the subclavian steal." N Engl J Med 265:912, 1961
22. Bornstein NM, Krajewski A, Norris JW: Basilar artery blood flow in subclavian steal. Can J Neurol Sci 15:417, 1988
23. Kesteloot H, Houte OV: Reversed circulation through the vertebral artery. Acta Cardiol 18:285, 1963
24. Lord RSA, Adar R, Stein RL: Contribution of the circle of Willis to the subclavian steal syndrome. Circulation 40:871, 1969
25. Fields WS, Lemak NA: Joint study of extracranial arterial occlusion. vii.subclavian steal: a review of 168 cases. JAMA 222:1139, 1972
26. Bornstein NM, Norris JW: Subclavian steal: a harmless hemodynamic phenomenon. Lancet 2:303, 1986
27. Gray H: The arteries. p. 561. In Goss CM (ed): Anatomy

of the Human Body. 29th Ed. Lea & Febiger, Philadelphia, 1973

28. Deutsch LS: Anatomy and angiographic diagnosis of extracranial and intracranial vascular disease. p. 1314. In Rutherford RB (ed): Vascular Surgery. WB Saunders, Philadelphia, 1989

29. Hennerici M, Klemm C, Rautenberg W: The subclavian steal phenomenon: a common vascular disorder with rare neurologic deficits. Neurology 38:669, 1988

30. Klingelhofer J, Conrad B, Benecke R, Frank B: Transcranial doppler ultrasonography of carotid-basilar collateral circulation in subclavian steal. Stroke 19:1036, 1988

31. Theron J, Melancon D, Ethier R: "Pre" subclavian steal syndromes and their treatment by angioplasty: hemodynamic classification of subclavian artery stenoses. Neuroradiology 27:265, 1985

32. Gray H: The Arteries. p. 561. In Goss CM (ed): Anatomy of the Human Body. 29th Ed. Lea & Febiger, Philadelphia, 1973

33. Diethrich EB: Normal cerebrovascular anatomy and collateral pathways. p. 51. In Zweibel WJ (ed): Introduction to Vascular Ultrasonography. Grune & Stratton, New York, 1982.

34. Matsushima Y, Inaba Y: The specificity of the collaterals to the brain through the study and surgical treatment of Moyamoya disease. Stroke 17:117, 1986

35. Fields WS, Lemak NA: Joint study of extracranial arterial occlusion-internal carotid artery occlusion. JAMA 235:2734, 1976

36. Barnett HJM: Delayed cerebral ischemic episodes distal to occlusion of major cerebral arteries. Neurology 28:769, 1978

37. Weinberger J, Robbins A, Jacobson J: Transient ischemic attacks with external carotid artery stenosis and a normal internal carotid artery. Angiology 34:764, 1983

38. Fogelholm R, Vuolio M: The collateral circulation via the ophthalmic artery in internal carotid artery thrombosis. Acta Neurol Scand 45:78, 1969

39. Diethrich EB, Liddicoat JE, McCutchen JJ et al: Surgical significance of the external carotid artery in the treatment of cerebrovascular insufficiency. J Cardiovasc Surg 9:213, 1968

40. Fields WS, Brustman ME, Wribel J: Collateral circulation of the brain. Monogr Surg Sci 2:183, 1965

41. Machleder HI, Barker WF: External carotid artery shunting during carotid endarterectomy: evidence for feasibility. Arch Surg 108:785, 1974

42. Schneider PA, Rossman ME, Bernstein EF et al: Noninvasive assessment of cerebral collateral blood supply through the ophthalmic artery. Stroke 22:31, 1991

43. Gertler JP, Cambria RP: The role of external carotid endarterectomy in the treatment of ipsilateral internal carotid occlusion: collective review. J Vasc Surg 6:158, 1987

44. Schuler JJ, Flanigan P, Debord JR et al: The treatment of cerebral ischemia by external carotid artery revascularization. Arch Surg 118:567, 1983

45. Zarins CK, DelBeccaro EJ, Johns L et al: Increased cerebral blood flow after external carotid revascularization. Surgery 89:730, 1981

46. McGuiness CL, Short DH, Kerstein MD: Subclavian-external carotid bypass for symptomatic severe cerebral ischemia from common and internal carotid artery occlusion. Am J Surg 155:546, 1988

7

Hemodynamic Considerations in Arterial Reconstruction

Robert M. Zwolak

Accurate application of hemodynamic principles underlies the ultimate success of arterial reconstruction. While the practicing vascular surgeon may not review Poiseuille's equation prior to each femoropopliteal bypass graft, the daily concerns of inflow stenosis, graft caliber, and the adequacy of outflow are clinical expressions of our involvement with hemodynamics. This chapter considers the concepts of hemodynamics as they relate to vascular bypass grafting. Issues discussed include graft caliber and length, blood flow velocity, geometry of graft anastomosis, shear stress, impedance, and the effects of graft pseudointima. However, hemodynamics cannot be considered in a biologic vacuum in the discussion of arterial reconstruction. The biology and biochemistry of the arterial wall, along with the enigmatic science of thrombosis, also impact dramatically on the success of arterial reconstructions.

ENERGY CONSIDERATIONS

Viscous Energy Losses and Shear Stress

The scientifically rigorous approach to hemodynamics begins with the analysis of energy transfer. In the arterial system, energy is imparted to blood through contraction of the left ventricle. Under normal conditions, the mean arterial pressure decreases only slightly as the blood approaches the periphery. However, in the presence of arterial occlusive disease, a stenosis involving the inflow, outflow, or bypass graft itself may reduce pressure and velocity sufficiently to place the graft at risk of thrombosis. Thus, a functional understanding of hemodynamic issues is paramount to the vascular surgeon. An accurate analysis of energy losses during pulsatile flow requires use of a complex set of differential equations (the Womersley equations), which are covered in a number of texts on hemodynamics.[1-4] However, through the use of Newtonian assumptions, including that of nonpulsatile laminar flow in a rigid tube, simple and far more intuitive relationships such as Poiseuille's equation may be used to describe frictional or viscous energy losses. As discussed in Chapter 4, Poiseuille's equation describes the loss of pressure as pressure energy is converted to heat in order to overcome the internal frictional resistance between the "sliding layers" of blood. This energy loss accounts for the greater part of the work that the heart must do in moving blood through the circulation.

Starting with the concept that viscous energy loss results in a pressure reduction (ΔP) equal to flow (Q) times resistance (R):

$$\Delta P = Q \cdot R$$

the Poiseuille equation defines the resistance term as

$$R = \frac{8L\eta}{\pi r^4}$$

where L is the conduit length, η is the fluid viscosity, and r is the conduit radius. Thus, all factors that contribute to viscous energy loss can be combined in a single equation:

$$\Delta P = Q \cdot \frac{8L\eta}{\pi r^4}$$

Since length and viscosity do not change significantly in the clinical setting, Poiseuille's equation indicates that radius and flow are the only variables likely to alter viscous energy losses in circulatory disorders. In large-caliber arteries or bypass grafts, the lumen diameter is generous with respect to the volume of flow traveling through it, and ΔP is essentially zero because r^4 is very much greater than any other term in the equation. Under these conditions, ΔP is insensitive to minor changes in r. However, in the presence of a severe stenosis, the value of r^4 decreases to a point at which any change in radius results in a large change in ΔP. Thus, the effect of changes in radius on ΔP may vary from negligible to very great, depending on the relative magnitude of Q and r^4. This relationship is best appreciated by consideration of the resistance curves in Figure 7-1.

While Poiseuille's equation describes the overall energy loss due to viscosity, the local effects of viscosity may be very important in biologic systems. When a layer of viscous fluid is set in motion by the application of a force, the motion is communicated to adjoining layers by the internal friction characterized as viscosity. At the blood-wall interface of an artery or bypass graft, this internal friction may represent an energy transduction system between the hemodynamic parameters of the flowing blood and the biological response of the adjacent vessel wall. Shear stress (S), expressed in dyn/cm², is the force (F) per unit area (A) that exists to overcome the viscous internal friction. It is proportional to the velocity gradient between layers of fluid (dv/dr), such that

$$S = F/A = \frac{\eta dv}{dr}$$

where dv/dr is the shear rate. For laminar flow in a circular tube, an analysis of Poiseuille's law shows that shear rate can be expressed in terms of the pressure gradient:

$$dv/dr = \frac{\Delta Pr}{2\eta}$$

allowing definition of shear stress as

$$S = \frac{\Delta Pr}{2}$$

Since r is the radius at any specified lamina, the shear stress is zero at the center line of the tube and maximal

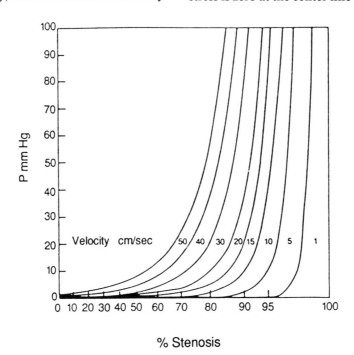

Figure 7-1 Relationship of the pressure drop across a stenosis to the degree of stenosis and flow velocity. Percentage stenosis refers to area reduction of the narrow region. Velocity refers to the value in the prestenotic segment. P is the change in pressure across stenosis. (Adapted from Strandness and Sumner,[13] with permission.)

at the blood-vessel wall interface.[3] Also, since shear represents a vector quantity oriented parallel to the axis of flow, the effect is unlikely to be detected more than a few microns deep to the fluid-wall interface. Thus, the endothelial cell lining of an artery or bypass graft is the only structural element likely to sense shear. Early experiments demonstrated that physical deterioration of canine aortic endothelial cells occurred when shear was increased and that prolonged exposure to elevated shear led to intimal fibrosis.[5,6] Other early data led to suggestions that low shear might be related to development of arterial pathology.[7] Since arterial bypass grafts constructed of autogenous vein contain a viable endothelial inner lining, it is reasonable to expect an effect of shear stress in these conduits as well. In fact, several experimental studies have shown an inverse correlation between shear stress and intimal hyperplasia.[8-12]

Kinetic Energy

Kinetic energy loss due to changes in velocity is another means by which blood pressure may dissipate in the vascular system. Since velocity is a vector quantity comprised of speed and direction, each curve and bifurcation in the arterial system results in kinetic energy loss. In addition, the changes in velocity brought about during each cardiac cycle also produce minute changes in kinetic energy. In simple terms, kinetic energy (W_K) may be expressed as

$$W_K = \tfrac{1}{2}\rho v^2$$

where ρ is mass, and v is the velocity vector. Although the total kinetic energy associated with blood flow is relatively small, energy loss in an arterial reconstruction may become significant at the anastomoses where entrance and exit effects are predicted to be of large magnitude (see Ch. 5).

HEMODYNAMICS OF GRAFT CONSTRUCTION
Prosthetic Graft Diameter

The vascular surgeon has little choice of graft caliber when using autogenous vein as the conduit for a vascular bypass, but a wide selection of conduit diameters is available when a prosthetic graft is used. Surprisingly few objective clinical or theoretical data exist regarding optimal diameter selection for vascular reconstructions. In commercially available aortic bifurcation prostheses, a hemodynamic mismatch exists between the primary tube and the secondary limbs, which are usually one-half the primary tube diameter. The area ratio is 0.25 for each limb, compared with the primary

tube, and the combined ratio is 0.5 for the two limbs. Thus, flow velocity in the secondary limbs is doubled, and each limb has a resistance 16 times that of the primary tube. In this situation, almost 50 percent of the incident pulsatile energy is reflected at the graft bifurcation.[13] If blood flow through the primary tube is near the vertical portion of the exponential radius-resistance relationship shown in Figure 7-1, the increased resistance in the secondary limbs will create a measurable reduction in blood pressure. However, if the capacity of the primary tube is well above that required for physiologic blood flow, the increase in resistance imposed by the secondary limbs will have no measurable effect. At least one clinical study and most surgeons' clinical experience would suggest this latter situation pertains with the available aortic bifurcation prostheses.

Schneider et al.[14] evaluated the effect of aortic graft diameter by comparing long-term patency of large diameter Dacron grafts (defined as 16- and 18-mm diameter) to that of smaller (12- and 14-mm diameter) aortobifemoral grafts used in patients with arterial occlusive disease. In general, graft size had been selected by the surgeon to match that of native arteries. Thus, the small-diameter grafts were used more often in women, but patient characteristics in the small and large diameter groups were otherwise comparable. Graft diameter did not influence life-table patency, which was 84 percent for small-diameter and 87 percent for large-diameter grafts at 3 years. In addition, there was no difference in postoperative ankle/brachial index (ABI) between patients with small-diameter and those with large-diameter grafts, suggesting no significant flow limitation at rest in the smaller-caliber conduits. Since clinical data such as this support the adequacy of outflow limbs even in small diameter bifurcation prostheses, there has been little effort on the part of graft manufacturers toward further optimization of the geometry of bifurcation grafts.

The axillobifemoral bypass graft provides another potentially limiting situation for graft and host artery diameter. This long bypass graft adds the blood flow demands of both lower extremities to that of the upper extremity which all must be supplied by a single subclavian artery. An axillofemoral graft limb is often constructed of 8- or 10-mm-diameter prosthetic conduit, and the femorofemoral segment is frequently smaller, either 6 or 8 mm in diameter. The hemodynamic performance of axillobifemoral grafts has been evaluated by comparison of postoperative ABIs with those following aortofemoral grafts in patients operated upon for aortoiliac occlusive disease.[15] Even after adjustment for severity of outflow disease, postoperative ABIs were much worse following axillobifemoral reconstruction. For patients with pure aortoiliac occlusive disease, postoperative ABIs would be predicted to equal 1.0 if the combination of host subclavian artery and prosthetic conduit provide resistance-free inflow. However, this was not found to be true. Thus, even in the absence of identifiable axillosubclavian occlusive disease, some axillobifemoral reconstructions may provide suboptimal lower extremity inflow. These clinical data support earlier theoretical predictions suggesting that a 6.3-mm-diameter conduit may be inadequate for lower-extremity blood flow.[16] Insufficient data exist to distinguish whether the native subclavian artery or the prosthetic conduit is the resistance producing element in these reconstructions. Thus, there is no clear clinical or theoretical conclusion regarding the optimal diameter for an axillobifemoral bypass.

Pseudointima Effect on Diameter

The preceding discussion of graft diameter assumed that the diameter of the conduit inserted by the vascular surgeon was the actual lumen diameter. However, in prosthetic grafts, a compact layer of fibrin and devitalized platelet debris called the *pseudointima* develops along the inner aspect of the conduit and reduces the cross-sectional area. Early studies reported pseudointima thickness in Dacron aortic bypass grafts measuring 0.5 to 3 mm.[17] Since a 1-mm-thick pseudointima reduces the luminal area of a 10-mm diameter graft by 19 percent, this reduction may have an important effect on resistance if blood flow places the graft near the ascending limb of the radius-resistance relationship (see Fig. 7-1). Does pseudointima thickness vary as a function of flow or diameter? Once again, few clinical data exist to answer this question.

Under experimental conditions, Kohler et al.[18] found that the inner lining that developed in PTFE grafts implanted in baboons was less thick when blood flow through the graft was enhanced by placement of a distal arteriovenous fistula. This inner lining remained responsive to volumetric flow, since flow reduction by fistula ligation 2 months after graft implantation resulted in a rapid increase in thickness. However, this experiment was performed in polytetrafluoroethylene (PTFE) conduits specially modified to increase porosity, and the inner lining, composed of viable smooth muscle cells under an endothelialized surface, was different from the nonviable pseudointima, which collects in human PTFE bypass grafts. While these data are not directly applicable to current clinical PTFE grafts, they may be relevant to ongoing research efforts to induce viable endothelial surface coverage in prosthetic bypass conduits.

Blood Velocity Effects

Blood flow velocity within a prosthetic conduit depends directly on the choice of conduit diameter as well as on many other less controllable variables, such as inflow pressure and outflow resistance. The current literature does not delineate the velocity range that would optimize long-term patency. Evaluation of several prosthetic grafts at controlled flow rates suggested that each had a characteristic threshold thrombotic velocity below which thrombus formation occurred rapidly.[19,20] Unfortunately, attempts to avoid thrombogenic low velocities by insertion of small caliber prostheses resulted in almost universal failure with currently available grafts at a diameter of 4 mm or less. Recent data in the thrombosis literature indicate that fibrin and platelets react differently to shear variation, and this finding may explain why both low and high blood velocity predispose to graft thrombosis. At low shear rates, human blood exposed to rabbit aorta subendothelium produced thrombus rich in fibrin, while only minimal fibrin deposition occurred at high shear rates. By contrast, the interaction of platelets with subendothelium was much more intense at high shear rates.[21] At high shear rates, human platelet adhesion to de-endothelialized rabbit aorta was mediated by glycoprotein IIb–IIIa and was independent of fibrinogen activity.[22] Platelet deposition at high shear rates in rabbits was enhanced in the presence of elevated plasma cholesterol levels.[23] These data form the basis for understanding how thrombosis may occur at regions of stasis and in tight stenoses in a prosthetic graft, and they imply that an optimal velocity range should exist to guide the choice of conduit diameter. While few objective data exist in this area, a standardized canine model has been recommended for the paired evaluation of flow and caliber, as well as other variables, such as length and the ability to withstand flexion.[24]

Vein Graft Diameter

Do these data imply that there is a lower functional limit for vein graft diameter? Authorities in vascular surgery have related vein graft failure to inadequacy of conduit diameter for decades, but the size considered to be minimally acceptable has decreased over time. In 1967 Darling et al.[25] reported poorer patency rates with veins less than 4 mm in diameter. In 1975 Strandness and Sumner[13] reported a theoretical basis for failure of venous conduits less than 4 mm in diameter, and they suggested that, if at all possible, vein grafts should exceed 4 mm in diameter even at their smallest end. They estimated that at 3-mm diameter, a 40-cm-long vein graft in the arterial circulation caused a pressure reduction of 8.8 mmHg at 100 ml/min blood flow, while a pressure gradient of 44 mmHg occurred along the same graft when blood flow was 500 ml/min. However, a decade later, Leather et al.[26] reported the long-term patency of in situ bypass grafts less than 3 mm in external diameter to be no different from that of grafts of 3.5-mm diameter or larger. Towne et al.[27] cited 2.0 mm as the minimal venous conduit diameter to be used successfully as an arterial bypass, and they suggested that the diameter of this type of graft was limited only by the technology of valve incision required for the in situ technique.

Despite the use of increasingly small venous grafts, few patients with patent bypass grafts complain of claudication. Thus, volumetric blood flow in these grafts must be adequate to satisfy metabolic demands during maximal ambulatory exercise, most likely a value less than the 500 ml/min calculated by Strandness and Sumner to produce a large pressure gradient. Actual duplex ultrasound determined volumetric blood flow in femoropopliteal and femorotibial bypass grafts at rest has been reported as 65 ml/min or greater,[28,29] while postocclusive hyperemic graft flow volumes have been reported in a range just greater than 200 ml/min.[28] For purposes of comparison, resting lower extremity blood flow has been measured by similar techniques in healthy young adults as 140 ± 11 ml/min in the popliteal artery and 16 ± 3 ml/min in the posterior tibial artery.[30]

Graft Length

Does the length of an arterial bypass graft impact on the durability of the reconstruction? Poiseuille's equation suggests that with an adequate caliber, the increment in vascular resistance provided by additional length should be minimal. Early clinical papers evaluating vein grafts were split between those claiming that shorter grafts had better patency[31] and those that found no relationship with length.[25] Recent papers also disagree. Andros et al.[32] noted a higher secondary patency of short venous bypass grafts compared to long grafts, but other investigators noted no patency differences that could be attributed to length.[26] Prosthetic graft patency is also difficult to relate directly to length. The superior patency of aortobifemoral reconstructions compared to axillofemoral grafts may involve the greater length of the latter procedure, but a multitude of other variables confound the analysis. Likewise, the superior patency of PTFE femoropopliteal reconstruc-

tions with an above-knee distal anastomosis compared to those with a below-knee anastomosis may be related to length, but the ability to withstand flexion across the knee cannot be isolated from length in the analysis.[24] It is likely that, under most circumstances, differences in patency for grafts of various lengths are more closely related to factors such as graft geometry and quality of distal runoff than to length as an independent variable.

Vascular Steal

When an extra-anatomic bypass is performed, a single donor inflow artery must supply several vascular runoff beds. Studies of crossover grafts in animal models have shown that the immediate effect of the graft is to double flow in the donor artery.[33,34] If this increase in flow shifts the flow-diameter relationship in the donor artery such that a pressure drop occurs, a vascular "steal" situation arises. Blood pressure in the limb ipsilateral to the donor artery is reduced, while pressure in the recipient limb may not improve as much as expected. In femorofemoral bypass grafts performed for claudication, the patient with postoperative vascular steal will report that the symptomatic limb is improved but the previously asymptomatic donor limb now has claudication. Experimental placement of an arteriovenous fistula in the recipient limb in animal crossover grafts increased graft flow by a factor of 10 without causing a steal from the donor limb, suggesting that steal symptoms should not occur in the absence of an inflow stenosis.[33] In fact, multiple pre-existing subcritical stenoses in the donor iliac artery, not evident on preoperative arteriograms, may provide the hemodynamic explanation of vascular steal syndrome when it occurs clinically.[35]

HEMODYNAMICS OF LATE GRAFT FAILURE

Late failure of many prosthetic bypass conduits, including aortofemoral and femoropopliteal reconstructions, is due to excessive intimal hyperplasia at the distal anastomoses.[36-39] Studies evaluating failed human grafts and experimental animal grafts documented the location of the intimal hyperplasia on the near wall of the recipient artery adjacent to the heel and the toe of the downstream anastomosis and on the far wall of the artery across the lumen from the anastomosis.[40-42] Biologic, biochemical, and hemodynamic mechanisms have all been proposed to explain the pathogenesis of anastomotic intimal hyperplasia.

Hemodynamic assessment has correlated the location of intimal hyperplasia with regions of high wall shear stress,[5] low wall shear stress.[41,8,43] boundary layer separation,[44] and high shear stress variation during the cardiac cycle.[43,45] Hemodynamic variables that may have a causal relationship include blood flow rate, graft-to-artery anastomotic angle, and graft-to-artery compliance mismatch.

Relationship of Flow to Intimal Hyperplasia

To identify the hemodynamic characteristics of the bloodstream adjacent to regions that develop intimal hyperplasia, Ojha et al.[46] used a nitrogen laser to monitor a photochromic tracer in a Plexiglass end-to-side 45-degree model anastomosis. For nonpulsatile flow, they found that rapidly moving fluid from the graft impacted the wall opposite the anastomosis creating a velocity profile that was skewed to the far wall just beyond the toe of the anastomosis. This thin, high-speed fluid layer persisted for 2.2 diameters along the far wall but, by 4 diameters downstream, a parabolic velocity profile had been re-established. The three-dimensional reconstruction showed the high velocity for wall flow swirling laterally in paired circumferential streams around the side walls towards the near wall (Fig. 7-2). Far wall analysis revealed a region of flow separation at the toe of the anastomosis which normal-

ized shortly thereafter. Pulsatile flow was established by superimposition of a sinusoidal wave on the steady flow conditions, resulting in flow patterns and velocity profiles that varied within each pulse. The peak effect of pulsatile flow occurred at midcycle, where a highly localized swirl was superimposed on the nonpulsatile flow pattern just beyond the toe of the anastomosis. This swirl limited the extent of flow separation.

In the pulsatile model, the maximal component of axial shear stress occurred shortly after peak flow on the far wall just beyond the toe of the anastomosis. The areas of low axial wall shear in the host vessel were identified along the near wall just proximal to the heel and just beyond the toe of the anastomosis. The bed of the host vessel where the entry flow was split into antegrade and retrograde components also had a focal region of low shear. However, the authors characterized that region as a complex area containing low shear, high shear, and high-frequency components due to movement of the stagnation point during the pulse cycle. Thus, these data support a low wall shear stress or flow separation pathogenesis at the toe and the heel of the anastomosis, but the region of intimal hyperplasia on the far wall of the artery was described as one of highly variable rather than low shear.

Bassiouny et al.[43] used bilateral iliofemoral saphenous vein and PTFE grafts in dogs to study anastomotic intimal hyperplasia. Flow visualization studies were then performed in transparent silicone models constructed from castings of the canine anastomoses. Two

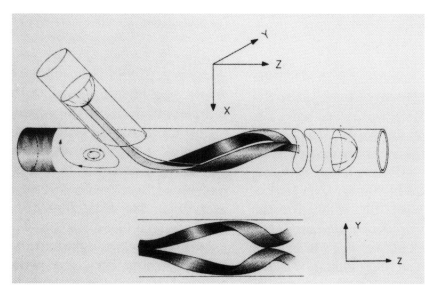

Figure 7-2 Pathline of the high inertia fluid seen under steady-state flow conditions, as well as for pulsatile flow near peak cycle flow: *(top)* side view, showing development of the double helix; *(bottom)* view from above. The high inertia fluid jet appeared at the far wall at 0.2 vessel diameters from the toe of the graft. At 2 diameters beyond the toe, the high inertia fluid appeared both at the far wall and the side walls. By 4 diameters downstream, parabolic flow was re-established. (Modified from Ojha et al.,[46] with permission.)

distinct regions of intimal thickening were identified. One occurred at the suture line and was greater in the PTFE grafts than the vein grafts. The authors interpreted this as a suture line healing response, and they suggested that compliance mismatch explained the greater effect of PTFE. The second hyperplastic region was on the arterial wall across from the hood of the graft, and the response was equal in vein and PTFE grafts (Fig. 7-3). At this location, the silicone model revealed flow oscillation and low shear. Thus, these authors agree with Ojha et al.[46] on the correlation of flow oscillation and low shear with the site of intimal thickening on the far arterial wall. However, disagreement exists regarding the nature and pathogenesis of thickening along the near wall adjacent to the anastomosis. Neither experiment offers data to support a causal relationship between shear effects and intimal hyperplasia.

Influence of Anastomotic Angle on Patency

The angle formed at the end-to-side distal anastomosis between bypass graft and native artery may influence the degree of intimal hyperplasia which develops by altering flow patterns and wall shear stress. Analyses of anastomotic angle have been performed in accurately defined rigid-wall in vitro models to minimize the uncontrollable variables associated with in vivo experiments. Crawshaw et al. studied flow patterns in clear plastic model end-to-side anastomoses constructed with inlet angles of 15 degrees and 45 degrees, using dye injection techniques, lateral pressure measurements, and laser Doppler velocity measurements. Flow disturbance was minimal with the 15-degree inlet angle and occlusion of the proximal outflow segment. Patency of the proximal outflow segment or a 45-degree inlet angle resulted in boundary-layer separation at the near wall adjacent to the toe of the anasto-

mosis.[47] Keynton et al.[48] performed similar studies at junction angles of 30, 45, and 60 degrees. Flow patterns were evaluated under nonpulsatile conditions at flow rates found in coronary and femoral arteries. As in the previous study, all flow was introduced through the "graft" limb of the anastomosis. Analysis revealed flow patterns similar to those already noted, with streamlines skewed toward the far wall and a stagnation point adjacent to the far wall where the incoming stream split into reverse shear upstream and forward shear downstream flow components. An elliptical vortex, called the recirculation (or separation) zone, was present just upstream from the stagnation point in the center plane of the native artery. The angle of anastomosis had a distinct effect on the location of the stagnation point, which was farther downstream at smaller angles. The size of the separation zone was larger at smaller angles. (Fig. 7-4). Lower flow rates produced less circumferential motion, a longer elliptical vortex, and an upstream movement of the stagnation point when compared to higher flow at each anastomotic angle. Based on the assumption that low shear at an anastomosis should be avoided, the authors concluded that a 45-degree distal anastomotic angle was most advantageous in the femoral region since the normalized shear rate in the separation zone was higher than at 30 or 60 degrees.

The analysis of anastomosis angle has been extended to include pulsatile flow in a model with inflow through a "stenotic" recipient artery as well as the graft.[49] Doppler color flow imaging was used to analyze the velocity profiles. A 60 percent stenosis in the recipient artery just proximal to the anastomosis created a strong central jet that impacted the flow from the graft and deflected the stagnation zone downstream. There was a region of low velocity upstream of the stagnation point and also between the near wall and the jet just downstream of anastomosis. The region of low velocity and the separation zones increased in size throughout the pulse cycle. As the anastomotic angle increased from 30 degrees to 45 and 60 degrees, the size of all the low

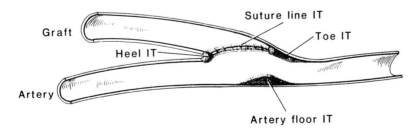

Figure 7-3 End-to-side anastomosis in sagittal section depicts sites of localization of intimal thickening (IT) at suture line and artery floor. Suture line thickening was found to be greatest with prosthetic grafts. It was concluded that the thickening represented vascular healing and might be influenced by compliance mismatch. Arterial floor thickening occurred with all graft types. It was most prominent in regions of low and/or oscillating shear stress. (From Bassiouny et al.,[43] with permission.)

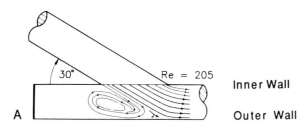

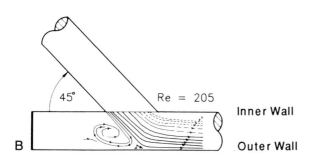

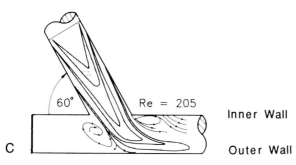

Figure 7-4 Effect of anastomosis angle on velocity profiles, stagnation point, and elliptical flow vortex. At 30 degrees (**A**), the stagnation point is further downstream along the recipient artery when compared to 45 degrees (**B**) or 60 degrees (**C**), and vortex size is greatest at low anastomatic angles. The Reynolds number (Re) is a representative value for the femoral artery. For all models, flow is nonpulsatile, and all inflow is from the graft limb. (Adapted from Keynton et al.,[48] with permission.)

velocity and separation zones increased (Fig. 7-4). This led the authors to conclude that in this model the 30-degree anastomosis would be most advantageous if reduction in separation zone area were the ultimate goal.

Influence of Compliance Mismatch on Patency

Is compliance mismatch important in the long-term patency of bypass grafts? Baird and Abbott presented a hypothesis in 1976, which suggested that the stiff or "incompliant" nature of small diameter vascular pros-

theses caused partial loss of the pulsatile component of left ventricular work, thereby increasing wave reflection and reducing the energy available for distal perfusion[50] (Fig. 7-5). Using compliance measurements (C) defined as

$$C = \frac{\Delta V}{V \cdot \Delta P}$$

where V is the initial volume of a vessel segment, ΔP is the pulse pressure, and ΔV is the change in volume induced by that pulse pressure, they found that Dacron grafts were slightly less compliant than canine autogenous vein grafts and that both were far less compliant than canine femoral artery.[51] In later studies, circumferential compliance (C), expressed as the percentage radial change per mmHg distending pressure, was determined according to the formula

$$C = (D_s - D_d)/[(P_s - P_d) \cdot D_d]$$

where D is the diameter, P is pressure, and subscripts s and d represent measurements taken during systole and diastole.[52] Using these parameters, several early publications provided experimental and clinical data

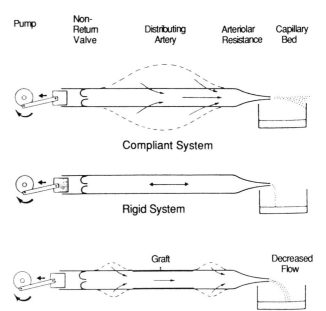

Figure 7-5 Effect of arterial and graft compliance on diastolic phase of pulsatile blood flow. Compliant distributing arteries (**A**) act as an elastic reservoir that stores energy and blood volume during systole and that provides antegrade downstream perfusion during diastole. A rigid system (**B**) is unable to sustain diastolic flow. Interposition of a noncompliant graft (**C**) would cause partial loss of the pulsatile component of the left ventricle external work, reduction of energy available for distal perfusion, and an increase in wave reflection. (Adapted from Baird and Abbott,[50] with permission.)

suggesting that "stiff" grafts had reduced patency compared to grafts with compliance that approximated that of the native artery.[52,53] When sequential measurements were taken longitudinally along the host artery and across an end-to-end anastomosis, compliance increased to a maximum just before the anastomosis, fell to a minimum at the anastomosis itself, then rebounded quickly toward mid-graft. The area of low compliance was called the "para-anastomotic hypercompliant zone," and this observation led to an hypothesis that the region of increased cyclic stretch promoted intimal hyperplasia near the anastomosis.[54]

In 1987, in a further effort to isolate compliance as a single variable, Abbott et al.[55] compared high to low compliance glutaraldehyde-fixed arterial autogenous grafts in 14 dogs. Grafts were identical except for the compliance variation produced by differential fixation. The grafts were considered "compliant" if their characteristics approached those of the host artery and "stiff" if the compliance was less than the artery (Fig. 7-6). At implantation, compliance in the graft and adjacent sections of artery differed significantly between

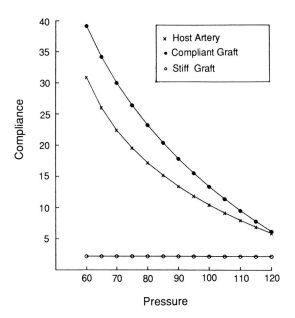

Figure 7-6 Compliance-pressure curves measured at implantation for host artery and compliant and stiff grafts implanted as femoral autografts in dogs. Stiff grafts were prepared by immersion in 10 percent gluteraldehyde for 1 hour, while compliant grafts were immersed in saline. Glutaraldehyde crosslinks elastin and collagen protein moieties, resulting in a biologic prosthesis with compliance similar to that of prosthetics. Compliance at 100 mmHg is used to calculate tubular compliance mismatch between artery and grafts. Units of pressure, mmHg; compliance, percentage radial change/mmHg × 10⁻². (From Abbott et al.,[55] with permission.)

groups (Fig. 7-7). By 3 months, eight stiff grafts and two compliant grafts had failed, for life-table 3-month patencies of 85 percent and 37 percent ($p < 0.05$). The authors concluded that a graft with less than 40 percent of host artery compliance is inconsistent with prolonged patency. Since gross inspection of the thrombosed grafts did not reveal subintimal thickening, intimal hyperplasia was considered an unlikely cause of graft failure. The authors believed that increased impedance, disturbed flow patterns, or pulsatile anastomotic mechanical stress were more likely pathophysiologic explanations for the increased thrombosis rate in the low-compliance grafts. Thus, while experimental and some clinical data compiled over two decades correlate graft failure with compliance mismatch, a causal relationship between anastomotic intimal hyperplasia and compliance mismatch has yet to be firmly established.[56,57]

Evaluation of the Arterial Runoff Bed and Effect on Patency

The ability to predict initial and late graft patency on the basis of preoperative or intraoperative assessment of the arterial runoff bed has been a goal of vascular surgeons for many years. Most attention in this area has been devoted to qualitative and quantitative runoff evaluation on preoperative arteriograms, but the ability to correlate arteriographic findings with early or late graft patency has been variably successful.[58-63] Intraoperative hemodynamic measurements of outflow resistance,[64-71] volumetric blood flow,[58,60] and flow waveform analysis[72] have also been studied, but none of these methods has been uniformly successful in the prediction of graft failure, nor have these hemodynamic parameters always correlated with arteriographic runoff scores.

Resistance Measurements

Ascer and co-workers have been proponents of intraoperative outflow resistance measurements as predictors of limb salvage during infrainguinal reconstructions.[64,65,68,69] Their method involved manual injection of 20 to 50 ml of normal saline solution through the bypass graft after the distal anastomosis had been completed. Pressure generated within the graft during the injection was measured through a needle placed in the graft and recorded.[65] The hydraulic analog of Ohm's law was used to determine outflow resistance:

$$R = P/F$$

where R is resistance (mmHg/ml/min), P is pressure

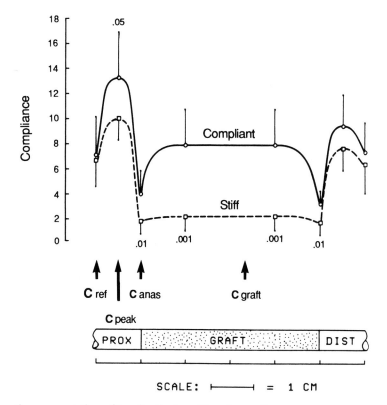

Figure 7-7 Schematic representation of longitudinal profiles of compliance near anastomoses adjacent to compliant and stiff grafts. C_{ref}, average compliance of host artery measured 9 and 10 mm from the anastomosis; C_{peak}, maximum compliance at a point between C_{ref} and the anastomosis (if compliance at C_{peak} was markedly greater than C_{ref}, the graft was said to have a "para-anastomotic hypercompliant zone"); C_{anas}, compliance at the anastomosis, was lower than C_{graft} in compliant grafts, while C_{anas} and C_{graft} were similar in stiff grafts. Data points are means ($\pm$ 1 SD). Numbers along the curve indicate p values associated with difference between compliant and stiff grafts were statistically significant. (From Abbott et al.,[55] with permission.)

(mmHg), and F is flow (ml/min). This equation can be integrated over the time of injection such that

$$R = \int_0^t Pdt/V$$

where V is the volume of fluid injected. An analog computer was used to integrate pressure over the time of injection. Backpressure from collateral flow was dealt with by electrically zeroing the recorder prior to saline injection. Proximal and distal outflow resistance were measured separately by alternate occlusion of the downstream and upstream outflow limbs. Vasospasm effects were evaluated by repeat measurements performed following injection of papaverine. Distal outflow resistance was measured in 101 lower-extremity reconstructions and found to be 0.46 ± 0.28 mmHg/ml/min in grafts which remained patent at 3 months, and 2.15 ± 1.07 mmHg/ml/min in grafts that had failed by 3 months. A critical value of 1.2 mmHg/ml/min was identified, above which all bypasses occluded

within 3 months and below which all bypasses remained patent. The response to papaverine injection was not predictive of bypass failure. Total outflow resistance decreased by a mean of 30 percent after papaverine injection and resulted in several false-negative outflow scores. Despite these impressive results, the authors recommended that resistance measurements not be used to abandon bypass operations in favor of amputation, since some bypasses with high distal resistance remained patent long enough to allow foot lesions to heal. A later retrospective analysis by this group studied the predictive value of outflow resistance based on distal anastomosis site and type of conduit.[68] Total outflow resistance measurements were not predictive when the distal anastomosis was at the popliteal level, but they were significantly predictive when the distal anastomosis was at the tibial level, where only 26 percent of 34 grafts with distal outflow resistance greater than 0.81 were patent at 1 year. Total and distal outflow resistance were predictive of infrainguinal

PTFE graft patency, but only distal outflow resistance was predictive of autogenous saphenous vein graft failure.[68]

Unfortunately, correlation of high outflow resistance with early graft failure has not been a universal finding. Peterkin et al.[70] measured runoff resistance in 80 consecutive patients with femoropopliteal and infrapopliteal bypass grafts, most of which were constructed with autogenous vein. Their method involved use of an infusion pump at a fixed flow rate, allowing direct use of the Ohm's law analog to calculate resistance, after pressure reached a plateau. After 12 months, there was no trend toward a difference in runoff resistance between those grafts that had failed and those that remained patent.[70] In addition, outflow resistance was compared with arteriographic runoff score by this group, and a correlation was found when the distal bypass site was the above-knee popliteal artery or the posterior tibial artery, but not for other distal anastomotic sites.[71] Thus, the predictive accuracy of outflow scores may depend on the method used for their determination and on the type of prosthesis employed, but no other firm conclusions may be reached at this time regarding their clinical value.

Flow Measurements

Intraoperative volumetric blood flow measurements are among the hemodynamic methods studied for their ability to predict bypass graft patency. Mundth et al.[58] used an electromagnetic flowmeter with circumferential probes to measure flow in 19 femoropopliteal reconstructions performed with saphenous vein. Mean graft flow was 79 ml/min in the entire group and 102 ml/min in the four bypass grafts that failed, an obviously nondiscriminatory result. Dean et al.[60] used a similar method to measure blood flow intraoperatively following completion of 98 femoropopliteal bypass grafts constructed with autogenous saphenous vein. All 16 grafts with a flow rate less than 70 ml/min failed within 30 days, while 18 percent of grafts with a flow rate greater than 70 ml/min also failed.[60] Based on these contradictory findings, as well as the difficulty encountered in calibrating electromagnetic flow probes, enthusiasm for intraoperative flow measurement has dwindled since these early reports. However, the measurement of bypass graft volumetric blood flow has been reported in postoperative graft surveillance protocols in which measurements taken both at rest or during postocclusive reactive hyperemia were sensitive for impending graft failure.[28,29] In these studies, mean blood velocity in the graft (V) was determined by electronic integration of transcutaneous Doppler ultrasound velocity spectra, and cross-sectional area of the bypass graft (A) was determined on B-mode ultrasound images. Volumetric blood flow (Q) is determined by the formula

$$Q = V \cdot A$$

expressed in milliliters per minute (ml/min). Finally, in addition to these quantitative estimates of volumetric flow, a qualitative method based on the analysis of intraoperative electromagnetic flowmeter derived waveforms has also been reported to be predictive of late bypass graft patency.[72] Further prospective investigation will be necessary to determine the true predictive value of these intraoperative or postoperative volumetric flow measurements.

Impedance Measurements

Vascular impedance is defined as the ratio of pulsatile pressure to pulsatile flow, and hence is analogous to resistance in a nonpulsatile system. Impedance considerations are important in hemodynamics because they give quantitative expression to the fact that pressure-flow relationships are largely a function of the physical properties of the blood vessels. Because impedance results from the frequency dependent oscillatory elements and reflected waves of the vascular system, it may have advantages over simple resistance measurements in the identification of failing bypass grafts.[73,74] One early report tested the predictive ability of impedance measurements performed intraoperatively,[73] while another form of impedance measurement, performed during postoperative graft surveillance, has been reported as a sensitive indicator of failing bypass grafts.[74]

Four different types of vascular impedance have been defined, and each provides a different expression of the relationship between pulsatile pressure and flow. Longitudinal impedance, expressed in dyn · s/cm⁵ per cm of vessel length, is the ratio of the pressure gradient to flow, and it is the most direct pulsatile analog of vascular resistance. Thus, resistance may be thought of as longitudinal impedance in a system when the pulse equals 0. Calculation of longitudinal impedance is based on the pressure gradient required to cross a segment of finite length; therefore, it depends primarily on the local properties of the vessel.

Input impedance is the ratio of pulsatile pressure to flow at any particular location along the vascular tree. Input impedance differs from longitudinal impedance in that it considers the energy of waves reflected from the entire downstream arterial outflow tract beyond the point of measurement. Since the diameter and physical properties of the vascular tree differ greatly from proximal to distal regions, a complex variety of reflected waves affects all more proximal segments. Thus, input impedance relates pressure to flow at a single point based on the energy influences beyond that point. Terminal impedance is defined as the input impedance at the end of a vessel, while the final impedance type, characteristic impedance, is the relationship between pressure and flow when pressure and flow waves are not influenced by wave reflection. Since actual pressure and flow waves contain both incident and reflected components, it is only possible to measure characteristic impedance directly in experimental models.

Most analyses of impedance assume that vessels are cylindrical and flow is laminar because analysis becomes very difficult under more complex conditions. To determine input impedance at a selected point in the circulation, real-time measurements of pulsatile pressure and flow are recorded simultaneously at the point, and the waveforms are subjected to a frequency analysis. Waves that are repeated regularly, such as those produced by the cardiac cycle, can be represented numerically as the sum of a unique set of sinusoidal waves whose frequencies are integral multiples of the frequency of the original wave. This set of sinusoidal curves is called a Fourier series, and the computation, a Fourier analysis, results in a series of input impedances at integral multiples of the heart rate. For example, at a heart rate of 60 beats/min the fundamental harmonic is 1 Hz, and the impedance is calculated at frequencies of 1, 2, 3, 4 ⋯ Hz. The data are then plotted as an impedance spectrum (in dyn/s/cm^5) on the ordinate, while frequency (in Hz) is on the abscissa[3] (Fig. 7-8).

Experimental measurements of impedance in living animals are inevitably affected by biologic "noise" that introduces a greater variability than the actual properties of blood flow or the physical limitations of the mechanical pressure and flow transducers. The point at which the signal/noise ratio becomes too small to give reliable results must be decided empirically under any

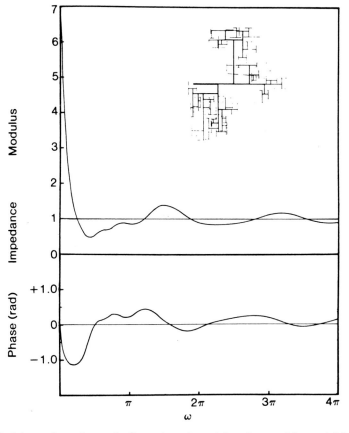

Figure 7-8 Theoretical input impedance *(ordinates)* at the origin of a model arterial bed, as a function of frequency *(abscissa)*. Model consists of eight generations of a branching system in which each tubular segment has a randomly assigned length *(scale diagram above)*. Elastic modulus increases in each generation; fluid viscosity is assumed to be zero. Terminal vessels end in pure resistances that yield a reflection factor of 0.6. Input impedances *(above)* and phases *(below)* calculated in accordance with Womersley's theory. (From Milnor,[3] with permission.)

set of experimental conditions but, in most situations, computation should be limited to frequencies lower than 25 Hz.

The report by Wyatt et al.[74] of impedance analysis to identify bypass grafts at risk of failure employed pulse volume recordings as a form of pressure measurement and Doppler velocity waveforms as flow measurements. An impedance curve was generated by Fourier waveform analysis and compared only over the first portion of the pulse cycle, to avoid the effect of reflected waves; thus, these data represent an attempt to determine characteristic impedance by noninvasive measurements. A discriminate impedance score was identified in a retrospective analysis, and this threshold score was then found to be predictive of incipient graft failure in a small prospective analysis.[74] While the attempt to employ impedance analysis represents a sophisticated approach to the hemodynamics of bypass graft surveillance, larger prospective studies will be necessary before firm conclusions can be drawn regarding the clinical validity of this method.

REFERENCES

1. Caro CG, Pedley TJ, Schroter RC et al: The Mechanics of the Circulation. Oxford University Press, New York, 1978
2. Fung YC: Biodynamics Circulation. Springer-Verlag, New York, 1984
3. Milnor WR: Vascular impedance. p. 167. In: Hemodynamics. 2nd Ed. Williams & Wilkins, Baltimore, 1989
4. Nichols WW, O'Rourke MF: McDonald's Blood Flow in Arteries. 3rd Ed. Lea & Febiger, Philadelphia, 1990
5. Fry DL: Acute vascular endothelial changes associated with increased blood velocity gradients. Circ Res 22:165, 1968
6. Fry DL: Responses of the arterial wall to certain physical factors. p. 93 In: Artherogenesis Initiating Factors. Ciba Foundation Symposium 12 (NS). Associated Scientific Publishers, Amsterdam, 1973
7. Caro CG, Fitz-Gerald JM, Schroter RC: Atheroma and arterial wall shear. Observation, correlation and proposal of a shear dependent mass transfer mechanism for atherogenesis. Proc R Soc Lond Biol 177:109, 1971
8. Berguer R, Higgins RF, Reddy DJ: Intimal hyperplasia: an experimental study. Arch Surg 115:332, 1980
9. Morinaga K, Okadome K, Kuroki M et al: Effect of wall shear stress on intimal thickening of arterially transplanted autogenous veins in dogs. J Vasc Surg 2:430, 1985
10. Dobrin PB, Littooy FN, Endean ED: Mechanical factors predisposing to intimal hyperplasia and medial thickening in autogenous vein grafts. Surgery 105:393, 1989
11. Galt SW, Zwolak RM, Wagner RJ et al: Differential response of arteries and vein grafts to blood flow reduction. J Vasc Surg 17:563, 1993
12. Dobrin PB: On the roles of deformation tension, and wall stress as critical stimuli eliciting myointimal/medial hyperplasia. J Vasc Surg 15:581, 1992
13. Strandness DE, Sumner DS: Grafts and grafting. p. 342. In: Hemodynamics for Surgeons. Grune & Stratton, Orlando, FL, 1975
14. Schneider JR, Zwolak RM, Walsh DB et al: Lack of diameter effect on short-term patency of size-matched Dacron aortobifemoral grafts. J Vasc Surg 13:785, 1991
15. Schneider JR, McDaniel MD, Walsh DB et al: Axillofemoral bypass: outcome and hemodynamic results in high risk patients. J Vasc Surg 15:952, 1992
16. Schultz RD, Hokanson DE, Strandness DE, Jr: Pressure-flow relations of the end-side anastomosis. Surgery 62:319, 1967
17. Wesolowski SA, Fries CC, Hennigar G et al: Factors contributing to long-term failures in human vascular prosthetic grafts. J Cardiovasc Surg 5:544, 1964
18. Kohler TR, Kirkman TR, Kraiss LW et al: Increased blood flow inhibits neointimal hyperplasia in endothelialized vascular grafts. Circ Res 69:1557, 1991
19. Sauvage LR, Berger KE, Mansfield PB et al: Future directions in the development of arterial prostheses for small and medium caliber arteries. Surg Clin North Am 54:213, 1974
20. Sauvage LR, Walker MW, Berger KE et al: Current arterial prostheses. Experimental evaluation by implantation in the carotid and circumflex coronary arteries of the dog. Arch Surg 114:687, 1979
21. Inauen W, Baumgartner HR, Bombeli T et al: Dose- and shear rate-dependent effects of heparin on thrombogenesis induced by rabbit aorta subendothelium exposed to flowing human blood. Arteriosclerosis 10:607, 1990
22. Weiss HJ, Hawiger J, Ruggeri ZM et al: Fibrinogen-independent platelet adhesion and thrombus formation on subendothelium mediated by glycoprotein IIb-IIIa complex at high shear rate. J Clin Invest 83:288, 1989
23. Badimon JJ, Badimon L, Turitto VT et al: Platelet deposition at high shear rates is enhanced by high plasma cholesterol levels. In vivo study in the rabbit model. Arteriosclerosis Thromb 11:395, 1991
24. Jones DN, Rutherford RB, Ikezawa T et al: Factors affecting the patency of small-caliber prostheses: observations in a suitable canine model. J Vasc Surg 14:441, 1991
25. Darling RC, Linton RR, Razzuk MA: Saphenous vein bypass grafts for femoropopliteal occlusive disease: a reappraisal. Surgery 61:31, 1967
26. Leather RP, Shah DM, Chang BB et al: Resurrection of the in situ saphenous vein bypass. 1000 cases later. Ann Surg 208:435, 1988
27. Towne JB, Schmitt DD, Seabrook GR et al: The effect of vein diameter on patency of in situ grafts. J Cardiovasc Surg 32:192, 1991
28. Kupinski AM, Stone MP, DePalma H et al: Is reactive hyperemia a reliable indicator of impending bypass failure? J Vasc Technol 14:163, 1990
29. Zwolak RM, Cronenwett JL, McDaniel MD et al: Vas-

cular laboratory detection of failing lower extremity arterial bypass grafts. J Vasc Surg 13:910, 1991

30. Field JP, Musson AM, Zwolak RM et al: Duplex arterial flow measurements in normal lower extremities. J Vasc Technol 13:13, 1989

31. DeWeese JA, Rob CG: Autogenous venous bypass grafts five years later. Ann Surg 174:346, 1971

32. Andros G, Harris RW, Salles-Cunha SX et al: Bypass grafts to the ankle and foot. J Vasc Surg 7:785, 1988

33. Ehrenfeld WK, Harris JD, Wylie EJ: Vascular "steal" phenomenon. An experimental study. Am J Surg 116:192, 1968

34. Shin CS, Chaudhry AG: The hemodynamics of extra-anatomic bypass grafts. Surg Gynecol Obstet 148:567, 1979

35. Flanigan DP, Tullis JP, Streeter VL et al: Multiple subcritical arterial stenoses: effect on poststenotic pressure and flow. Ann Surg 186:663, 1977

36. Imparato AM, Bracco A, Kim GE et al: Intimal and neointimal fibrous proliferation causing failure of artrial reconstructions. Surgery 72:1007, 1972

37. DeWeese JA: Anastomotic intimal hyperplasia. p. 147. In PN Sawyer and MJ Kaplitt (eds): Vascular Grafts. Apple-Century-Crofts, New York, 1978

38. Madras PN, Ward CA, Johnson WR et al: Anastomotic hyperplasia. Surgery 90:922, 1981

39. Echave V, Koornick AR, Haimov M et al: Intimal hyperplasia as a complication of the use of the polytetrafluoroethylene graft for femoral-popliteal bypass. Surgery 86:791, 1979

40. Sottiurai VS, Yao JST, Flinn WR et al: Intimal hyperplasia and neointima: an ultrastructural analysis of thrombosed grafts in humans. Surgery 93:809, 1983

41. Rittgers SE, Karayannacos PE, Guy JF et al: Velocity distribution and intimal proliferation in autologous vein grafts in dogs. Circ Res 42:792, 1978

42. LoGerfo FW, Quist WC, Nowak MD et al: Downstream anastomotic hyperplasia. A mechanism of failure in Dacron arterial grafts. Ann Surg 197:479, 1983

43. Bassiouny HS, White S, Glagov S et al: Anastomotic intimal hyperplasia: mechanical injury or flow induced. J Vasc Surg 15:708, 1992

44. LoGerfo FW, Soncrant T, Teel T et al: Boundary layer separation in models of side-to-end arterial anastomoses. Arch Surg 114:1369, 1979

45. Okadome K, Yukizane T, Mii S et al: Ultrastructural evidence of the effects of shear stress variation on intimal thickening in dogs with arterially transplanted autologous vein grafts. J Cardiovasc Surg 31:719, 1990

46. Ojha M, Ethier CR, Johnston KW et al: Steady and pulsatile flow fields in an end-to-side arterial anastomosis model. J Vasc Surg 12:747, 1990

47. Crawshaw HW, Quist WC, Serrallach E et al: Flow disturbance at the distal end-to-side anastomosis. Arch Surg 115:1280, 1980

48. Keynton RS, Rittgers SE, Shu MC: The effect of angle and flow rate upon hemodynamics in distal vascular graft anastomoses: an in vitro model study. J Biomech Eng 113:458, 1991

49. Rittgers SE, Bhambhani GH: Hemodynamics within leiofemoral graft anastomosis models. Video J Color Flow Imag 2:153, 1992

50. Baird RN, Abbott WM: Pulsatile blood-flow in arterial grafts. Lancet 2:948, 1976

51. Baird RN, Kidson IG, L'Italien GJ et al: Dynamic compliance of arterial grafts. Am J Physiol 233:H568, 1977

52. Kidson IG, Abbott WM: Low compliance and arterial graft occlusion. Circulation, suppl. 1. 58:I-1, 1978

53. Walden R, L'Italien GJ, Megerman J et al: Matched elastic properties and successful arterial grafting. Arch Surg 115:1166, 1980

54. Hasson JE, Megerman J, Abbott WM: Increased compliance near vascular anastomoses. J Vasc Surg 2:419, 1985

55. Abbott WM, Megerman J, Hasson JE et al: Effect of compliance mismatch on vascular graft patency. J Vasc Surg 5:376, 1987

56. Okuhn SP, Connelly DP, Calakos N et al: Does compliance mismatch alone cause intimal hyperplasia? J Vasc Surg 9:35, 1989

57. Abbott WM, Megerman J: Does compliance mismatch alone cause neointimal hyperplasia? (Letter to the Editor.) J Vasc Surg 9:507, 1989

58. Mundth ED, Darling RC, Moran JM et al: Quantitative correlation of distal arterial outflow and patency of femoropopliteal reversed saphenous vein grafts with intraoperative flow and pressure measurements. Surgery 65:197, 1969

59. McCurdy JR, Lain KC, Allgood RJ et al: Angiographic determinants of femoropopliteal bypass graft patency. Ten-year experience. Am J Surg 124:789, 1972

60. Dean RH, Yao JST, Stanton PE et al: Prognostic indicators in femoropopliteal reconstructions. Arch Surg 110:1287, 1975

61. Nicholas GG, Latshaw RF: Femoropopliteal bypass grafting: predictive value of preoperative angiography. Am J Surg 138:672, 1979

62. Rutherford RB, Flanigan DP, Gupta SK et al: Suggested standards for reports dealing with lower extremity ischemia. J Vasc Surg 4:80, 1986

63. Karacagil S, Almgren B, Bergström R et al: Postoperative predictive value of a new method of intraoperative angiographic assessment of runoff in femoropopliteal bypass grafting. J Vasc Surg 10:400, 1989

64. Ascer E, Veith FJ, Morin L et al: Quantitative assessment of outflow resistance in lower extremity arterial reconstructions. J Surg Res 37:8, 1984

65. Ascer E, Veith FJ, Morin L et al: Components of outflow resistance and their correlation with graft patency in lower extremity arterial reconstructions. J Vasc Surg 1:817, 1984

66. Menzoian JO, LaMorte WW, Cantelmo NL et al: The preoperative angiogram as a predictor of peripheral vascular runoff. Am J Surg 150:346, 1985

67. LaMorte WW, Menzoian JO, Sidawy A et al: A new method for the prediction of peripheral vascular resistance from the preoperative angiogram. J Vasc Surg 2:703, 1985

68. Ascer E, Veith FJ, White-Flores SA et al: Intraoperative outflow resistance as a predictor of late patency of femoropopliteal and infrapopliteal arterial bypasses. J Vasc Surg 5:820, 1987

69. Ascer E, White SA, Veith FJ et al: Outflow resistance measurement during infrainguinal arterial reconstructions: a reliable predictor of limb salvage. Am J Surg 154:185, 1987

70. Peterkin Ga, LaMorte WW, Menzoian JO: Runoff resistance and early graft failure in infrainguinal bypass surgery. Arch Surg 123:1199, 1988

71. Peterkin GA, Manabe S, LaMorte WW et al: Evaluation of a proposed standard reporting system for preoperative angiograms in infrainguinal bypass procedures: angiographic correlates of measured runoff resistance. J Vasc Surg 7:379, 1988

72. Okadome K, Eguchi H, Yukizane T et al: Long-term results of arterial reconstruction of lower extremities determined by flow waveform analysis. J Cardiovasc Surg 30:64, 1989

73. Cave FD, Walker A, Naylor GP et al: The hydraulic impedance of the lower limb: its relevance to the success of bypass operations for occlusion of the superficial femoral artery. Br J Surg 63:408, 1976

74. Wyatt MG, Muir RM, Tennant WG et al: Impedance analysis to identify the at risk femorodistal graft. J Vasc Surg 13:284, 1991

Physiology of Venous Obstruction and Valvular Incompetence

The venous system over the years has had a less "distinguished" position than its arterial counterpart in the fields of vascular surgery and interventional radiology. Occlusive arterial lesions presented problems that were directly amenable to a variety of diagnostic and therapeutic efforts. On the venous side of the circulation, the role of the radiologist was largely confined to the use of venography to detect deep venous thrombi. Less frequently, the same or modified diagnostic procedures were used to document the location and extent of chronic venous obstruction and valvular damage and incompetence.

Interestingly, it was the development of the labelled fibrinogen method that provided us with most of our information about the localization of thrombi in the deep venous system, when they developed, and how propagation might take place. Even though the labelled fibrinogen method had serious drawbacks, it also served as a suitable marker for evaluating methods of prophylaxis, and was the method through which most of our information on effective forms of prophylaxis emerged.

Until the past few years, the treatment of chronic venous insufficiency was largely related to the proper fitting and wearing of graduated compression hose. This form of therapy was designed to prevent edema and hopefully to forestall the development of the long-term complications of pigmentation and ulceration.

Surgical approaches were largely confined to the treatment of primary varicose veins and the late complications of chronic venous insufficiency. Surgical methods varied from ligation and stripping of the saphenous system to a more vigorous attempt to also interrupt the key communicating veins that were found in the gaiter area of the lower leg. Unfortunately, there is no proof as to which approaches are the most effective in either preventing or treating the long-term complications of this very common disorder because proper randomized trials of these forms of therapy have never been carried out.

In order to understand the pathophysiology of both acute deep vein thrombosis and the postthrombotic syndrome, it is necessary to know the anatomy and the physiology of venous function. The venous system is in many respects more complicated than its arterial counterpart. The reasons for this will become evident upon review of Chapters 8 to 10. The place of a clear understanding of the relevant physiology becomes even more evident when the role of valve replacement and valvuloplasty is reviewed. It is not only necessary to understand valve function; methods must be also employed to study how valves work at all levels of the venous circulation.

The first two chapters in this section, Chapters 8 and 9, will review the anatomy and physiology of the venous system with slightly different points of emphasis. Attention will be paid to not only the large and medium sized veins but also the blood supply of the skin, which is the final target area for the chronic alterations in venous flow that occur during the chronic phase of venous insufficiency. Most discussions of the postthrombotic syndrome do not take into account the final target area—the skin. In the review of these chapters, one will find some minor overlaps and perhaps slightly different views, but this is healthy given our current lack of knowledge. For example, it is assumed that all communicating veins have valves, which may not be true as shown by Dr. Cheatle in Chapter 10, Anatomy and Physiology of the Veins of the Lower Limb. Is this indeed true, and if so what does this mean in terms of venous function after an episode of acute deep vein thrombosis? This raises several important questions. For example, can one have normal venous function when the key and constant perforating veins may not have valves? Is the absence of or loss of valve function in the communicating veins essential for the development of the advanced skin changes associated with the postthrombotic syndrome? These questions and many others, which only time and more research can answer, emerge from these chapters.

Since acute deep vein thrombosis is so common and potentially dangerous, it is important to review the current status of our knowledge in this area. It is clear that there are many facets to the problem that relate to not only contributing risk factors but also the extent of deep venous involvement. The proper treatment of the deep venous thrombosis and long-term outcome is dependent on both the location of the thrombi and, as we now know, the degree to which spontaneous thrombolysis with recanalization occurs. It has been thought that the recanalization was an infrequent event, with resulting chronic obstruction being a very common endpoint. It is now clear from long-term duplex ultrasound studies that spontaneous lysis is very common, with the long-term outcome depending upon the extent to which valve function is preserved. While there is no doubt that this process is less efficient than we would like, it does help explain why up to one-third of patients with an episode of deep vein thrombosis will never experience any of the sequelae of the postthrombotic syndrome.

The material in this section will set the stage for the later chapters that deal with the therapeutic aspects of both acute and chronic venous disease.

8

Applied Physiology of the Venous System

D. Eugene Strandness, Jr.

The venous system is much more complicated than its arterial counterpart. This is because (1) the veins are collapsible, (2) valves are found at all levels of the venous circulation, (3) it is a relatively low-pressure system, (4) the effect of gravity is important in terms of function, and (5) events on the right side of the heart can influence venous return.

While there are structural differences in the arteries supplying various organs and levels of the limb, the differences on the venous side are more complex. Without some comprehension of the anatomy of the venous system, it is impossible to understand its function, the control mechanisms, and how it is affected by disease. Before considering the physiology of the venous system, the pertinent anatomy is briefly reviewed.

ORGANIZATION OF THE VENOUS SYSTEM

The major components of the venous system can be divided into the three major elements: the superficial system, the communicating veins, and the deep venous system. The division between the superficial and deep system is the deep fascia. The superficial system collects the blood from the skin and subcutaneous tissue, ultimately delivering it to the deep veins, which convey the blood back to the right heart.

The two major channels of the superficial system are the greater and lesser saphenous veins, which are, in effect, the largest perforating veins in the body. The superficial and deep systems are connected by a range of perforating veins that are relatively constant in some areas and not so in others. Those perforating veins thought to be the most important from a clinical standpoint are shown in Figure 8-1. There is a common misconception that these perforating veins in the gaiter area communicate directly with the greater saphenous vein. These communicate with the posterior arch vein, which lies posterior to the greater saphenous but joins it at about the knee level (Fig. 8-2).

From a physiologic standpoint, the most important structural elements in the venous system are the valves. These are found in increasing numbers, with the smallest number found in the iliac veins and the greatest number in those veins below the knee. These are bicuspid in design with a fine connective tissue skeleton covered by endothelium. The concave surfaces are directed centrally, facilitating flow toward the heart and at the same time are very effective in preventing reflux. Valves are also found in the communicating veins, which normally permit flow only from the superficial

103

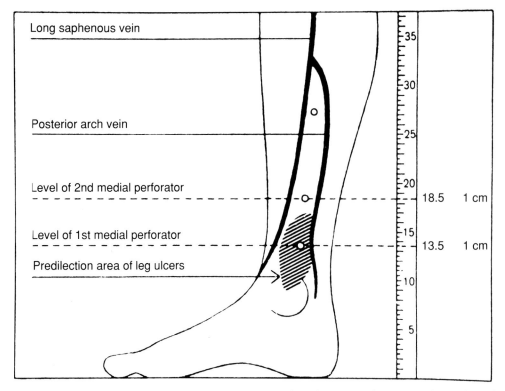

Figure 8-1 Location of the most important communicating veins of the lower limb and their relationship to the site at which pigmentation and ulceration most commonly occur. (From Hobbs,[47] with permission.)

to the deep venous system. This is shown schematically in Figure 8-3.

Since many of the functional tests are designed to test valve competence, it is important to have an appreciation of the valve numbers by location in the venous system. These can be summarized as follows[1,2]:

1. The average number of valves in the deep system from the inguinal ligament to the knee is five.
2. A valve is commonly found in the deep femoral vein approximately 2 cm from its termination in the common femoral vein.
3. Another common site for a valve to be found is in the superficial femoral vein at the level of the adductor hiatus.
4. The distribution of valves in the common femoral and iliac system can be seen in Figure 8-4. As is noted it is not uncommon for regions above the inguinal ligament to be devoid of valves.

PROPERTIES OF THE VENOUS WALL

On the arterial side of the circulation, the distribution of elastin, collagen, and smooth muscle is extremely variable, depending on the site within the system. For example, the aorta is dominated by elastin, but its amount and the amount of collagen tend to reverse as one proceeds distally; that is, the arteries become stiffer. In addition, in contrast to the veins, the arteries are not collapsible.

Another feature of the venous system is its ability to undergo remarkable changes in volume with very few changes in transmural pressure. This is important, in terms of the capacitance function of the venous system. The venous wall is approximately one-third to one-tenth as thick as the systemic arteries.[3] The veins contain relatively little elastin and consist largely of smooth muscle. The veins of the foot contain 60 to 80 percent smooth muscle, as compared with 5 percent for the axillary vein.[4] It is not well appreciated that the materials in the wall of the vein are stiffer per unit of cross section as compared with arteries at the same distending pressure. This is true because of the relative paucity of elastin and the prominent adventitia, which is largely collagen.

PRESSURE AND FLOW RELATIONSHIPS

One of the fascinating aspects of both the arterial and venous systems is the dramatic differences that are present, even though both have as their major function

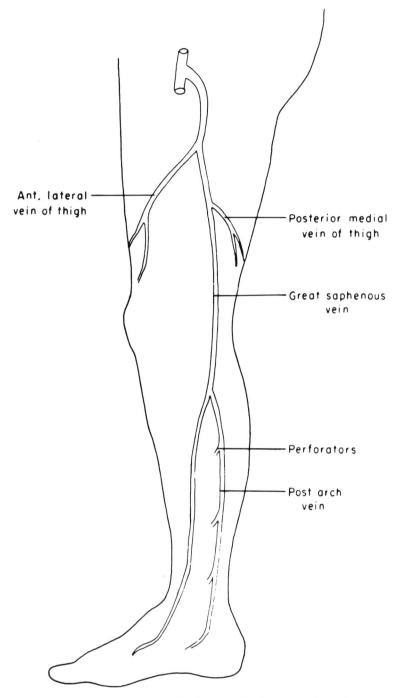

Ant. lateral
vein of thigh

Posterior medial
vein of thigh

Great saphenous
vein

Perforators

Post arch
vein

Figure 8-2 Relationship between the posterior arch vein to which the perforating veins connect and the greater saphenous vein. (From Strandness and Thiele,[48] with permission.)

transport of blood from the heart to the tissues and back again. These relationships are very complex, but understanding them will give the reader a better understanding of how these systems can function both in the normal state and when affected by disease.

In order to understand the pressures involved, it is first necessary to consider the effects of gravity on the hydrostatic pressure in the upright "dead" man as shown in Figure 8-5. As noted in the open tube, the pressure at the top of the tube would be atmospheric or zero. In the body, however, there are two systems of tubes with different properties that are connected. The volume to fill the entire system is not there so the veins that are collapsible will do so under the influence of

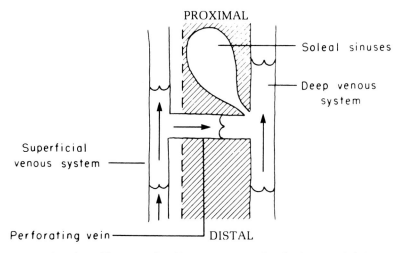

Figure 8-3 Position and direction of flow permitted by competent valves in the superficial, deep, and communicating veins of the lower leg. (From Strandness and Thiele,[48] with permission.)

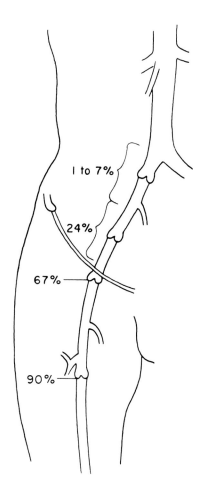

Figure 8-4 Frequency and distribution of valves in the iliac and common femoral veins. (From Basmajian,[1] with permission.)

atmospheric pressure at the upper end. The point of collapse is the zero point. The pressure in the rigid tube (the artery) above the zero point will be negative, as shown.

The changes in the pressures in the system with the addition of a pulsatile pump are shown in Figure 8-6. Here, the pressures are affected not only by gravity but also by the presence of the pump itself and by the resistance to flow offered by the various parts of the circuit. The resistance offered can be noted by the gradients between various points in the arteries and also in the veins. However, there is a very large pressure drop across the arterioles which reflects the very high resistance of these small arteries. There is also a rather large drop across the diaphragm, possibly due to the collapse of the vena cava in this location.[5]

With the assumption of the upright position, there are dramatic changes in pressure. The only point at which the pressure remains constant is the hydrostatic indifferent point (HIP), just below the diaphragm. All pressures distal to this point are increased due to the weight of the blood but the arteriovenous pressure gradient remains the same (83 mmHg). With the arm extended, the perfusion pressure drops, changing the pressure gradient across the arterioles to 31 mmHg. Thus, the blood flow to the hand would fall, as might be expected with the arm in the position above the head.[6]

The fact that the transcapillary pressure gradient is the same in the supine position as when the subject stands up does not imply that gravity does not have an effect. In fact, when assuming the upright position, there is an accumulation of approximately 500 ml of blood, largely due to reflux.[7] There is some loss of fluid into the tissues, which is picked up by the lymphatics.

Hydrostatic pressure (mmHg)

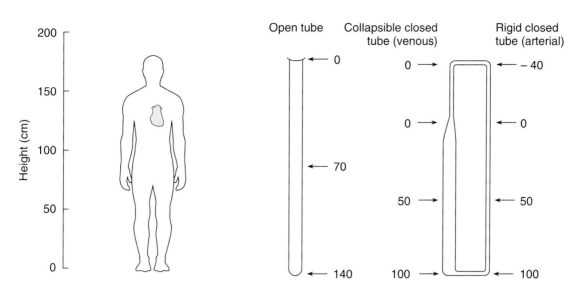

Figure 8-5 Hydrostatic pressures that would be present in the upright "dead" man. Pressures in the open tube are those expected with a rigid tube. Pressures on the right would be found in a parallel series of tubes that are collapsible on the venous side and not on the arterial side. (From Strandness and Sumner,[49] with permission.)

In addition, quiet standing will result in a gradual increase in tissue volume, which could account for a blood volume reduction of at least 15 percent.

The changes and sequence of events necessary to ensure venous valve closure are schematically depicted in Figure 8-7. In order for valve closure to occur, there must first be a reversal of the normal transvalvular pressure gradient. A pressure and generated velocity of flow exceeding 30 cm/s leads to valve closure.

The role of the venous valves while quietly standing is not well understood. Ludbrook[8] found the pressures in the superficial and deep veins to be essentially the same during quiet standing. Arnoldi[9] found that the pressure in the posterior tibial vein to be 1 mmHg

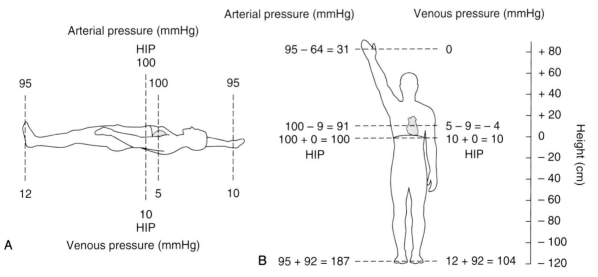

Figure 8-6 Pressures found in the normal arterial and venous system in the **(A)** horizontal and **(B)** upright position. HIP represents the hydrostatic indifferent point, located just below the diaphragm. (From Strandness and Sumner,[49] with permission.)

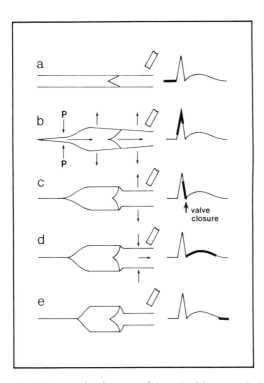

Figure 8-7 Schematic diagram of the velocities recorded distal to a valve during the phases of valve closure. **(A)** baseline with valve open. **(B)** With rise in proximal pressure (P), there will be some reflux as the diameter of the vein increases. **(C)** Valve closure. **(D)** Recoil of vein wall. **(E)** Cessation of flow. (From van Bemmelen et al.,[50] with permission.)

higher, which would tend to keep the valves in the perforating veins closed. The role of the venous valves during exercise is intuitively obvious. Since their major purpose is to promote antegrade flow, the changes that take place to prevent reflux from occurring are very important (Fig. 8-7). The other essential parts of the circuit are patent outflow veins and an active and functioning calf muscle pump. The actual changes that occur with a single step (Fig. 8-8) have been characterized by cinephlebography. The venous pressure changes at the level of the foot that occur with this single step are shown in Fig. 8-9.

Calf muscle contraction will empty the soleal sinuses and gastrocnemial veins into the posterior tibial and popliteal veins. As relaxation occurs, the veins of the normal limb are nearly empty and can fill from both the proximal venous segments by reflux and antegrade via blood coming from the capillary network. It also appears that the superficial veins empty into the deep system during the phase of muscular relaxation.

The volumes of blood and the pressures generated by calf muscle contraction have been estimated. It has been estimated that the volume of the two soleal si-

nuses is on the order of 8 ml. The volume of the proximal half of the intermuscular veins is also not large and is probably within the range of 30 ml, which is close to the stroke volume of the calf during active standing.[10] The pressures generated are in the range of 100 to 200 mmHg.[19]

Venous flow patterns are dependent on the site of interrogation, body position, and the phase of the respiratory cycle. This is clearly illustrated in Figure 8-10, where simultaneous recordings were made from the subclavian and femoral veins with the patient supine and upright. It should be noted that the change in position results in a phase shift in the timing of flow in the femoral vein. In the supine position, it is antegrade during expiration. In the vertical position, the opposite is true for the femoral vein.

Since nearly all of the major problems that we deal with clinically are in the lower limbs, it is important that we come to understand the flow patterns, how they are generated and how they may be influenced by disease. Moneta et al.[11] studied a series of normal subjects to determine the relationship between body position and femoral venous flow velocity. The dramatic effect of gravity can be seen in the diameters of femoral vein, when a normal subject is moved from −10 to +30 degrees. In the −10-degree position, the mean common femoral vein diameter corrected for body surface area was 0.447 ± 11 cm/m², as compared with 0.90 ± 016 cm/m² in the +30-degree position. This represents a nearly 92 percent increase. There is also a dramatic change in flow rate in the femoral vein with a change in position. At −10 degrees, the mean flow velocity was 41 ± 10 cm/s, as compared with 13 ± 5 cm/s in the +30-degrees position (p < 0.001). There also appeared to be a linear relationship between the mean diameter of the femoral vein and the mean peak velocity (R = −0.99).

Moneta et al.[11] also evaluated the relationship between body position, respiration and the events on the right side of the heart. With the body in −10 degrees, the blood flow is largely dependent on cardiac events (Fig. 8-11). There is a marked increase in flow during diastole, with flow essentially coming to zero during systole. As the position changed to a more upright one, the flow events come to be dominated more by the events of the respiratory cycle (Fig. 8-12).

VENOUS SYSTEM AS A RESERVOIR

It has been estimated that 60 to 75 percent of the blood in the body is to be found in the veins.[12] Of this total volume, about 80 percent is contained in veins of less than 200 μm in diameter.[13] It is important to ex-

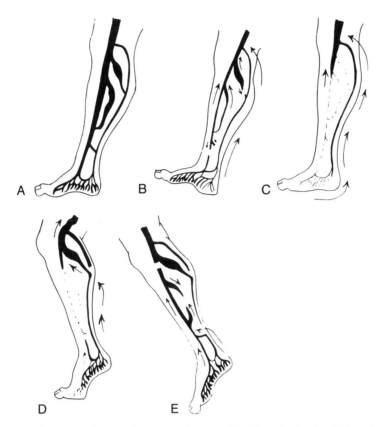

Figure 8-8 Sequence of volume changes that occur in the calf with a single step: **(A)** resting; **(B)** heel pressed against support (early contraction); **(C)** entire foot pressed against support (fully contracted); **(D)** knee flexed (forefoot compressed to floor, soleus contracted, gastrocnemius relaxed); **(E)** all muscles relaxed. (From Almen and Nylander,[51] with permission.)

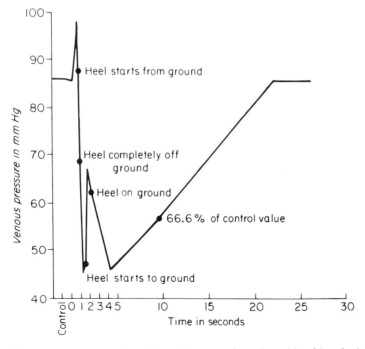

Figure 8-9 Changes in the mean pressure from the saphenous vein at the ankle with a single step. (From Pollack and Wood,[52] with permission.)

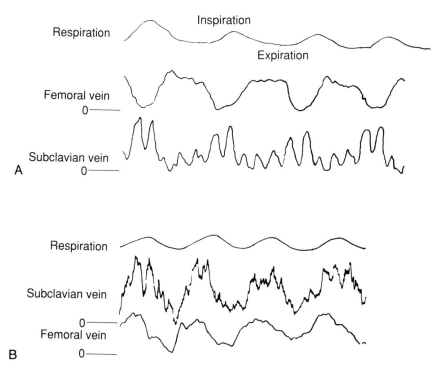

Figure 8-10 Simultaneous velocity tracings made from the subclavian and femoral veins in the **(A)** supine and **(B)** upright positions. (From Lewis et al.,[53] with permission.)

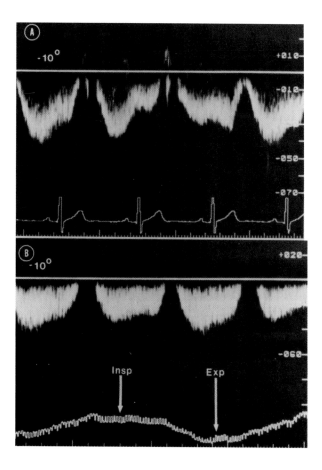

Figure 8-11 Femoral venous flow velocities as a function of position. **(A)** Cardiac events. **(B)** The relationship to events of the respiratory cycle. insp, inspiration; exp, expiration. (From Moneta et al.,[11] with permission.)

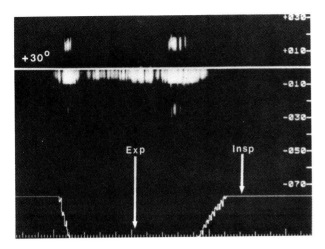

Figure 8-12 Femoral venous flow velocity patterns with the subject at +30 degrees. In this position, the respiratory cycle is the dominant factor affecting venous flow. Exp, expiration; Insp, inspiration. (From Moneta et al.,[11] with permission.)

amine the reservoir function as it is related to the major components. The splanchnic and skin are richly supplied by sympathetic fibers with the muscular veins have little or none. The veins in skeletal muscle are very responsive to catecholamines.[14]

METHODS OF STUDYING VENOUS FUNCTION

In the clinical assessment of acute and chronic venous problems, an assortment of methods are currently available, each of which will provide some insight into particular aspects of venous function. Function is closely tied to the anatomy of the venous system, so it is only natural that attempts would be made to depict the anatomy and relate this to outcome. The one imaging method designed for this purpose is phlebography. This method was first studied exhaustively by Bauer in 1940,[15] who must be given credit for its acceptance and introduction into clinical medicine. Since it could permit visualization of the major venous channels, the valve sites and the venous collaterals, it did provide indirect evidence concerning function. However, its major role was to assist in the diagnosis of acute deep venous thrombosis.

Plethysmography in a variety of forms has been used very successfully to evaluate many aspects of venous function (see Ch. 13). The strain gauge method in conjunction with venous occlusion methods could be used to measure venous capacitance and maximal venous outflow, both of which may be altered by both acute

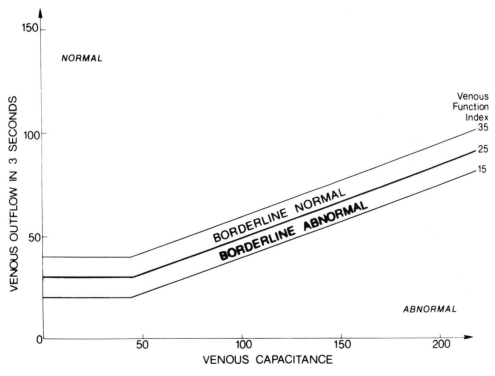

Figure 8-13 Scheme used for characterizing the relationship between venous outflow within 3 seconds and venous capacitance expressed in millimeters of paper deflection. In 83 percent of patients with acute deep venous thrombosis, the venous function index was in the 0 to 14 range. Sixteen percent were in the 15 to 24 range, with only 1 percent above 25. (From Strandness and Thiele,[48] with permission.)

and chronic venous disease. The mercury strain gauge plethysmographic method found its greatest use in physiologic studies and is still useful for documenting the venous volume and flow changes that occur in patients with venous claudication.[16-18]

The impedance plethysmographic method was developed primarily as a screening test for acute deep venous thrombosis.[19-20] This method, which was simple to use, could not be quantitated in the same way as the strain gauge method but was very useful and widely tested as a screening method. More recently, the air plethysmograph has been introduced as a method of studying many aspects of venous function.[21]

The air plethysmograph (APG) is a pneumatic volume system that can be calibrated. The inflatable cuff extends from the ankle to the knee. The cuff is inflated to a pressure of 6 mmHg, ensuring contact with the calf. The cuff is calibrated by injecting 100 ml of air from a calibrated syringe. The study procedure is designed to study the parameters relevant to venous function:

1. *Venous filling index.* As the patient moves from the supine to the upright position, the volume increase is a reflection of the amount of reflux.
2. *Ejection fraction (volume of blood expelled).* This is a measurement of the amount of volume decrease that accompanies a single tiptoe maneuver.
3. *Residual volume fraction.* This is the volume of the calf achieved by muscular contraction, as compared with that obtained by leg elevation.

This new method has the potential for describing many aspects of venous physiology that cannot be obtained with other methods. Since venous function is a complex interrelationship between the status of the venous valves and the ability of the calf muscle pump to work both in normal patients and in patients with various stages of chronic venous disease.

While impedance plethysmography became widely used as a screening method for acute deep venous thrombosis, the mercury strain gauge method has not found a place in the clinical practice of physicians interested in venous problems. They require a great deal of care in performing the procedure, and the information would not appear in many cases to make a difference in clinical management.

What was needed were methods that were easily applicable to most patient situations and at the same time, provided useful clinical data. The two methods most widely applied are continuous wave (CW) Doppler and photoplethysmography (PPG).[22-25]

CW Doppler was used for two major purposes-to assess the presence or absence of acute venous obstruction and secondly, to determine the location and extent of venous valvular incompetence.[23] The Doppler method is highly dependent on the skill of the examiner. Another drawback is that it is difficult if not impossible in some cases to be certain of the site(s) from which the venous velocity signals were obtained. This problem has been overcome by the development of duplex scanning (see Ch. 11).

The use of CW Doppler for the detection of reflux is in theory straightforward but is dependent on two basic methods of inducing reflux—the Valsalva maneuver and limb compression. The inadequacies of this approach are covered in Chapter 11. It will be noted that standing testing using the cuff method is much more reliable for detecting valvular incompetence at all levels of the superficial and deep veins of the lower limbs.

One of the major attractions of PPG is that it provides information on reflux, which appears to be very similar to that obtained by the assessment of venous pressure. The venous pressure changes with a single step have been well characterized. It is also well known that with loss of normal valve function, these pressure changes are drastically altered. The pressures with ambulation do not fall as low, and the recovery time is greatly shortened.[24] For example, if one accepts the time course of the changes with the PPG as similar to those obtained by direct measurement of venous pressure, the physiologic alterations are clearly evident. The time to recovery after five rhythmic compressions of the calf is 24 ± 12 seconds in limbs that are free of acute deep vein thrombosis. With damage to the valves of the deep system, this is in the range of 10 seconds.[24]

While both direct venous pressure measurements and the PPG results reflect abnormalities in valvular function, they do not predict the location for the valve defects that are responsible for the abnormal test results.[26] Van Bemmelen et al.[26] noted that an abnormal PPG is often associated with multilevel valvular reflux and skin changes in the gaitre zone of the lower leg. The PPG was compared with the results of duplex scanning and the cuff method of documenting reflux in both the superficial and deep venous systems. In an interesting study of PPG, Rosfors[27] was able to show that the results obtained were greatly influenced by regional hemodynamics. In addition, the results with PPG were most often found to be related to superficial rather than deep venous insufficiency.[28]

The only method that appears to be acceptable for investigation of valvular competence at all levels of the limb (superficial and deep) is duplex scanning using the cuff method described by van Bemmelen et al.[29,30] This method and its application is covered in detail in Chapter 66.

PHYSIOLOGIC CHANGES WITH VENOUS OBSTRUCTION

During the acute phase of venous obstruction secondary to venous thrombosis, venous pressure will be elevated, as the collaterals channels will have a higher than normal resistance to flow. It is also apparent from the strain gauge and impedance plethysmographic studies that venous emptying is impaired which is the sole basis for the diagnosis by this method. The data can be expressed in many ways, but the most useful is to plot the venous outflow against venous capacitance as shown in Figure 8-13. With the mercury strain gauge method, it is possible to express the capacitance and outflow values in quantitative terms. However, as noted in Figure 8-13, this is not possible with the impedance method, which uses chart paper deflection, rather than absolute numbers. As the venous collaterals improve and thrombus lysis begins, the maximal venous outflow will improve.

Acute venous occlusion also alters the flow velocity patterns observed. Obviously, in the sites of venous thrombosis, there will be no flow at all. The alterations in flow patterns are best seen in those veins distal to the site(s) of obstruction. Flows in the venous side of the circulation with the patient supine are dominated primarily by respiratory events. These are normally described as spontaneous and phasic. Spontaneous refers to flow detected without requiring augmentation to bring it out. This must always be present in the larger proximal veins (popliteal to inferior vena cava). Below the knee, spontaneous venous flow may not be detected if the ambient room temperature is low and there is marked vasoconstriction. When there is an occlusion proximal to the examination site, the venous flow is often continuous and not affected by respiration. However, as collateral function improves, the velocity patterns will again become spontaneous and phasic with respiration.

A large number of studies have been performed during the chronic phase after an episode of DVT. These have been very helpful in defining the status of the venous system and how it was affected by the DVT. Before considering some of these studies in detail, let us review some of the commonly held concepts that are not entirely true.

1. Venous thrombi rarely extend while the patient is on treatment. This is not true, as has been shown by more than one investigator.[31,32]
2. Recanalization is rare and often incomplete. While this is true to some degree, this is not the picture that we have been able to discern from our long-term studies.[31,32]
3. There is a good relationship between the extent of the original thrombosis and outcome. This is only partially true and this view will have to be modified to more closely fit the facts.[33-35]
4. Intrinsic fibrinolysis is ineffective in preventing the long-term sequelae of acute DVT. This is only partially true, since some patients with extensive DVT may have no future trouble at all.[34-36]
5. The popliteal valve is the key to preservation of reasonable venous function. This is not exactly true since it is the valves below the knee that bear the brunt of the potential directional changes in blood flow that accompany calf muscle contraction.[37,38]
6. Venous valvular reflux occurs months to years after an episode of acute DVT. This is not true as has been shown by prospective follow-up studies.[31,33,34]

Each of the above items is extremely important and has a direct bearing on outcome both with an episode of DVT and in the long term. The current status of each of these items in terms of the physiology and physiologic consequences will be dealt with separately.

Extension of Venous Thrombi

If the diagnosis of DVT is made, the only way that extension of the thrombus would be discovered is if a repeat imaging study were carried out, be it phlebography or duplex scanning. In most cases, the assumption is made that heparin—properly given—will prevent extension of the thrombus. Evidence for extension is as one might expect skimpy at best. Hirsh et al.[39] made the following statement with regard to heparin therapy—"ideally the amount of heparin given to a patient with thromboembolism should be the smallest dose that prevents thrombus extension, but precise data on this dose are not yet available for human thrombotic disease." In one of the few phlebographic studies, Marder et al.[40] showed that up to 20 percent of patients with deep venous thrombosis will get worse on heparin. In the duplex study conducted by Krupski et al.,[32] 38 percent of patients with proven DVT had thrombus progression on heparin. Only one-third of patients were not considered adequately anticoagulated.

In the study by Killewich et al.,[31] patients with DVT were followed at regular intervals of time by duplex scanning after diagnosis to assess the status of the veins, the level of recanalization and the prevalence of extension. In the study group of 21 patients, 3 (14 percent) extended during the first week, with 4 (19 percent) extending in the time interval of 30 to 180 days.

From a physiologic standpoint, it is difficult to know

what this means, particularly in terms of valve function. We do know that even with extension, intrinsic lysis still will occur. However, the earlier the lysis takes place, the more likely it is that venous valve function will be preserved.[34] Until more complete studies of this problem are done, it will be difficult to determine the significance of the extension and how it may affect long-term venous function.[41]

Recanalization After Deep Venous Thrombosis

Another interesting and fascinating aspect of DVT is the rate and extent to which intrinsic fibrinolysis may occur and how this may affect outcome. Before the availability of duplex scanning, short of phlebography, there was not a satisfactory method of documenting recanalization. While spontaneous thrombolysis is commonly observed in the pulmonary circuit, the extent to which it occurred in the leg was not well known or appreciated. In one of the earliest studies to use duplex scanning, Killewich et al.[31] found that up to 53 percent of patients with DVT would have recanalization of all involved segments by 90 days after presentation.

In a similar study, van Ramshorst et al.[42] carried out prospective follow-up of 20 legs in 18 patients. Recanalization was observed in 21 of the 31 initially occluded venous segments and occurred during the first 6 weeks after the diagnosis was made in 20 of 23 segments. As with the study by Killewich et al.,[31] these investigators also noted extension of the thrombi in seven of the patients.

It would appear that the intrinsic fibrinolytic system and its ability to clear the venous system of thrombi, as imperfect as it might be, can in some patients be extensive enough to not only restore patency but also preserve valve function. This may be why Browse et al.[35] was unable to predict on the basis of phlebographic appearance, the long-term outcome after an episode of DVT. The naturally occurring process might be aided and speeded up by the administration of a lytic agent such as Urokinase. Markel et al.[43] examined the potential for thrombolytic therapy in 209 patients who had DVT at the University of Washington Medical Center in Seattle. Of this group a contraindication to thrombolysis was present in 94 percent of the patients. Recent surgery was the most common contraindication for this form of therapy. Nonetheless, it would appear that thrombolysis may be of value in preserving valve function if it is given soon enough after the event, considered to be 7 days or less.

Key Valves

Since valves are found throughout the venous system is there any valve or set of valves that are critically important for proper venous function? Obviously they all play a role in preventing reflux during muscle contraction and relaxation and for this reason play an additive role in preventing ambulatory hypertension from developing. In order to put this problem into proper perspective, it is necessary to consider what the residual venous volumes and pressures are during walking. There are three basic patterns that can be postulated:

1. *Incompetence of the superficial system.* The residual venous volume within the superficial veins will remain high, and the mean venous pressure will not fall with walking.[44]
2. *Incompetence of the deep venous system.* The residual venous volume in the deep system remains high, with no fall in either the peak systolic pressure or the mean venous pressure during exercise.
3. *Combined superficial and deep incompetence.* There is an assumption that the communicating veins are also incompetent. In this case the residual volume remains high in both systems with the higher systolic pressures associated with contraction of the calf muscles transmitted to the superficial veins via the perforating veins.[45]

THERAPY FOR POSTTHROMBOTIC SYNDROME

In a study by van Bemmelen et al.,[38] 42 patients with chronic venous disease were studied by duplex scanning. The groups included 12 patients with ulceration who had a history of DVT, 13 patients with ulceration who gave no prior history of DVT, 10 patients with a history of DVT but no ulceration, and seven patients with varicose veins, no history of DVT and no ulceration. The findings in this study can be summarized as follows:

1. In all patients with varicose veins, no history of DVT, and no ulceration, the deep venous system distal to the level of the common femoral vein was competent.
2. In the 22 limbs with ulceration, venous valvular incompetence was found in 22 limbs at levels that communicated with the ulcer bearing area.
3. In the 17 limbs with DVT but normal ankle skin, there were only two instances where a single segment of posterior tibial vein in the midcalf was found to be incompetent. However, incompetence at more proximal levels of the venous system was common further lending support to the importance of valves below the knee in the preservation of skin integrity.

4. One of the striking findings in this study related to the status of the greater and lesser saphenous veins. In the group with a previous history of DVT and ulceration, reflux was found in the greater and lesser saphenous veins in 15 of the 25 limbs. By contrast, in the 10 limbs without ulceration but a positive history of DVT, the greater and lesser saphenous veins were competent.

The findings in the study by van Bemmelen et al.[38] raise several questions relevant to the issue of the posthrombotic syndrome, how it leads to ulceration, and what findings could be of importance in planning therapy. Why the greater and lesser saphenous veins became incompetent in some patients with ulceration is not known. It is doubtful that this occurred secondary to thrombosis followed by recanalization since concomitant thrombosis of the deep system plus the greater and lesser saphenous systems is very rare. Do these superficial veins become incompetent over time as a percentage of the venous volume below the knee is now shunted into the superficial venous system via the perforating veins?[46] The answer to this question will only be found by long-term sequential study of the status of the greater and lesser saphenous veins by duplex scanning in patients with DVT.

Do the findings of the van Bemmelen et al.[38] study have any relevance to the form of therapy that might be used for patients with chronic venous insufficiency? For the patients with primary varicose veins and a patent and competent deep venous system, the answer would appear to be straightforward. Removal of the incompetent superficial veins would be all that is needed.

For patients with ulceration, the problem would appear to be much more complex. In this setting, we now have incompetence of the deep system below the knee, in the popliteal region and in the greater and lesser saphenous veins. While one could remove perhaps the greater and lesser saphenous veins, this would leave the deep system untouched which would not appear to work since it was here that the problem took its origin. If one were to propose a valvuloplasty, what might be required and would be left untouched?

1. Valvuloplasty might be applied to 18 of 25 limbs with reflux in the superficial femoral veins, but this would leave 19 of 25 limbs with an incompetent popliteal vein.
2. If it were possible to correct the problem at both the superficial femoral and popliteal vein level, 16 of the 25 limbs with reflux would still be below the knee in the posterior tibial veins.
3. Without some attention to the veins below the knee, the perforating veins would also remain incompetent.

Perhaps one would have to entertain the following

therapy based on the findings in the study by van Bemmelen et al.[38]:

1. Removal of the incompetent superficial veins
2. Interruption of the incompetent perforating veins in the lower leg
3. Restoration of valve competence for those areas currently accessible where there is a prospect for success

The only areas where the latter seems reasonable, or is feasible at the moment, is in the superficial femoral and popliteal veins. For the critical area below the knee, where multiple levels of incompetence are frequent, valvuloplasty or replacement are not yet feasible and have not been tried. One of the major problems with venous valve surgery for the patient with advanced changes and ulceration is that compression hose is needed as well. It is clear that there are no answers to this problem short of a very large and perhaps randomized clinical trial to determine which form of therapy is most successful.

REFERENCES

1. Basmajian JV: Distribution of valves in the femoral, external iliac and common iliac veins and their relationship to varicose veins. Surg Gynecol Obstet 95:537, 1952
2. Cockett FB, Dodd H (eds): The Pathology and Surgery of the Veins of the Lower Limb. Churchill Livingstone, Edinburgh, 1976
3. Learoyd BM, Taylor MG: Alterations with age in the viscoelastic properties of human arterial walls. Circ Res 18:278, 1966
4. Kugelen Ab: Uber des Verhaltnis von Ringmuskulatatur an Innendruck in menschlichen grossen Veren. Z Zellforsch Mikrosk Anat 127:278, 1955
5. Gauer OH, Thron HL: Postural changes in the circulation. p. 2409. In Hamilton WF, Dow P (eds): Handbook of Physiology. Section 2: Circulation. Vol. III. American Physiological Society, Washington, D.C., 1965
6. Holling HE, Verel D: Circulation in the elevated forearm. Clin Sci 16:197, 1957
7. Henry JP, Slaughter OL, Greiner T: A medical massage suit for continuous wear. Angiology 6:482, 1955
8. Ludbrook J: Functional aspects of the veins of the leg. Am Heart J 64:796, 1962
9. Arnoldi CC: Venous pressures in the leg of healthy human subjects at rest and during muscular exercise in the nearly erect position. Acta Chir Scand 130:570, 1965
10. van Bemmelen PS, Bergan JJ: Physiology and Pathophysiology. p. 13. In: Quantitative Measurement of Venous Incompetence. RG Landes, Austin, TX, 1992
11. Moneta GL, Bedford G, Beach KW et al: Duplex ultrasound assessment of venous diameters, peak velocities and flow patterns. J Vasc Surg 8:286, 1988

12. Shepherd JT: Role of the veins in the circulation. Circulation 33:484, 1966

13. Knisely WH, Mahaley MS, Jr, Jett HH: Approximation of total vascular space and its distribution in three sizes of blood vessels in rats by plastic casts. Circ Res 6:20, 1958

14. Shepherd JT: Muscle pumping and the dependent leg. Circ Res 19:180, 1978

15. Bauer G: A venographic study of thromboembolic problems. Acta Chir Scand, suppl 61, 1940

16. Baumgartner I, Franzewck UK, Bollinger A: Venous claudication evaluated by ambulatory plethysmography. Phlebology 7:2, 1992

17. Cramer M, Langlois Y, Beach KW et al: Standardization of venous flow measurement by strain gauge plethysmography: the definition of normality. Bruit 7:33, 1983

18. Whitney RJ: The measurement of volume changes in human limbs. J Physiol (Lond) 121:1, 1953

19. Hull R, Hirsh J, Sackett DJ et al: Combined use of leg scanning and impedance plethysmography using the occlusive cuff technique in the diagnosis of venous thrombosis: an alternative to venography. N Engl J Med 296:1497, 1977

20. Wheeler HB: Diagnosis of deep vein thrombosis: symposium on deep vein thrombosis. Am J Surg 150:7, 1985

21. Christopoulos D, Nicolaides A, Szendro G: Venous reflux quantification and correlation with clinical severity of chronic venous disease. Br J Surg 75:352, 1988

22. Abramowitz HB, Queral LA, Flinn WR et al: The use of photoplethysmography in the assessment of venous insufficiency: a comparison to venous pressure measurements. Surgery 86:434, 1979

23. Barnes RW: Doppler ultrasonic diagnosis of venous disease. p. 724. In Bernstein EF (ed): Noninvasive Diagnostic Techniques in Vascular Disease. 3rd Ed. CV Mosby, St. Louis, 1985

24. Killewich LA, Martin R, Cramer M et al: An objective assessment of the physiologic changes in the postthrombotic syndrome. Arch Surg 120:424, 1985

25. van Bemmelen PS, Bergan JJ: Photoplethysmography and LRR. p. 37. In: Quantitative Measurement of Venous Incompetence. RG Landes, Austin, TX, 1992

26. van Bemmelen PS, van Ramshorst B, Eikelboom B: Photoplethysmography reexamined: lack of correlation with duplex scanning. Surgery 112:544, 1992

27. Rosfors S: Venous photoplethymography: relationship between transducer position and regional distribution of venous insufficiency. J Vasc Surg 11:436, 1990

28. Rosfors S: A methodological study of venous valvular insufficiency and musculovenous pump function of the lower leg. Phlebology 7:12, 1992

29. van Bemmelen PS, Bedford G, Beach K, Strandness DE, Jr: Quantitative segmental evaluation of venous valvular reflux with duplex ultrasound scanning. J Vasc Surg 10:425, 1989

30. van Bemmelen PS, Bergan JJ: Segmental duplex reflux examination and color flow imaging. p. 51. In Quantitative Measurement of Venous Incompetence. RG Landes, Austin, TX, 1992

31. Killewich LA, Bedford GR, Beach KW, Strandness DE, Jr: Spontaneous lysis of deep venous thrombi: rate and outcome. J Vasc Surg 9:89, 1989

32. Krupski WC, Bass A, Dilley RG et al: Propagation of deep venous thrombosis identified by duplex ultrasonography. J Vasc Surg 12:467, 1990

33. Markel A, Manzo RA, Bergelin RO, Strandness DE, Jr: Valvular reflux following deep vein thrombosis: incidence and time of occurrence. J Vasc Surg 15:377, 1992

34. Meissner MH, Manzo RA, Bergelin RO, Strandness DE, Jr: Deep venous insufficiency: relationship between lysis and subsequent reflux. J Vasc Surg (in press)

35. Browse NL, Clemenson G, Thomas ML: Is the postphlebitic leg always postphlebitic? Relation between phlebographic appearance and late sequelae. Br Med J 281:1167, 1981

36. Strandness DE, Jr, Langlois YE, Cramer MM et al: Long-term sequelae of acute venous thrombosis. JAMA 250:1289, 1983

37. Shull KC, Nicolaides AN, Fernandes e Fernandes J, Miles C et al: Significance of popliteal reflux in relation to ambulatory venous pressure and ulceration. Arch Surg 114:1304, 1979

38. van Bemmelen PS, Bedford G, Beach K, Strandness DE, Jr: Status of the valves in the superficial and deep venous system in chronic venous disease. Surgery 106:730, 1991

39. Hirsh J, Marder VJ, Salzman EW, Hull RD: Treatment of venous thromboembolism. p. 1270. In Colman RW, Hirsh J, Marder VJ, Salzman EW (eds): Hemostasis and Thrombosis: Basic Principles and Clinical Practice. JP Lippincott, Philadelphia, 1987

40. Marder VJ, Sooulen RL, Atichartakarn V et al: Quantitative venographic assessment of deep vein thrombosis in the evaluation of streptokinase and heparin therapy. J Clin Lab Med 89:1018, 1977

41. Strandness DE, Jr: Thrombus propagation and level of anticoagulation—an editorial. J Vasc Surg 12:497, 1990

42. van Ramshorst B, Bemmelen PS, Hoeneveld H et al: Thrombus regression in deep venous thrombosis: quantification of spontaneous thrombolysis with duplex scanning. Circulation 86:414, 1992

43. Markel A, Manzo RA, Strandness DE, Jr: The potential role of thrombolytic therapy in venous thrombosis. Arch Intern Med 152:1265, 1992

44. Hjelmstedt A: Pressure decrease in the dorsal pedal veins on walking in patients with and without thrombosis. Acta Chir Scand 134:309, 1968

45. Bjordal RI: Simultaneous pressure and flow recording in varicose veins of the lower extremity. A hemodynamic study of venous dysfunction. Acta Chir Scand 136:309, 1970

46. Cockett FB, Jones DFW: The ankle blow out syndrome, a new approach to the varicose ulcer problem. Lancet 1:17, 1953

47. Hobbs JT: Anatomy of leg veins. p. 18. In Haeger K (ed): The Treatment of Venous Disorders. JB Lippincott, Philadelphia, 1977

48. Strandness DE, Jr, Thiele BL (eds): Venous anatomy of the lower limb. p. 1. In: Selected Topics in Venous Disor-

ders: Pathophysiology, Diagnosis and Treatment. Future, Mt. Kisco, NY, 1981

49. Strandness DE, Jr, Sumner DS: Venous hemodynamics and control of venous capacity. p. 120. In: Hemodynamics for Surgeons. Grune & Stratton, Orlando, FL, 1975

50. van Bemmelin PS, Beach KW, Bedford G, Strandness DE, Jr: The mechanism of venous valve closure: its relationship to the velocity of reverse flow. Arch Surg 125:617, 1990

51. Almen T, Nylander G: Serial phlebography of the normal leg during muscular contraction and relaxation. Acta Radiol 57:264, 1962

52. Pollack AA, Wood EH: Venous pressure in the saphenous vein at the ankle in man during exercise and changes in posture. J Appl Physiol 1:649, 1949

53. Lewis J, Hobbs J, Yao J: Normal and abnormal femoral vein velocities. p. 51. In Roberts VP (ed): Blood Flow Measurement. Williams & Wilkins, Baltimore, 1972

9

Pathology of Deep Venous Thrombosis

Timothy R. Cheatle

DEFINITIONS

A deep venous thrombosis (DVT) occurs when a thrombus is formed within the veins running in the subfascial compartment of the lower limb, the iliac veins, or the inferior vena cava. The much less common situation of upper limb venous thrombosis is not discussed in this chapter.

Thrombophlebitis occurs when there is a marked inflammatory response to a thrombosis. It is most commonly seen in the superficial veins, where, as the name implies, the pathology lies superficial to the deep fascia of the leg. While there is a spectrum, DVT is not considered a truly inflammatory disorder. For that reason, the term *thrombophlebitis* is reserved for the problem that occurs in the superficial veins of the legs and arms.

NATURAL HISTORY

Venous thromboses consist of an adherent nidus at the site of formation, with coralline thrombus superimposed on it. A "red tail" is attached to the coralline thrombus and points in the direction of blood flow. Structurally the tail is composed of a loose mesh of fibrin and erythrocytes, with white lines (the "lines of Zahn") spaced throughout it at regular intervals. These represent layers of platelets deposited on the red thrombus and act as a stimulus to the deposition of further thrombus. Platelets are not plentiful at the site of origin of the thrombus and probably play a minor role in their pathogenesis (see p. 123).

When the thrombus fills the vein, it will adhere to the wall, making it relatively safe from the risk of embolization. The thrombus will then contract (generally about 5 days after formation), and recanalization will begin. Valves within the thrombosed vein may be destroyed, but this is not invariable. This process describes the type of DVT most commonly seen. It is likely that many small thrombi will lyse completely without adverse consequences.

SCALE OF THE PROBLEM

Few would disagree that the problem of DVT, together with its potentially catastrophic sequelae of pulmonary embolism (PE) and the post-thrombotic limb, is a major one. Despite many studies, the precise incidence and prevalence remain unknown. This is largely due to the difficulty in making a reliable clinical diagnosis of both DVT and PE. Many patients suspected of having a DVT will not have the disorder, while many true DVTs remain silent. The same applies to PE.

Therefore, clinical estimates of prevalence cannot be

viewed as reliable. Nonetheless, the large surveys, as imperfect as they are, provide the only data against which we can gauge the magnitude of the problem. Coon et al.[1] have arrived at a figure of over 250,000 clinical DVTs per annum in the United States, with a prevalence of 500,000 to 1,000,000 active or healed venous ulcers. Gjores, in Sweden, estimated on clinical grounds that 2 to 3 percent of the Swedish population had suffered a DVT at some period of their life.[2] As many as 100,000 to 200,000 people die each year in the United States from PE,[3] while roughly 2,000,000 work days are lost annually in the same country because of post-thrombotic symptoms.[4]

More accurate and objective methods of determining the presence or absence of DVT tend to be applied to selected groups of subjects, making population-wide conclusions hard to estimate. Patients clinically thought to be suffering from DVT, or at high risk of developing DVT, will comprise such studies. Autopsy-based studies suffer from the same problem.

Some estimates of the incidence of DVT have been made using venography. Nylander and Olivecrona,[5] basing their study on the catchment area of their hospital in Malmo, found 231 positive venograms in one year from a population of 263,000 and derived an incidence of 0.9/1,000/year. Although this study eliminates false negatives (assuming venography to be 100 percent sensitive), it does not by its nature detect DVT that occur without symptoms. Kakkar[6] has shown that one-third of patients undergoing venography for a suspicion of DVT will have normal deep veins. Conversely, one-half of patients diagnosed as having a DVT by iodine 125 (^{125}I) fibrinogen test are asymptomatic.

Autopsy data tend to give strikingly high estimates of DVT prevalence. A number of studies carried out in patients dying in hospital have shown a prevalence of DVT ranging from 34 to 72 percent.[7-11] Such thrombi may develop in the late stages of the terminal illness, making it very difficult to extrapolate these data to the general population.

For surgeons, it is the DVT that develops during the postoperative period that are of particular importance. Here more definitive data are available. This was made possible by the ^{125}I fibrinogen uptake test, developed by Hobbs and Davies in 1960.[12] This method has provided prospective information on the incidence of DVT in the surgical patient.

Colditz et al.[13] have examined the published literature and found an overall DVT incidence of 29 percent for patients undergoing general surgical procedures without any form of prophylaxis. This is close to the figure of 35 percent found by Flanc et al.[14] For individual subgroups of patients the risk may be much higher, especially in the orthopedic patients or in those with malignant disease. A 75 percent incidence of DVT has been found for patients undergoing repair of a pertrochanteric fracture, for example.[15] A number of studies have indicated high rates of DVT following vascular procedures.[16-18] This is surprising, given the liberal usage of heparin during the performance of these procedures. However, it should be kept in mind that studies using ^{125}I uptake are likely to have a high rate of false-positive results in such patients. Wounds and bruising in the leg will cause the isotope to be taken up within the area, thus giving a false-positive result. The relative risks of developing DVT in different surgical sub-groups have been reviewed by Browse et al.[19]

PREDISPOSING FACTORS

Apart from surgery, a number of variables are associated with an increased (sometimes decreased) likelihood of developing DVT. Some of these associations are rather tenuous, some more convincing. In nearly all cases, the reason for the association remains poorly understood.

Age

Many series have shown that the incidence of DVT increases with age.[17,20-22] A ^{125}I fibrinogen uptake study of postoperative DVT, conducted by Kakkar et al.,[23] showed that the condition was almost twice as common in the over-60 group of patients (46 percent) as in the under-60 group (24 percent).

DVT is uncommon in childhood, although postoperative DVT has been reported.[24] Pulmonary embolism has been reported more often, usually in association with cachexia, infection or chronic wasting conditions.[25]

Sex

Most series do not show a significant sex difference in the incidence of DVT. Women are sometimes said to be at higher risk, but the evidence is not convincing. Pregnancy-related factors may lead to a higher DVT rate, but being a woman per se does not seem to be a risk factor.

Race

When assessing racial differences regarding the incidence of DVT it is difficult to separate local geographic and cultural factors, such as climate and diet, from true ethnic variability. In addition, in many poorer regions of the world, objective investigative techniques such as the ^{125}I fibrinogen uptake test are less readily available. Epidemiologic studies will then have to rely on clinical diagnosis which is an unreliable marker for DVT. Allowing for these caveats, racial variation does seem to occur. A number of reports have indicated a lower incidence of postoperative DVT in the Far East and Africa,[26-30] although a rigorous South African study using ^{125}I fibrinogen uptake and venography did not confirm interracial differences.[31] Burkitt[32] reported that DVT is rare among primitive tribes.

Obesity

Obese people have higher plasma fibrinogen levels and lower plasma fibrinolytic activity than do normal persons.[33,34] Most studies indicate a higher incidence of DVT among the obese.

Oral Contraception

That there is a significantly higher risk of the development of DVT among users of the contraceptive pill than among nonusers is now incontrovertible.[35] The risk of the development of a postoperative DVT is less for women using a preparation containing less than 100 μg of estrogen than among those using a higher-strength preparation.[36] Possible mechanisms have been reviewed by Ogston.[37] In particular, a fall in the inhibitory activity of factor Xa has been postulated as the mode of action.[38] There does not appear to be a higher incidence of DVT among women taking low-dose estrogen preparations to relieve menopausal symptoms.[39]

Pregnancy

Although the increased development of DVT during and shortly after pregnancy is well known, most studies will be based on clinical evaluation alone, making them less accurate. There is an understandable unwillingness to subject expectant mothers to the possible risks of x-rays or radioactive isotopes. However, in the few studies to use such techniques, the risk of developing DVT may have been overestimated; using venography, Kierkegaard found an incidence of less than one DVT per 1000 pregnant women.[40] Nevertheless, a 1982 government report found PE to be the single most common cause of maternal death in pregnancy and the puerperium.[41]

Inactivity and Body Position

In addition to prolonged bed rest,[8] DVT is generally recognized as being associated with any activity entailing prolonged immobility, such as sitting continuously during long-haul flights. A celebrated example in the United Kingdom was the sharp rise in DVT and PE that occurred early in World War II, when Luftwaffe bombing raids led to large numbers of civilians taking shelter in underground air-raid shelters, often in awkward positions and for long periods.[42]

Blood Group

There is some evidence that blood group O is protective against DVT and PE.[43,44]

Other Diseases

Malignancy,[45] paraplegia,[46] fractures of the lower limb,[47] myocardial infarction,[48] polycythaemia rubra vera,[49] ulcerative colitis,[50] Behçet syndrome,[51] homocystinuria,[52] and sickle cell disease[53] are all associated with an increased incidence of DVT and PE. A full review and discussion of the possible mechanisms in various disease states has been given by Ogston.[54]

Previous DVT

People who have already had a DVT are at higher risk of the development of another.[23]

Smoking

DVT has repeatedly been shown to be less common among cigarette smokers than among nonsmokers or pipe smokers.[55-57]

Drugs

Apart from the oral contraceptive, a number of drugs have been described as leading to an increased risk of developing DVT. In all cases, the risk appears to be small and does not justify withholding the drug when its use is thought to be necessary. Corticosteroids have been associated with DVT, but it seems likely that, in most cases, the DVT could equally be ascribed to the underlying illness and associated immobility for which the drug was prescribed. Decreased levels of serum plasminogen activator activity have been described in healthy volunteers taking prednisolone.[58] At least one report has described a significantly increased incidence of DVT in renal transplant patients taking cyclosporine compared with patients taking alternative forms of immunosuppression.[59] Four cases of DVT occurring in women who had recently started taking tamoxifen were reported in 1978.[60] However, three were suffering from metastatic breast cancer, itself a predisposing factor. No link between the drug and DVT has subsequently been confirmed. Paradoxically, heparin is associated with an increased incidence of recurrent venous thrombosis, related to its propensity to cause thrombocytopenia by a process of platelet aggregation. This has been termed the heparin-induced thrombosis-thrombocytopenia syndrome (HITTS).[61]

FORMATION OF THROMBI

Site of Origin

Most DVTs start in the calf. A small proportion then propagate proximally, leading to the more serious entity of iliofemoral thrombosis. However, thrombi may originate in the proximal veins (popliteal to inferior vena cava) without extension from the calf.

The earliest studies to address the question of site of origin involved autopsy dissections. Originally it was thought that most thrombi had their origin in the iliofemoral veins[62] but at about mid-century the opposite view appeared.[7,8] More recent techniques such as the ^{125}I-fibrinogen test and postmortem intraosseous venography have tended to confirm this concept.[14,63] The soleal sinusoids are the commonest single site of origin. It must be stressed, however, that DVTs may form de novo in the more proximal larger veins. Browse and Lea-Thomas found, using venography, that in one third of examined limbs with DVT, the site of origin was proximal to the calf.[64] Another study of 535 DVTs showed a rather lower proportion (8 percent) starting in the proximal veins.[65] All these patients were, naturally, being examined on clinical suspicion of DVT; screening with the ^{125}I-fibrinogen test indicates that if subclinical silent DVTs are included, the proportion swings back in favor of a distal origin. Nevertheless, a significant proportion of patients with clinically significant DVT will have normal calf veins.

DVTs can also originate in valve sinuses. The stasis and turbulence one might anticipate in sinuses has been confirmed using cineradiography and cinemicrography[66,67] and postmortem evidence for this site of formation has been known for many years.[68] Intermittent pneumatic compression of the foot has been shown by videphlebography to cause increased blood flow in the valve pockets,[69] probably the basis of its prophylactic action against DVT formation.

A number of studies have shown a slight preponderance of left-sided DVT. This has been explained by Cockett as being due to two factors: the slightly greater angle of the left common iliac vein vis-à-vis the inferior vena cava, and, perhaps more importantly, its tendency to be compressed by the right common iliac artery, which crosses it.[70]

Mechanism of Initiation

The relative importance of the three factors making up Virchow's triad has still to be settled. He suggested that venous thrombosis was initiated by changes in the vein wall, the flow of blood, and the constituents of the blood. Although it is highly unlikely that any one of these is solely responsible for the development of DVT, it is possible to discuss the relative importance of these elements and their potential contribution to the problem.

Vein Wall

The most convincing clinical evidence of the importance of endothelial damage in DVT pathogenesis is to be found in the very high incidence of femoral vein DVT following hip surgery for trauma.[47,71] It is the proximity of the DVT to the site of injury in such cases that implies a local effect on the vessel wall.

There have been two problems associated with the investigation of the importance of endothelial changes in DVT production, one technical and one due to methodologic error. Until the advent of electron microscopy, investigators relied on conventional transmission electron microscopy to search for endothelial abnormalities in vessels affected by DVT. The fact they were generally unable to find any may be ascribed to the inadequacy of the technique, rather than to the integrity of the vessels. The methodologic error has been in the manner in which experimental trauma has been applied to veins in an attempt to create a model for DVT formation. Thrombi in the venous system typically contain plentiful fibrin, with many enmeshed red cells. Platelets are relatively scarce in contrast to arterial thrombi, which are plentiful. Many of the models used to study DVT have involved the infliction of massive endothelial damage with the subsequent production of platelet-rich thrombi. These do not relate closely to the situation seen in patients where such damage is unusual. A more realistic model is that of Ashford and Freiman,[72] who found that gentle pinching of the rat femoral vein (causing some edema but no bleeding) could lead to endothelial desquamation and the subsequent deposition of a fibrin mesh containing relatively few platelets. This corresponds both to the degree of vein wall damage likely in patients suffering trauma to adjacent structures and also to the type of thrombosis seen in this situation.

Over the past two decades, Stewart has been responsible for much of the work on the integrity of the venous endothelium in DVT. She demonstrated that direct injury was not a prerequisite for the development of vein wall damage. A combination of local stasis and distant trauma was sufficient to cause endothelial desquamation in the wall of a large vein. This was brought about by white blood cell adherence to, and migration through, the vein wall, with slight separation of the endothelial cells, as shown by electron microscopy. This exposure of subendothelial structures was the trigger for activating the coagulation process.[73] She also showed that migrating white blood cells tended to bind fibrin and suggested that they may be responsible for anchoring fibrin to the vein wall.[74]

Another possible mechanism by which endothelial damage may occur without direct trauma has been suggested by Hamer.[75] He measured the PO_2 within valve pockets and showed that when flow within them became stagnant, the partial pressure of oxygen fell to levels that resulted in damage to the cells of the vein wall. This explanation may be a factor leading to the development of thrombi within the valve sinuses.

Another important area for the genesis of DVT may be related to the endothelium itself. We now realize that the endothelium is far from being a simple layer lining blood vessels. The endothelial cell is a dynamic structure synthesizing a number of compounds that are crucial to the balance between coagulation and fibrinolysis. Tissue plasminogen activator (tPA), prostacyclin, and glycosoaminoglycans (which are mainly in the form of heparan sulfate, a weak anticoagulant) are all found in the vein wall and all tend to counter the tendency toward thrombosis. Reduced levels of tPA in particular have been associated with familial DVT,[76] and a proportion of patients with DVT have an increased plasma level of plasminogen activator inhibitor.[77] Attempts to correlate the preoperative levels of tPA inhibitor with subsequent DVT development, have met with some success.[78] The concept of endothelial cell dysfunction as a factor in DVT pathogenesis has been discussed more fully by Browse et al.[19]

Stasis

Reviews of the pathogenesis of DVT often start any discussion of the role of stasis by quoting Hewson's 1771 experiment, in which he showed that blood isolated in a segment of vein between ligatures took several hours to clot.[79] This was often taken to decry the importance of stasis as compared to the other components of Virchow's triad. Nevertheless, the blood does

clot, and it is likely that simple stasis is the single most important factor contributing to DVT formation in certain patient groups. For example, there is a much higher incidence of DVT in the paralyzed leg of patients who have suffered a stroke than in the contralateral leg.[80] PE is also a common necropsy finding among such patients.[81] The rate of venous blood flow is demonstrably slower in such limbs,[82] as it is in the limbs of patients undergoing general anaesthesia,[83] where stasis is exacerbated by the vasodilatory properties of anaesthetics such as halothane. Selective venography has demonstrated that stasis in the horizontal leg is particularly marked in the soleal sinusoids,[84] generally accepted as the most common site of origin of DVT. Stasis of blood would also seem to be the overriding factor in DVT formation where there is mechanical extrinsic venous compression, such as in pregnancy or venous obstruction by a transplanted kidney.[85,86]

It is also true to say that stasis is inextricably bound to endothelial damage, with hypoxia as the responsible agent, and that it is a potent catalyst to the formation of thrombi when the third member of Virchow's triad, increased blood coagulability, is present. Its importance must not be overlooked.

Changes in Blood Constituents

Changes in the constituents of blood may be conveniently divided into platelets and the coagulation and fibrinolytic pathways. Unlike the situation in arteries, platelets probably do not play an important role in the pathogenesis of DVT. A study by Sevitt[87] indicated that platelets were only numerous in the propagated parts of small DVTs (the "lines of Zahn") and that the distal portions, where the thrombi started, were relatively platelet poor. This is in opposition to traditional teaching which states that the coralline thrombus is formed principally of platelets. It has subsequently been shown that platelets are not required in order for fibrin to be deposited at low flow rates.[88]

It has been known for many years that platelet activity rises appreciably following trauma,[89] but attempts to correlate this rise with an increased susceptibility to DVT have not been successful.[90] Clinical trials of antiplatelet agents have not shown any benefit in reducing postoperative DVT,[91] and there is evidence that heparin, the most widely used prophylactic agent, actually increases platelet adhesiveness.[92] Smoking, which appears to protect against DVT formation, is also known to promote both platelet adhesiveness and platelet aggregation.[93,94] Therefore, it seems unlikely that platelets play a major role in the initiation of DVT. Since platelets are vital to normal hemostasis by virtue of their propensity to adhere to damaged endothelium and subendothelial structures, this might be thought to argue against a significant role for endothelial damage as a major factor in DVT formation.

Changes in the Coagulation and Fibrinolytic Pathways

There is a general consensus that patients predisposed to DVT formation harbor a poorly defined "hypercoagulable" state. Much of the thrombosis research of recent years has been aimed at defining exactly which components of the clotting and fibrinolytic systems are abnormal in patients with DVT.

The rise in plasma fibrinogen after surgery is a constant feature that might promote DVT formation. This is probably largely due to its effect on blood viscosity, as demonstrated by Dormandy.[95]

Wessler was the first to show how activated clotting factors, augmented by local stasis, were potent stimuli for intravascular thrombosis.[96] How are such factors activated in the circumstances that led to DVT formation? (See Ch. 18 for a detailed discussion of the coagulation mechanism.) Briefly, blood coagulation can be initiated in two ways. There is an "intrinsic" pathway in which circulating factor XII (Hageman factor), kininogen, prekallikrein, and factor XI are activated upon contact with, typically, collagen. They then interact to activate factor IX, precipitating a cascade of reactions culminating in the polymerisation of fibrinogen to fibrin. Thus, it can be seen how trauma (e.g., surgery) can activate coagulation by exposing blood elements to subendothelial or extravascular structures and setting the intrinsic pathway in motion. Circulating activated factors may then cause thrombosis at a distant site where local stasis is present, such as the soleal sinuses.

The extrinsic system is activated on cell surfaces, the initial step being the binding of tissue factor to factor VII in the presence of calcium. This leads to the activation of factor X and, through a further cascade, to the formation of fibrin. Tissue factor is a membrane glycoprotein that is expressed on cell surfaces. Its distribution throughout the body has been mapped immunohistochemically.[97] It tends to be present in high quantities in regions in which bleeding would be particularly destructive, such as the cerebral cortex, but is absent from synovial membrane, which is thought to influence the site of bleeding in hemophilia. It tends to be located on the adventitial rather than the intimal surfaces of blood vessels but, crucially, it can also be expressed on the surface of activated circulating monocytes. Its expression is stimulated by specific agonists, which include endotoxin, interleukin-1 (IL-1), and tumor necrosis factor (TNF).[98] Thus, one can postulate a second mechanism for the initiation of DVT.

Schmid-Schonbein has shown that the likelihood of a leukocyte adhering to a vessel wall is inversely proportional to the shear force exerted on it, and thus to its velocity.[99] Monocytes, being the largest species of white cell, marginate preferentially. As mentioned above, Stewart has shown conclusively how white blood cells adhere to venous endothelium in large numbers when venous stasis is allied to distant trauma. The subsequent monocyte activation leads to the release of IL-1 and TNF, (both known to be released by activated monocytes.[100,101] These cytokines stimulate the expression of tissue factor, triggering activation of the extrinsic pathway of coagulation. This model would also help to explain the tendency of nontrauma patients with septicemia or malignancy to develop DVT, where high circulating levels of endotoxin or cytokines, or both, may be responsible.

If these are the mechanisms by which the coagulation pathways may initiate venous thrombosis when predisposing factors are present, are there any common abnormalities of these pathways which in themselves lead to DVT formation? An increasing body of research would suggest that there are. Plate et al.[102] examined a number of coagulation and fibrinolytic parameters in 69 patients who had suffered an iliofemoral DVT, most requiring surgical thrombectomy. The studies were carried out at least 6 months after the illness, in an attempt to offset any residual effects of the illness itself or consequent surgery. Significant abnormalities were found in 51 percent of those examined. The most common were defective fibrinolysis (usually increased tPA inhibitor levels) and increased factor VIII levels.[102] Of particular interest was the finding that 15 of the 21 patients who had developed an "idiopathic" thrombosis (i.e., one without significant predisposing factors) had coagulation abnormalities.

A fuller study by Felez reached similar conclusions,[98] although with a rather smaller proportion of clotting abnormalities. Of 578 unselected patients with a DVT, 92 (16 percent) had a demonstrable coagulopathy. Again, an increased tPA inhibitor level was the single most common aberrancy, and again abnormalities tended to be more common in those suffering from idiopathic thromboses. This study went on to examine relatives of those patients found to have abnormal coagulation and found large numbers to be affected (with the exception, interestingly, of those with increased tPA). This would seem to indicate that the observed abnormalities were the cause rather than the effect of DVT in the patient group. A full review of the congenital abnormalities of coagulation and fibrinolysis that may predispose to DVT has been given by Ogston[54] (see Ch. 18). Ideally, improved knowledge of the factors underlying the development of DVT will help us to predict accurately which patients are at greatest risk and to take the appropriate prophylactic action. There is evidence that protocols to predict those at risk are becoming more accurate.[103] Until such time as we can accurately predict who will develop DVT, it remains essential to remain alert to the potential risk of DVT. This will permit the application of effective prophylactic measures to prevent the development of this potentially lethal disease.

REFERENCES

1. Coon WW, Willis PW III, Keller JB: Venous thromboembolism and other venous disease in the Tecumseh community healthy study. Circulation 48:839, 1973
2. Gjores J-E: The incidence of venous thrombosis and its sequelae in certain districts of Sweden. Acta Chir Scand, suppl. 206:1, 1956
3. Dalen JE, Albert JS: Natural history of pulmonary embolism. Prog Cardiovasc Dis 17:259, 1975
4. Browse NL, Burnand KG: The post-phlebitic syndrome: a new look. In Bergan JJ, Yao JST (eds): Venous Problems. Year Book Medical Publishers, Chicago, 1978
5. Nylander G, Olivecrona H: The phlebographic pattern of acute leg thrombosis within a defined urban population. Acta Chir Scand 142:505, 1976
6. Kakkar VV: Medical treatment of deep vein thrombosis. Br J Hosp Med 6:741, 1971
7. Hunter WC, Krygrer JJ, Kennedy JC, Sneedon VD: Etiology and prevention of thrombosis of the deep leg veins. Surgery 17:178, 1945
8. Gibbs NN: Venous thrombosis of the lower limbs with particular reference to bed rest. Br J Surg 45:209, 1957
9. Sevitt S, Gallagher NG: Venous thrombosis and pulmonary embolism: a clinicopathological study in injured and burned patients. Br J Surg 48:475, 1961
10. Roberts GH: Venous thrombosis in hospital patients: a post mortem study. Scott Med J 8:11, 1963
11. Havig O: Deep vein thrombosis and pulmonary embolism: an autopsy study with multiple regression analysis of possible risk factors. Acta Chir Scand, Suppl. 478:1, 1977
12. Hobbs JT, Davies JWL: Detection of venous thrombosis with ^{131}I-labelled fibrinogen in the rabbit. Lancet 2:134, 1960
13. Colditz GA, Tuden RA, Oster G: Rates of venous thrombosis after general surgery: combined results of randomized clinical trials. Lancet 2:143, 1968
14. Flanc C, Kakkar VV, Clarke MB: The detection of venous thrombosis of the legs using ^{125}I labelled fibrinogen. Br J Surg 55:742, 1968
15. Field ES, Nicolaides AN, Kakkar VV, Crellin RQ: Deep vein thrombosis in patients with fractures of the femoral neck. Br J Surg 59:377, 1972
16. Hamer JD: Investigation of oedema of the lower limb following successful femoro-popliteal bypass surgery:

the role of phlebography in demonstrating venous thrombosis. Br J Surg 59:979, 1972
17. Nicolaides AN, Irving D: Clinical factors and the risk of deep venous thrombosis. p. 193. In Nicolaides AN (ed): Thromboembolism. MTP, Lancaster, 1975
18. Belch JJF, Lowe GDO, Pollock JG et al: Subcutaneous heparin in the prevention of venous thrombosis after elective aortic bifurcation graft surgery. Thromb Haemost 42:303, 1979
19. Browse NL, Burnand KG, Lea Thomas M: Diseases of the Veins. Arnold, London, 1988
20. Barker NW, Nygard KK, Walters W, Priestley JT: A statistical study of postoperative venous thrombosis and pulmonary embolism. II. Predisposing factors. Proc Mayo Clin 16:1, 1941
21. Towbin A: Pulmonary embolism: incidence and significance. JAMA 156:209, 1954
22. Coon WW, Coller FA: Some epidemiological considerations of thromboembolism. Surg Gynecol Obstet 109:487, 1959
23. Kakkar VV, Howe CT, Nicolaides AN et al: Deep vein thrombosis of the leg: is there a "high risk" group? Am J Surg 120:527, 1970
24. Joffe S: Postoperative deep vein thrombosis in children. J Pediatr Surg 10:539, 1975
25. Zuschlag E: Infarction of the lung in children. Am J Dis Child 74:399, 1947
26. Chumnijarakij T, Poshyachinda V: Postoperative thrombosis in Thai women. Lancet 1:1357, 1975
27. Tso SC, Wong V, Chan V et al: Deep vein thrombosis and changes in coagulation and fibrinolysis after gynaecological operations in Chinese: the effect of oral contraceptives and malignant disease. Br J Haematol 46:603, 1980
28. Cunningham IGE, Yong DNK: The incidence of deep vein thrombosis in Malaysia. Br J Surg 61:482, 1974
29. Thomas WA, Davies JNP, O'Neal RM, Dimakulangan AA: Incidence of myocardial infarction correlated with venous and pulmonary thrombosis and embolism: a geographic study based on autopsies in Uganda, East Africa and St. Louis, USA. Am J Cardiol 5:41, 1960
30. Hassan MA, Rahman EA, Rahman IA: Prostatectomy and deep vein thrombosis in Sudanese patients. Br J Surg 61:650, 1974
31. Joffe SN: Racial incidence of postoperative deep vein thrombosis in South Africa. Br J Surg 61:982, 1974
32. Burkitt DP: Varicose veins, deep vein thrombosis and haemorrhoids: epidemiology and suggested aetiology. Br Med J 2:556, 1972
33. Balleisen L, Bailey J, Epping P-H et al: Epidemiological study on factor VII, factor VIII and fibrinogen in an industrial population. 1. Baseline data on the relation to age, gender, body-weight, smoking, alcohol, pill-using, and menopause. Thromb Haemost 54:475, 1985
34. Ogston D, McAndrew GM: Fibrinolysis in obesity. Lancet 2:1205, 1964
35. Royal College of General Practitioners' Oral Contraception Study: Oral contraceptives, venous thrombosis, and varicose veins. J Roy Coll Gen Pract 28:393, 1978

36. Stolley PD, Tonascia JA, Tockman MS et al: Thrombosis with low-estrogen oral contraceptives. Am J Epidem 102:197, 1975

37. Ogston D: The Physiology of Haemostasis. Croom Helm, London, 1983

38. Wessler S, Gitel SN, Wan LS, Pasternack BS: Estrogen-containing oral contraceptive agents: a basis for their thrombogenicity. JAMA 236:2179, 1976

39. Boston Colaborative Drug Surveillance Program: Surgically confirmed gallbladder disease, venous thromboembolism, and breast tumors in relation to postmenopausal estrogen therapy. N Engl J Med 290:15, 1974

40. Kierkegaard A: Incidence and diagnosis of deep vein thrombosis associated with pregnancy. Acta Obstet Gynecol Scand 62:239, 1983

41. Department of Health and Social Security (UK): Report on confidential enquiries into maternal deaths in England and Wales, 1976–1978. Her Majesty's Stationary Office, DHSS 26, London, 1982

42. Simpson K: Shelter deaths from pulmonary embolism. Lancet 2:744, 1940

43. Talbot S. Wakley EJ, Ryrie D, Langman MJS: ABO blood groups and venous thromboembolic disease. Lancet 1:1257, 1970

44. Mourant AE, Kopec AC, Domaniewska-Sobczak K: Blood groups and blood-clotting. Lancet 1:223, 1971

45. Barker NW, Nygard KK, Walters W, Priestley JT: A statistical study of postoperative venous thrombosis and pulmonary embolism. I. Incidence in various types of operation. Proc Mayo Clin 15:769, 1940

46. Myllynen P, Kammonen M, Rokkanen P et al: Deep venous thrombosis and pulmonary embolism in patients with acute spinal cord injury: a comparison with non-paralyzed patients immobilized due to spinal fractures. J Trauma 25:541, 1985

47. Montrey JS, Kistner RL, Kong AYT et al: Thromboembolism following hip fracture. J Trauma 25:534, 1985

48. Maurer BJ, Wray W, Shillingford JP: Frequency of venous thrombosis after myocardial infarction. Lancet 2:1385, 1971

49. Fitts WT, Erde A, Peskin GW, Frost JW: Surgical implications of polycythemia vera. Ann Surg 152:548, 1960

50. Edwards FC, Truelove SC: The course and prognosis of ulcerative colitis. III: Complications. Gut 5:1, 1964

51. Chajek T, Fainaru M: Behçet's disease: report of 41 cases and a review of the literature. Medicine 54:179, 1975

52. Carson NAJ, Dent CE, Field CMB, Gaull GE: Homocystinuria: clinical and pathological review of ten cases. J Pediat 66:565, 1965

53. Diggs LW: Sickle cell crises. Am J Clin Path 44:1, 1965

54. Ogston D: Venous Thrombosis. Wiley, Chichester, 1987

55. Pollock AV, Evans M. Cigarette smoking and postoperative deep vein thrombosis. Br Med J 3:637, 1978

56. Clayton JK, Anderson JA, McNicol: Effect of cigarette smoking on subsequent postoperative thromboembolic disease in gynaecological patients. Br Med J 2:402, 1978

57. Prescott RJ, Jones DRB, Vasilescu C et al: Smoking and risk factors in deep vein thrombosis. Thromb Haemost 40:128, 1978

58. Isacson S: Effect of prednisone on the coagulation and fibrinolytic systems. Scand J Haem 7:212, 1970

59. Vanrenterghem Y, Roels L, Lerut T et al: Thromboembolic complications and hemostatic changes in cyclosporin-treated cadaveric kidney allograft recipients. Lancet 1:999, 1985

60. Nevasaari K, Heikkinen M, Taskinen PJ: Tamoxifen and thrombosis. Lancet 2:946, 1978

61. Arthur CK, Isbister JP, Aspery EM: The heparin induced thrombosis-thrombocytopenia syndrome (H.I.T.T.S.). Pathology 17:82, 1985

62. Homans J: Thrombosis of deep veins of the lower leg causing pulmonary embolism. N Engl J Med 211:933, 1934

63. Diener L: Origin and distribution of venous thrombi studied by postmortem intraosseous phlebography. p. 149. In Nicolaides AN (ed): Thromboembolism. MTP, Lancaster, 1975

64. Browse NL, Lea-Thomas M: Source of non-lethal pulmonary emboli. Lancet 1:258, 1974

65. Stamatakis JD, Kakkar VV, Lawrence D, Bentley PG: The origin of thrombi in the deep veins of the lower limb: a venographic study. Br J Surg 65:449, 1978

66. McLachlin AD, McLachlin JA, Jory TA, Rawling EG: Venous stasis in the lower extremities. Ann Surg 152:678, 1960

67. Karino T, Motomiya M: Flow through a venous valve and its implication for thrombus formation. Thromb Res 36:245, 1984

68. McLachlin J, Paterson JC: Some basic observations on venous thrombosis and pulmonary embolism. Surg Gynecol Obstet 93:1, 1951

69. Gardner AMN, Fox RH: The Return of Blood to the Heart. John Libbey, London, 1989

70. Cockett RB, Lea-Thomas M, Negus D: Iliac vein compression: its relation to iliofemoral thrombosis and the post-thrombotic syndrome. Br Med J 2:14, 1967

71. Stamatakis JD, Kakar VV, Sagar S et al: Femoral vein thrombosis and total hip replacement. Br Med J 2:223, 1977

72. Ashford TP, Freiman DG: The role of the endothelium in the initial phases of thrombosis. Am J Path 50:257, 1967

73. Stewart GJ: The role of the vessel wall in deep venous thrombosis. In Nicolaides AN (ed): Thromboembolism. MTP, Lancaster, 1975

74. Stewart GJ, Ritchie WGM, Lynch PR: Venous endothelial damage produced by massive sticking and emigration of leucocytes. Am J Path 74:507, 1974

75. Hamer JD, Malone PC, Silver IA: The PO_2 in venous pockets: its possible bearing on thrombogenesis. Br J Surg 68:166, 1981

76. Stead NW, Bauer KA, Kinney TR et al: Venous thrombosis in a family with defective release of vascular plas-

10

Anatomy and Physiology of the Veins of the Lower Limb

Timothy R. Cheatle

The venous anatomy of the lower limb can be conveniently classified into four main categories: the foot, the superficial and the deep axial systems, and the perforating (or communicating) veins. An understanding of the pathologic changes that occur in the skin when venous hypertension is present requires a knowledge of the normal skin anatomy and microcirculatory pattern.

Veins differ from arteries in a number of ways. They have thinner walls with very little muscle and are, as a result, both distensible and collapsible. Unlike arteries, veins can be divided into deep and superficial systems. Deep veins are very thin walled and below the knee, tend to be arranged in pairs accompanying the axial arteries (venae comitantes). Superficial veins have slightly more muscle in their walls and tend to run singly, spatially separated from the arterial tree. The two systems are connected by short communicating veins, also known as perforating veins.

VEINS OF THE FOOT

The venous anatomy of the foot has attracted little interest in the medical community. Recent anatomic and physiologic work indicates that the foot may not be the inert unimportant appendage as previously thought; rather, it may have an active role in the return of blood from the limb.

Each toe has two plantar and two dorsal digital veins. These join in the web space to form the dorsal metatarsal veins,[1] which then unite to form the superficial dorsal venous arch. This is normally visible. The medial end of this arch travels up anterior to the medial malleolus, to become the long saphenous vein, while the lateral end drains into the short saphenous system.

The veins of the sole of the foot are less well described but probably have crucial functional importance. They comprise the plantar cutaneous arch and the deep plantar veins, joined by many valveless communicating veins. The plantar cutaneous arch drains into the lateral and medial marginal veins, which in turn empty into the short and long saphenous system. The deep plantar veins, stretching from the fourth metatarsal to the medial malleolus, have an especially capacious central portion, far in excess of the functional capacity necessary to drain the foot, and which has been likened to a concertina.[2] These deep plantar veins drain preferentially into the posterior tibial veins although communications exist with the superficial venous system.

The anatomy and functional significance of the pedal veins have been comprehensively reviewed by Gardner and Fox.[3]

MAJOR SUPERFICIAL VEINS OF THE LOWER LIMB

The major superficial veins of the lower limb comprise the long and short saphenous veins. The long saphenous vein (LSV) is formed in front of the medial malleolus by the junction of the medial marginal vein and the medial end of the superficial dorsal arch. It runs in the superficial fascia along the medial side of the leg, where it is closely applied to the saphenous nerve. This sensory branch of the femoral nerve can easily be damaged when the vein is stripped below the knee. The vein runs behind the femoral condyles at the level of the knee before running forward again to lie medially in the thigh. The LSV terminates by leaving its superficial plane in the groin, where it pierces the cribriform fascia at the foramen ovale and enters the femoral vein. Almost invariably, a valve is present in the mouth of the LSV at this point, and many other valves are usually present along its length.

The tributaries of the LSV are important. Negus[4] has likened the most constant to two inverted tridents, one below the knee and one at the groin. Below the knee, the anterior superficial tibial and posterior arch veins enter the LSV at approximately the same level. At the groin, the two largest and most important tributaries are the anterolateral and posteromedial veins of the thigh, which form the two lateral prongs of the "trident." The first of these, in particular, may be larger than the LSV itself and can easily be mistaken for it by the unwary. Other tributaries of the LSV are less constant, the principal ones being the superficial epigastric, circumflex iliac, and superficial and deep external pudendal veins. All must be divided if the vein-stripping operation is to be performed successfully. Anatomic variants are common at this site. Any of the tributaries can drain directly into the femoral vein and, on occasion, the LSV may be duplicated. Browse et al.[5] estimate this latter variation to be present in about 5 percent of all limbs. High or low insertion of the LSV into the femoral vein may be confusing to the surgeon who is unaware of this possibility; luckily, these variations are relatively rare. Perhaps the most common variant is to find the superficial external pudendal artery running in front of, rather than behind, the LSV. This vessel can be safely divided, but recognition of its presence obviously demands careful dissection.

The short saphenous vein (SSV) starts at the lateral end of the superficial dorsal venous arch, behind the lateral malleolus. (This contrasts with the LSV which, of course, runs in front of its respective malleolus.) Running back toward the midline posteriorly, it drains the posterolateral aspect of the leg. It pierces the deep fascia relatively low in the calf (a fact originally observed by Gay, then generally forgotten until recently reemphasized by Negus[4], runs upward, and enters the popliteal vein at a level traditionally described as lying between the two heads of the gastrocnemius muscle. It is important to realize, however, that this arrangement only holds true in about 60 percent of cases. In 30 percent of cases, the SSV continues up the thigh to join either the LSV, the profunda femoris vein, or, occasionally a branch of the iliac system, while in the remaining 10 percent it ends in the calf by draining into either the LSV or a gastrocnemius vein.[6] This wide anatomic variability reflects the evolutionary history of the vein, when it acted as the postaxial vein of the hindlimb and drained into the internal iliac vein. As regards the practical significance of such variability, when surgery on the short saphenous system becomes necessary, preoperative imaging of the anatomy is essential, to avoid failure at operation. This is now easily performed using duplex ultrasound, but conventional venography will suffice where this is unavailable.

DEEP VEINS OF THE LOWER LIMB

The deep veins of the lower limb run in the muscular compartments of the leg and thigh. Below the knee, they comprise two anterior tibial, two posterior tibial, and two peroneal veins. These run with the similarly named arteries, of which they are venae comitantes. They have many valves and join at the lower end of the popliteal fossa to form the popliteal vein. Short vessels, known as sinusoids, run from the calf muscles to join these veins. Those leaving the soleus muscle generally lack valves and are rather baggy and inconstant in position, while those coming from the gastrocnemius are usually thinner and often valved and tend to be arranged in two pairs.

The popliteal vein, lying deep to the popliteal nerve but superficial to the artery, courses its way upward and medially through the adductor hiatus, where it enters the subsartorial canal and changes its name to the superficial femoral vein. In the femoral canal, it receives the profunda femoris vein and becomes the common femoral vein. Lying medially in the canal, this runs upward under the inguinal ligament to leave the lower limb and become the external iliac vein. There are fairly constant valves at the mouths of the deep and superficial femoral veins as they merge, while in two-thirds of cases a valve is found in the common femoral vein.[7] Distally, valves are present but tend to be inconstant in position and number.

COMMUNICATING VEINS

The communicating veins link the axial veins of the deep and superficial systems together; they are often referred to as "perforators," since they traverse the deep fascia of the leg. There are more than 100 of these veins in most limbs, mainly less than 2 mm in diameter. Traditionally they are described in groups, often named after their discoverers.

Unnamed communicating veins exist in the foot, connecting the deep and superficial venous arches. In the gaiter region of the leg, there are an important group of perforators running between the posterior arch vein and the posterior tibial vein. These are short and large and are often referred to as Cockett's veins.[8] There are usually three or four principal veins in this group, situated approximately a hand's-breadth apart. Linton[9] was also responsible for our appreciation of the importance of these communicating veins. When incompetent, the reflux through the communicating veins leads to localized venous hypertension on the medial side of the lower leg. As Linton pointed out, the perforators in this region are relatively unsupported by connective tissue compared with those elsewhere in the leg. This could make them more vulnerable to dilatation and subsequent valvular incompetence.[10] The operation bearing his name, which involves radical extirpation of the medial communicating veins, has been used successfully in the treatment of some cases of intractable ulceration.[11,12] On the lateral aspect of the leg, an inconstant perforating vein of less functional importance links the short saphenous to the peroneal veins.

Farther up the calf, more tortuous and inconstant vessels are found joining the LSV and SSV to the veins within the gastrocnemius muscle.[13] Just below the level of the knee joint, a fairly major and constant perforator runs between the LSV and the posterior tibial vein, often referred to as Boyd's vein.[14] In the thigh, a number of perforators connect the LSV to the superficial femoral vein; these have been named after both Dodd[15] and Hunter.[16]

A description of the communicating veins would be incomplete without addressing the question of valves within them. It is commonly believed that perforators have valves that permit blood to flow from the superficial to the deep system. Only when the valves become incompetent can blood flow occur in the reverse direction, leading to local cutaneous venous hypertension, with its pathologic consequences. However, it is by no means certain that the majority of perforators do in fact have valves. Anatomic dissections have only shown their presence in the larger communicating veins.[17] In a study of 25 fresh postmortem limbs, Hadfield[18] exam-

ined the perforators and found no valves in any of the smaller vessels and only rudimentary valvular structures in the larger. This discovery confirmed the earlier findings of Barber and Shatara,[19] who reported that perforating veins less than 1 mm in diameter have no valves. These investigators also reported finding perforators with valves constructed in such a way as only to allow blood to flow from deep to the superficial system, a rather startling finding.

A recent study by Sarin et al.[20] has examined the question of flow direction in normal perforating veins in the gaiter region. Through the use of color duplex ultrasound, 29 perforating veins were identified in 20 limbs without clinical or ultrasound evidence of venous disease. When 60 mmHg pressure with a pneumatic cuff was applied to the foot, flow in the communicating vein was from the deep to superficial system in 6 (21 percent). In patients with proven superficial venous incompetence, outward flow was only seen in 7 percent of perforating veins during this maneuver. With deep venous incompetence, 37 percent of perforators showed outward flow. Thus, flow from the deep to the superficial system can be observed in normal limbs.

VEINS OF THE LOWER LIMB: PHYSIOLOGY

Pressure within the normal veins of the leg is dependent on two principal factors: the hydrostatic pressure and the "vis à tergo." The latter is the term (literally, "force from behind") used to describe the remnants of the arterial pressure wave after it has passed through the capillary bed (the capillary venous filling pressure). This is normally in the region of 15 mmHg.

In the supine position, pressure in a foot vein is largely the capillary venous filling pressure. On standing, however, the pressure will be increased by the hydrostatic pressure. This is the pressure exerted by the column of blood due to gravity and is equivalent to the vertical distance between the right atrium and the foot. This rise in venous pressure is also accompanied by an equivalent increase in arterial pressure. Hence, even in the upright position, the transcapillary pressure gradient remains unchanged.

This simple picture can be modified by the capacitance function of the venous system. Veins are capable of accommodating at least 70 percent of the total blood volume. This is made possible by their distensible walls. With a low volume, a typical vein is elliptical in cross-sectional area but, as the amount of blood entering it increases, the vein gradually becomes more circular, with very little corresponding rise in venous pressure. Thus, venous pressure will only begin to rise when venous filling is already well advanced. In the erect posture, about 250 ml of blood is shifted from the central venous circulation to each leg. The veins become filled and circular in outline. Any further rise in venous volume in this situation is accompanied by a significant rise in pressure, since the limit of venous expansion has been reached.

An important concept in considering venous pressure is the concept of transmural pressure. The brief outline above considers intraluminal venous pressure; transmural pressure is this pressure minus the extraluminal pressure exerted by the supporting tissues. This parameter is fundamental to understanding how compression therapy works.

Normal extraluminal pressure is about 5 mmHg. Since, in the supine position, the vis à tergo is approximately 15 mmHg, the net transmural pressure is 10 mmHg. If the extraluminal pressure is increased by 10 to 15 mmHg, as it is by anti-embolism stockings, the transmural pressure falls to zero. The cross-sectional venous area falls, venous flow velocity will increase, and venous emptying is enhanced. Transmural pressure is greatly increased in the dependent position, because of the gravitational effects. The effect of raising the extraluminal pressure by 15 mmHg in these circumstances with antiembolism stockings becomes negligible.

Finally, at issue is the question of oncotic pressure inside and outside the capillary lumen. This is the pressure exerted by the number of macromolecules in a particular compartment, and is important in the process of edema formation in venous disease and other conditions. The tendency of fluid to pass in or out of the capillaries as a result of osmotic change is described by Starling's hypothesis, which details those factors that affect the flow of fluid across the walls of capillaries.[21] The equation describing these forces takes the form

$$P_c + O_{if} - P_{if} - O_c = P_{TC}$$

where P_c and P_{if} represent the hydrostatic pressures inside and outside the capillaries, respectively, and O_c and O_{if} represent the osmotic pressures of the same two compartments. P_{TC} represents the net transcapillary pressure. When venous hydrostatic pressure rises, as during standing, pressure is transmitted back to the venular end of the capillary loop; this leads to a rise in P_c and a resultant rise in P_{TC}. This process is augmented by the concomitant rise in arteriolar pressure, so-called *venous priming*. The relationship in the venule between hydrostatic pressure, leading to outward movement of fluid, and osmotic pressure, and then to fluid resorption—a relationship normally favoring the latter—is altered in favor of the former. The effect is to cause fluid to move out of the capillary into the interstitium with edema the result. Normally, this is protected against by the anti-edema reflex, which causes contraction of the pre-arteriolar sphincter[22] and by the calf muscle venous pump, which will be discussed below. Starling's hypothesis explains edema formation both due to increased venous pressure and to decreased intravascular oncotic pressure.

STRUCTURE OF THE SKIN

The skin comprises the epidermis and the dermis. Its basic functions can be categorized as protective, sensory, thermoregulatory, and excretory. Most of these are in fact functions of the epidermis or its appendages, which include the sweat glands, and nerve endings.

The epidermis is an avascular layer 40 to 200 μm thick, depending on the site, consisting of five layers. The deepest of these is the stratum basale, contiguous with the dermal papillae that project into the epidermis. This is composed of a single layer of undifferentiated cells from which cell division occurs. About 10 percent of the cells in this layer undergo mitosis every day. New cells move upward into the stratum spinosum, so called because of the light microscopic appearance of prickles covering the surface of cells in this layer. These represent intercellular bridges that bind the cells together; they do not represent cytoplasmic continuity, as was formerly thought. These bridges disappear as the cells move superficially into the stratum granulosum. The granules after which this layer is named, are formed of a precursor of keratin, which is the principal constituent of cells in the strata lucidum and corneum. The cells in these strata are dead and contribute principally to the protective function of the integument.

Cells take 10 to 14 days to pass from the stratum basale to the skin surface, from which they are shed. Although the vast majority of cells in the epidermis are keratinocytes, others are also found, principally, melanocytes; Langerhans cells, which play a role in antigen recognition and which may also aid in control of keratinocyte proliferation; and Merkel cells, which transduce sensory stimuli into nervous impulses.

The dermis is traditionally thought of as playing a mere supporting role in the architecture of the skin. It is a viscoelastic tissue weighing up to 20 percent of the total body weight. Its principal constituents are collagen, elastin, reticulin, and ground substance. It is traversed by blood vessels, nerves, lymphatic channels, and the epidermal appendages. It can be separated into two main subdivisions: the papillary region, close to the epidermis; and the deeper reticular region, superficial to the subcutaneous fat. These two regions are clearly demarcated in some parts of the body, less so in others. In general, the papillary region is far richer in blood vessels, nerves, and extravascular leucocytes. Inflammatory reactions in the skin take place mainly in the papillary region. The reticular dermis, by contrast, contributes more to the structural support and elasticity of the skin. Both parts of the dermis act as significant reservoirs of body water.

The epidermis is separated from the dermis by a basement membrane. This is joined to the plasma membranes of the cells of the stratum basale by a series of microfilaments, which are thought to assist in epidermal stability. Focal breaks in it are associated with preinvasive carcinoma.[23] A separate system of microfibrils attaches the basal lamina to the underlying dermis. These are joined to the extracellular network of elastic fibers. The basement membrane, which is composed of collagen and glycoprotein, is permeable to macromolecules and to cells which include the Langerhans cells, lymphocytes, mast cells and granulocytes all of which can cross the basement membrane under normal conditions.

BLOOD SUPPLY TO THE SKIN

Much of the basic work in elucidating the anatomy of the skin circulation was done during the 1920s by Spalteholz in Germany. His contributions have been reviewed by Champion.[24] Generally, it is agreed that a number of different plexuses exist within the blood supply to the skin. Nonetheless, there is a great deal of overlap and interconnection between these vascular beds. These plexuses are arranged in strata throughout the dermis and are linked by vertical vascular channels.

The deepest of these is the "internal vascular belt" described by Moretti,[25] which lies at the junction of the subcutaneous tissues and dermis. Vessels run vertically from this plexus through the reticular dermis before spreading out horizontally to form the subpapillary plexus. From here, capillary loops project into the papillae themselves to follow the course of the dermo-epidermal junction. In addition, there are individual plexuses around hair follicles and exocrine sweat glands. However, as Montagna and Ellis have pointed out, "It will be noted that current studies place too much emphasis on the apparently predictable geometric distribution of cutaneous vessels. Although plexuses of sorts do exist, they are all interconnected by vessels which completely riddle the dermis." [26]

At the microscopic level, a knowledge of some of the ultrastructural features of the skin capillaries is necessary for an understanding of many of the abnormalities seen in venous disease. Microcirculatory units in the skin, as elsewhere, comprise the precapillary arteriole, the capillary and the postcapillary venule. Each capillary loop is approximately 0.2 to 0.4 mm in height. Capillary loops are found principally in the papillary portion of the dermis and project up the papillae toward the epidermis. The electron microscopic studies of Yen and Braverman[27,28] have provided precise detail concerning the structure of these vessels.

In tracing the course of arterioles through the dermis, Yen and Braverman demonstrated that, as the vessel diameter falls from approximately 30 to 15 μm, it loses its muscular coat, except for the precapillary sphincter. The elastin layer, which normally lies between the muscular layer and the endothelium, thus becomes more peripheral, until it too is lost when the vessel tapers to less than 12 to 15 μm in diameter. Below this level are the true capillaries, composed only of an endothelial tube, a basement membrane, and occasional individual pericytes. Pericytes resemble poorly developed smooth muscle cells, having less well-developed dense bodies, scattered cytoplasmic mitochondria, and fewer microfilaments. They form tight junctions with the endothelium through breaks in the basal membrane. The internal diameter of the capillary is 4 to 6 μm. Pinocytotic vesicles in both the endothelium and the pericytes are common. Weibal-Palade bodies, which contain von Willebrand factor, are scanty.

At the apex of the papilla, the endothelial cells become attenuated, and the diameter of the capillary is at its narrowest. The gaps between individual endothelial cells are approximately 20 nm, except on the luminal side, where the cells are apparently contiguous. Pericytes are scarce.

In the descending limb of the capillary loop, the principal structural change involves the basement membrane. It becomes laminated; Yen and Braverman suggest that this structural appearance should be taken as representing the transition from capillary to postcapillary venule. Pericytes reappear, especially as the vessel leaves the papilla, and veil cells (fibroblasts) are also seen. Gradually a thin muscular coat develops; the ratio of luminal diameter to muscle coat thickness in these vessels is about 100:1. The microanatomy of the venous capillaries and venules has been comprehensively described by Rhodin.[29] Functionally, these vessels are of fundamental importance in the control of total resistance and capillary pressure, hence capillary filtration. They comprise the main part of the subpapillary plexus, where they are responsible for normal skin color. From this plexus, larger venules run down through the reticular dermis into the internal vascular belt and on into the large collecting veins in the subcutaneous tissues.

Recently, the arrangement of contractile cells around the microvessels of the skin has been further elucidated by three-dimensional computer reconstructions from serial electron micrographs.[30] These have shown more clearly the way in which the smooth muscle cells of the terminal arteriole act as sphincters. They tend to have cytoplasmic "wings" encircling the endothelial tube and often overlap one another. In the postcapillary venule, pericytes are shown to form large numbers of contact points with the endothelium, holding the venule in a vicelike grip. It is suggested that they may have a true contractile role to play in the determination of systemic resistance at this site, unlike the case in the larger venules, where they have less contact points and probably act as an architectural support.

It can be seen that the blood supply to the skin is greatly in excess of its nutritive requirement, especially considering that the skin has one of the lowest metabolic rates of any organ. Temperature control is the generally accepted reason, based on the presence of numerous arteriovenous shunts at the interface of dermis and subcutaneous tissues. These communications, known as Sucquet-Hoyer canals, are muscular and are under sympathetic innervation. They are particularly numerous in the feet, hands, lips, nose, and ears; elsewhere, less specialized arteriovenous communications are found, in fewer numbers.

Under normal conditions, of only moderate sympathetic tone, the shunts are at least partially open, and there is free flow to the dermis, permitting heat radiation through the skin. However, in cold conditions, the shunts will close under intense sympathetic stimulation with blood bypassing the dermis to conserve heat. As the nutritive requirements of the skin are low, skin damage is unusual unless exposure to cold is prolonged and severe. Normal skin blood flow is approximately 250 ml/m²/min. It is only when flow falls below about 30 ml/m²/min that skin damage might follow. Conversely, in hot conditions, the shunts are fully relaxed, and flow to the skin is greatly increased, reaching values as high as 2 L/m²/min.

The mechanism described above also indicates another benefit consequent to the excessive vascularity of the skin. Sympathetic outflow is increased in conditions of shock (e.g., hypovolemic shock). By closure of the shunts and vasoconstriction of the arterioles, a considerable volume of blood is diverted to vital organs.

Special considerations apply to the situation in the leg. At birth, the lower limb capillary pattern is the same in the leg as elsewhere.[31] Ryan and Cherry[32] pointed out that the disproportionate increase in limb growth compared with the face or trunk leads to an increase in skin surface area with which the dermal capillaries fail to keep pace, so the number of capillary loops in the skin of the leg is less than that in other sites. The capillaries themselves tend to be elongated and more convoluted than elsewhere; a change that is exacerbated in the presence of venous hypertension. Thus, even in health, there is a tendency towards uneven perfusion of the skin of the leg.

A universal characteristic of skin blood flow is the presence of "vasomotion"—spontaneous changes in diameter of small arterioles and their branches, which occur several times a minute. The phenomenon was fully described by Chambers and Zweifach in bat's wing tissue[33] and has also been described in cat mesentery,[34] rat kidney,[35] rat testis,[36] and bone.[37] The precise underlying mechanism is not entirely clear. It is generally thought to be a function of spontaneous contractile activity in the muscular layer of the precapillary arterioles,[38] but it has also been suggested that a local feedback mechanism may be at work by which the local buildup of metabolites or hypoxia induces regular contraction and dilatation.[39]

In the skin, vasomotion has been studied by Salerud et al.[40] using laser Doppler velocimetry. These investigators found that regular waxing and waning of skin blood flow occurred at all sites, with a frequency of 5 to 10 rhythmic variations per minute. The rate of variation differed from one site to another in the same patient, as well as at the same site from one patient to another. Vasomotion was unaffected by regional anesthesia but was abolished by direct application of anaesthetic skin paste—a finding that would tend to support the hypothesis that vasomotion is the result of the spontaneously contractile properties of vascular smooth muscle cells. Vasomotion was reduced by local heating, as overall flow increased. Inspiration of 100 percent oxygen did not affect the frequency of vasomotion—further evidence that hypoxia is not a controlling factor in the cause of the phenomenon. The vasomotive characteristics of the skin microcirculation have been shown to be markedly abnormal in the presence of lipodermatosclerosis due to venous hypertension, a finding that may shed light on the mechanism by which skin damage occurs in venous disease.[41]

REFERENCES

1. Kuster G, Lofgren EP, Holinshead WH: Anatomy of the veins of the foot. Surg Gynecol Obstet 127:817, 1968
2. Gardner AMN, Fox RH: The venous pump of the human foot. Bristol Med Chir J 98:109, 1983
3. Gardner AMN, Fox RH: The Return of Blood to the Heart. John Libby & Co., London, 1989

4. Negus D: Leg Ulcers. Butterworth–Heinemann, Oxford, 1991
5. Browse NL, Burnand KG, Thomas ML: Diseases of the Veins. Edward Arnold, London, 1988
6. Hobbs JT: A new approach to short saphenous varicosities. p. 301. In Bergan JJ, Yao JTS (eds): Surgery of the Veins. Grune & Stratton, Orlando, FL, 1985
7. Basmajian JV: The distribution of valves in femoral, external iliac and common iliac veins and their relationship to varicose veins. Surg Gynecol Obstet 95:537, 1952
8. Cockett FB: The pathology and treatment of venous ulcers of the leg. Br J Surg 43:260, 1955
9. Linton RR: The post-thrombotic ulceration of the lower extremity; its etiology and surgical treatment. Ann Surg 138:415, 1953
10. Linton RR: The communicating veins of the lower leg and the operative technic for their ligation. Ann Surg 107:582, 1938
11. Field P, van Boxel P: The role of the Linton flap procedure in the management of stasis dermatitis and ulceration in the lower limb. Surgery 70:920, 1971
12. Wilkinson GE, Maclaren IF: Long term review of procedures for venous perforator insufficiency. Surg Gynecol Obstet 163:117, 1986
13. Thomson H: The surgical anatomy of the superficial and perforating veins of the lower limb. Ann R Coll Surg Engl 61:198, 1979
14. Boyd AM: Discussion on primary treatment of varicose veins. Proc R Soc Med 41:633, 1948
15. Dodd H: The varicose tributaries of the superficial femoral vein passing into Hunter's canal. Postgrad Med J 35:18, 1959
16. Papadakis K, Christodolou C, Christopoulos D et al: Number and anatomical distribution of incompetent thigh perforating veins. Br J Surg 76:581, 1989
17. Cockett FB, Elgan-Jones DE: The ankle blow-out syndrome. Lancet 1:17, 1953
18. Hadfield JIH: The anatomy of the perforating veins of the leg. p. 4. In The Treatment of Varicose Veins by Injection and Compression. Stoke Mandeville Symposium, Hereford, 1971
19. Barber RF, Shatara FI: The varicose disease. NY State J Med 25:162, 1925
20. Sarin S, Scurr JH, Coleridge Smith PD: Medial calf perforators in venous disease: the significance of outward flow. J Vasc Surg 16:40, 1992
21. Sumner DS: Applied physiology in venous problems. p. 3. In Bergan JJ, Yao JST (eds): Surgery of the Veins. Grune & Stratton, Orlando, FL, 1985
22. Levick JR, Michel CC: The effects of position and skin temperature on capillary pressures in the fingers and toes. J Physiol (Lond) 274:97, 1978
23. Breathnach AS, Wolff K: Structure and development of the skin. p. 41. In Fitzpatrick TB, Eisen AZ, Wolff K et al. (eds): Dermatology in General medicine. 2nd Ed. McGraw-Hill, New York, 1979
24. Champion RH: Blood vessels and lymphatics of the skin. In Champion RH, Gillman T, Rook AJ, Sims RT (eds): An Introduction to the Biology of the Skin. Blackwell, Oxford, 1970
25. Moretti G: The blood vessels of the skin. p. 491. In Gans O, Steigleder GK (eds): Jadassohn's Handbuch der Haut —und Geschlechtskrankheiten. Vol 1/1. Springer-Verlag, Berlin, 1968
26. Montagna W, Ellis RA (eds): Advances in Biology of the Skin Vol. II. Pergamon, Oxford, 1961
27. Yen A, Braverman IM: Ultrastructure of the human dermal microcirculation: the horizontal plexus of the papillary dermis. J Invest Dermatol 66:131, 1976
28. Braverman IM, Yen A: Ultrastructure of the human dermal microcirculation. II. The capillary loops of the dermal papillae. J Invest Dermatol 68:44, 1977
29. Rhodin JAG: Ultrastructure of mammalian venous capillaries, venules and small collecting veins. J Ultrastruct Res 25:452, 1968
30. Braverman IM, Sibley J: Ultrastructural and three-dimensional analysis of the contractile cells of the cutaneous microvasculature. J Invest Dermatol 95:90, 1990
31. Perera P, Kurban AK, Ryan TJ: The development of the cutaneous microvascular system in the newborn. Br J Dermatol, suppl. 5. 82:86, 1970
32. Ryan TJ, Cherry GW: The assessment of vascular abnormalities of the leg. p. 87. In Champion RW (ed): Recent Advances in Dermatology. Vol. 7. Churchill Livingstone, Edinburgh, 1986
33. Chambers R, Zweifach BW: Functional activity of the blood capillary bed, with special reference to visceral tissue. Ann NY Acad Sci 46:683, 1944
34. Johnsson PC, Wayland H: Regulation of blood flow in single capillaries. Am J Physiol 212:1405, 1967
35. Eggart P, Weiss C: Periodic microflow pattern measured with a new microflow probe within the rat kidney cortex. Pflugers Arch 383:223, 1980
36. Damber J-E, Lindahl O, Selstam G, Tenland T: Testicular blood flow measured with a laser Doppler flowmeter: acute effects of catecholamines. Acta Physiol Scand 115:209, 1982
37. Hellem S, Jacobsson L, Nilsson GE, Lewis DH: Measurement of microvascular blood flow in cancellous bone using laser Doppler flowmetry and 133 Xe-clearance. Int J Oral Surg 12:165, 1982
38. Intaglietta M: Vasomotor activity, time-dependent fluid exchange and tissue pressure. Microvasc Res 21:153, 1981
39. Guyton AC, Ross JM, Carrier O, Walker JR: Evidence for tissue oxygen demand as the major factor causing autoregulation. Circ Res, Suppl. 1. 15:60, 1964
40. Salerud EG, Tenland T, Nilsson GE, Oberg PA: Rhythmical variations in human skin blood flow. Int J Microcirc Clin Exp 2:91, 1983
41. Cheatle TR, Shami SK, Stibe ECL et al: Vasomotion in venous disease. J R Soc Med 84:261, 1991

Section IV

Diagnostic Techniques in Vascular Repair

The diagnostic approaches to patients with suspected vascular disease have undergone a dramatic evolution during the past 20 years. While arteriography and venography evolved to become the principal methods used, it was apparent that due to their invasive nature they had serious limitations. During this same time frame, we become aware of the fact that the standard history and physical examination, while essential components to the patient evaluation, also had serious drawbacks. Because of the need for greater precision, an intensive search began for methods that were both noninvasive and objective enough to provide the physician with data relative to both the location of disease and its effect on function.

Most of the early noninvasive methods that were employed were indirect, obtaining physiological information from externally placed sensors. These methods that become widely used still occupy an important place in the field although they have been replaced to some degree by the emergence of duplex scanning.

The major change that took place with regard to noninvasive testing was the introduction of duplex scanning in 1974, which has revolutionized the entire field. For the first time it was possible to generate flow information from precise locations within the vascular system. This method is now the standard method used in most vascular laboratories today. It has great utility not only as an initial screening method but also as a means to provide natural history information that cannot be obtained by any other diagnostic tests.

The newest modality to appear on the scene is magnetic resonance arteriography. While many of its applications are still under study, it is clear that perhaps in combination with ultrasound, it will have a major impact in the field. Since it is noninvasive, it may well with more time and experience become the standard method of carrying out arteriography. If this were to occur, it would be a major advance for the field, since the complications related to the invasive procedures could be avoided.

The conventional angiographic methods remain with us and will for the foreseeable future. Arteriography, particularly in conjunction with interventional methods, remains a necessity. The situation on the venous side of the circulation is different. At the moment, venography for the diagnosis of acute and chronic venous disease has been largely replaced by duplex scanning.

In this section, the currently available and widely used methods will be considered in some detail. It should become clear that we now have the capability of examining the vascular system with a degree of precision that was not considered feasible just a few years ago.

11

Indirect Noninvasive Testing

D. Eugene Strandness, Jr.

Until the mid- to late 1960s the essential ingredients for evaluation of peripheral vascular problems were perceived to be the history, the physical examination, and angiography. There is no doubt that this approach led to many of the spectacular advances in the treatment of arterial and venous disorders. Yet as the surgical community began to examine the role of the above approaches, it was clear that additional information, particularly as it related to the functional status of the patient, would be worthwhile. In order to obtain this information it was necessary to develop noninvasive methods that could be used to evaluate pressure and flow in the limbs.

On the arterial side of the circulation, it would seem logical that volume blood flow would be the most useful information that might be obtained. Surprisingly, as noted in numerous studies, this has not proved to be the case. For example, in patients with occlusion of the major inflow arteries to the limb, there is no reduction in the level of calf blood flow.[1] This means that the collateral circulation is ample to supply the needs of the limb at rest. While there is no doubt that blood flow measured during exercise (a period of increased demand) would be lower in patients with intermittent claudication, it is difficult to make these measurements.[2]

Since volume blood flow measurements proved to be of little diagnostic value, it became necessary to look for other parameters that might be important clinically. The two variables found to be most important were blood pressure and velocity of flow.[3] The methods to measure these two variables were developed during the 1960s and remain in use even today. As noted in Section II, limb blood pressures and flow patterns in both normal subjects and patients with arterial narrowing and occlusion are well understood.

While indirect testing has been replaced in some areas by duplex scanning, it remains useful for the evaluation of both arterial and venous disorders.

METHODS OF MEASUREMENT

Blood Pressure

While it would interesting to obtain measurements of both systolic and diastolic blood pressure from all levels of the arterial circulation, this is not feasible. Systolic and diastolic pressures can only be obtained when an intra-arterial catheter is used; in practice such measurements are largely limited to the aortoiliac segments at the time an arteriogram is performed.[4] It is difficult to measure intra-arterial pressures in the upper limb distal to the subclavian artery and in the lower limb distal to the inguinal ligament. While a catheter may be guided into the arteries of the arm and leg, this is not routinely done for the estimation of the pressure gradient that may be present across suspected areas of disease. There is a problem in medium-sized arteries because if the catheter is large relative to the diameter of the artery, it may produce a partial obstruction that is significant enough to produce a pressure gradient.

A common method for measuring systolic pressure in both the arm and leg is based on the reappearance of a palpable pulse as the pressure in an occluding cuff is gradually reduced from suprasystolic levels. This method will work only if there are no occlusive lesions proximal to the recording site. One must be able to feel the peripheral pulses in order to use this method. However, it is the principle of pulse reappearance during cuff deflation that is the basis for the indirect noninvasive methods of measuring limb blood pressure.

The sensors first used to measure systolic limb blood pressure were of the plethysmographic type.[5] The earliest models employed sealed plastic cups that were placed over the terminal digits and used to sense the volume changes that occurred during cuff deflation. With the cup sealed at the base of the digit to make it air tight, a change in the volume of the digit could be detected by the displacement of air to a sensing transducer. A later device, which is still in use today, is the mercury-in-Silastic strain gauge.[6] This very simple device, which can detect minute changes in length, is placed about the distal phalanx, where it can detect the volume pulses that occur with each heart beat (Figs. 11-1 and 11-2). In addition, the return of pulses during deflation of a cuff at a level proximal to the sensor is a sensitive method of measuring systolic blood pressure.[7]

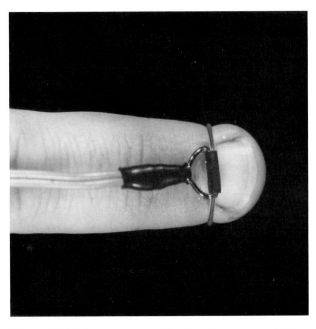

Figure 11-1 The mercury-in-Silastic strain gauge plethysmograph can detect small changes in the circumference of the digit. These can be amplified to present the digit volume pulse that occurs with each heart beat. They can also be made long enough to fit about the calf for measurements of calf blood flow and venous outflow.

A photoplethysmograph may also be used in a similar manner to measure systolic blood pressure.[8]

Regardless of the type of sensing device used, the procedure for measuring systolic blood pressure is the same. A cuff placed at any point proximal to the sensor is rapidly inflated to pressures well above the systolic pressure level. When this is done, digit volume pulses will disappear and the volume of the digit will decrease.[7] As the pressure in the cuff is slowly decreased, digit pulses and the volume of the digit itself will increase at the point where the pressure in the cuff is below systolic levels. The point at which the volume pulses appears and/or the digit volume increases is taken as the opening or systolic blood pressure for that level of the limb at which the pneumatic cuff has been placed.

The most commonly used method for measuring limb blood pressures today is continuous wave (CW) Doppler.[9] The return of the arterial velocity signal from the tibial and peroneal arteries is the endpoint taken to measure the systolic blood pressure (Fig. 11-3).

Volume Changes

It is well known that arterial narrowing and/or occlusion will change both the pressures distal to the sites of involvement and the manner in which the volume of the limb or digits responds to the volume of blood entering the limb with each heart beat.[10] Normally the pressure pulses in the arteries of the limb have as their major components a sharp systolic peak with a well-defined dicrotic wave on the downslope. When the pressure is decreased distal to a hemodynamically significant arterial stenosis or occlusion, the volume pulse loses its sharp systolic peak and the dicrotic wave is no longer seen.[7] This is commonly referred to as a *damped* pulse (Fig. 11-2). This change in the contour of the volume pulse is identical to that observed in the arteries at the site of the measurement. To document these volume changes, a variety of sensors have been developed and used.

The most commonly used volume change detectors are the simple pneumatic cuff and the mercury-in-Silastic strain gauge.[11] When a pneumatic cuff is used to measure the volume changes, it is filled with a fixed amount of air and connected to a transducer, which makes possible monitoring of the phasic changes in limb volume that occur with each heart beat. Since the cuffs can be placed at the upper thigh, above the knee, below the knee, and at the ankle, it is possible to evaluate the volume pulses at these levels, which can be related to the location and extent of the arterial disease (Fig. 11-4). While the cup method can be applied to the

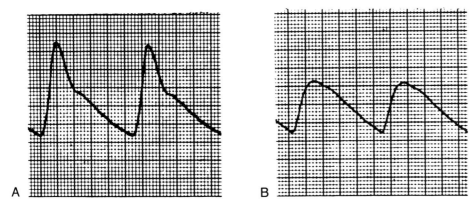

Figure 11-2 The digit volume pulses shown in **(A)** are normal with a sharp systolic peak and dicrotic wave on the downslope. With arterial obstruction **(B)**, the sharp systolic peak and dicrotic wave are lost. (From Strandness,[65] with permission.)

digits to obtain this pulse information, the mercury-in-Silastic strain gauge or photoplethysmograph is much simpler to use at this level. Although the photoplethysmograph does not measure a volume change of the entire digit, it is a sensitive to changes in the volume of blood in the dermis of the skin. It has been shown that the waveforms detected by this method are very similar in contour to those obtained with the pneumatic cuffs and the mercury-in-Silastic strain gauge.

Velocity Changes

An important advance in the field of noninvasive testing was the introduction of Doppler methods to blood flow velocity measurement. Satomura in 1959 was the first to demonstrate that ultrasound could be transmitted through the skin to detect the frequency shifts that occur when flowing blood is insonated by ultrasound.[12] The magnitude of the frequency shifts (positive and negative) that occur are directly related to the velocity of flow. The following considerations apply to Doppler measurements of blood flow velocity.[3]

1. Frequency shifts are affected by the direction as well as the velocity and direction of blood flow. In the usual case in which the transducer is angled in the direction of flow, the frequency shift is positive. During the phase in which reverse flow occurs, the frequency shift is in the negative direction. It is possible to take advantage of this in producing an analogue output of the velocity patterns (Fig. 11-5).

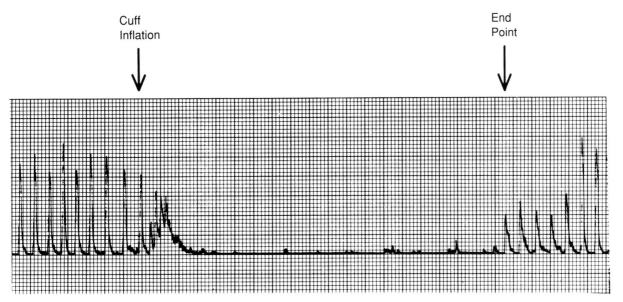

Figure 11-3 Obliteration of arterial velocity waveforms with rapid cuff inflation proximal to the site of the transducer placement. The point at which the pulses return is taken as the opening or systolic pressure at that level. (From Strandness,[66] with permission.)

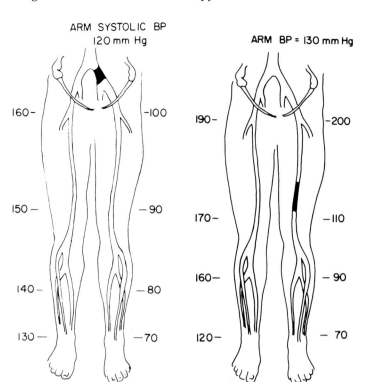

Figure 11-4 Pressure gradients detected by measurement of systolic pressures at the levels shown. The pressure falls distal to the site or occlusion. Note that the upper thigh pressures are artifactually high due to the discrepancy in size between the cuff used and the circumference of the thigh. (From Strandness,[7] with permission.)

2. The higher the transmitting frequency, the higher the frequency shift for the same velocity of flow. If the transmitting frequency is doubled, the recorded frequency shift will also be doubled. It is also well known that the cosine of the angle of incidence of the sound beam with the vessel influences the recorded frequency shift. The maximal frequency shift is noted at zero degrees, which is never possible to achieve when the method is used transcutaneously. In practice one should attempt to use the CW Doppler system at the same angle of insonation with the blood vessel as a matter of routine. For nearly all peripheral arteries, a 5-MHz transmitting frequency is adequate for reaching arteries of interest. It is important to realize that the depth of penetration is improved by using lower transmitting frequencies.

3. CW Doppler will provide an audio output signal that is useful in distinguishing normal and abnormal patterns of flow.

4. CW Doppler can be used to detect flow in all major arteries and veins outside the abdomen, thorax, and skull. In practice it is useful to use the companion artery or vein for proper identification and as a landmark. For example, if one were interested in examining the superficial femoral artery, one would identify its companion vein as the initial step. This would ensure that the vessel being insonated was in fact the correct one. Likewise, if one is searching for the superficial femoral vein, it is helpful to first identify the adjacent artery.

5. For some applications the observer may want to document the velocity changes with a permanent record. This can be achieved by using a fast Fourier transform (FFT) system, which will display all the important information in the Doppler spectrum. To determine blood flow velocity in absolute terms, it is necessary to know the angle of incidence of the sound beam with the vessel.

6. A major advantage of CW Doppler is that it can be used both to screen major peripheral arteries to assess their velocity patterns and to measure the limb systolic blood pressure at several levels of the limb, as noted earlier.[3,9] In practice, flow is detected and lower limb pressures are measured in the posterior tibial and dorsalis pedis arteries at the level of the ankle. To measure segmental pressures, the cuffs are placed at the ankle, below the knee, above the knee, and at upper thigh. In using CW Doppler for measuring pressure, it is important to rapidly inflate the pressure in the cuff to suprasystolic levels. It is unwise to measure the pressure at that point where flow disappears during cuff inflation. The recorded pressures are more accurate and reproducible when the pressure is measured at the point where flow is restored during slow cuff deflation (Fig. 11-3).

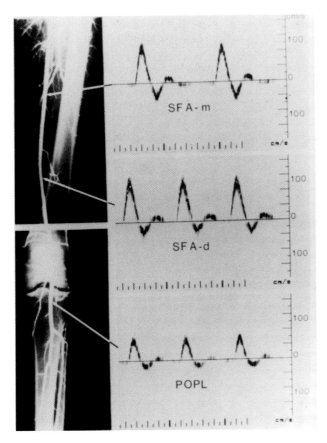

Figure 11-5 Velocity waveform obtained from a normal superficial femoral artery (SFA) and popliteal artery (POPL). These were obtained with a pulsed Doppler system. (From Strandness,[28] with permission.)

CLINICAL APPLICATIONS

Peripheral Arterial Disease

Narrowing and occlusion of peripheral arteries is most commonly secondary to atherosclerosis; this is referred to as *arteriosclerosis obliterans* (ASO). It tends to be a disease of branch points and bifurcations, frequently sparing those segments of the arterial system in which the vessels are relatively straight and have few branches.[13] Another interesting aspect of the disease is that it rarely involves the arteries of the arm distal to the origin of the subclavian artery. The reasons for this are poorly understood, since all commonly accepted risk factors, such as cigarette smoking, hypertension, and high lipid levels, act on the walls of these arteries as well.

In the nondiabetic patient, the most commonly involved arterial segments include the aortoiliac area and the superficial femoral artery in the adductor canal.[14] It is important to realize that patients with diabetes mellitus have a different pattern of disease involvement. They have a lower incidence of aortoiliac disease and the same amount of involvement of the superficial femoral artery, but a much higher incidence of occlusions in the tibial and peroneal arteries.[14,15] In addition, when the disease develops it is more extensive (Fig. 11-6).

There are two other problems commonly seen in the type 2 diabetic patient that must be understood. The first is the development of medial calcification (Mönckeberg's medial sclerosis). This process bears no relationship to the atherosclerosis that develops.[13] In an unselected population of diabetic patients, it will be found in about 2 percent,[16] but among patients who are referred to a vascular clinic for evaluation, the prevalence of medial calcification will be in the range of 15 percent. The calcification is generally limited to the tibial and peroneal arteries but in some cases may extend above the knee to involve the superficial femoral artery. Since medial calcification does not restrict blood flow, it has no clinical significance. However, its presence may make measurement of systolic pressure

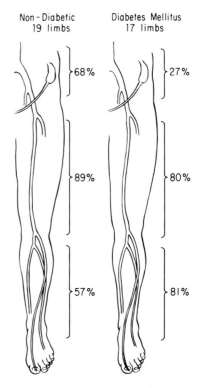

Figure 11-6 Differences in site of occlusion between diabetic and nondiabetic patients with arteriosclerosis obliterans. In each instance the extent of involvement below the knee was documented by dissection of the amputated limb.

impossible.[16,17] The calcified arteries may not be compressible, which results in values of systolic pressure that are falsely high. When this situation is encountered, it is necessary to measure the blood pressures in the toes, where medial calcification of the digital arteries is not seen.[17]

Another problem unique to type 2 diabetics is the development of a peripheral neuropathy.[15] When this occurs, the patient loses the ability to appreciate deep pain sensation. From a physiologic standpoint, this complication results in an "autosympathectomy," which results in permanent denervation with a warm foot and dry skin. This condition is found in 30 to 40 percent of type 2 patients who are being evaluated for the presence or absence of peripheral arterial disease.[14] This loss of sympathetic tone also results in loss of the normal respiratory reflexes that affect peripheral arterial tone. For example, a normal person will undergo vasoconstriction during the course of taking a deep breath; this reflex is lost with a neuropathy, as can be documented by noting the digit volume changes associated with respiration. The vasoconstriction that follows a deep inspiration will be seen as a decrease in the amplitude of the digit volume pulse recorded by a plethysmographic system.[6]

Clinical Presentation

Since arteriosclerosis obliterans results in progressive narrowing and total occlusion, it produces symptoms and signs that are directly related to the level and extent of the involvement. From a clinical standpoint, it is important to note that the patients will fall into one or both of two categories. The most commonly encountered patients are those who present with exercise-induced pain (intermittent claudication)[18]; the second important group of patients consists of those who present with limb-threatening ischemia.[19] This distinction and separation in manner of presentation is important to appreciate when the patient is seen for a vascular laboratory evaluation.

While the vascular laboratory evaluation can stand alone as a set of measurements, it is important to review the symptoms and/or signs that are used in making the diagnosis. Intermittent claudication can be recognized by the walk-pain-rest cycle that occurs and the constant nature of the cycle from day to day.[18] Patients with this problem do not have good and bad days—their days are always the same. Other important features include the fact that the pain is always made worse by increasing the work load (walking up a grade). When the pain occurs, it is relieved by simply stopping the walk and standing for periods of seconds to a few minutes. The patient never has to sit or lie down for relief.

In contrast, there is a large group of patients who develop pain in their limbs that is related to exercise but not secondary to arterial disease. These patients are considered to have *pseudoclaudication* secondary to degenerative joint disease, spinal stenosis, herniated nucleus pulposus, or in rare cases, spinal cord tumors.[20] These patients have a walk-pain-rest cycle that varies from day to day and—in contrast to those with arterial disease—will have good days. In addition, it is not at all uncommon for symptoms to develop when the patient is simply standing. When these patients develop symptoms with exercise, they may be required to lie or sit down for pain relief.

When the patient presents with both arterial disease and neurospinal involvement, determination of which of the two entities is most important in causing the symptoms can be difficult. The role of the vascular laboratory in making this distinction will be covered in the section on exercise testing.

The threatened limb is recognized by the characteristic presentation of pain in the toes and foot that is present at rest. In mild cases the pain is relieved by dependency. It is often referred to as *nocturnal rest pain,* since the patient will first experience it at night after retiring. It is at this time that the patient first notices that the pain is decreased or relieved by hanging the leg over the side of the bed.

In far advanced cases the pain at rest may be accompanied by development of ulceration and/or gangrene. The prospects for tissue loss increase the gravity of the situation, since even restoration of flow may not permit preservation of the toes or forefoot. The diabetic who presents with advanced ischemia may not have pain as a component of the clinical presentation because a peripheral neuropathy when present may keep the patient pain-free even in the presence of ischemia and ulceration.[14,15]

Physical Examination

Since the history is the major source of important diagnostic information, the physical examination is used to confirm the initial impression and provide information as to the most proximal level of occlusion. An examination of the limbs is considered to be an integral part of the vascular laboratory evaluation. Inspection is helpful for noting changes in color, hair patterns, and nail growth and the presence or absence of ulceration or gangrene. It must be noted, however, that short of far advanced tissue changes, inspection alone provides little information concerning the extent of arterial involvement.

The two most important aspects of the physical examination are palpation for pulses and the listening for bruits. The sites of examination include the abdominal aorta, the iliac arteries, the common femoral and popliteal arteries, and the tibial arteries at the ankle. Examination of the abdomen is particularly important since the patient may have an abdominal aortic aneurysm. If an aneurysm is found or suspected, it should further be investigated by either ultrasound or computed tomographic (CT) scanning.

There is little doubt that pulse detection is important, but even if accurate, it provides information only about the most proximal level of involvement. For example, if only a femoral pulse is palpable, the observer knows that the superficial femoral and/or the popliteal artery is significantly narrowed or occluded, but the status of the tibial and peroneal arteries is not known. The sites most difficult to examine are the popliteal artery and the tibial arteries at the ankle. Variability in detection of pulses is not at all uncommon. This is one reason why measurement of ankle systolic pressure has become such a critical and standard part of patient evaluation.

Bruit detection may provide important clues concerning the status of the arterial circulation. A bruit represents vibration of the arterial wall due to the turbulence that develops secondary to narrowing of the arterial lumen. It is important to be aware that (1) bruits are never transmitted upstream from the area of stenosis and (2) they are transmitted downstream from the site of narrowing for a variable distance. When listening for bruits the physician must realize that the bruit will be loudest at/or just distal to the site of the narrowing. When the bruit is heard for a considerable distance downstream, this is proof that the artery is patent at the levels where the bruit is heard.

Limb Blood Pressures and Volume Pulse Detection

It is now standard practice to measure limb blood pressures with or without the assessment of the limb volume pulses.[17,21] These will assist the physician in confirming the diagnosis as well as providing information concerning the extent of the involvement.

The systolic arterial pressure is normally amplified as one progresses from the level of the abdominal aorta to the tibial arteries at the ankle.[22] This means that the systolic pressure at the ankle will be higher than that recorded from the aorta and the arm. Since systemic blood pressures vary, the convention that has been adopted is to express ankle systolic pressures as a ratio.[23] This ratio (the ankle/arm index) in the normal subject should be equal to or greater than 1.0. With an index at this level, a hemodynamically significant lesion cannot be present proximal to the ankle. However,

it is possible to have a stenosis that only becomes hemodynamically significant with the increase in flow that occurs with exercise.[24] As the flow velocity increases through a moderate stenosis, a pressure drop may develop that is significant and a cause of intermittent claudication. As noted earlier, limb blood pressures may not be measurable at the ankle level in patients with diabetes owing to the medial calcification that makes the arteries below the knee incompressible.[16,17] The prevalence of this finding is in the range of 15 percent in diabetics with peripheral arterial disease.

If the systolic pressures cannot be measured at the ankle because of medial calcification of the tibial arteries, it is possible to measure them from the toes.[25] This requires use of either a strain gauge plethysmograph or a photoplethysmograph as the sensing element. Since the digital arteries are rarely calcified, it is generally possible to measure the systolic pressures. At the level of the toe, the systolic pressure should normally be 60 percent or more of the arm systolic blood pressure.[17]

Segmental Limb Studies

If one wishes to further estimate the level and extent of the arterial disease, it is possible to measure the systolic pressures at the level of the calf, lower thigh, and upper thigh.[3] It has been shown that segmental pressures can provide diagnostic information if one compares the pressures between similar sites of the two limbs and the gradients between the limb segments. Normally, the gradient between adjacent segments should be 20 mmHg or less. The pressures recorded from the thigh, particularly the upper thigh, will be falsely high owing to the discrepancy between the width of the cuff used to measure the pressure and the circumference of the limb. This fact must be kept in mind when interpreting the results (Fig. 11-4).

With use of a pulse volume recorder it is possible to record the volume pulses from the same limb segments at which the pneumatic cuffs have been placed to measure the segmental pressure.[11] The major use of these pulses is to examine the shape of the recorded volume pulse change. Normally, the limb volume pulses should have a sharp systolic peak with a prominent dicrotic wave on the downslope. When there is an arterial occlusive lesion proximal to the cuff, the volume pulses are damped, with loss of the sharp systolic peak and the dicrotic wave (Fig. 11-2).

While it is difficult to generalize about the role of these measurements in clinical practice, the following guidelines are helpful.

1. The ankle systolic pressures confirm the status of the arteries proximal to the recording site.

2. The ankle/arm ratio may serve as the baseline value for future comparison. It is known that the variability in measurement will fall in the ±0.15 range.[26] This is important since the systolic pressure can be used for monitoring both the status of the disease and the extent to which it is modified by surgical and endovascular methods designed to improve flow.

3. The ankle/arm index can also provide the observer with indirect clues as to the extent of involvement. For example, if the ankle/arm ratio is higher than 0.50, it is likely that only one major arterial segment is narrowed or occluded; if the ratio is less than 0.50, more than one major arterial segment is probably involved. The ankle/arm ratio reflects the pressure drops across the collateral circuits that are in series[1] (i.e., those that are additive). This information can be of value as the surgeon attempts to predict at the initial visit which form of therapy will most likely be needed to improve the circulation.

4. The absolute levels of the ankle systolic blood pressure provide indirect information on the status of the perfusion. In general, with systolic pressures above 50 mmHg nutritional flow to the digits is adequate. Levels below 50 mmHg are worrisome, particularly if an ulcer is present.[27] Under these circumstances healing might be a serious problem.

Velocity Waveform Analysis

CW Doppler is the quickest and most accurate method of measuring limb systolic pressures[9] but also permits assessment of the arterial velocity flow patterns at several levels of the limb. The areas that cannot be insonated include the major vessels within the thorax and those inside the skull. While access to the basal arteries of the brain is now possible by the use of transcranial pulsed Doppler, this requires a separate device, whose applications are different from those for the peripheral arteries. The transmitting frequency employed with CW Doppler is in the 5- to 7.5-MHz range. These transmitting frequencies are adequate for reaching most arteries and veins of interest.

In order to determine the effect of arterial and venous disease on flow patterns, it is necessary to identify with certainty the vessels being studied. In the leg it is possible with CW Doppler to study the external iliac artery and vein but not the common iliac artery and aorta. This is due to the depth of these arteries and the uncertainty of the source of the backscattered signal. As discussed in Chapter 12, this problem has been overcome by using duplex scanning, which has both imaging and pulsed Doppler as a part of its function. On the other hand, useful information can be obtained with CW Doppler for those arteries distal to the inguinal ligament.

Since the velocity patterns that are observed vary with the organ or tissue being studied, it is important for the user to be aware of the patterns observed.

1. *Low-resistance organs,* which include the brain, liver, and kidney,[28] demand a high level of blood flow for proper function. While the level of blood flow varies, these organs do not show the same wide swings in levels of flow that are seen with some other organs or tissues. Their vascular beds are characterized by a high end-diastolic velocity, which varies little with activity or from day to day.

2. In *variable-resistance organs and tissues* flow is entirely dependent upon level of activity at the time of the study. For example, flow in the superior mesenteric artery is at its lowest point under fasting conditions, reflecting the low metabolic activity of the organ.[29] At this time reverse flow may often be seen and end-diastolic flow is low. However, within 20 minutes of eating, this pattern changes as resistance to flow decreases. During the maximal vasodilatory phase, the peak systolic and end-diastolic flows will dramatically increase, providing a velocity pattern that is very similar to that seen with the low-resistance organs.

The same applies to the arms and legs, where the observed normal velocity patterns are dependent upon activity at the time of study. In the legs the flow patterns of the large and medium-sized arteries (named vessels) under resting conditions is of the high-resistance type, with a prominent reverse flow component[30] (Fig. 11-5). However, with the vasodilation of exercise, the pattern changes dramatically. Flow reversal disappears, and peak systolic and end-diastolic flows increase. The upper extremities are more variable in their level of resistance to flow under resting conditions. The following sequence of steps in the examination is recommended.

1. The initial interrogation should be at the groin level. Here it is possible to assess the velocity patterns in the distal external iliac and common femoral arteries. The normal arterial signal has a triphasic waveform (forward flow, reverse flow, and late forward flow); if this pattern is not present, one can be assured that there is a problem proximal to the examination site. If there is a hemodynamically significant stenosis or occlusion proximal to the common femoral artery, the velocity waveform will lose its sharp systolic peak and reverse flow component becoming, a monophasic waveform.

2. While it would be desirable to also study the profunda femoris artery by this approach, this is impossible with CW Doppler. It is necessary to use the duplex scanner to identify and accurately study the flow patterns in this important collateral artery.[31]

3. Since the superficial femoral artery is a common site for the development of arteriosclerotic narrowing and occlusion, it is important to survey this vessel throughout its length. In order to accurately identify this artery, it is useful to use the adjacent superficial femoral vein as a landmark. The velocity waveforms should be the same as those observed in the common femoral artery. If a stenosis is encountered, the peak systolic velocity will dramatically increase.[9] However, one caveat is in order. If the artery is totally occluded and the Doppler beam happens to detect

flow in a collateral at its site of origin, the peak systolic velocity may appear to suddenly increase, when in fact only a sudden change in the angle of incidence of the sound beam with the vessel has occurred. If, for example, the angle of insonation were to suddenly approach or become zero, this would result in an apparent dramatic increase in velocity.

4. The popliteal artery, for reasons that are poorly understood, is considerably less subject to atherosclerotic involvement than is the superficial femoral artery.[13] The most suitable position of the patient for examining the popliteal artery is prone with the lower leg elevated on a pillow.

5. With CW Doppler, it is not possible to scan the entire length of the tibial and peroneal arteries. Routinely, these arteries are examined at the level of the ankle at those points where the arterial velocity signals are used to measure the ankle systolic pressures. If no signals are detected in the tibial arteries, the peroneal artery should be looked for at the point where it curves around the lateral malleolus. It can become an important collateral artery to the foot.

When the pressures have been measured and the velocity patterns surveyed, the observer has important preliminary information as to the site(s) of involvement. Other methods, including the pulsatility index (PI)[32] and Laplace transform analysis (LTA),[33] have been used to complement the audible interpretation of the velocity signal. These have been developed as methods for evaluating the status of the common iliac artery by analyzing the recorded velocity signal from the common femoral artery.

The PI is a dimensionless number that is calculated by measuring the peak-to-peak height of the waveform and dividing this by the mean height of the waveform. In most available systems the PI can be automatically calculated by the computer software in the spectrum analyzer system that is used. It is important to realize that the PI is independent of the angle the sound beam makes with the artery. Normally, the value of the PI increases as one moves from the femoral artery to the tibial arteries at the ankle. For example a normal value for the PI of the femoral artery would be 13.0, increasing to 18.0 at the ankle.[32] From the PI values it is possible to calculate the inverse damping factor (DF), which is the ratio of the PI in the popliteal and tibial arteries to the proximal PI. The following examples illustrate typical values of these indices for the major arterial segments.

1. In normal subjects
   a. Common femoral, PI 13.0
   b. Popliteal, PI 16.7, DF 1.3
   c. Posterior tibial and dorsalis pedis, PI 17 to 18.0, DF 1.1
2. With an iliac artery occlusion
   a. Common femoral, PI 2.4
   b. Popliteal, PI 2.7, DF 1.1

   c. Dorsalis pedis and posterior tibial, PI 4.6–5.6, DF 2.1
3. With an occlusion of the superficial femoral artery
   a. Common femoral, PI 6.1
   b. Popliteal, PI 4.4, DF = 0.72.
   c. Dorsalis pedis and posterior tibial, PI 4.6 to 5.6, DF 1.3
4. With combined disease-iliac artery and superficial femoral occlusion
   a. Common femoral, PI 3.1
   b. Popliteal, PI 2.4, DF 0.78
   c. Dorsalis pedis and posterior tibial, PI 3.1 to 3.7, DF 1.5

It has been noted by Johnston and Kassam[34] that the PI recorded from the femoral artery decreases as the degree of involvement increases. For stenoses that narrow the iliac artery by more than 50 percent, it is not unusual to have PIs in the 1 to 4 range. With total occlusions this value often falls even further. The femoral-popliteal DF also decreases as a function of the degree of involvement as noted by arteriography. High-grade stenoses and total occlusions result in values in the 0 to 1.0 range.

When the PI and DF results have been compared with arteriographic studies, the following results[34,35] have been noted:

1. For the femoral artery with use of a cutoff value of 5.5 for the PI, the sensitivity for detecting a stenosis that is 50 percent or greater is 82 percent, with a specificity of 99 percent. When the DF is used for the detection of femoro-popliteal disease and a cutoff level of 1.0 is chosen, the sensitivity is 86 percent and the specificity is 95 percent.

2. If the cutoff point of 1.0 is used for the tibial DF, the sensitivity for severe tibial disease is 88 percent with a specificity of 98 percent.

Johnston[35] also investigated the relationship between PI and the aortofemoral pressure gradient measured at the time of arteriography. When the gradient was equal to or greater than 10 mmHg, the PI had an overall accuracy of 95 percent.

In 1980 Skidmore and Woodcock[33] introduced the (LTA) method, which processes the velocity waveform into the frequency domain. The theory behind this approach is based upon the prediction that the coefficients of the transform are related to (1) the proximal stenosis (D or damping factor), (2) the arterial wall stiffness (WO), and (3) the distal impedance (G). This relationship can be expressed as

$$H(S) = 1/(S^2 + 2DWO + WO^2)(S + G)$$

The solution of the equation yielded two complex poles related to D and WO and a real pole related to G, all of which can be expressed on an Argand diagram. A significant proximal iliac stenosis would reduce both D and W, shifting the poles from X1 to X2. Normal values of D ranged from 0.20 to 0.40. Increasing degrees of stenosis proximally resulted in an increase in

D, and with severe damping of the waveform, the complex poles became real and D reached a maximum of 1.0. WO was related to the stiffness of the proximal arterial walls, normal arteries having a value above 15 with lower values resulting from proximal stenosis. G was related to the radius of the distal runoff system. The model predicted that D and WO would be independent of distal impedance and would therefore not be affected by disease of the superficial femoral artery.

Baker et al.[36] evaluated the arteriograms for a series of 148 limbs in 101 patients to determine the status of the aortoiliac and femoropopliteal arteries. The aortoiliac segments were categorized by the degree of stenosis. The superficial femoral arteries were simply classified as patent or occluded vessels. For stenoses that exceeded 50 percent in terms of diameter reduction, the best threshold value for D was found to be 0.60 (sensitivity of 92 percent, specificity of 94 percent with use of instantaneous mean velocities). When a peak velocity detector was used for the same patients, the sensitivity was 87 percent, and the specificity of 98 percent. The results of such studies and the receiver operating characteristic (ROC) curves for the data are shown in Figure 11-7.

Exercise Testing

Since the most common problem that develops in patients with arterial occlusive disease is intermittent claudication, it is only natural that an exercise stress test should be used to document its severity. In the normal subject exercise is followed by a dramatic increase in skeletal muscle blood flow to meet the needs of the working muscle groups. The major features of the normal hemodynamic response are the expected dramatic and nearly instantaneous increase in flow and the following short period of recovery, when the blood flow rapidly returns to the pre-exercise levels (period of postexercise hyperemia).[1] Because of the difficulty of measuring blood flow during exercise, it has been necessary to make the measurements before exercise and immediately after the exercise has been completed.

When arterial narrowing of a significant degree develops proximal to the exercising muscle mass, the situation is dramatically changed, since flow is now directed around the area(s) of obstruction via the collaterals. These important arteries have three major zones, namely the stem vessels, the midzone, and the reentry channels. From a functional standpoint the most important vessels are those found in the midzone, where they are normally very small.[37] As these vessels increase in size, they connect with the reentry vessels, where flow is now reversed in direction.[38] An example of a critical collateral circuit is the profunda femoris artery, which is a stem artery in cases of occlusion of the superficial femoral artery. The midzone vessels are those in the midthigh that connect with the geniculate arteries, which are now serving as the reentry channels.

Since the collaterals have higher than normal resistance to flow, there is a larger than normal pressure drop

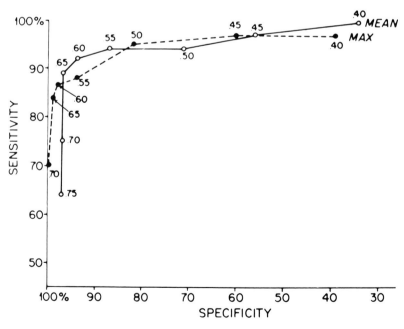

Figure 11-7 Receiver-operator curves for the damping factor (0) determined by LaPlace transform analysis of Doppler recordings from the common femoral artery. The 0.60 cutoff point was found to be best for detection of a greater than 50 percent stenosis of the common iliac artery. (From Baker et al.,[36] with permission.)

across these arteries. This results in a lower perfusion pressure to the exercising muscles in addition to the restriction in the actual volume of blood that the collaterals are able to provide to the muscle during exercise. Unfortunately, with exercise and subsequent vasodilation, the perfusion pressure in the arteries supplying the muscle progressively falls. This further limits the amount of flow that can be provided to the muscle during its time of maximal need. This vicious circle is reversed only when the exercise is terminated.

The hemodynamic changes that are of interest in the patient with claudication are as follows (Fig. 11-8):

1. The peak blood flow levels to muscle is below normal.[1]
2. The arterial perfusion pressure falls from its pre-exercise level to a much lower level.
3. The time of the postexercise hyperemia is greatly prolonged.[1]

The major features of the exercise response that can be evaluated in the vascular laboratory include the

baseline ankle systolic blood pressure, the walking time on the treadmill, and the postexercise ankle blood pressure. While it would appear desirable to measure calf muscle blood flow in addition to pressures, this is not practical and most importantly, not necessary. The reason for this is that the response of the ankle systolic blood pressure to exercise is an accurate reflection of the hemodynamic deficit and is much simpler to measure.[1] The procedure used for such studies is as follows.

1. It is preferable to use a treadmill to control the walking speed and elevation.[39] While there are differences in the walking speed and elevation that are used, we prefer a speed of 2 mph with an elevation of 12 degrees. We have arbitrarily set a walking time limit of 5 minutes, since times beyond that add no diagnostic information. Furthermore, if a patient can walk for 5 minutes, this represents very mild claudication, which rarely requires interventional therapy.
2. The arm and ankle systolic pressures are measured in the supine position before starting the exercise. The ankle

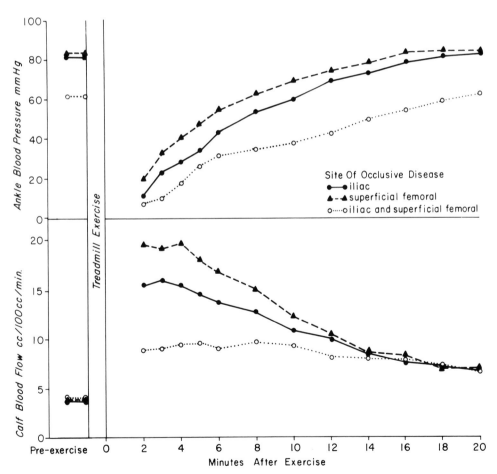

Figure 11-8 Ankle systolic blood pressures and calf blood flow measured before and after exercise in patients with arteriosclerosis obliterans and intermittent claudication. It should be noted that there is an inverse relationship between the calf blood flow and the ankle systolic pressure. (From Sumner and Strandness,[1] with permission.)

blood pressure cuffs are left in place during the walking period on the treadmill.

3. It is important for the technologist to carefully observe the walking pattern and record the time of onset of the pain, the site at which the pain develops, and its pattern of radiation. The patient is urged to walk as long as possible. An additional advantage of the stress test is that if other symptoms, such as shortness of breath or angina pectoris, appear under this modest work load, this can also be noted.

4. After the exercise is completed, the patient immediately resumes the supine position, and the ankle systolic pressures are again measured. It is important to realize that ankle systolic pressure may be so low initially that it cannot be recorded; however, the pressure will slowly increase to reach the baseline. The time required for the return of the ankle pressure to the pre-exercise level may exceed 15 minutes in some patients. While it is a common practice to also record the arm systolic pressures after exercise, this need not be done, since it adds nothing to the evaluation. Normally, the arm systolic pressures increase by an amount related to the work load. It is not necessary to record the postexercise changes as the ankle/arm ratio, since the most important findings are the magnitude of the drop in ankle systolic pressure and the time required to return to baseline.

5. The duration of the walking time is relevant. Patients with severe claudication will not be able to walk for more than 1 minute and will have a dramatic fall in ankle systolic pressure even with this low work load. Patients with walking times in the range of 1 to 3 minutes are moderately disabled but are generally able to carry out their usual activities; however, for those who must walk for their occupation this time may be insufficient. Patients with mild claudication will be able to walk longer than 3 minutes.

The exercise test not only permits objective documentation of the walking time and its physiologic response but is also very helpful in sorting out other causes of leg discomfort that may be difficult to evaluate on the basis of the history and physical examination alone.

Peripheral Venous Disease

The Problem

Among all the diseases of the vascular system, acute thrombosis of the deep venous system (DVT) remains a common and perplexing problem. It is in fact, the only vascular disease whose etiology appears to be related to acute and chronic illness and injury. The original triad described by Virchow in 1856 — stasis, intimal injury, and hypercoagulability — still appears to contain the essential elements for development of this problem.[40] Each element of the triad is very difficult to define in quantitative terms, but theoretically these elements appear to be necessary for the disease to occur.

For example, the relationship between bed rest and the development of DVT is well known. *Stasis* is defined as the persistence of blood in contact with the intima for abnormally long periods of time. The sites at which this has been demonstrated include the soleal sinusoids and the sinuses of the venous valves.[41] While there must be an element of local hypercoagulability for thrombosis to develop, this has not been firmly documented. Short of the recently demonstrated importance of proteins C and S and antithrombin III, it is impossible in most patients to find any evidence of a systemic coagulopathy. Some changes in the intima at the site of thrombosis must occur, but in the absence of direct trauma to the vein, we have little information concerning the exact role of this third element in Virchow's triad.

A problem that has plagued the medical profession is that acute DVT does not, except in rare circumstances, give rise to symptoms and signs that are specific enough to make the diagnosis.[42] Except in the patient with massive iliofemoral thrombosis (phlegmasia cerulea dolens), the clinical picture is nonspecific. The massive total leg swelling, pain, and coolness of the involved limb in a patient with acute iliofemoral thrombosis are difficult to confuse with the indications of any other disease.

Since acute DVT is difficult to assess accurately at the bedside, it is only natural that noninvasive methods would be developed to evaluate the status of the deep venous system. In this regard it is important to recognize that the problem we are discussing does not include superficial thrombophlebitis, which is a distinct and separate entity with a distinctive inflammatory component that is not difficult to recognize at the bedside. Although the term *thrombophlebitis* has also been applied to acute DVT, this is not appropriate, since neither infection nor inflammation is a prominent part of its pathophysiology.

While venography remains the "gold standard" for the diagnosis of acute DVT, it has not been widely applied. This is due to the fact that the test is painful and costly and can be associated with the development of serious complications in a small percentage of patients. Between 2 and 10 percent of patients who undergo this procedure develop a contrast material-induced phlebitis that needs to be treated.[43]

Disease Localization

Before reviewing the indirect tests that are of value in the diagnosis of acute DVT, it is necessary to review the sites at which the disease occurs, the problems it creates, and the strategies that are necessary to recognize its presence. Interest in localization and progression of deep venous thrombi came following the introduction of the iodine 125-labeled fibrinogen method by Hobbs.[44] This method permits the detection and localization of venous thrombi in their earliest stages. After the ^{125}I fibrinogen is injected, it becomes incorporated in the forming thrombus, setting up site(s) of increased radioactivity that can be detected externally by scintillation counters. Numerous studies using this method have shown that the earliest site for development of thrombi is within the sinuses of the soleus muscle. If untreated, 80 percent of the thrombi will resolve by lysis and produce no problems.[45] On the other hand, in the remaining 20 percent of patients thrombus propagation will occur that may extend to the level of the popliteal vein and even higher. Unfortunately, the ^{125}I method is insensitive to thrombi at more proximal levels such as the superficial femoral, common femoral, and iliac veins. This method has been used primarily for prospective studies in which it was possible to also test the role of prophylactic measures designed to prevent DVT from occurring.

When thrombi remain confined to the calf, few problems are likely to occur. Pulmonary emboli are uncommon and rarely serious. When thrombi involve the major proximal veins (popliteal to inferior vena cava), serious problems may develop acutely and chronically.

Since the venous thrombi that develop in the proximal veins are the most dangerous, it is for these segments that the indirect noninvasive tests have had their greatest utility and success. The methods that have been used for screening the major proximal veins have involved either CW Doppler or some method of plethysmography.[46-49]

Diagnostic Approaches

Continuous Wave Doppler Evaluation

The principles behind the use of CW Doppler to interrogate the major deep veins are very similar to those that apply to the study of the arterial circulation. For the lower limbs, a 5-MHz system is adequate for reaching all the major veins from the level of the posterior tibial at the ankle to the external iliac vein.[46] No attempt is made to study the flow in the common iliac vein or the inferior vena cava, since without the benefit of imaging it is not possible to be certain which veins are being insonated. When studying the veins below the knee, the anterior tibial and peroneal veins are not evaluated by CW Doppler for two reasons: first, the anterior tibial vein is rarely the site of acute DVT, and second, it is very difficult to precisely identify the peroneal vein in the calf.

In practice, the adjacent large or medium-sized artery is used as the landmark for identification of its accompanying vein. This provides some assurance that the CW transducer has been placed in the proper position for detecting venous flow from the appropriate vessel. The procedures that must be followed in studying the deep venous system are as follows.

1. The same sites in the two limbs must be examined and compared. While bilateral venous obstruction secondary to DVT can occur, it is relatively uncommon.
2. The procedure should be the same for each study. It is preferable to start in the groin and from that point move sequentially down the limb to the posterior tibial veins at the ankle. The popliteal vein is best studied with the patient in the prone position with the feet supported by a pillow.
3. For the proximal veins (popliteal to external iliac), normal venous flow should be spontaneous and vary with respiration. During inspiration, flow will diminish when the intra-abdominal pressure exceeds that in the inferior vena cava.[50] For the posterior tibial veins, spontaneous flow may not be present. This is due to the fact that flow velocity in this vein may be very low and below the threshold of CW Doppler. In this circumstance it is necessary to use augmentation maneuvers to increase venous flow to a detectable level. For example, compression of the foot will result in a surge of venous flow that is easily heard.
4. When a major vein is occluded, no flow is detected from that vein. One must be very careful in this situation, since collateral veins in the path of the sound beam may give the impression that the vein is indeed patent. However, flow in a collateral vein in these circumstances is usually continuous and not phasic with respiration. In fact, the finding of continuous venous flow in one limb and not in the other is good evidence that acute DVT is present.

When CW Doppler studies have been compared with venography, the results have been satisfactory. Overall, sensitivity should be in the range of 87 percent, with a specificity of 88 percent.[51] While the method is best for the major proximal veins, it is also possible to use it to detect abnormal flow patterns below the knee. The problem here is that the false positive rate for below-the-knee findings with CW Doppler is quite high. This is due to the fact that other conditions can alter the flow patterns in this area in a manner similar to that found with DVT. Any inflammatory condition in the limb will cause venous flow patterns to become continuous.

One of the major problems associated with use of CW Doppler is its dependence on the skill of the examiner. It requires a great deal of experience as well as some knowledge of regional anatomy and the venous flow patterns associated with the development of acute DVT.

Plethysmography

Since venous thrombosis leads to total occlusion of the involved segments in most instances, it is only natural that methods designed to measure venous outflow from the lower extremity would be applied to the problem of detecting acute DVT. If flow is diverted through high-resistance collateral vessels, the venous outflow from that limb should be lower than that from the unaffected limb. The methods that have been employed to make this determination include use of the mercury-in-Silastic strain gauge and impedance plethysmography. To test the rate at which the venous collaterals can drain the limb following a period of transient venous occlusion, a cuff is placed about the thigh and rapidly inflated to 50 mmHg. Since venous capacitance is related to venous outflow, it is necessary to keep the cuff inflated until the limb volume increase has stabilized. This requires 2 to 3 minutes. After the calf volume increase has stabilized, the cuff is rapidly deflated, which gives rise to the venous outflow curve for the limb. This information can be handled in several ways.

1. If a mercury-in-Silastic strain gauge is used, the actual volume change over time can be calculated. This was originally done by taking the maximal slope of the line as the value of what became known as the *maximal venous outflow*. While this worked fairly well, there were some problems with this measurement.
   a. The exact initial slope of the outflow curve was not always easy to determine.
   b. Because the venous outflow rate is related to the venous capacitance, the venous outflow should be plotted against capacitance, which is defined as the volume change that occurs after the thigh cuff is inflated. As noted earlier, the time required to reach maximal calf volume is usually 2 to 3 minutes.
   c. With the impedance plethysmograph, in contrast to the mercury-in-Silastic strain gauge, the values for the volume increase and the venous outflow cannot be expressed in quantitative terms. Nonetheless, it is possible to compare the amplitude of the deflection that occurs during the phase of the volume increase with the amplitude of the fall at 2 seconds after cuff deflation. By plotting these two values against a discriminant line, it is possible to classify the test result as normal or abnormal.
   d. Since the volume sensor is on the calf of the leg, the values obtained will reflect the patency of the venous segments proximal to this level. It has been shown that the plethysmographic methods are sensitive for the detection of acute thrombi that develop in the proximal veins.

The plethysmographic methods have been extensively tested against venography. For proximal venous thrombosis (popliteal to inferior vena cava), the reported results can be summarized as follows[51]:

1. Strain gauge plethysmography: sensitivity 97 percent; specificity 83 percent; positive predictive value 86 percent; negative predictive value, 96 percent.
2. Impedance plethysmography: sensitivity 90 percent; specificity 93 percent; positive predictive value 83 percent; negative predictive value 96 percent.

It has been shown that if a screening test is negative, the patient need not have a venogram, and furthermore, anticoagulation can be withheld. Although the plethysmographic methods cannot detect DVT that develops below the knee, data suggest that thrombi confined to the calf and missed by this method will not have serious immediate consequences for the patient. Pulmonary emboli of a serious nature rarely occur from calf vein thrombi.

However, there are questions relative to calf DVT that need to be answered. Three approaches can be used: (1) venography, which will settle the issue of suspected disease in this region; (2) duplex scanning, which has been shown to be as accurate as venography and is becoming the standard for the field[52,53]; and (3) empiric treatment based upon the clinical findings, which is not the best alternative given the poor correlation between the clinical impression and the results of objective testing.

Extracranial Cerebrovascular Disease

Because of the importance of the carotid bifurcation as a site for the development of atherosclerosis and its role in the production of ischemic cerebral events, it is only natural that a great deal of attention would be paid to the development of noninvasive tests for this area. The tests that were first introduced to study the carotid arteries were CW Doppler and, subsequently, plethysmography. These methods have been extensively tested against arteriography, so we know how they can and should be used.

Diagnostic Approaches

Periorbital Doppler

As the disease at the carotid bifurcation becomes progressively more severe, a point is reached at which flow will be diverted in greater volume through the available collateral circulation. One pathway is provided by the external carotid artery, which communicates with the ophthalmic artery in the orbit by the medial frontal and supraorbital arteries. Normally, blood flows out of the orbit via these vessels to supply the forehead. The direction of flow in the medial frontal and supraorbital arteries will depend upon the pressure gradient that exists between the external and the internal carotid arteries distal to the carotid bifurcation.

The procedure requires a direction-sensing CW Doppler scanner that will permit accurate documentation of the direction of flow in the medial frontal and supraorbital arteries.[54] When a hemodynamically significant stenosis develops in the internal carotid artery, the flow in the medial frontal and supraorbital arteries may be reversed. In addition, compression of the superficial temporal artery will result in cessation of flow in these periorbital vessels, signifying that the external carotid artery is now serving as a collateral source to the hemisphere on the side of the stenosis. This test has serious limitations but still may be of some value in certain circumstances. Its problems relate to the fact that it cannot distinguish between high-grade stenosis and total occlusion. In addition, if other collateral pathways are the primary feeding channels to the brain, the periorbital studies may not detect the problem. One of the simplest applications of this approach is its use in the perioperative period after carotid endarterectomy. If a patient awakes from anesthesia with a deficit or develops one very early, it may be possible to use this test to determine if an internal carotid occlusion has developed.

Oculoplethysmography

The oculoplethysmographic (OPG) system developed by Gee is a simple indirect method that uses cups applied to the sclera of the eye and placed under a negative pressure sufficient to stop blood flow to the eye.[55] As the pressure in the system is gradually reduced, a point is reached at which ocular pulsations return. It is possible to relate the pressure in the ophthalmic artery to this point. This test is in principle similar to the periorbital Doppler method in that it is most useful in detecting of stenoses and occlusions that are sufficiently severe to reduce pressure and flow. The OPG method is unable to distinguish between a tight stenosis and a total occlusion. In addition, once the test becomes positive, further changes in the status of the disease cannot be evaluated. In theory, one of its advantages could be the detection of a tight siphon lesion that would be missed by duplex scanning.

While this method is useful, it has largely been superseded by duplex scanning. As noted in Chapter 12, duplex scanning has the great advantage of being able to assess not only the carotid bifurcation but also the vertebral arteries. In addition, the availability of transcranial Doppler now makes it possible to investigate the status of the basal arteries and the carotid siphon. While the place of OPG is yet to be determined, it will provide an additional method that may be of value in specific circumstances.

Transcranial Doppler

With the availability of transcranial Doppler it is now feasible to examine the basilar arteries to the brain through the intact skull, the orbit, and the foramen magnum. The transmitting frequencies used are lower than in most systems used in transcutaneous applications. For example, a transmitting frequency of 2.0 MHz is most often employed.[56] In order for the sound to penetrate through the skull, it has been necessary to increase the acoustic intensity to more than 100 mW/cm^2, and the sample volume size has been increased as well. The current systems operate at a maximum acoustic power of 266 mW/cm^2, with a sample volume size of 14 × 7 mm. The temporal bone window is the site commonly used for access to the middle cerebral artery, but owing to the thickness of this bone, it is impossible to penetrate the skull in up to 13 percent of subjects. It is important to realize that when this method uses the transorbital approach to the anterior cerebral arteries, the acoustic power must be dramatically reduced to 10 percent of that used to gain access to the middle cerebral artery.

The applications of this method have been the following:

1. Confirmation of the presence of extracranial arterial disease[57]
2. The subclavian steal syndrome[58]
3. Intracranial arterial occlusive disease[59]
4. Cerebral vasospasm secondary to subarachnoid hemorrhage[60]
5. Intracranial arteriovenous malformations[61]
6. The diagnosis of brain death[62]
7. Intraoperative monitoring during carotid endarterectomy[63]

The velocity signals obtained from the normal intracranial vessels are similar to those obtained by conventional duplex scanning in the neck. The velocity patterns have a high end-diastolic velocity, reflecting the low resistance of the brain. When there is a lesion proximal to the recording site, peak systolic velocities decrease. In addition, if the collateral circulation is involved owing to a hemodynamically significant carotid or vertebral lesion, the direction of flow in one or more of the basilar arteries should be noted. For example, a high-grade stenosis or occlusion of an internal carotid artery will be followed by a reversal of flow in the ipsilateral anterior communicating artery. This will, of course, be accompanied by an increase in flow in the contralateral anterior communicating artery. Likewise, flow via the posterior communicating artery can increase to become another important source of collateral input via the posterior cerebral artery. When there is associated disease in the carotid siphon that is not detectable by duplex studies of the neck, transcranial Doppler evaluation may be the only way of detecting this with certainty.

The subclavian steal syndrome remains a challenging situation to evaluate. While reversal of flow in the vertebral artery distal to a subclavian stenosis or occlusion is common, it is rarely the cause of symptoms and/or signs.[64] Transcranial Doppler can permit the examiner to directly examine the direction of flow, not only in the vertebral artery but in the basilar artery as well. Whether this capability will add materially to the identification of patients with this problem remains to be demonstrated.

Another potentially attractive feature of the transcranial approach is the detection of stenoses and/or occlusions of the intracranial arteries. In the Western world at least, lesions at this level as a cause of transient or permanent neurologic deficits are very uncommon. It has been shown that the method is capable of detecting such lesions, but the numbers of patients studied is relatively small, and it is yet uncertain when this type of screen is needed for the patients who present with cerebral ischemic events.[59]

One use of the method that appears to be most widely accepted is in detecting and following the course of events after an episode of subarachnoid hemorrhage. It is well known that this problem develops in some patients, leading to a worsening of their neurologic status. When this occurs, there is an increase in flow velocity in the middle cerebral artery, which can become progressive. It is important to note that the changes in velocity will precede the appearance of new symptoms, providing the treating physician an opportunity of intervening prior to the development of irreversible changes.[60]

Since it is possible that a perioperative event such as a stroke can develop secondary to inadequate performance of a shunt, transcranial Doppler has been used as for continuous monitoring of flow during operation. It has been suggested that peak systolic velocity after cross-clamping may be indicative of the adequacy of cerebral perfusion; the values that are proposed vary between 10 and 30 cm/s.[63] The problem here is that the incidence of perioperative events in most series is reported to be between 1 and 5 percent. To determine whether transcranial Doppler criteria can be used to lower this even further would require a very large randomized series of patients.

Since the brain is normally a low-resistance circuit, change in the end-diastolic velocity of flow in the basilar arteries has been proposed as an accurate method of recognizing brain death.[62] The conversion of this normally high end-diastolic velocity to one in which flow reversal is seen is believed to be a good indicator of brain death, particularly if it persists over several days of observation.

REFERENCES

1. Sumner DS, Strandness DE Jr: The relationship between calf blood flow and ankle systolic blood pressure in patients with intermittent claudication. Surgery 65:763, 1969
2. Strandness DE Jr, Sumner DS: Measurement of blood flow. p. 31. In Strandness DE Jr, Sumner DS (eds): Hemodynamics for Surgeons. Grune & Stratton, New York, 1975
3. Knox RA, Strandness DE Jr: Ultrasound techniques for evaluation of lower extremity arterial occlusion. Semin Ultrasound 2:264, 1981
4. Castaneda-Zuniga W, Knight L, Formanek A et al: Hemodynamic assessment of obstructive aortoiliac disease. AJR 127:559, 1976
5. Winsor T: Influence of arterial disease on the systolic blood pressure gradients of the extremity. Am J Med Sci 220:117, 1950
6. Strandness DE Jr: Peripheral vascular disease. Diagnosis and objective evaluation using a mercury strain gauge. Ann Surg, suppl. 161:S1, 1965
7. Strandness DE Jr: The physiology of arterial narrowing and occlusion. p. 20. In Strandness DE Jr (ed): Peripheral Arterial Disease. Little, Brown, Boston, 1969
8. Sumner DS: Volume plethysmography in vascular disease: an overview. p. 97. In Bernstein EF (ed): Noninvasive Diagnostic Techniques in Vascular Disease. 3rd Ed. CV Mosby, St. Louis, 1985
9. Strandness DE Jr, Schultz RD, Sumner DS et al: Ultrasonic flow detection: a useful technique in the evaluation of peripheral vascular disease. Am J Surg 113:311, 1967
10. Strandness DE Jr: The effect of arterial obstruction on the physiology of exercise. p. 61. In Strandness DE Jr (ed): Peripheral Arterial Disease. Little, Brown, Boston, 1969
11. Raines JK: The pulse volume recorder in peripheral arterial disease. p. 563. In Bernstein EF (ed): Noninvasive Diagnostic Techniques in Vascular Disease. 3rd Ed. CV Mosby, St. Louis, 1985
12. Satomura S: Study of blood flow patterns in peripheral arteries by ultrasonics. J Acoust Soc Jpn 199:326, 1959
13. Lindbom A: Arteriosclerosis and arterial thrombosis in the lower limb: a roentgenologic study. Acta Radiol Suppl (Stockh) 80:1, 1950
14. Strandness DE Jr, Priest RE, Gibbons GE: A combined clinical and pathologic study of diabetic and nondiabetic peripheral arterial disease. Diabetes 13:366, 1964
15. Wheelock FC Jr: Transmetatarsal amputations and arte-

rial surgery in diabetic patients. N Engl J Med 264:316, 1961

16. Marinelli MR, Beach KW, Glass MJ et al: Noninvasive testing vs. clinical evaluation of arterial disease. JAMA 241:2031, 1979

17. Carter SA: Role of pressure measurements in vascular disease. p. 513. In Bernstein EF (ed): Noninvasive Diagnostic Methods in Vascular Disease. 3rd Ed. CV Mosby, St. Louis, 1985

18. Strandness DE Jr: Intermittent claudication. p. 53. In Brest AN (ed): Peripheral Vascular Disease. FA Davis, Philadelphia, 1971

19. Strandness DE Jr: Traditional methods of evaluation. p. 25. In Strandness DE Jr (ed): Duplex Scanning in Vascular Disorders. Raven Press, New York, 1991

20. Goodreau JJ, Greasy JK, Flanigan DP et al: Rational approach to the differentiation of vascular and neurogenic claudication. Surgery 84:74, 1978

21. Strandness DE Jr, Sumner DS: Measurement of arterial and venous pressure. p. 21. In Strandness DE Jr, Sumner DS (eds): Hemodynamics for Surgeons. Grune & Stratton, Orlando 1975

22. McDonald DA: Blood Flow in Arteries. Williams & Wilkins, Baltimore, 1960, Ch. 11

23. Yao JST, Hobbs JT, Irvine WT: Ankle systolic pressure measurements in arterial disease affecting the lower extremities. Br J Surg 56:676, 1969

24. Carter SA: Response of ankle systolic pressure to leg exercise in mild or questionable arterial disease. N Engl J Med 287:578, 1972

25. Carter SA, Lezack JD: Digital systolic pressures in the lower limbs in arterial disease. Circulation 43:905, 1971

26. Baker DJ, Dix D: Variability of Doppler ankle pressures with arterial occlusive disease: an evaluation of ankle index and brachial-ankle pressure gradient. Surgery 89:135, 1981

27. Strandness DE Jr: Noninvasive tests in vascular emergencies. p. 103. In Bergan JJ, Yao JST (eds): Vascular Surgical Emergencies. Grune & Stratton, Orlando, 1987

28. Strandness DE Jr: Hemodynamics of the normal arterial and venous system. p. 38. In Strandness DE Jr (ed): Duplex Scanning in Vascular Disorders. Raven Press, New York, 1991

29. Moneta GL, Taylor DC, Helton WS et al: Duplex ultrasound measurement of postprandial intestinal blood flow: effect of meal composition. Gastroenterology 95:1294, 1988

30. Jager KA, Phillips DA, Martin RL et al: Noninvasive mapping of lower limb arterial lesions. Ultrasound Med Biol 11:515, 1985

31. Kohler TR, Nance DR, Cramer MM et al: Duplex scanning for diagnosis and evaluation of aortoiliac and femoropopliteal disease: a prospective study. Circulation 76:1074; 1987

32. Gosling RG, Dunbar G, King DH et al: The quantitative analysis of occlusive arterial disease by a noninvasive ultrasonic technique. Angiology 22:52, 1971

33. Skidmore R, Woodcock JP: Physiological interpretation of Doppler-shift waveforms: theoretical considerations. Ultrasound Med Biol 6:7, 1980

34. Johnston KW, Kassam MS: Processing Doppler signals and analysis of peripheral arterial waveforms: problems and solutions. p. 40. In Bernstein EF (ed): Noninvasive Diagnostic Techniques in Vascular Disease. 3rd Ed. CV Mosby, St. Louis, 1985

35. Johnston KW: Peripheral arterial Doppler blood flow-velocity waveform analysis. p. 154. In Kempczkinski RF, Yao JST (eds): Practical Noninvasive Vascular Diagnosis. 2nd Ed. Year Book Medical Publishers, Chicago, 1987

36. Baker JD, Skidmore R, Cole SEA: LaPlace transform analysis of femoral artery Doppler signals: the state of the art. Ultrasound Med Biol 15:9, 1989

37. Longland CJ: The collateral circulation to the limb. Ann R Coll Surg Engl 13:161, 1953

38. Winblad JN, Reemstma K, Vernhet JL: Etiologic factors in the development of collateral circulation. Surgery 45:105, 1959

39. Strandness DE Jr, Zierler RE: Exercise ankle pressure measurements in arterial disease. p. 575. In Bernstein EF (ed): Noninvasive Diagnostic Techniques in Vascular Disease. 3rd Ed. CV Mosby, St. Louis, 1985

40. Virchow R: Gesammelte Abhandlungen zur Wissenschaftlichen Medizin. p. 219. Medinger Sohn, Frankfurt, 1856

41. Nicolaides AN, Gordon-Smith I: The prevention of deep venous thrombosis. p. 211. In Hobbs JT (ed): The Treatment of Venous Disorders. JB Lippincott, Philadelphia, 1977

42. Haeger K: Problems of acute deep venous thrombosis: the interpretation of signs and symptoms. Angiology 20:219, 1969

43. Athanasoulis CA: Phlebography for diagnosis of deep leg vein thrombosis and pulmonary embolism. DHEW Publ, NIH #76-866, 1975

44. Hobbs JT: External measurement of fibrinogren uptakes in experimental venous thrombosis and other pathological states. Br J Exp Pathol 43:48, 1962

45. Kakkar VV, Howe CT, Flanc C, Clarke UB: Natural history of postoperative venous thrombosis. Lancet 2:230, 1969

46. Barnes RW: Doppler ultrasonic diagnosis of venous disease. p. 724. In Bernstein EF (ed): Noninvasive Diagnostic Techniques in Vascular Disease. 3rd Ed. CV Mosby, St. Louis, 1985

47. Cramer M, Langlois Y, Beach KW et al: Standardization of venous flow measurement by strain gauge plethymography in normal subjects. Bruit 7:33, 1983

48. Hull R, Hirsh J, Sackett DL et al: Combined use of leg scanning and impedance plethysmography using the occlusive cuff technique in the diagnosis of venous thrombosis: an alternative to venography. N Engl J Med 296:1497, 1977

49. Wheeler HB: Diagnosis of deep vein thrombosis. Review of clinical evaluation and impedance plethysmography. In Symposium on Deep Vein Thrombosis. Am J Surg 150:7, 1985

50. Moneta GL, Bedford G, Beach KW et al: Duplex ultrasound assessment of venous diameters, peak velocities, and flow patterns. J Vasc Surg 8:286, 1988

51. Moneta GL, Strandness DE Jr: Basic data concerning noninvasive vascular testing. Ann Vasc Surg 3:190, 1989

52. Killewich LA, Bedford GR, Beach KW, Strandness DE Jr: Diagnosis of deep venous thrombosis: a prospective study comparing duplex scanning to contrast venography. Circulation 79:810, 1989

53. Lensing AWA, Prandoni P, Brandjes D et al: Detection of deep vein thrombosis by real time B-mode ultrasonography. N Engl J Med 320:342, 1989

54. Barnes RW, Russell HE, Bone GE et al: Doppler cerebrovascular examination: improved results with refinements of technique. Stroke 8:468, 1977

55. Gee WG: Ocular pneumoplethysmography. Surv Ophthalmol 29:121, 1985

56. Fujioka K, Kuehn K, Sola-Pierce N, Spencer M: Transcranial Doppler for evaluation of cerebral arterial hemodynamics. J Vasc Tech 13:89, 1989

57. Lindegard KF, Bakke SJ, Grolimund P et al: Assessment of intracranial hemodynamics in carotid artery disease by transcranial Doppler. J Neurosurg 63:890, 1985

58. Hennerici M, Klemm C, Rautenberg W: The subclavian steal phenomenon: a common vascular disorder with rare neurologic deficits. Neurology 38:669, 1988

59. Spencer MP, Whisler D: Transorbital Doppler diagnosis of intracranial stenosis. Stroke 17:916, 1986

60. Aaslid B, Huber P, Nornes H: Evaluation of cerebrovascular vasospasm with transcranial Doppler ultrasound. J Neurosurg 60:37, 1984

61. Lindegard KF, Grolimund P, Aaslid R, Nornes H: Evaluation of AVM's using transcranial Doppler ultrasound. J Neurosurg 65:335, 1986

62. VanVelthoven V, Calliauw L: Diagnosis of brain death. Transcranial Doppler as an additional method. Acta Neurochir (Wien) 95:57, 1988

63. Padayachee TS, Gosling RG, Lewis RR et al: Transcranial Doppler assessment of cerebral collateral during carotid endarterectomy. Br J Surg 74:260, 1987

64. Bornstein NM, Norris JW: Subclavian steal: a harmless hemodynamic phenomenon. Lancet 2:303, 1986

65. Strandness DE Jr: Mercury strain gauge plethysmography: evaluation of patients with acquired arteriovenous fistula. Arch Surg 85:215, 1962

66. Strandness DE Jr: Techniques in the evaluation of vascular disease. Surg Annu Vol 3:181, 1971

12

Duplex Scanning

David L. Dawson
D. Eugene Strandness, Jr.

Ultrasound duplex scanning combines real-time two dimensional B-mode imaging of vessels and their surrounding structures with pulsed Doppler ultrasound evaluation of blood flow. Duplex scanning, by combining sonographically derived imaging and hemodynamic information, takes advantage of the strengths of each modality and avoids many of the problems inherent in the use of imaging or flow studies alone.

Real-time B-mode ultrasound displays an image of a two-dimensional plane, or "slice," through the scanned structure. This method of sonographic imaging provides anatomic information about the size, orientation, course, and structural characteristics of blood vessels. While modern ultrasound scanners display detailed images with depth resolution as fine as 0.2 mm, imaging as a sole modality has a number of drawbacks. Image quality is affected by the depth of insonation, tissue refraction, acoustic shadowing by high-impedance materials (such as tissue calcifications), instrument features, and other factors. In addition, it is difficult to accurately characterize complex three-dimensional structures, such as atherosclerotic plaques, with a scanning plane that displays only two dimensions.

In duplex ultrasound systems, the Doppler scanner provides physiologic information. The frequency shift produced when ultrasound is scattered by moving reflectors (flowing blood) is the Doppler frequency. Either a broad or a narrow band of frequency shifts may be produced, depending on the uniformity of the moving reflectors. These signals are processed and the derived flow information can be presented as an audio output, a spectral waveform, or a two-dimensional color display "superimposed" on the gray-scale B-mode image. Information about the characteristics and velocity of flowing blood (obtained from the Doppler signal) is much more useful when the precise site of sampling is known. Without concomitant imaging there is no way to be certain which vessel is being interrogated. The angle of insonation cannot be determined (this is necessary for standardizing examinations and the calculation of the flow velocities). Flow patterns specific to certain locations may not be recognized (such as those that may occur at bifurcations, adjacent to vessel walls, or with pathology, such as aneurysms).

The past two decades have seen the development of the hardware and techniques of ultrasound duplex scanning (Fig. 12-1). This approach has become the definitive method for screening purposes as well as for long-term studies in both arterial and venous diseases.

ADVANTAGES

Duplex scanning has emerged as the principal testing modality in the noninvasive vascular laboratory.[1-3] It is a direct method of vascular assessment. In contrast to indirect methods such as plethysmography or blood

157

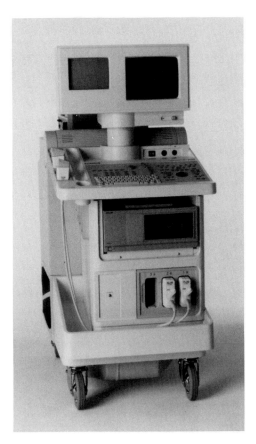

Figure 12-1 Duplex scanner. (Courtesy of Siemens Quantum, Inc.)

laboratory can perform cerebrovascular, peripheral arterial, venous, and intra-abdominal diagnostic studies.

Traditionally, noninvasive diagnostic methods were primarily designed as screening studies, with contrast angiography providing the definitive diagnoses. However, since the accuracy of many duplex scanning applications now approaches or equals that of contrast studies, it has supplanted them in selected cases. For example, a duplex scan diagnosis of lower extremity deep venous thrombosis (DVT) is sufficient for anticoagulation to be initiated. Duplex scanning may also be used to plan operative procedures such as carotid endarterectomy. There is evidence that in some cases endarterectomy may be performed without prior arteriography.[10,11] This is possible only if the quality of the duplex scan has been confirmed, an appropriate lesion is found, and the clinical presentation is not unusual.[12]

Duplex scan findings can also complement the findings of contrast studies. For example, duplex scanning can determine if an anatomic lesion identified by arteriography is hemodynamically significant.[13] This can be especially useful when biplanar views and direct intra-arterial pressure measurements are not available.

In many cases the risks, discomfort, or cost of contrast studies precludes their use, and noninvasive tests provide the only diagnostic option. Arteriography is seldom appropriate for testing asymptomatic individuals, for follow-up of known lesions, or for serial evaluation of the result of an operation or other interventional procedure.

pressure measurements, duplex scanning permits specific examination of any vessel segment at nearly any location in the body. It thereby avoids much of the uncertainty of the indirect testing methods, which do not provide site-specific findings. For example, in carotid artery testing, pneumatic oculoplethysmography (OPG-Gee) is an accurate means of detecting a hemodynamically significant unilateral carotid stenosis, but it has no ability to distinguish a high-grade stenosis from a total occlusion.[4–6] Duplex scanning, on the other hand, can both detect and localize lesions, and it can categorize their severity.[7–9] The duplex scan may also permit detection of mild to moderate disease, and it can be used to follow disease progression.

Although initially duplex scanning was only applied to the extracranial carotid arteries, it can now be applied to nearly every vascular bed except those in the chest, where the air-containing lung limits ultrasound transmission. Higher transmitting powers have even allowed transcranial duplex scanning and color-flow imaging. The versatility of duplex scanning adds to its cost effectiveness. With a single scanner, a vascular

DISADVANTAGES

Although duplex scanning has become the noninvasive method of choice for most vascular examinations, it is not without deficiencies. The greatest problem with duplex scanning is that it is operator-dependent; accurate studies require well trained and experienced technologists to operate the equipment. Instrument setup, adjustment, and operation must be individualized for each examination. Although excellent diagnostic accuracy can be obtained with duplex scanning, significant variability between institutions may exist, and therefore each vascular laboratory must establish its accuracy for each examination it offers.

Other factors must be considered when comparing the results reported from different vascular laboratories. Ultrasound systems have different capabilities and strengths. One machine may have a better Doppler system than another, and image processing systems also vary. The type of transducers used makes a great difference for some applications. In addition, the interpretation criteria used may vary, thus adding another layer of uncertainty, which limits direct comparison of different centers' results.

One criticism of duplex scanning is that interpretation of examination results may vary among observers. The problem of interobserver variability is not unique to duplex scanning, however. In the process of validating duplex scanning methods against arteriography, it was observed that two experienced radiologists reading the same sets of arteriograms would not necessarily agree on how to categorize the severity of a stenosis. This observation provided an example of the fact that variability is inherent in any diagnostic testing, even when the diagnostic standard is being considered.[7] Interobserver variability in the interpretation of a single arteriogram exceeded that observed when comparing a duplex scan with a single arteriographer's interpretation.

The most important variable in evaluating the results of duplex scanning is the interest and dedication of the particular laboratory performing the tests. The techniques are often demanding and can be time-consuming. For example, renal artery studies or complete lower extremity arterial mapping may require up to 2 hours. In some busy offices or laboratories this time investment is not seen as practical. In settings in which appropriate time and energies are not invested, the value of a duplex scan may be limited.

Cost savings are relative. As compared with the hardware, software, and control systems required for angiography or magnetic resonance imaging, ultrasound equipment is quite inexpensive; the price of a fully equipped scanner is in the $100,000 to $200,000 range. However, this expense is an order of magnitude greater than that required to set up a laboratory to do simple indirect testing.

HISTORICAL PERSPECTIVE

Early Development of Doppler Ultrasound Systems

In 1959 Satomura reported that information about blood flow could be derived from Doppler-shifted echoes of ultrasound transmitted through intact skin.[14] The first usable continuous wave Doppler system became available in the mid-1960s. Initially, only the audio output of the system was used for the detection of flow. It was found to be useful for the measurement of limb systolic pressures and proved simpler than the plethysmographic methods previously used for this purpose.[15,16] The audible Doppler signal also permitted a subjective assessment of velocity flow patterns at multiple sites in the upper and lower limbs.

The need for an analog display of the velocity pattern was evident early. The first signal processor employed a differentiator and low-pass filter.[17] This removed the higher carrier frequency of the transmitted ultrasound and detected the frequencies of the Doppler-shifted signal. However, this method was nondirectional and provided only an "envelope" of the backscattered Doppler information.

From animal studies with electromagnetic flowmeters, it was known that velocity patterns in peripheral arteries had a complicated forward-reverse-forward pattern of flow during each pulse cycle. To record the directional information from continuous wave ultrasound required a method for separating the positive and negative Doppler frequency shifts associated with changes in flow direction.[18,19] By comparing the received ultrasound to two quadrature reference signal channels (one reference wave shifted by a quarter of a wave from the other), upper and lower sidebands could be isolated from the echo's signal. The flow components in each direction could be displayed on different channels or presented on a differential display. With this method both the direction and the phasic nature of the flow patterns could be displayed on a strip chart recorder.

The ability to localize the site at which flow is detected is limited with continuous wave Doppler systems. Every moving object within the path of the sound beam will produce a Doppler shift. With continuous wave systems it is not possible to ascertain the sites from which the detected velocities come.

To permit sampling from specific tissue depths, pulsed Doppler systems had to be developed.[20] By pulsing the ultrasound and time-gating the receiver, sampling could be limited to a specific depth in the tissue. Since the speed of ultrasound in tissue is nearly constant, the depth from which the signal is obtained could be determined. A pulsed Doppler system can operate with single or multiple gates; therefore it can be used to assess flow from a selected point or a number of positions along the scan line.

Development of Ultrasound Imaging

An ultrasound echo has both amplitude and frequency characteristics. Ultrasound vascular imaging systems can use information from either the phase shift or amplitude of a returning echo. Imaging systems based on each of these characteristic have been developed. By mapping the origins of Doppler-shifted echoes regions with flowing blood can be demonstrated. Alternatively, physical structures such as the arterial wall can be localized by the echogenicity of their interfaces with luminal blood or the surrounding anatomy.

Doppler flow information can be used to generate a flow image, yielding a picture similar to that obtained with arteriography. Devices for "ultrasonic arteriography" have been used with either continuous wave (without depth resolution)[21,22] or pulsed Doppler systems.[23,24] The transducers for these systems were mounted on a position-sensing arm that translated the position of the detected flow information to the signal processing and display system. The image was then displayed in either a transverse or longitudinal view. However, acoustic shadowing from plaques or low-velocity flow would result in a weak or absent Doppler signal and therefore an overestimation of stenosis severity from the image. In addition to generating a map showing where flow occurred, these systems made it possible to selectively sample the flow velocity at any point within the vessel. Analysis of this velocity information provided the hemodynamic data necessary to reliably determine the presence or characterize the severity of arterial lesions.[25]

Sonographic imaging of static structures such as vessel walls and atherosclerotic plaque uses the amplitude information from the ultrasound pulse. The simplest application of this pulse-echo information is amplitude modulation, or A-mode, which displays the strength of a return echo signal as a vertical deflection on the horizontal time (depth) base of an oscilloscope screen. This only allows distance measurements along a single line (Fig. 12-2). While A-mode can give a noninvasive measurement of arterial luminal diameter,[26] it provides little other anatomic information.

Display of a recognizable image of the anatomy became possible with the development of the brightness modulation method, or B-mode, in which amplitude information at each point along the scan line is represented by the brightness of a dot. The first such instruments were bistable, showing each point as either a black or a white dot of uniform brightness.[27] The introduction of the analog scan converter permitted gray-scale displays.[28] With the broader dynamic range in these systems, low- and high-amplitude echo signals could be displayed in a single scan image. This markedly improved the ability to visualize structures that differ little in echogenicity.

Early B-scan generation of static two-dimensional images required moving a transducer assembly on an articulated arm across the scan plane. Information from multiple transducer locations was accumulated to form a single image. Improvements in scanhead design and image processing led to the development of real-time scanners. By rapidly acquiring and updating image data, video output to the display is frequently updated. Display frame rates exceeding 15 frames per second appear continuous, and the physiologic movement of tissues is visualized.

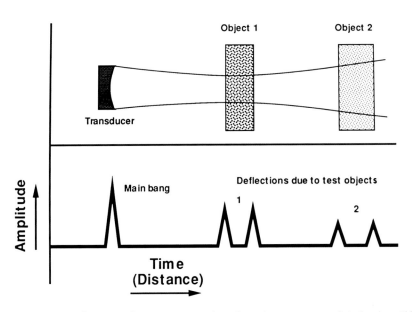

Figure 12-2 Ultrasound is reflected as it passes across interfaces between materials having different acoustic impedances (e.g., the surfaces of a test object). The time between the transmission of the ultrasound pulse and the echo's return is a function of the distance between the transducer and the reflector. The amplitude of returning pulses decreases with increasing distance between transducer and reflector.

Technical Evolution of Duplex Scanning

Duplex scanning is a melding of pulsed Doppler and B-mode technologies. In the early 1970s at the University of Washington, experiments with a prototype real-time ultrasonic B-mode scanning device pointed out the problems associated with imaging alone and led to the development of the first duplex scanner.[29,30] Images with this scanning system displayed crude but recognizable views of vessels in cross-sectional or longitudinal views. One of the first patients studied was found to have clearly imaged common, internal, and external carotid arteries, and all three branches appeared patent. Subsequent arteriography, however, demonstrated that the internal carotid artery was occluded. Because the thrombus in the internal carotid artery had acoustic properties similar to those of flowing blood, it could not be recognized on the basis of the image alone. The addition of a Doppler flow detector to the scanning system solved the problem of assessing the patency of an imaged vessel.[29,30]

Initially, Doppler information was added to the image simply to differentiate occluded from patent vessels, but progress in signal processing electronics and transducer design led to the ability to generate on-line spectral analysis of Doppler information. Honeywell Corporation engineers Langenthal and Gessert developed a fast Fourier transform (FFT) analyzer that could accurately display the information in the Doppler spectrum in real time.[31] With this signal analysis method it was possible to display frequency intensities and the pattern of flow velocities within the imaged blood vessel. Since vessels are found at various depths, addition of a wide range of operating frequencies became necessary. With the introduction of low-frequency (2- to 3-MHz) transducers, the visceral and renal arteries became accessible to interrogation with Doppler ultrasound.

The addition of color Doppler displays came later. Color has become a useful tool for identifying areas in an image in which flow is present, facilitating accurate placement of the pulsed Doppler sample volume.

Clinical Acceptance

The carotid artery was the first vessel of major clinical importance to be studied with duplex scanning. Even today, it is the most frequent arterial study performed in most laboratories.

The need for reliable tests to assess the carotid artery was prompted by the growing recognition of the importance of carotid bifurcation atherosclerosis as a cause of stroke. Clinical evaluation of carotid artery disease is woefully inadequate. The traditional "gold standard" for definitive carotid artery evaluation is contrast arteriography. However, the risks and costs of arteriography preclude its widespread use as a primary screening method.[32-37] The finding of a bruit is a poor predictor of the presence or the severity of a stenosis[38]; therefore arteriography is not appropriate as a first-line test for the evaluation of a patient with a bruit. Of patients with strokes or symptoms suggesting transient hemispheric ischemia, only those who are candidates for carotid endarterectomy need arteriography. It is now well established that patients having significant carotid stenoses as the source of their symptoms will benefit from carotid endarterectomy.[39] Only these symptomatic patients need arteriography, as patients with minimal carotid disease do not have a similar risk for future symptoms.[40] Thus, for both asymptomatic and symptomatic patients with suspected carotid artery disease, some noninvasive means is needed to select those who warrant further evaluation with an arteriogram.

The grading system for carotid artery diagnosis was the first to be developed. Categories of stenosis severity were empirically determined by prospectively comparing duplex scan information with multiplanar contrast arteriograms.[7,41] The arteriographic assessment of stenosis severity involved comparing the diameter of the residual lumen with the estimated diameter of the carotid bulb. Since patients thought to have significant carotid stenoses frequently underwent arteriography, it was relatively easy to correlate the results of duplex scanning with those of invasive studies. Furthermore, because arteriography routinely examines both sides, normal and moderately diseased arteries were also available for comparison. In the course of evaluating the accuracy of duplex scanning, it was also possible to test both the intra- and interobserver variability in arteriographic estimations of the degree of stenosis. This was found to be more significant than previously expected; a variability in this "gold standard" measurement of ±20 percent is not unusual.

For evaluating arterial stenoses, the emphasis has remained focused on Doppler signal analysis. Even with modern imaging systems, B-mode alone is not as good as arteriography for assessing significant carotid artery stenoses.[42] While it is a sensitive means of detecting early atherosclerotic changes in the arterial wall,[43-45] the B-mode image has not been found to be an optimal means of quantitating significant stenoses. Several features of diseased arteries interfere with quality imaging: (1) plaque calcifications may obscure ultrasound transmission; (2) irregular luminal contours may present different sectional appearances depending on the imaging plane used; and (3) hypoechoic plaque or thrombus may not be recognized.

Doppler signal evaluation is a more reliable and robust method for grading stenosis severity than imaging alone. Stenoses are graded by examining the flow velocity changes caused by the stenosis. A significant stenosis is always associated with a change in the velocity and character of blood flow, and even when the image or Doppler signal is suboptimal, these velocity patterns can be recognized. Furthermore, there is a relationship between the degree of stenosis and clinical outcome.[46,47]

After the application of duplex scanning to the carotid artery was established, many of the lessons learned were applied to other vascular beds. Findings characteristic of carotid stenoses, including increasing Doppler frequency shift (increased flow velocity), spectral broadening (flow disturbance), and poststenotic turbulence, were also detectable with other arterial stenoses. Lower extremity and visceral artery scanning, however, were only made practical with the introduction of better ultrasound equipment and a wider range of ultrasound transmitting frequencies. The same process of empirical arteriographic comparison was carried out for each arterial bed, and criteria for grading disease were thereby defined.

BASIC PRINCIPLES OF ULTRASOUND PHYSICS

An understanding of the fundamental physical and physiologic principles upon which duplex scanning is based is important if one is to apply this modality clinically. This familiarity is needed both for proper operation of the duplex scanner and for interpretation of the studies. Errors in diagnosis are avoided by appreciation both of the limitations of duplex scanning and of factors that potentially cause artifacts in the image or flow displays.

The imaging and Doppler functions of a duplex scanner both utilize a pulse-echo system. An ultrasonic piezoelectric transducer acts as both an ultrasound generator and a receiver. Transmission of an electric pulse to the piezoelectric crystal causes it to generate an ultrasonic vibration. The duration of the vibration, and therefore the spatial pulse length, is shortened by mounting a damping material behind the crystal. After the brief pulse is emitted, the crystal becomes inactive, and until the pulse repetition time passes, it awaits the return of echoes. Each ultrasound pulse propagates through the tissue, and a small part of the ultrasound energy is reflected by interfaces in the tissue. When the ultrasound returns to the transducer, the crystal vi-

brates at the frequency of the returning ultrasound, and this produces a voltage change. The amplitude of the voltage generated is proportional to the strength of the returning echo. The frequency with which this pulse-echo cycle repeats is the *pulse repetition frequency* (PRF).

Ultrasound actually travels through different tissues at different speeds, depending on the density and elasticity of the tissue. (Table 12-1). A value of 1540 m/s is commonly used for an average velocity in soft tissue. By using this value, the depth of an ultrasound reflector (distance from the transducer) can be calculated by determining the time required for a pulse to return as an echo.

$$\text{Time for echo to return} = \frac{\text{round trip distance}}{\text{speed of ultrasound}}$$

$$\text{round trip distance} = 2 \times \text{depth}$$

$$\text{depth (d)} = \frac{\text{time} \times \text{speed}}{2}$$

With a focused pulse transmitted in a known direction, this depth information gives spatial localization of the ultrasound reflector. Information from a discrete volume in space can be selected by time-gating the receiver to detect only those echoes from a selected depth. The size of this sample volume is defined by the breadth of the ultrasound beam and the time for which the receiver gate is open. While the former is defined by the transducer design, the latter can be adjusted by the operator.

B-Mode Ultrasound Imaging

Two-dimensional B-mode generates an image of tissue structures from the echoes within the scan plane. In analogy with the ability of an optical lens to focus light rays (another type of propagated wave), an acoustic lens in front of the ultrasound transducer can focus

Table 12-1 Ultrasound and Tissue Properties

Medium	Wave propagation speed (C) m/s	Ultrasound Impedance (Z) rayls (kg/m²s)
Air	330	430
Water	1490	1,490,000
Blood	1570	1,620,000
Liver	1550	1,630,000
Muscle	1580	1,640,000
Bone	3360	4,800,000

the sound energy. Alternately, focusing of the ultrasound beam can be achieved by shaping the transducer itself or by electronic means. Focusing the ultrasound pulses into a scan line defines one axis of a reflector's position. The duration of the pulse-echo cycle gives the distance of the reflector from the transducer. Registration, or the positioning of reflectors on the display, is accomplished by defining specific points on the scan lines with these geometric data.

A scan plane is generated by one of two methods. With mechanical sector scanning transducers, the piezoelectric crystal is rotated and the line of transmission sweeps across the scan plane. Points are localized by the angular position of the scan line and depth. Multiple transducer elements can also be arrayed in a linear or curved row, thus providing imaging across a plane without requiring a moving system. Linear arrays of elements can be operated by sequentially applying a voltage to groups of elements (linear switched array) or by applying voltage to all elements, but with small time differences (linear phased array). A linear array can be simultaneously operated as both a switched and a phased array, which allows scanning, steering, and shaping of the beam. Transducers may also be constructed with an array of concentric ring-shaped elements (annular array). Phased annular arrays may be focused electronically, but beam steering is mechanical (manual).

As echo data are acquired, they are sent to the scan converter. This device receives data at the scanning rate of the transducer and then provides that information to a video circuit at a different rate. Analog devices have been superseded in current ultrasound scanners by digital scan converters. These digitize the image data and store it in memory, with values at each memory address describing the location and amplitude of each image element. In addition, the data can be processed both before and after their conversion to a video signal. This pre- and postprocessing can enhance the appearance of the display.

Video output from the scan converter is displayed on a monitor. Each point of the scan plane image (picture element, or pixel) is correspondingly displayed. The brightness of each pixel reflects the amplitude of the returning echo from each location in the scan plane. Thus, the B-mode image is a three-axis display, providing depth and lateral spatial localization of the echo source and gray-scale representation of the echogenicity of the reflector. The range of values of echo amplitude (dynamic range) represented in the gray-scale display can be selected. A lower dynamic range makes it easier to discriminate between reflectors with similar echogenicity, but much of the echo information from stronger or weaker echo sources will be lost.

A few physical principles are important for the understanding of ultrasound imaging. Acoustic impedance (Z) is a function of the physical properties of the medium through which the sound travels and is a measure of how easily longitudinal acoustic waves can be formed. It is defined as the product of the velocity of sound propagation (C) and the density (ρ) of the propagating medium:

$$Z = C\rho$$

As ultrasound encounters interfaces between tissues having different acoustic impedances, some is reflected and some is refracted. The nature of the reflection depends on the characteristics of the tissue interfaces (Table 12-1). When the irregularities of the reflecting surface are large with respect to the wavelength of the ultrasound, a specular reflection results. A mirror or a smooth surface of water is a specular light reflector. Examples of specular reflectors for ultrasound include the smooth interface between dissimilar impedances that exists when a Lucite block is immersed in a water bath or the interface between blood in the lumen of a vessel and the intima of the vessel wall (Plate 12-1). Specular reflectors produce the strongest ultrasound echoes, but the amount of ultrasound energy returning to the transducer will depend on the angle of incidence at which the ultrasound strikes the reflector. When this angle approaches 90 degrees (normal incidence), a strong echo will return. At angles less than 90 degrees, most of the reflected ultrasound energy will be directed away from the transducer. Diffuse reflectors, on the other hand, have irregularities in the reflecting surface that are small in relation to the wavelength, and they produce lower-amplitude echoes. Much of the reflected ultrasound energy is scattered (Fig. 12-3).

Imaging *resolution* refers to the ability of the system to visualize two reflectors as separate (resolution is the minimum separation distance required to see the reflectors as distinct). Longitudinal (also known as depth, axial, or range) resolution is relatively constant for a given transducer. Reflectors must be separated by at least half of the spatial length of the ultrasound pulse. Spatial pulse length is a function of the number of cycles in the pulse and the wavelength of the ultrasound. On the other hand, lateral (also known as transverse, angular, or azimuthal) resolution varies with the depth and position of the reflector. The best lateral resolution is approximated by the diameter of the ultrasound beam. This varies with the focus and depth, as well as with the accuracy of the imaging system's angular localization of the beam direction.

The ultrasound intensity from a simple disc transducer increases as the beam converges in the near field. The length of the near field, or Fresnel zone, depends

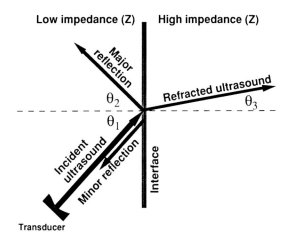

Low impedance (Z)   High impedance (Z)

Figure 12-3 Reflections and refractions are generated as ultrasound passes into a medium with a different acoustic impedance. These effects are the best defined with a specular reflector, which has a smooth and distinct boundary between the media. Ultrasound reflected (at angle θ_2) from a specular reflector has the greatest intensity when the angle of incidence (θ_1) is zero. This is why structures such as vessel walls are most clearly imaged when the ultrasound beam is at a right angle to the structure. The angle of refraction (θ_3) depends on both θ_1 and the relative speed of ultrasound propagation in the different media. Lateral distortion from refraction is minimized when θ_1 is zero.

on both the transducer diameter (d_T) and the frequency or wavelength λ of the ultrasound:

$$\text{Near zone length} = \frac{(d_T)^2}{\lambda}$$

In the transition zone between the near field and the far field lies the region of greatest ultrasound intensity and transducer sensitivity. Beyond this region of natural

focus, in the far field (Fraunhofer zone), the beam becomes divergent and lateral resolution degrades (Fig. 12-4). Focusing a transducer lengthens the transition zone and brings it closer to the transducer face (Fig. 12-5); it also results in a widened beam in the far field (Fig. 12-6).

As ultrasound crosses an interface between different acoustic impedances (other than at right angles), the direction of wave propagation is altered; this is refraction. The magnitude of the refractive bending of the sound waves depends on the relative speed of ultrasound in the different materials or tissues. The relationship of the angle of incidence to the angle of refraction is described by Snell's law. Refraction is another factor limiting the lateral resolution of ultrasound imaging, as accurate correction for the lateral bending of the beam is not feasible. Depth, or distance, measurements are unaffected by tissue refraction.

Because tissues absorb ultrasound energy, echoes returning from deeper sites in the tissue have less of the original ultrasound pulse's energy. Tissue attenuation causes the amplitude and intensity of the ultrasound signal to decay in an inverse exponential fashion with depth. The energy lost is dissipated as heat. The tissue attenuation factor (a) depends somewhat on the type of tissue being insonated; ultrasound is less attenuated by blood than by fat and less by fat than by muscle. The attenuation of ultrasound in tissue is inversely related to the frequency of the ultrasound (Fig. 12-7), Ultrasound of 10-MHz frequency has twice the attenuation of 5-MHz ultrasound. The expected attenuation for a given tissue can be calculated as

$$Ee^{-2aFd}$$

E being the intensity of the incident ultrasound with frequency F. The negative value of the exponent makes

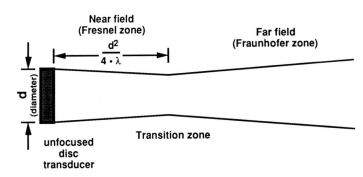

Figure 12-4 The width of an ultrasound beam (and therefore the lateral resolution limit) varies with distance from the transducer. The width of a beam from a single, unfocused (flat) disc transducer decreases in the near field such that the beam's intensity (and resolving power) is greatest in the transition zone (point of natural focus). Near-field length is a function of the transducer's diameter and the wavelength of the ultrasound. The beam is divergent in the far field.

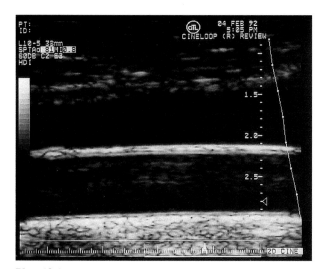

Plate 12-1

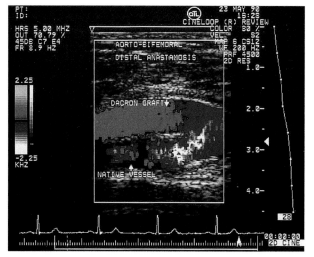

Plate 12-2

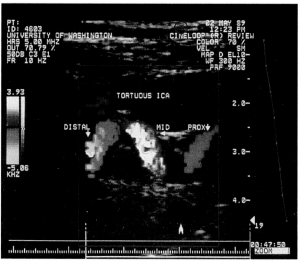

Plate 12-3

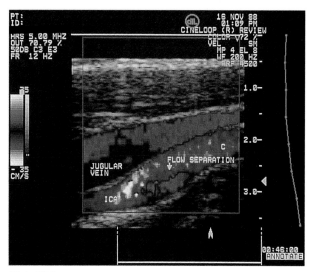

Plate 12-4

Plate 12-1 The blood–intima interface at the wall of a normal artery can act as a specular reflector. In this example, a normal common carotid artery is imaged with the ultrasound beam at a right angle to the vessel wall. The double-line appearance of the arterial wall (best seen in the deep wall), is from a second strong reflection in the outer media. The width of the double line correlates with pathologic measurements of the combined thickness of the intima and media.

Plate 12-2 Color is assigned to pixels based on direction and velocity of flow at each point. The color bar on the far left shows the color assignment. The curvature of this aortofemoral graft results in an abrupt change in the color representing blood flow from red to blue. This is because the left part of the image has flow velocity vectors directed towards the transducer; on the right they are away from the transducer.

Plate 12-3 Color-flow imaging can be quite useful to identify the course of a tortuous vessel, such as this internal carotid artery (ICA). As the orientation of the vessel (and direction of flow) changes with respect to the transducer, the color assignment changes.

Plate 12-4 Color-flow imaging demonstrates flow separation (flow reversal in blue) at peak-systole in the carotid bulb where boundary layer separation occurs. ICA, internal carotid artery. (Courtesy of Advanced Technology Laboratories, Bothell, WA.)

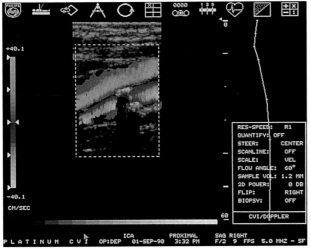

Plate 12-5

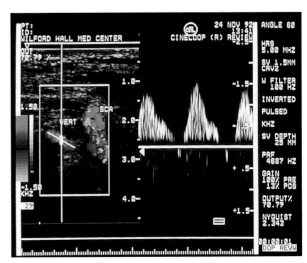

Plate 12-6

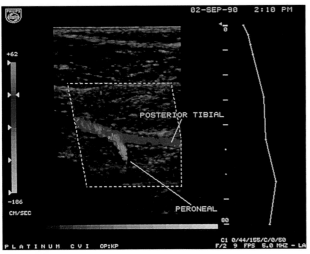

Plate 12-7

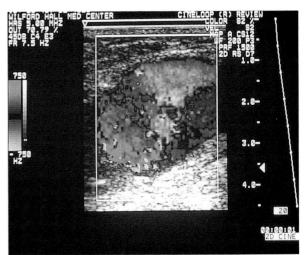

Plate 12-8

Plate 12-5 This calcified plaque blocks ultrasound transmission, and shadowing is evident with absence of both image and Doppler information deep to the plaque. (Courtesy Philips Medical Systems, Santa Ana, CA.)

Plate 12-6 Vertebral artery is seen near its origin from the subclavian artery in the base of the neck.

Plate 12-7 Color-flow imaging facilitates identification of infragenicular vessels. This is the bifurcation of the tibioperoneal trunk, imaged from a medial approach. (Courtesy of Philips Medical Systems, Santa Ana, CA.)

Plate 12-8 Study performed to evaluate a groin mass after cardiac catheterization. The finding of a hypoechoic mass (see Fig. 12-6) is consistent with a simple hematoma, but by demonstrating the presence of blood flow the diagnosis of pseudoaneurysm is made.

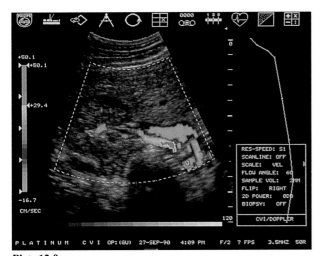

Plate 12-9

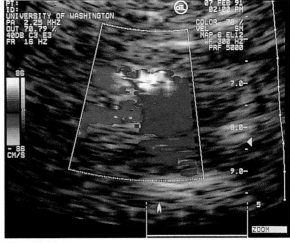

Plate 12-10

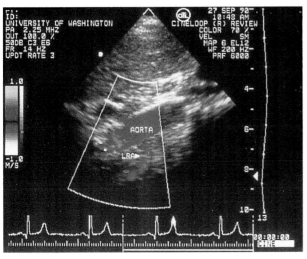

Plate 12-11A

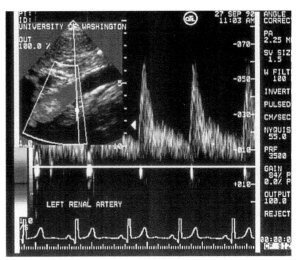

Plate 12-11B

Plate 12-9 Right kidney and right renal artery and vein. (Courtesy of Philips Medical Systems, Santa Ana, CA.)

Plate 12-10 Multiple renal arteries can occasionally be demonstrated with duplex scanning (shown here), but small accessory renal arteries can be missed.

Plate 12-11 (A) From a flank approach, both renal artery origins can be seen. (B) A normal spectral waveform, demonstrating high diastolic flow (low outflow resistance), is demonstrated.

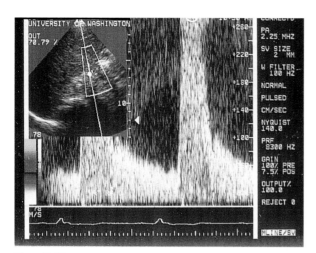

Plate 12-12

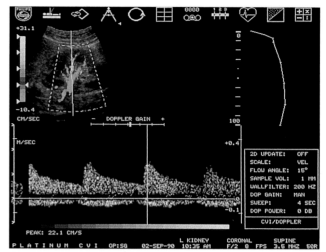

Plate 12-13

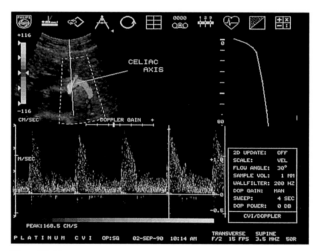

Plate 12-14

Plate 12-12 Spectral waveform from a stenotic renal artery.

Plate 12-13 Normal hilar signal from the left kidney. (Courtesy of Philips Medical Systems, Santa Ana, CA.)

Plate 12-14 The low vascular resistance of the spleen and liver result in continuous forward diastolic flow in the celiac artery. (Courtesy of Philips Medical Systems, Santa Ana, CA.)

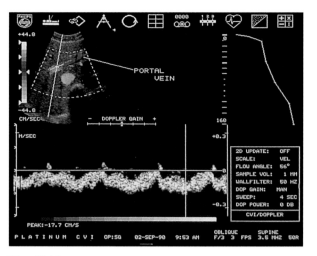

Plate 12-15

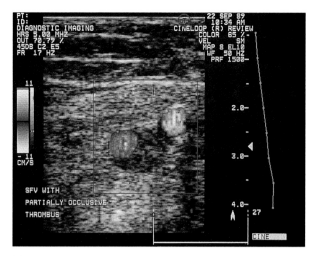

Plate 12-16

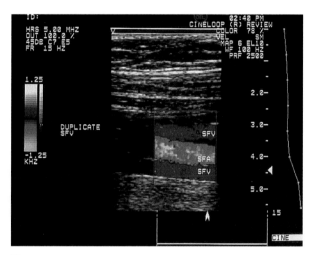

Plate 12-17

Plate 12-15 The portal vein is seen lying anterior to the inferior vena cava in the color-flow image. Normal hepatopetal flow is demonstrated. (Courtesy of Philips Medical Systems, Santa Ana, CA.)

Plate 12-16 Thrombus in veins can be seen with the gray-scale B-mode image. However, in this example of deep venous thrombosis the thrombus is only partially occluding and some venous flow (with a reduced diameter flow channel) can be seen with color-flow image.

Plate 12-17 Duplicated superficial femoral veins (SFV) are uncommon, but are readily identifiable with duplex scanning. One vein is noted on either side of the superficial femoral artery. Thrombosis of a single vein of a paired trunk could be identified by duplex scanning, but would not be recognizable with plethysmography or venography.

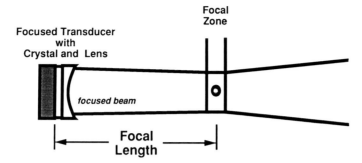

Figure 12-5 The point of greatest intensity of a focused ultrasound beam in a nonattenuating medium is the *focal point.* The *focal length* is the distance from the center of the transducer to the focal point. The *focal zone,* which extends axially on either side of the focal point, is defined as the region in which the amplitude of a reflection from a standard reflector is reduced by ≤ 6 dB.

this a decay function, dependent on the round-trip distance for the ultrasound pulse ($2 \times d$). Low-frequency ultrasound penetrates to deeper tissues more readily than high-frequency ultrasound. Higher transmitting power (stronger intensity) is required to image deeper structures (as in an intra-abdominal application) or for imaging through tissues that have strong attenuating properties (as in transcranial duplex scanning). Table 12-2 lists some of the properties of ultrasound that vary with frequency.

To depict both superficial and deeper structures on the B-mode display, signals from deeper echoes are amplified appropriately to compensate for the expected signal attenuation with depth. Because anatomic structures being examined do not have uniform tissue composition or a single constant attenuation factor, most instruments also allow the operator to change the amplifier gain and to selectively control the signal amplification from different depths [time gain compensation (TGC)].

Blood is a weak ultrasound reflector. Red blood cells cause scattering of a small fraction of the ultrasound energy, the amount of scattering depending on the frequency of the ultrasound. This scatter occurs because the ultrasound wavelength (0.3 mm for 5-MHz ultrasound) is much greater than the size of the reflectors (the 7- to 8-μm red blood cells). Backscatter increases with the fourth power of the ultrasound frequency, more ultrasound being reflected as the wavelength shortens. Thus, the longer-wavelength, low-frequency ultrasound that is more effective at greater depths returns weaker echo signals from its interaction with blood. Since backscatter from blood cells represents only a small part of the total ultrasound energy returning to the transducer, blood appears hypoechoic in images, but because of the Doppler frequency shift in this part of the echo signal, flow velocity information can be easily detected.

Pulsed Doppler

While the pulse-echo B-mode system uses the amplitude information from the returning pulse to generate the image, the pulse-echo Doppler system uses the phase information in the echo. An ultrasound pulse backscattered by flowing blood is phase-shifted as compared with the transmitted ultrasound waves; this is the Doppler effect.

The Doppler equation describes the rate of phase shift between pulses, or the magnitude of the frequency shift in the returning echoes, as a function of the closing speed of the ultrasound transducer and the ultrasound reflector. The resultant Doppler frequency is the difference between the transmitted and the receiver ultra-

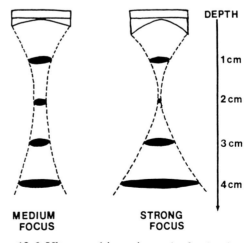

Figure 12-6 Ultrasound intensity at the focal point can be increased by focusing the ultrasound transducer. However, this shortens the focal zone, and ultrasound intensity diminishes more rapidly in the far field.

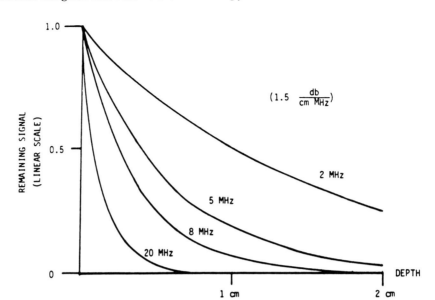

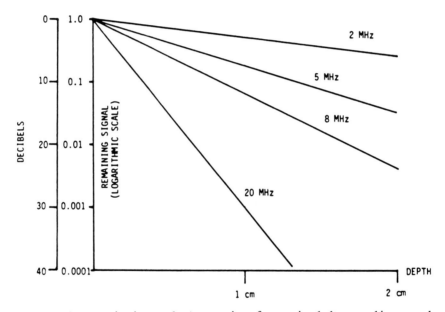

Figure 12-7 Ultrasound attenuation in muscle. Attenuation of transmitted ultrasound increases logarithmically with increasing depth. Higher frequencies are more rapidly attenuated. (From Beach and Phillips,[193] with permission.)

sound frequencies, expressed in reciprocal seconds (Hz). It is an expression of the rate at which the round-trip distance between the probe and the moving object is changing. An ensemble of several cycles is transmitted with each ultrasound pulse, and the phase change between returning pulses is divided by the time between pulses to yield the Doppler frequency; faster-moving reflectors produce a larger phase shift and therefore a higher Doppler frequency f_D. The rate of phase change between pulses is equal to twice the speed (S) at which the reflector is moving toward or away from the transducer, divided by the ultrasound wavelength λ. This is the Doppler equation:

$$f_D = \frac{2 \times S}{\lambda}$$

Since

$$\lambda = \frac{C \text{ (speed of ultrasound in tissue)}}{F \text{ (ultrasound frequency)}}$$

substitution yields

$$f_D = \frac{2 \times S \times F}{C}$$

Table 12-2 Effects of Ultrasound Frequency Selection

High Ultrasound Transmission Frequency	Low Ultrasound Transmission Frequency
Higher Doppler frequency for a given blood velocity (V) and angle of insonation (θ)	Lower Doppler frequency for a given blood velocity (V) and angle of insonation (θ)
More backscattering from blood cells	Less backscattering from blood cells
Poorer depth penetration	Better depth penetration
Narrow ultrasound focus	Wide ultrasound focus
Shorter required duration of pulsed Doppler ultrasound bursts	Longer required duration of pulsed Doppler ultrasound bursts

This relationship between reflector speed S and Doppler frequency f_D assumes that the reflector is moving directly in line with the direction of ultrasound transmission and reflection. To apply this to the problem of vascular diagnosis requires that the direction of blood flow be exactly toward or away from the transducer. In most situations this arrangement is impractical. Blood flow velocity is a vector quantity, with both magnitude (speed) and direction. If the ultrasound beam insonates the blood flow within a vessel at any angle less than 90 degrees, there will be some vector component of flow velocity in the direction of insonation. By fixing this Doppler angle, obtained Doppler frequencies may be compared between individuals or between successive examinations. Alternatively, by using the trigonometric relationship between the angle of insonation (θ) and the magnitude of the flow vector in line with the ultrasound beam (S), the angle-adjusted flow velocity (V) can be calculated:

$$\cos \theta = \frac{S}{V}$$

Substitution into the Doppler equation yields

$$f_D = \frac{2 \times F \times V \times \cos \theta}{C}$$

or

$$V = \frac{f_D \times C}{F \times 2 \times \cos \theta}$$

When θ exceeds 70 degrees (and cos θ approaches zero) small changes in θ have relatively larger effects on f_D or V. By keeping a consistent Doppler angle of 60 degrees or using angle-adjusted velocities with θ less than 70 degrees, errors can be reduced.

Accurate determination of flow velocity requires that the Doppler angle between the ultrasound beam and the flow direction be accurately known. In duplex scanning applications, the flow direction is assumed to be along the longitudinal axis of the vessel. While this may be valid in a long, straight vessel, away from bifurcations or branches, it is not the case in many clinically important situations in which bifurcations or vessel curvature may create helical, nonaxial flow. In these cases the true value for θ may not be known and substituting V · cos θ to obtain the angle-adjusted velocity adds an additional element of variability[48] (Fig. 12-8).

Using typical ultrasound frequencies in the megahertz range to examine flowing blood, which normally moves at speeds of less than 150 cm/s, yields Doppler frequencies in the audible (kilohertz) range. For example, using a 5-MHz transducer and insonating at 60 degrees to the vessel axis to examine flow in a common femoral artery with a peak-systolic flow velocity of 115 cm/s would give a peak f_D of

$$f_D = \frac{2 \times 5 \times 10^6 \text{ cycles/s} \times 115 \text{ cm/s} \times \cos 60 \text{ degrees}}{1540 \text{ cm/s}}$$

$$= 373,377 \text{ cycles/s}$$

$$f_D = 373 \text{ kHz}$$

Directly converting this signal to an audio output is the simplest way to present the frequency shift. The pitch of the audio output corresponds to velocity and the loudness to signal strength (amplitude).

Repeated pulses of ultrasound are required to adequately characterize flow in the selected sample volume. To ensure that each transmitted pulse and each received echo is correctly paired, the echo from each transmission must be received before the next is transmitted. Because the time for an echo to return increases with the depth of the ultrasound reflector, the rate at which the pulses can be repeated will be a function of depth (Fig. 12-9). The maximum pulse repetition frequency (PRF) at a given depth in tissue is

$$PRF_{max} = \frac{C}{2 \times d}$$

Limiting the PRF limits the magnitude of the velocity that can be examined. It should be recalled that the Doppler frequency is the phase change in the returning ultrasound waves divided by the time between pulses. To accurately describe the larger phase changes that occur when echoes return from a fast-moving reflector, the pulses must be close together (i.e., the PRF must be high). This may be thought of as describing a dynamic process in terms of a number of discrete samples. To correctly describe the returning ultrasound wave's peaks and valleys there must be at least one sample for each peak or valley (half-wave). If the PRF, or sampling rate, is too low, the wave describing these sampling points will appear to have lower frequency than it really

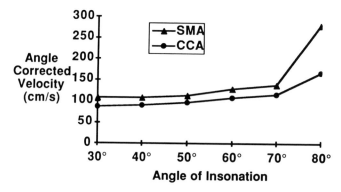

Figure 12-8 Data from normal common carotid (CCA) and superior mesenteric (SMA) arteries show that changing the angle of insonation (Doppler angle values [θ]) introduces variability in the values of the calculated peak systolic velocities. This graph shows the most dramatic change in derived peak systolic velocities (calculated by the Doppler equation $V = \dfrac{c \cdot f_{D}}{2 \cdot F \cdot \cos\theta}$) as the Doppler angle exceeds 70 degrees. (Adapted from Rizzo et al.,[194] with permission.)

does. A simple photographic analogy is the appearance of a wagon wheel in a motion picture. When the frame exposure rate of the camera is slow with respect to the rate at which the position of the wheel spokes changes, the wheel may appear to be moving slowly, or even in reverse. To accurately depict the wheel's movement, either the wheel must be moving slowly or a high-speed camera must be used.

Because a sample must be obtained from each half-wave, the highest Doppler frequency that can be de-scribed with the pulsed Doppler will be half of the PRF. This frequency is referred to as the *Nyquist limit.* If the highest velocities being examined produce a Doppler frequency greater than the Nyquist limit (half the PRF), there can be loss of information, with incorrect representation of the direction and rate of blood flow; this is called *aliasing.* Sampling at a PRF that is less than twice the Doppler frequency means that each wave may be insufficiently characterized to define both the magnitude and direction of the phase shift. For

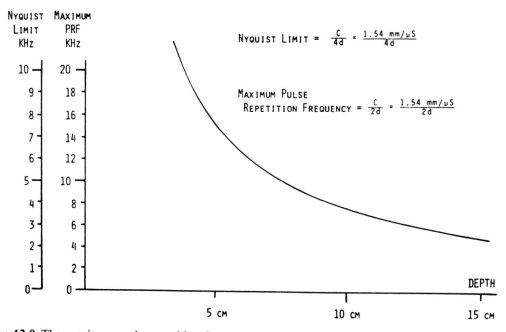

Figure 12-9 The maximum pulse repetition frequency (PRF) at any depth is limited. The maximum pulse repetition period is the time required for the round trip of an ultrasound pulse. (From Beach and Phillips,[193] with permission.)

example, a positive phase shift of three-fourths of a wave has the same value as a negative phase shift of one-fourth of a wave. When a pulsed Doppler signal aliases, the direction of flow will appear to reverse abruptly. (Fig. 12-10).

Doppler Signal Processing

The Doppler shift provides information about the speed and flow pattern of blood within the examined vessel.

First, it must be recognized that the movement of blood cells is nonuniform, both in time and in space. Flow events in arteries change with cardiac systole and diastole. In veins it is the respiratory events and the associated venous pressure changes that determine the flow pattern. However, even at a single point in time, the movement of the cells within the pulsed Doppler sampler volume is not uniform. Each red blood cell within the sample volume has a velocity vector, with both magnitude and direction. For each, there is a velocity vector component in the direction of the vessel's axis. These vectors will not have exactly the same value;

"Nyquist limit"

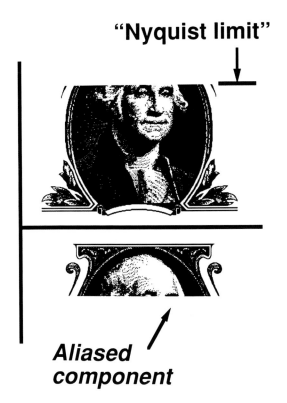

Aliased component

Figure 12-10 Aliasing can be illustrated with a familiar image. With a Doppler spectral waveform, aliasing "cuts off" the top of the waveform and assigns an opposite sign (direction) to the highest values. This places the top of the waveform at the bottom of the display.

rather there will be a number of values distributed between a minimum and a maximum. In a statistical sense, blood cell flow vectors within a sample volume can be thought of as a sample population. Flow velocity within the sample can be characterized in a number of ways: by the single highest or lowest values, by how broad a range of values is included, by an "average" value (which could be the mean, median, or mode), or by the statistical variance within the sample. When blood flow is laminar, and the sample volume is small with respect to the vessel, most of the cells in the sample volume will have similar velocities so that there is a narrow range of values, tightly distributed around the mean. When flow is disturbed, blood cells within a specified volume may be moving in different directions at different speeds and the velocity vector values will have a broad distribution with a less well-defined mean.

When a pulse of ultrasound is backscattered by flowing blood, a spectrum of Doppler frequencies is produced, which, within the sample volume selected, correlates with the distribution of flow velocity vectors. The Doppler shift in the echo received by the transducer is a composite of these frequencies. By analyzing the echo for the strength of its composite frequencies, the nature of the blood flow in the sample volume can be characterized.

The Doppler-shifted ultrasound backscattered to the transducer by flowing blood can be analyzed in a variety of ways. The first Doppler systems provided only an audio output, and the frequency analyzer was the operator's ear.[49] This audible Doppler signal is still useful to the examiner using a duplex scanner. The audible signal can be used to discriminate arterial from venous flow and to select this from background noise, as well as to recognize the velocity pattern associated with disease.[17]

Because assessment of the audio output of the Doppler signal is subjective and operator-dependent, systems for analyzing and recording the velocity data were developed. In current duplex scanners this is usually accomplished by a real-time digital frequency analyzer using the fast Fourier transform (FFT).[50] The Fourier transform is a means of analyzing periodic signals for their frequency content. The received echo produces a signal that is a sum of a number of Doppler shifts reflecting the distribution of different velocity vectors within the sample volume. The Fourier transform separates the composite frequencies and assesses their relative intensities.

Digital signal processing rapidly accomplishes this function. Digitized signals are resistant to noise and may be more easily stored in the processor's memory. Large amounts of digital information can be held in a buffer and manipulated or replayed off-line. The first task, digitization of the analog audio frequency Doppler signal, is performed with rapid, continuous real-time sampling. The concept of representing a complex analog waveform by sampling a set of discrete points is familiar; this is how music is recorded on a digital compact disc. At regular brief intervals the signal voltage is measured, and its magnitude and sign (direction) are recorded as a binary value. To avoid aliasing around the sampling rate of the duplex scanner's frequency analyzer, the frequency analyzer must sample as fast as or faster than the pulsed Doppler system.

The spectrum analyzer repeatedly examines the Doppler signal data over short periods of time, typically around 10 ms. For each period, the digitized samples are "sorted" by frequency, and the strength of each frequency is assessed. The result of this analysis can be represented by a two-dimensional plot of amplitude as a function of frequency, but since flow events are dynamic, a time dimension is needed. This three-dimensional display is accomplished by using a gray scale to represent the amplitude of each component frequency when frequency is plotted as a function of time. The highest value for a given point in time represents the maximal Doppler shift at that time; the brightest point is the mode frequency.

The resultant display is a spectral waveform. This is a time-dependent display of the Doppler frequencies (or flow velocities) in the sample volume. Time (and therefore the point in the cardiac cycle) is represented on the abscissa. The frequency range shown on the ordinate equals the PRF, or twice the Nyquist limit. By convention, frequency shifts from velocities toward the transducer are displayed above the baseline, while velocities away from the transducer are displayed below the baseline. A strong Doppler signal may also be produced by tissue motion, such as the pulsation of the arterial wall. A high-pass filter excludes Doppler frequencies near zero to allow the lower-intensity blood flow signal to be discerned. The wall filter, however, can also cause loss of Doppler signals from low-velocity flow. Low-velocity flow, such as that distal to a tight stenosis or in the venous circulation, may be important.[51]

Spectral analysis has several advantages over methods of characteristic frequency analysis of the Doppler information. With characteristic frequency analysis only the predominant Doppler frequency is identified. The most commonly used device of this type is the zero crossing detector.[52] Spectral analysis is a relatively robust technique for signal analysis, as it is usable even if the signal-to-noise ratio is low and it is not amplitude-dependent. High-velocity jets can be more sensitively identified by spectral analysis because all the Doppler frequencies are displayed. A weak high-frequency signal is not lost in a stronger midrange signal. With characteristic frequency analysis no information about the strength of the signal or the number of composite frequencies that it contains is available.

Doppler Color-Flow Imaging

Color-flow imaging is another method of displaying the same velocity information that is represented in the spectral waveform. The two-dimensional image is essentially a real-time color-coded display of regions with flow, superimposed on the conventional gray-scale anatomic image of the pulse-echo B-mode scan. For each pulse-echo cycle, multiple sample gates on each scan line acquire Doppler information at a range of depths. To minimize sampling error, several pulses (a pulse ensemble) are used to generate each color scan line. A single frequency value for each point is color coded and displayed. Alternatively, the displayed pixel's color can represent the variance within the Doppler sample volume. Color-flow systems, therefore, discard some of the information from each sample volume. They differ in this respect from spectral waveform analyzers, which display the intensity of up to 128 Doppler frequencies for each point in time.

Color assignment can be determined by one of several techniques. The most common is based on an average value from an FFT analysis, but other methods, including detection of phase changes between adjacent echoes, time-domain analysis, and power analysis are also used. The sign, average velocity, and variance of the composite Doppler frequencies are calculated for each sample volume. These data are assigned a pixel color by using a preselected scheme, which is illustrated as a color bar or "map." Positive and negative Doppler frequencies are assigned to colors on opposite sides of the color map. The magnitude of the Doppler frequency can be represented by gradation in hue (the color perceived), color saturation (the amount of color present in a mix with white), or luminance (the brightness of the hue and saturation presented). The color bar can display a range of frequencies depending on the PRF used, and the values at the ends of the color bar represent the Nyquist limit.

While a color-flow image can be set up to have red represent arterial flow and blue venous flow, this assignment is arbitrary. Also, it is important to realize that pixel color assignment is based on the flow velocity relative to the transducer. Small changes in the direction of the flow vectors can have a large effect on the resultant Doppler frequency; this is why color changes in the flow stream cannot be used to define hemodynamic streamlines. Angle effects can also result in the displayed flow within a single vessel changing colors if the direction of flow changes with respect to the insonating Doppler ultrasound (Plates 12-2 and 12-3).

While color-flow imaging displays the same Doppler information that the spectral waveform contains, velocity data from each point on the color-flow image are not directly comparable with velocities determined by spectral waveform analysis. The color display value represents an average (rather than peak) velocity. Also, because of the large amount of data from multiple sample volumes that need to be acquired and displayed, the display rate for each set of values (the image from rate) is limited. Therefore, spectral waveform analysis is better than color-flow imaging for detecting and quantitating time-dependent features of blood flow.

Color-flow images are subject to spatial and temporal distortion, since events in the circulation may be faster than the acquisition of a frame of color-flow data. The color Doppler image lines are sequentially generated, sweeping across the image plane. Flow events depicted on one side of the image have occurred earlier than those depicted on the other. For example, the forward flow in late systole and the reverse flow of early diastole can occasionally be seen in the same image frame.

Although quantitative assessment with color-flow imaging has not been found to be practical, many of the features of the color-flow examination make it a useful complement to the standard duplex scan. With color flow, vascular structures are readily identified and arteries are easily differentiated from veins. Flow events are simultaneously displayed over a large area and in multiple vessels. Flow velocity and direction changes and areas with flow disturbances are distinctly seen. These features help the technologist to identify and follow the course of vessels, as well as facilitating appropriate placement of the Doppler sample volume to obtain spectral waveforms. This reduces the requirement for interrogating multiple sites to search for flow disturbances. The additional qualitative information from the color-flow image may increase the overall diagnostic accuracy of the duplex scan.

Since color-flow imaging systems are pulsed Doppler instruments, they are subject to the same limitations as other Doppler instruments.[53] The apparent flow velocity is angle-dependent, with a small Doppler frequency detected as the Doppler angle approaches 90 degrees. Doppler frequencies greater than twice the PRF produce aliasing. In color systems this is displayed as the transition of adjacent pixels from a color at one end of the color assignment map to a color at the opposite end.

DOPPLER ULTRASOUND AND HEMODYNAMICS

Doppler ultrasound examinations provide direct assessment of the physiologic or pathologic features of blood flow. For the most part, the diagnoses of vascular disease by duplex scanning involves noting the hemodynamic changes that deviate from normal. Understanding the hemodynamics of normal and abnormal flow patterns is prerequisite for duplex scan interpretation. The following sections review a few principles of arterial and venous hemodynamics and their application in the interpretation of duplex scans.

Characteristics of Arterial Blood Flow

Arterial blood flow patterns are complex and vary depending on the part of the arterial tree that is being considered. Normal flow in a straight, branchless segment of artery is considered to be laminar. Flow profiles are directed in the direction of the vessel axis. Interaction between blood and the vessel wall causes blood close to the wall to move more slowly than blood farther away from the wall. The slowest flow is in the boundary layer, immediately adjacent to the vessel wall. The fastest flow is in the center of the artery (Fig. 12-11).

These relationships can be demonstrated with duplex scanning. The fastest flow velocities are expected to be in the center of the artery, where, by convention, the Doppler sample volume is normally positioned. With a small sample volume and undisturbed flow, a narrow spectral waveform will be obtained. Distur-

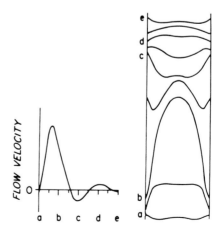

Figure 12-11 Velocity profile across a normal peripheral artery.

bances in the laminar flow patterns will lead to spectral broadening in the Doppler signal. This simply reflects the fact that the velocities within the sample volume do not all have the same value. If the sample volume is large or it is near the vessel wall, spectral broadening will also be observed.[54]

Axial laminar flow patterns can also be disrupted by the presence of bifurcations or branches or by directional changes in the artery. For example, in the carotid bulb the boundary layer separates from the wall, and focal areas of stasis or flow reversal will develop.[55,56] This is demonstrable with pulsed Doppler spectral waveforms and color-flow imaging[57,58] (Fig. 12-12 and Plate 12-4). The flow pattern near the apical flow divider is antegrade throughout the entire cardiac cycle, but sampling along the lateral aspect of the bulb detects lower velocity flow with both forward and reverse flow components. This complex flow pattern was not recognized as normal in the early experience with carotid duplex scanning and it resulted in a lower specificity until its true nature was appreciated.[57] Now that flow separation is appreciated to be a normal hemodynamic pattern, documentation of its presence confirms that the carotid bulb is free of disease.

The relationship of arterial pressure to flow depends on the resistance and arterial wall characteristics of the peripheral runoff bed. Two normal patterns are seen. Organs with a requirement for continuous, high blood flow rates (e.g., brain, liver, kidney) have a low vascular resistance (or more correctly, vascular *impedance,* as the arterial system has pulsatile flow[59]). Flow velocity waveforms in low-resistance systems have a more gradual acceleration phase, a rounded peak, and continuous forward flow in diastole.

Flow to high-resistance runoff beds, as in lower extremity arteries under resting flow conditions, occurs principally during systole. The compliance and elasticity of the arterial wall, along with reflections of pulse waves from branch points, result in triphasic or biphasic arterial velocity waveforms. Velocity waveforms show a steeper rise with systolic acceleration, followed by a rapid fall in velocity to zero as the pulse pressure wave passes. Dissipation of energy transferred to the arterial wall in systole results in a brief phase of reverse flow in early diastole, which can in turn be followed by a brief period of low-velocity forward flow. This normal triphasic waveform in peripheral arteries may be accentuated in younger individuals. Sometimes flow reversal can be noted again in late diastole, contributing a fourth component to the flow velocity waveform.

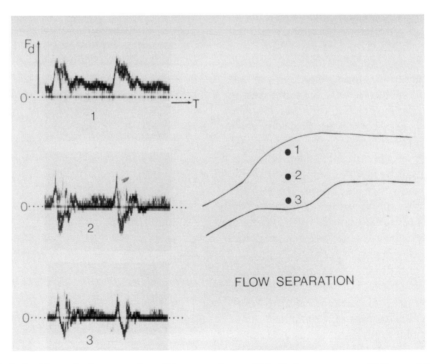

Figure 12-12 Pulsed Doppler interrogation of the normal carotid bulb demonstrates: *(1)* forward flow throughout the cardiac cycle along the surface of the proximal flow divider; *(2)* complicated forward and reverse flow with the sample volume positioned to include the boundary layer (separated from the wall); and *(3)* low-velocity, complicated flow patterns in the separation zone along the opposite wall.

Flow hemodynamics associated with arterial stenoses produce the velocity waveform features that are the basis for duplex scan diagnosis of arterial disease. The increase in flow velocity has long been noted to be a feature of more severe lesions (this is detectable with even simple continuous wave Doppler instruments.[60] The character of the flow pattern is also important. As flow accelerates through the stenotic segment, it expands and contracts at the inlet and outlet of the stenosis. This disrupts laminar flow, producing flow vortices with less severe stenoses and highly disturbed flow (turbulence) with more severe stenoses. This is displayed as spectral broadening in the velocity waveform. The tendency for laminar flow to become turbulent is described by the Reynolds number Re, which is defined by

$$Re = \frac{\rho \times d \times V}{\eta}$$

where ρ is blood density, d is the vessel diameter, V is flow velocity, and η is the viscosity of the blood. Turbulence is more marked with tighter stenoses and higher velocities.

The hemodynamic effects of irregularities in the vessel wall or projections into the vessel lumen depends not only on the Reynolds number but also on the profile of the lesion. Turbulence develops downstream from a sharp-edged atherosclerotic plaque if

$$\frac{h}{r} \geq \frac{4}{Re}$$

where h is the lesion height and r is the artery radius. Smooth stenoses, such as a recurrent carotid artery stenosis from intimal hyperplasia, cause less turbulence (and less spectral broadening) than irregular atherosclerotic lesions that produce the same degree of luminal narrowing.

A stenosis is termed *critical* when it produces a significant reduction in pressure or flow.[61] Generally, this occurs when a stenosis narrows the lumen diameter by 50 percent or more (thus reducing the cross-sectional area by at least 75 percent). Because the actual pressure drop across a lesion depends on the distal resistance and the flow across the lesion, it is difficult to predict the hemodynamic significance of a lesion on the basis of diameter narrowing alone.

Fluid energy is rapidly lost across a critical stenosis. At the site of a severe stenosis high velocities and turbulence can be noted. This loss of fluid energy changes the spectral waveform distally. The systolic rise time of the spectral waveform is prolonged, and the waveform peak is rounded. To compensate, peripheral resistance decreases.[59] The combination of fluid energy loss and lowering of outflow resistance results in the disappearance of the diastolic reverse flow component of the peripheral arterial velocity waveform.

Characteristics of Venous Blood Flow

Flow in the venous side of the circulation is influenced by multiple factors, including respiration, right heart filling pressures, position, arterial inflow, and activity of the muscle pump. Because the effects of the cardiac and respiratory cycles are different in the upper and lower body, venous flow patterns differ by location. Close to the right atrium, cardiac events have a pronounced effect on venous flow, with antegrade flow decreased in systole. As the diaphragm descends with inspiration, intrathoracic pressure drops and intra-abdominal pressure rises. Inspiration therefore increases centripetal flow in the upper body and decreases antegrade flow in the lower body.

Doppler shifts due to venous flow are of lower frequency and are phasic with respiration. In the abdomen or in the central veins of the upper torso and neck, cessation of flow with systole may be evident, with venous flow appearing pulsatile.[62,63] With obstruction of the normal venous channels, the phasic nature of venous flow may be absent, and flow through higher-resistance collateral beds will be more continuous in nature.

Valves, which are unique to the venous circulation, affect the nature of venous blood flow. They maintain antegrade flow, and in the extremities they prevent flow from the deep to the superficial veins. The term *reflux* as used in reference to the venous system describes pathologic reverse flow when venous valves are damaged or absent. Duplex scanning, however, can normally demonstrate brief reversal of flow in veins with intact valve function, as valve closure requires reversal of the normal pressure gradient. In a study of subjects in a supine position, valve closure was achieved only after reverse velocities exceeded 30 cm/s. In over 95 percent of normal subjects the valves close in less than 0.5 seconds when this reverse transvalvular gradient develops.[64]

Because of the capacitance function of the venous system, venous dimensions can change dramatically. Veins collapse when empty, and venous filling is positional. In normal subjects common femoral vein diameters increase by almost 100 percent with a change in position from 10 degrees Trendelenburg to 30 degrees reverse Trendelenburg. Concomitant with this increase in cross-sectional area is a decrease in flow velocity. Phasic changes in venous flow with respiration are more noticeable when the veins are distended; cardiac events are more noticeable when the veins are fully distended.[65] For venous duplex scanning, it is important to consider the physiologic effects of position and intravascular volume status.

APPLICATIONS

The clinical uses of duplex scanning continue to expand. Other chapters review the natural history of specific vascular problems and outline diagnostic approaches. The role of duplex scanning in common applications will be discussed here.

Cerebrovascular Disease

Stroke, which affects 500,000 Americans each year, is the third leading cause of death in the United States.[66] The most common mechanism by which strokes occur is embolism of atheromatous material and thrombotic debris from atherosclerotic lesions of the carotid bifurcation and bulb. These emboli result in distal occlusion of intracranial branch vessels, producing ischemic brain injury in the distribution of the involved vessel. Since collateral circulation and autoregulatory abilities can compensate for most unilateral carotid artery lesions, reduction of hemispheric cerebral flow from carotid artery narrowing is a less important cause of neurologic symptoms in the pathophysiology of this disease than is atheroembolism. Thromboembolism, however, is closely associated with the presence of a hemodynamically significant stenosis.

Finding a significant lesion in the carotid artery is important, as surgical therapy can reduce the risk of stroke in selected patients. Carotid endarterectomy has proven efficacy in reducing this risk in patients who present with stroke, transient ischemic attack, or retinal artery embolization that produces transient monocular blindness (amaurosis fugax). The North American Symptomatic Carotid Endarterectomy Trial (NASCET) found that symptomatic patients with internal carotid artery stenoses that narrowed the arterial lumen by more than 70 percent had a 24 percent incidence at 2-year follow-up of fatal or nonfatal ipsilateral stroke when given optimal medical management (including antiplatelet therapy). This was significantly higher than the 7 percent stroke rate in the surgically treated group.[39] "Prophylactic" endarterectomy is also useful in preventing neurologic events in asymptomatic patients who have very high-grade carotid artery stenoses (with ≥ 80 percent diameter reduction).[46] In general, the greater the degree of narrowing of the internal carotid artery, the greater the risk of stroke.

The principal goal of the vascular diagnostic laboratory is identification of patients at increased risk for neurologic events, so that timely surgical intervention can reduce the threat of death or disability from stroke. Although carotid artery lesions that cause only mild to moderate narrowing of the arterial lumen do occasionally ulcerate and embolize, most lesions that produce symptoms reduce the lumenal diameter by 50 percent or more. Not only are the plaques in these lesions more extensive, accumulating larger amounts of atherosclerotic debris,[67] but the flow disturbances that they produce result in areas of stasis and altered wall shear forces, which in turn may play a causative role in further plaque formation and platelet deposition.[68]

Cerebrovascular testing is the most commonly performed arterial duplex scan study. It is safe and accurate and is the noninvasive method of choice for the diagnosis of cerebrovascular disease.[2] The techniques and methods of interpretation of duplex scanning evolved from the initial experience with carotid testing.

Indications

The usual indications for cerebrovascular testing in the vascular laboratory are evaluation of a cervical bruit, screening of selected high-risk patients undergoing cardiac or other major surgery, evaluation of potentially embolic neurologic symptoms, and postoperative evaluation after carotid endarterectomy.[69] Thromboemboli from carotid artery disease can lead to hemispheric transient ischemic attacks, anterior or middle cerebral artery distribution of cerebral infarcts, or retinal embolization (producing Hollenhorst plaques and/or symptoms of amaurosis fugax). In addition, screening of older patients with peripheral artery disease may be appropriate, as they have a significant incidence of asymptomatic carotid artery disease.[70]

Technique

Duplex scanning can evaluate the carotid arteries from the base of the neck to just above the angle of the mandible. In addition, the subclavian arteries and the proximal portions of the vertebral arteries can be studied to provide some indication of the status of the blood supply to the posterior circulation. The patient is examined supine, with the head turned slightly to the opposite side. A 5-MHz Doppler transducer is the standard for cerebrovascular studies, but either a 5- or a 7-MHz imaging transducer gives adequate imaging depth to evaluate the relatively superficial vascular structures of the neck. The basic method of scanning is the same with or without color.

The B-mode image is useful to identify the vessels of interest, but an examination of flow characteristics is sometimes needed to avoid confusing the internal and external carotid arteries. The internal carotid artery has a low outflow resistance; its waveform has an end-diastolic frequency well above the zero baseline. The external carotid artery, supplying the face and scalp, has a higher outflow resistance and a waveform more like that of a peripheral artery. Flow in diastole is usually at or near zero, and the resistance can vary with ambient temperature and the state of cutaneous vasodilatation. In addition, the presence of branches helps to distinguish the external carotid artery.

In some ways B-mode imaging and arteriography provide similar information: they can localize atherosclerotic plaques, measure residual lumen width, and identify vessel wall irregularities. Arteriography, however, provides only a picture of the luminal surface, whereas ultrasound can identify some of the changes in the arterial wall resulting from developing atherosclerosis.[71] The B-mode image can identify the presence of arterial wall thickening or focal plaque. This is helpful in recognizing early arterial disease, as the flow disturbance from minimal lesions may be subtle or absent.

For more prominent plaques, a general description of the nature of the lesion is appropriate.[72] Plaques can be described as homogenous or heterogeneous by their characteristic echo pattern. Heterogeneous plaques have nonuniform echoes and anechoic areas within the lesion, as well as calcifications, which result in acoustic shadowing (Fig. 12-13 and Plate 12-5). Also, surfaces can be graded as smooth or irregular. Many authors have postulated that ulceration in carotid artery plaques is important in the pathogenesis of thromboembolic disease and that the detection of arterial ulcers would be useful diagnostically. However, evidence to support this assertion is lacking. In multicenter trials, B-mode imaging (and arteriography) were found lacking in their ability to accurately detect plaque ulceration (identified in specimens removed at operation).[39,71,73]

Pulsed Doppler spectral waveforms are obtained from multiple locations. The sample volume is kept as small as possible (usually 1.5 mm long) and is positioned in the centerline of the vessel. Spot readings are insufficient; a complete survey of the vessels is necessary to avoid missing a focal lesion. Any stenosis should be completely delineated with prestenotic, stenotic, and poststenotic velocity waveforms. The highest values of the peak-systolic and end-diastolic Doppler frequencies should be used for interpretation.

In examining the carotid arteries it is important to

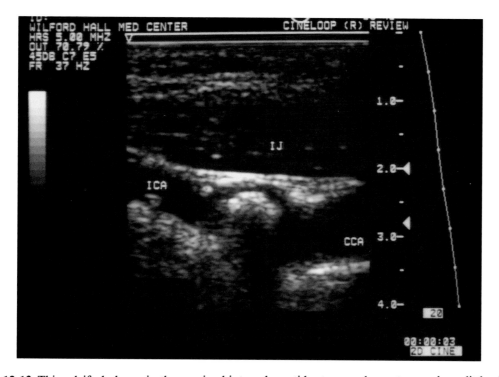

Figure 12-13 This calcified plaque in the proximal internal carotid artery produces strong echoes; little ultrasound energy is transmitted through. Acoustic shadowing (dark area without echoes) is present deep to the plaque. This shadowing obscures the features of the opposite arterial wall.

obtain Doppler spectra for the common carotid artery as far proximally as possible as well as in the midportion of the vessel. Common carotid artery lesions are frequently located near the vessel's origin. In the internal carotid artery spectral waveforms should be examined in the bulb, in the midportion of the imaged artery, and as far distal as possible. A Doppler angle of 60 degrees to the long axis of the artery should be maintained whenever possible. In addition to the presence of a stenosis, higher-frequency Doppler signals may result from changes in the angle (due to vessel tortuosity, nonaxial flow, etc.). The presence or absence of post-stenotic turbulence (spectral broadening) can help to determine whether an increased Doppler frequency is due to a stenosis.

Flow in the vertebral arteries is assessed qualitatively (Plate 12-6). Patency can be established if flow is detected and the direction of flow can be determined. Flow patterns can be characterized as disturbed if a significant stenosis is present, but there are no criteria for grading the degree of stenosis. Some segments of the subclavian arteries can be interrogated, but their curvature and position behind the clavicles may interfere with accurate quantitative assessment. Continuous wave Doppler measurement of blood pressures in each arm is part of a complete cerebrovascular examination. A brachial pressure differential of 20 mmHg or more is suggestive of a subclavian stenosis or occlusion.

The use of color-flow imaging can facilitate the examination but there are no useful means for classifying cerebrovascular disease on the basis of color-flow findings. For the most part, color is an aid to vessel identification, definition of the anatomy, and rapid recognition of those areas where flow disturbances are to be found.

Interpretation Criteria and Validation

The criteria for grading the severity of internal carotid artery stenoses are based on the hemodynamic effects of the lesions.[7,9,74,75] Stenoses that narrow the bulb by less than 50 percent are diagnosed by the presence and severity of the disruption of axial laminar flow. Significant stenoses, which reduce the diameter by 50 percent or more, are recognized by an increase in the peak-systolic velocity. They are further stratified into categories of 50 to 79 percent or more than 80 percent by the magnitude of the end-diastolic velocity.[41] These criteria are summarized in Table 12-3 and Figure 12-14.

These criteria have been found to be 99 percent sensitive in detecting significant ($\geq$ 50 percent diameter-reducing) lesions and to correctly identify completely normal (category A) arteries with 84 percent specificity (overall accuracy 93 percent).[7,9,74,75] The accuracy of the determination that a significant stenosis (associated with an elevated peak systolic velocity) has reduced the vessel diameter by 80 percent or more is 87 percent (sensitivity of 83 percent, specificity of 86 percent).[41] Variability in the duplex scan categorization of stenosis

Table 12-3 Duplex Scan Classification of Internal Carotid Artery Stenosis

Class	Lumen Diameter Reduction[a]	Peak Systole Frequency Shift (Velocity)	End Diastole[b] Frequency Shift (Velocity)	Spectral Waveform Characteristics
A	None	<4 kHz (<125 cm/s)		Minimal or no spectral broadening; boundary layer separation present in the bulb[c]
B	1–15%	<4 kHz (<125 cm/s)		Spectral broadening during deceleration phase of systole[d]
C	16–49%	<4 kHz (<125 cm/s)		Spectral broadening throughout systole
D	50–79%	>4 kHz (>125 cm/s)		Marked spectral broadening[e]
D+	80–99%	>4 kHz (>125 cm/s)	>4.5 kHz (>140 cm/s)	Marked spectral broadening
E	100% (total occlusion)			No flow in internal carotid artery; flow to zero in ipsilateral common carotid artery

[a] These classifications were based upon arteriographic measurements of stenosis, using methods that compared residual internal carotid artery lumen diameter with the estimated diameter of the carotid bulb.

[b] End-diastolic frequency or velocity values are only used to distinguish class D (50–79%) from D+ (80–99%) stenoses.

[c] The technologist's notes should include comment if normal boundary layer separation is noted in the bulb.

[d] Minimal to moderate spectral broadening is normal after carotid endarterectomy, even without residual stenosis.

[e] In cases of contralateral internal carotid artery occlusion, if the peak systolic frequency shift is $\leq$ 4 kHz but spectral broadening is absent or minimal, a comment should be recorded to the effect that the stenosis may be overestimated.

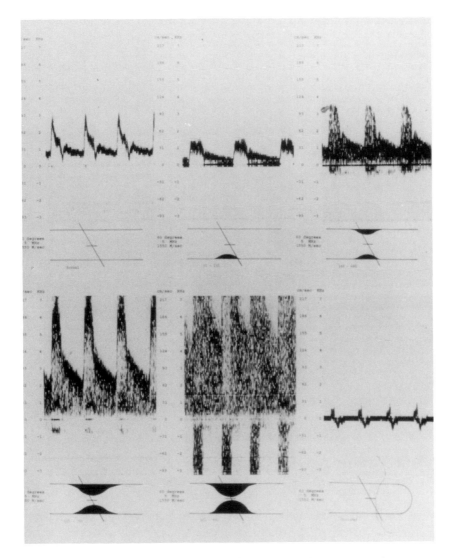

Figure 12-14 Waveform characteristics of the categories of internal carotid artery stenosis. Percent stenosis refers to reduction of luminal diameter as compared with estimated diameter of the carotid bulb. From left, top: 0% (normal); 1–15% (minimal disease); 16–49% (moderate disease). Bottom row: 50–79%; 80–99%; total occlusion.

severity is greatest for stenoses of less than 50 percent because of both the variability in arteriographic measurements and the use of subjective criteria for assessment of the Doppler flow patterns. While distinguishing minimally from moderately severe stenosis is usually not a clinical concern, recognition of normal flow separation patterns in the carotid bulb has further improved the specificity.[75,76]

The arteriographic definition of stenosis severity used to validate these criteria was based on a comparison of the residual lumen with the estimated bulb diameter. The percent of stenosis calculated by this method is slightly greater than the value that would be obtained by comparing the diameter of the residual arterial lumen with the diameter of an undiseased segment of the more distal internal carotid artery. The former recognizes that atherosclerosis in the bulb may be present although not severe enough to narrow the flow channel to a diameter less than that of the distal internal carotid artery. The shortcoming of the method is that the true bulb dimension cannot always be known with certainty, which thus adds an element of variability to the arteriographic measurement. These criteria are valid for lesions of the first 3 cm of the internal carotid artery. Their accuracy for characterizing lesions of the common and external carotid arteries have not been determined.

The use of other velocity criteria to define high-grade

internal carotid artery stenoses has been evaluated. In the NASCET study, stenoses were graded by arteriography, the narrowest luminal diameter being compared with the diameter of the distal normal internal carotid artery.[39] Results for symptomatic patients with diameter-reducing stenoses of 70 percent or greater were published in the initial NASCET report, and these confirmed the superiority of surgery over medical therapy. The use of an alternate duplex scan standard to define the presence of a high-grade stenosis has been proposed to correlate better with the NASCET stenosis definition. Moneta et al.[77] found that a 4.2 or higher ratio of the peak-systolic velocity in the internal carotid artery to that in the common carotid artery corresponds to a 70 percent or greater stenosis. The sensitivity and specificity of this value (ICA PSV/CCA PSV $\geq$ 4.2) were 90 and 87 percent respectively, with a positive predictive value of 77 percent.

Velocities through a stenosis in an internal carotid artery can be affected by the extent of disease in the contralateral artery; there will be a compensatory increase in flow if the contralateral internal carotid artery contains an occlusion or a high-grade stenosis.[78-80] Modified criteria have been proposed for cases of contralateral carotid occlusion.[81] A moderate elevation in peak-systolic frequency (4.0 to 4.5 kHz), but with absent or less pronounced spectral broadening, should be considered suggestive of a 16 to 49 percent diameter-reducing lesion, and the end-diastolic frequency cutoff for the diagnosis of more than 80 percent stenosis is 5.0 kHz.

The grading of internal carotid artery stenoses that narrow the bulb diameter by less than 50 percent is more subjective. Since peak-systolic velocities do not increase, the examiner must assess the degree of waveform spectral broadening. In addition to judging spectral broadening, the amount of atherosclerotic plaque seen on B-mode imaging may be considered in distinguishing between minimal and moderate disease. Boundary layer separation and the presence of a separation zone in the carotid bulb, opposite the flow divider, characterize the normal carotid bifurcation.[58,76]

A potential error is classification of a very high grade stenosis of the internal carotid artery as an occlusion.[51,82] The very narrow flow channel may be missed. In addition, the very low frequency signals from slow flow distal to a very tight stenosis may fall below the Doppler detection threshold, being removed by the high-pass wall filter. The duplex scan diagnosis of internal carotid artery occlusion should be based on a combination of findings: (1) no pulsed Doppler or color-flow evidence of flow in the internal carotid artery; (2) diastolic flow approaching zero in the common carotid artery; (3) increased velocities in the external

carotid artery; and (4) an audible "thump" at the stump of the occluded internal carotid artery (Fig. 12-15).

The B-mode depiction of plaque morphology is of interest but has limited value in making clinical decisions. Examining specimens removed at the time of carotid endarterectomy, Reilly et al.[22] found that 91 percent of heterogeneous lesions had intraplaque hemorrhage and 100 percent of the ulcerated lesions had a heterogeneous ultrasound appearance. In 82 percent of specimens (41 of 50), ultrasound correctly identified the presence or absence of intraplaque hemorrhage. However, it must be recognized that large amounts of lipid in the lesions can mimic the appearance of intraplaque hemorrhage. Bluth and co-workers[83] found similar results when they prospectively evaluated the ability of ultrasound to detect intraplaque hemorrhage in carotid lesions. The correlation of the sonographic and pathologic findings (heterogeneous appearance and intraplaque hemorrhage) with the presence of embolic symptoms, however, was poor. Of the patients with heterogeneous plaques, 65 percent had symptoms, but 52 percent of those with homogenous plaques were also symptomatic. Thus, to date, plaque features as assessed by ultrasound have not been of great importance in clinical decision making. Stenosis severity as determined by velocity changes remains the best predictor of which carotid lesions are most likely to be associated with clinical events.[46]

Clinical Uses

Although arteriography is the accepted standard for preoperative assessment prior to endarterectomy,[84] duplex scanning has been found to provide similar information about the anatomy of the cervical carotid artery, the severity of stenoses, and the extent of disease. Because the carotid artery is superficial, it is easily imaged, and because atherosclerosis of the carotid artery is frequently localized to the region of the bifurcation, the diagnostic information from the ultrasound study is usually satisfactory. In these cases, subsequent arteriography may not change the clinical management decisions that were based on the results of the duplex scan.[12,85]

Although diagnostic errors occur with every type of study, technical limitations or sources of error with duplex scanning are generally identifiable at the time of the examination. Failure to obtain clear images or velocity waveforms in patients with a short neck, a high carotid bifurcation, or densely calcified vessels, unusual anatomic features (such as coils or kinks) causing flow disturbances, and marked abnormalities of inflow, as with a severe common carotid lesion, can interfere with accurate classification of the carotid

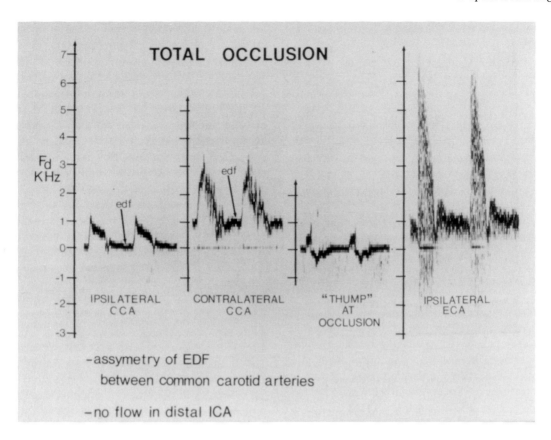

Figure 12-15 Spectral waveform features of internal carotid artery occlusion include: absence of detectable flow in a visualized internal carotid artery (ICA); flow to zero [low or absent end-diastolic forward flow (EDF)] in the common carotid artery (CCA), with increased velocities in the contralateral common carotid artery as it carries collateral flow; preocclusive "thump"; and increased flow velocities in the ipsilateral external carotid artery (ECA).

disease. All these situations are recognizable with experience. For the most part, an experienced technologist will be able to assess the general reliability of an examination. In cases of diagnostic uncertainty arteriography should be performed.

In addition to its use prior to operation in the assessment of patients with carotid artery disease, duplex scanning can also be used for postoperative evaluation after carotid endarterectomy.[86,87] In the perioperative period, duplex scanning can be used to assess patency of the internal carotid artery when a patient develops new neurologic symptoms. The techniques of scanning and the interpretation of duplex scan findings after endarterectomy are similar to those used for preoperative studies, but there are some differences.

After endarterectomy, the proximal end point of the endarterectomy in the distal common carotid artery can be identified. The intima-media "double-line"[88] is abruptly interrupted, and there is often a small shelf or "step-off" where the plaque has been removed. The

distal endarterectomy end point is difficult to image. Myointimal hyperplasia can develop in the region where the plaque has been removed. This problem, which develops in 10 to 20 percent of patients, usually occurs within the first few months. The process is usually complete in the first year.[87,89]

The velocity criteria for grading postoperative stenoses are similar to those used for preoperative diagnosis. Recurrent stenosis after endarterectomy occurs more frequently in arteries found to have a significant flow disturbance by postoperative duplex scanning.[90]

The need for regular postoperative surveillance is controversial. The finding of an asymptomatic recurrent stenosis would not prompt endarterectomy, as lesions secondary to myointimal hyperplasia seem to have a lower risk of thromboembolic complications.[89,91] Although duplex scanning may be useful for following known contralateral asymptomatic disease or evaluating patients with recurrent symptoms, its routine clinical use to identify patients with asymptomatic restenosis after carotid endarterectomy may be unnecessary and not cost-effective.[92,93]

Aortoiliac and Lower Extremity Arterial Disease

Duplex scanning has several important roles in the evaluation and follow-up of patients with lower extremity arterial occlusive disease. It can identify and characterize stenoses and occlusions from the level of the aortic bifurcation to the tibial vessels at the ankle.[94] The use of duplex scanning is not limited to the initial diagnostic assessment and preoperative planning; its application for postoperative graft evaluation has also proved to be of great value.

Indications

Noninvasive testing can be of assistance in planning the arteriographic technique, in selecting the approach, and in the timing of injection and runoff filming. Anatomic regions of particular interest are localized before the procedure. Also, the velocity data are helpful in determining the hemodynamic significance of detected lesions. Arteriograms, while considered the "gold standard," inadequately assess the degree of arterial narrowing unless multiple projections are obtained.[95] The findings from duplex scanning and arteriography are often complementary.

A subset of patients with lower extremity ischemic problems who have short segmental stenoses are candidates for transluminal angioplasty (TLA). Duplex scanning is 100 percent sensitive and 95 percent specific for identifying lesions amenable to TLA. Routine duplex scanning prior to TLA not only allows better planning of the arteriographic approach but also provides both the radiologist and the patient with important information concerning the likely course of intervention to be followed.[96]

Performing duplex scans before and after TLA can also be useful for assessing the adequacy of the technical result of the procedure. Not only does this allow a more objective assessment of success (both early and late),[97,98] but it may also help with the clinical management of some patients after TLA. For example, TLA of a proximal iliac artery stenosis may be performed prior to a femorofemoral or infrainguinal bypass procedure. A subsequent duplex scan can help to establish the adequacy of the inflow, and thus avoid problems with the steal phenomenon or subsequent graft failure.

Technique

A complete lower extremity arterial examination includes the aortoiliac, femoropopliteal, and tibial segments. In general, scanning begins proximally and proceeds in the direction of flow. Because of the depth of the aortoiliac segment, a low-frequency (2- to 3-MHz) transducer is used for the abdominal and pelvic portions of the examination. Scanning of this region is facilitated by an overnight fast to reduce the amount of image-obscuring bowel gas. Below the inguinal ligament a 5.0- or 7.5-MHz scanhead can be used. The femoral artery can be followed for most of its course through the anteromedial thigh, but it may be difficult to evaluate it in the distal thigh where it enters the adductor canal. Most of the examination is performed with the patient supine, but the popliteal artery may be more easily imaged with the patient prone. Visualization of plaques can identify the presence of arterial disease, but quantitative assessment of the degree of narrowing is best accomplished by pulsed Doppler analysis of the velocities across the suspected areas of narrowing.

Color-flow imaging can be helpful in rapidly identifying vessels, especially below the knee.[99] The time of the examination can be reduced. Minimizing the size of the color box will increase the frame rate, allowing rapidly changing flow features to be observed. The pattern of color filling readily distinguishes arterial from venous flow. The use of color-flow imaging can help to rapidly and accurately identify areas of flow disturbance or occlusion.[100] Useful color findings that may identify the presence of a significant stenosis or occlusion include the presence or absence of triphasic flow, poststenotic turbulence, bruits, and prominent collateral vessels.[101] In the color-flow image, triphasic flow appears as a color change from red to blue to red during a single cardiac cycle. Bruits represent tissue motion adjacent to a significant stenosis, producing low-frequency color Doppler speckling outside of the vessel during systole. Color assignment outside the vessel from excessive color Doppler gain settings will be present in both systole and diastole.

Interpretation Criteria and Validation

Criteria for the grading of lower extremity arterial stenoses were developed by Jäger and colleagues[94,102] and prospectively validated with arteriographic comparisons[103] (Table 12-4). Unlike the interpretation of carotid duplex scans, there is no absolute velocity that discriminates a significant stenosis from less severe lesions. The peak-systolic flow velocity in extremity arteries will normally decrease as one proceeds distally[102] (Table 12-5). In peripheral arteries it is the magnitude of the focal increase in peak-systolic velocity that categorizes the degree of stenosis. An increase of 100 percent or more in the peak-systolic velocity from one segment of artery to the next signifies the presence of a 50 percent or greater diameter-reducing stenosis.

Table 12-4 Duplex Scan Classification of Lower Extremity Arterial Stenosis

Lumen Diameter Reduction	Peak Systolic Velocity (PSV)	Spectral Waveform Characteristics
None (normal)	No defined normal velocity[a]	Triphasic waveform, spectral broadening minimal or absent
1–19%	<30% increase in PSV as compared with closest proximal normal arterial segment	Triphasic waveform, minimal to moderate spectral broadening in late systole
20–49%	30–100% increase in velocity as compared with proximal normal arterial segment	Preservation of reverse flow components of the waveform, increased spectral broadening throughout systole
50–99%	Twice the velocity in the proximal adjacent arterial segment or PSV >200 cm/s	Reverse flow component absent; poststenotic turbulence in segment immediately beyond stenosis; waveform just beyond the stenosis usually monophasic with reduced systolic velocity (but normalized triphasic waveforms may appear distal to stenosis)
Occlusion	No flow in the imaged artery	Monophasic, preocclusive "thump" proximal to occlusion; diminished distal velocities and monophasic distal waveforms

[a] Normal peak systolic velocity varies through the arterial tree, generally decreasing distally. Stenoses are graded by changes in velocity across diseased segment; relative, rather than absolute values, are of principal interest.

While the magnitude of the end-diastolic frequency is used to classify high-grade stenoses in the carotid artery, this approach does not appear applicable to peripheral arteries.[13] The absence of flow reversal is a good indication of a significant proximal stenosis or occlusion. The loss of reverse flow in a narrowed segment has been correlated with a greater than 15 mmHg systolic pressure gradient, which would be clinically significant.[13]

For detection of lower extremity arterial stenoses that are shown by arteriography to reduce the lumen diameter by 50 percent or more, duplex scanning has a sensitivity of 82 percent, a specificity of 92 percent, a positive predictive value of 80 percent, and a negative predictive value of 93 percent.[103] Color-flow arterial mapping appears to improve the specificity of the examination.[100] It particularly facilitates the detection of deeper and smaller vessels (Plate 12-7).

With careful imaging techniques, color-flow imaging as a sole modality can detect hemodynamically signifi-

cant lesions (50 percent or greater diameter-reducing stenosis or occlusion) in the superficial femoral and popliteal arteries with sensitivities of 85 and 100 percent and specificities of 97 and 92 percent, respectively. For the anterior and posterior tibial arteries, the sensitivities are 86 and 79 percent and the specificities are 96 and 100 percent, respectively.

The best results are obtained by combining color-flow imaging with pulsed Doppler waveform analysis. This yields reproducible, quantifiable data (velocities) and is less sensitive than color-flow imaging alone to subtle changes in technique or instrument settings that can significantly affect the displayed color-flow image.

Postoperative Graft Surveillance

Postoperative assessment of patients who have had infrainguinal bypasses has been markedly improved by the use of duplex scanning. Anatomic abnormalities in grafts that lead to graft failure can be accurately de-

Table 12-5 Normal Arterial Dimensions and Flow Velocities in Lower Extremity Arterial Segments

Arterial Segment	Diameter ± SD (cm)	V_{sys} ± SD (cm/s)	V_{rev} ± SD (cm/s)	V_{dias} ± SD (cm/s)
External iliac	0.79 ± 0.13	119.3 ± 21.7	−41.5 ± 10.7	18.2 ± 7.5
Common femoral	0.82 ± 0.14	114.1 ± 24.9	−40.6 ± 9.2	16.4 ± 8.3
Superficial femoral (proximal)	0.60 ± 0.12	90.8 ± 13.6	−35.8 ± 8.2	14.5 ± 7.2
Superficial femoral (distal)	0.54 ± 0.11	93.6 ± 14.1	−35.0 ± 9.8	14.6 ± 6.7
Popliteal	0.52 ± 0.11	68.6 ± 13.5	−27.8 ± 9.2	9.8 ± 6.0

Abbreviations: V_{sys}, peak systolic velocity; V_{rev} peak velocity of reverse flow component; V_{dias}, peak forward diastolic flow velocity; SD, standard deviation. (From Jäger et al.,[94] with permission.)

tected. This is important because clinical assessment alone is insensitive for detecting lesions within a vein graft.

Routine graft surveillance can identify grafts at risk for thrombosis and can prolong graft function by prompting elective revision before the graft occludes. Grafts that are failing, whether because of lesions intrinsic to the graft or because of progression of atherosclerotic disease in the native arteries, can be salvaged if surgery is performed prior to thrombosis. The long-term results of saphenous vein grafts can be improved if the lesions that may lead to graft thrombosis are corrected. Secondary patency of infrainguinal bypass grafts at 5 years is 85 percent when revision with patch angioplasty is undertaken electively. In marked contrast is the 19 percent 5-year patency rate following thrombectomy of an occluded graft.[104] Duplex scanning can also identify residual arteriovenous fistulae or intact valve cusps left after in situ grafting. Residual arteriovenous fistulae with low flows can be observed serially, and if they persist, they can be selectively ligated.[105]

Duplex scanning is also useful in the evaluation of suspected operative complications, both early and late. Perigraft fluid collections can be identified, and with the use of Doppler or color-flow imaging, anastomotic pseudoaneurysms can be differentiated from other causes of postoperative groin masses[106,107] (Fig. 12-16, Plate 12-8).

The ankle/arm index (AAI) is not particularly sensitive for detecting impending graft failure. The rate of unexpected failure despite surveillance with AAIs is difficult to establish; the reported incidence ranges from 4 to 44 percent.[108–110] The use of the AAI alone to monitor graft status also lacks specificity. Noting a drop in the AAI does not localize the site of the pressure-reducing lesion, nor can it help to differentiate a single major lesion from serial minor lesions.

Graft stenoses in the first postoperative year occur most frequently from myointimal hyperplasia. These lesions most commonly occur in the proximal or distal extremes of the graft, close to but not involving the anastomoses.[111] Graft surveillance examinations should occur at 3-month intervals during this first year. An abnormal duplex study of a graft in a patient with normal or unchanged AAIs should prompt arteriography, although in some cases a discrete lesion identified by duplex scanning can be repaired on the basis of this information alone.

Changes in the velocity waveform are useful in detecting lesions within a graft that have not yet reduced pressure; AAI changes greater than 0.15 were absent in 38 percent of graft stenoses (> 50 percent diameter reduction) in one series.[112] Peak-systolic velocity in infrainguinal grafts has been useful in predicting outcome. Early graft occlusion has been associated with low peak-systolic velocities (< 40 to 45 cm/s) and the

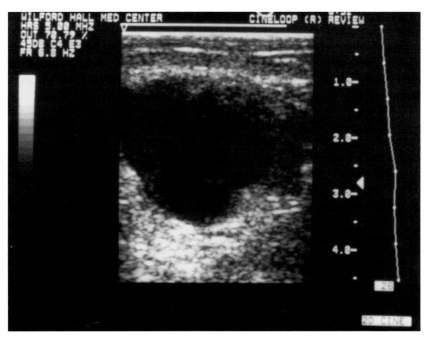

Figure 12-16 Study performed to evaluate a groin mass after cardiac catheterization. The finding of a hypoechoic mass is consistent with a simple hematoma, but by demonstrating the presence of blood flow (see Plate 12-8) the diagnosis of pseudoaneurysm is made.

absence of diastolic forward flow (indicative of high outflow resistance).[113] A highly phasic ("staccato") configuration velocity waveform, with a narrow spectrum and brief reverse diastolic flow, is indicative of an almost completely obstructing distal occlusive lesion.[108] A decrease in a previously satisfactory peak-systolic velocity to less than 40 to 45 cm/s correlates well with the development of problems that could be in the inflow artery, the graft itself, or the outflow vessels. The specificity of a low flow velocity in a graft is low, however. Low peak-systolic velocities can occur without the risk of impending graft thrombosis in a large-diameter ($\geq$6-mm) vein graft anastomosed to a smaller-caliber artery.[114] The degree of luminal narrowing is quantified on the basis of velocity measurements and the characteristics of the pulsed Doppler spectral waveforms. Duplex scanning categorization of bypass graft stenoses correlates well with angiographic findings.[112,115] Criteria for duplex scan grading of graft stenoses are outlined in Table 12-6.

Identification of grafts with velocity-reducing lesions followed by prophylactic intervention has yielded a 4-year patency rate of 81 percent, which is comparable with the 86 percent 4-year patency rate of primary reconstructions not found to have occlusive lesions.[116]

The addition of color-flow imaging can be helpful. Areas of flow disturbance can be easily identified and then graded by pre- and poststenotic peak-systolic velocity.[117,118] This may substitute for the more time-consuming process of sampling velocities through the entire graft length by the pulsed Doppler technique. There are caveats to the use of color. Subtle flow disturbances may not be displayed with color if the PRF is set too high. Also, as color-flow imaging displays *mean* velocity information, it is less sensitive to the moderate lesions that cause spectral broadening and increase peak systolic velocities by only a small amount. Finally, to avoid incorrectly diagnosing the presence of a stenosis, it is important to use the pulsed Doppler to measure velocities in those areas where disturbed flow is detected by the color-flow image. However, there will be velocity changes and flow disturbances at a distal graft anastomosis if the graft and recipient artery are mismatched for size. Differentiating this situation from an anastomotic stricture is important.

Because the finding of high-grade stenoses usually prompts graft revision, the natural history of asymptomatic diameter-reducing lesions in bypass grafts (or the proximal or distal arteries) is not known.[109] The finding of a significant focal graft stenosis correlates with increased graft failure risk but is not specific.[119] Criteria used for the elective revision of infrainguinal grafts are not uniformly established, but pressure-reducing lesions (those that produce an interval decrease in AAI of 0.15), lesions responsible for new ischemic symptoms, or those that progress to a more than 75 percent diameter reduction should be considered for elective revision. It does appear that increasing stenosis severity correlates with increasing risk of graft thrombosis.[120]

Table 12-6 Duplex Scan Classification of Stenoses in Lower Extremity Arterial Bypass Grafts

Lumen Diameter Reduction	Peak Systolic Velocity (PSV)	Spectral Waveform Characteristics
None (normal)	$\geq$ 45 cm/s	No spectral broadening, waveform usually triphasic
1–19% (wall irregularity)	$\leq$ 30% increase in PSV as compared with proximal site; PSV $\geq$ 45 cm/s	Minimal to moderate spectral broadening during systole
20–49%	30–100% increase in velocity as compared with the proximal (normal) arterial segment	Preservation of reverse flow components of the waveform; increased spectral broadening throughout pulse cycle
50–99%	Velocity, as compared with the proximal adjacent graft segment, increased by $\geq$ 100% in focal segment of graft[a] or PSV > 200 cm/s	Reverse flow component absent; poststenotic turbulence in segment immediately beyond stenosis; waveform just beyond the stenosis usually monophasic with reduced systolic velocity (but normalized triphasic waveforms may appear distal to stenosis)
Occlusion	No flow in the imaged artery	Monophasic, preocclusive "thump" proximal to occlusion; distal velocities diminished and distal waveforms monophasic

[a] PSV $\leq$ 45 cm/s or decreased by 20 cm/s compared to prior bypass graft duplex scan are considered signs of impending graft thrombosis.

Renal Artery Duplex Scanning

Renal artery stenosis is the most common cause of secondary hypertension and is an important cause of renal dysfunction.[121] Renal artery stenoses can be effectively treated by endarterectomy or bypass or if the lesion does not involve the vessel's origin, by percutaneous transluminal renal angioplasty. High-grade renal artery stenoses, if untreated, tend to progress to occlusion, with permanent loss of renal function in the affected kidney.[122-124] Revascularization of an ischemic kidney, on the other hand, can improve creatinine clearance and increase renal size.[125]

Identifying candidates for surgical revascularization or angioplasty requires both identifying a renal artery stenosis and establishing that it is physiologically significant.[126] Renal artery duplex scanning is an excellent screening test, as it can provide anatomic information (presence or absence of a stenosis, size of the affected kidney) as well as physiologic information (hemodynamic significance of a stenosis, pattern of parenchymal perfusion and renovascular resistance). In addition, it is as accurate as arteriography for identifying the location of a stenosis, which is important for the selection of therapeutic modalities.[127]

Indications

Duplex scanning for renal artery disease is indicated for the evaluation of patients with significant hypertension or renal insufficiency who are candidates for renal artery reconstruction or transluminal angioplasty. Renovascular hypertension may be suspected in (1) young patients with severe hypertension; (2) patients with rapidly accelerating hypertension; (3) patients with malignant hypertension or flash pulmonary edema; (4) patients whose blood pressure is particularly difficult to control; and (5) patients with concomitant hypertension and renal insufficiency.[128] It is also useful for serial observation of identified renal artery lesions and follow-up after surgical or transcatheterization intervention.[124,129-131] It can also detect renal artery stenosis in transplanted kidneys.[132,133]

Technique

Renal artery duplex scanning requires a low-frequency (2- to 3-MHz) transducer. Patients are prepared for scanning with an overnight fast to minimize the amount of bowel gas present. Scanning the supine patient from a midline approach accesses the aorta, visceral vessels, and the proximal and midsegments of both main renal arteries. The left renal vein crossing the aorta is a landmark for identifying the location of the renal arteries, which typically originate directly posterior to the left renal vein. The origin of the right renal artery is slightly more anterior than that of the left, and the right renal artery is behind the inferior vena cava (Plate 12-9). Occasionally both arteries can be seen in the same transverse scan plane.

Color-flow imaging can help in renal artery identification. The color PRF is set to avoid aliasing (3 to 5 kHz), and the baseline may be shifted down (since there is no reverse flow component that needs to be displayed). The color sector or box should be limited in size to the specific region being examined. This color setup is needed for this deep examination; otherwise the frame rate will be low and temporal distortion will result.

The pulsed Doppler study confirms the identification of the renal arteries. The kidney offers a low-resistance outflow bed with a characteristic renal artery Doppler signal associated with high diastolic flow. If possible, a Doppler angle of 60 degrees should be maintained while the velocity spectra are being recorded. Doppler signals are obtained from the aorta at the level of the superior mesenteric artery and in the renal arteries from their origins to the renal hila.

The presence of multiple renal arteries or smaller accessory branches is not uncommon, occurring in 10 to 20 percent of kidneys. Significant renovascular hypertension can occur when only one of a kidney's supplying arteries is stenotic. If only the nonstenotic renal artery is identified, a false-negative result (missing a diagnosis of renal artery stenosis) may be obtained. Duplex scanning, even with color-flow imaging, has not proved reliable in detecting accessory renal arteries (Plate 12-10).

Flow in the parenchyma and segmental renal arteries can be assessed from a lateral approach. Flow characteristics in the distal arterial branches are altered if there is a hemodynamically significant stenosis in the main renal artery. These flow signals can be analyzed by measuring the duration of systolic acceleration or by determining the ratio of the peak-systolic velocity to the diastolic velocity. Since these measurements and calculations are not dependent on the absolute value of the Doppler frequency or velocity, they can be determined without Doppler angle correction.

Imaging can provide useful information about the end-organ effects of renal artery disease, specifically, kidney size. Measuring the length of the kidney is a means of assessing renal mass, and, by inference, the number of functional nephrons. Renal mass appears to decrease in the presence of a high-grade renal artery stenosis.[123,124] In the setting of renal artery occlusion the kidney length is often less than 9 cm. Kidney length should be measured with the scan plane in the sagittal plane of the organ. This is accomplished by imaging from the flank, with the patient in either the decubitus or prone position.

The renal veins and inferior vena cava should also be examined in a renal duplex study. With renal vein thrombosis, thrombus may be visualized in the renal vein and there will be no Doppler signal. Large venous collaterals may be noted.

Interpretation Criteria and Validation

Normal renal artery peak-systolic velocities are 104 ± 25 cm/s on the right and 93 ± 19 cm/s on the left[134] (Plate 12-11). An increase in the renal artery peak-systolic velocity is a reliable indicator for discriminating between a normal and a diseased artery. By using a value of above 180 cm/s as the criterion, renal artery disease can be detected with 95 percent sensitivity and 90 percent specificity[127] (Plate 12-12). As noted above, the normal variability in renal artery velocities is not inconsequential. To minimize the effect of this variability on diagnostic end points, renal artery velocities are indexed against aortic velocities. The ratio of the peak-systolic velocity of the renal artery to that of the aorta is used for the detection of high-grade lesions; This value is the renal/aortic ratio (RAR):

$$RAR = \frac{\text{renal artery peak-systolic velocity}}{\text{aortic peak-systolic velocity}}$$

The criteria for classifying the severity of renal artery disease are listed in Table 12-7. These criteria were initially established by retrospective comparison of duplex scans with arteriography[135] and were subsequently validated with prospective studies. In these prospective studies a RAR of 3.5 or higher was found to be 84 to 92 percent sensitive and 62 to 97 percent specific in the diagnosis of a hemodynamically significant (≥ 60 per-cent diameter-reducing) renal artery stenosis (93 percent accuracy).[127,136] The lower value of 62 percent for specificity reflects a disagreement between the arteriogram and duplex scan with respect to lesion severity, not the presence or absence of a lesion.[127] If the RAR is less than 3.5, a renal artery peak-systolic velocity of 180 cm/s or higher suggests a 1 to 59 percent diameter-reducing renal artery stenosis.

The diagnosis of renal artery occlusion is made when the renal artery is adequately visualized but no Doppler flow signal can be obtained. The diagnosis of occlusion is further supported by the findings of a small (< 9 cm long) kidney and a low-amplitude velocity signal in the renal parenchyma.

Aortic dimensions and velocities should be noted. Peak-systolic velocities may be as low as 20 cm/s in an aortic aneurysm or large aortic graft. High aortic velocities may be present if there is significant atherosclerotic disease involving the juxtarenal aorta. If the aortic velocities are lower than 40 cm/s or higher than 100 cm/s, the RAR should not be used. The presence of a renal artery stenosis may still be inferred from the presence of focal increases in renal artery flow velocities (≥ 180 cm/s), recognition of poststenotic turbulence, or hilar signal analysis.

Spectral broadening is not used for grading less severe renal artery stenoses as it is in carotid artery examinations. The depth of the examined structures, the lower ultrasound frequency used, and movements with respiration require a larger Doppler sample volume for renal artery examinations. As the sample volume includes the entire artery width, some spectral broadening will normally be seen in the renal artery Doppler waveforms. However, the finding of marked spectral broadening distal to a segment of high-velocity flow suggests poststenotic turbulence and corroborates the diagnosis of a significant renal artery stenosis.

Table 12-7   Duplex Scan Classification of Renal Artery Stenosis

Lumen Diameter Reduction	Renal/Aortic Ratio[a]	Renal Artery Peak Systolic Velocity
None (normal)	<3.5	<180 cm/s
$<60\%$ diameter reduction	<3.5	≥ 180 cm/s
60–99% diameter reduction[b]	≥ 3.5	
Occlusion	—	No detectable flow in any segment of main renal artery[c]

[a] Angle corrected (60 degrees) renal artery peak systolic velocity (PSV) divided by aortic PSV. This value may be unreliable if there is aneurysmal dilation of the aorta.

[b] Hemodynamically significant stenosis.

[c] Parenchymal flow signals may be present despite renal artery occlusion. If collateral circulation has maintained some renal blood flow, low-amplitude, low-velocity Doppler signals may be detected.

One of the problems with renal artery duplex scanning is that the examination is technically inadequate in 10 to 15 percent of cases.[135,136] The proximal and midportions of the main renal arteries may be difficult to visualize from an anterior approach. Obesity, bowel gas, and respiratory movements can make it difficult to accurately identify the location of the renal arteries, which is necessary to sweep the sample volume along the course of the vessels. Alternately, arterial signals can be acquired from a flank or translumbar approach. These approaches image the kidney without overlying gas, but signals cannot be obtained from the proximal renal artery.

Analysis of distal renal artery flow signals from segmental or interlobular arteries in the hilum of the kidney has been proposed as an indirect means of detecting proximal renal artery stenosis.[137-139] It has been advocated both as a more rapid means of detecting significant renal artery stenoses and as a way to obviate the difficulties associated with scanning from an anterior abdominal approach (Plate 12-13). Hilar signals can be obtained in 98 to 99 percent of subjects, typically in 15 to 30 minutes.[138-140]

Hilar Doppler signals are analyzed for the acceleration time (AT), acceleration index (AI) and acceleration time ratio (ATR). The AT is the time from the onset of systole to the peak-systolic velocity. When there is a "notch" in the velocity profile, the first peak is used. The AI is the slope of the systolic upstroke and ATR is the ratio of the renal artery AT to the AT the juxtarenal aorta. With renal artery stenoses of 50 percent or more, the velocity waveform is blunted, showing a more gradual upstroke. ATs of 0.07 seconds[137,138] and 0.10 seconds[139,140] have been used as cutoff points for AT by different investigators. AIs of 291 cm/s² or less have been correlated with the presence of significant stenoses.

The proper role for hilar signal analysis is yet to be established. In prospective comparisons against arteriographically defined renal artery stenoses of 50 percent or more, the AI has been reported to be 87 to 100 percent sensitive and 93 to 94 percent specific.[138,139] The AT sensitivity and specificity were found to be 87 to 100 and 83 to 98 percent, respectively.[138,139] In a subsequent duplex scanning controlled study that used a RAR of 3.5 or higher (corresponding to ≥ 60 percent stenosis) as the basis of comparison, the sensitivity and specificity of AI were 62 and 79 percent and the sensitivity and specificity of AT were 62 and 89 percent, respectively.[140] This suggested that hilar studies alone are inadequate as a screening tool to detect hemodynamically renal artery stenoses. Furthermore, since hilar signal analysis is an indirect test, it cannot differentiate between stenosis and occlusion, nor can it localize a lesion along the course of the artery.

The pulsatility of the Doppler waveform in the cortex and medulla is used as a marker for small vessel disease. The diastolic/systolic frequency (DRS) ratio (also referred to as the end-diastolic ratio) is a function of the renovascular resistance in the parenchyma.

$$DSR = \frac{\text{end-diastolic velocity of parenchymal waveform}}{\text{peak-systolic velocity of parenchymal waveform}}$$

In canine models a drop in the DSR correlates well with increased renovascular resistance induced by microsphere injections. In human studies, an increase in the estimated renovascular resistance as compared with controls is seen in age-matched hypertensive and atherosclerotic patients.[141] A low DSR (high resistance) is seen with increasing serum creatinine, even in the absence of renal artery stenosis (Fig. 12-17). The DSR, therefore, may be a marker for renal parenchymal disease. This can include, but is not specific to, ischemic nephropathy.

In a normal kidney, the DSR is 0.3 or higher. A DSR of 0.2 to 0.3 is consistent with an intermediate increase in renovascular resistance, while a DSR of 0.2 or lower suggests high renovascular resistance.

Evaluation of the Transplanted Kidney

The techniques of renal duplex scanning are useful for the early and late evaluation of the transplanted kidney. The transplanted kidney is relatively superficial in its iliac fossa location, and therefore it may be easier to study than a native kidney. In addition to the examination of vascular structures with imaging and Doppler, the B-mode imaging capabilities of the scanner can be used to detect anatomic problems such as perigraft fluid or dilatation of the ureter and collecting system.

The renal artery in a transplanted kidney should have flow characteristics similar to those of a normal renal artery. The normal velocity waveform pattern is one of a high-flow, low-resistance vessel. There is a rapid systolic upstroke, gradual descent in diastole, and continued high diastolic flow.

The development of hypertension or worsening azotemia can be the result of a significant stenosis in the renal artery of the transplanted kidney. The renal artery to the graft is evaluated for a stenosis in a similar fashion to that used in examination of a native kidney.[132,133,142] Stenoses are most common at or just distal to the anastomosis. The findings of a focal velocity increase and poststenotic spectral broadening identify a stenosis. A renal artery/external iliac artery peak-systolic velocity ratio of 3.0 or higher is predictive of graft renal artery stenosis.[143]

A technical complication or hyperacute rejection may result in early postoperative thrombosis of the

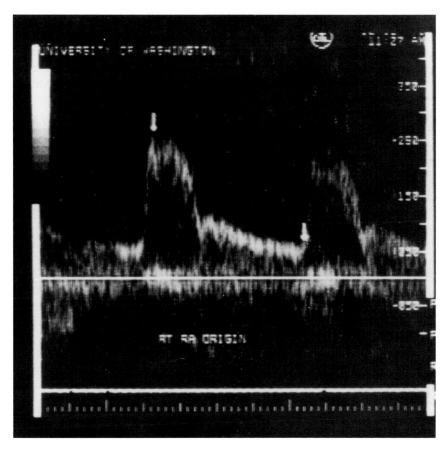

Figure 12-17 In the renal artery the ratio of the end-diastolic velocity *(right arrow)* to the peak systolic velocity *(left arrow)* gives a measurement of renovascular resistance. The diastolic/systolic ratio here is 0.33 (normal). This waveform is from a renal artery with <60% stenosis.

graft renal artery or vein. Postoperative evaluation of an anuric transplant patient can establish this diagnosis. Occlusion is suggested by the absence of Doppler signals in the visualized artery or vein. A large sample volume and a low wall filter setting should be used to avoid missing areas of low flow. Because of the tissue ischemia, the B-mode image of the graft may show a noticeable increase in kidney echogenicity. Color-flow imaging is useful to identify areas of perfusion and ischemia and may also define areas of segmental renal infarction.

Renal vein thrombosis is diagnosed by the absence of flow in the renal vein, but this vein may be difficult to image in the early postoperative period. With renal vein thrombosis, examination of the renal artery flow signals may show spiking of the systolic velocity waveform, shortening of the systolic rise time, and reverse flow in diastole, which is consistent with high outflow resistance.[142,144] Transplant renal vein thrombosis is usually accompanied by thrombosis of the ipsilateral iliac vein.

Identifying the cause of renal dysfunction in first days or weeks after transplantation is necessary if ap-

propriate therapy is to be instituted. For example, drugs used to treat rejection (such as cyclosporine) could aggravate renal injury from ischemia or drug toxicity. Differentiating these causes often requires a kidney biopsy, an invasive procedure associated with risks of infection, hematoma, or graft injury.

Acute vascular rejection of a renal allograft is the result of a proliferative endovasculitis. Increasing renovascular resistance, with a low diastolic/systolic ratio (≤2.0 to 2.5), has been noted to be a feature of acute vascular rejection, but it is not seen with acute interstitial (cellular) rejection or with chronic rejection (until very late).[143,145–148] The segmental arteries appear to be the most sensitive sites for detecting the flow changes associated with acute rejection.[146] Azotemia from cyclosporine nephrotoxicity is not usually associated with a change in the renovascular resistance.[143,145,147]

Distinguishing acute rejection from acute tubular necrosis (ATN) by duplex scanning has its limitations.[149] Studies seeking to differentiate rejection from ATN have used another indicator of the renovascular resistance, namely the Pourcelot, or resistive index (RI):

$$RI = \frac{\text{peak-systolic frequency} - \text{end-diastolic frequency}}{\text{peak-systolic frequency}}$$

A resistive index of 0.80 or higher has been proposed as an indication of acute rejection.[149,150] This cutoff value is only 69 percent sensitive and 86 percent specific. Furthermore, one-third of patients with ATN fall into this RI range. Use of an RI of 0.9 or higher is 100 percent specific for acute rejection, but only 13 percent sensitive.[150] Currently, high resistance in the graft can be used as a good marker for pathologic change. Very high resistance suggests acute rejection, but intermediate increases in resistance could be due to either ATN or rejection.

Mesenteric Circulation

The arterial supply to the gut includes the celiac artery, the superior mesenteric artery (SMA), and the inferior mesenteric artery. Duplex scanning can be used to study the celiac, splenic, hepatic, and superior mesenteric arteries. The inferior mesenteric artery is more difficult to evaluate, but the availability of color-flow imaging has made such evaluation possible in some patients.

Indications

Duplex scanning is of limited value in the diagnosis of acute mesenteric ischemia. Even if the celiac artery and the SMA are visualized and have flow demonstrated in their proximal portions, the possibility of a more distal occlusion cannot be excluded with assurance. The urgent nature of the problem mandates a rapid and definitive diagnosis. A delay in revascularizing severely ischemic bowel results in irreversible intestinal infarction.

On the other hand, chronic intestinal ischemia is appropriately investigated with duplex scanning. It is often a difficult problem to diagnose. Classically, the patient develops abdominal pain associated with eating (intestinal angina), diarrhea, and weight loss. Because the symptoms are progressive and nonspecific, the correct diagnosis is seldom considered early. The finding of an epigastric bruit on examination suggests intra-abdominal arterial disease but gives little additional information. Once the diagnosis is suspected, lateral aortography is the definitive test for documenting the blood supply to the small intestine. Duplex scanning is the best available noninvasive diagnostic method for the detection of lesions in the celiac and superior mesenteric arteries that could be responsible for the patient's complaints.

The diagnosis of chronic mesenteric ischemia is supported by the finding of significant stenosis or occlusion of two or more of the major arteries supplying the small bowel. As collaterals are usually well developed in the mesenteric circulation, chronic occlusive disease of a single artery will not produce symptoms. If the duplex scan is normal or if only one artery is involved, the diagnosis of chronic mesenteric ischemia can be excluded.

Postoperative duplex scanning can also be useful in documenting the technical result of intra-abdominal arterial procedures. It can be used to document graft patency both early and late.[130] After liver transplantation, it can document patency of the hepatic artery, a feature critical to success of the graft.[151]

Technique

Duplex scans of the visceral vessels are best done after the patient has fasted overnight. Low-frequency (2- to 3-MHz) transducers are typically used, but a 5-MHz transducer may be useful in a very slender patient. Patients with chronic mesenteric ischemia are thin, which makes the examination easier.

The aorta and the origins of the celiac axis and the SMA can be visualized by scanning the upper midabdomen with the patient supine (Fig. 12-18). Celiac branches are best identified with a transverse scan plane. Normal celiac artery velocities are 90 to 100 cm/s; if a high-velocity celiac artery signal is obtained, the vessel should be rescanned as the patient takes a

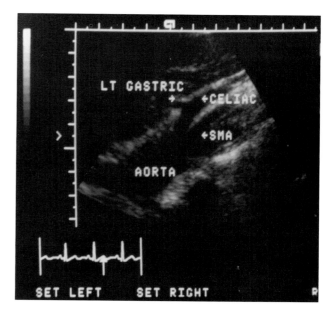

Figure 12-18 The celiac axis and the superior mesenteric artery (SMA) originate within 1 to 2 cm of each other from the anterior aspect of the aorta.

deep breath. Normalization of a high-velocity celiac artery signal with inspiration suggests extrinsic compression by the median arcuate ligament rather than intrinsic disease of the artery.[152] The SMA arises 1 to 2 cm distal to the celiac axis and is directed caudad, roughly in the plane of the aorta. In fasting patients peak-systolic velocities are 100 to 120 cm/s. As in other Doppler examinations, the velocity data are angle-dependent. The Doppler angle should be constant between examinations, and it is preferably kept at 60 degrees. The variability introduced in the velocity measurements by changing the Doppler angle is even greater in the SMA than in the carotid artery.[153]

Color-flow imaging facilitates vessel identification. Focal stenoses can be recognized by the appearance of flow disturbances and increases in velocity.

Interpretation Criteria and Validation

Spectral waveforms from the celiac axis show constant forward diastolic flow owing to the low resistance of the splenic and hepatic arterial beds. (Plate 12-14).

The small intestine has a variable metabolic and functional status, depending on its digestive activity. In the fasting state the SMA has a high resistance pattern, with little or no forward diastolic flow. There is usually a diastolic flow reversal, producing a triphasic velocity waveform similar to that seen in lower extremity arteries[154] (Fig. 12-19). After a meal the resistance to flow decreases and the flow in the SMA increases dramatically. In a study of 20 normal subjects, the SMA peak-systolic velocity rose from an average of 120 to 190 cm/s after ingestion of a standard meal.[155] Subsequent

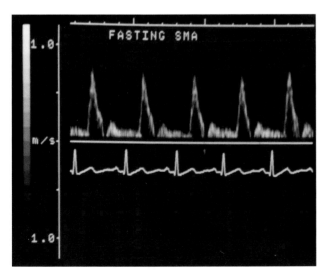

Figure 12-19 In the fasting subject the superior mesenteric artery (SMA) has a velocity waveform characteristic of high resistance outflow.

studies have revealed that diastolic forward flow shows the greatest postprandial change from baseline in normal subjects.[156] This hemodynamic response can be reproduced by administration of glucagon.[157]

The increases seen in SMA flow after a meal are blunted in patients with occlusive disease affecting the mesenteric artery.[156] However, the blunting of the postprandial response is not specific for the presence of a proximal mesenteric artery stenosis, as this response is also altered in diabetics with autonomic neuropathy.[158]

The degree of luminal diameter reduction in the mesenteric arteries that produces a pressure gradient is not known, but it has been suggested that a 70 percent diameter reduction will probably reduce flow and pressure. Retrospective studies have suggested that the duplex scan findings that correlate with the presence of a 70 percent or greater stenosis or occlusion of the SMA are a peak-systolic velocity of 275 cm/s or greater in the SMA or the absence of a flow signal in an adequately visualized vessel. In the celiac artery, a 70 percent or greater stenosis or occlusion is associated with a peak-systolic velocity of 200 cm/s or higher or no flow. Prospective, blinded studies comparing these duplex scan findings with arteriographic results have found these criteria to be accurate. The sensitivity, specificity, and positive and negative predictive values for the SMA were 100, 96, 81, and 100 percent, respectively; the corresponding values for the duplex scan diagnosis of 70 percent or more celiac axis stenosis or occlusion were 91, 80, 63, and 96 percent, respectively.[159] The reasons for the lower accuracy in the celiac axis are not hard to appreciate. This artery has a very short trunk before branching into the common hepatic, left gastric, and splenic arteries. There is no straight segment without major branches, and it is difficult to obtain a 60-degree Doppler angle with the celiac artery. Abnormal hepatic artery flow characteristics, including retrograde flow, turbulence, and diminished pulsatility are indirect indications of the presence of a significant celiac artery stenosis or occlusion.[160]

Because of its location and smaller size, the inferior mesenteric artery is not routinely visualized with duplex scanning, although some instances of SMA occlusion or severe stenosis, it can be markedly enlarged and easy to scan. There are no published criteria for characterizing inferior mesenteric artery disease.

Portal Vein Duplex Scanning

The portal vein is imaged in the right upper quadrant or from an anterior midline approach. The walls of the portal vein are relatively echogenic because of the surrounding fibrous tissue in the porta hepatis (Fig.

12-20). The normal portal vein spectral waveform has continuous flow with low peak and mean velocities. Flow is mildly turbulent, and phasic variation is seen with respiration and events of the cardiac cycle (Plate 12-15). Velocities will normally vary with posture, activity, and prandial state.

Duplex scanning can help to establish or confirm the diagnosis of portal hypertension. Sonographic criteria for the diagnosis of portal hypertension include: portal vein diameter greater than 13 mm, dilatation of other splanchnic veins, patency and dilatation of the umbilical vein, visualization of dilated collateral veins, splenomegaly with dilatation of splenic vein radicles, and disappearance of normal respiratory variations in splanchnic vein caliber.[161]

It is important to demonstrate portal and splenic vein patency and direction of flow if operative intervention is being considered. Partial or complete portal vein thrombosis is a contraindication to portacaval shunting. Also, the direction of flow in the portal vein is important in planning shunt strategies.[162] Portal vein thrombus can be visualized with B-mode imaging, and the pulsed Doppler scan can determine direction of flow.

After portacaval shunting, duplex scanning can assess patency of the shunt. Direct indications of shunt patency include B-mode visualization of the anastomosis and pulsed Doppler findings of flow disturbance across the shunt and reversed portal vein flow. Indirect criteria suggesting shunt patency include the findings of a normal portal vein diameter with respiratory variation in its caliber, dilatation of the inferior vena cava at the level of the shunt, and the disappearance of periportal collaterals.[163]

Extremity Veins

Acute deep venous thrombosis (DVT) affects as many as 800,000 patients annually in the United States, of whom as many as one-third may develop pulmonary embolism. The clinical diagnosis of DVT is notoriously poor—roughly equal in sensitivity and specificity to a coin flip.[164] It is important to make an accurate diagnosis of DVT, as therapy should be started without delay. In addition, treatments such as anticoagulation or thrombolytic therapy carry potential risks and should not be given without clear indications.

Chronic venous insufficiency is another common problem; 6 to 7 million Americans have demonstrable signs of lower extremity venous disease. Severe venous disease with ulceration has a prevalence of 1 percent in all adults and 3 to 4 percent in those over 65 years of age.[165] Commonly, venous valvular insufficiency follows an episode of DVT (often by many years). Fibrotic or immobilized valve cusps no longer function properly, and ambulatory venous hypertension results. Because veins usually recanalize after an episode of DVT, venous obstruction is rarely a major contributor to the pathophysiology of the postthrombotic syndrome. Reflux, especially in the popliteal vein and venous segments below the knee, is frequently associated with the development of venous ulceration after an episode of DVT.[166]

Indications

Patients with symptoms or clinical findings that suggest DVT should be evaluated with duplex scanning. These include (1) patients for whom a clinical suspicion of DVT exists; (2) those with suspected or proven pulmonary emboli; (3) those with unexplained leg swelling after orthopedic, pelvic, or vascular surgery; and (4) those with chronic leg swelling of undetermined cause. Duplex scanning can also document the status of the deep venous system after the acute phase of the DVT has passed. This can help determine the need for elastic support. Duplex scanning is an excellent tool for defining the incidence of DVT in high-risk populations (such as hospitalized patients with acute spinal cord injury or those undergoing neurosurgery or hip surgery),[167] but it is not currently recommended as routine in the absence of a clinical indication of DVT.[69]

After the diagnosis of DVT is established, duplex scanning is helpful in the evaluation of patients who

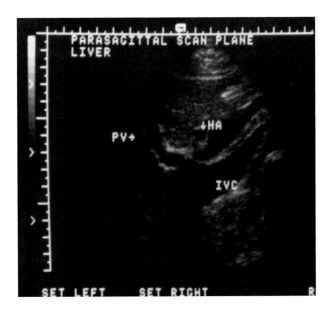

Figure 12-20 Intrahepatic portions of the portal vein (PV) (left) characteristically have an echogenic appearance. This is due to the fibrous tissue that surrounds the vein. The retrohepatic inferior vena cava (IVC) and a hepatic artery branch (HA) are also noted in this B-mode image.

vein or upper extremity cephalic or basilic veins. Most of the examination relies on the B-mode image, although the pulsed Doppler flow information can be complementary, and the Doppler scan can be important in confirming venous occlusion (Fig. 12-21). Color-flow imaging can be helpful in following or finding a small vein and can aid the identification of branches or tributaries. Criteria for the acceptability of a vein for use as a bypass graft typically include internal diameter 2.0 mm or larger; vein free of thrombus; no occluded or atretic segments; and absence of major truncal varicosities.

In prospective studies B-mode assessment of GSVs was 93 to 96 percent sensitive in selecting a vein that was confirmed to be adequate at operation. The positive predictive value of the test was equally high.[188,189] The specificity of B-mode imaging was, however, only 65 to 67 percent. Vein segments with diameters marginally less than 2.0 mm, segments with localized presence of chronic thrombus, and small double segments that communicate with each other have been successfully used after being deemed unsatisfactory by preoperative B-mode assessment.[190] In the absence of a better alternative, marginal segments of vein should be explored surgically before abandoning attempts at the harvest of autogenous vein.

The upper extremity should not be ignored as a source of venous conduit for bypass. Cephalic and basilic veins approximate the GSV in length, although injury from prior phlebotomy or intravenous lines may make segments unsuitable for use. B-mode

imaging of arm vein has an 88 percent positive predictive value.[191]

Imaging for superficial vein mapping requires a scanner with good high-resolution B-mode capabilities. A high-frequency (7- to 10-MHz) transducer and a light touch are needed. Linear array transducers have the advantage of imaging a longer segment of superficial veins in each field. The use of a standoff to aid near-field imaging is optional. The following maneuvers to augment venous distension facilitate the examination: (1) positioning of the patient standing, in the reverse Trendelenburg position, or with the examined extremity dependent; (2) exercise, reactive hyperemia, or heating to increase flow; and (3) occlusion of venous return with a tourniquet. Superficial veins are imaged over their entire length. Wall thickening or incompressibility during cross-sectional imaging suggest a chronically diseased vein.

A duplex examination for vein mapping requires only 20 to 30 minutes per extremity. The course of the vein, sites of tributaries and branches, and double segments are marked on the skin with an indelible marker.[192] The luminal diameter of the vein is recorded at several locations. If the marks are to be used by the surgeon to plan the location of the incision, it is critically important that marking be done with the extremity positioned as it will be for surgery. Repositioning, especially with obese patients, can move the skin in relation to deeper subcutaneous structures. Accurate mapping helps to avoid unnecessary dissection and creation of undermined skin flaps at the time of opera-

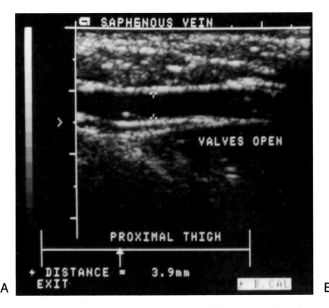
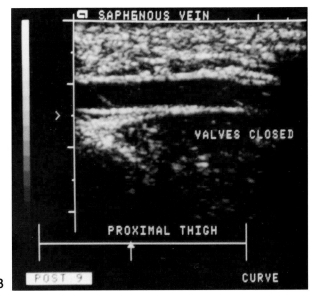

Figure 12-21 Features of superficial extremity veins can be seen with B-mode imaging. Valve leaflets in this segment of the greater saphenous vein can be seen opening (**A**) and closing (**B**).

tion, actions that increase the risk of wound complications.

CONCLUSIONS

Duplex scanning is most useful when the examination and interpretation are done by individuals who have a sound background in vascular anatomy and physiology and who understand the basics of ultrasound physics. By appreciating the potential pitfalls in the use of duplex scanning, errors can be avoided.

Like other technologies, duplex scanning continues to evolve. Newer instrument packages and transducers provide improved imaging and allow deeper structures, as well as very small and superficial structures, to be examined. Still, the biggest advances in noninvasive vascular testing with duplex scanning result from the gradual acquisition of knowledge about the pathophysiology and natural history of vascular diseases.

REFERENCES

1. Bergamini TM: Indications and uses of the noninvasive vascular laboratory: extremity or visceral arterial evaluation. J Ky Med Assoc 89:220, 1991
2. Kempczinski RF, Thiele BL, Strandness DE Jr, Bandyk DF: Accreditation of vascular laboratories. J Vasc Surg 12:629, 1990
3. O'Keeffe ST, Persson AV: Use of noninvasive vascular laboratory in diagnosis of venous and arterial disease. Cardiol Clin 9:429, 1991
4. Ginsberg MD, Greenwood SA, Goldberg HI: Limitations of quantitative oculoplethysmography and of directional Doppler ultrasonography in cerebrovascular diagnosis: assessment of an air-filled OPG system. Stroke 12:27, 1981
5. Riles TS, Eikelboom BC, Pauliukas P et al: Ocular pneumoplethysmography (OPG-Gee) in noninvasive evaluation of carotid artery stenosis. Angiology 34:724, 1983
6. Ellis MR, Greenhalgh RM: Management of asymptomatic carotid bruit. J Vasc Surg 5:869, 1987
7. Langlois Y, Roederer GO, Chan A et al: Evaluating carotid artery disease. The concordance between pulsed Doppler/spectrum analysis and angiography. Ultrasound Med Biol 9:51, 1983
8. Kohler TR, Langlois Y, Roederer GO et al: Variability in measurement of specific parameters for carotid duplex examination. Ultrasound Med Biol 13:637, 1987
9. Taylor DC, Strandness DE Jr: Carotid artery duplex scanning. JCU 15:635, 1987
10. Moore WS, Ziomek S, Quiñones-Baldrich WJ et al: Can clinical evaluation and noninvasive testing substitute for arteriography in the evaluation of carotid artery disease? Ann Surg 208:91, 1988
11. Gelabert HA, Moore WS: Carotid endarterectomy without angiography. Surg Clin North Am 70:213, 1990
12. Dawson DL, Zierler RE, Strandness DE Jr et al: The role of duplex scanning and arteriography before carotid endarterectomy: a prospective study. J Vasc Surg [in press] 1993
13. Kohler TR, Nicholls SC, Zierler RE et al: Assessment of pressure gradient by Doppler ultrasound: experimental and clinical observations. J Vasc Surg 6:460, 1987
14. Satomura S: Study of flow patterns in peripheral arteries by ultrasonics. J Acoust Soc Jpn 15:151, 1959
15. Winsor T: Influence of arterial disease on the systolic blood gradients of the extremity. Am J Med Sci 220:117, 1950
16. Strandness DE Jr, Bell JW: Peripheral vascular disease: diagnosis and objective evaluation using a mercury strain gauge. Ann Surg, suppl. 161:51, 1965
17. Strandness DE Jr, McCutcheon EP, Rushmer RF: Application of a transcutaneous Doppler flowmeter in evaluation of occlusive arterial disease. Surg Gynecol Obstet 122:1039, 1966
18. Nippa JH, Hokanson DE, Lee DR et al: Phase rotation for separating forward and reverse blood velocity signals. IEEE Trans Sonics Ultrasonics SU-22:340, 1975
19. McLeod FD Jr: Progress report, directional Doppler blood flow meter. NRG 33-010-074, Cornell University, May 1969
20. Baker DW: Pulsed ultrasonic Doppler blood flow sensing. IEEE Trans Biomed Eng 17:170, 1970
21. Spencer MP, Brockenbrough EC, Davis DL, Reid JM: Cerebrovascular evaluation using Doppler continuous wave ultrasound. Ultrasound Med Biol 3:1291, 1977
22. Reilly LM, Lusby RJ, Hughes L et al: Carotid plaque histology using real-time ultrasonography. Clinical and therapeutic implications. Am J Surg 146:188, 1983
23. Hokanson DE, Mozersky DJ, Sumner DS, Strandness DE Jr: Ultrasonic arteriography: a new approach to arterial visualization. Biomed Eng 6:420, 1971
24. Mozersky DJ, Hokanson DE, Strandness DE Jr: Ultrasonic arteriography. Arch Surg 72:253, 1971
25. Barnes RW, Bone GE, Reinertson J et al: Noninvasive ultrasonic carotid angiography. Prospective validation by contrast arteriography. Surgery 80:328, 1976
26. Goldberg B, Ostrum BJ, Isard HJ: Ultrasonic aortography. JAMA 198:119, 1966
27. Leopold G: Ultrasonic abdominal aortography. Radiology 96:9, 1975
28. Kosoff G: Gray scale echography in obstetrics and gynecology. Report No. 60, Commonwealth Acoustic Laboratories, Sydney, Australia, 1973
29. Barber FE, Baker DW, Nation AWC et al: Ultrasonic duplex echo Doppler scanner. IEEE Trans Biomed Eng 21:109, 1974
30. Barber FE, Baker DW, Strandness DE Jr et al: Duplex scanner II for simultaneous imaging of artery tissues and flow. Ultrasonics Symp. Proc IEEE, 1974
31. Phillips DJ, Powers JE, Eyer MK et al: Detection of

peripheral artery disease using the duplex scanner III. Ultrasound Med Biol 6:205, 1980

32. Dion JE, Gates PC, Fox AJ et al: Clinical events following neuroangiography: a prospective study. Stroke 18:997, 1987

33. Earnest F, Forbes G, Sandok BA et al: Complications of cerebral angiography: prospective assessment of risk. AJR 142:247, 1984

34. Hankey GJ, Warlow CP, Molyneux AJ: Complications of cerebral angiography for patients with mild carotid territory ischaemia being considered for carotid endarterectomy. J Neurol Neurosurg Psychiatry 53:542, 1990

35. Mani RL, Eisenberg RL, McDonald EJ et al: Complications of catheter cerebral arteriography: analysis of 5000 procedures. I. Criteria and incidence. AJR 131:61, 1978

36. Mani RL, Eisenberg RL: Complications of catheter cerebral arteriography: analysis of 5000 procedures. II. Relation of complication rates to clinical and arteriographic diagnoses. AJR 131:867, 1978

37. Mani RL, Eisenberg RL: Complications of catheter cerebral arteriography: analysis of 5000 procedures. III. Assessment of arteries injected, contrast medium used, duration of procedure, and age of patient. AJR 131:871, 1978

38. Kartchner MM, MacRae LP: Noninvasive evaluation of the asymptomatic carotid bruit. Surgery 82:840, 1977

39. North American Symptomatic Carotid Endarterectomy Trial Collaborators: Beneficial effect of carotid endarterectomy in symptomatic patients with high-grade carotid stenosis. N Engl J Med 325:445, 1991

40. Zierler RE, Kohler TR, Strandness DE Jr: Duplex scanning of normal or minimally diseased carotid arteries: correlation with arteriography and clinical outcome. J Vasc Surg 12:447, 1990

41. Roederer GO, Langlois YE, Jäger KA et al: A simple spectral parameter for accurate classification of severe carotid disease. Bruit 8:174, 1984

42. O'Leary DH, Bryan FA, Goodison MW et al: Measurement variability of carotid atherosclerosis: real-time (B-mode) ultrasonography and angiography. Stroke 18:1011, 1987

43. Handa N, Matsumoto M, Maeda H et al: Ultrasonic evaluation of early carotid atherosclerosis. Stroke 21:1564, 1990

44. Persson J, Stavenow L, Wikstrand J et al: Noninvasive quantification of atherosclerotic lesions. Reproducibility of ultrasonographic measurment of arterial wall thickness and plaque size. Arterioscler Thromb 12:261, 1992

45. O'Leary DH, Polak JF, Wolfson SK Jr, et al: Use of sonography to evaluate carotid atherosclerosis in the elderly: The Cardiovascular Health Study. Stroke 22, 1155, 1991

46. Roederer GO, Langlois YE, Jäger KA et al: The natural history of carotid arterial disease in asymptomatic patients with cervical bruits. Stroke 15:605, 1984

47. Moneta GL, Taylor DC, Zierler RE et al: Asymptomatic high-grade internal carotid artery stenosis: is stratification according to risk factors or duplex spectral analysis possible? J Vasc Surg 10:475, 1989

48. Phillips DJ, Beach KW, Primozich J, Strandness DE Jr: Should results of ultrasound Doppler studies be reported in units of frequency or velocity? Ultrasound Med Biol 15:205, 1989

49. Reneman RS, Spencer MP: Local Doppler audio spectra in normal and stenotic carotid arteries in man. Ultrasound Med Biol 5:1, 1979

50. Cochran WT, Cooley JW, Favin DL et al: What is the fast Fourier transform? IEEE Trans Audio Electroacoust AU-15:45, 1967

51. Bornstein NM, Beloev ZG, Norris JW: The limitations of diagnosis of carotid occlusion by Doppler ultrasound. Ann Surg 207:315, 1988

52. Reneman RS, Clarke HF, Simmons N, Spencer MP: In vivo comparison of electromagnetic Doppler flowmeters with special attention to the processing of the analogue Doppler flow signal. Cardiovasc Res 7:557, 1973

53. Kremkau FW: Principles of color flow imaging. J Vasc Tech 15:104, 1991

54. Knox RA, Phillips DJ, Breslau PJ et al: Empirical findings relating sample volume size to diagnostic accuracy in pulsed Doppler cerebrovascular studies. JCU 10:227, 1982

55. Gutstein WH, Schneck DJ, Marks JO: In vitro studies of local blood flow disturbance in a region of separation. Atherosclerosis 8:381, 1968

56. Ku DN, Giddens DP, Phillips DJ, Strandness DE Jr: Hemodynamics of the normal human carotid bifurcation: in vitro and in vivo studies. Ultrasound Med Biol 11:13, 1985

57. Phillips DJ, Green FM, Langlois Y et al: Flow velocity patterns in the carotid bifurcation of young, presumed normal subjects. Ultrasound Med Biol 9:39, 1983

58. Zierler RE, Phillips DJ, Beach KW et al: Noninvasive assessment of normal carotid bifurcation hemodynamics with color-flow ultrsound imaging. Ultrasound Med Biol 13:471, 1987

59. Strandness DE Jr, Sumner DS: Hemodynamics for Surgeons. Grune & Stratton, Orlando, 1975

60. Strandness DE Jr, Schultz RD, Sumner DS: Ultrasonic flow detection: a useful technic in the evaluation of peripheral vascular disease. Am J Surg 113:311, 1967

61. Buerguer R, Hwang NHC: Critical arterial stenosis: a theoretical and experimental solution. Ann Surg 180:183, 1974

62. Smith HJ, Grottum P, Simonsen S: Ultrasonic assessment of abdominal venous return. I. Effect of cardiac action and respiration on mean velocity pattern, cross-sectional area and flow in the inferior vena cava and portal vein. Acta Radiol 26:581, 1985

63. Smith HJ, Grottum P, Simonsen S: Ultrasonic assessment of abdominal venous return. II. Volume blood flow in the inferior vena cava and portal vein. Acta Radiol 27:23, 1986

64. Van Bemmelen PS, Beach K, Bedford G, Strandness DE Jr: The mechanism of venous valve closure. Its relationship to the velocity of reverse flow. Arch Surg 125:617, 1990

65. Moneta GL, Bedford G, Beach K, Strandness DE Jr: Duplex ultrasound assessment of venous diameters, peak velocities, and flow patterns. J Vasc Surg 8:286, 1988

66. Heart Facts. American Heart Association, Dallas, 1983, p. 15

67. Dempsey RJ, Diana AL, Moore RW: Thickness of carotid artery atherosclerotic plaque and ischemic risk. Neurosurgery 27:343, 1990

68. Glagov S, Zarins C, Giddens DP, Ku DN: Hemodynamics and atherosclerosis. Insights and perspectives gained from studies of human arteries. Arch Pathol Lab Med 112:1018, 1988

69. Strandness DE Jr, Andros G, Baker JD, Bernstein EF: Vascular laboratory utilization and payment: report of the Ad Hoc Committee of the Western Vascular Society. J Vasc Surg 16:163, 1992

70. Ahn SS, Baker JD, Walden K, Moore WS: Which asymptomatic patients should undergo routine screening carotid duplex scan? Am J Surg 162:180, 1991

71. Ricotta JJ, Bryan FA, Bond MG et al: Multicenter validation study of real-time (B-mode) ultrasound, arteriography, and pathologic examination. J Vasc Surg 6:512, 1987

72. Baker JD, Rutherford RB, Bernstein EF et al: Suggested standards for reports dealing with cerebrovascular disease. Subcommittee on Reporting Standards for Cerebrovascular Disease, Ad Hoc Committee on Reporting Standards, Society for Vascular Surgery/North American Chapter, International Society for Cardiovascular Surgery J Vasc Surg 8:721, 1988

73. Edwards J, Krichell I, Riles T, Imparato A: Angiographically undetected ulceration of the carotid bifurcation as a cause of embolic stroke. Radiology 132:369, 1979

74. Fell G, Phillips DJ, Chikos PM et al: Ultrasonic duplex scanning for disease of the carotid artery. Circulation 64:1191, 1981

75. Zierler RE: Carotid artery evaluation by duplex scanning. Semin Vasc Surg 1:9, 1988

76. Nicholls SC, Phillips DJ, Primozich JF et al: Diagnostic significance of flow separation in the carotid bulb. Stroke 20:175, 1989

77. Moneta GL, Edwards JM, Chitwood RW et al: Correlation of North American Symptomatic Carotid Endarterectomy Trial (NASCET) angiographic definition of 70% to 99% internal carotid artery stenosis with duplex scanning. J Vasc Surg 17:152, 1993

78. Hayes AC, Johnston KW, Baker WH et al: The effect of contralateral disease on the carotid Doppler frequency. Surgery 103:19, 1988

79. Cato FR, Bandyk DF, Livigni D et al: Carotid collateral circulation decreases the diagnostic accuracy of duplex scanning. Bruit 10:68, 1986

80. Spadone DP, Barkmeier LD, Hodgson KJ et al: Con-

tralateral internal carotid artery stenosis or occlusion: pitfall of correct ipsilateral classification — a study performed with color-flow imaging. J Vasc Surg 11:642, 1990

81. Fujitani RM, Mills JL, Wang LM, Taylor SM: The effect of unilateral internal carotid arterial occlusion upon contralateral duplex study: criteria for accurate interpretation. J Vasc Surg 16:459, 1992

82. Maiuri F, Gallicchio B, Cinalli G: Diagnosis of carotid artery occlusion by duplex scanning. Neurol Res 12:75, 1990

83. Bluth EI, Kay D, Merritt CR et al: Sonographic characterization of carotid plaque: detection of hemorrhage. AJR 146:1061, 1986

84. Moore WS, Mohr JP, Najafi H et al: Carotid endarterectomy: practice guidelines. Report of the Society for Vascular Surgery and the North American Chapter of the International Society for Cardiovascular Surgery. J Vasc Surg 15:469, 1992

85. Dawson DL, Zierler RE, Kohler TR: Role of arteriography in the preoperative evaluation of carotid artery disease. Am J Surg 161:619, 1991

86. Bodily KC, Zierler RE, Marinelli MR et al: Flow disturbances following carotid endarterectomy. Surg Gynecol Obstet 151:77, 1980

87. Zierler RE, Bandyk DF, Thiele BL, Strandness DE Jr: Carotid artery stenosis following endarterectomy. Arch Surg 117:1408, 1982

88. Pignoli P, Tremoli E, Poli A et al: Intimal plus medial thickness of the arterial wall: a direct measurement with ultrsound imaging. Circulation 74:1399, 1986

89. Nicholls SC, Phillips DJ, Bergelin RO et al: Carotid endarterectomy. Relationship of outcome to early restenosis. J Vasc Surg 2:375, 1985

90. Bandyk DF, Kaebnick HW, Adams MB, Towne JB: Turbulence occurring after carotid bifurcation endarterectomy: a harbinger of residual and recurrent carotid stenosis. J Vasc Surg 7:261, 1988

91. Green RM, McNamara J, Ouriel K, DeWeese JA: The clinical course of residual carotid arterial disease. J Vasc Surg 13:112, 1991

92. Mattos MA, Shamma AR, Rossi N et al: Is duplex follow-up cost-effective in the first year after carotid endarterectomy? Am J Surg 156:91, 1988

93. Cook JM, Thompson BW, Barnes RW: Is routine duplex examination after carotid endarterectomy justified? J Vasc Surg 12:334, 1990

94. Jäger KA, Phillips DJ, Martin RL et al: Noninvasive mapping of lower limb arterial lesions. Ultrasound Med Biol 11:515, 1985

95. Bruins Slot HCK, Strijbosch L, Greep JM: Interobserver variability in single plane arteriography. Surgery 90:497, 1981

96. Edwards JM, Coldwell DM, Goldman ML, Strandness DE Jr: The role of duplex scanning in the selection of patients for transluminal angioplasty. J Vasc Surg 13:69, 1991

97. Dawson DL, Zierler RE, Strandness DE Jr: Duplex scan diagnosis of arterial injury from angioplasty:

unusual and specific findings. J Vasc Tech 15:260, 1991

98. Kinney EV, Bandyk DF, Mewissen MW et al: Monitoring functional patency of percutaneous transluminal angioplasty. Arch Surg 126:743, 1991

99. Caster JD, Cummings CA, Moneta GL et al: Accuracy of tibial artery duplex mapping (TADM). J Vasc Tech 16:63, 1992

100. Cossman DV, Ellison JE, Wagner WH et al: Comparison of contrast arteriography to arterial mapping with color-flow duplex imaging in the lower extremities. J Vasc Surg 10:522, 1989

101. Hatsukami TS, Primozich JF, Zierler RE et al: Color Doppler imaging of infrainguinal arterial occlusive disease. J Vasc Surg 16:527, 1992

102. Jäger KA, Ricketts HJ, Strandness DE Jr: Duplex scanning for the evaluation of lower limb arterial disease. p. 619. In Bernstein EF (ed): Noninvasive Techniques in Vascular Disease. 3rd Ed. C.V. Mosby, St. Louis, 1985

103. Kohler TR, Nance DR, Cramer MM et al: Duplex scanning for diagnosis of aortoiliac and femoropopliteal disease: a prospective study. Circulation 76:1074, 1987

104. Whittemore A, Clowes A, Couch N, Mannick J: Secondary femoropopliteal reconstruction. Ann Surg 193:35, 1981

105. Chang BB, Leopold PW, Kupinski AM et al: In situ bypass hemodynamics. The effect of residual A-V fistulae. J Cardiovasc Surg 30:843, 1989

106. Mitchell DC, Grasty MS, Stebbings WS et al: Comparison of duplex ultrasonography and venography in the diagnosis of deep venous thrombosis. Br J Surg 78:611, 1991

107. Helvie MA, Rubin JM, Silver TM, Kresowik TF: The distinction between femoral artery pseudoaneurysms and other causes of groin masses: value of duplex Doppler sonography. AJR 150:1177, 1988

108. Bandyk DF: Postoperative surveillance of infrainguinal bypass. Surg Clin North Am 70:71, 1990

109. Barnes RW, Thompson BW, MacDonald CM et al: Serial noninvasive studies do not herald postoperative failure of femoropopliteal or femorotibial bypass grafts. Ann Surg 210:486, 1989

110. Green RM, McNamara J, Ouriel K, DeWeese JA: Comparison of infrainguinal graft surveillance techniques. J Vasc Surg 11:207, 1990

111. Mills JL, Fujitani RM, Taylor SM: The characteristics and anatomic distribution of lesions that cause reversed vein graft failure: a five-year prospective study. J Vasc Surg 17:195, 1993

112. Bandyk DF, Seabrook GR, Moldenhauer P et al: Hemodynamics of vein graft stenosis. J Vasc Surg 8:688, 1988

113. Bandyk DF, Cato RF, Towne JB: A low flow velocity predicts failure of femoropopliteal and femorotibial bypass grafts. Surgery 98:799, 1985

114. Barry R, Pienaar C, Nel CJ: Accuracy of B-mode ultrasonography in detecting carotid plaque hemorrhage and ulceration. Ann Vasc Surg 4:466, 1990

115. Grigg MJ, Nicolaides AN, Wolfe JH: Detection and grading of femorodistal vein graft stenoses: duplex velocity measurements compared with angiography. J Vasc Surg 8:661, 1988

116. Bandyk DF, Schmitt DD, Seabrook GR et al: Monitoring functional patency of in situ saphenous vein bypasses: the impact of a surveillance protocol and elective revision. J Vasc Surg 9:286, 1989

117. Londrey GL, Hodgson KJ, Spadone DP et al: Initial experience with color-flow duplex scanning of infrainguinal bypass grafts. J Vasc Surg 12:284, 1990

118. Polak JF, Donaldson MC, Dobkin GR et al: Early detection of saphenous vein arterial bypass graft stenosis by color-assisted duplex sonography: a prospective study. AJR 154:857, 1990

119. Mattos MA, van Bemmelen PS, Hodgson KJ et al: Does correction of stenoses identified with color duplex scanning improve infrainguinal graft patency? J Vasc Surg 17:54, 1993

120. Idu MM, Blankenstein JD, de Gier P et al: Impact of a color-flow duplex surveillance program on infrainguinal vein graft patency: a five-year experience. J Vasc Surg 17:42, 1993

121. Gifford RW: Epidemiology and clinical manifestations of renovascular hypertension. p. 77. In Stanley JC, Ernst CB, Fry WJ (eds): Renovascular Hypertension. WB Saunders, Philadelphia, 1984

122. Wollenweber J, Sheps SG, David DG: Clinical course of atherosclerotic renovascular disease. Am J Cardiol 21:60, 1968

123. Schreiber MJ, Pohl MA, Novick AC: The natural history of atherosclerotic and fibrous renal artery disease. Urol Clin North Am 11:383, 1984

124. Guzman RP, Zierler RE, Isaacson JA et al: Progressive renal atrophy in hypertensive patients with > 60% renal artery diameter reduction: a prospective duplex evaluation. Circulation [in press] 1993

125. Dean RH, Englund R, Dupont WD: Retrieval of renal function by revascularization: study of preoperative outcome predictors. Ann Surg 202:367, 1985

126. Pickering TG: Diagnosis and evaluation of renovascular hypertension. Indications for therapy. Circulation 83(Suppl 2): I147, 1991

127. Hoffmann U, Edwards JM, Carter S et al: Role of duplex scanning for the detection of atherosclerotic renal artery disease. Kidney Int 39:1232, 1991

128. Strandness DE Jr: Duplex scanning in diagnosis of renovascular hypertension. Surg Clin North Am 70:109, 1990

129. Taylor DC, Moneta GL, Strandness DE Jr: Follow-up of renal artery stenosis by duplex ultrasound. J Vasc Surg 9:410, 1989

130. Sandager G, Flinn WR, McCarthy WJ et al: Assessment of visceral arterial reconstruction using duplex scan. J Vasc Tech 11:13, 1987

131. Eidt JF, Fry RE, Clagett GP et al: Postoperative follow-up of renal artery reconstruction with duplex ultrasound. J Vasc Surg 8:667, 1988

132. Reinitz ER, Goldman MH, Sais J et al: Evaluation of

transplant renal artery blood flow by Doppler sound-spectrum analysis. Arch Surg 118:415, 1983

133. Taylor KJW, Morse SS, Rigsby CM et al: Vascular complications in renal allografts: detection with duplex Doppler. Radiology 162:31, 1987

134. Strandness DE Jr: Duplex Scanning in Vascular Disorders. Raven Press, New York, 1990

135. Kohler TR, Zierler RE, Martin RL et al: Noninvasive diagnosis of renal artery stenosis by ultrasonic duplex scanning. J Vasc Surg 4:450, 1986

136. Taylor DC, Kettler MD, Moneta GL et al: Duplex ultrasound scanning in the diagnosis of renal artery stenosis: a prospective evaluation. J Vasc Surg 7:363, 1988

137. Handa N, Fukunaga R, Uehara A et al: Echo-Doppler velocimetry in the diagnosis of hypertensive patients: the renal artery Doppler technique. Ultrasound Med Biol 12:945, 1986

138. Handa N, Fukunaga R, Etani H et al: Efficacy of echo-Doppler examination for the evaluation of renovascular disease. Ultrasound Med Biol 14:1, 1987

139. Martin RL, Nanra RS, Wlodarczyk J et al: Renal hilar Doppler analysis in the detection of renal artery stenosis. J Vasc Tech 15:173,1991

140. Zierler RE, Isaacson JA, Strandness DE Jr: Noninvasive screening for renal artery stenosis: comparison of renal artery and renal hilar duplex scanning. Presented at the 10th Annual Meeting of the Pacific Northwest Vascular Society. Tacoma, WA, November 1992

141. Norris CS, Pfeiffer JS, Rittgers SE, Barnes RW: Noninvasive evaluation of renal artery stenosis and renovascular resistance. Experimental and clinical studies. J Vasc Surg 1:192, 1984

142. Neumeyer MM, Gifford RRM, Yang HC, Thiele BL: Applications of duplex ultrasound/color flow imaging for the evaluation of renal allografts. J Vasc Tech 15:156, 1992

143. Peterson L, Blackburn D, Astleford P et al: Duplex evaluation of renal transplant perfusion. J Vasc Tech 13:79, 1989

144. Sorrell K, Blacksher B, Fogle M: Diagnosis of occlusive renal vein thrombosis in renal allografts by duplex ultrasonography. J Vasc Tech 16:3, 1992

145. Buckley AR, Cooperberg PL, Reeve CE, Magil AB: The distinction between acute renal transplant rejection and cyclosporine nephrotoxicity: value of duplex sonography. AJR 149:521, 1987

146. Rigsby CM, Burns PN, Weltin GG et al: Doppler signal quantitation in renal allografts: comparison in normal and rejecting transplants, with pathologic correlation. Radiology 162:39, 1987

147. De Gaetano AM, Boldrini G, Nanni G et al: Noninvasive surveillance of allografted kidneys by ultrasonic duplex scanning. Angiology 40:705, 1989

148. Akiyama T, Ishii T, Nishioka T et al: Renal transplant blood flow evaluation by ultrasonic duplex scanning. Hinyokika Kiyo 34:1733, 1988

149. Genkins SM, San Filippo FD, Carroll BA: Duplex Doppler sonography of renal transplants: lack of sensi-tivity and specificity in establishing pathologic diagnosis. AJR 152:535, 1989

150. Rifkin DM, Needleman L, Pasto ME et al: Evaluation of renal transplant rejection by duplex Doppler examination: value of resistive index. AJR 148:759, 1987

151. Letourneau JG, Day DL, Frick MP et al: Ultrasound and computed tomographic evaluation in hepatic transplantation. Radiol Clin North Am 25:323, 1987

152. Taylor DC, Moneta GL, Cramer MM, Strandness DE Jr: Extrinsic compression of the celiac artery by the median arcuate ligament of the diaphragm: diagnosis by duplex ultrasound. J Vasc Tech 11:236, 1987

153. Rizzo RJ, Sandager G, Astleford P et al: Mesenteric flow velocity variations as a function of angle of insonation. J Vasc Surg 11:688, 1990

154. Moneta GL, Taylor DC, Helton WS et al: Duplex ultrasound measurement of postprandial intestinal blood flow: effect of meal composition. Gastroenterology 95:1294, 1988

155. Jäger K, Bollinger A, Valli C, Ammann R: Measurement of mesenteric blood flow by duplex scanning. J Vasc Surg 3:462, 1986

156. Nicholls SC, Kohler TR, Martin RL, Strandness DE Jr: Use of hemodynamic parameters in the diagnosis of mesenteric insufficiency. J Vasc Surg 3:507, 1986

157. Lilly MP, Harward TR, Flinn WR et al: Duplex ultrasound measurement of changes in mesenteric flow velocity with pharmacologic and physiologic alteration of intestinal blood flow in man. J Vasc Surg 9:18, 1989

158. Best IM, Pitzele A, Green A et al: Mesenteric blood flow in patients with diabetic neuropathy. J Vasc Surg 13:84, 1991

159. Moneta GL, Lee RW, Yeager RA et al: Mesenteric duplex scanning: a blinded prospective study. J Vasc Surg 17:79, 1993

160. LaBombard FE, Musson A, Bowersox JC, Zwolak RM: Hepatic artery duplex as an adjunct in the evaluation of chronic mesenteric ischemia. J Vasc Tech 16:7, 1992

161. Bolondi L, Mazziotti A, Arienti V et al: Ultrasonographic study of portal venous system in portal hypertension and after portosystemic shunt operation. Surgery 95:261, 1984

162. Henderson JM, Warren WD: Current status of the distal splenorenal shunt. Semin Liver Dis 3:251, 1983

163. Helton WS, Montana MA, Dwyer DC, Johansen K: Duplex sonography accurately assesses portacaval shunt patency. J Vasc Surg 8:657, 1988

164. Cranley JJ, Canos AJ, Sullivan WJ: The diagnosis of deep vein thrombosis. Arch Surg 111:34, 1976

165. Coon WW, Willis PW, Keller JB: Venous thromboembolism and other venous disease in the Tecumseh community health study. Circulation 48:839, 1973

166. Van Bemmelen PS, Bedford G, Beach K, Strandness DE Jr: Functional status of the deep venous system after an episode of deep venous thrombosis. Ann Vasc Surg 4:455, 1990

167. Barnes RW, Nix ML, Barnes CL et al: Perioperative

asymptomatic venous thrombosis: role of duplex scanning versus venography. J Vasc Surg 9:251, 1989
168. Wingo JP et al: Duplex evaluation of inferior vena caval patency: a prospective study of patients with the Greenfield filter. J Vasc Tech 9:167, 1987
169. Guglielmo FF, Kurtz AB, Wechsler RJ: Prospective comparison of computed tomography and duplex ultrasonography in the evaluation of recently inserted Kimray-Greenfield filters into the vena cava. Clin Imaging 14:216, 1990
170. Markel A, Goldman ML, Coldwell DM et al: Follow-up of percutaneously placed vena cava filters by duplex scanning. J Vasc Tech 162:74, 1992
171. Gooley NA, Sumner DS: Relationship of venous reflux to the site of venous valvular incompetence: implications for venous reconstructive surgery. J Vasc Surg 7:50, 1988
172. Van Bemmelen PS, Bedford G, Beach K, Strandness DE Jr: Quantitative segmental evaluation of venous valvular reflux with duplex ultrasound scanning. J Vasc Surg 10:425, 1989
173. Van Bemmelen PS, Bedford G, Strandness DE Jr: Visualization of calf veins by color flow imaging. Ultrasound Med Biol 16:15, 1990
174. Nix ML, Troilett RD: The use of color in venous duplex examination. J Vasc Tech 15:123, 1991
175. Talbot SR: Use of real-time imaging in identifying deep venous obstruction: a preliminary report. Bruit 6:41, 1982
176. Sullivan ED, Peter DJ, Cranley JJ: Real-time B-mode ultrasound. J Vasc Surg 1:465, 1984
177. Langsfeld M, Hershey FB, Thorpe L et al: Duplex B-mode imaging for the diagnosis of deep venous thrombosis. Arch Surg 122:587, 1987
178. Lensing AWA, Prandoni P, Brandjes D et al: Detection of deep vein thrombosis by real-time B-mode ultrasonography. N Engl J Med 320:342, 1989
179. Killewich LA, Bedford GR, Beach KW, Strandness DE Jr: Diagnosis of deep venous thrombosis. A prospective study comparing duplex scanning to contrast venography. Circulation 79:810, 1989
180. Cochlo JCU, Sigel B, Ryva RC et al: B-mode sonography of blood clots. JCU 10:323, 1982
181. Alanen A, Kormano M: Correlation of the echogenicity and structure of clotted blood. J Ultrasound Med 4:421, 1985

182. Raghavendra BN, Horii SC, Hilton S et al: Deep venous thrombosis: detection by probe compression of veins. J Ultrasound Med 5:89, 1986
183. Cronan JJ, Dorfman GS, Scola FH et al: Deep venous thrombosis: US assessment using vein compression. Radiology 162:191, 1987
184. Kerr TM, Smith JM, McKenna P et al: Venous and arterial anomalies of the lower extremities diagnosed by duplex scanning. Surg Gynecol Obstet 175:309, 1992
185. Karmody AM, Leather RP, Shah DM, Corson JD: The in situ saphenous vein arterial bypass: current problems and solutions. p. 561 In Bernhard VM, Towne JB (eds): Complications in Vascular Surgery. 2nd Ed. Grune & Stratton, Orlando, 1985
186. Shah DM, Chang BB, Leopold PW et al: The anatomy of the greater saphenous venous system. J Vasc Surg 3:273, 1986
187. Rutherford RB, Sawyer JD, Jones DN: The fate of residual saphenous vein after partial removal or ligation. J Vasc Surg 12:422, 1990
188. Ruoff BA, Cranley JJ, Hannan LA et al: Real-time duplex ultrasound mapping of the greater saphenous vein before in situ infrainguinal revascularization. J Vasc Surg 6:107, 1987
189. Bagi P, Schroeder T, Sillisen H, Lorentzen JE: Real-time B-mode mapping of the greater saphenous vein. Eur J Vasc Surg 3:103, 1989
190. Leather RP, Kupinski AM: Preoperative evaluation of the saphenous vein as a suitable graft. Semin Vasc Surg 1:51, 1988
191. Salles-Cunha SX, Andros G: Preoperative duplex scanning prior to infrainguinal revascularization. Surg Clin North Am 70:41, 1990
192. Magee TR, Leopold PW, Campbell WB: Vein marking through ultrasound coupling gel. Eur J Vasc Surg 4:491, 1990
193. Beach KW, Phillips DJ: Doppler instrumentation for the evaluation of arterial and venous disease. p. 11. In Jaffe CC (ed): Vascular and Doppler Ultrasound. Churchill Livingstone, New York, 1984
194. Rizzo RJ, Sandager G, Astleford P et al: Mesenteric flow velocity variations as a function of angle of insonation. J Vasc Surg 11:688, 1990

13

Angiographic Assessment in Peripheral Vascular Disease

Anne C. Roberts

John A. Kaufman

Stuart C. Geller

Peripheral vascular disease is a common problem that is becoming increasingly important as the population continues to age. Physicians treating patients with vascular disease need to be knowledgeable of the angiographic procedures their patients will undergo and to be familiar with the angiographic appearance of the various vascular diseases. A properly performed angiographic procedure will provide the information required to determine appropriate surgical or percutaneous therapy. In addition, the outcome of various therapies may be assessed with angiographic studies. As with any complex diagnostic procedure, careful technique is essential to optimal results.

PREANGIOGRAPHIC EVALUATION

Angiography is an invasive procedure associated with some risk to the patient. Before an angiogram is performed, the patient should be evaluated with the appropriate noninvasive studies. The patient should be evaluated for factors that increase the risk of the procedure, such as evidence of renal insufficiency, allergies, and severe cardiac disease. To maximize the informa-

tion obtained and minimize any risk to the patient, an evaluation is done to determine the proper study and study approach. This allows a tailored approach to each patient. Adherence to guidelines for the performance of diagnostic angiography will ensure optimal examination and enhance the safety of angiographic studies.[1]

The vascular or interventional radiologist is an integral member of a team caring for patients with peripheral vascular disease. The vascular radiologist should act as a consultant in the evaluation of a patient and in the determination of what, if any procedure, is most appropriate for a given patient. The angiographer must be familiar with the patient's clinical history and physical examination findings and be informed of the results of any noninvasive tests that have been performed. The clinical history obtained usually focuses on vascular risk factors, a list of current medications, and cardiovascular symptoms. The duration and extent of symptoms related to the patient's peripheral vascular disease should be assessed. Aspects of the patient's clinical history that influence the performance of angiography include a history of allergies, particularly to contrast medium; cardiac disease, such as a recent myocardial infarction, congestive heart failure, or hypertension;

renal dysfunction; dehydration; diabetes; advanced age; previous operations, particularly any peripheral vascular surgery or transcatheter intervention; and a history of infectious processes, such as hepatitis or human immunodeficiency virus (HIV) infection.

The patient is examined, including a general assessment to exclude significant concurrent illnesses. A complete pulse examination should be performed and the anticipated puncture site(s) evaluated. If an axillary approach is contemplated, the axillary, brachial, upper-extremity, and carotid pulses are evaluated and blood pressure obtained in each arm. In evaluating the lower extremities, at a minimum, ankle/brachial indices are obtained. Segmental pressure measurements or pulse volume recordings may be helpful in defining the level of disease and in planning the angiographic approach.

Laboratory evaluation includes measurement of renal function (BUN and creatinine), hematocrit, and bleeding parameter, for the patient on anticoagulation therapy or in whom these values may be abnormal. Electrolyte concentrations are checked if there is some reason to suspect that they may be abnormal.

The angiographic procedure and any possible percutaneous therapeutic options are explained to the patient. There should be a frank discussion of possible complications, including hematoma, allergic reactions, and damage to arteries, such as dissection, thrombosis, or embolism. The alternatives and benefits of the procedure are discussed and documented. Informing the patient about the anticipated sequence of events will help allay fears regarding the procedure. Education, instructions, suggestions, and encouragement are useful in decreasing patient anxiety.[2] Appropriate patient preparation for angiography includes adequate hydration to minimize the nephrotoxic effects of contrast. Premedication should include sedatives and narcotics.[3,4] Other premedications are tailored to the specific medical condition of the patient.[5,6]

BASIC CATHETERIZATION TECHNIQUES

The basic approach for all angiographic procedures involves the Seldinger technique. This technique consists of puncturing an arterial wall with a needle and placing a guidewire through the needle to obtain access into the arterial system; after the needle is removed, a catheter is placed over the guidewire and manipulated into position for the appropriate study.

Transfemoral Approach

The transfemoral approach to catheterization is the one used most commonly. With this approach, it is possible to obtain diagnostic information on any segment of the arterial tree. Contraindications to this approach include severe atherosclerotic disease, specifically occlusion, of the aorta, iliacs vessels, or common femoral artery, precluding catheterization. Groin infections, recent surgery, and femoral artery aneurysms are other contraindications. Careful localization of the puncture site is essential. Ideally, the common femoral artery is punctured over the femoral head.

In the vast majority of patients, the common femoral artery runs over the medial third of the femoral head. Particularly in obese patients, the inguinal crease may have descended considerably lower than the common femoral artery.[7] In these patients, often it is necessary to make the skin incision substantially higher than the inguinal crease. Fluoroscopic localization of the femoral head avoids low punctures, which may lead to inadvertent catheterization of either the superficial or the deep femoral artery. Puncturing the artery above the inguinal ligament may lead to a difficult compression and to retroperitoneal hematoma.[8,9] With a low puncture, the femoral head is not available to support the arterial compression, and pseudoaneurysm formation may develop.[9,10] Puncturing the profunda femoral artery also increases the risk of arteriovenous fistulae.[11]

Antegrade puncture of the common femoral artery is indicated for diagnostic studies of the lower extremity, as well as for interventional procedures, such as angioplasty and embolization. As with retrograde femoral catheterization, the puncture site must be below the inguinal ligament, to avoid retroperitoneal hematoma. However, the entrance site should be relatively high in the common femoral artery to allow room to negotiate into the superficial femoral artery.

Transaxillary Approach

The usual axillary artery approach is, in fact, a high brachial artery puncture. The location for the puncture is just distal to the lateral axillary fold. At this location, the artery is usually quite easy to palpate, slightly more removed from the brachial plexus, and relatively easy to compress against the humerus.

For peripheral vascular studies, the left axillary artery is preferred. This approach avoids manipulation across the origins of the great vessels. If the ascending aorta is to be studied or if the left-sided approach is unavailable, the right axillary approach is used. The primary indication for an axillary approach is lack of femoral access. The greater morbidity of this approach precludes its use on a routine basis. However, brachial arteriography with puncture of the artery at the antecubital fossa has been used for routine diagnostic angiography, especially for outpatient studies. Wider acceptance of this approach has been facilitated by the availability of smaller and safer catheter systems.[12,13]

Contraindications to this approach include a decreased brachial artery blood pressure, absent pulses, the presence of a supraclavicular bruit, or infection in the region of the puncture site. Relative contraindications include a bleeding diathesis, uncontrolled hypertension, and subclavian artery bypass grafts.

Translumbar Approach

Although the translumbar approach was one of the original routes of access to the vascular system, it has largely been abandoned in favor of the femoral and axillary approaches, which permit greater flexibility for catheterization and percutaneous therapy. The translumbar approach is still used when no other access is available and if intravenous digital subtraction angiography (IV-DSA) does not give adequate delineation of the vascular anatomy.

Contraindications to the translumbar approach include severe hypertension, a bleeding diathesis, abdominal aortic aneurysm, aortic dissection, or an aortic graft in the region of the puncture. Patients who have difficulty lying prone for several hours because of respiratory difficulties, cardiac problems, or obesity are not good candidates for this procedure. Puncture of the aorta in obese patients is also difficult because of the length of the needle needed to reach the aorta.

INTRAPROCEDURAL ASPECTS OF CARE

Patient Monitoring

All patients should be monitored during a procedure with continuous electrocardiography (ECG), intermittent blood pressure, and pulse oximetry. Pulse oximetry is mandatory for the patient receiving sedation; in such cases, appropriately trained personnel should be available to monitor the patient. Documentation of intraprocedural care, including frequent vital signs (heart rate, blood pressure, and oxygen saturation); of drugs administered; and of any complications and ap-

propriate actions taken in response to these complications is essential.

All equipment needed to support the patient should be available. There should be ready access to such emergency drugs as atropine, epinephrine, lidocaine, naloxone (Narcan), and Benadryl. Oxygen, suction equipment, and a defibrillator should be available. An emergency cart with instruments and medication for resuscitation should be immediately available.

Contrast Administration

Certain basic considerations apply when administering intravascular contrast material; both the appropriately trained medical personnel, and emergency medical equipment and medication required to treat any adverse reactions should be readily available. All patients referred for contrast examination should be appropriately screened for the presence of risk factors that might increase the likelihood of adverse reactions. If significant risk factors are present, alternative diagnostic procedures should be considered. All patients should be adequately hydrated and appropriate premedication given, when indicated.

A decision must be made about the type of contrast material to be used. Two categories of contrast material are currently available: higher osmolality contrast agents (HOCA) and lower osmolality contrast agents (LOCA).

HOCA have been used for many years and are considered both safe and effective. Some discomfort and risk are associated with their use. Some evidence suggests that pretreatment with steroids (a two-dose steroid pretreatment regimen) before the administration of HOCA may decrease contrast reactions.[14]

LOCA have a lower rate of severe adverse reactions and are associated with less, but not complete absence of, discomfort. Some institutions have switched to LOCA for all patients; others have adopted selective use of LOCA. The following guidelines have been recommended for selective use of LOCA[15]:

1. Patients with a history of a previous adverse reaction to contrast material, with the exception of a sensation of warmth, flushing, or a single episode of nausea or vomiting
2. Patients with a history of asthma or allergy
3. Patients with known cardiac dysfunction, including recent or potentially imminent cardiac decompensation, severe arrhythmias, unstable angina pectoris, recent myocardial infarction, and pulmonary hypertension
4. Patients with generalized severe debilitation
5. Patients in whom there is a specific indication for the use of LOCA—for example, sickle cell disease, those at risk of

aspiration, those who are very anxious about the procedure, those in whom risk factors cannot be ascertained because communication cannot be established, and those who request LOCA

ANGIOGRAPHIC FILMING

All peripheral vascular procedures require recording of the findings. Several different modalities can be used for acquiring images. An angiographic facility should have a high-resolution imaging intensifier, television chain, and standard arteriographic filming capabilities. The standard imaging technique is cut film, which requires a mechanical rapid film changer capable of obtaining rapid serial images of at least 14 inches in diameter.[16] Power injectors, capable of delivering large volumes of contrast over precise time intervals, are also required.

Several techniques can be used; a thorough evaluation requires visualization of the entire vasculature in the area of interest. Patients with vascular disease may have slow filling of the extremity arteries; serial filming, often with prolonged delays, is necessary to avoid errors in diagnosis. Single-film or "one-shot" arteriograms, limited field-of-view image intensifiers, and manual injections of small volumes of contrast are not suitable for diagnostic purposes. Permanent recording of the angiographic study should be of high quality. Cineradiographic or video recordings are generally suboptimal for diagnostic purposes. Biplanar imaging is optimal for evaluation of the aorta and is frequently of value in the pelvis. At a minimum, multiple oblique views are necessary for complete scrutiny of complex vascular structures. Single-plane straight anteroposterior filming will often miss significant lesions. Tortuous arteries and vascular bifurcations are areas requiring careful and complete visualization. Multiple views are more readily achieved with less contrast volumes since the advent of digital subtraction angiography (DSA).

DSA has proved a valuable adjunct to angiographic procedures. This technique permits digitization of a fluoroscopic image and computer manipulation of the data. A "mask" image without contrast is subtracted from images containing contrast to remove background structures, thus enhancing the structures containing contrast. DSA permits detection of a significantly lower concentration of contrast material than is possible with cut-film techniques. Improved imaging chains have allowed for increased resolution when using DSA technique. Large image intensifiers are now available (14 to 16 inches), for extended anatomic coverage. Newer machines have a 1024×1024 image matrix, with filming rates of up to 30 frames per second. As manufacturers continue to refine the technology, it is likely that eventually digital systems will totally replace film-screen arteriography; indeed, this is occurring to a significant degree in Europe. Unfortunately, DSA is very sensitive to motion artifact, limiting its usefulness in the abdomen and chest and requiring patient cooperation in lower-extremity studies.

Although intravenous DSA was once promoted as a replacement for conventional angiography, it has not found an extensive role and remains a technique of limited clinical value. IV-DSA requires administration of a significant volume of contrast material and bolus transmission of the contrast through the circulation. Venous DSA generally requires a central venous contrast injection (superior vena cava or right atrium). Thus, patients with congestive heart failure, poor cardiac output, or poor renal function are not good candidates for this technique. Motion artifact is particularly troubling with IV-DSA; these studies should be attempted only for patients who can cooperate during the examination. Decreased contrast concentration produces significantly degraded resolution. The primary indication for this technique is to document severe aortic disease occlusion in patients with poor arterial access (Fig. 13-1).

Intra-arterial DSA has several advantages. A smaller amount of contrast material is used, which is beneficial in patients with renal dysfunction or cardiac dysfunction, or both. The image quality is significantly better than with IV-DSA. Motion artifact is still a problem but is not as serious as with IV-DSA. In patients with renal disease or with an allergy to contrast material, intra-arterial DSA in conjunction with the administration of intra-arterial CO_2 may provide adequate evaluation of the peripheral vascular system (Fig. 13-2). Carbon dioxide is absorbed and excreted within minutes. It should not be used in the region of the great vessels, as it may affect the respiratory center of,[17] but it has no known side effects in the periphery.

PHARMACOLOGIC ADJUNCTS

Pharmacologic agents that have been used in the vascular system are usually divided into vasoconstricting and vasodilating agents. In the peripheral vascular bed, the vasodilating agents are used most commonly.

The vasoconstricting agents include epinephrine and angiotensin. Both drugs cause vasoconstriction of normal blood vessels but do not affect tumor vascularity, improving visualization of these abnormal arteries. Epinephrine is used most often in the visceral and renal arteries. Angiotensin is used occasionally in the pelvic

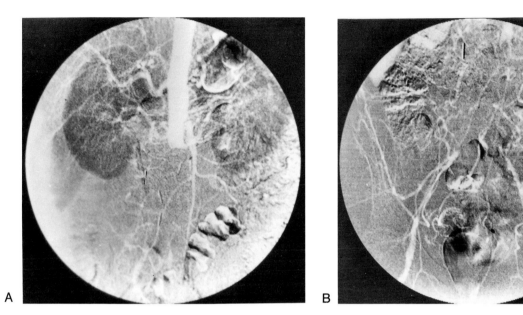

Figure 13-1 **(A)** Intravenous digital subtraction angiogram (DSA) demonstrating complete occlusion of the abdominal aorta below the level of the renal arteries. Resolution is significantly less than with intra-arterial digital or standard arteriography but permits documentation of the site of occlusion. **(B)** Intravenous DSA of the pelvic vessels demonstrates reconstitution of the iliac arteries at the common iliac bifurcations. In this patient, intravenous DSA was sufficient to allow operative planning.

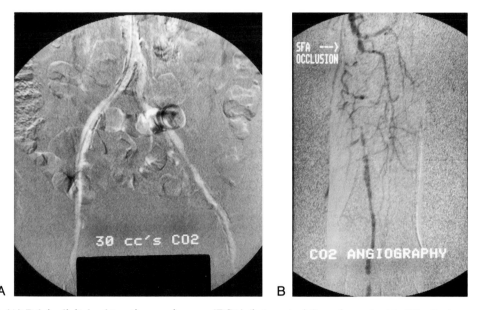

Figure 13-2 **(A)** Pelvic digital subtraction angiogram (DSA) (intra-arterial) performed with CO_2. Patient with severe renal insufficiency. CO_2 was used to avoid the risk of further deterioration of renal function. **(B)** DSA at the level of the lower femur documenting superficial femoral artery occlusion. Note reconstitution of the distal popliteal artery. Breakup of the contrast of the gaseous contrast material can lead, however, to artifacts that may simulate occlusion.

and extremity arteries for evaluation of hypovascular tumors.

Vasodilating drugs include priscoline (Tolazoline), nitroglycerin, nifedipine, papaverine, and reserpine. Vasodilating drugs are used to relieve spasm in arteries, increase blood flow in the extremities to enhance visualization of the distal arteries, and to assess possible reversibility of spasm in vasospastic diseases.

Priscoline (Tolazoline) is frequently used as a vasodilating drug in the peripheral vascular system. It acts directly on the vascular smooth muscle to produce a vasodilating effect. An injection of 10 to 25 mg of priscoline immediately before contrast injection in the extremities will increase visualization of the distal vasculature. It is also used as a provocative test to assess the hemodynamic significance of arterial stenoses. Nitroglycerin also acts on the arterial smooth muscle to produce its vasodilating effects. This short-acting agent is particularly useful in treating catheter-induced spasm. It has a less profound systemic effect than priscoline and, due to its brief half-life, can be used repeatedly. Doses range from 100 to 300 μg. Nitroglycerin can also be used to produce peripheral vasodilatation for improved opacification of arterial structures and to provoke a hemodynamic gradient during intra-arterial pressure measurements. Its relative lack of significant side effects has led to its increased utilization as the preferred vasodilating agent during arteriography. Nifedipine and other calcium channel blockers can be used to cause peripheral vasodilatation and to treat patients with peripheral vasospastic disease. Papaverine is a smooth muscle relaxant used to treat vasospastic disorders or spasm associated with trauma or surgical manipulation. Reserpine produces sustained peripheral vasodilatation and has been used to evaluate and treat peripheral vasospastic disease; however, it is no longer available.

Other pharmacologic agents used in peripheral studies include lidocaine and heparin. Lidocaine can be mixed with ionic contrast material to decrease the discomfort of the injection.[18,19] Heparin is usually placed in the flush solution, but some investigators advocate routine administration of heparin during the procedure.[20-22]

PRESSURE MEASUREMENTS AND HEMODYNAMICS

The hemodynamics of the arterial system are very important in evaluating atherosclerotic disease as well as the results of bypass grafts or angioplasty therapy.

Noninvasive examinations can be performed for a baseline assessment and to assess the patient's response to therapy. A complete discussion of noninvasive techniques can be found in Ch. 11.

Direct intra-arterial hemodynamics are of vital importance in determining the significance of a stenosis and in evaluating the results of transcatheter therapy. A pressure gradient is an important indicator of the hemodynamic significance of a lesion. A resting peak systolic pressure gradient greater than 10 to 15 mmHg systolic is considered significant. If the gradient is less than 10 to 15 mmHg, a provocative maneuver may be employed. Ischemic hyperemia or administration of a vasodilator, such as nitroglycerin or priscoline, may be used to simulate exercise and determine the severity of the stenosis.

Several methods are available to determine intra-arterial hemodynamics. The easiest method is to place a catheter beyond the stenosis, obtaining a pressure measurement above the stenosis, and then pulling the catheter back, obtaining a second measurement on the downstream side of the stenosis. A straight end hole catheter is used to obtain these pressure measurements.

If a second catheter is in place (i.e., in both femoral arteries), one catheter can be placed in the aorta and the other distal to the obstructing lesion, to obtain simultaneous pressure measurements. This technique is particularly helpful if a vasodilator is being used, as the latter may decrease the aortic pressure, which could produce a factitious pressure gradient without simultaneous measurement of the aortic pressure.

The pressures obtained can be recorded on a recorder as a waveform (Fig. 13-3). Systolic, diastolic, and mean pressure measurements also should be recorded and maintained as part of the permanent record. Intra-arterial pressure measurements should be obtained whenever the hemodynamic significance of a lesion is in question. It is of particular value in the iliac arteries, where pressure can be readily measured as a routine part of a peripheral vascular examination.

ANGIOGRAPHIC TECHNIQUE

A variety of disease processes can affect the extremities. These include atherosclerotic disease, thromboembolic disease, trauma, vasculitides, arteriovenous malformations, tumors, and compression syndromes. A complete angiographic study must be obtained to establish the proper diagnosis and effect proper therapy.

An adequate study for the evaluation of the extremi-

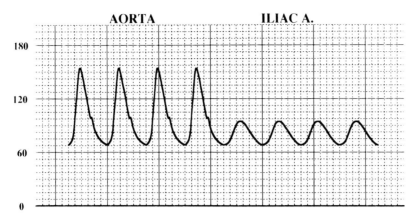

Figure 13-3 Intra-arterial pressure measurements during catheter withdrawal from the aorta to the iliac artery across an area of stenosis (after intra-arterial nitroglycerine). Drop-in pressure was 155 mm systolic to 95 mm. As an alternative to "pullback" pressures, two catheters, one positioned above and one below the stenosis, can be used.

ties will call into play many of the elements that have been discussed earlier. The proper preparation of the patient; appropriate monitoring; the correct selection of approach, equipment, drugs, and contrast agent — all are important for obtaining a complete study in a safe and expeditious manner.

The extremities can be accessed by a transfemoral, transaxillary, or translumbar approach. The transfemoral approach is the approach of choice. In most cases, the groin with the best femoral pulse is used for the puncture. Catheterizing the patient's least symptomatic side is preferable, to allow full evaluation of the symptomatic side. Catheterizing the diseased artery may lead to further compromise, necessitating urgent intervention, before a full diagnostic study is complete. If an intervention is to be performed, the lesion may be approached from either an antegrade or a retrograde approach.

If a single extremity is to be examined, a contralateral approach is preferred, as this allows antegrade injection of contrast agent and better opacification. It also leaves the groin of the abnormal leg untouched, providing full access if surgery or intervention is needed.

Most patients undergo lower-extremity angiography for atherosclerotic peripheral vascular disease. A study of the lower extremities would generally includes an abdominal aortogram, a runoff examination, and bilateral oblique pelvic angiograms, for a comprehensive survey of the major vessels that may require surgical or transcatheter therapy. Studies must be individualized for each patient undergoing a procedure, with further oblique views and intra-arterial pressure measurements as necessary.

ATHEROSCLEROTIC DISEASE

Occlusive Atherosclerotic Disease

Atherosclerosis is a disease affecting the intima of the major arteries that leads to narrowing of the lumen by plaque and superimposed thrombus. The arterial bifurcations are frequently involved, a propensity believed to result from hydrostatic and shear forces arising from turbulent flow.[23] Some of the resulting lesions are simple narrowings, but many are more complicated lesions. Complicated lesions are irregular in appearance, frequently representing ulcerated plaques, and may be associated with thrombus, subintimal hemorrhage, and calcification.

Atherosclerotic disease affects primarily older patients, particularly men over the age of 50 years and postmenopausal women. Predisposing factors include smoking, hyperlipidemia, hypercholesteremia, diabetes, hypertension, obesity, family history, and genetic factors.

Intermittent claudication is the most common symptom. Patients describe an aching sensation, fatigue, cramping, or pain in their legs associated with walking. Usually, the most distal muscle groups are affected first, followed by the more proximal ones. Other symptoms include impotency, paresthesias, and limb weakness. Because the disease is slowly progressive, collateral channels have time to develop, explaining why many patients with considerable disease have only mild symptoms. Acute exacerbation of symptoms is commonly caused by occlusion of a pre-existing stenosis. Claudication is associated with progression to more severe symptoms in a minority of patients (25 to 30 percent).[24]

The differential diagnosis for claudication includes a number of diseases: arterial dissection, emboli, adventitial cystic disease of popliteal artery, metabolic diseases such as gout, neurologic disorders such as amyotrophic lateral sclerosis (ALS), or multiple sclerosis; popliteal entrapment syndrome, and vasospastic disorders.

Critical ischemia characterized by rest pain, ulceration, necrosis, and gangrene requires a very different therapeutic approach. Ischemic symptoms are a harbinger of impending or coexisting tissue loss, requiring prompt intervention to reverse or stabilize the ischemic state. Ischemic neuropathy can develop as a sequela of long-standing severe ischemia. This is characterized by a sensation of numbness or burning, disuse atrophy,

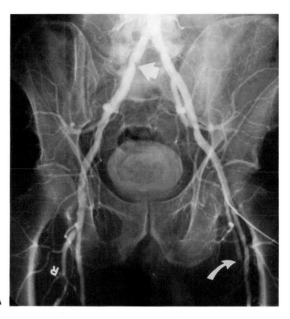

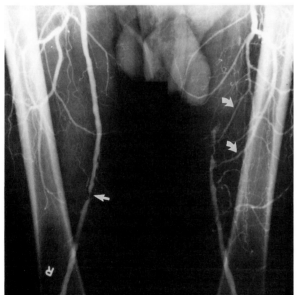

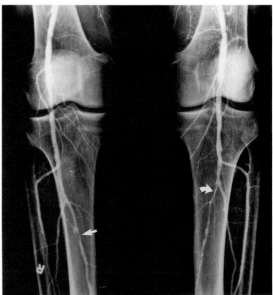

Figure 13-4 Typical atherosclerotic peripheral vascular disease in an elderly male smoker with bilateral claudication. **(A)** Pelvic angiogram demonstrating a mild right common iliac stenosis *(straight arrow)* and left superficial femoral artery (SFA) occlusion *(curved arrow)*. **(B)** Distal right SFA disease with a focal stenosis *(straight arrow)*. The left SFA is reconstituted by profunda femoris artery (PFA) collaterals in the mid-thigh *(curved arrows)*. **(C)** Intact distal runoff with a focal proximal stenosis in the right posterior tibial artery *(straight arrow)*, and diffuse narrowing of the left posterior tibial artery *(curved arrow)*.

loss of muscle mass, and reflex sympathetic dystrophy.[25]

The angiographic appearance of occlusive disease includes narrowing of the arteries, particularly in areas of bifurcation and in regions in which the arteries undergo mechanical stress (Fig. 13-4). Such regions include the adductor canal, the popliteal space, and the hiatus of the interosseous membrane. Mural plaques, ulcerated plaques, or complete occlusions may be present. Occlusions result from the slowing of blood flow to such a degree that thrombosis occurs. The thrombosis then extends to the level of the most proximal and distal collaterals. Collaterals can develop in response to the obstruction because the slow progression of atherosclerotic disease allows sufficient time for collaterals to form. The pattern of atherosclerotic disease may be diffuse or focal.

A specific subset of atherosclerotic disease is known as "atherosclerotic coarctation,"[26] or the small aorta syndrome[27] (Fig. 13-5). The syndrome occurs in women, typically those with a small frame and a long history of cigarette smoking. The arteriographic findings are of a discrete stenosis of the distal abdominal aorta. The distal vessels are small and usually without significant stenosis.

An arteriographic examination should define the location and extent of the arteriosclerotic disease. Evaluation usually includes the infrarenal aorta, the iliac arteries, and the lower-extremity runoff from the groin to the forefoot. Oblique views may be necessary to evaluate the origins of the iliac vessels and of the superficial and deep femoral arteries. In some cases demonstrating poor distal runoff, pharmacologic or ischemic hyperemia may be necessary to increase the opacification of the distal vessels. Opacification of the tibial and pedal vessels is particularly important in patients with severe occlusive disease that may require distal bypass. Pressure measurements are useful to determine the significance of stenoses.

Atherosclerotic disease is less of a problem in the upper extremities, although these arteries can be involved. Symptoms of intermittent claudication can occur in the upper extremity when the arteries are stenotic or occluded. The subclavian artery is involved more commonly than the distal vessels. If the proximal subclavian is involved, a subclavian steal syndrome can occur (Fig. 13-6). This syndrome results from reversal of flow in the vertebral artery, as it supplies collateral flow in the subclavian artery distal to the occlusion. The change in flow dynamics may lead to symptoms of vertebrobasilar insufficiency, including vertigo, syncope, and paresthesias.

Dissection

Dissections are usually associated with atherosclerotic disease, the diseased intima acting as the substrate for the dissection. Other pathologic processes predisposing to dissection include fibromuscular dysplasia or cystic medial necrosis. Systemic hypertension is an important etiologic factor. The dissection plane usually occurs within the media proper or between the media and external elastic layers of the arterial wall. Medium to small muscular arteries are frequently affected by dissection, with the site of dissection close to the arterial origin from the aorta. Isolated dissection of the abdominal aorta or iliac arteries is rare.[28-30] Dissection involving these major arteries is more commonly the result of the abdominal extension of a type III thoracic aortic dissection (Fig. 13-7). Dissection can be secondary to trauma, usually iatrogenic from catheter manipulation, angioplasty, or endarterectomy,[28] or it can occur as a result of blunt or penetrating trauma.[31]

The usual angiographic appearance is one of an intimal flap—a linear radiolucency in the opacified lumen, with contrast material on either side of the flap. The arterial lumen may be compressed by the false channel, or the intimal flap may occlude the lumen. Angiographic evaluation defines the location and extent of the dissection. Evaluation of the inflow and outflow is performed to guide surgical therapy.

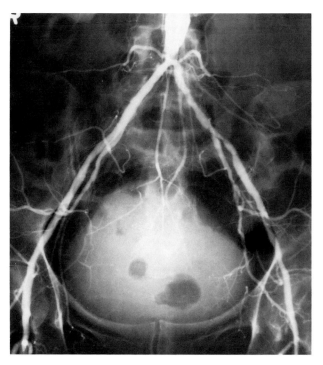

Figure 13-5 "Small aorta" syndrome. Small distal aorta with superimposed atherosclerosis in a middle-aged diabetic woman.

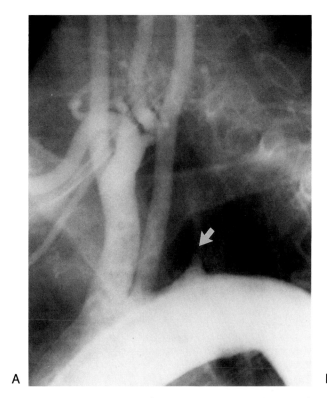
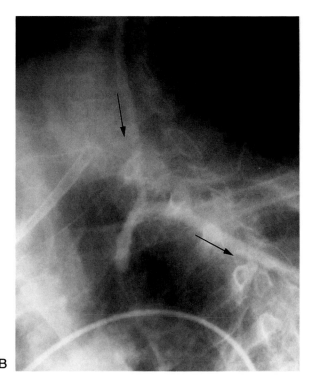

A   B

Figure 13-6 Subclavian steal syndrome. **(A)** Early film from an aortic arch injection demonstrating atherosclerotic occlusion of the left subclavian artery and normal left carotid and inominate arteries. **(B)** Retrograde
flow down the left vertebral reconstituting the left subclavian artery *(arrows)* on a late film from the same
injection.

Aneurysms

An aneurysm is defined as a permanent localized
(i.e., focal) dilatation of an artery with at least a 50
percent increase in diameter as compared with the expected normal diameter of the artery.[32] Among the
numerous causes of aneurysms, the most common in
the Western world is atherosclerosis. Other causes include congenital or developmental aneurysms; mechanically induced aneurysms, such as poststenotic
dilatation, and aneurysms associated with arteriovenous fistulae; traumatic aneurysms from either blunt
or penetrating trauma; inflammatory (noninfectious)
aneurysms; infectious aneurysms; and anastomotic
pseudoaneurysms.

Congenital or developmental aneurysms arise from
defects in the arterial wall.[33] Commonly these are due
to a generalized disorder of arterial tissue, such as a
connective tissue disorder with associated cystic medial
necrosis. Cystic medial necrosis involves degeneration
of medial elastic fibers with replacement by collagen
and mucoid material.[34] This entity is most commonly
seen in Marfan and Ehlers-Danlos syndromes, both
manifesting typical arterial lesions and the pathologic

changes distinctive of cystic medial necrosis.[35] A focal
defect of the arterial wall unassociated with vessel wall
degeneration has been reported.[35] Such rare defects
have been found in conjunction with intracranial berry
aneurysms.[36] The absence or poor development of the
tunica media results in the aneurysm formation.

Traumatic aneurysms are usually false aneurysms.
The wall of a false aneurysm or pseudoaneurysm does
not contain all three layers that make up an arterial
wall. Most false aneurysms have a wall formed only by
adventitia and perivascular tissue. Traumatic aneurysms commonly involve the thoracic aorta and are a
result of a deceleration injury, but penetrating trauma
can lead to pseudoaneurysm formation as well.

Inflammatory noninfectious processes may result in
aneurysm formation. Chronic inflammation with destruction of elastic fibers, vessel wall necrosis, and fibrosis is found with these aneurysms.[36] Such aneurysms are seen in a variety of disorders, including
Takayasu's disease, Behçet's disease,[37] Kawasaki disease, polyarteritis, ankylosing spondylitis, relapsing
polychondritis, and periarterial inflammatory disease,
such as pancreatitis. Polyarteritis nodosa has been associated with multiple aneurysms throughout the arte-

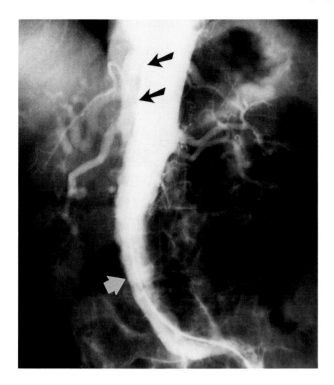

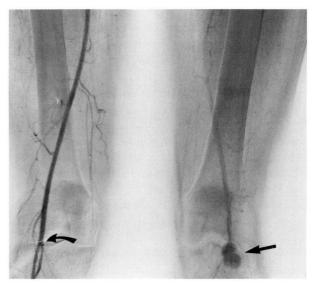

Figure 13-8 Mycotic aneurysm. Mycotic aneurysm in the left popliteal artery in a patient with postpartum sepsis *(straight arrow)*. An anomalous high origin of the anterior tibial artery is present *(curved arrow)*.

Figure 13-7 Aortic dissection occluding the right common iliac artery. Abdominal aortagram from the left femoral approach demonstrating a dissection flap *(black arrows)* in the upper abdominal aorta that occludes the right common iliac artery origin *(white arrow)*. Note that the right and left renal arteries fill from different lumens.

rial system, most commonly in the renal and visceral vessels.[36] Giant cell arteritis has mixed cellular infiltrates with giant cells and destruction of the normal wall architecture.[35,36] Kawasaki disease usually involves the coronary arteries but has also been described in the axillobrachial and iliofemoral vessels.[35]

A variety of infectious agents, including bacterial, fungal, and spirochetal, can cause mycotic aneurysms. These aneurysms result from the destruction of the arterial wall by hematogenous seeding of microbes into the artery (Fig. 13-8). This seeding occurs as a consequence of a systemic infection, such as endocarditis or bacteremias.[35] Direct invasion by a paravascular infection, such as an adjacent abscess, usually produces a false aneurysm.[35] *Salmonella, Staphylococcus,* and *Escherichia coli* are commonly associated with bacteremia-induced aneurysms. Aneurysms caused by spread from adjacent infection often indicate such etiologic agents as *Salmonella, Staphylococcus, Mycobacterium,* and fungus. Mycotic aneurysms of the femoral artery are particularly common in drug abusers.[38] Umbilical artery catheters have been implicated in mycotic aneurysm formation in neonates.[36] Syphilis

causes an inflammatory process of the vasavasorum, leading to a slow degeneration of muscle fibers and weakening of the arterial wall.[39]

The clinical aspects of atherosclerotic aneurysms show a substantial male preponderance. In various series, men predominate by a factor of 3:1 to 8:1.[40] This is particularly true with popliteal and femoral artery aneurysms.[39,40] Aneurysms tend to be multiple, and aortic aneurysms often are associated with iliac artery and femoropopliteal aneurysms. Abdominal aortic aneurysms show a familial predisposition, a family history of aneurysm is seen in 6 to 20 percent of patients with aneurysms. The importance of genetic factors in the pathogenesis of aneurysms is supported by animal and human data.[40,41] A strong correlation exists between smoking and hypertension, or both, in the development of abdominal aortic aneurysms. The incidence of hypertension in patients with aneurysms is 40 to 70 percent.[40,41] Abdominal aortic aneurysms were eight times more frequent among smokers than among nonsmokers; one study found that 86 percent of patients with abdominal aortic aneurysms were smokers.[40,41]

Biochemical factors may also be important in the pathogenesis of aneurysms. Elastin and collagen deficiencies have been found in the walls of aneurysms.[40,42] Proteolytic enzymes such as collagenase or elastase have been postulated to be present in abnormal concentrations.[40,42] The nutritional supply of the abdominal aorta wall has also been implicated; the abdominal aorta has relatively little vasavasorum, and its nourishment depends on diffusion from the lumen. Diffusion of nutrients may be compromised when the subendothelial region becomes thickened by atherosclerosis.[42]

Complications of aneurysms include rupture, arteriovenous fistula, inflammatory aneurysms, atheroembolism, and thrombosis (Fig. 13-9). Atheroembolism from an abdominal aortic aneurysm is a well-described entity estimated to be the source of approximately 10 percent of peripheral emboli. The emboli can either be thrombus from the lumen of the aneurysm or cholesterol microemboli from the intima of the aneurysm.[43] Thrombosis of an aneurysm is another complication associated with aneurysms. Thrombosis is more common in the smaller arteries, such as the popliteal and femoral arteries, but it can also occur in abdominal aortic aneurysms.

Multiple imaging modalities can be used for evaluation of aneurysms. The morphologic aspects of an aneurysm that should be identified include its dimensions, its shape, and its relationship to branch vessels.[32]

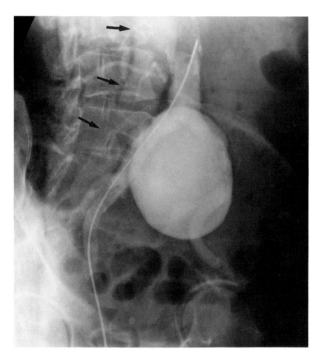

Figure 13-9 Atherosclerotic common iliac aneurysm. Left posterior oblique pelvic angiogram demonstrating a large atherosclerotic aneurysm arising from the left common iliac artery and simultaneous faint opacification of the iliac veins and the inferior vena cava *(arrows)* due to spontaneous rupture of the aneurysm into the iliac vein. The patient presented with a pulsatile abdominal mass and congestive heart failure.

Ultrasound

The accuracy of ultrasound for identifying the presence or absence of an abdominal aneurysm approaches 100 percent.[44] It is a relatively inexpensive technique, requires no ionizing radiation, and is an excellent method for following patients, as the measurements are highly reproducible.[44] Ultrasound examination is excellent for making the diagnosis and determining the size and the presence or absence of thrombus but does have its limitations. Ultrasound presents difficulty in determining the relationship of aneurysms to branch vessels, is often unable to diagnosis aneurysms in the iliac arteries, and cannot diagnosis associated occlusive disease.

Computed Tomography

Computed tomography (CT) is a more comprehensive method of evaluating aortic aneurysms. It can diagnose aneurysms and determine size very accurately. It can also identify extent. Iliac artery aneurysms can be identified. However, associated occlusive disease cannot be assessed, and the relationship between aneurysms and branch vessels is also difficult.

Magnetic Resonance Imaging

Magnetic resonance imaging (MRI) is an excellent means of evaluating aneurysms, as it shows inherent contrast between flowing blood and adjacent structures without the need for intravenous contrast material.[45] It is superior to CT in determining extent of aneurysms and can identify iliac artery aneurysms. MRI does not reliably assess associated occlusive disease, although with magnetic resonance angiography (MRA), visualization of associated occlusive disease is improving. Multiple renal arteries often are not identified. No ionizing radiation is required for the examination. However, MRI is an expensive modality and some patients may have problems with claustrophobia during the examination.

Angiography

There is debate in the literature as to the need for routine aortography for abdominal aortic aneurysms.[46,47] However, it has been, and continues to be, the "gold standard" for staging of aortic aneurysms. In one series, aortography was found to influence therapeutic decisions in 75 percent of cases evaluated.[48] It allows the surgeon to plan the operative procedure and avoid surprises in the operating room. An angiogram is excellent for obtaining information on extent and identifying associated aneurysms (e.g., iliac, renal, popliteal). It also permits identification of multiple renal arteries or other aberrant vessels. In addition, associated occlusive disease is easily evaluated. Complications of aneurysms, such as dissection, thrombosis, and aortovenous fistula, can be evaluated. Aortography is clearly indicated when the patient has associated occlusive iliofemoral disease, renovascular hypertension, evidence of mesenteric ischemia, suspicion of a horseshoe kidney or other renal anomaly, or the presence of femoral or popliteal aneurysms. It does require radiation, contrast material, and catheter manipulation. Angiography is not accurate in determining the size or presence of the aneurysm because the presence of thrombus may give the appearance of normal arterial caliber. In such cases, other evidence of the aneurysm, such as the occlusion of the lumbar arteries and mural calcification, should be sought.

The vast majority of iliac artery aneurysms are atherosclerotic in origin, although infection, iatrogenic trauma (hip replacement and lumbar disc surgery), and pregnancy have been reported as causative factors.[49] Aneurysms of isolated iliac arteries are far less common than abdominal aortic aneurysms.[49,50] Most iliac artery aneurysms are continuations of, or associated with, an abdominal aortic aneurysm. Most patients with isolated iliac artery aneurysms either are asymptomatic or have such nonspecific complaints that the diagnosis is delayed or erroneous.[49] Iliac artery aneurysms, particularly internal iliac artery aneurysms, may produce unusual symptoms because of their location. The anatomic proximity to the bladder and ureters results most frequently in manifestations falsely attributed to the genitourinary system.[51] Other erroneous diagnoses include diverticulitis, appendicitis, and neoplastic adenopathy.[49] Internal iliac artery aneurysms tend to be larger than common iliac artery aneurysms when detected[49] (Fig. 13-10). These aneurysms have a higher rate of rupture, with a reported incidence of 14 to 70 percent.[49] This probably relates to the rarity, the difficulty in detecting these lesions, and their large size at discovery.[49] CT scanning is the best screening tool for evaluating these aneurysms, as the pelvic arteries are relatively inaccessible for sonographic evaluation owing to intestinal gas, vessel tortuosity, and deep location.[51] MRI has similar advantages to those of CT.

Atherosclerosis is responsible for the most aneurysms of the femoral arteries. Aneurysms can develop in the common femoral artery, profunda femoris artery, or the superficial femoral artery in the region of the adductor canal. Other aneurysms arising in these areas include anastomotic aneurysms occurring after aortofemoral bypass grafts, traumatic aneurysms, and

mycotic aneurysms from drug abuse,[37] penetrating trauma, or as a result of an infected hematoma. Ultrasound is an excellent aid to diagnosis. Arteriography is used to examine the extent of the aneurysm and to evaluate the runoff before surgery.

The popliteal artery is the most common site for the development of a peripheral atherosclerotic aneurysm[52] (Fig. 13-11). These aneurysms are most frequently located in the popliteal artery just distal to the adductor hiatus.[53] There is a marked male predominance.[54] There is a frequent association with aneurysms in other arteries; 78 percent of patients with popliteal artery aneurysms had a second aneurysm, 64 percent with an aortoiliac aneurysm.[55] Popliteal artery aneurysms are bilateral in 38 to 58 percent of cases[56] and, when bilateral, are even more frequently associated with aneurysms elsewhere. Popliteal aneurysms rarely rupture.[56] The most frequent complications are thrombosis and distal embolization, which have been reported in 18 to 77 percent of patients.[57-59] The most frequent presentation of a popliteal aneurysm is severe limb ischemia resulting from thrombosis of the aneurysm or embolization. Less commonly, local pain, swelling, or chronic popliteal artery occlusion is the presenting complaint.[60] Patients whose presenting signs are of thrombosis or embolization have an amputation rate of 20 to 50 percent.[60] Because of these limb-threatening complications, elective resection usually is recommended,[58-60] although the treatment of asymptomatic popliteal aneurysms remains somewhat controversial.[54] Ultrasound and CT are excellent means of establishing the diagnosis of a popliteal artery aneurysm.[54,61] Angiography is useful in evaluating the extent of the aneurysm and the runoff before surgical therapy. The runoff examination is particularly important because of the high rate of embolism. The presence and size of popliteal aneurysms can be underestimated angiographically if intra-aneurysmal thrombus is present.[61]

Aneurysms involving the upper extremity are very unusual. Atherosclerotic aneurysms occasionally involve the subclavian artery[62] and have been reported in aberrant right subclavian arteries.[63] Upper-extremity aneurysms most frequently result from arterial trauma and are actually pseudoaneurysms (Fig. 13-12). Other rare causes include cystic medial necrosis,[64] inflammatory aneurysms associated with arteritis,[65] or mycotic aneurysms.

Angiography for aneurysms is tailored to the type of aneurysm being evaluated and should be performed in such a way as to provide all the information needed to perform the surgical repair. In the aorta this would include evaluation of the celiac and superior mesen-

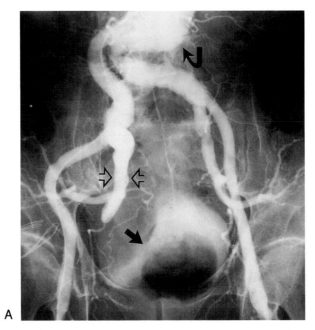

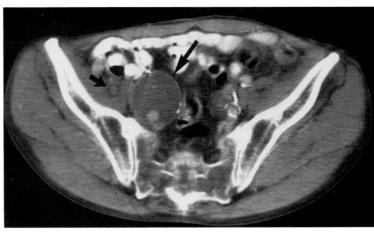

Figure 13-10 Internal iliac artery aneurysm. **(A)** Pelvic angiogram demonstrating an ectatic right hypogastric artery *(open arrows)* and an abdominal aortic aneurysm *(curved arrow)*. A pelvic mass is suggested by the deformity of the bladder *(solid straight arrow)*. **(B)** Computed tomography (CT) of the pelvis with oral and intravenous contrast revealing the pelvic mass to be a large right hypogastric artery aneurysm *(large arrow)* lined with thrombus. The residual lumen appears only slightly enlarged. The *small arrow* identifies the external iliac artery.

teric artery origins, using biplane filming. The extent of the aneurysm; whether it is suprarenal, juxtarenal, or infrarenal; and involvement of the iliac arteries should be determined. The number, position, and relationship of the renal arteries to the aneurysm must be assessed. Associated occlusive disease of the renal arteries, iliac arteries, and femoral arteries is evaluated. This should include the origins of the internal iliac, deep femoral, and proximal superficial arteries. Unusual presentations such as aortocaval fistulae, aortoenteric fistulae,

associated horseshoe kidney, or crossed fused ectopia may be discovered.

Iliac artery aneurysms should be evaluated in terms of inflow and outflow. The contralateral iliac artery should also be evaluated, which is particularly important in assessing internal iliac artery aneurysms. Evaluation of the femoral and popliteal arteries should also include the extent of the aneurysm and the status of inflow and outflow. Evaluation of outflow is especially crucial for popliteal artery aneurysms because of the

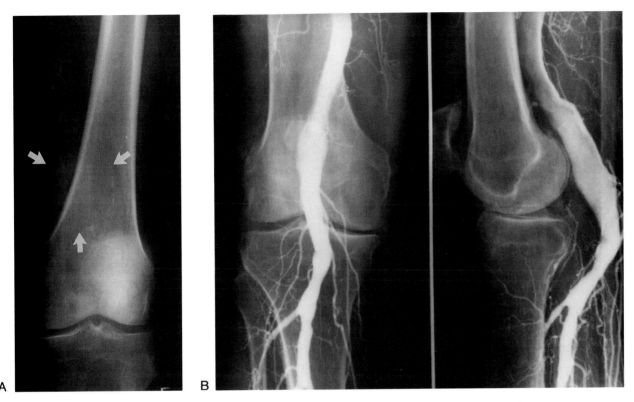

Figure 13-11 Popliteal artery aneurysm. **(A)** Calcified popliteal artery aneurysm on a plain film *(arrows)*. **(B)** Angiogram from a different patient with a popliteal artery aneurysm.

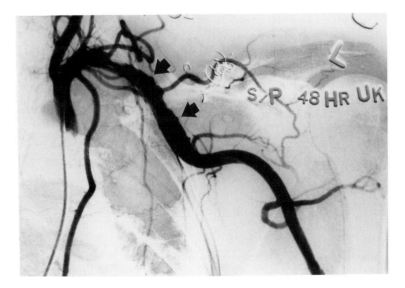

Figure 13-12 Post-traumatic subclavian artery aneurysm. Left subclavian artery aneurysm in a patient with a history of left clavicular fracture and non-union despite multiple surgical repairs (note the wire fragments in the vicinity of the fracture). The irregular contour of the aneurysm is due to mural thrombus *(arrows)*. The patient had presented 48 hours earlier with distal embolization requiring lytic therapy.

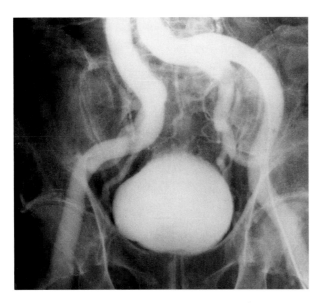

Figure 13-13 Arteriomegaly. Enlargement and tortuosity of the pelvic arteries without focal aneurysm formation.

high rate of distal embolism. Both lower extremities should be examined because bilateral aneurysms are common. In the upper extremities, the inflow and outflow should be examined, especially outflow, because symptomatic emboli are common.[66]

Arteriographic findings that should be determined include the morphology, which may be fusiform or saccular, and the dimensions of the aneurysm. Atherosclerotic aneurysms tend to be fusiform although they may be saccular. Mycotic and traumatic aneurysms are usually saccular. Occluded aneurysms will have an abrupt termination of the main artery and may show draping of branches around the thrombosed aneurysm. If thromboembolism has occurred, the arteries distal to the aneurysm may terminate abruptly, and filling defects may be visualized. Large aneurysms may require higher volumes of contrast material and slower filming because of the size of the vessel and the slow flow. Oblique views may be required to visualize arterial bifurcations and the origins of branch vessels.

Arteriomegaly

Arteriomegaly is defined as diffuse arterial enlargement involving several arterial segments (i.e., nonfocal) with increase in diameter of greater than 50 percent over the expected normal diameter[32] (Fig. 13-13). In most cases, there is diffuse dilatation of the aortoiliac system and of the femoropopliteal system. The arteries are dilated, elongated, and tortuous. The pathologic abnormality appears to be diffuse loss of medial elastic tissue.[67] Often blood flow is slow, probably owing to the increased luminal diameter. Angiographic evaluation requires increased volume of contrast medium and prolonged filming time. If arterial occlusions are seen with this entity, the occlusions are usually complications of aneurysmal disease, including thrombosis or embolism.[68]

Thromboembolic Occlusion

The causes of peripheral arterial occlusion include embolism that is most commonly cardiac in origin. Other sources of emboli include aneurysms, ulcerated plaques,[69] cholesterol showers from catheter manipulation,[70] blunt trauma, tumor,[71] or surgery. Atheroembolism can be associated with the use of anticoagulants and thrombolytic agents.

The diagnosis of acute embolic occlusion is not difficult. The classic presentation of acute arterial occlusion is described by the six p's: pain, pallor, paresthesias, pulselessness, paralysis, and polar (cold). There is an abrupt onset of ischemic symptoms. Patients with acute emboli will often have a history of heart problems, such as previous myocardial infarction, atrial fibrillation, or other arrhythmias.[72] The differential diagnosis is embolism versus a sudden thrombotic occlusion of an atherosclerotic artery. A history of intermittent claudication and the more gradual onset of symptoms will help with the differential diagnosis. The opposite leg is frequently abnormal in patients with underlying peripheral vascular disease and superimposed thrombosis. Although most patients with emboli will have sudden development of symptoms, occasionally symptoms will gradually develop and, in a few patients, peripheral embolization may be silent.[73] In some patients with emboli a profound irreversible ischemia will develop, characterized by absent capillary refill, profound muscle weakness with paralysis (rigor), profound anesthesia, and inaudible arterial and venous Doppler signal. This constellation of findings is associated with a very high amputation rate and a high mortality rate.[74,75]

Emboli can affect all peripheral vessels. They commonly lodge at bifurcations or at areas of pre-existing stenoses and then break up, with smaller emboli migrating distally. The femoral artery is the most common site of occlusion in the lower extremity (Fig. 13-14). Emboli to the upper extremity commonly originate from the heart[76] and are a frequent cause of acute vascular ischemia, particularly in the elderly. Most emboli to the upper extremities lodge in the proximal arteries, usually in the brachial artery.[76]

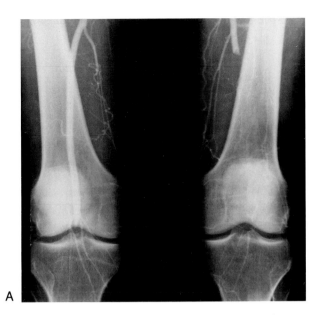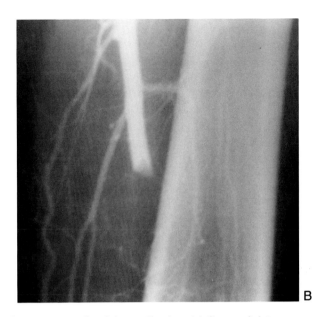

A   B

Figure 13-14 Peripheral emboli. **(A)** Emboli from a cardiac source to the right popliteal and left superficial femoral arteries (SFA). There is little of opacification of the distal vessels due to the paucity of collateral vessels in acute occlusions. **(B)** Closeup of the left SFA illustrating the typical convex filling defect seen with emboli.

Blue toe syndrome represents end-artery embolism, usually due to atheromatous microemboli. The patient has blue toes and acute livedo reticularis. Livedo reticularis is a red-blue mottling of the skin occurring in a netlike fashion and is a common manifestation of atheromatous emboli. It is not pathognomonic of atheroemboli, however, as it may occur spontaneously or in other conditions. Progression to gangrene of the digits or patchy gangrene of the skin may occur. In some cases, the entire extremity may be lost because of the severe diffuse ischemia. A classic finding with atheromatous microemboli is the presence of palpable pedal pulses.[69]

In most cases of suspected embolism, angiography is employed in the evaluation. Angiography permits localization of the embolus and definition of the arterial anatomy, in particular, the distal circulation. An abrupt occlusion of artery, with the notable absence of collaterals around the obstruction, is a common finding. A meniscus sign, with a superiorly convex meniscus, is considered pathognomonic. If the embolus is not completely occluding the artery, it may be outlined with contrast and appears as a filling defect. Proximal and distal to occlusion, the vessel will appear normal. In some cases, the vessel may be widened by the presence of the embolus.

Thrombosis of pre-existing aneurysms or stenoses may cause acute symptoms and simulate an acute embolic occlusion. Angiographically, a thrombosis may exhibit tapering of the artery in the region of the stenosis and the presence of numerous well-developed collaterals. Examination of the contralateral extremity may demonstrate symmetric atherosclerotic disease. These findings permit differentiation between embolism and sudden occlusion of an atherosclerotic stenosis. It is important to differentiate between acute thrombosis and embolism.[77] Acute thrombosis superimposed on a chronic stenosis will not respond well to embolectomy and requires a definitive revascularization procedure.

The performance of angiography includes a biplane aortogram and oblique views of the pelvis to identify localized ulcerated plaques in the aorta, or in the iliac or femoral arteries, which might represent the source of the embolus. A bilateral leg runoff examination is performed to look for evidence of contralateral peripheral vascular disease, which might indicate that thrombosis, rather than embolism, is responsible for the ischemia. The runoff should be examined for evidence of other, possibly asymptomatic, emboli. If the emboli are in the upper extremity, the thoracic aorta and the proximal vessels should be examined for evidence of aneurysm, ulcerated plaque, or a thoracic outlet syndrome, which may give rise to an atherosclerotic intimal lesion, poststenotic dilatation, or aneurysm in the subclavian.[78] Magnification views of feet and hands may be obtained to demonstrate filling defects or abrupt occlusion from small emboli. If lower-extremity emboli are present but no source of embolism is found on abdominal aortogram and runoff, and no other clinical source such as cardiac origin is found, a biplane thoracic aortogram should be performed to evaluate this region as a potential source.

Trauma

Emergency arteriography is indicated in patients with diminished or absent pulses, distal ischemia, a bruit, an expanding hematoma, a history of pulsatile bleeding, shotgun wounds, or a proximity injury that cannot be accurately followed clinically, such as possible injury to the subclavian artery, aorta.[79] Elective arteriography is indicated in patients with proximity injuries and normal arterial pulses, although the likelihood of discovering major occult arterial injury will be very low, on the order of 1 to 10 percent.[79-82] Arteriography may be necessary to evaluate the late manifestations of arterial trauma, the most common of which are the development of an arteriovenous fistula and pseudoaneurysm formation.[83]

The causes of penetrating trauma include knife and gunshot wounds; glass or metal shards from motor vehicle or industrial accidents; and iatrogenic injuries, such as femoral artery punctures,[84,85] angioplasty,[86] intra-aortic balloon pump insertion,[87] balloon thrombectomy,[88] and orthopaedic procedures.[89,90] Blunt trauma is primarily seen with motor vehicle accidents, often associated with fractures, but can also be due to falls[91] or crush injuries. Mechanisms of arterial injury in the extremities from blunt trauma include stretch injury, focal arterial spasm, intimal disruption, medial tears, and arterial thrombosis. Penetrating injuries may result in laceration or transection of an artery, which may have the consequent thrombosis, formation of a pseudoaneurysm, or an arteriovenous fistula (Fig. 13-15).

The entire peripheral vascular system can be affected by trauma. In patients in whom injury to the abdominal aorta is suspected, physicians are usually concerned about the possibility of injury to other abdominal structures, and the patient will often be taken directly to surgery. If arteriography is indicated to localize and evaluate the extent of the injury, a flush aortogram with biplane filming is used for evaluation.[93]

Injuries to the iliac arteries are caused primarily by blunt trauma, usually motor vehicle accidents resulting in severe pelvic fractures. The internal iliac branches are involved most commonly. A flush pelvic arteriogram is usually the first examination, but selective internal iliac arteriography may be necessary to demonstrate bleeding. Arteriographic findings include extravasation, pseudoaneurysms, occlusion, and arteriovenous fistulae. Penetrating trauma is less common but has similar findings.

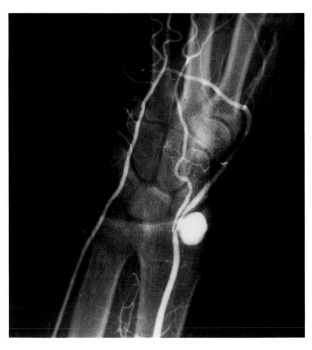

Figure 13-15 Post-traumatic pseudoaneurysm. Radial artery pseudoaneurysm after arterial blood gas sampling.

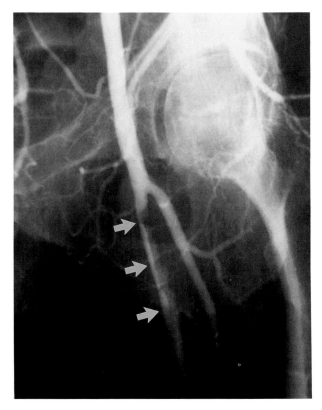

Figure 13-16 Catheter-induced trauma. Intimal defects and associated mural thrombus *(arrows)* in the superficial femoral artery after attempted arterial line placement.

The femoral artery is one of the most frequently injured vessels. This is commonly an iatrogenic injury resulting from arterial punctures,[9] intra-aortic balloon pump insertion, and orthopedic misadventures[93,94] (Fig. 13-16). Injuries to the common femoral artery can often be diagnosed with duplex ultrasound. Duplex ultrasound is particularly good for pseudoaneurysm diagnosis[95,96] Occasionally blunt trauma to the thigh will result in vascular injury to the superficial or deep femoral arteries.[97]

Injury to the popliteal artery has a poor prognosis if not recognized and treated promptly. Popliteal vascular injuries are associated with a high risk of lower extremity amputation.[98,99] Posterior knee dislocation is an injury likely to cause an isolated local disruption of the artery proximal to the trifurcation[100] (Fig. 13-17). Prompt diagnosis and repair are important for successful treatment of this injury, because the critical factor in determining limb survival is the period of ischemia.[101] In one study, 28 percent of patients with knee dislocations had popliteal artery injuries; one-half of these patients eventually lost the injured limb.[102] To exclude blunt arterial injury, arteriography is recommended in all patients with knee dislocations, knee instability after

acute blunt trauma, displaced fractures near the knee with circulatory deficits that resolve after reduction, compression injuries from automobile bumpers, or fractures near the knee requiring surgery.[103]

Tibial and peroneal arteries injuries are most often due to blunt trauma, usually associated with fractures (Fig. 13-18). Occasionally penetrating trauma will involve the tibial arteries; iatrogenic injuries from Fogarty catheters have also been reported.[104] Injuries of a single artery may not be apparent because collaterals maintain distal pulses. Arteriography is recommended for penetrating wounds that traverse the central leg and for severely displaced or comminuted tibial fractures.[103] Reconstruction is required for wounds involving the tibial peroneal trunk or when more than one artery is involved.[103] In reported military experience, single tibial artery injuries were associated with limb loss in 14 percent, and injury to two tibial arteries was associated with 70 percent limb loss if reconstruction was not performed.[105] This experience has led some authorities believe that if the anterior or posterior tibial is injured in blunt trauma, it should be repaired immediately; however, an isolated peroneal injury can be kept under observation. Two-vessel injuries should be

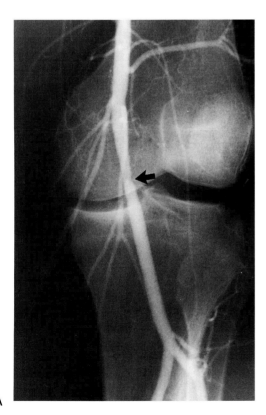
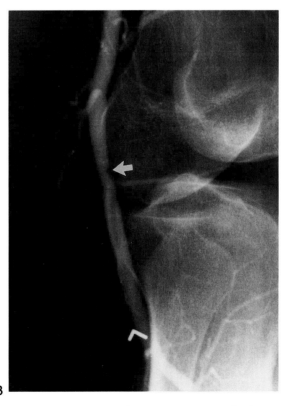

A   B

Figure 13-17 (A & B) Popliteal trauma. Two views of the popliteal artery in a patient who had a posterior knee dislocation and normal pulses. The angiogram revealed nonocclusive spasm and a small intimal tear *(arrows).*

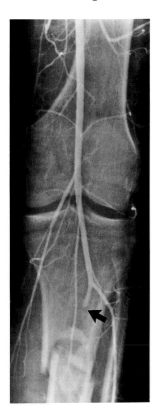

Figure 13-18 Blunt trauma. Comminuted tibial fracture with associated occlusion of the tibial-peroneal trunk *(arrow)*.

repaired immediately.[105] Delayed reconstruction tends to be more difficult than early repair because of scar formation, tissue defects, and loss of runoff.

Arterial injuries of the upper extremities are very common.[106] Both penetrating trauma and blunt

trauma can give rise to arterial injury. Penetrating trauma tends to be more common than blunt trauma in the upper extremities.[107] Traumatic injury to the subclavian and axillary arteries may be accompanied by damage to the brachial plexus, which can result in significant and permanent neurological deficits.[108] Blunt trauma that causes stretching of the brachial plexus may be associated with arterial injury (Fig. 13-19). The development of a hematoma or pseudoaneurysm in the region of the brachial plexus, caused by penetrating trauma, may compress the nerves, producing a neurologic deficit.[108] Because of the abundant collateral supply of the upper extremity, the pulses may be normal or only slightly diminished, even with significant arterial injury. The result may be delayed recognition of arterial injury.[108]

Elbow dislocations are analogous to knee dislocations and are associated with arterial injury.[109] They are usually the result of a stretch injury, but if the dislocation is accompanied by fractures, laceration of the artery can occur.[110]

A unique injury in the upper extremity is the hypothenar hammer syndrome (Fig. 13-20). This entity results from repetitive blunt trauma to the palm of the hand. The position of the ulnar artery in the hypothenar eminence crossing the hamate bone makes it vulnerable to such trauma. The arterial lesion may appear angiographically as spasm, occlusion, aneurysm, or a combination of these entities. Aneurysm development may lead to embolization of the digital arteries.[111,112]

Angiographic appearance[113] in trauma includes arterial narrowing, a smooth narrowing over a relatively long segment. This appearance may be the result of arterial spasm, extrinsic compression, or subintimal hematoma. A long segment of narrowing with slow

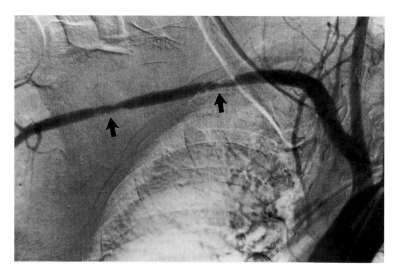

Figure 13-19 Stretch injury. Focal subclavian and axillary artery spasm and severe intimal irregularity *(arrows)* in a patient with a traction injury to the right upper extremity sustained while falling out of a tree.

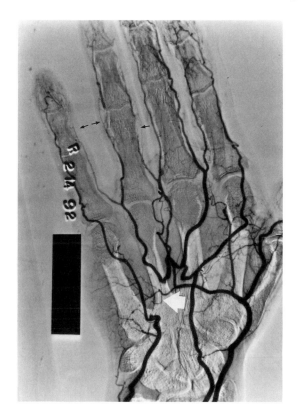

Figure 13-20 Hypothenar hammer syndrome. Occlusion of the ulnar artery over the hypothenar emminence *(white arrow)* with embolii to the 4th and 5th proper palmar digital arteries *(small black arrows).* The patient was a 35-year-old right-handed auto mechanic.

arterial flow and absent filling of small muscular branches may represent a compartment syndrome.[113] Arterial occlusion may be caused by arterial transection with secondary vaso-occlusion or intimal injury with secondary thrombosis.[113] Arterial occlusion of the proximal vessels is likely to be reconstituted by collaterals, whereas occlusion of the distal vessels is less likely to demonstrate reconstitution. Other angiographic findings of trauma include intraluminal filling defects, which may represent intraluminal thrombus or intimal flaps. Intimal flaps often appear as thin lucent strips in the contrast column. Pseudoaneurysms are represented by focal widening of the lumen and are the result of damage to the arterial media. Other findings associated with laceration of an artery are contrast extravasation and arteriovenous fistulae, resulting from transmural injury. Arteriovenous fistulae exhibit communication into the adjacent vein and are unusual in acute trauma but are more common as a late manifestation of trauma (Figs. 13-21 and 13-22). Blunt trauma is manifested as an arterial laceration, thrombosis, dissection, or false aneurysm formation; penetrating

trauma appears as occlusion, arteriovenous fistula, false aneurysm, or laceration with extravasation of contrast material.

The angiographic examination should be performed to include the entire region of interest. The entrance and exit sites should be marked so that the whole area of possible vessel damage is included in the examination. In performing the angiographic examination, it is important to take into account the cavitation effect, which can cause damage at a considerable distance from the path of the missile. This type of effect is seen with high-velocity missiles and shotgun blasts.[114] Administration of a vasodilator may help visualize distal vessels in trauma patients who may have previously been in shock or who may be cold, and therefore vasoconstricted.

Trauma arteriography is used to exclude the presence of a vascular injury in a patient who otherwise has no indication for operative exploration, to detect a lesion that was not exposed by other techniques, such as physical examination or noninvasive examinations (e.g., ankle-arm measurements), or to plan the operative management of a patient with a major vascular injury.

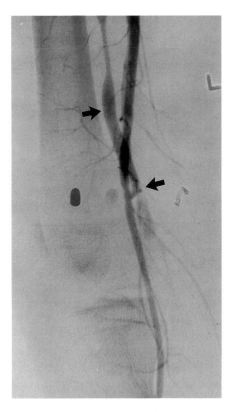

Figure 13-21 Arteriovenous fistula (AVF). Traumatic AVF between the popliteal artery and vein *(arrows)* due to gunshot wound.

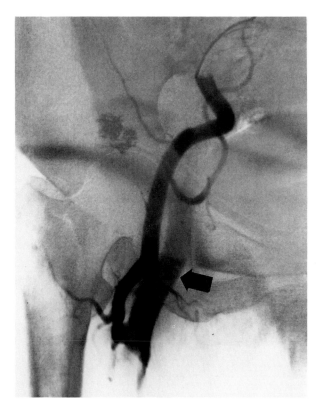

Figure 13-22 Arteriovenous fistula (AVF) between the profunda femoris artery and vein *(arrow)* after cardiac catheterization.

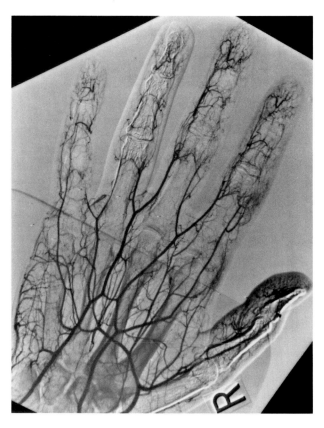

Figure 13-23 Vasculitis. Multiple digital artery occlusions in a 22-year-old woman with digital ulcers and systemic lupus erythematosus (SLE). There was no change after injection of a vasodilating agent.

Vasculitis

Vasculitis is a moderately common disease entity requiring angiographic evaluation. It is usually present in the upper extremities, but the lower extremities may be involved, particularly with Buerger's disease. Vasculitis is seen in multiple collagen vascular disorders, including scleroderma, periarteritis nodosa, lupus erythematosus, rheumatoid arthritis, dermatomyositis, and giant cell arteritis. The disease process primarily affects small and medium arteries (Fig. 13-23). Vasculitis is associated with the deposition of antigen-antibody immune complexes on the endothelium, followed by the development of arterial wall damage.[115] Thrombosis, aneurysm formation, hemorrhage, or arterial occlusion all may follow or accompany the transmural inflammatory arterial damage.[68] Arterial vasoconstriction associated with vasculitis may be either localized or diffuse. If the vasospasm is of short duration, no tissue changes will result. However, if the vasospasm is prolonged, tissue damage may result. The arterial ischemia secondary to vasculitis often is manifested by gangrene, tissue loss, or ulceration of the fingers.

Clinically, the patient may have Raynaud's phenomenon, characterized by episodic attacks of discoloration of the digits induced by cold or at times by emotional stimuli (Fig. 13-24). Raynaud's disease may be primary, without known underlying disease, or it may be secondary, occurring in association with an underlying systemic disease. Causes of Raynaud's phenomenon include arterial occlusive disease, collagen vascular disease, trauma, and ergotism. The syndrome usually involves the upper extremity; isolated lower-extremity involvement is very rare.[116]

Patients may have intermittent claudication, tissue loss, gangrene, or ulceration of the fingers. The angiographic appearance includes focal areas of arterial spasm and occlusion involving small and medium arteries. All connective tissue disorders affect primarily the digital vessels of the upper extremity, although the digital vessels of the feet can also be involved. Involvement of tibial arteries is relatively common. Occasionally the superficial femoral artery or popliteal artery is involved. Involvement of the major limb arteries may

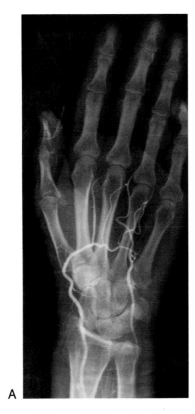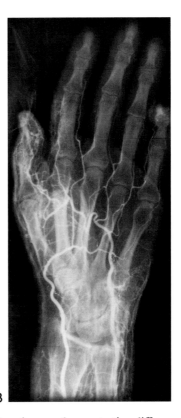

A   B

Figure 13-24 Raynaud's disease. **(A)** Late film from a hand angiogram demonstrating diffuse spasm and under-filling of the distal arteries. **(B)** After intra-arterial injection of a vasodilator (priscoline), the spasm is partially reversed. Venous shunting is present in the thumb.

be due to lupus erythematosus, giant cell arteritis, or rheumatoid arteritis.[117]

Buerger's Disease

Buerger's disease, or thromboangiitis obliterans, is an inflammatory disease of unknown cause. Tobacco use is the sole known etiologic factor[118,119] and is thought to trigger the disease through an autoimmune mechanism.[120] Histologically, this is a non-necrotizing panarteritis, mostly involving the medium and small arteries of the extremities. The walls of the arteries or veins, or both, are swollen with a moderate cellular infiltrate of the adventitia and media. The lumen is occluded by a highly cellular thrombus. This thrombus contains characteristic microabscesses.[121] Although considered primarily an arterial disorder, venous involvement is often present. A histologic examination of an artery or vein is required for a definite diagnosis. Some patients thought to have Buerger's disease actually have premature atherosclerotic disease or a form of collagen vascular disease.

The typical patient is a young adult man, a heavy smoker, whose presenting symptom is pain in the distal aspect of the extremities. The disease rarely occurs in women (less than 2 percent), although a 10-fold increase in the prevalence of Buerger's disease among women has recently been reported. This increase is presumably due to the increased prevalence of smoking in the female population.[120]

Bilateral leg claudication is a common presenting symptom; this may be limited to the foot or calf. Usually two or more limbs are affected at presentation. Pedal pulses may be present, but usually they are diminished or absent.[121] Other symptoms include rest pain, ulceration, and gangrene. Superficial migratory phlebitis may be part of the clinical presentation.

Angiographically, the small vessels of the calf and the foot are most frequently affected.[122-124] Predominantly involved are the small arteries, such as the anterior tibial, posterior tibial, or peroneal arteries or the plantar arteries of the foot. Popliteal artery involvement is less frequent. The vessels proximal to the popliteal artery are virtually always normal arteriographically. In the upper extremity, the palmar, digital, ulnar, and radial arteries are affected (Fig. 13-25).

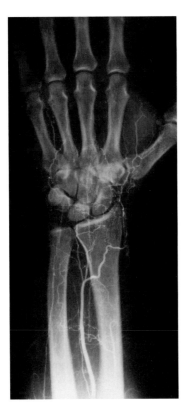

Figure 13-25 Buerger's disease. Upper-extremity angiogram demonstrating occlusion of the radial and ulnar arteries in the forearm and the named hand vessels. The interosseus artery supplies only small collateral vessels distal to the wrist.

Bilateral, focal, or often multifocal segmental occlusions are seen with abrupt transition from a normal-caliber vessel to a very diseased vessel or an occlusion. The lumen above the thrombosed segments is smooth and narrow, without evidence of arterial wall irregularity. An extensive tortuous collateral system is present. The collaterals often are described as "corkscrew" or "corrugated" collaterals. Although frequently described in the literature, they do not appear to be pathognomonic of Buerger's disease and have been seen in other diseases with diffuse arterial narrowing and occlusions. Areas of arterial spasm also may be identified.

Vascular Malformations

An arteriovenous fistula is an abnormal communication between an artery and a vein, without any interposed capillary system. Arteriovenous fistulae represent a single direct communication between an artery and a vein. These communications usually are secondary to trauma but can be the result of an aneurysm or chronic inflammation. Arteriovenous mal-

formations have multiple communications between arteries and veins in the same area. These communications are believed to be congenital in origin. (For a detailed discussion of arteriovenous malformations and their embryology, diagnosis, and treatment, see Ch. 81.)

Neoplasms

The role of angiography in the evaluation of neoplasms has decreased with the advent of CT and MRI scanning. These newer modalities are better able to determine the extent of tumor and can usually delineate involvement of major vessels.[125,126] Angiography is indicated if CT or MRI imaging does not clearly demonstrate the relationship of the neoplasm to major vascular structures. Angiography can also be used to better define tumor vascularity and origin of the tumor's vascular supply.[127,128] Angiography also may demonstrate the need for, and be used to perform, preoperative embolization or intra-arterial chemotherapy.

The angiographic appearance of neoplasms is variable. The normal course and appearance of major arteries are often altered. The arteries may be displaced, bowed, or stretched. Alteration of the diameter of the vessels and abrupt changes in caliber indicate vascular encasement. Arteries and veins may be narrowed or completely occluded. Small fine vasculature with irregular vessels showing abrupt changes in direction and in caliber with loss of the normal arterial arborization pattern is characteristic of neovascularity (Fig. 13-26). However, it may not be possible to distinguish tumor neovascularity from the neovascularity seen in inflammatory conditions, postoperative healing, and benign tumors.[129] A hypervascular tumor will have increased flow, leading to a tumor "stain" or "blush." Arteriovenous shunting, with the presence early draining veins, is common. Parasitization of blood supply from neighboring arterial sources may be identified. Other findings include pooling of contrast medium in vascular lakes and venous invasion.

Pharmacoangiography can be used to aid the diagnosis of tumor vascularity. Pharmacologic agents can be divided into those that produce vasodilatation and those that produce vasoconstriction. Tolazoline (Priscoline, Ciba Pharmaceuticals) is a commonly used vasodilator[130] that improves visualization of lesions and of venous structures. Angiotension (Hypertensin, Ciba Pharmaceuticals) causes vasoconstriction in the periphery; epinephrine is used more frequently in visceral vessels. The lack of contractile elements in the walls of the tumor arteries makes the tumor vasculature less responsive than normal vessels to vasoconstriction.[129] Thus, after administration of vasocon-

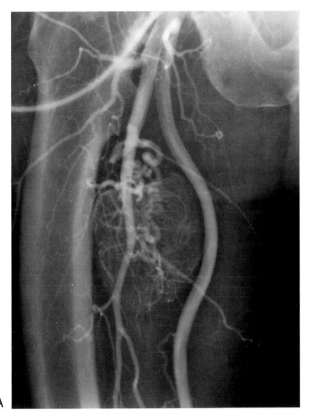

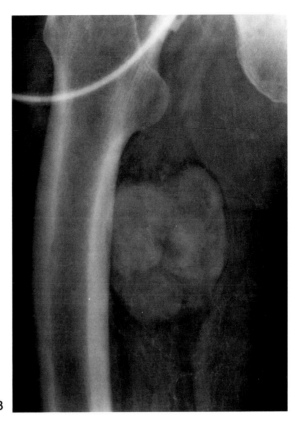

A   B

Figure 13-26 Tumor. **(A)** Angiogram of a hemangiopericytoma of the thigh demonstrating mass effect on the superficial femoral artery (SFA), hypertrophy of the feeding profunda femoris branches, and neovascularity within the mass. **(B)** The tumor remains densely opacified on a late image from the same injection.

stricting agents, the tumor vessels appear more prominent.

Entrapment Syndromes

Popliteal Artery Entrapment Syndrome

In popliteal artery entrapment, the popliteal artery may have an abnormal course in the popliteal fossa with an associated abnormal attachment of the medial head of the gastrocnemius or popliteus muscle. The syndrome is characteristically seen in young athletes with intermittent claudication and has often been described in young military personnel.[131,132] Males are affected more frequently than females.[133] The onset of symptoms is frequently acute, with the sudden development of a cold leg as the patient's initial symptom. Alternatively, the patient may complain of progressively increasing intermittent claudication. Some older patients with isolated disease of the popliteal artery may in fact have a popliteal entrapment syndrome.[134] The disease is bilateral in 20 to 67 percent.[134,135] Pulses may be normal, diminished or absent. If pulses are

present, passive plantar flexion of the foot will diminish or obliterate the pulse.

Classifications of this syndrome are based on the relationship of the popliteal artery to the gastrocnemius muscle attachment to the femur, and other normal structures of the popliteal fossa. Five types are described[136]:

Type I. The popliteal artery deviates medially around the medial head of the gastrocnemius muscle, which compresses it. The gastrocnemius muscle arises in a normal position.

Type II. The popliteal artery deviates around the medial head of the gastrocnemius muscle, but there is less deviation of the artery position than in type I. The medial head of the gastrocnemius arises more laterally than usual.

Type III. The popliteal artery is entrapped beneath an accessory slip of the medial head of the gastrocnemius muscle. The artery is normally positioned in the popliteal fossa.

Type IV. The popliteal artery is compressed by the popliteus muscle or a deep fibrous band. The artery may follow a normal course or may have a medially deviated course.

Type V. The artery and vein are both displaced medially and compressed by a normal medial gastrocnemius muscle.

Characteristically the angiogram demonstrates medial deviation of the popliteal artery. However, in type III, the course of the artery is in its usual position, and in type II and type IV, the artery may be only slightly deviated. With extreme passive dorsiflexion or active knee extension and foot plantar flexion, the artery is compressed by the muscle or fibrous bands. Thus, if arteriography with the leg in a neutral position is not diagnostic, stress arteriography with the foot in plantar flexion will demonstrate compression or occlusion of the popliteal artery[137] (Fig. 13-27).

Other arteriographic findings include premature atherosclerotic changes, presumably due to repeated trauma,[138] segmental occlusion, aneurysmal dilatation,[139] or poststenotic dilatation of the popliteal artery. The distal vessels should be evaluated for the possibility of emboli.[140]

CT can be used for diagnosis. It gives excellent delineation of the soft tissue, vascular, and bony structures. The abnormal relationship between the popliteal artery and the gastrocnemius muscle can be well seen.[141] Even if the artery is thrombosed, CT can show an abnormal muscle band that establishes the diagnosis of popliteal entrapment.[142] MRI can also be used to evaluate the popliteal fossa structures. It can demonstrate the muscular anatomic features and the course of the artery as well as its patency.[133] The ability of MRI to provide longitudinal views permits better definition of the anatomy than is possible with CT.

Thoracic Outlet Syndrome

The etiology of thoracic outlet syndrome involves the compression of structures passing through the area known as the thoracic outlet. The structures include the brachial plexus, the subclavian artery, and the subclavian vein. These structures can be compressed in the region of the interscalene triangle, bounded by the anterior and medial scalene muscles and the first rib; the costoclavicular space, formed by the clavicle and the first rib; and the pectoralis minor triangle, formed by the insertion of the pectoralis minor muscle and the coracoid process. Any anomaly that encroaches on these spaces can cause compression of the artery, vein, and nerves. The anomalies that can produce compression include cervical ribs; abnormalities of the scalenus anterior muscle, either hypertrophy or abnormal insertions; or abnormalities of the clavicle, first rib, or cervical vertebral bodies, such as fractures or malignancies.[143,144]

Patients commonly have neurologic symptoms, including pain, numbness of the hand and fingers, and paresthesias. Vascular presentations include emboli, claudication, and Raynaud's phenomenon (which may be unilateral).[145]

Indications for angiography include evidence of ischemia or embolism. Arteriography is performed first with the arm in the neutral position and then with the shoulder hyperabducted and the face turned toward the opposite shoulder. After the views of the subclavian artery are obtained, the distal vasculature is examined

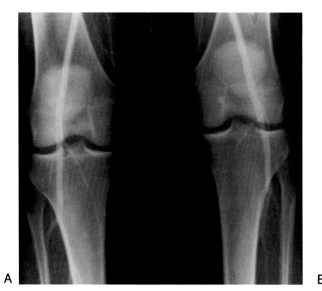
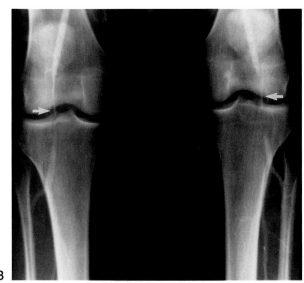

Figure 13-27 Popliteal entrapment. **(A)** Bilateral popliteal angiograms with the feet in neutral position in a young male with bilateral calf claudication. **(B)** Repeat injection with the feet in plantar flexion demonstrating compression of the popliteal arteries *(arrows).*

for evidence of emboli. An upper-extremity venogram is also performed with the patient's arm in the neutral and abducted position.

Arteriographic findings of poststenotic dilatation of the distal subclavian artery (the most common finding) with the arm in the neutral position, and compression of the artery between the clavicle and first rib when the arm is in the hyperabducted position, are diagnostic. Other findings include focal stenosis or occlusion of the subclavian, axillary, or brachial arteries, aneurysms, mural thrombus, distal embolization, and prominent collaterals (Fig. 13-28). Venous findings include dilation of the subclavian vein, and collaterals and compression or obstruction of the venous flow when the arm is in the hyperextended position.

MISCELLANEOUS VASCULAR DISEASES

Adventitial Cystic Disease

The etiology of adventitial cystic disease is unknown. A mucin-containing cyst arises in the outer tunica media or subadventitial layer of the arterial wall and then expands into the adventitia. The cyst may involve only part of the wall or totally surround the artery.[146] The buildup of mucin within the cyst causes external compression of the artery.

Various mechanisms have been proposed to explain this disorder, including (1) microtrauma, (2) ganglion formation in the adventitia because the cysts are found in arteries in the region of joints, (3) myxomatous degeneration in the adventitial coat, or (4) the presence of synovial cell rests sequestered within the arterial wall.[146] The cyst may be uniloculated or multiloculated and usually contains clear fluid, although hemorrhagic fluid has been reported.[147]

Advential cystic disease should be in the differential diagnosis of intermittent claudication in young patients. Clinically, patients have abrupt onset of cramplike calf pain, followed by progressively worsening intermittent claudication. The degree of stenosis and the presence of collaterals determine the severity of the symptoms. The popliteal and distal pulses are diminished or absent. Men are affected more frequently than women.[146] The most commonly involved artery is the popliteal artery, but the condition has been reported in other arteries, including the radial, ulnar, brachial, iliac, and femoral arteries.[146,148] The same pathologic process has also been reported in the walls of veins.[148,149]

The angiographic appearance is that of localized segmental stenosis with a normal artery proximal and distal to the lesion. The stenosis is characteristically a smooth filling defect, which may be eccentric, concentric, or spiral shaped (Fig. 13-29). If the cyst is on one side of the artery, a curvilinear scimitar sign is seen. An

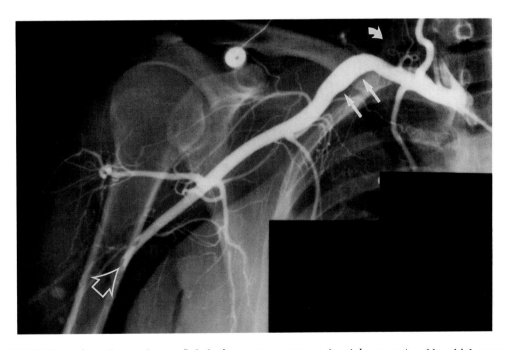

Figure 13-28 Thoracic outlet syndrome. Subclavian artery aneurysm *(straight arrows)* and brachial artery embolus *(open arrow)* in a patient with a cervical rib *(curved arrow)*.

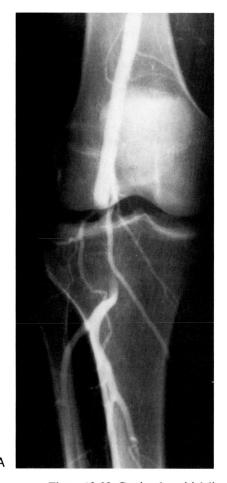
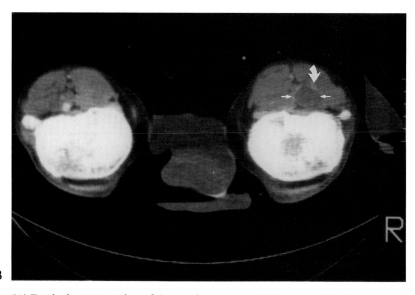

A   B

Figure 13-29 Cystic adventitial disease. **(A)** Extrinsic compression of the popliteal artery. **(B)** Contrast CT of the popliteal fossae with the patient supine. A low attentuation mass *(small arrows)* compresses the popliteal artery *(curved arrow)* on the right. A normal popliteal artery is present on the left.

hourglass configuration may be seen if the cyst encircles the artery. Segmental occlusion of the popliteal artery can occur.

CT scanning can be used to visualize the cyst[150] and will demonstrate compression of the popliteal artery lumen by a cystic structure with a low attenuation value (between that of water and muscle). The cyst may appear septated and multiloculated. Although the rim may enhance with contrast medium, the cyst contents do not demonstrate enhancement.[151] MRI has also been used to evaluate cystic disease.[152]

Surgical removal, often with bypass grafting, has been the standard therapy for these cysts. Surgical enucleation of the cyst[153] and aspiration of cysts under CT guidance[154] have been described. Spontaneous resolution[155] and spontaneous rupture[152] have also been reported.

Fibromuscular Dysplasia

Fibromuscular dysplasia (FMD) is an uncommon disease described most frequently in the renal arteries but found in all arterial beds, including those of the cervical arteries, visceral arteries, and extremities.[147] All the peripheral vessels, including the iliac, superficial femoral, popliteal, tibial, subclavian, and axillary arteries, have been reported to have FMD involvement.[156,157] The lesion typically arises in the middle or distal arterial segments, sparing the orificial or bifurcation sites where atherosclerotic disease would typically be found.

Classification of this entity into three main types is based on the layers of the vessel wall involved[158]: intimal, medial, and periarterial. An additional classification includes intimal fibroplasia, medial hyperplasia, medial fibroplasia, perimedial fibroplasia, and periarterial fibroplasia. Of the three main types, medial FMD is the most frequent, accounting for 70 to 95 percent of all FMD lesions.[156] The cause of FMD is unknown and various theories proposed to explain the disease implicate genetic,[159] mechanical, toxic, and hormonal factors.[147,156] The disease occurs primarily in women, usually younger than would ordinarily be affected by atherosclerotic disease.

Involvement of the subclavian artery is frequently found in patients with systemic FMD.[156] Severe lesions may cause weakness of the arm, claudication, and paresthesias; in addition, subclavian steal may occur. In the lower extremities, the lesions are frequently asymptomatic, but patients can demonstrate claudication, ischemia, microembolism, or dissection.[156,160] In older patients, the superimposition of atherosclerotic disease on asymptomatic FMD may lead to the development of symptoms. The angiographic appearance of FMD is classically described as a "string of pearls" (Fig. 13-30). Other findings are aneurysmal dilatation, smooth focal stenoses, long tubular stenoses, or complete occlusion.[161]

Ergotism

Ergot compounds produce intense vasoconstriction; these agents act both as an α-adrenergic antagonist and as a partial agonist on α-receptors in the arterial wall.

Vasoconstriction leads to the development of arterial spasm and ischemic neuropathy. During the Middle Ages, ergotism was caused by ingestion of ergot alkaloids produced by fungus in contaminated rye. Today the cause of ergotism is primarily iatrogenic.[162] Ergotamine tartrate, dihydroergotamine (DHE), and methysergide maleate (a semisynthetic drug) are commonly used for migraine headaches but also are used as oxytocic agents for the control of postpartum hemorrhage, as pressor agents to control postural hypotension, and for the prophylaxis of deep venous thrombosis. All these agents are known to be associated with vascular ischemia.[162-165]

The symptoms of ergotism are a burning pain, primarily in the extremities, as well as intermittent claudication, rest pain, and occasionally gangrene. Most of the patients are young women, probably reflecting the higher prevalence of migraine headaches in women. On physical examination, the peripheral arterial pulses are found to be severely diminished or absent, and the

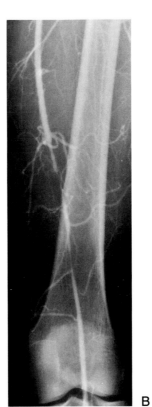
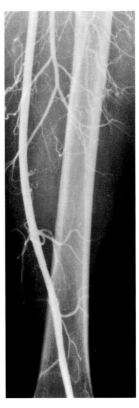
A B

Figure 13-31 Ergotism. **(A)** Diffuse vascular spasm with a long stenosis of the distal left superficial femoral artery (SFA) and proximal popliteal in a patient with severe headaches and left leg claudication. **(B)** Same patient 5 days later. The only intervention has been withdrawal of ergotamines, with resolution of the claudication.

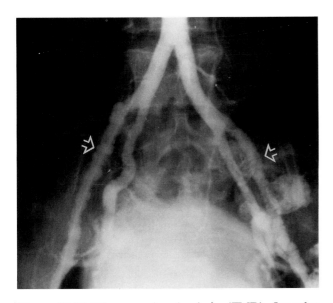

Figure 13-30 Fibromuscular dysplasia (FMD). Irregular asymmetric "string-of-pearls" appearance of medial FMD in both external iliac arteries *(arrows)*.

extremities are cool and pale, with slight mottling. Any vessel, including the coronary, mesenteric, renal, carotid, digital, and ophthalmic arteries, can be affected. However, the lower-extremity arteries are most usually affected by ergot preparation.

The angiographic appearance is one of generalized intense spasm of the arteries, usually bilateral and symmetrical in distribution (Fig. 13-31). The caliber of the vessel may decreased abruptly, but with a smooth-walled, long, string-like narrowing. Diffuse or focal spasm may be seen. The superficial femoral artery, popliteal artery, and distal tibial vessels are involved most often but larger, more proximal arteries, including the aorta, also may be affected. In cases of chronic ergot use, extensive collaterals are present. With acute overadministration of ergot, collaterals are less common. Infrequently, thrombosis of the arteries may be present. After discontinuation of the ergot preparation, the follow-up arteriogram often demonstrates the return to a normal appearance.

Treatment for ergotism includes discontinuation of the ergot preparation; administration of nitroglycerin, papaverine, and nitroprusside either intravenously or intraarterially; or administration of nifedipine given sublingually.[166]

MISCELLANEOUS ANGIOGRAPHIC APPEARANCES

Corrugated arteries, stationary waves, and standing arterial waves are terms used to describe regular, periodic, symmetric transverse striations in the contrast column within an artery[117,167] (Fig. 13-32). These standing waves occur commonly in the muscular vessels, such as the femoral, popliteal, and tibial arteries. The cause of this phenomenon is unclear, and multiple theories have been proposed, including circular muscle spasm,[168] pulse-pressure wave phenomenon,[169] or transient arterial spasm due to forceful injection of the contrast media. Whatever the cause, the finding usually disappears when a vasodilator is given, and it has no apparent significance.

Early filling of veins is often seen in patients with varicose veins and chronic deep venous insufficiency. This may be due to abnormally high arterial pressure, resulting in the formation of an arteriovenous fistula.[170] Microfistulae have been cited as the reasons for

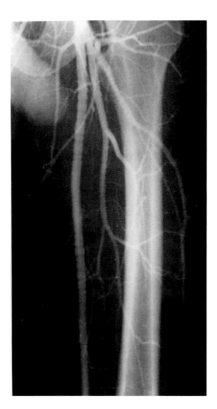

Figure 13-32 Standing waves. Regular symmetric beading of the superficial femoral artery (SFA) and profunda femoris artery (PFA) typical of standing waves (see Fig. 13-30).

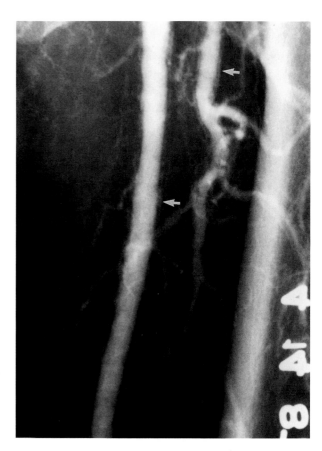

Figure 13-33 Monckeberg sclerosis. Fine linear calcification in the media of the superficial femoral artery (SFA) and profunda femoris artery (PFA) *(arrows).*

the visualization of thigh or calf veins in the early phases of arteriography.

Marked arterial calcification is seen in Monckeberg sclerosis, which represents calcification involving the tunica media of large and medium arteries[171] (Fig. 13-33). Monckeberg sclerosis tends to involve only muscular arteries of medium to small size.[172] This is in contradistinction to the calcification associated with atherosclerotic disease. Atherosclerotic calcification involves the intima and the aorta and arteries of the extremities particularly over the joints are affected. Other causes of significant arterial calcification include chronic renal failure,[173] arteriosclerosis obliterans, and a rare condition of idiopathic infantile arterial calcification with calcification affecting all the blood vessels.[174]

REFERENCES

1. Spies JB, Bakal CW, Burke DR et al: Standards for diagnostic arteriography in adults. JVIR 4:385, 1993
2. Egbert LD, Battit GE, Turndorf H, Beecher HK: The value of the preoperative visit by an anesthetist. JAMA 185:553, 1963
3. Cragg AH, Smith TP, Berbaum KS, Nakagawa N: Randomized double-blind trial of midazolam/placebo and midazolam/fentanyl for sedation and analgesia in lower-extremity angiography. AJR 157:173, 1991
4. Miller DL, Wall RT: Fentanyl and diazepam for analgesia and sedation during radiologic special procedures. Radiology 162:195, 1987
5. Dripps RD, Eckenhoff JE, Vandam LD: Premedication and preparation for anesthesia. p. 37. In Dripps RD, Vandam LD (eds): Introduction to Anesthesia. The Principles of Safe Practice. 7th Ed. WB Saunders, Philadelphia, 1988
6. Stoelting RK, Miller RD: Preoperative medication. p. 115. In: Basics of Anesthesia. Churchill Livingstone, New York, 1984
7. Lechner G, Jantsch H, Waneck R, Kretschmer G: The relationship between the common femoral artery, the inguinal crease, and the inguinal ligament: a guide to accurate angiographic puncture. Cardiovasc Intervent Radiol 11:165, 1988
8. Lang EK: A survey of the complications of percutaneous retrograde arteriography: Seldinger technique. Radiology 81:257, 1963
9. Altin RS, Flicker S, Naidech HJ: Pseudoaneurysm and arteriovenous fistula after femoral artery catheterization: association with low femoral punctures. AJR 152:629, 1989
10. Rapoport S, Sniderman DW, Morse SS et al: Pseudoaneurysm: a complication of faulty technique in femoral arterial punctures. Radiology 154:529, 1985
11. Marsan RE, McDonald V, Ramamurthy S: Iatrogenic femoral arteriovenous fistula. Cardiovasc Intervent Radiol 13:314, 1990
12. Gritter KJ, Laidlaw WW, Peterson NT: Complications of outpatient transbrachial intraarterial digital subtraction angiography. Radiology 162:125, 1987
13. Grollman JH, Marcus R: Transbrachial arteriography: technique and complications. Cardiovasc Intervent Radiol 11:32, 1988
14. Lasser EC, Berry CC, Talner LB et al: Pretreatment with corticosteroids to alleviate reactions to intravenous contrast material. N Engl J Med 317:845, 1987
15. Committee on Drugs and Contrast Media, Commission on Education: Manual on Iodinated Contrast Media. American College of Radiology, Reston, VA, 1991
16. Standards of Practice Committee of the Society of Cardiovascular and Interventional Radiology: Standards for interventional radiology. J Vasc Interrvent Radiol 2:59, 1991
17. Weaver FA, Pentecost MJ, Yellin AE et al: Clinical applications of carbon dioxide/digital subtraction arteriography. J Vasc Surg 13:266, 1991
18. Widrich WC, Singer RJ, Robbins AH: The use of intraarterial lidocaine to control pain due to aortofemoral arteriography. Radiology 124:37, 1977
19. Guthaner DF, Silverman JF, Hayden WG, Wexler L: Intraarterial analgesia in peripheral arteriography. AJR 128:737, 1977
20. Wallace S, Medellin H, de Jongh D, Gianturco C: Systemic heparinization for angiography. AJR 116:204, 1972
21. Thomson KR, Goldin AR: Angiographic techniques in interventional radiology. Radiol Clin North Am 17:375, 1979
22. Miller DL: Heparin in angiography: current patterns of use. Radiology 172:1007, 1989
23. Zarins CK: Hemodynamics in atherogenesis. p. 86. In Moore WS (ed): Vascular Surgery: A Comprehensive Review. WB Saunders, Philadelphia, 1991
24. Kannel WB, Shurteff O: The natural history of arteriosclerosis obliterans. Cardiovasc Clin 3:37, 1971
25. Wilbourn AJ, Furlan AJ, Hulley W, Roschhaupt W: Ischemic monomelic neuropathy. Neurology 33:447, 1983
26. Raaf JH, Shannon J: Atherosclerotic coarctation of the abdominal aorta in women. Surg Gynecol Obstet 150:715, 1980
27. Yao JST, Neiman HL: Aorta and iliac artery. p. 57. In Neiman HL, Yao JST (eds): Angiography of Vascular Disease. Churchill Livingstone, New York, 1985
28. Graham D, Alexander JJ, Franceschi D, Rashad F: The management of localized abdominal aortic dissections. J Vasc Surg 8:582, 1988
29. Azodo MVU, Gutierrez OH, DeWeese JA: Abdominal aortic dissection with retrograde extension into the thoracic aorta: case report. Cardiovasc Intervent Radiol 12:317, 1990
30. Becquein JP, Deleuze P, Watelet J et al: Acute and chronic dissections of the abdominal aorta: clinical features and treatment. J Vasc Surg 11:397, 1990
31. Hewitt RL, Grablowsky OM: Acute traumatic dissect-

ing aneurysm of the abdominal aorta. Ann Surg 171:160, 1970

32. Subcommittee on Reporting Standards for Arterial Aneurysms: Suggested standards for reporting on arterial aneurysms. J Vasc Surg 13:444, 1991

33. Sterpetti AV, Hunter WJ, Schultz RD: Congenital abdominal aortic aneurysms in the young. J Vasc Surg 7:763, 1988

34. Orron DE, Kim D: Arteriographic evaluation of peripheral aneurysmal disease. p. 141. In Kim D, Orron DE (eds): Peripheral Vascular Imaging and Intervention. Mosby Year Book, St. Louis, 1991

35. Sarkar R, Coran AG, Cilley RE et al: Arterial aneurysms in children: clinicopathologic classification. J Vasc Surg 13:47, 1991

36. Sarkar R, Cilley RE, Coran AG: Abdominal aneurysms in childhood: report of a case and review of the literature. Surgery 109:143, 1991

37. Bartlett ST, McCarthy WJ, Palmer AS et al: Multiple aneurysms in Behçet's disease. Arch Surg 123:1004, 1988

38. Boike GM, Gove N, Dombroswki MP et al: Mycotic aneurysms in pregnancy. Am J Obstet Gynecol 157:340, 1987

39. Spittel JA, Spittel PC: Aneurysms. p. 307. In Young JR, Graor RA, Olin JW, Bartholomew JR (eds): Peripheral Vascular Diseases. CV Mosby, St. Louis, 1991

40. Reilly JM, Tilson MD: Incidence and etiology of abdominal aortic aneurysms. Surg Clin North Am 69:705, 1989

41. Johnston KW, Scobie TK: Multicenter prospective study of nonruptured abdominal aortic aneurysms. I. Population and operative management. J Vasc Surg 7:69, 1988

42. Dobrin P: Pathophysiology and pathogenesis of aortic aneurysms. Surg Clin North Am 69:687, 1989

43. Bower TC, Cherry KJ, Pairolero PC: Unusual manifestations of abdominal aortic aneurysms. Surg Clin North Am 69:745, 1989

44. Quill DS, Colgan MP, Sumner DS: Ultrasonic screening for the detection of abdominal aortic aneurysms. Surg Clin North Am 69:713, 1989

45. La Roy LL, Cormier PJ, Matalon TA et al: Imaging of abdominal aortic aneurysms. AJR 152:785, 1989

46. Nuno IN, Collins GM, Bardin JA et al: Should aortography be used routinely in the elective management of abdominal aortic aneurysm? Am J Surg 144:53, 1982

47. Brewster DC, Retana A, Waltman AC et al: Angiography in the management of aneurysms of the abdominal aorta. N Engl J Med 292:822, 1975

48. Rosch J, Keller FS, Porter JM et al: Value of angiography in the management of abdominal aortic aneurysm. Cardiovasc Radiol 1:83, 1978

49. Richardson JW, Greenfield LJ: Natural history and management of iliac aneurysms. J Vasc Surg 8:165, 1988

50. Brunkwall J, Hauksson H, Bengtsson H et al: Solitary aneurysms of the iliac arterial system: an estimate of their frequency of occurrence. J Vasc Surg 10:381, 1989

51. Krupski WC, Bass A, Rosenberg GD et al: The elusive isolated hypogastric artery aneurysm: novel presentations. J Vasc Surg 10:557, 1989

52. Szilagyi DE, Schwartz RL, Reddy DJ: Popliteal artery aneurysms: their natural history and management. Arch Surg 116:724, 1981

53. Bouhoutsos J, Martin P: Popliteal aneurysm: a review of 116 cases. Br J Surg 61:469, 1974

54. Farina C, Cavallaro A, Schults RD et al: Popliteal aneurysms. Surg Gynecol Obstet 169:7, 1989

55. Flanigan DP: Aneurysms of the peripheral arteries. p. 325. In Moore WS (ed): Vascular Surgery: A Comprehensive Review. WB Saunders, Philadelphia, 1991

56. Bowyer RC, Cawthorn SJ, Walker WJ et al: Conservative management of asymptomatic popliteal aneurysm. Br J Surg 77:1132, 1990

57. Shortell CK, DeWeese JA, Ouriel K et al: Popliteal artery aneurysms: a 25-year surgical experience. J Vasc Surg 14:771, 1991

58. Dawson I, van Bockel H, Brand R et al: Popliteal artery aneurysms: long-term follow-up of aneurysmal disease and results of surgical treatment. J Vasc Surg 13:398, 1991

59. Lilly MP, Flinn WR, McCarthy WJ et al: The effect of distal arterial anatomy on the success of popliteal aneurysm repair. J Vasc Surg 7:653, 1988

60. Schellack J, Smith RB, Perdue GD: Nonoperative management of selected popliteal aneurysms. Arch Surg 122:372, 1987

61. Rizzo RJ, Flinn WR, Yao JST et al: Computed tomography for evaluation of arterial disease in the popliteal fossa. J Vasc Surg 11:112, 1990

62. Engel A, Adler OB, Carmeli R: Subclavian artery aneurysm caused by cervical rib: case report and review. Cardiovasc Intervent Radiol 12:92, 1989

63. Austin EH, Wolfe WG: Aneurysm of aberrant right subclavian artery with a review of the literature. J Vasc Surg 2:571, 1985

64. Barabas AP: Vascular complication in the Ehlers-Danlos syndrome with special reference to the "arterial type" or Sack's syndrome. J Cardiovasc Surg 13:160, 1969

65. Kadir S: Arteriography of the upper extremity. p. 172. In Kadir S: Diagnostic Angiography. WB Saunders, Philadelphia, 1986

66. Hobson RW, Isreal MR, Lynch TG: Axillosubclavian arterial aneurysms. p. 435. In Bergan JJ, Yao JST (eds): Aneurysms Diagnosis and Treatment. Grune & Stratton, Orlando, Fl, 1982

67. Randall PA, Omar MM, Rohner R et al: Arteria magna revisited. Radiology 132:295, 1979

68. Porter JM, Taylor LM, Harris EJ: Nonatherosclerotic vascular disease. p. 97. In Moore WS (ed): Vascular Surgery: A Comprehensive Review. WB Saunders, Philadelphia, 1991

69. Adamson AS, Pittam MR, Darke SG: Atheroembolism presenting as selective muscle embolization. J Cardiovasc Surg 32:705, 1991

70. Henderson MJ, Manhire AR: Case report: cholesterol

embolization following angiography. Clin Radiol 42:281, 1990

71. Ramchandani P, Morris MC, Zeit RM: Acute limb ischemia due to arterial embolism of tumor. Cardiovasc Intervent Radiol 13:372, 1990

72. Rubin BG, Barzilai B, Allen BT et al: Detection of the source of arterial emboli by transesophageal echocardiography: a case report. J Vasc Surg 15:573, 1992

73. Abbott WM, Maloney Rd, McCabe CC et al: Arterial embolism: a 44 year perspective. Arch Surg 143:460, 1982

74. Blaisdell FW, Steele M, Allen RE: Management of acute lower extremity arterial ischemia due to embolism and thrombosis. Surgery 84:822, 1978

75. Yeager RA, Moneta GL, Taylor LM et al: Surgical management of severe acute lower extremity ischemia. J Vasc Surg 15:385, 1992

76. Savelyev VS, Zatevakhin II, Stepanov NV: Artery embolism of the upper limbs. Surgery 81:367, 1977

77. Cambria RP, Abbott WM: Acute arterial thrombosis of the lower extremity: its natural history contrasted with arterial embolism. Arch Surg 119:784, 1984

78. Cormier J, Amrane M, Ward A et al: Arterial complications of the thoracic outlet syndrome: fifty-five operative cases. J Vasc Surg 9:778, 1989

79. Dennis JW, Frykberg ER, Crump JM et al: New perspectives on the management of penetrating trauma in proximity to major limb arteries. J Vasc Surg 11:85, 1990

80. Lipchik EO, Kaebick HW, Beres JJ et al: The role of arteriography in acute penetrating trauma to the extremities. Cardiovasc Intervent Radiol 10:202, 1987

81. Weaver FA, Yellin AE, Bauer M et al: Is arterial proximity a valid indication for arteriography in penetrating extremity trauma? Arch Surg 125:1256, 1990

82. Reid JD, Redman HC, Weigelt JA et al: Wounds of the extremities in proximity to major arteries: value of angiography in the detection of arterial injury. AJR 151:1035, 1988

83. Feliciano DV, Cruse PA, Burch JM et al: Delayed diagnosis of arterial injury. Am J Surg 154:579, 1987

84. Roberts SR, Main D, Pinkerton J: Surgical therapy of femoral artery pseudoaneurysm after angiography. Am J Surg 154:676, 1987

85. Oweida SW, Roubin GS, Smith RB, Salam AA: Postcatheterization vascular complications associated with percutaneous transluminal coronary angioplasty. J Vasc Surg 12:310, 1990

86. Moran CG, Ruttley MST: Development of a false aneurysm following percutaneous transluminal angioplasty. Br J Surg 74:652, 1987

87. Skillman JJ, Kim D, Baim DS: Vascular complications of percutaneous femoral cardiac interventions. Arch Surg 123:1207, 1988

88. Cronenwett JL, Walsh DB, Garrett HE: Tibial artery pseudoaneurysms: delayed complication of balloon catheter embolectomy. J Vasc Surg 8:483, 1988

89. Beck DE, Robison JG, Hallett JW: Popliteal artery pseudoaneurysm following arthroscopy. J Trauma 26:87, 1986

90. McAuley CE, Steed DL, Webster MW: Arterial complications of total knee replacement. Arch Surg 119:960, 1984

91. White RA, Scher LA, Samson RH, Veith FJ: Peripheral vascular injuries associated with falls from heights. J Trauma 27:411, 1987

92. Brunsting LA, Ouriel K: Traumatic fracture of the abdominal aorta with minimal trauma. J Vasc Surg 8:184, 1988

93. Shoenfeld NA, Stuchin SA, Pearl R, Haveson S: The management of vascular injuries associated with total hip arthroplasty. J Vasc Surg 11:549, 1990

94. Giacchetto J, Gallagher JJ: False aneurysm of the common femoral artery secondary to migration of a threaded acetabular component: a case report and review of the literature. Clin Orthop 231:91, 1988

95. Mitchell DG, Needleman, Bezzi M et al: Femoral artery pseudoaneurysms: diagnosis with conventional duplex and color doppler US. Radiology 165:687, 1987

96. Coughlin BF, Paushter DM: Peripheral pseudoaneurysms: evaluation with duplex US. Radiology 168:339, 1988

97. Norris CS, Zlotnick R, Silva WE, Wheeler HB: Traumatic pseudoaneurysm following blunt trauma. J Trauma 26:480, 1986

98. Cone JB: Vascular injury associated with fracture-dislocation of the lower extremity. Clin Orthop 243:30, 1989

99. Downs AR, MacDonald P: Popliteal artery injuries: civilian experience with sixty-three patients during a twenty-four year period (1960–1984). J Vasc Surg 4:55, 1986

100. Shields L, Mital M, Cave EF: Complete dislocation of the knee: experience at the Massachusetts General Hospital. J Trauma 9:3, 1969

101. Green NE, Allen BL: Vascular injuries associated with dislocations of the knee. J Bone Joint Surg 59A:236, 1977

102. Lefrak EA: Knee dislocation. Arch Surg 111:1021, 1976

103. Snyder WH: Popliteal and shank arterial injury. Surg Clin North Am 68:787, 1988

104. Davidson JT: Peroneal arteriovenous fistula: a complication of Fogarty catheter thromboembolectomy. Am Surg 55:616, 1989

105. Shah DM, Corson JD, Karmody AM et al: Optimal management of tibial artery trauma. J Trauma 28:228, 1988

106. Borman KR, Snyder WH, Weigelt JA: Civilian arterial trauma of the upper extremity. an 11 year experience in 267 patients. Am J Surg 148:796, 1984

107. Myers SI, Harward TR, Maher DP et al: Complex upper extremity vascular trauma in an urban population. J Vasc Surg 12:305, 1990

108. McCready RA, Procter CD, Hyde GL: Subclavian-axillary vascular trauma. J Vasc Surg 3:24, 1986

109. Linscheid RL, Wheeler DK: Elbow dislocations. JAMA 194:1171, 1965
110. Kadir S: Arteriography of the upper extremity. p. 172. In Kadir S (ed): Diagnostic Angiography. WB Saunders, Philadelphia, 1986
111. Conn J, Bergan JJ, Bell JL: Hypothenar hammer syndrome: posttraumatic digital ischemia. Surgery 68:1122, 1970
112. Latshaw RF, Weidner WA: Ulnar artery aneurysms: angiographic considerations in 2 cases. AJR 131:1093, 1978
113. Rose SC, Moore EE: Angiography in patients with arterial trauma: correlation between angiographic abnormalities, operative findings, and clinical outcome. AJR 149:613, 1987
114. Armstrong K, Sfeir R, Rice J et al: Popliteal vascular injuries and war: are Beirut and New Orleans similar? J Trauma 28:836, 1988
115. Fauci AS, Haynes BF, Katz P: The spectrum of vasculitis. Ann Intern Med 89:660, 1978
116. Porter JM, Snider RL, Bardana EJ et al: The diagnosis and treatment of Raynaud's phenomenon. Surgery 77:11, 1975
117. Yao JST, Neiman HL: Occlusive arterial disease below the inguinal ligament. p. 109. In Neiman HL, Yao JST (eds): Angiography of Vascular Disease. Churchill Livingstone, New York, 1985
118. Lie JT: Buerger's disease and inflammatory aspects of atherosclerosis. Curr Opinion Rheumatol 2:76, 1990
119. Matsushita M, Shionoya S, Matsumoto T: Urinary cotinine measurement in patients with Buerger's disease —effects of active and passive smoking on the disease process. J Vasc Surg 14:53, 1991
120. Abdullah AN, Keczkes K: Thromboangiitis obliterans (Burger's disease) in a woman—a case report and review of the literature. Clin Exp Dermatol 15:46, 1990
121. Giblin WJ, James WDE, Benson PM: Buerger's disease. Int J Dermatol 28:638, 1989
122. Hagen B, Lahse S: Clinical and radiological aspects of Buerger's disease. Cardiovasc Intervent Radiol 7:283, 1984
123. Kadir S: Arteriography of the lower extremity vessels. p. 254. In: Diagnostic Angiography. WB Saunders, Philadelphia, 1986
124. Lie JT: The rise and fall and resurgence of thromboangiitis obliterans (Buerger's disease). Jpn Soc Pathol 39:153, 1989
125. Demas BE, Heelan RT, Lane J et al: Soft-tissue sarcomas of the extremities: comparison of MR and CT in determining the extent of disease. AJR 150:615, 1988
126. Sundaram M, McGuire MH, Herbold DR et al: Magnetic resonance imaging in planning limb salvage surgery for primary malignant tumors of bone. J Bone Joint Surg 68A:809, 1986
127. McLean G, Freiman DB: Angiography of skeletal disease. Orthop Clin North Am 14:257, 1983
128. Mitty HA, Hermann G, Abdelwahab IF et al: Role of angiography in limb-tumor surgery. Radiographics 11:1029, 1991
129. Kadir S: Neoplasms and neoplasm-like conditions of the extremities, shoulders, and pelvis. p. 323. In: Diagnostic Angiography. WB Saunders, Philadelphia, 1986
130. Kadir S, Athanasoulis CA, Waltman AC: Tolazoline augmented arteriography in the evaluation of bone and soft tissue tumors. Radiology 133:792, 1979
131. Love JW, Whelan TJ: Popliteal artery entrapment syndrome. Am J Surg 109:620, 1965
132. Greenwood LH, Hallett JW, Yrizarry JM et al: The angiographic evaluation of lower-extremity arterial disease in the young adult. Cardiovasc Intervent Radiol 8:183, 1985
133. Persky JM, Kempczinski RF, Fowl RJ: Entrapment of the popliteal artery. Surg Gynecol Obstet 173:84, 1991
134. Collins PS, McDonald PT, Lim RC: Popliteal artery entrapment: an evolving syndrome. J Vasc Surg 10:484, 1989
135. Biemans RGM, van Bockel JH. Popliteal artery entrapment syndrome. Surg Gynecol Obstet 144:604, 1977
136. Rich NM, Collins GJ, McDonald PT et al: Popliteal vascular entrapment: its increasing interest. Arch Surg 114:1377, 1979
137. Hallett JW, Greenwood LH, Robison JG: Lower extremity arterial disease in young adults: a systematic approach to early diagnosis. Ann Surg 202:647, 1985
138. Berg-Johnsen J, Holter O: Popliteal entrapment syndrome. Acta Chir Scand 150:493, 1984
139. McDonald PT, Easterbrook JA, Rich NM et al: Popliteal artery entrapment syndrome: clinical, non-invasive and angiographic diagnosis. Am J Surg 139:318, 1980
140. Fong H, Downs AR: Popliteal artery entrapment syndrome with distal embolization. J Cardiovasc Surg 30:85, 1989
141. Muller N, Morris D, Nichols DM: Popliteal artery entrapment demonstrated by CT. Radiology 151:157, 1984
142. Rizzo RJ, Flinn WR, Yao JST et al: Computed tomography for evaluation of arterial disease in the popliteal fossa. J Vasc Surg 11:112, 1990
143. Kadir S: Arteriography of the upper extremity. p. 172. In: Diagnostic Angiography. WB Saunders, Philadelphia, 1986
144. Yao JST, Bergan JJ, Neiman HL: Arteriography for upper-extremity and digital ischemia. p. 353. In Neiman HL, Yao JST (eds): Angiography of Vascular Disease. Churchill Livingstone, New York, 1985
145. Cormier J, Amrane M, Ward A et al: Arterial complications of the thoracic outlet syndrome: fifty-five operative cases. J Vasc Surg 9:778, 1989
146. McAnespey D, Rosen RC, Cohen JM et al: Adventitial cystic disease. J Foot Surg 30:160, 1991
147. Gray BH, Young JR, Olin JW: Miscellaneous arterial diseases. p. 379. In Young JR, Graor RA, Olin JW, Bartholomew JR (eds): Peripheral Vascular Diseases. CV Mosby, St. Louis, 1991
148. Ishikawa K: Cystic adventitial disease of the popliteal artery and of other stem vessels in the extremities. Jpn J Surg 17:221, 1987
149. Paty PSK, Kaufman JL, Koslow AR et al: Adventitial

cystic disease of the femoral vein: a case report and review of the literature. J Vasc Surg 15:214, 1992

150. Jasinski RW, Masselink BA, Partridge RW et al: Adventitial cystic disease of the popliteal artery. Radiology 163:153, 1987

151. Wilbur AC, Woelfel GF, Meyer JP et al: Adventitial cystic disease of the popliteal artery. Radiology 155:63, 1985

152. Lossef SV, Rajan S, Calcagno D et al: Spontaneous rupture of an adventitial cyst of the popliteal artery: confirmation with MR imaging. JVIR 3:95, 1992

153. Melliere D, Ecollan P, Kassab M et al: Adventitial cystic disease of the popliteal artery: treatment by cyst removal. J Vasc Surg 8:638, 1988

154. Wilbur AC, Spigos DG: Adventitial cyst of the popliteal artery: CT-guided percutaneous aspiration. J Comput Assist Tomogr 10:161, 1986

155. Owen ERTC, Speechly-Dick EM, Kour NW et al: Cystic advential disease of the popliteal artery—a case of spontaneous resolution. Eur J Vasc Surg 4:319, 1990

156. Luscher TF, Lie JT, Stanson AW et al: Arterial fibromuscular dysplasia. Mayo Clin Proc 62:931, 1987

157. Iwai T, Konno S, Hiejima K et al: Fibromuscular dysplasia in the extremities. J Cardiovasc Surg 26:496, 1985

158. Harrison EJ, McCormack LJ: Pathologic classification of renal arterial disease in renovascular hypertension. Mayo Clin Proc 46:161, 1971

159. Rushton AR. The genetics of fibromuscular dysplasia. Arch Intern Med 140:233, 1980

160. van denDungen JJAM, Oosterhuis JW: Femoropopliteal arterial fibrodysplasia. Br J Surg 77:396, 1990

161. Walter JF, Stanley JC, Mehigan JT et al: External iliac artery fibrodysplasia. AJR 131:125, 1978

162. Bongard O, Bounameaux H: Severe iatrogenic ergotism: incidence and clinical importance. Vasa 20:153, 1991

163. Schulman EA, Rosenberg SB: Claudication: an unusual side effect of DHE administration. Headache 31:237, 1991

164. Seifert KB, Blackshear WM, Cruse CW et al: Bilateral upper extremity ischemia after administration of dihydroergotamine-heparin for prophylaxis of deep venous thrombosis. J Vasc Surg 8:410, 1988

165. Tanner JR: St. Anthony's fire, then and now: a case report and historical review. Can J Surg 30:291, 1987

166. Ashenburg RJ, Phillips DA: Ergotism as a consequence of thromboembolic prophylaxis. Radiology 170:375, 1989

167. Wickbom I, Bartley O: Arterial "spasm" in peripheral arteriography using the catheter method. Acta Radiol 47:433, 1957

168. Koehler R: Regular alternating changes in arterial width in lower limb angiograms. Acta Radiol 3:529, 1965

169. Mayall GF: A model for the study of stationary arterial waves. Clin Radiol 17:84, 1966

170. Vallance R, Quin RO, Forrest H: Arterio-venous shunting complicating atherosclerotic peripheral vascular disease. Clin Radiol 37:389, 1986

171. Silbert S, Lippmann HI: Monckeberg's arteriosclerosis. JAMA 151:1176, 1953

172. Lachman AS, Spray TL, Kerwin DM et al: Medial calcinosis of Monckeberg. Am J Med 63:615, 1977

173. Wilkinson SP, Stewart WK, Parham DM, Guthrie W: Symmetric gangrene of the extremities in late renal failure; a case report and review of the literature. Q J Med 67:319, 1988

174. Moran JJ: Idiopathic arterial calcification of infancy: a clinicopathologic study. Pathol Annu 10:393, 1975

14

Imaging of Acquired Thoracic and Abdominal Aortic Disease

Janette D. Durham

John A. Kaufman

Aortography has been established as the "gold standard" for imaging acquired diseases of the aorta because of its accuracy in detecting vascular disease. The invasive nature of the procedure and its cost have prompted a search for less invasive tests, both to screen patients for vascular disease prior to aortography and to replace aortography. Chest radiography, ultrasound, computed tomography (CT), and magnetic resonance imaging (MRI) all have some potential value in diagnosing aortic aneurysm, traumatic aortic rupture (TAR), aortic dissection, and aortic occlusive disease. Prospective comparative investigations of accuracy, cost, and morbidity of imaging modalities to diagnose aortic disease are scarce, however, and the ultimate role of each imaging technique has yet to be defined.

In the absence of these data, we summarize here our preliminary impressions of the appropriateness of various imaging tests for aortic disease using the following information: the pathophysiology of the suspected disease; the patient's clinical presentation and need for intervention; the imaging information needed to initiate therapy; and the potential for an imaging test to yield an accurate diagnosis and answer the necessary questions to direct therapy.

IMAGING TECHNIQUES

Radiography

The first suspicion of aortic pathology frequently arises when, during evaluation of patients for other medical problems, chest or abdomen films are obtained that suggest aortic disease. Despite the low sensitivity and specificity of plain radiographs for aortic disease, the low patient risk (Table 14-1), short time requirement (Table 14-2), and low dollar cost (Table 14-3) of radiographs, combined with the ability to look for associated cardiopulmonary or abdominal disease that may affect subsequent evaluation, make radiography a reasonable first step. To evaluate the aorta, two perpendicular projections are obtained, typically posteroanterior and lateral views. The examination is limited to the evaluation of the contour of the aorta, calcification in the aortic wall, adjacent structures, and associated soft tissue.

Ultrasound

Evaluation of the aorta can not be performed by a single ultrasound technique; a combination of transab-

Table 14-1   Incidence of Morbidity with Aortic Imaging Studies

Imaging Modality	Risks

Radiographs
  AP chest
	Radiation exposure
	  10–15 mR

Lateral chest	35–60 mR
AP abdomen	400–600 mR
Ultrasound Transabdominal	None
Transthoracic	None
Transesophageal	Cardiac arrhythmias during placement of endoscope

Computed tomography	Radiation exposure: 1–2 rads uniform through slice
	Intravenous contrast
	  Renal failure, 2%
	
	  Reactions:
	    All, 2–14%
	    Severe, including death, 0.01–0.1%

Magnetic resonance imaging
Aortography
	None
	Radiation exposure
	  Conventional, 2–3 R
	  Digital, 8–24 R
	
	Intra-arterial contrast
	  Renal failure, 2%
	  Reactions: same as or less than with IV contrast
	
	Transfemoral access complications: hematoma, arterial thrombosis, arteriovenous fistula, pseudoaneurysm, amputation, 0.47–1.7%
	
	Systemic complications: cardiac, neurologic, seizures, 0.55–0.91%
	
	Death, 0.03–0.09%

dominal, transthoracic (TTE), and transesophageal (TEE) echocardiographic techniques is used to evaluate the aorta in its entirety. Transabdominal ultrasound is restricted to the evaluation of the infrarenal aorta in most patients, as the iliac arteries are usually not visualized. When bowel gas obscures the retroperitoneum or the patient is obese, visualization of the abdominal aorta may also be limited. TTE can be used to evaluate the ascending aorta; the extent of aorta that can be evaluated depends on the acoustic window through the thorax. This window is obscured by an abnormal chest wall configuration, narrow intercostal spaces, obesity, pulmonary emphysema, and mechanical ventilation. The descending aorta is not well visualized by TTE, but the recent addition of TEE has vastly

Table 14-2   Time for Completion of Emergency Examination

Imaging Modality	Minutes
Radiographs	10
Transabdominal ultrasound	15–30
Transesophageal ultrasound	15
Computed tomography	15–60
Magnetic resonance imaging	30–60
Aortography	
Conventional	70
Digital	40

Table 14-3   Relative Cost of Imaging Modalities

Modality	Cost ($)
Radiographs	100
Transabdominal ultrasound	300
Transesophageal ultrasound	700
Computed tomography	800
Magnetic resonance imaging	1000
Aortography	1000

improved the sensitivity of ultrasound for aortic pathology involving the descending aorta. TEE allows evaluation of the ascending and descending thoracic aorta, except for a small segment of the aorta that is obscured by the trachea and proximal left bronchus. The abdominal aorta cannot be visualized by this technique. TEE is somewhat more invasive than the other ultrasound examinations since esophageal intubation is required. The patient is mildly sedated for the examination, and cardiac arrhythmias account for minimal morbidity.

More than any other aortic imaging test that has been described, ultrasound is operator-dependent. Diagnostic examinations and accurate diagnoses require highly skilled operators, both technologists and physicians, who must have considerable ultrasound and vascular expertise to provide accurate diagnoses. The variability in this aspect of the examination must be kept in mind when considering an imaging approach to a specific clinical situation.

Computed Tomography

The decreased scanning times of new-generation CT machines allows rapid evaluation of the entire chest in patients with dissection and aortic rupture or of the chest and abdomen in patients with aortic aneurysm. Evaluation is performed by dynamic incremental scanning with 5- to 10-mm scan collimation 15 to 30 seconds after mechanical injection of 1 to 2 ml/s of ionic or nonionic contrast agent.

Although CT is less operator-dependent than ultrasound, patient cooperation is critical to a good study, and patient movement must be minimized. As many as 10 percent of studies in trauma patients may be inadequate, due primarily to motion artifacts. Apparatus exterior to the chest or abdomen, including chest leads, nasogastric tubes, and respiratory equipment should be removed and the arms positioned above the head to avoid artifacts. Accurate interpretation requires viewing of the images at multiple window and level settings in order to optimally evaluate calcification, thrombus, and contrast enhancement. This is particularly important in the evaluation of aortic dissection.

A major disadvantage of CT is the need for intravenous contrast administration, which adds the risk of renal failure and contrast reaction to an imaging study.[1-3] The ability to image in the axial plane only introduces errors due to volume averaging and limits the sensitivity and specificity of the examination. As the quality of computer reconstructions of other imaging planes improves, this limitation will decrease in importance.

Magnetic Resonance Imaging and Magnetic Resonance Angiography

While magnetic resonance techniques, including both MRI and magnetic resonance angiography (MRA), are still in their infancy, their role in the diagnosis of aortic disease is evolving rapidly. Axial spin echo image acquisition is used most frequently to evaluate the aorta. Imaging in oblique, sagittal, and coronal planes allows large-field-of-view imaging, with better examination of the aortic root and proximal descending aorta than can be accomplished with CT. Gradient echo image acquisition can be used to enhance flow velocities and help distinguish slow flow from thrombus. Cardiac gating is employed to eliminate phase-encoding artifacts from cardiac motion and breathing. Examination time is dependent on the number of acquisitions obtained, but 30 to 60 minutes is typical.

Pacemakers, intracranial aneurysm clips, and intraocular metallic fragments are absolute contraindications to MRI. Patient motion, inability to cooperate, and cardiac arrhythmias detract from the examination. MRI involves no risk to a patient being studied electively. Because of logistical issues regarding the narrow diameter of most MRI scanner bores and strong magnetic fields, MRI evaluation at the present time is restricted to stable patients, who do not require cardiac or respiratory monitoring. The cost of MRI in most institutions approaches or exceeds that of aortography, so its usefulness as a *screening* test will depend on the frequency with which aortography is avoided.

Aortography

Conventional aortography is performed most often from a femoral approach using 5 to 7 French catheters. In patients with extensive iliac occlusive disease, a transaxillary or transbrachial route is chosen. Translumbar aortography is reserved for the rare patient with occlusion of all peripheral access, since translumbar access more frequently results in suboptimal studies and tends to increase patient discomfort.

Two views of the aorta are routinely obtained in order to visualize all borders of the aorta en face. The thoracic aorta is most commonly imaged by using 45-degree right posterior oblique and straight anteroposterior (AP) or 10-degree left posterior oblique projections, following injection of 60 to 70 ml of ionic or nonionic contrast. The abdominal aorta is imaged in AP and lateral projections by using 40 to 60 ml of contrast. In most patients filming must be done at the rate of three films per second or higher to adequately visualize the thoracic aorta and two films per second to visualize the abdominal aorta. Flow through aneurysms may be dramatically slow and extended filming programs and larger volumes of contrast may be required.

Intra-arterial digital aortography has replaced conventional filming in many situations, reducing the required catheter size to 4 to 5 French, reducing contrast volume to 30 to 50 ml, and increasing the speed of examination. Although digital imaging results in some loss of resolution and is further compromised by patient movement, it may replace or complement conventional aortography in many cases, depending on the need for fine detail. Intravenous digital aortography has been abandoned as a routine approach because of inferior resolution and the large volume of contrast required as compared with arterial studies. Digital subtraction imaging after venous injection may allow adequate visualization of anatomy in patients who have no peripheral arterial access and in whom translumbar access is contraindicated. This technique depends on adequate cardiac function and is not well tolerated in patients with coronary ischemia.

Catheterization complications, even in the hands of radiologists in training, are surprisingly infrequent (2 to 3 percent). Puncture site hematomas, the most frequent complication, are most often inconsequential. If an axillary approach is used, local complications may have more impact because of the possibility of a compressive neuropathy of the brachial plexus. Contrast-induced renal failure is the most common serious adverse outcome following aortography and can be expected in 2 to 5 percent of patients.

AORTIC ANEURYSMS

A bulge in the wall of a blood vessel, whether localized or diffuse, is an aneurysm. *True* aneurysms histologically retain all three layers of vessel wall, including intima, media, and adventitia. Enlargement occurs symmetrically as a result of weakening of the media and is either fusiform or cylindrical. *False* aneurysms have an incomplete wall owing to disruption of one or more of the three layers; they tend to be localized, enlarge asymmetrically, and are described as saccular. The term *dissecting* aneurysm is a misnomer. Aortic dissection occurs when blood obtains access to and dissects the medial layer of an artery, resulting in two parallel vascular channels. Although enlargement of the false channel may result in overall enlargement of the aortic diameter, the etiology, structural abnormality, and treatment of aortic dissection are distinct from those of aneurysmal disease (Figs. 14-1 and 14-2).

The most common etiology for aneurysms is atherosclerosis or medial degeneration of unknown etiology with superimposed atherosclerosis.[4,5] Trauma, discussed separately, is the second most common etiology; medial cystic degeneration, infection, and syphilis are less common. Both the configuration and the location of aneurysms help in determining etiology.[6]

Atherosclerotic aneurysms most frequently involve the infrarenal aorta, typically in elderly men. Thoracic aortic aneurysms are much less common and occur in the descending aorta distal to the left subclavian artery. These patients commonly have associated abdominal aneurysms. Atherosclerotic aneurysms tend to be fusiform in configuration, although they may have a saccular appearance in up to 20 percent of patients. When dense perianeurysmal fibrosis surrounds a thickened aneurysmal wall, the aneurysm is described as inflammatory, a finding that complicates surgical repair.[7]

A focal aneurysm of the proximal descending aorta at the aortic isthmus is typically a chronic traumatic aneurysm from remote blunt chest trauma. With time, these initially irregular, false aneurysms develop secondary atherosclerosis, resulting in smooth intimal calcification. The saccular, localized appearance, the location at the aortic isthmus, and a history of trauma help to identify the etiology.[8]

Aneurysms of the aortic sinus and tubular ascending

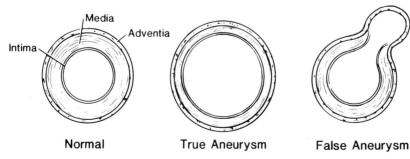

Figure 14-1 The media in a true aneurysm becomes atrophic, allowing the entire wall to dilate. When the aortic wall is disrupted, a false aneurysm, contained by adventitial or surrounding soft tissue, results. Aortic dissection results in overall vascular enlargement because blood dissects and distends the media, with compression of the true aortic lumen. (Adapted from LaRoy et al.,[12] with permission.)

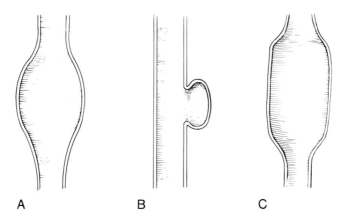

Figure 14-2 The common shapes of aortic aneurysms are **(A)** fusiform, **(B)** saccular, and **(C)** cylindrical.

aorta are usually the result of cystic medial necrosis, either of genetic etiology, due to Marfan's or Ehlers-Danlos syndrome, or idiopathic. Typically fusiform enlargement of the ascending aorta is present, with sparing of the arch. These true aneurysms have little calcification, involve the sinuses of Valsalva symmetrically, and often result in aortic insufficiency. They are frequently complicated by dissection.

Infectious aneurysms occur when injured intima secondary to atherosclerosis, trauma, surgery, or catheterization is exposed to bacteria. Patients who are immunocompromised, those who use intravenous drugs, and those with bacterial endocarditis are at risk. Infection occurs by embolization, contiguous spread from an extra- or intravascular source, or lymphangitic spread. The infection eventually destroys the elastic lamella, media, and adventitia. Infectious aneurysms may be true or false aneurysms, depending on the degree of wall destruction. They are commonly saccular and are located in the ascending aorta in proximity to an infected heart valve.

Syphilitic aneurysms are uncommon inflammatory aneurysms, which develop 10 to 30 years after infection. They are thick-walled true aneurysms resulting from chronic inflammation, which weakens the media. They tend to be asymmetric, saccular aneurysms with "pencil-line" thin calcification of the aortic wall and perianeurysmal fibrosis. The intima has a characteristic irregular appearance termed *tree barking.* The ascending aorta, arch, and proximal descending aorta are involved with equal frequency. The aortic sinuses can be involved asymmetrically.

Indications for Imaging

Imaging of nontraumatic thoracic aortic aneurysms is performed for four indications: diagnosis and surveillance of asymptomatic aneurysms, preoperative evaluation of asymptomatic aneurysms prior to elective repair, preoperative evaluation of symptomatic aneurysms prior to urgent or emergent repair, and follow-up after surgery for postoperative complications.

Diagnosis and Surveillance

Most patients with aortic aneurysms either are asymptomatic or have mild symptoms secondary to compression of adjacent structures. Diagnosis may be made on the basis of physical examination or during imaging performed for other indications. Specifically directed imaging is then performed to confirm the diagnosis; obtain an accurate aortic diameter; determine the configuration, location, and extent of the aneurysm; and assess for complications such as rupture. Surveillance imaging is conducted to identify enlargement of the aneurysm or complications that would prompt repair.

Elective Operative Repair

Elective repair of asymptomatic aneurysms is justified by the large difference in operative mortality between patients who undergo elective repair of unruptured aneurysms and those who undergo emergent surgery after rupture—5 versus 30 to 70 percent, respectively.[5,9] Furthermore, the risk of rupture rises substantially with increased aneurysm size.[10] In the ascending aorta, operative repair is recommended when an aneurysm becomes larger than 6 cm in diameter (i.e., twice the size of the adjacent aorta) or when there is a rapid increase in size. Abdominal aortic aneurysms are electively repaired when they reach 4 to 5 cm in diameter.[5,10]

Preoperative imaging is performed to ensure successful treatment with low morbidity and mortality. In order to plan the time of operation, the surgical approach, and the method of reconstruction, the following questions about the aneurysm must be answered: (1) What is its exact cranial and caudal extent? (2) What is the location with respect to the branch vessels, including the coronary, carotid, subclavian, mesenteric, and renal arteries? (3) What is the status of the aortic valve? (4) What is the size and the extent of mural thrombus? (5) What is the status of the downstream vessels? (6) What is the wall integrity? (7) Is there fluid or fibrosis in the periaortic space? (8) What other conditions or anatomic anomalies are present that might complicate surgery?

Urgent or Emergent Repair of Symptomatic Aneurysms

A symptomatic aneurysm implies complications or expansion heralding imminent or existent rupture. Complications of aneurysms include cardiac ischemia, aortic insufficiency, tracheal or esophageal compression, bone erosion, infection, and embolization.[11] Ascending aortic aneurysms rupture most commonly into the pericardium and pleural space, descending aortic aneurysms rupture into the pleural space, and abdominal aortic aneurysms rupture into the pararenal and perirenal spaces.[12]

Postoperative Complications

Postoperative complications following aneurysm repair include graft infection, false aneurysm formation, graft-enteric fistulae, and graft occlusion. Graft infections are usually subacute in nature but devastating in consequence, as cure requires excision of the contaminated prosthesis. False aneurysms may appear at any time, characteristically at anastomotic suture lines. Graft-enteric fistulae are difficult to image, presenting as episodic massive gastrointestinal bleeding. Graft occlusion may indicate an underlying structural abnormality or loss of adequate distal outflow. Late graft complications include aneurysmal degeneration of the graft itself, usually 10 or more years after placement.

Imaging Tests

Radiographs

Aneurysms of the thoracic aorta produce mediastinal masses, resulting in mediastinal widening. An ascending aortic aneurysm causes the right superior mediastinum to have a convex contour on frontal radiographs and fills the retrosternal space on lateral radiographs. Involvement of the aortic root is often not apparent. An arch aneurysm may result in an aortico-pulmonary window mass on a frontal projection,

which can be localized in the AP dimension on the lateral projection. A descending aortic aneurysm produces a mass to the left of the spine on frontal radiographs, widening and displacing the left paraspinal line to the left (Fig. 14-3). Intimal calcification helps identify the aortic wall. On the lateral chest radiograph, both borders of the descending aorta may be surrounded by lung, allowing visualization and measurement of the aortic diameter. Intimal calcification can be detected on abdominal radiographs in more than half of abdominal aneurysms. Complications of aneurysms, such as left ventricle enlargement from aortic insufficiency, tracheal compression, and bone erosion suggest the diagnosis.[12-14]

Ultrasound

Aneurysms of the ascending aorta can be visualized in most patients by TTE.[15] In addition, the aortic valve can be studied for vegetations, dilatation, or insufficiency. Pericardial fluid is reliably detected. A combination of TEE and TTE should improve the usefulness of ultrasound in diagnosis of descending thoracic aortic aneurysms, but to date experience is limited.

Infrarenal abdominal aortic aneurysms are easily identified, accurately measured, and readily followed in a cost-effective manner with transabdominal ultrasound, except when bowel gas obscures visualization or the patient is obese. Echogenic thrombus can be separated from the echolucent aortic lumen, and wall thickness can be measured (Fig. 14-4). The proximal and distal extent of the aneurysm is difficult to assess because of poor visualization of the descending aorta, suprarenal aorta, and iliac vessels. Although mesenteric and main renal artery origins can often be recognized, coexistent aneurysmal or occlusive disease is poorly assessed.[16,17]

Computed Tomography

Aneurysms are identified on CT images by focal or diffuse aortic dilatation extending over a variable length. Thrombus forms a circumferential crescent around the patent lumen and may be distinguished from the aortic lumen after contrast administration. The exact size at which the thoracic aorta becomes aneurysmal is somewhat arbitrary. Published normal measurements for the thoracic aorta by CT are 3.6 cm at the valve ring, 3.5 cm in the tubular ascending aorta, 2.6 cm in the proximal descending aorta, and 2.4 cm in the distal descending aorta.[18] An infrarenal abdominal aorta greater than 3 cm (normal range 1.6 to 1.9 cm) is considered aneurysmal by most authors.[19] A simplistic approach is the recognition that the aorta should de-

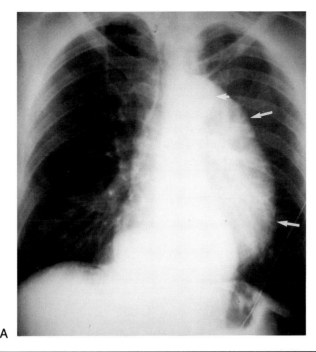

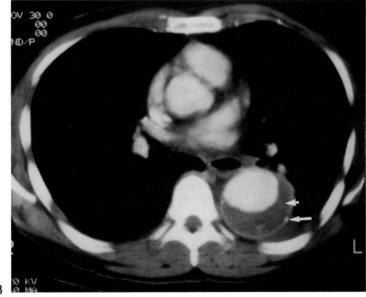

Figure 14-3 (**A**) An anteroposterior (AP) chest radiograph reveals a mediastinal mass *(arrows)*, which obliterates the left paraspinal line and the descending aorta. The aortic arch is distinct *(arrowhead)*. (**B**) A contrast-enhanced CT image reveals a large thoracoabdominal aneurysm. There is peripheral calcification in the aortic wall *(arrow)* and a large amount of intraluminal thrombus *(arrowhead)*. The ascending aorta is normal in size.

crease in size as it proceeds distally and any enlargement is pathologic. The diameter of the aorta may be overestimated on CT when aortic tortuosity results in the measured segment obliquely traversing the scan plane. Thin slices and long axis reconstructions can help overcome this limitation.[8]

CT is more sensitive than radiographs for intimal calcification. Localization of calcification peripherally helps to exclude the diagnosis of aortic dissection and strengthen the case for aneurysm. Displacement of intimal calcification centrally suggests dissection. Punctate calcification within aneurysm thrombus can confuse this distinction, and other findings must be used to make the differentiation.[8]

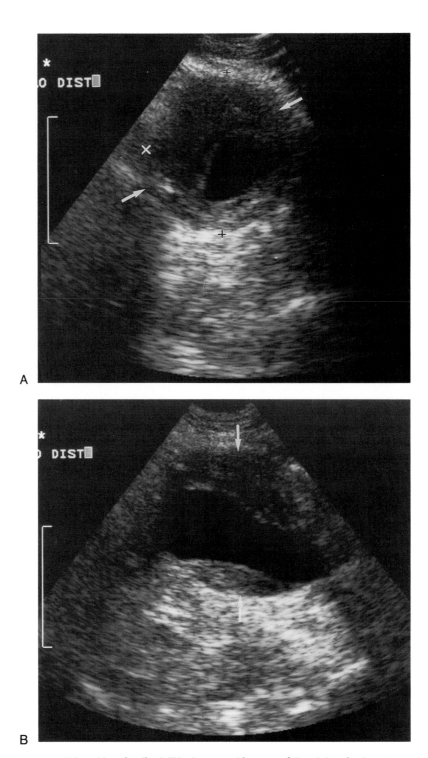

Figure 14-4 Transverse **(A)** and longitudinal **(B)** ultrasound images of the abdominal aorta reveal an infrarenal aneurysm. The crosshairs on the transverse image mark the AP (+) and transverse (x) diameters. There is a large amount of echogenic thrombus *(arrow)* surrounding the echolucent aortic lumen.

and distal extent of aneurysms with reference to branch vessels; however, aortic tortuosity resulting in oblique scan planes may make this finding problematic. Often the neck of the aneurysm cannot be confidently identified in relation to branch vessels, especially in suprarenal, juxtarenal, and thoracic aneurysms.[16] In the case of the rare ascending aortic aneurysm, the competence of the valve and the involvement of the coronary arteries cannot be assessed by CT. Similarly, extension of aneurysmal disease into the downstream vessels or concomitant occlusive disease of the iliac arteries cannot be diagnosed reliably. Significant improvements in

CT is superior to ultrasound in defining the proximal

CT evaluation of aneurysmal disease may be possible with dynamic scanning and three-dimensional volumetric reconstruction. This promising new technique may obviate the need for other imaging studies including aortography in many patients (Fig. 14-5).

Currently, the most important role of CT is evaluation of the periaortic space. CT allows the diagnosis of inflammatory, infected, or ruptured aneurysms by the demonstration of perianeurysmal soft tissue, fluid, and gas (Fig. 14-6).[20] Abnormalities of other retroperitoneal structures that can complicate surgery, such as congenital anomalies of the vena cava and kidneys, are also well demonstrated.

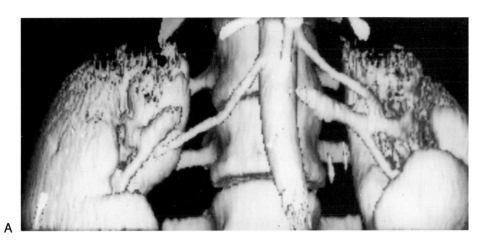

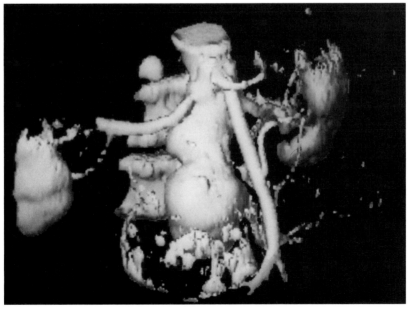

Figure 14-5 **(A)** Spiral computed tomography (CT) volumetric reconstruction demonstrates a relatively normal aorta, with a single renal artery on the right and two left renal arteries. There is an ostial stenosis of the lower pole, renal artery. **(B)** Spiral CT reconstruction shows an abdominal aortic aneurysm with mural thrombus and calcification of the outer wall. The superior mesenteric artery (SMA) crosses anteriorly over the aneurysm. The neck of aneurysm and its relationship to the renal arteries is well demonstrated. (Illustrations courtesy of Michael Dake, M.D., Stanford University.)

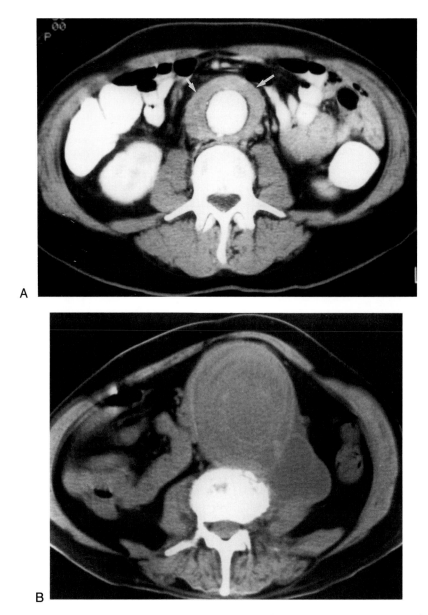

Figure 14-6 Axial computed tomography (CT) images in three patients demonstrate three different retroperitoneal processes: **(A)** smooth, concentric periaortic soft tissue that enhances *(arrows),* characteristic of an inflammatory aneurysm; **(B)** contained periaortic fluid, consistent with blood from a ruptured infrarenal aneurysm; *(Figure continues.)*

Magnetic Resonance Imaging

No large comparative studies are available that demonstrate a clear advantage of MRI over CT in the diagnosis and surveillance of aortic aneurysms; however, small aneurysms, missed by axial CT images, may be more accurately demonstrated by sagittal MRI views. The aortic root and ascending aorta are better visualized with MRI than with CT[21,22] (Fig. 14-7). A disadvantage of MRI is the loss of signal in the presence of calcification, an important distinguishing characteristic between aneurysms and dissection. MRA of aortic aneurysms is currently an investigational technique that holds promise of allowing not only accurate evaluation of the size and location of aneurysms but also demonstration of the inflow and outflow vasculature.

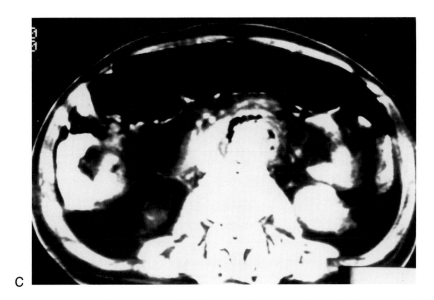

Figure 14-6 *(Continued.)* **(C)** gas and fluid surrounding an aortic graft, diagnostic of infection.

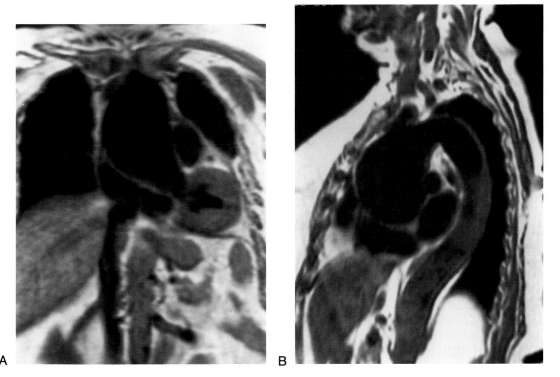

Figure 14-7 T_1-weighted **(A)** coronal and **(B)** sagittal magnetic resonance image (MRI) of a large ascending aortic aneurysm. There is excellent visualization of the aortic root, an area difficult to visualize with axial computed tomography (CT) imaging.

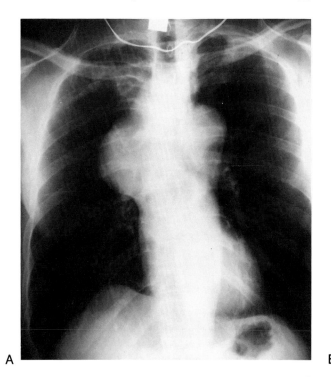
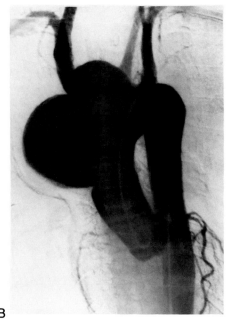

A

B

Figure 14-8 (A) An AP chest radiograph demonstrates a right mediastinal mass. **(B)** Aortography reveals a saccular aneurysm of the tubular ascending aorta, away from the valve. The appearance and location suggest the correct diagnosis, a syphilitic aneurysm.

Aortography

An aneurysm is demonstrated by aortography as a widened aortic lumen, either fusiform, cylindrical, or saccular (Fig. 14-8). Aortic plaque and thrombus result in irregularity of the vessel lumen. The angiographic size of the aneurysm can be misleading because only the patent lumen is demonstrated. Unopacified thrombus lining the aneurysm can mask its true size or obscure the aneurysm entirely. Identification of calcification in the aortic wall suggests the true diameter. Magnification, intrinsic to the technique, can be of the order of 30 percent.

Aortography provides a "road map" of the aorta, precisely displaying the extent and location of the aneurysm.[16,23,24] The origins of the coronary arteries, great vessels, and mesenteric and renal arteries are readily evaluated for involvement in the aneurysm. Absence of normal expected branch vessels, even if the aortic lumen is normal in size, can signal an aneurysm. Thoracic aneurysms such as those of the lumbar or intercostal arteries, are frequently associated with abdominal aneurysms, and abdominal aneurysms are associated with iliac and femoral aneurysms. Complete angiographic evaluation of the downstream vessels is necessary to determine the extent of reconstruction re-

quired.[16] In thoracic aneurysms, selective angiography of spinal cord blood supply is advocated by some to allow preoperative assessment of the risk of cord injury with surgery.[25]

Recommendations for Imaging Aortic Aneurysms

Diagnosis and Surveillance

Plain radiographic diagnosis is confirmed by axial imaging with ultrasound, CT, or MRI. The sensitivity, availability, and low cost of ultrasound support its use as the primary imaging test for this indication. When the clinical presentation or location suggests a complex aneurysm, CT or MRI should be performed to better define the aneurysm's extent and the periaortic space.

Preoperative Imaging of Asymptomatic Aneurysms

The tendency for atherosclerotic aneurysms to be confined to the infrarenal aorta, with only 2 to 7 percent of abdominal aneurysms extending to the juxtarenal or suprarenal area, has encouraged several authors to promote a selective approach to aortography in preoperative assessment.[26-28] Angiograms are obtained in addition to CT only in patients considered to be at high-risk (i.e., those with supra- or juxtarenal abdominal aortic aneurysms that are poorly evaluated by CT alone) and those who present with hypertension, renal dysfunction, visceral ischemia, or occlusive peripheral myocardial vascular disease. Complete cardiovascular evaluation at the time of operation is required; this should include stress or dipyridamole thallium studies, cardiac catheterization if indicated, noninvasive peripheral vascular testing, and Doppler evaluation of colon perfusion. With this approach aortography is required in only 10 to 20 percent of patients undergoing operation.[26-29] Despite unexpected findings in 7 percent of patients, reported morbidity is acceptably low, and a nonoptimal surgical approach — one that would have been changed if aortography had been performed — is only infrequently chosen.[27]

In our experience a combined approach with cross-sectional imaging (CT or MRI) and angiography affords the most complete preoperative evaluation and eliminates the morbidity, time, and expense of unexpected findings at the time of operation. As enumerated above, CT and angiography are complementary tests, with little overlap in the information that they provide. CT evaluates the size of the aneurysm, the amount of thrombus, and the periaortic space for complications and anatomic anomalies. It also directs the surgical approach and the timing of the operation. Aortography directs the type of surgical reconstruction performed by demonstrating the extent of the lesion, the status of the aortic valve, the involvement of branch vessels, and the downstream vasculature.[27,30]

MRI with MRA may soon replace CT and angiography in most instances for preoperative evaluation of aneurysms, for this one modality has the potential to supply all the necessary preoperative information.[22] Three-dimensional dynamic CT may also fill this role.

Preoperative Imaging of Symptomatic Aneurysm

The mortality associated with aneurysm rupture necessitates a rapid evaluation that enhances operative survival without unjustifiably delaying treatment. The ready availability of CT and its ability to assess the pericardial and periaortic space for blood permits its use prior to operative repair to confirm the clinical impression of rupture[31] (Fig. 14-9). In the case of the abdominal aorta, clinical misdiagnosis of rupture may be as high as 50 percent, resulting in unnecessary emergent surgery that is fraught with morbidity.[32] CT to rule out rupture is clinically most useful in an imaging environment that can provide CT evaluation in 15 to 30

minutes. If time permits and the patient is hemodynamically stable, aortography can be performed to supply more detailed information prior to reconstruction.

Postoperative Complications

Graft occlusion and false aneurysm can be diagnosed by ultrasound, CT, MRI, or aortography. When infection is suspected, CT or MRI is indicated.[33] Graft infection, manifested by failure of graft incorporation and perigraft abscess, alters the periaortic tissues and is best detected by axial imaging in combination with functional studies (scintigraphy). Perigraft gas 7 weeks postoperatively on CT or perigraft fluid 3 months postoperatively on CT or MRI suggests infection[34,35] (Fig. 14-10). CT-guided fine-needle aspiration of fluid for culture can be performed for confirmation of infection.[36] Duodenal wall thickening, perivascular fluid, and perigraft gas suggest a graft-enteric fistula (Fig. 14-11), while development of focal dilatation at an anastomosis suggests a false aneurysm. Angiography, except for the confirmation of a false aneurysm and the infrequent demonstration of a graft-enteric fistula on lateral aortography, contributes little to the diagnosis but may be required for planning reconstruction (Fig. 14-12).

TRAUMATIC AORTIC RUPTURE

A small fraction (15 percent) of patients who sustain blunt chest trauma from sudden deceleration will survive TAR and present for medical evaluation.[37,38] Although autopsy specimens reveal that isthmic tears account for only 50 percent of injuries, 95 percent of patients who survive to undergo aortography have tears that occur at the aortic isthmus between the left subclavian artery and the ligamentum arteriosum.[39-41]

Angiographic documentation of rupture of the ascending aorta above the aortic valve, the descending aorta, or one of the proximal great vessels is much less frequently found.

The mechanism for aortic rupture is unknown, but most frequently is explained as the result of torsion of the mobile ascending and descending aorta on the relatively fixed aortic isthmus and heart base during rapid deceleration.[42] A recent hypothesis suggests that compression of the bony thorax results in an "osseous pinch" of the aorta, which causes laceration.[43] Whatever the mechanism, the outcome is a false aneurysm involving disruption of the intima, the intima and media, or all layers of the aortic wall, with the hematoma contained by surrounding mediastinal tissues.

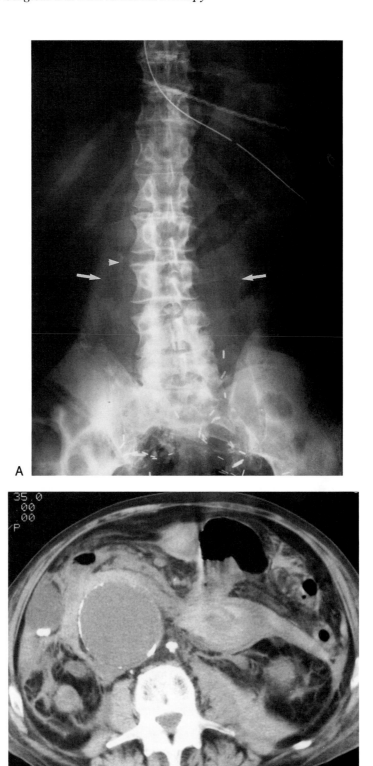

Figure 14-9 On the abdomen film **(A)** the psoas margins are obliterated by soft tissue *(arrows)*. Calcification can be seen to the right of the spine *(arrowhead)*. Although this is suggestive of a ruptured abdominal aortic aneurysm, the diagnosis is rapidly confirmed by computed tomography (CT) prior to operation **(B)**. There is uncontained rupture into the anterior and posterior pararenal spaces.

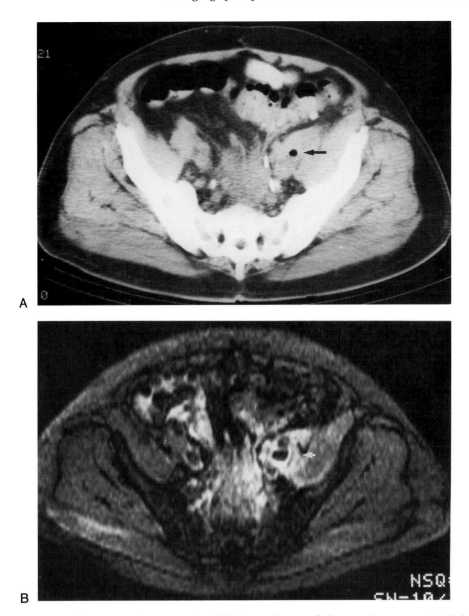

Figure 14-10 **(A)** A pelvic computed tomography (CT) image shows soft tissue and gas around an infected left limb of an aortofemoral graft (arrow). **(B)** Increased signal on a magnetic resonance image (MRI) at the same level more conspicuously displays the perigraft fluid *(arrowhead)*.

Clinical findings in patients with TAR are frequently absent, subtle, or unreliable. The suspicion of aortic injury is raised by the mechanism of injury suffered and confirmed by aortography. Surgical repair or replacement of the injured aorta is necessary for survival, with only 5 percent of untreated patients surviving 4 months.[37] Imaging is performed for diagnosis and preoperative planning. The information that must be obtained prior to surgical repair includes the presence of aortic rupture, the location of the tear, and the presence of associated injury of the great vessels, coronary arteries, and aortic valve.

Imaging Tests

Radiographs

In patients who have undergone a deceleration injury, the presence of mediastinal hematoma suggests severe chest trauma and raises the possibility of TAR. A chest radiograph that demonstrates a widened mediastinum with loss of the aortic contour is the most sensitive predictor of TAR and the most frequent indication for aortography.[44-48] The sensitivity of a widened mediastinum for TAR is 92 to 100 percent, but the speci-

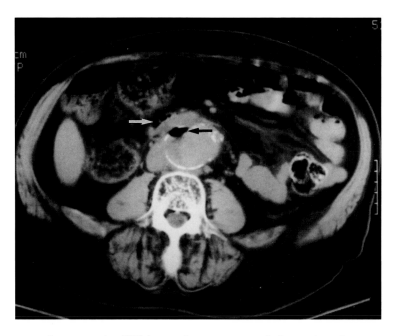

Figure 14-11 A computed tomography (CT) image demonstrates an infrarenal aortic aneurysm. Immediately anterior to the heavily calcified aortic wall is the duodenum. Extraduodenal gas *(arrow)* is diagnostic of aortoduodenal fistula, more commonly found following aortic grafting but also complicating native aortic aneurysms.

ficity is only 10 to 67 percent.[45,46,48] In older patients the mediastinum is more difficult to evaluate because of aortic ectasia and tortuosity and is less useful in predicting TAR. Numerous accessory radiographic findings have been described as predictive of aortic injury, including loss of the aortopulmonary window, rightward deviation of the trachea and/or nasogastric tube, left bronchus depression, widened left paraspinous stripe, apical cap, hemothorax, first and second rib and clavicle fractures, and pulmonary contusion.[39] Unfortunately, many of these findings are prevalent in trauma patients in general and are useful only to support a suspicion of significant chest trauma.

The incidence of normal chest radiographs in patients with TAR is unknown but is believed by most authors to be low.[49] In Raptopoulos et al.'s investigation reported in 1992, TAR was found in 2 (1 percent) of 199 patients with negative chest radiographs,[50] and in a literature review by Woodring,[51] 48 (7.3 percent) of 656 patients were found to have a significant vascular injury and a radiographically normal mediastinum.[51]

Computed Tomography

The possibility of false negative chest radiographs has liberalized the indication for aortography to mechanism of injury alone without chest radiographic abnormality, with a resultant increase in the use of aortography, so that in our experience TAR is found in

only 5 percent of those patients studied. In order to decrease this seeming overutilization of aortography, investigators have sought more specific screening tests. CT, as discussed below, has undergone the most extensive evaluation. MRI might be superior to CT in demonstrating TAR, but at present logistics make MRI inappropriate in critically ill patients.

Dynamic incremental contrast-enhanced scanning protocols to evaluate for aortic rupture have been described, which use contiguous 5- or 10-mm scan collimation through the upper mediastinum and aortic arch, with mechanical injection of 1 ml/s of contrast agent following a short scan delay. Technically inadequate or equivocal scans can be expected in 10 percent of patients.[52]

Criteria for diagnosis of TAR, originally described by Heiberg et al.,[53] have been used in subsequently published investigations. Direct signs of injury include false aneurysm; an intimal tear, indicated by a linear lucency within the opacified aortic lumen resulting from the torn edge of the aorta; and marginal irregularity of the opacified aortic lumen. Indirect signs include intramural or periaortic hematoma. Most authors have broadened these criteria to include any mediastinal hematoma—intraluminal, periaortic or remote[54-57] (Fig. 14-13).

The superiority in resolution and speed of modern scanners strongly influences the feasibility and success of CT in diagnosing subtle aortic pathology. Table 14-4

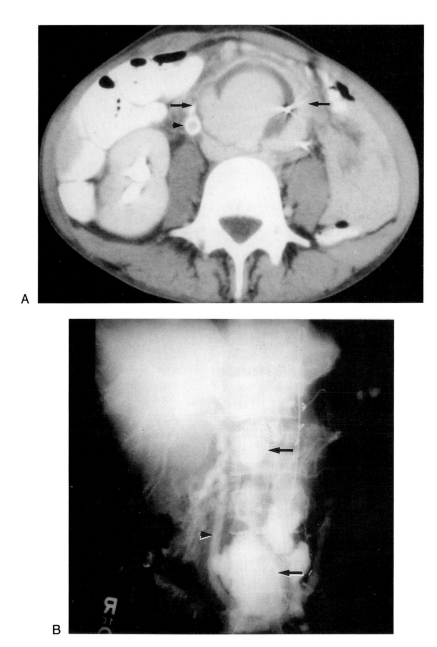

Figure 14-12 **(A)** An axial computed tomography (CT) image **(A)** of the infrarenal aorta reveals a large false aneurysm *(arrows)* in a patient who 10 years previously had undergone aortic replacement for a large thoracoabdominal aneurysm. His right kidney was revascularized with an iliac-to-renal graft *(arrowhead)*. **(B)** Aortography more clearly shows the relationship of the large right anastomotic aneurysm *(bottom arrow)* to the renal bypass graft *(arrowhead)*. The left anastomosis is also aneurysmal. Coils are seen in the midabdomen just superior to a second collection of contrast medium, a recurrent mesenteric pseudoaneurysm *(topmost arrow)*. The coils had been placed 1 year previously when the mesenteric reimplantation site developed a pseudoaneurysm, which was bypassed but still filled postoperatively.

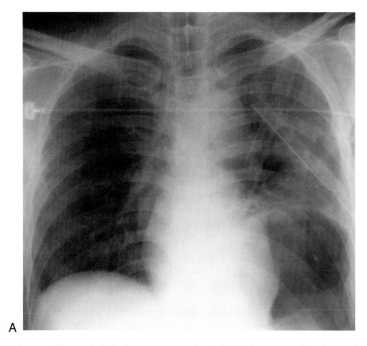

Figure 14-13 An AP chest radiograph **(A)** demonstrates the left diaphragm to be elevated, with left lung base atelectasis (traumatic diaphragmatic hernia). The aortic arch is indistinct, and the aorticopulmonary window is full. *(Figure continues.)*

shows the results of the most recent prospective series.[50,52,54,58,59] In these studies unstable patients and patients believed to be at high risk for TAR were excluded, and all patients underwent subsequent abdominal CT to evaluate abdominal injuries. Selection criteria varied between reports with respect to chest radiographic findings, and therefore the likelihood of injury varied from low probability of injury in patients with normal chest radiographs to moderate probability of injury in those with equivocal or positive chest x-rays. The sensitivity and specificity calculated from a combination of these data are 82 and 85 percent, respectively. Miller et al.[54] reported the only false negative examinations, including two cases of missed TAR and three cases of missed great vessel injury. One missed TAR was due to an error in diagnosis in a case in which mediastinal hematoma was missed; the other case was technically inadequate. None of the great vessel injuries required repair. Raptopoulos et al.[50] evaluated all patients undergoing abdominal CT despite

Table 14-4   Traumatic Aortic Rupture: Results of Computed Tomography

Author (Year)	No. of Patients	Chest X-ray	CT Results Versus Aortography/ Surgical/Clinical Follow-up[a]			
			TP	FN	TN	FP
Miller et al.[54] (1989)	104	P	6	5	62	31
Maydayag et al.[58] (1991)	93	N	1	0	83	9
Richardson et al.[52] (1991)	90	E	4	0	63	23
Raptopoulos et al.[50] (1992)	326	P&N	10	0	272	44
Morgan et al.[59] (1992)	160	N	1	0	152	7
Total	773		22	5	632	114

Abbreviations: P, positive; N, negative; E, equivocal; TP, true positive; FP, false positive; TN, true negative; FN, false negative.
[a] Sensitivity = TP/TP + FN; specificity = TN/TN + FP.

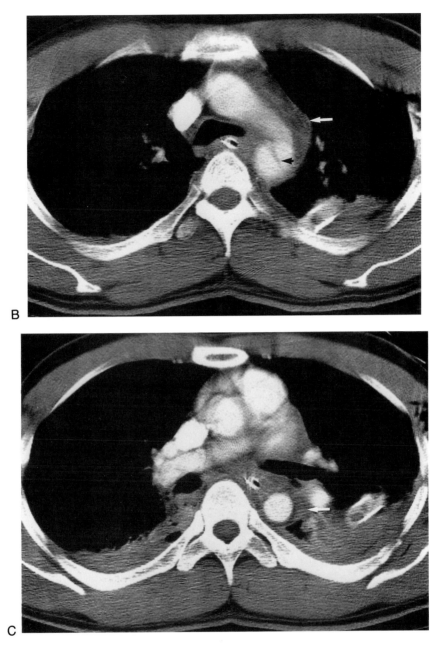

Figure 14-13 *(Continued.)* **(B)** Computed tomography (CT) images reveal fluid *(arrow)* surrounding the aortic arch. The proximal descending aorta is enlarged, and there is a filling defect (intimal flap) traversing the lumen *(arrowhead).* **(C)** Lower scan at level of descending aorta demonstrates fluid around aorta *(arrow).* These findings are direct evidence for aortic rupture. The diagnosis was confirmed by aortography. (Courtesy of Marsha Henig, M.D., Ph.D., Denver General Hospital, Denver, CO.)

chest x-ray findings and reported the largest experience, 326 patients. They found CT to have a sensitivity for TAR of 100 percent and specificity of 86 percent, as compared with 80 and 62 percent for chest radiography. Two patients with normal chest radiographs had abnormal CT studies and subsequent positive aortography, supporting the view that mechanism of injury

may be more predictive of TAR than chest radiography.

Several authors have attempted to address the impact of CT on aortography, although no cost studies have been completed. Morgan et al.[59] evaluated 28 patients with abnormal chest x-rays, who were believed to be at low risk for aortic injury. They were able to exclude mediastinal hemorrhage in 22 (78 percent), and 19 (68 percent) were treated without aortography. Richardson et al.,[52] who selected patients with equivocal or technically inadequate chest x-rays, found no hematoma on CT in 77 percent of patients, who were treated without aortography. Raptopoulos et al.[50] found that when CT was used as an adjunct to chest radiography to screen patients prior to aortography, use of aortography fell by 56 percent.

Several questions remain unanswered: Can a CT scan be normal in the presence of aortic laceration or great vessel injury? Is there a role for CT screening in high-risk patients? And can CT direct patients to surgery without aortography? Obviously large numbers of patients with TAR will need to be studied to determine the true incidence of false negative examinations or the sensitivity of CT in detecting rare great vessel injuries. No investigator has attempted to use CT to study patients at high risk for TAR in whom mediastinal hemorrhage is evident on chest radiographs. The number of positive CT studies that have been found to date is therefore small, making the false negative rate more difficult to evaluate and leaving the role of CT for high-risk patients unknown. All authors recommend aortography prior to surgical exploration, since most positive CT examinations demonstrate only mediastinal hematoma, not actual vascular injury; in fact, 80 to 90 percent of patients with abnormal CT scans (those with mediastinal hematomas) have no aortic injury.[50,52,54,58,59]

Administration of additional contrast agent to trauma patients who may require subsequent aortography is the major medical risk of performing CT. The investment in time to obtain a scan is the second concern. Obviously, a patient who is hemodynamically unstable should not undergo a CT examination of any kind. The addition of this step to the workup of stable patients largely depends on an imaging department that is organized to efficiently investigate critical patients. CT examination of the aorta can easily be added to CT evaluation of the head or abdomen, requiring only 15 to 20 additional minutes.[56]

Ultrasound

The use of TEE for screening patients with TAR has recently been suggested by Sparks et al.,[60] who studied a series of 11 patients with chest trauma, including 6 patients with arteriographic demonstration of TAR. They identified TAR in three patients and excluded it in three patients with false positive aortograms; one of these exclusions was confirmed surgically and two were confirmed clinically. This preliminary experience represents a selected group of patients likely to have aortic injury, and investigators were aware of aortographic findings at the time of evaluation; however, TEE is a

test worthy of future investigation as a screening test for aortic rupture.

Aortography

Arteriographically, the torn edges of the intima can be seen as sharp, transverse linear defects (Figs. 14-14 and 14-15). Intimal injuries may be multiple and discontinuous. Changes in the outer aortic wall may be absent, with intimal injury the only evidence of laceration, or may range from subtle irregularity of the aortic contour to a false aneurysm. Extravasation of contrast medium through the injured wall is rare. Injuries at the isthmus are associated with injuries of the great vessels in 5 percent of cases, including stenosis or thrombosis secondary to intimal injury, as well as rupture with false aneurysm.[61] Tears of the ascending aorta may be associated with cardiac, coronary artery, and aortic valve injuries.

Conventional aortography has been reported to have a 100 percent sensitivity and 99 percent specificity for the diagnosis of TAR, with a positive predictive value of 97 percent and a negative predictive value of 100 percent.[62] The 1 to 2 percent false positive rate necessitates a rare negative exploration. The most common reason for an equivocal or false positive aortogram is an atypical ductus bump. Although the ductus usually forms gentle obtuse angles at its junction with the aortic wall, a few patients will have an acute angle superiorly, which can cause uncertainty. The absence of an intimal flap helps distinguish this normal variant.[63]

A report of two patients with TAR who died during aortography underscores the importance of avoiding any catheter manipulation in the region of the potentially injured aorta.[64] Other reported complications have been rare, despite the critical nature of the patient population being studied. Administration of contrast to hemodynamically compromised or at-risk patients is the greatest concern. In general, the risk of contrast-induced acute renal failure (usually reversible) is outweighed by the potential morbidity of an unrecognized aortic transection. Aortography for this indication takes an average of 70 minutes, including 30 minutes of preparation and postangiography care. Digital imaging can reduce the time required for acquiring images from 40 to 20 minutes.[65] Patients who are comatose, intoxicated, or otherwise uncooperative may be difficult to study by digital image acquisition.

Recommendations for Imaging Traumatic Aortic Rupture

Despite its poor specificity, chest radiography remains the most widely used screening test for aortic injury. The use of CT to screen for TAR is still investi-

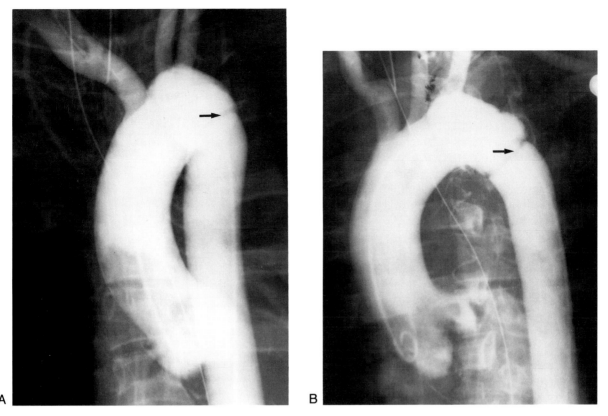

Figure 14-14 **(A)** AP and **(B)** right posterior oblique aortograms demonstrate a sharp linear defect crossing the aortic lumen horizontally, the inferior site of the intimal tear *(arrow)*. The oblique view best demonstrates a pseudoaneurysm beginning at the subclavian artery and extending to the intimal tear. The upper edge of the tear is obscured by the pseudoaneurysm.

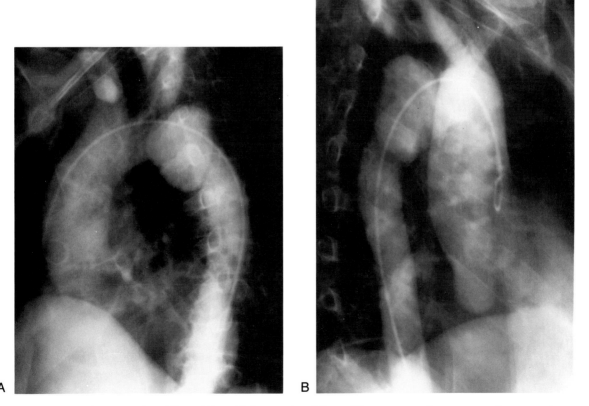

Figure 14-15 Right posterior oblique **(A)** and left posterior oblique **(B)** aortograms demonstrate a large pseudo-aneurysm at the aortic isthmus in a patient with aortic rupture.

gational; currently, it is appropriate only in institutions where CT can be provided in expeditious fashion and where CT is indicated for evaluation of abdominal or other trauma. Aortography remains the most direct and accurate diagnostic test for TAR, with little patient risk, and is required in all patients undergoing operative repair. The cost and personnel required to provide emergency aortography, a study that may have a positive rate as low as 5 to 10 percent, provide the motivation for seeking a more specific screening examination.

The multiplicity of injuries resulting from high-speed trauma demands a rapid diagnostic plan. If chest radiography suggests aortic injury and the patient cannot be stabilized, thoracotomy without imaging tests of any kind is indicated. In hemodynamically stable patients who have suffered a deceleration injury and whose chest radiographs demonstrate mediastinal hemorrhage or suggest aortic injury, aortography should be performed immediately.

Patients with normal chest x-rays who are believed to be at high risk because of the mechanism of injury, as well as patients at low or moderate risk who have equivocal or technically inadequate chest x-rays, can be screened with chest CT prior to abdominal CT. If a mediastinal hematoma or any direct evidence of TAR is present, the patient proceeds to aortography. If the mediastinum is normal, the patient is observed clinically and followed with serial chest radiography. When patients present with chest radiographs or other imaging tests suggesting chronic aortic lacerations, MRI can be used to confirm the diagnosis, with aortography reserved for patients in whom surgical repair is anticipated (Fig. 14-16).

AORTIC DISSECTION

Aortic dissection is most commonly thought to occur as a result of a structural defect in or degeneration of the aortic media, which allows blood to gain entry to the media and dissect the aortic wall. Patients with aortic dissection who are younger than 40 frequently have genetic cystic medial necrosis (Marfan's syndrome); older patients are likely to have smooth muscle degeneration related to aging and hypertension.[66] The recognition of medial dissections that occur in the absence of intimal injury supports a structural abnormality of the media as the etiologic factor. Although isolated medial dissection without intimal tear has been reported in only 5 percent of surgical and autopsy series, recent recognition of this condition by MRI and CT suggests a higher incidence.[67] Bleeding from the vasa vasorum into the media is suspected to be an initiating event. An alternative theory of the cause of aortic dissection proposes intimal trauma as the primary injury that allows blood to enter and then dissect the media. This theory is supported by the prevalence of the supravalvular ascending aorta and the aortic isthmus as entry points in dissection, the same locations at which TAR occurs.

Aortic dissection results in the development of two aortic channels—a native or true channel is compressed by an abnormal medial or false channel; the two channels being separated by the intima. The false channel spirals around the true channel from the right anterior ascending aorta to the superior posterior arch to the left posterior descending aorta. With time, the false channel endothelializes and the wall may calcify.

After gaining entry into the media, blood may reenter the true lumen, come to a halt, or erupt into the pericardium, pleural space, or periaortic tissues. Communications between the true and false channel can be multiple. Most often dissection occurs in an antegrade direction, but retrograde dissection from an intimal injury at the aortic isthmus also occurs. The arch and the iliac arteries are involved in half and renal arteries in one-fourth of autopsied patients, but these involvements are less frequently found in survivors.[68]

Since prognosis and treatment depend on the segment of involved aorta, classification is based on location. Two classification schemes are commonly used. In the Stanford scheme any dissection involving the ascending aorta is type A, while a dissection beginning distal to the left subclavian artery and limited to the descending aorta is type B.[69] The DeBakey classification differentiates type A lesions into DeBakey I lesions, which extend from the ascending aorta to involve the descending aorta, and DeBakey II lesions, which are confined to the ascending aorta. A DeBakey III lesion is similar to a Stanford B lesion.[70] The incidence of DeBakey I, II, and III dissections is 51, 6, and 42 percent, respectively.[71] Dissections that present within 2 weeks of the event are considered acute, the rest chronic.

Medical treatment is directed toward immediate and long-term control of hypertension and reduction of pulse pressure. This is the standard therapy for uncomplicated Stanford B dissections. Surgery for B dissections is necessary when complications develop, including rupture, vascular compromise, pain, extension of dissection, or aneurysmal enlargement of the false channel.[66] Stanford A dissections require immediate surgery because of the tendency for rupture, coronary artery occlusion, and acute aortic insufficiency. Surgical treatment, aimed at preventing extension of the dissection to the aortic root and preventing rupture, includes correction of aortic insufficiency, either by valve replacement or resuspension; replacement, or

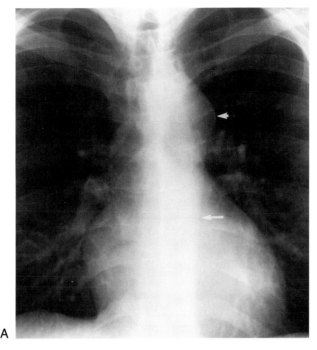

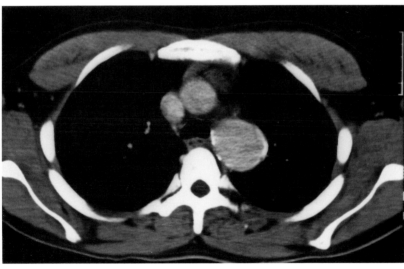

Figure 14-16 (A) An AP chest radiograph demonstrates a mass in the aorticopulmonary window, with peripheral calcification *(arrowhead)*. The left border of the descending aorta is distinct *(arrow)*. (B) CT confirms the impression that there is an aortic aneurysm of the proximal descending aorta. The heavily calcified aortic wall and the characteristic location raise the possibility of a chronic traumatic aneurysm. *(Figure continues.)*

less commonly, repair of the ascending aorta to prevent communication between the false channel and the aortic root; and coronary artery reconstruction if needed.[72,73] The persistence of a patent false channel due to multiple communications between the true and false lumina following successful operative repair suggests that repair of the proximal intimal injury site may not be mandatory as long as the injury is separated from the aortic valve by an aortic interposition graft.[74,75]

A recently recognized complication of penetrating atherosclerotic thoracic aortic ulcer is rupture into the media (Fig. 14-17). These ulcers occur most commonly within the proximal descending thoracic aorta in elderly hypertensive men. Frequently an atherosclerotic aneurysm is present. Symptoms of severe intrascapular back pain, mimicking dissection, may indicate hemorrhage into the media or impending transmural rupture. This propensity for rupture necessitates repair.[76,77]

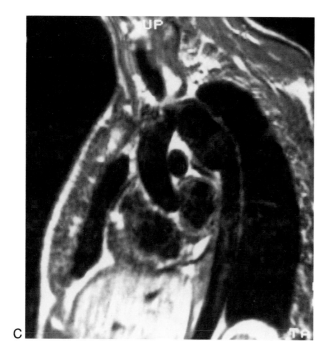

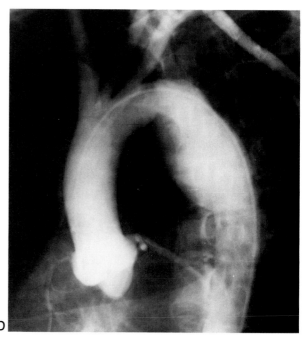

Figure 14-16 *(Continued.)* **(C)** T₁-weighted magnetic resonance image (MRI) in a sagittal plane demonstrates the aneurysm configuration clearly and its relationship to the subclavian artery. **(D)** Aortography was performed prior to surgical repair.

Indications for Imaging

There are two indications for imaging in patients with suspected or known aortic dissection: diagnosis and preoperative imaging of acute aortic dissection and surveillance of postoperative and chronic aortic dissection.

Diagnosis and Preoperative Imaging of Acute Aortic Dissection

Imaging in the setting of suspected acute dissection is performed to confirm the diagnosis and to localize the aortic injury in order to direct therapy. Other important information includes the competency of the aortic valve and the involvement of the coronary arteries, great vessels, and abdominal vessels when there is evidence of visceral or renal ischemia. Correct identification of the site of intimal tear and of other communications between the true and false channels (entry and reentry points) may not be important if the surgical approach to be employed focuses on proximal reconstruction and valve replacement rather than on correction of the intimal injury.[54,66]

Surveillance of Postoperative and Chronic Aortic Dissection

Following surgical therapy for type A dissection, 40 percent of patients may require repeat operation for complications.[74] Indications for reoperation of type A aortic dissection or operative repair of type B aortic dissection include an enlarging thoracic false channel, pseudoaneurysm formation, redissection, extension of dissection, dilatation of a sinus of Valsalva, persistence of mediastinal or pericardial fluid, and ischemia resulting from branch vessel involvement.[74,75]

Imaging Tests

Radiographs

Although routine chest radiographs tend to be abnormal, with evidence of a widened mediastinum, this finding is nonspecific and common in a population of elderly men; 25 percent of patients with acute aortic dissection will have normal chest radiographs.[68] The finding of mediastinal widening is most helpful when previous radiographs reveal that this finding is acute.

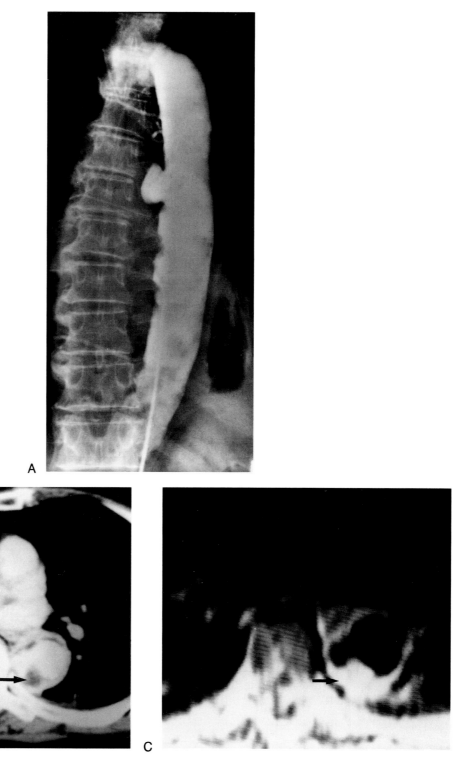

Figure 14-17 **(A)** An AP aortogram demonstrates a medial atherosclerotic ulcer. **(B)** Axial imaging with computed tomography (CT) demonstrates the ulcer in a transverse plane. There is periaortic fluid, which looks like thrombus *(arrow)*. **(C)** Magnetic resonance image (MRI) demonstrates a high signal in this soft tissue, which is characteristic of acute hemorrhage *(arrow)*. Penetrating thoracic ulcer represents aortic rupture and requires surgical repair. (Courtesy of E. Kent Yucel, M.D., Massachusetts General Hospital, Boston, MA.)

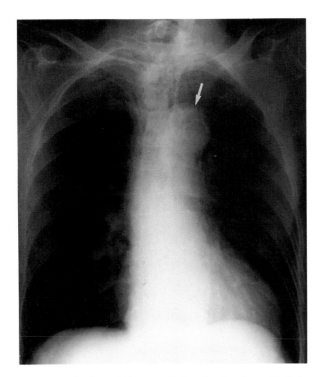

Figure 14-18 There is heavy calcification in the wall of the transverse aorta. Soft tissue peripheral to this calcification raises the possibility of aortic dissection *(arrow).*

Internal displacement of calcification from the peripheral wall of the aorta and disparity in the size of the ascending and the descending aorta are other suspicious signs (Fig. 14-18).

Ultrasound

TTE has been used to screen patients for aortic dissection with a sensitivity ranging from 77 to 80 percent.[78] Its successful use depends on an appropriate window to the ascending aorta through the thorax. The descending aorta is not well visualized in 30 percent of cases, making diagnosis of type B lesions difficult.[15] Diagnostic criteria include identification of two lumina with a separating intimal flap; detection of a thrombosed lumen, with displaced intimal calcification or separation of intimal layers by thrombus; and identification of intimal tears by disruption in the continuity of the flap, with fluttering of the ruptured intimal borders.

Hashimoto et al.[79] evaluated TEE in comparison with TTE and CT in a series of 22 patients with aortic dissection, which had been surgically confirmed in 12. TEE successfully made the diagnosis of aortic dissection and identified the involved aortic segment in all patients and identified the site of intimal tear in 17.

TTE failed to make the diagnosis in 7 patients, failed to accurately localize the involved aortic segment in 11, and failed to diagnose the site of intimal tear in 17. CT, although as successful as TEE in identifying the intimal flap and localizing the involved aortic segment, was unable to diagnose the site of intimal tear in any patient. TTE and TEE were successful in identifying aortic regurgitation in 12 of the 17 patients in whom this complication was confirmed by aortography.

A comparative study by Erbel et al.[78] determined the sensitivity and specificity of combined TTE and TEE as compared with CT and aortography in 164 patients with suspected aortic dissection, 71 patients with autopsy or surgical proof of aortic dissection, and 82 patients with proof by two or more imaging tests. The sensitivity of TTE and TEE (98 percent) was superior to that of both CT (83 percent) and aortography (88 percent). False positive examinations by TEE occurred in two patients with aortic ectasia because of reverberation artifact in the ascending aorta, and a false negative examination occurred in one patient with a small localized tear of the aortic root, missed also by aortography and subsequently detected at surgery.

These data suggest that the presence and location of dissection and the site of intimal tear are diagnosed more frequently with TEE than with TTE, CT, or even the "gold standard" aortography. In addition, TEE allows detection of complications of aortic dissection, including aortic regurgitation, pericardial effusion, left pleural effusion, abnormal cardiac wall motion, and compression of cardiac structures.[71] TEE cannot evaluate the coronary arteries and great vessels, and angiography is still necessary prior to surgical repair.

Computed Tomography

Presently CT is the most widely used screening test for aortic dissection because of its availability. Diagnosis depends on the demonstration of the true and false channels separated by an intimal flap, within the aortic lumen, following administration of contrast medium (Fig. 14-19). Aortic wall thickening, widening of the aorta, clotted blood in the false lumen, inward displacement of intimal calcification, and compression of the true lumen support the diagnosis. Pleural, mediastinal, and pericardial fluid suggest rupture and herald death.

Accurate diagnosis relies on high-quality examinations with appropriately timed contrast medium administration. Initial protocols used dynamic nonincremental scanning at three levels through the arch during the administration of contrast. Decreased scanning times now allow the entire ascending aorta to be imaged during mechanical contrast injection, with 5-

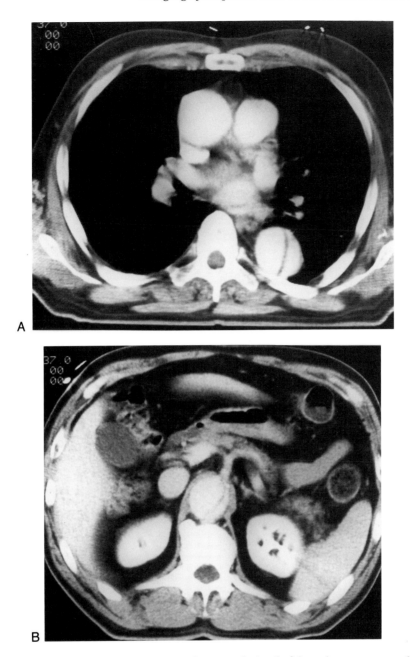

Figure 14-19 (A) Axial computed tomography (CT) image at the level of the pulmonary artery shows a normal ascending aorta. The descending aorta is transected by a linear flap, the intima, which separates two aortic channels. This represents a type III aortic dissection. (B) Scan at the level of the celiac artery demonstrates the flap extending to this level and involving the origin of the celiac artery.

to 10-mm scan collimation. Images must be reviewed at multiple window and level settings in order to avoid missing subtle differences in enhancement between the true and false channels and also to visualize the intimal flap.

Extensive experience has been obtained with the use of CT for evaluation of acute aortic dissection. The sensitivity and specificity of CT range from 83 to 100 percent and from 96 to 100 percent.[80-83] False negative studies have been reported when simultaneous or equal opacification of the true and false channels occurs or when there is complete thrombosis of the false lumen, making differentiation from aortic aneurysm difficult.[84,85] The aortic root and the proximal descending aorta are difficult to evaluate because of artifact and volume averaging in these areas.

Although CT is sensitive for the presence of aortic dissection and can separate type A and B lesions, it does not evaluate the aortic valve, the coronary arteries, or the great vessels. Similarly, CT rarely establishes the entry site. Therefore any patients requiring surgery, including those with type A or symptomatic B lesions, must subsequently undergo aortography. CT is adequate for the evaluation of patients with asymptomatic B lesions who will be managed medically. The increased dose of contrast agent when CT is used prior to aortography may increase the risk of both studies. Direct referral to aortography is indicated in patients with highly suspicious clinical presentations.

Magnetic Resonance Imaging

The inherent contrast between flowing blood and soft tissue allows visualization of the intimal flap as a linear structure of medium signal intensity surrounded by signal void in the true and false channels on spin-echo MRI (Figs. 14-20 and 14-21). In MRI, unlike CT, similar flow in the true and false channels does not mask the flap. Gradient echo acquisition can be used to enhance flow velocities and identify entry sites, as well as to distinguish slow flow in the false channel from thrombus. MRI is valuable in the diagnosis of intramural hemorrhage without intimal tear secondary to vasa vasorum rupture within the wall. This results in medial hematoma, demonstrated by high signal intensity on T_1 images. This finding cannot be visualized at aortography. Fruehwald et al.[86] reported a comparative study of MRI, TTE, CT, and aortography, which demonstrated a sensitivity of MRI for aortic dissection of 100 percent, as compared with 44 percent for TTE, 83 percent for CT, and 77 percent for aortography. Aortography results in this study were compromised by performance of intravenous digital examinations in 20 percent of patients.

Frequently anatomic and artifactual findings mimic aortic dissection, including the left brachiocephalic vein, arch artery origins, superior pericardial recess, aortic plaque, apposition of the azygos vein and descending aorta, mediastinal fibrosis, subacute thrombus on gradient echo images, and motion in the phase-

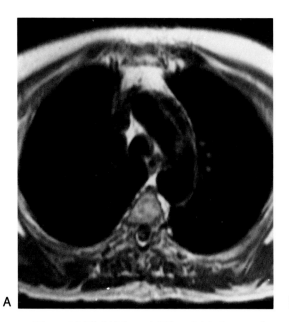

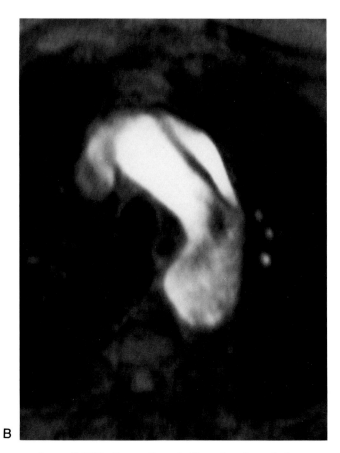

A   B

Figure 14-20 **(A)** An axial T_1-weighted magnetic resonance image (MRI) of a type I aortic dissection through the transverse aorta reveals an intimal flap separating two lumina. **(B)** The signal characteristics on a time-of-flight magnetic resonance angiography (MRA) image are reversed. The intimal flap is devoid of signal *(black)* and the patent aortic lumina have a high-intensity signal *(white)*.

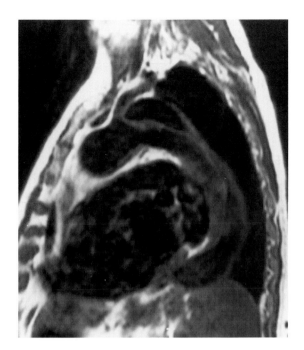

Figure 14-21 A sagittal T_1-weighted image demonstrates a type III dissection.

encoding direction.[87] As experience with this technique grows, the impact of these findings should diminish.

Just as with CT, the coronary arteries, great vessels, and aortic valve are not evaluated by standard MRI sequences. Therefore acute type A dissections and symptomatic B dissections will need subsequent aortography prior to surgery. MRI is sufficient for evaluation of acute type B dissections and has several advantages over CT, including direct multiplanar imaging, better visualization of the aortic root, improved sensitivity, and no requirement for intravenous contrast.

Aortography

Visualization of the intimal flap separating the true and false channels is the hallmark of dissection on aortography. Other signs of aortic dissection include narrowing and compression of the true lumen by the nonopacified false lumen, an abnormal catheter position separated from the outer wall of the aorta, differential opacification of the two channels, occluded branch vessels, aortic wall thickening, and aortic regurgitation (Fig. 14-22). To date aortography is the only

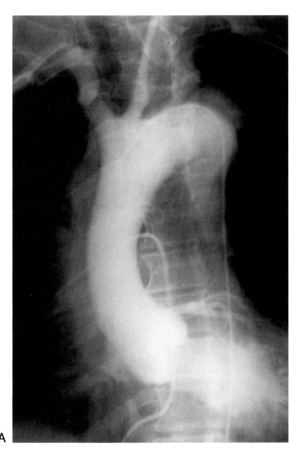

A

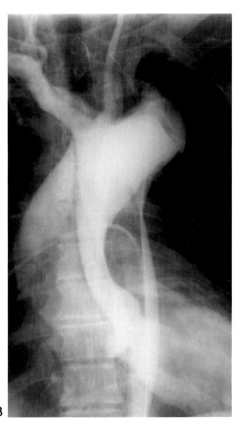

B

Figure 14-22 **(A)** Right posterior oblique aortogram (early phase) demonstrates a type I aortic dissection. The false channel is large and compresses the true channel. The left coronary artery fills from the true lumen. **(B)** Later phase. Contrast is now seen in the false lumen; there is severe aortic insufficiency; and the dissection extends into the great vessels.

imaging method that is able to define the involvement of the coronary arteries and branch vessels and to assess the involvement and function of the aortic valve. The exact site of entry and reentry can be demonstrated in some but not all cases.

Angiographic pitfalls include failure to opacify a thrombosed false lumen, necessitating the radiographic recognition of aortic wall thickening to make the diagnosis (Fig. 14-23). When simultaneous opacification of both channels occurs, the intimal flap may be hidden. Small, localized dissections near the aortic root can be missed even when views are obtained in multiple projections. Careful examination of all images and rigorous technique are important to avoid missing subtle dissections. Subtraction views and delayed films may be necessary to demonstrate the false channel. Aortography cannot diagnose dissection that occurs without intimal injury.

Because coronary arteriography may be necessary prior to surgical repair, cineangiography may be performed rather than conventional or digital aortography. The ability to image at 30 frames per second makes cineangiography well suited to evaluate the dynamic action of the aortic valve, the motion of an intimal flap, and entry and reentry sites in the ascending aorta.[88,89] The trade-off for improved temporal resolution is a loss of spatial resolution when the descending aorta is panned as a bolus of contrast proceeds down the aorta. This hinders the diagnosis of dissection and limits the understanding of branch vessel involvement in the abdomen.

Recommendations for Imaging Aortic Dissection

Diagnosis and Preoperative Imaging of Acute Aortic Dissection

At present TEE appears to be the most appealing screening test for acute aortic dissection because it determines quickly and accurately, with minimal morbidity, which patients require aortography and surgery. If a type A lesion is found by TEE, aortography is pursued. Type B dissections found by TEE require further evaluation by CT or MRI to confirm the diagnosis and provide a baseline examination. When TEE is not available, CT may be used in its place; however if there is a high suspicion for type A aortic dissection, immediate aortography is more expeditious and avoids the large volume of contrast medium required to perform both examinations. In this case conventional aortography, followed by coronary angiography if needed, is the best strategy to confirm the diagnosis and localize the injury. CT or MRI is adequate for surveillance of chronic and postoperative dissections, with aortography reserved for preoperative evaluation when complications develop.

Surveillance of Postoperative and Chronic Aortic Dissection

Either CT or MRI can be used to survey patients with chronic or postoperative aortic dissection. Changes in the features of the true and false lumina including size, patency, thrombosis, and calcification, are well demonstrated by these modalities.[74,90] CT surveillance has added to our understanding of the usual postoperative course, including the persistence of the false channel in 70 to 90 percent of patients owing to multiple fenestrations between the two lumina that may persist after surgery.[74,91,92] The persistence of the false lumen in postoperative and chronic aortic dissection emphasizes the importance of the investigation of vital arteries threatened by ischemia.[8,92]

AORTIC OCCLUSIVE DISEASE

Arterial occlusive disease is best demonstrated by arteriography. Ultrasound, CT, and MRI, except in the carotid location, have had limited success in visualizing

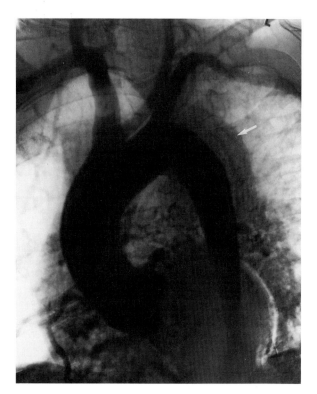

Figure 14-23 A compressed aortic lumen directs attention to the soft tissue lateral to the descending aorta *(arrow)*, which represents a thrombosed false channel of a type III dissection.

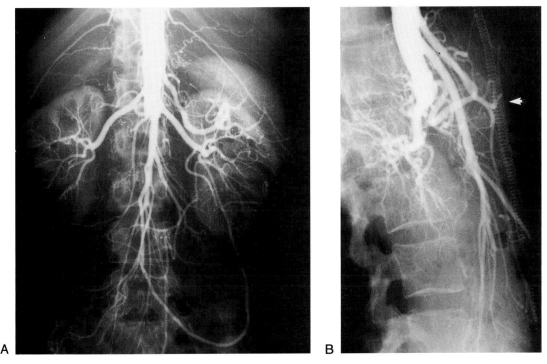

Figure 14-24 AP (**A**) and lateral (**B**) abdominal aortograms demonstrate occlusion of the aorta just below the left renal artery. Enlarged intercostal and middle colic arteries help to collateralize the pelvis. The metallic rings of an extra-anatomic graft is seen anteriorly on the lateral aortogram *(arrowhead)*.

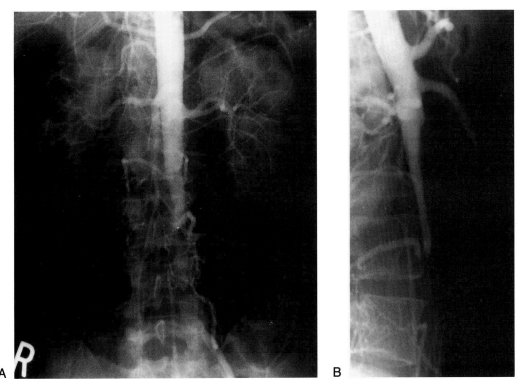

Figure 14-25 AP (**A**) and lateral (**B**) aortograms in a female patient with infrarenal aortic occlusion demonstrate an occlusion distal to the renal arteries at the third lumbar artery.

the disease adequately for surgical planning. Diagnostic algorithms for imaging occlusive disease of the aorta are therefore straightforward. If clinical symptoms and noninvasive laboratory measurements suggest arterial occlusive disease and surgical therapy is contemplated, aortography is performed prior to intervention.

Atherosclerotic occlusive disease may involve the branch vessels of the aorta, including the coronary, innominate, subclavian, carotid, and visceral arteries. The thoracic aorta itself, perhaps because of its large diameter, does not itself become occluded secondary to atherosclerosis; therefore, when narrowing or occlusion of the thoracic aorta is discovered, a different etiology must be suspected. Narrowing and occlusion of the infrarenal aorta from atherosclerosis does occur. Leriche syndrome (buttock claudication, absent femoral pulses, impotence, and cool lower extremities) results from infrarenal aortic occlusion in men (Fig. 14-24). Occlusion is generally just below the renal arteries. Although women may have a similar aortographic picture, more commonly the site of aortic occlusion is several centimeters below the renal arteries, with an enlarged lumbar artery pair providing the terminal runoff (Fig. 14-25). This difference in occlusive pattern may be secondary to an increased frequency of hypoplastic aorta or small infrarenal aorta in women as compared with males. In either case aortic occlusion in most cases presents after gradual progression of symptoms, and large intercostal, lumbar, and epigastric collaterals proximally reconstitute internal and external iliac, femoral, and profunda vessels distally.

Two nonatherosclerotic causes of aortic occlusion are adult coarctation and arteritis. Adult coarctation of the aorta results from a congenital obstruction of the aortic arch at or just past the ligamentum arteriosum, produced by an internal diaphragm or ridge of tissue composed of intima and media. Unlike preductal, infantile coarctation, this disease may not be detected until late childhood or early adulthood. Patients present with chest pain and lower extremity claudication. Clinical findings include upper extremity hypertension, diminished lower extremity pulses, and heart failure. The diagnosis is suggested by chest radiography, the findings of which include left ventricular hypertrophy, poststenotic dilatation of the proximal descending aorta immediately beyond the coarctation, an indistinct aortic arch, and rib notching. Because patients have hypertension, asymmetric pulses, and other clinical findings that mimic aortic dissection, aortography may be requested emergently for clarification. In less dramatic presentations the chest radiographic diagnosis can be confirmed by demonstrating aortic narrowing and multiple arterial collaterals with MRI,

aortography being reserved for preoperative planning[93] (Fig. 14-26).

Takayasu's arteritis, a granulomatous vasculitis involving the thoracic and abdominal aorta and its large branch arteries,[94] may result in thoracic aortic stenosis or occlusion. The disease is most prevalent in 20- to 30-year-old women. Cardiovascular or nonspecific systemic symptoms and an elevated sedimentation rate may suggest the diagnosis, but depending on the presenting complaints, asymmetric pulses may again suggest acute aortic dissection. Aortography reveals focal, smooth symmetric narrowing of the aorta and multiple branch vessel stenosis or occlusions (Fig. 14-27).

CONCLUSIONS

At present most patients with aortic pathology ultimately come to aortography for final preoperative planning. The role of noninvasive imaging modalities

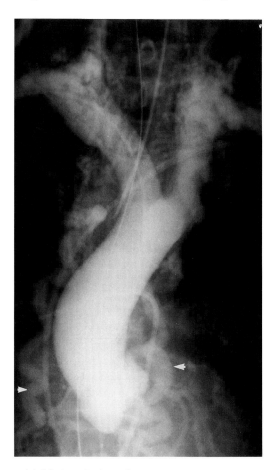

Figure 14-26 An AP thoracic aortogram shows aortic occlusion just past the left subclavian artery in a patient with adult coarctation of the aorta. The large internal mammary arteries *(arrowheads)* reconstitute the distal aorta.

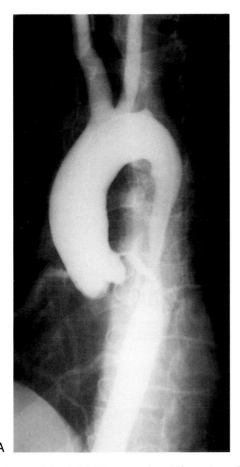
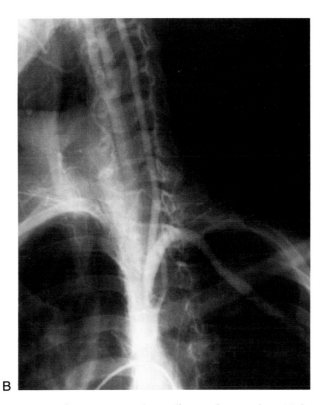

A   B

Figure 14-27 **(A)** Right posterior oblique thoracic aortogram demonstrates a descending aortic stenosis and left subclavian occlusion in a patient with Takayasu's arteritis. **(B)** The subclavian artery fills on a later image by reversed flow in the left vertebral artery.

to screen patients for aortic pathology is expanding as new techniques are developed and validated. Prospective comparative studies of imaging tests and combinations of tests are needed to determine the safest and most cost-efficient algorithms for diagnosis. In the meantime diagnostic strategies, particularly for critically ill patients, must be adapted to the environment in which they are conducted and to the available imaging expertise and must be based on a thorough knowledge of the suspected disease and its therapy. As with many vascular disorders, this requires a cooperative effort between the vascular radiologist and the surgeon.

REFERENCES

1. Katayama H, Yamaguchi K, Kozuka T et al: Adverse reactions to toxic and nonionic contrast media: a report from the Japanese Committee on the Safety of Contrast Media. Radiology 175:621, 1990

2. Palmer FJ: The R.A.C.R. survey of intravenous contrast media reactions: a preliminary report. Australas Radiol 32:8, 1988

3. Hessel SJ, Adams DF, Abrams HL: Complications of angiography. Diagn Radiol 138:273, 1981

4. Crawford ES: Replacement of the thoracic aorta. p. 336. In Grillo HC, Austen WG, Wilkins EW et al (eds): Current Therapy in Cardiothoracic Surgery. BC Decker, Philadelphia, 1989

5. Hollier LH, Taylor LM, Ochsner J: Recommended indications for operative treatment of abdominal aortic aneurysms. J Vasc Surg 15:1046, 1992

6. Posniak HV, Demos TC, Marsan RE: Computed tomography of the normal aorta and thoracic aneurysms. Semin Roentgenol 24:7, 1989

7. Goldstone J: Inflammatory aneurysms of the aorta. Semin Vasc Surg 1:165, 1988

8. Godwin JD: Conventional CT of the aorta. J Thorac Imaging 5:18, 1990

9. Mannick JA, Whittemore AD: Management of ruptured or symptomatic abdominal aortic aneurysms. Surg Clin North Am 68:377, 1988

10. Nevitt MP, Ballard DJ, Hallett JJ: Prognosis of abdominal aortic aneurysms. A population-based study. N Engl J Med 321:1009, 1989

11. Akins CW: Composite aortic valve and aortic root replacement in aneurysmal disease. p. 381. In Grillo HC, Austen WG, Wilkins EW et al (eds): Current Therapy in Cardiothoracic Surgery. BC Decker, Philadelphia, 1989

12. LaRoy LL, Cormier PJ, Matalon TA et al: Imaging of abdominal aortic aneurysms. AJR 152:785, 1989

13. Guthaner DF: The plain chest film in assessing aneurysms and dissecting hematomas of the thoracic aorta. In Taveras JM, Ferrucci J, Buonocore E, Elliot LP (eds): Radiology. Diagnosis—Imaging—Intervention. Vol. 2. 2nd Ed. JB Lippincott, Philadelphia, 1990

14. Daves ML: Aortic "aneurysms". In Daves ML (ed): Cardiac Roentgenology. Shadows of the Heart. Year Book Medical Publishers, Chicago, 1981

15. Bruno L, Prandi M, Colombi P, La Vecchia L: Diagnostic and surgical management of patients with aneurysms of the thoracic aorta with various causes. Echocardiography and contrast enhanced computed tomography in prophylactic replacement of the ascending aorta. Br Heart J 55:81, 1986

16. Papanicolaou N, Wittenberg J, Ferrucci JJ et al: Preoperative evaluation of abdominal aortic aneurysms by computed tomography. AJR 146:711, 1986

17. Pavone P, Di Cesare E, Di Renzi P et al: Abdominal aortic aneurysm evaluation: comparison of US, CT, MRI, and angiography. Magn Reson Imaging 8:199, 1990

18. Aronberg DJ, Glazer HS, Madsen K, Sagel SS: Normal thoracic aortic diameters by computed tomography. J Comput Assist Tomogr 8:247, 1984

19. Horejs D, Gilbert PM, Burstein S, Vogelzang RL: Normal aortoiliac diameters by CT. J Comput Assist Tomogr 12:602, 1988

20. Vogelzang RL, Sohaey R: Infected aortic aneurysms: CT appearance. J Comput Assist Tomogr 12:109, 1988

21. Link KM, Lesko NM: The role of MR imaging in the evaluation of acquired diseases of the thoracic aorta. AJR 158:1115, 1992

22. Dinsmore RE, Liberthson RR, Wismer GL et al: Magnetic resonance imaging of thoracic aortic aneurysms: comparison with other imaging methods. AJR 146:309, 1986

23. Larsson E-M, Albrechtsson U, Christenson JT: Computed tomography versus aortography for preoperative evaluation of abdominal aortic aneurysm. Acta Radiol 25:95, 1984

24. Vowden P, Wilkinson D, Ausobsky JR, Kester RC: A comparison of three imaging techniques in the assessment of an abdominal aortic aneurysm. J Cardiovasc Surg (Torino) 30:891, 1989

25. Williams GM, Perler BA, Burdick JF et al: Angiographic localization of spinal cord blood supply and its relationship to postoperative paraplegia. J Vasc Surg 13:23, 1991

26. Friedman SG, Kerner BA, Krishnasastry KV et al: Abdominal aortic aneurysmectomy without preoperative angiography. A prospective study. N Y State J Med 90:176, 1990

27. Todd GJ, Nowygrod R, Benvenisty A et al: The accuracy of CT scanning in the diagnosis of abdominal and thoracoabdominal aortic aneurysms. J Vasc Surg 13:302, 1991

28. Bandyk DF: Preoperative imaging of aortic aneurysms. Conventional and digital subtraction angiography, computed tomography scanning, and magnetic resonance imaging. Surg Clin North Am 721, 1989

29. Couch NP, O'Mahoney J, McIrvine A et al: The place of abdominal aortography in abdominal aortic aneurysm resection. Arch Surg 118:1029, 1983

30. Williams LR, Flinn WR, Yao JST et al: Extended use of computed tomography in the management of complex aortic problems: a learning experience. J Vasc Surg 4:264, 1986

31. Kucich VA, Vogelzang RL, Hartz RS et al: Ruptured thoracic aneurysm: unusual manifestation and early diagnosis using CT. Radiology 160:87, 1986

32. Zarnke MD, Gould HR, Goldman MH: Computed tomography in the evaluation of the patient with symptomatic abdominal aortic aneurysm. Surgery 103:638, 1988

33. Vogelzang RL, Limpert JD, Yao JS: Detection of prosthetic vascular complications: comparison of CT and angiography. AJR 148:819, 1987

34. Auffermann W, Olofsson PA, Rabahie GN et al: Incorporation versus infection of retroperitoneal aortic grafts: MR imaging features. Radiology 172:359, 1989

35. O'Hara PJ, Borkowski GP, Hertzer NR et al: Natural history of periprosthetic air on computerized axial tomographic examination of the abdomen following abdominal aortic aneurysm repair. J Vasc Surg 1:429, 1984

36. Katz BH, Black RA, Colley DP: CT-guided fine needle aspiration of a periaortic collection. J Vasc Surg 5:762, 1987

37. Parmley LF, Mattingly TW, Manion WC, Jahnke EJ: Nonpenetrating traumatic injury of the aorta. Circulation 17:1086, 1958

38. Greendyke RM: Traumatic rupture of aorta. JAMA 195:119, 1966

39. Fisher RG, Hadlock F, Ben-Menachem Y: Laceration of the thoracic aorta and brachiocephalic arteries by blunt trauma: report of 54 cases and review of the literature. Radiol Clin North Am 19:91, 1981

40. Fishbone G, Robbins DI, Osborn DJ, Grnja V: Trauma to the thoracic aorta and great vessels. Radiol Clin North Am 11:543, 1973

41. Daniels DL, Maddison FE: Ascending aortic injury: an angiographic diagnosis. AJR 136:812, 1981

42. Lundevall J: The mechanism of traumatic rupture of the aorta. Acta Pathol Microbiol Scand 62:34, 1964

43. Crass JR, Cohen AM, Motta AO et al: A proposed new mechanism of traumatic aortic rupture: the osseous pinch. Radiology 176:645, 1990

44. Clark DE, Zeiger MA, Wallace KL et al: Blunt aortic trauma: signs of high risk. J Trauma 30:701, 1990

45. Barcia TC, Livoni JP: Indications for angiography in blunt thoracic trauma. Radiology 147:15, 1983
46. Gundry SR, Burney RE, Mackenzie JR et al: Assessment of mediastinal widening associated with traumatic rupture of the aorta. J Trauma 23:293, 1983
47. Sefczek DM, Sefczek RJ, Deeb ZL: Radiographic signs of acute traumatic rupture of the thoracic aorta. AJR 141:1259, 1983
48. Kram HB, Wohlmuth DA, Appel PL, Shoemaker WC: Clinical and radiographic indications for aortography in blunt chest trauma. J Vasc Surg 6:168, 1987
49. Ayella RJ, Hankins JR, Turney SZ, Crowley RA: Ruptured thoracic aorta due to blunt trauma. J Trauma 17:199, 1977
50. Raptopoulos V, Sheiman RG, Phillips DA et al: Traumatic aortic tear: screening with chest CT. Radiology 182:667, 1992
51. Woodring JH: The normal mediastinum in blunt traumatic ruptures of the thoracic aorta and brachiocephalic arteries. J Emerg Med 8:467, 1990
52. Richardson P, Mirvis SE, Scorpio R, Dunham CM: Value of CT in determining the need for angiography when findings of mediastinal hemorrhage on chest radiographs are equivocal. AJR 156:273, 1991
53. Heiberg E, Wolverson MK, Sundaram M, Shields JB: CT in aortic trauma. AJR 140:1119, 1983
54. Miller FB, Richardson JD, Thomas HA et al: Role of CT in diagnosis of major arterial injury after blunt thoracic trauma. Surgery 106:596, 1989
55. Mirvis SE, Bidwell JK, Buddemeyer EU et al: Imaging diagnosis of traumatic aortic rupture. A review and experience at a major trauma center. Invest Radiol 22:187, 1987
56. Fenner MN, Fisher KS, Sergel NL et al: Evaluation of possible traumatic thoracic aortic injury using aortography and CT. Am Surg 56:497, 1990
57. Ishikawa T, Nakajima Y, Kaji T: The role of CT in traumatic rupture of the thoracic aorta and its proximal branches. Semin Roentgenol 24:38, 1989
58. Maydayag MA, Kirshenbaum KJ, Nadimpalli SR et al: Thoracic aortic trauma: role of dynamic CT. Radiology 179:853, 1991
59. Morgan PW, Goodman LR, Aprahamian C et al: Evaluation of traumatic aortic injury: does dynamic contrast-enhanced CT play a role? Radiology 182:661, 1992
60. Sparks MB, Burchard KW, Marrin CAS et al: Transesophageal echocardiography. Preliminary results in patients with traumatic aortic rupture. Arch Surg 126:711, 1991
61. Magilligan DJ, Jr, Davila JC: Innominate artery disruption due to blunt trauma. Arch Surg 114:307, 1979
62. Sturm JT, Hankins DG, Young G: Thoracic aortography following blunt chest trauma. Am J Emerg Med 8:92, 1990
63. Morse SS, Glickman MG, Greenwood LH et al: Traumatic aortic rupture: false-positive aortographic diagnosis due to atypical ductus diverticulum. AJR 150:793, 1988
64. LaBerge JM, Jeffrey RB: Aortic lacerations: fatal complications of thoracic aortography. Radiology 165:367, 1987
65. Pozzato C, Fedriga E, Donatelli F, Gattoni F: Acute posttraumatic rupture of the thoracic aorta: the role of angiography in a 7-year review. Cardiovasc Intervent Radiol 14:338, 1991
66. DeSanctis RW, Doroghazi RM, Austen WG, Buckley MJ: Aortic dissection. N Engl J Med 317:1060, 1987
67. Yamada T, Tada S, Harada J: Aortic dissection without intimal rupture: diagnosis with MR imaging and CT. Radiology 168:347, 1988
68. Demos TC, Posniak HV, Marsan RE: CT of aortic dissection. Semin Roentgenol 24:22, 1989
69. Dailey PO, Trueblood HW, Stinson EB et al: Management of acute aortic dissection. Ann Thorac Surg 10:237, 1970
70. DeBakey ME, Henly WS, Cooley DA et al: Surgical management of dissecting aneurysms of the aorta. J Thorac Cardiovasc Surg 49:130, 1965
71. Wechsler RJ, Kotler MN, Steiner RM: Multimodality approach to thoracic aortic dissection. Cardiovasc Clin 17:385, 1986
72. Crawford ES, Svensson LG, Coselli JS et al: Aortic dissection and dissecting aortic aneurysm. Ann Surg 208:254, 1988
73. Wolfe WG, Oldham HN, Rankin JS, Moran JF: Surgical treatment of acute ascending aortic dissection. Ann Surg 197:738, 1983
74. Yamaguchi T, Guthaner DF, Wexler L: Natural history of the false channel of type A aortic dissection after surgical repair: CT study. Radiology 170:743, 1989
75. Guthaner DF, Miller DC, Silverman JF et al: Fate of the false lumen following surgical repair of aortic dissections: an angiographic study. Radiology 133:1, 1979
76. Cooke JP, Kazmier FJ, Orszulak TA: The penetrating aortic ulcer: pathologic manifestations, diagnosis and management. Mayo Clin Proc 63:718, 1988
77. Yucel EK, Steinberg FL, Egglin TK et al: Penetrating aortic ulcers: diagnosis with MR imaging. Radiology 177:779, 1990
78. Erbel R, Daniel W, Visser C et al: Echocardiography in diagnosis of aortic dissection. Lancet 1:457, 1989
79. Hashimoto S, Kumada T, Osakada G et al: Assessment of transesophageal Doppler echography in dissecting aortic aneurysm. J Am Coll Cardiol 14:1253, 1989
80. Thorsen MK, San Dretto MA, Lawson TL et al: Dissecting aortic aneurysms: accuracy of computed tomographic diagnosis. Radiology 148:773, 1983
81. Landtman M, Kivisaari L, Standertskjöld-Nordenstam C-G, Taavitsainen M: Computed tomography in pre- and postoperative evaluation of aortic dissection. Acta Radiol 27:273, 1986
82. Vasile N, Mathieu D, Keita K et al: Computed tomography of thoracic aortic dissection: accuracy and pitfalls. J Comput Assist Tomogr 10:211, 1986
83. Oudkerk M, Overbosch E, Dee P: CT recognition of acute aortic dissection. AJR 141:671, 1983

84. Mügge A, Daniel WG, Laas J et al: False-negative diagnosis of proximal aortic dissection by computed tomography or angiography and possible explanations based on transesophageal echocardiographic findings. Am J Cardiol 65:527, 1990

85. St. Amour TE, Gutierrez FR, Levitt RG, McKnight RC: CT diagnosis of type A aortic dissections not demonstrated by aortography. J Comput Assist Tomogr 12:963, 1988

86. Fruehwald FXJ, Neuhold A, Fezoulidis J et al: Cine-MR in dissection of the thoracic aorta. Eur J Radiol 9:37, 1989

87. Solomon SL, Brown JJ, Glazer HS et al: Thoracic aortic dissection: pitfalls and artifacts in MR imaging. Radiology 177:223, 1990

88. Archiniegas JG, Soto B, Little WC, Papapietro SE: Cineangiography in the diagnosis of aortic dissection. Am J Cardiol 47:890, 1981

89. Gutierrez FR, Gowda S, Ludbrook PA, McKnight RC: Cineangiography in the diagnosis and evaluation of aortic dissection. Radiology 135:759, 1980

90. White RD, Ullyot DJ, Higgins CB: MR imaging of the aorta after surgery for aortic dissection. AJR 150:87, 1988

91. Mathieu D, Keita K, Loisance D et al: Postoperative CT follow-up of aortic dissection. J Comput Assist Tomogr 10:216, 1986

92. Hendrix P, Rieder P, Prokop M et al: Intravenous DSA and dynamic computed tomography for postoperative follow-up of type A aortic dissections. Eur J Radiol 9:158, 1989

93. Gomes AS, Lois JF, George B et al: Congenital abnormalities of the aortic arch: MR imaging. Radiology 165:691, 1987

94. Procter CD, Hollier LH: Takayasu's arteritis and temporal arteritis. Ann Vasc Surg 6:195, 1992

15

Carotid Angiography

Jill V. Hunter
J. K. Chin

Carotid angiography, using iodinated contrast media, continues to be the "gold standard" for diagnosing cerebrovascular disease. Its status, however, is being challenged by noninvasive techniques such as pulsed color-flow Doppler and magnetic resonance angiography (MRA). There is no doubt that under certain circumstances, successful surgery is currently being performed on the basis of these noninvasive studies.[1] Ultimate determination of the role of these various modalities must await further evaluation.

Current indications for carotid angiography are many and varied: they include the display of causes of arterial insufficiency, such as atheroma, fibromuscular hyperplasia, vasculitis (including Takayasu's disease), and dissection; the demonstration of tumor circulation; and the diagnosis or exclusion of aneurysm in the workup of subarachnoid hemorrhage. Arteriography of the carotid circulation is also an integral part of therapeutic neuroradiology in that it displays anatomy before and during interventional procedures, such as the closure of caroticocavernous fistulae and other vascular malformations, embolization with liquid or particle therapy, and thrombolytic treatment.

Conventional angiography is required to demonstrate extra- and intracranial vascular stenoses, occlusions, and ulcerated plaques. Patterns of collateral blood flow are delineated by angiography.

While arteriography is currently the study of choice for full evaluation of cerebrovascular disease, it should only be used in those patients in whom management will be altered thereby. A full discussion of every cerebrovascular pathology in which angiography plays a role is beyond the scope of this chapter, which does not include nonoperative abnormalities but rather addresses only those conditions that are amenable to surgical correction, concentrating mainly on the diagnosis of cervical carotid disease.

HISTORY

Moniz[2] introduced cerebral angiography using surgical exposure of the carotid artery, thereby revolutionizing radiologic diagnosis of neurologic disease. This technique subsequently evolved into direct percutaneous carotid angiography.[3,4] Following the introduction of the Seldinger technique of catheterization, the transfemoral placement of angiographic catheters into the great vessels of the aorta became the standard procedure for the evaluation of extracranial and intracranial carotid disease.[5] Although the transfemoral approach has been the most popular, other entry sites have been used, including the brachial and axillary arteries and even the abdominal aorta through a translumbar route.[6,7]

In addition to direct puncture techniques and selective catheterization of the carotid and vertebral arteries, nonselective retrograde brachial artery injections were also performed for the evaluation of the right carotid and bilateral vertebral arteries.[8] This permitted relatively safe examination of these vessels and their intracranial supply without the increased risk of selective catheterization; however, it did result in increased contrast load, as well as decreased opacification of the vessels. The advent of digital subtraction angiography, as well as improvements in catheter technology, with smaller French size catheters now routinely available, has improved the safety and quality of selective and nonselective angiographic studies.

INDICATIONS

Extracranial Carotid Evaluation

Although the pathophysiology of transient ischemic events and stroke is still incompletely understood, the general implications of the North American Symptomatic Carotid Endarterectomy Trial (NASCET)[9] and European Carotid Surgery Trial (ECST)[10] results are that in patients with severe (70 to 99 percent) carotid stenosis, a large proportion of ipsilateral ischemic strokes in subsequent years are due to atherothrombosis at the carotid bifurcation, with complicating embolism and/or low flow. Furthermore, these studies found that the majority of these strokes could prevented by "apparently successful" carotid endarterectomy. In the ECST, the percent reduction in diameter of the relevant carotid artery was measured from the angiographic view that showed the maximum disease at the origin of the internal carotid artery (ICA) or if more stenosed, the distal portion of the common carotid artery (CCA).

Patients presenting with a transient ischemic attack (TIA) with symptoms lasting less than 24 hours or with an evolving or fixed neurologic deficit will usually be evaluated by noninvasive Doppler imaging or MRA prior to consideration of conventional angiography. This will prevent the performance of unnecessary contrast angiography and allow a more individualized examination once the decision to proceed with angiography is made.

Angiography is therefore used alone or in conjunction with suspicious or discordant noninvasive studies to demonstrate anatomy at the carotid bifurcation, including variants such as webs and idiopathic aneurysmal dilatation, as well as plaques, stenosis, dissection, occlusion, and possibly ulceration or outpouchings. In addition to the diagnosis of bifurcation disease prior to carotid endarterectomy (CEA), postoperative follow-up angiography may be required if symptoms recur.

Evaluation of the Intracranial Circulation

Intracranial atherosclerosis occurs in the elderly but is also seen in younger diabetic or hypertensive patients. Severe narrowing of the cavernous portion of the carotid artery (carotid siphon) may be found, as well as irregularity of the proximal and distal intracranial branches. Therefore in evaluating the patient with suspected carotid disease for possible surgery, it is important to assess the intracranial circulation for severe disease distal to the common carotid bifurcation. Sometimes unexpected pathology such as an aneurysm, venous angioma, or arteriovenous malformation is demonstrated, which may alter the proposed management.

Atherosclerotic disease of the cervical carotid is considered the most common etiology of symptomatic vascular problems involving the carotid circulation,[11] but emboli can also originate from the flap of a carotid dissection or can have a more proximal source, including the heart. The majority of emboli in the carotid system flow into the territory of the middle cerebral artery. When the patient is studied early following the neurologic event, abrupt cutoff of vessels may be seen. While these patients often have severe neurologic deficits that may be thought to preclude angiography, recent interest in aggressive neurointerventional treatment may lead to an expanded role for angiography in these patients. At some centers direct application of thrombolytic therapy via a microcatheter is being evaluated in patients seen within a few hours of onset of their deficit.[12]

If a patient with a minor embolic event is studied later in the course of the disease, no occlusions may be seen because of fragmentation and lysis of the emboli; in a more major event, however, one can see continued occlusion, residual emboli in peripheral branches, narrowing of arterial caliber, mass effect, or capillary blush.[13] The vascular blush and occasional early arteriovenous shunting that one can see in stroke patients reflects loss of vascular autoregulation in the area of infarction and surrounding brain.[14,15]

Angiography is not recommended routinely in the acute stroke patient unless it is going to alter immediate management, as there is anecdotal evidence, at least, of possible worsened morbidity following the early introduction of iodinated contrast agent.[16]

Collateral Supply

With internal carotid artery occlusion or a hemodynamically severe stenosis, one can see collateral supply to the distal intracranial circulation via a number of pathways. These include the anterior and posterior communicating arteries, as well as external carotid artery (ECA) to ICA communications. There may be retrograde filling of the ophthalmic artery from ECA branches, with opacification of the carotid siphon. Typical ECA collaterals include the superficial temporal, anterior deep temporal, middle meningeal, and facial arteries. Evidence of collateral supply confirms the severity of the hemodynamic compromise, and this information is important in planning medical or surgical therapy.

Vertebrobasilar Assessment

If vertebrobasilar circulation symptoms are present, the vertebral arteries should be studied, with attention to the vertebral origins and the vertebrobasilar junctions. As part of an evaluation for carotid artery disease, the intracranial posterior circulation should be investigated to document collateral supply to the anterior circulation in cases of severe bilateral carotid disease or cases of severe unilateral disease with possible insufficient cross-circulation through the anterior communicating artery. If the cerebral hemisphere appears truly "isolated" from contralateral or posterior collateral supply, aggressive therapy may be warranted. Vertebral artery catheterization can be more difficult than selection of the common carotid arteries, and complications that arise can affect the brain stem in addition to the visual cortex.[17] In cases in which selection of the vertebral artery is difficult, a subclavian artery injection with an inflated blood pressure cuff on the arm may provide the necessary information.

Trauma

Both penetrating and blunt trauma to the neck may require angiographic evaluation to determine the need for surgical intervention. In large metropolitan hospitals in the United States, 60 to 80 percent of penetrating carotid injuries are due to gunshot wounds, with stab wounds accounting for 20 to 30 percent.[18] The most common injury is laceration of the artery, but other findings include spasm, fistulae (including caroticocavernous fistulae), pseudoaneurysms, sometimes presenting late, arterial occlusions, and embolization of bullets. Blunt injuries, such as those due to karate chops, usually result in carotid dissection. The clinical presentation of the patient and the location of the injury will determine the need for angiography versus immediate surgery or observation.[19] Preoperative angiography should be performed, however, whenever feasible to allow for optimal surgical planning. Angiog-

raphy can determine the site and extent of arterial injury, the need for operative intervention, and the presence of secondary (branch) injuries; finally, it may identify injuries amenable to interventional treatment (e.g., embolization).

Tumors

Tumors of the head and neck region may involve the carotid artery at presentation or subsequent to surgery and/or radiation therapy (Fig. 15-1). Cross-sectional imaging can give important information about proximity to and possibly about the involvement of the vessels, but angiography may be the only modality to accurately determine tumor invasion. Irregularity of the arterial wall or intraluminal filling defects are usually the findings if there is tumor involvement. However, even in the absence of overt signs of tumor involvement by angiography, excision of the tumor without carotid artery sacrifice may not be possible. Balloon test occlusion of the carotid artery, with or without induced hypotension, can be useful in those circumstances in which sacrifice of the carotid is a possible therapeutic maneuver.

Head and neck cancer patients can also present with sentinel hemorrhages from necrotic tumor beds; these bleeds may herald a major hemorrhage from carotid disruption. Angiography is necessary to demonstrate the site of hemorrhage for therapy, whether by surgery or embolization. We have found in a number of such patients that the site of hemorrhage was not the CCA or the ICA but instead branches of the ECA. This type of hemorrhage can be treated by embolization without the need for sacrifice of the ICA, with its attendant risk of stroke.

Angiography is necessary in the evaluation of possible hypervascular tumors such as chemodectomas. In these cases angiography not only provides diagnostic information but also can be a prelude to preoperative embolization.

TECHNIQUE

Carotid angiography should be performed in appropriately equipped angiography suites by angiographers with the requisite skills and training. C- or U-arm fluoroscopic stands with capabilities of high-speed multiple film sequences and magnification are required.

Biplane filming capability is useful to decrease the contrast material load administered to the patient, and to reduce the overall procedure time. A biplane digital subtraction angiography (DSA) facility further shor-

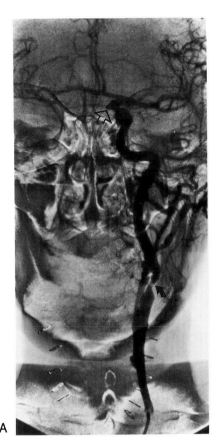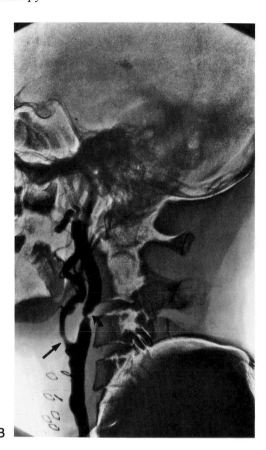

A   B

Figure 15-1 This 63-year-old man with known occlusion of the right common carotid artery had prior surgery and radiation therapy to the neck for laryngeal carcinoma. **(A)**, Anteroposterior (AP) view, left common carotid artery (CCA) injection. There is moderately severe focal stenosis of the left (ICA) *(curved arrow)*. Additionally noted is an aneurysm of the left ophthalmic artery *(open arrow)*. There is good collateral cross-filling to the right ICA via the anterior communicating artery. **(B)** Lateral view, same injection. Stenosis of the ICA *(curved arrow)* is profiled; in addition, there is some mild narrowing *(straight arrow)* of the proximal external carotid artery (ECA) *(Figure continues.)*

tens the procedure; immediate subtraction information is obtained and image processing time is minimized.

DSA has dramatically improved the safety and ease of carotid angiography. Digital road mapping allows the angiographer to proceed through very tortuous vasculature with more control. The acquisition matrix for DSA has now progressed to 1024 × 1024 pixels. Images produced by such angiographic units approach those obtained by film-screen combination with respect to clinical utility if not actually with respect to resolution. State-of-the-art DSA may replace film-screen angiography in almost all instances of clinical practice involving carotid artery disease, although many still believe that film-screen angiographic capabilities are requisite for ultimate small vessel resolution. DSA can be significantly degraded by even slight motion artifacts, which mandates cooperative or sedated patients. Neither condition may apply to patients requiring carotid angiography, as patients with ongoing

stroke or other neurologic processes may be uncooperative or may present a high risk for sedation in the absence of an anesthesiologist.

The advent of DSA and the availability of nonionic contrast media have raised hopes of performing carotid angiography from an intravenous approach. It has been shown that intravenous DSA produces fewer neurologic complications as compared with intra-arterial DSA or conventional carotid angiography.[20] However, the image quality is severely limited. The availability of duplex and magnetic resonance angiography have surpassed venous DSA even as a screening tool owing to their greater safety and cost effectiveness.

Contrast Material

Despite the continuing controversy regarding the use of low-osmolarity contrast material, we have switched to the use of only nonionic media for carotid and verte-

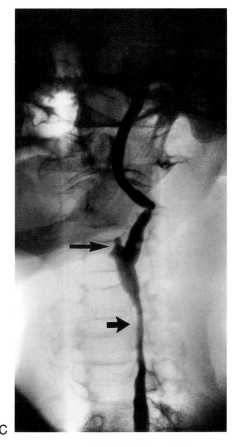
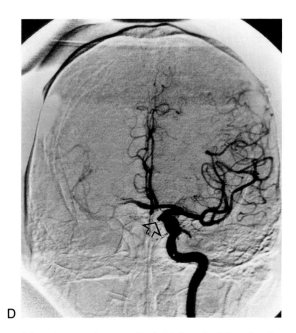

Figure 15-1 *(Continued)* **(C)** Oblique left common carotid angiogram 4 years after initial study. There has been progressive disease in the common carotid artery *(short arrow)* and occlusion of the left ECA, with an irregular stump *(long arrow)*. The stenosis of the ICA remains unchanged (confirmed with further views). **(D)** Digital subtraction angiogram, left carotid artery, AP view, also 4 years after initial study. There is continued cross-filling of the right cerebral hemisphere via the anterior communicator, as well as persistence of the ophthalmic artery aneurysm *(open arrow)*.

bral angiography. This is especially important if multiple vertebral injections are planned, with their attendant risk of cortical blindness.[21] These media are also more comfortable for those patients undergoing selective ECA angiography. There may also be benefits to patients with borderline renal function, for whom the total amount of contrast administered needs to be restricted. In these patients, aggressive prior hydration and administration of intravenous mannitol can be of value in ameliorating the nephrotoxic effects of contrast. Low-osmolarity contrast agents also decrease the dehydrating effects of high-osmolarity contrast and cause fewer adverse cardiovascular (and potentially neurologic) changes in compromised patients.

In vitro, a greater thrombosis-causing tendency of the newer nonionic iodinated contrast media as compared with ionic contrast has been observed. As a result, some centers now routinely heparinize nonionic contrast, using approximately 5 units of heparin per milliliter of contrast agent.

Angiographic Approaches

Direct-puncture carotid angiography cannot be justified for routine diagnostic purposes; it continues to play a limited role in neurointerventional procedures. Its use in diagnostic angiography should be considered appropriate only in the unusual circumstance in which no other arterial access is available. The major morbidity of the procedure other than arterial trauma is compromise of the airway by a large hematoma. This may require intubation or even emergency tracheotomy if sufficiently severe.[4]

Direct Brachial Puncture

Retrograde brachial angiography is a safe, if rarely used, method of demonstrating the cerebral vasculature without risking direct trauma to the cerebral vessels. This is a nonselective technique, producing opacification of both carotid and vertebral arteries with resultant limited image quality. The technique is better for evaluation of the vertebrobasilar circulation; although the right carotid artery can be evaluated by a right brachial injection in the majority of cases, this is a very limited method for the study of the left carotid artery.[8] As with direct carotid puncture, routine use of this technique cannot be justified. Complications include local hematoma, loss of the radial pulse, and damage to the median nerve. In Chase et al.'s series of 200 patients, there were more than 300 examinations, with five lost radial pulses and no limb ischemia.[22]

Use of the brachial artery as a site for selective catheter access is preferred to the nonselective brachial techniques. This approach has been advocated for outpatient carotid angiography with use of arch injections and DSA.[23] The axillary artery can also be used for selective or nonselective catheter access, but the greater potential for neurologic complications due to proximity to the brachial plexus makes this a less desirable approach. From either a brachial or axillary approach, catheters can be manipulated selectively into the right-sided arch vessels and even into those on the left.[6,24]

Potential complications include hematoma and specifically, damage to the brachial plexus. Close monitoring of these patients is required after the procedure in case surgical decompression is required. The need for surgery should be based on progressive neurologic symptoms, and operation, if necessary, should be promptly undertaken to avoid irreversible damage. The hematoma may not be palpable on physical examination.

The femoral route is the preferred approach for all arterial studies. Smaller-caliber angiographic catheters allow safe outpatient studies in the majority of patients, and this access provides the greatest flexibility for selective cerebrovascular catheterization.

In the event that selective catheterization is not possible, nonselective injections can be made especially with the use of DSA to obtain the necessary information. The evaluation of the intracranial circulation tends to be less than optimal but can still be satisfactory.

Complications

The reported complication rate for carotid angiography has ranged from less than 1 to 20 percent, varying with the patient population and the experience of the operator.[25-27] An overview of the results suggests that the risk of a neurologic complication is about 4 percent and that a permanent neurologic deficit (disabling stroke) occurs in about 1 percent.[28] The mortality rate is less than 0.1 percent. Previously, complication rates

included complications related to use of noncatheter techniques, specifically percutaneous entry into the carotid arteries. In these cases the local complications, such as large neck hematomas, could be devastating.

Even experienced angiographers can expect a finite incidence of complications from contrast carotid angiography; this complication rate is even higher in a patient population with a high incidence of atherosclerotic disease. The complications of contrast angiography are related to the catheterization of the vessel as well as to the adverse effects of the contrast material. Catheter-related events are due to dislodged embolic material, emboli from thrombus formation on the catheter[29] or guidewire, and intimal injury from the catheter tip or injection jet. A constant infusion of heparanized saline through the catheter by means of a pressure pump may prevent formation of intraluminal clot.[30]

PATHOLOGY

Atherosclerosis

Carotid Stenosis

Hemodynamically significant lesions in the ICA origin may result from gradual enlargement of the atherosclerotic plaque or from sudden subintimal hemorrhage. These plaques are found predominantly in the region of the CCA bifurcation and extending into the origin of the ICA (Fig. 15-2) on its posterior wall.[31,32] Other sites for atheroslerotic disease include the proximal common carotid artery as well as the more distal ICA.

The evaluation of significant stenoses involves actual measurement of the residual lumen if the magnification factor is known or if a radiopaque standard is used (a lead bead or a catheter of known diameter); alternatively, the percentage of stenosis can be determined relative to the unaffected distal ICA taken as the norm. At our institution we rely on actual measurements, with a residual luminal diameter of 2 mm or less considered to be significant. With a residual luminal diameter of 1 mm or less, one can see delayed filling of the intracranial circulation relative to the ECA branches (assuming no significant disease involving the origin of the ECA).

Ulcerated Plaque

Neurologic events due to embolic phenomena may develop from ulcers within plaques that do not cause hemodynamic compromise. The emboli that form

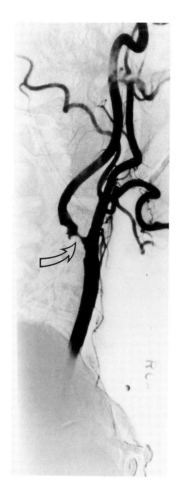

Figure 15-2 Preoperative (coronary artery bypass graft) angiogram of 72-year-old man with a right carotid bruit. There is severe stenosis of the proximal ICA *(arrow)*. Significant irregularity just distal to the stenosis is consistent with ulceration.

may consist of platelet aggregates, atherosclerotic debris, or thrombus that develops on a disrupted intimal surface. The diagnosis of an ulcerated plaque is usually straightforward, but it is important to always obtain at least two views of the common carotid bifurcation. There has been some recent evidence to suggest that spiral computed tomography (CT) may be a useful device with which to study ulcerated plaque. The majority of the ulcers are found on the posterior wall of the carotid bifurcation and carotid bulb and are best seen on the lateral view (Fig. 15-3). The ulcers are usually small, measuring 4 to 5 mm in diameter, but occasionally they may be as large as 1.5 cm.[33]

Although it is usually possible to identify ulcerated lesions, a subintimal hematoma may mimic the appearance of an ulcer but possess a smooth intimal surface.[34] Small symptomatic ulcers that had been missed

on preoperative angiography have also been identified at the time of surgery.[35,36]

Subintimal Hematoma

Subintimal hematomas were found by Edwards et al.[34] in 24 percent of carotid bifurcations during surgery for repeated TIAs in a single hemispheric distribution; only 33 percent were associated with ulcerations. The typical angiographic appearance was a sharply marginated, rounded, and eccentric filling defect located near the carotid bifurcation; occasionally such a defect may simulate a typical smooth or even ulcerated atherosclerotic plaque. Hemorrhage into an atherosclerotic plaque may convert a nonstenosing lesion into one with critical stenosis, with clinical sequelae. This appeared to be the case in many patients studied by Edwards et al.[34] who showed high-grade stenosis without ulceration. Hemorrhage in a plaque has also been observed to be associated with a rupture of the intima. The resulting exposure of the underlying basement membrane can lead to platelet adhesion with formation of thrombus and possibly subsequent embolization, which constitutes another mechanism for neurologic changes resulting from subintimal hematomas.

Carotid Occlusion

Total occlusion of the ICA at its origin with thrombus extending above the skull base is not readily amenable to surgical treatment; however, a severe stenosis with a distal trickle of blood can be opened by endarterectomy. It is therefore very important to differentiate these two entities by careful angiography with a prolonged filming sequence. The greater contrast sensitivity of DSA techniques may allow for easier identification of a minute remaining lumen. Carotid occlusion may result from thrombus formation of a critically stenotic atherosclerotic plaque or from subintimal hematoma.

Trauma

Closed injury to the neck can result in trauma to the ICA at the high cervical level opposite the highest cervical vertebrae. The injuries range from spasm to intimal tear with thrombus formation, medial tear, and aneurysm formation.[37] Intimal injuries may be very subtle and require meticulous attention to technique. Penetrating injuries can result in arterial laceration, total occlusion (Fig. 15-4), or aneurysm formation (false aneurysms).[18] Careful attention to entrance and exit sites of injury will facilitate thorough evaluation (Fig. 15-5).

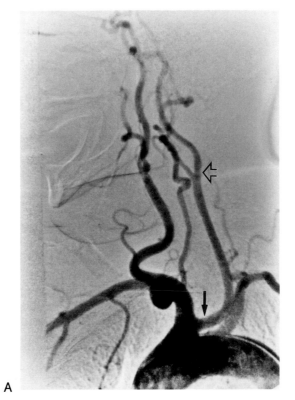

A

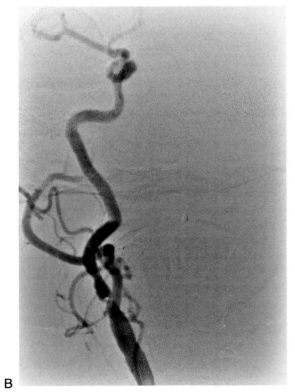

B

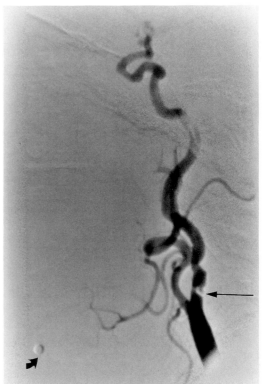

C

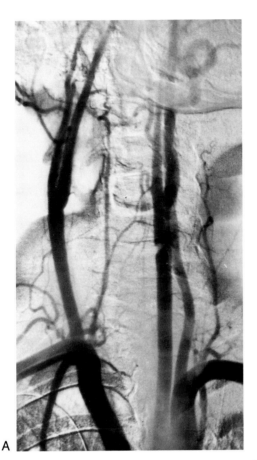 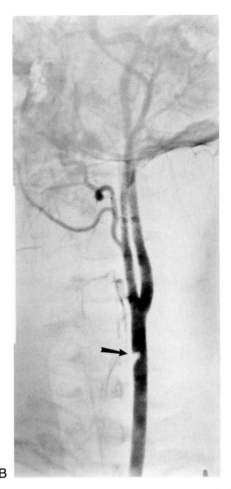

Figure 15-4 Patient with gunshot wound to the neck. (A) Nonselective arch injection demonstrates some intimal irregularity of the left common carotid artery. (B) Selective left common carotid injection better shows the defect projecting into the lumen of the artery *(arrow)*.

Carotid Dissection

Dissection of the extracranial ICA may develop either as an idiopathic process[38] or from known trauma or neck manipulation. The trauma may be blunt, as from a motor vehicle accident, or may be penetrating in nature with direct vascular injury.[39] Conditions that predispose toward developing carotid dissection include fibromuscular dysplasia and cystic medial necrosis. A spontaneous dissection may arise in what appears to be a normal artery, although histologic investigation may suggest medial degeneration.[40]

Figure 15-3 Digital subtraction angiogram of 59-year-old woman with right-sided transient ischemic attacks. (A) The left common carotid artery arises from the innominate *(straight arrow)*, a common anatomic variant. The left internal carotid artery is mildly diseased *(open arrow)* with loss of the normal bulb. There is irregularity noted in the right ICA proximally; however, this nonselective study does not allow complete evaluation. (B) AP view, right CCA injection. The right ECA is projected over the proximal ICA. There is suggestion of a severe stenosis of the ICA proximally, with a mild stenosis just beyond this. The remainder of the ICA to the carotid siphon appears patent. (C) Lateral projection. The high-grade stenosis of the right ICA is well visualized *(long arrow)*. Central collection of contrast within this indicates ulceration. Notice the size of the residual lumen as compared with the 3-mm metal marker *(curved arrow)* in the anterior aspect of the film. The milder stenosis more distally is also appreciated. The remainder of the ICA is well visualized to the carotid siphon. Multiple projections may be necessary to fully evaluate an arterial segment and to ensure that all stenoses have been optimally defined.

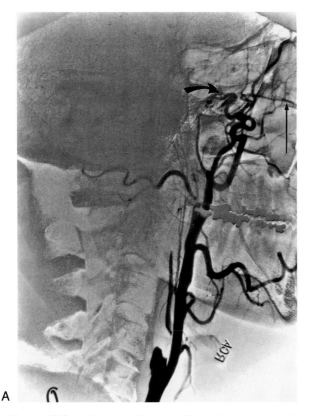
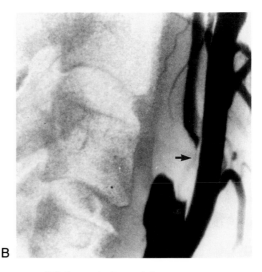

Figure 15-5 A 44-year-old man with right neck pain after trauma. **(A)** Lateral view, right common artery projection. There is a severe stenosis with near total occlusion (string sign) of the proximal internal carotid artery shortly past its origin. There is filling of the cavernous carotid *(curved arrow)* via retrograde flow from the opthalmic artery *(long arrow)*. The opthalmic artery is filling via the external carotid artery collaterals. **(B)** Closeup view at the carotid bifurcation. The minimal antegrade filling of the ICA is marked *(arrow)*. Careful attention to angiographic technique is necessary to differentiate near total occlusions such as this from complete occlusions. This differentiation may be difficult or impossible with Doppler.

ICA dissections usually start in the middle to upper cervical carotid artery, although they may be seen near its origin. The angiographic appearance is usually that of a markedly tapered narrowing (Fig. 15-6), which extends distally up to the petrous portion of the carotid but may extend even more distally. If there is circumferential involvement of the vessel, the appearance of the opacified vessel may be string-like.[44] The resulting stenosis can be very severe, with little antegrade flow into the intracranial circulation; symptoms can be due to hemodynamic compromise or to emboli from the damaged portion of the artery. However, complete occlusion can occur, with resulting intravascular thrombosis and formation of emboli from this thrombus. The presenting event may be a dense hemiplegia.

If a patent lumen is present and the patient can be treated by anticoagulation, the vessel may return to normal appearance after weeks to months of therapy. Sometimes the follow-up angiogram demonstrates residual narrowing or aneurysmal dilatation of the vessel.

Continued embolic neurologic events despite coagulation should prompt follow-up angiographic studies. We have treated one patient in whom angiography 1 year after the initial presentation demonstrated aneurysmal dilatation at the site of the dissection. Thrombus forming within this aneurysm was believed to be the source of his continued emboli. Balloon occlusion of the ICA was performed for definitive management of this problem.

Extracranial Aneurysms

Aneurysms of the extracranial carotid artery are uncommon.[42] Syphilis and local infection were the common etiologic factors in the early 1950s but are rare in the present era.[43] Arteriosclerosis, trauma, and previous surgery account for the majority of extracranial carotid artery aneurysms today; atherosclerosis is the most common etiology, with severe hypertension as a compounding factor.[44] Rupture is rare; more com-

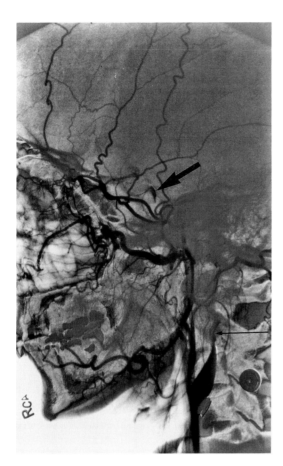

Figure 15-6 A 43-year-old woman with a right middle cerebral artery territory infarct 11 days earlier. Lateral angiogram after right CCA injection. There is a tapered occlusion of the right internal carotid artery *(small arrow)* originating approximately 2 cm distal to the carotid bifurcation. Minimal opacification of the cavernous carotid *(large arrow)*. This filled via external collaterals from the temporal, supra-orbital and supratrochlear arteries. The location and tapered occlusion are consistent with recent carotid dissection.

monly, thromboembolic events occur. Although painful swelling is the most common symptom, neurologic dysfunction is the most ominous. Those aneurysms caused by metastatic disease or trauma commonly arise at the base of the skull and represent complicated management problems.

There are two morphologic types of extracranial aneurysms. Those of the more common type are fusiform, apparently atherosclerotic, and develop in the carotid artery bifurcation.[45] They have a bilateral predilection. Examples of the second type of aneurysm are saccular, usually unilateral, and often located in the midsegment of the ICA or the CCA trunk (Fig. 15-7). They may be of congenital origin or associated with fibromuscular dysplasia of the carotid artery, but most are post-traumatic or postsurgical. The postsurgical

aneurysms are usually false aneurysms and occur most commonly following those carotid endarterectomies in which prosthetic patch material is used.[42]

Aneurysmectomy with arterial reconstruction is the treatment of choice.

Vasculitis

Takayasu's Arteritis

Although Takayasu's arteritis is generally a vasculitis involving the proximal great vessels, the disease can affect the distal carotid system.[46,47] There is luminal compromise due to infiltration of the adventitia by inflammatory cells, and there be may associated constitutional symptoms such as myalgia and fever.

An aortic arch injection will demonstrate the diffuse narrowing and occlusion of the brachiocephalic vessels at their origins from the aorta. These vascular changes may extend distally. In contrast to atherosclerotic disease, the lumen is smooth (Fig. 15-8). Neurologic symptoms may be seen in the patient in the chronic

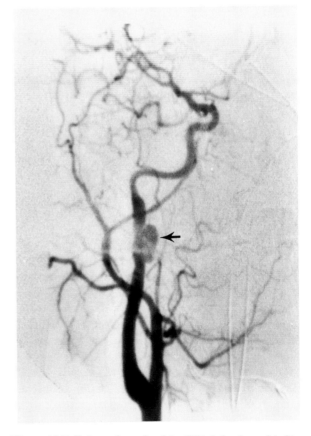

Figure 15-7 Subtraction of a right CCA injection with filming from the common carotid bifurcation to the carotid siphon. There is a saccular aneurysm of the internal carotid artery just at the skull base *(arrow)*.

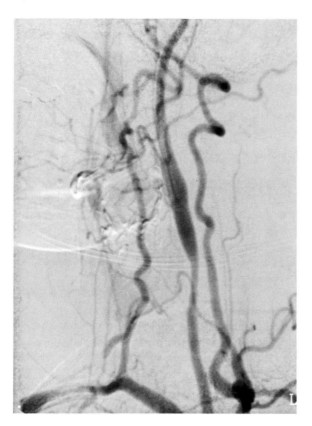

Figure 15-8 Arch aortogram of a young female with Takayasu's disease. There is complete occlusion of the right CCA, fusiform narrowing of the left CCA. Note also the severe narrowing of the right subclavian. The vertebral arteries are spared.

stage of Takayasu's arteritis of the ascending aorta and its branches.[42] These patients pose a difficult surgical problem owing to the diffuse nature of the disease, and bypass with autologous or prosthetic material has been considered the best approach.[48] Alternatively, there has been interest in the use of angioplasty, with or without stenting.[46]

Fibromuscular Dysplasia

Connett and Lansche in 1965 described involvement of the ICA by fibromuscular dysplasia.[49] Involvement of the carotid artery is second in frequency only to involvement of the renal artery. Fibromuscular dysplasia primarily affects older women and may be an incidental finding; it may, however, lead to ischemic problems and can predispose to carotid dissection. The disease, the etiology of which is unknown, has a predilection for small- to medium-sized vessels. It usually involves the ICA 3 to 4 cm distal to the origin, approximately at the C2 vertebral[50] level (Fig. 15-9), and is

frequently bilateral. There is a frequent association with renal fibromuscular dysplasia as well as with intracranial aneurysms.

Cerebrovascular fibromuscular dysplasia accounts for 25 to 30 percent of the published cases. Three main types of fibromuscular dysplasia have been identified: intimal fibroplasia, medial fibromuscular dysplasia, and periarterial or periadventitial fibroplasia. Lesions involving the media may be further subclassified into medial fibroplasia, perimedial fibroplasia, and medial hyperplasia.[51] The differential diagnosis of fibromuscular dysplasia includes arteriosclerosis, inflammatory vascular diseases such as Takayasu's arteritis, and vascular lesions of neurofibromatosis. Certain types of inherited connective tissue diseases, such as Ehler-Danlos syndrome, can mimic the aneurysmal type of fibromuscular dysplasia.

An association between fibromuscular dysplasia and intracranial aneurysms was first raised by Palubinskas and Newton.[52] Others have noted an incidence as high as 51 percent, with some cases involving multiple aneurysms.[51] The aneurysms are noted in the intracranial portion of the ICA and the middle cerebral artery. In a review of 284 patients with cerebrovascular fibromuscular dysplasia, intracranial aneurysms were found in 21 percent; two-thirds of the patients had multiple aneurysms.[51] In view of these findings, the evaluation of a patient with carotid fibromuscular dysplasia should include cerebral angiography; the renal arteries should also be studied.

There are three characteristic angiographic patterns, the most common is the "string of beads" appearance, found in 80 percent.[53] A second, much less common, pattern is unifocal or multifocal tubular stenosis. The third type, which has been called "atypical fibromuscular dysplasia" by Houser et al.,[50] usually involves only one wall of the segment and demonstrates a diverticulum-like smooth or corrugated outpouching, which can evolve and become a true saccular aneurysm. Typical cases of fibromuscular dysplasia demonstrate alternating zones of widening and narrowing of the arterial lumen, which is smooth. Distinguishing characteristics include dilatations that are always wider than the normal arterial lumen and are separated from one another by ring-like bands of luminal constriction.[50]

Miscellaneous

Tortuosity of the ICA may be seen without clinical sequelae. Coils and kinks of the carotid arteries have been reported to occur in between 5 and 16 percent of arteriograms.[54] With the development of atherosclero-

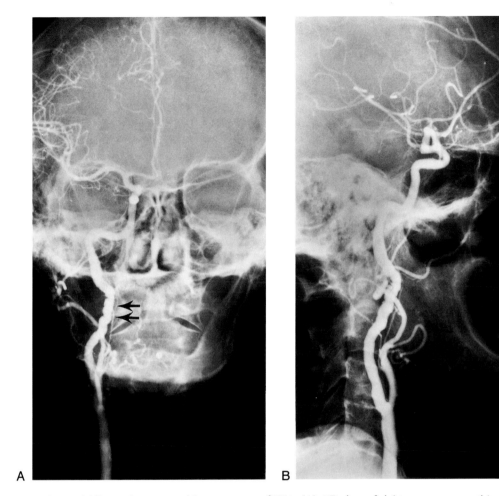

Figure 15-9 A middle-aged woman with symptoms of TIA. **(A)** AP view of right common carotid angiogram with characteristic "string of beads" appearance of fibromuscular dysplasia in the ICA *(arrows).* **(B)** Lateral view, same injection. Fibromuscular disease is less apparent. Note minor irregularity of the carotid bulb, which may represent coexistent atherosclerotic plaque.

sis, there may be further elongation of the artery, with increasing angulation at the kink; this may result in hemodynamic compromise, especially with head turning. The evaluation of such a patient should include angiography with the head so positioned that symptoms could occur.

CONCLUSION

Contrast angiography using catheter techniques still provides necessary information for the management of extracranial carotid artery disease. In this era of increasingly sophisticated noninvasive vascular imaging, it is especially important that proper indications be met before proceeding to catheterization. Complete familiarity with the appropriate indications and techniques for the various available imaging studies should allow

for optimal evaluation of each patient. Rather than viewing these as competitive, a more productive and useful perspective is to consider them as complementary and to individualize their use according to the clinical need.

REFERENCES

1. Gaudier JH, Lamparello PJ, Riles TS et al: Is duplex scanning sufficient evaluation before carotid endarterectomy? J Vasc Surg 9:193, 1989
2. Moniz E: L'encéphalographie artérielle, son importance dans la localisation des tumeurs cérébrales. Rev Neurol 2:72, 1927
3. Scheinberg P, Zunker E: Complications in direct percutaneous carotid arteriography. Arch Neurol 8:676, 1963
4. Bauer J, Salazar JL, Sugar O, Pawl RP: Direct percutane-

ous cerebral angiography in neurosurgical practice. J Neurosurg 52:525, 1980

5. Seldinger SI: Catheter replacement of the needle in percutaneous arteriography. Acta Radiol 39:368, 1953

6. Lin JP: Techniques of cerebral angiography. Radiol Clin North Am 12:223, 1974

7. Maxwell SJ, Kwon OJ, Millan VG: Translumbar carotid arteriography. Radiology 148:851, 1983

8. Ostrowski AZ, Hardy WG, Lindner DW et al: Retrograde brachial vertebral-basilar angiography. Arch Neurol 4:608, 1961

9. Barnett HJM, North American Symptomatic Carotid Endarterectomy Trial Collaborators: Beneficial effects of carotid endarterectomy in symptomatic patients with high-grade carotid stenosis. N Engl J Med; 325:445, 1991

10. European Carotid Surgery Trialists' Collaborative Group: MRC European Carotid Surgery Trial: interim results for symptomatic patients with severe (70–99%) or with mild (0–29%) carotid stenosis. Lancet 337:1235, 1991

11. Gomez CR: Carotid plaque morphology and risk for stroke. Stroke 21:148, 1990

12. Leclerc X, Rondepierrre R, Henon H, et al: Thrombolysis in severe ischemic strokes. Presented at 78th Scientific Assembly and Annual Meeting, Radiological Society of North America, Chicago, Illinois, November 29–December 4, 1992. Radiology 185 (suppl):248, 1992

13. Irino T, Taneda M, Minami T: Angiographic manifestations in postrecanalized cerebral infarction. Neurology 27:471, 1977

14. Leeds NE, Goldberg HI: Abnormal vascular patterns in benign intracranial lesions: pseudotumors of the brain. AJR 118:576, 1973

15. Lassen NA: The luxury-perfusion syndrome and its possible relation to acute metabolic acidosis localised within the brain. Lancet 2:1113, 1966

16. Hankey GJ, Warlow CP, Sellar RJ: Cerebral angiographic risk in mild cerebrovascular disease. Stroke 21:209, 1990

17. Howieson J, Megison LC Jr: Complications of vertebral artery catheterization. Radiology 91:1108, 1968

18. Pearce WH, Whitehill TA: Carotid and vertebral arterial injuries. Surg Clin North Am 68:705, 1988

19. Richardson JD, Simpson C, Miller FB: Management of carotid artery trauma. Surgery 104:673, 1988

20. Stevens JM, Barter S, Kerslake R, Schneidau A, Barber C, Thomas DJ. Br J Radiol 62:813, 1989

21. Studdard WE, Davis DO, Young SW: Cortical blindness after cerebral angiography. Case report. J Neurosurg 54:240, 1981

22. Chase N, Hass HK, Ransohoff J: Modified method for percutaneous brachial angiography. Arch Neurol 8:632, 1963

23. McCreary JA, Schellhas KP, Brant ZM et al: Outpatient DSA in cerebrovascular disease using transbrachial arch injections. AJR 145:941, 1985

24. Westcott JL, Taylor PT: Transaxillary selective four-vessel arteriography. Radiology 104:277, 1972

25. Chynn KY: Transfemoral carotid and vertebral angiography. Acta Radiol 9:244, 1969

26. Earnest F4, Forbes G, Sandok BA et al: Complications of cerebral angiography: prospective assessment of risk. AJNR 4:1191, 1983

27. Hankey GJ, Warlow CP, Molyneux AJ: Complications of cerebral angiography for patients with mild carotid territory ischaemia being considered for carotid endarterectomy. J Neurol Neurosurg Psychiatry 53:542, 1990

28. Waugh JR, Sacharias N: Arteriographic complications in the DSA era. Radiology 182:243, 1992

29. Cronqvist S, Efsing HO, Palacios E: Embolic complications in cerebral angiography with the catheter technique. Acta Radiol 10:97, 1970

30. Epstein BS: The use of a constant pressure pump for maintaining the patency of catheters and needles during angiography. AJR 113:572, 1971

31. Simmons CR, Tsao E, Smith LL et al: Angiographic evaluation in extracranial vascular occlusive disease. Arch Surg 107:785, 1973

32. Kerber CW, Cromwell LD, Drayer BP, Bank WO: Cerebral ischemia. I. Current angiographic techniques, complications, and safety. Roen AJR 130:1097, 1978

33. Kishore PR: The significance of the ulcerative plaque. Radiol Clin North Am 12:343, 1974

34. Edwards JH, Kricheff II, Gorstein F et al: Atherosclerotic subintimal hematoma of the carotid artery. Radiology 133:123, 1979

35. Edwards JH, Kricheff II, Riles T, Imparato A: Angiographically undetected ulceration of the carotid bifurcation as a cause of embolic stroke. Radiology 132:369, 1979

36. Eikelboom BC, Riles TR, Mintzer R et al: Inaccuracy of angiography in the diagnosis of carotid ulceration. Stroke 14:882, 1983

37. Batzdorf U, Bentson JR, Machleder HI: Blunt trauma to the high cervical carotid artery. Neurosurgery 5:195, 1979

38. Fisher CM, Ojemann RG, Roberson GH: Spontaneous dissection of cervico-cerebral arteries. Can J Neurol Sci 5:9, 1978

39. Fabian TC, George SJ, Croce MA et al: Carotid artery trauma: management based on mechanism of injury. J Trauma 30:953, 1990

40. Anderson RM, Schechter MM: A case of spontaneous dissecting aneurysm of the internal carotid artery. J Neurol Neurosurg Psychiatry 22:195, 1959

41. Ojemann RG, Fisher CM, Rich JC: Spontaneous dissecting aneurysm of the internal carotid artery. Stroke 3:434, 1972

42. Smullens SN: Surgically treatable lesions of the extracranial circulation, including the vertebral artery. Radiol Clin North Am 24:453, 1986

43. Busuttil RW, Davidson RK, Foley KT et al: Selective management of extracranial carotid arterialaneurysms. Am J Surg 140:85, 1980

44. Rhodes EL, Stanley JC, Hoffman GL et al: Aneurysms of extracranial carotid arteries. Arch Surg 111:339, 1976

45. Kaupp HA, Haid SP, Jurayj MN et al: Aneurysms of the extracranial carotid artery. Surgery 72:946, 1972

46. Hodgins GW, Dutton JH: Transluminal dilatation for Takayasu's arteritis. Can J Surg 27:355, 1984

47. Hodgins GW, Dutton JH: Subclavian and carotid angioplasties for Takayasu's arteritis. Can Assoc Radiol J 33:205, 1982

48. Bloss RS, Duncan JM, Cooley DA et al: Takayasu's arteritis: surgical considerations. Ann Thorac Surg 27:574, 1979

49. Connett MC, Lansche JM: Fibromuscular hyperplasia of the internal carotid artery: report of a case. Ann Surg 162:59, 1965

50. Houser OW, Baker HLJ: Fibromuscular dysplasia and other uncommon diseases of the cervical carotid artery: angiographic aspects. AJR 104:201, 1968

51. Luscher TF, Lie JT, Stanson AW et al: Arterial fibromuscular dysplasia. Mayo Clin Proc 62:931, 1987

52. Palubinskas AJ, Newton TH: Fibromuscular hyperplasia of the internal carotid arteries. Radiol Clin Biol 34:365, 1965

53. Osborn AG, Anderson RE: Angiographic spectrum of cervical and intracranial fibromuscular dysplasia. Stroke 8:617, 1977

54. Mukherjee D, Inahara T: Management of the tortuous internal carotid artery. Am J Surg 149:651, 1985

16

Magnetic Resonance Angiography

E. Kent Yucel

In recent years magnetic resonance angiography (MRA) has moved from the investigational realm into the clinical practice of vascular imaging. As newer pulse sequences are developed and as more clinical studies into imaging protocols and specific vascular disease applications are initiated, we may expect this trend to continue and even to accelerate in the near future.

BASIC PRINCIPLES

MRA images depend on the production of contrast between blood within vessels and the surrounding tissue. Unlike x-ray angiography, in which this contrast is produced by the injection of a contrast medium directly into the vessels one wishes to image, MRA relies on the physical properties of hydrogen atoms in the blood as they move through magnetic field gradients to elicit contrast between moving blood and stationary soft tissue. Two basic approaches have been employed to detect this motion: the time of flight (TOF) and method the phase contrast (PC) method. All clinical MRA techniques employed today are based on variations of one of these two basic methods.

Time of Flight MRA

TOF angiography relies on the fact that tissue sections undergoing the repetitive applications of radio-frequency pulses that are used to produce magnetic resonance (MR) images become "saturated," so that they are unable to produce as strong an MR signal as in their unperturbed state. Blood flowing through such a saturated section of tissue is capable of producing a stronger signal than the surrounding stationary tissue because it has not experienced the preceding radiofrequency pulses. The gradient echo imaging technique used for the production of MRA images depends on the production of the MR signal or "echo" by gradient reversal rather than by application of additional 180-degree refocusing radiofrequency pulses.

The features that must be manipulated to produce high-quality TOF MRA images include the repetition time (TR) of the radiofrequency pulses and the flip angle. The TR is generally chosen to be less than 50 ms in order to keep imaging time short and to maintain adequate stationary tissue saturation. Saturation increases with decreasing TR and increasing flip angle. The actual values chosen must be adjusted according to the velocity and orientation of the flow being imaged.

Two additional factors must be kept in mind to

maintain an adequate signal within vessels: echo time (TE) minimization and gradient moment nulling. Hydrogen atoms, or spins, moving through magnetic field gradients undergo phase shifts that are proportional to their velocity. In most vessels parabolic flow is present, with a range of velocities across the vessel cross section. This results in a range of phase shifts and in cancellation of signal due to intravoxel phase dispersion. The longer the TE, or time to gathering the MR signal, the greater the resulting phase dispersion. Therefore a designer of pulse sequences for use in MRA goes to great lengths to minimize TE, including use of asymmetric echo acquisitions to maximize the intravascular signal.

Gradient moment nulling, or flow compensation, uses additional lobes in the gradient waveforms to refocus, or compensate for the phase shifts due to constant velocity motion. Additional lobes can be applied to compensate for higher orders of motion, such as acceleration and "jerk." However, gradient moment nulling does increase the TE, which tends to diminish the blood vessel signal, partially negating the effects of gradient moment nulling. For physiologic flows, application of first-order flow compensation for constant velocity has been found to be helpful despite the increase in TE. However, the potential benefits of higher orders of flow compensation are negated by the resulting prolongation in TE, and these have not been found helpful in practice.

TOF MRA slices may be obtained in one of two modes, sequential single slice (two-dimensional) or volume (three-dimensional). In the two-dimensional mode[1] each slice is obtained individually before moving on to the next. The plane of acquisition depends on the orientation of the blood vessels being evaluated. The contrast between blood and stationary tissue is maximized when blood flow is perpendicular to the plane of the slice. For rapid flow perpendicular to the imaged slice, the TR is kept short and the flip angle high (up to 90 degrees) to maximize stationary tissue saturation. However, for slow flow and in-plane flow, TR and flip angle must be adjusted to prevent saturation of the flowing spins while maintaining contrast between blood and stationary tissue. The time to image a single slice is given by multiplying the TR by the y-axis matrix size, and the number of excitations. Thus, with a TR of 50 ms, a 256×128 matrix size, and one excitation, a slice can be obtained in 0.05 second $\times 128 \times 1 = 6.4$ seconds). This value must be multiplied by the total number of slices to obtain the total imaging time. (A small additional time factor is introduced by the time required to move from one slice to the next.) The advantages of the two-dimensional mode include sensitivity to a wide range of flow velocities, the capability of obtaining slices within a single breath-hold, and the

ability to image as large a portion of the body as desired, the only limiting factor being available imaging time (Fig. 16-1).

In the three-dimensional mode[2,3] an entire volume is imaged in a single acquisition and displayed as 28 to 64 partitions or slices. Acquisition time is determined by the same factors as in two-dimensional mode with the result multiplied by the number of partitions or slices. Therefore a typical three-dimensional acquisition with the same parameters as in the preceding paragraph and 60 partitions would require 6.4 seconds $\times 60 = 384$ seconds, or 6.4 minutes. Contrast still depends of the inflow of unsaturated blood into the imaged volume, which is partially saturated. However, in the three-dimensional mode the flowing blood itself becomes saturated as it moves through the imaged volume. Slowly moving blood, such as venous flow or flow distal to an obstruction, becomes rapidly saturated and may not be visualized. Even for relatively fast flows, the TR must be increased or the flip angle decreased relative to two-dimensional acquisition in order to minimize saturation of the blood as it moves through the imaged volume. Therefore, contrast between moving blood and stationary tissue is not as high as in the two-dimensional mode. Furthermore, after a certain number of partitions all blood will become saturated unless gadolinium is administered. This limits the effective distance over which flowing blood can be visualized. The major advantage of the three-dimensional mode is its higher spatial resolution, allowing isotropic voxel size with submillimeter resolution.

Multislab three-dimensional acquisition is a recently developed hybrid technique, which combines aspects of both two-dimensional and three-dimensional imaging.[4] In this method multiple, thin, overlapping three-dimensional slabs are acquired. A postprocessing program then eliminates the overlapping slices and reorders the slices from each slab into a set of contiguous thin slices. This method has the high spatial resolution of the three-dimensional mode, but because each individual slab is quite thin, saturation effects are minimized. As in the two-dimensional mode, any desired distance may be imaged by adding on additional slabs, the limited only limitation being available imaging time (Fig. 16-2). As compared with two-dimensional imaging, however, a substantial time penalty is incurred by the requirement of substantial overlap between the slabs (up to 50 percent) to eliminate so-called venetian blind artifacts on the final angiograms.

Once slices are acquired by either the two-dimensional, three-dimensional, or multislab three-dimensional techniques, they are stacked and then postprocessed to produce projectional images. These projections may be in planes orthogonal to the original

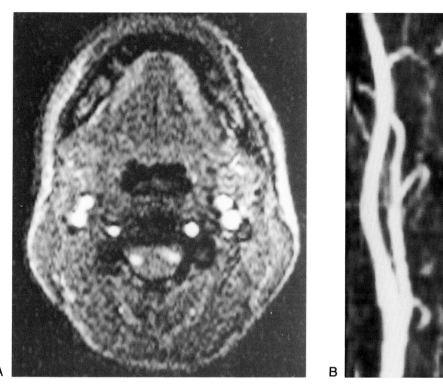

A   B

Figure 16-1 (A) Single axial gradient echo slice through the neck, with superior presaturation demonstrating the carotid bifurcations and vertebral arteries bilaterally. **(B)** MR angiogram produced by applying the maximum intensity pixel (MIP) algorithm to multiple slices like that in Fig. A. (From Yucel,[47] with permission.)

acquisition (e.g., sagittal or coronal projections from an axial set of slices) or they may be in the same plane as the original slices giving what is commonly referred to as a *collapsed* image. The method most commonly used to process the individual slices is the maximum intensity pixel (MIP) algorithm. In this method a ray is passed along the axis desired in the final projection

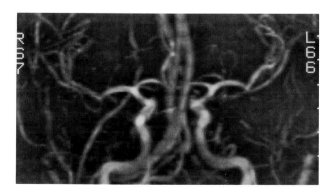

Figure 16-2 Multiple overlapping thin slab angiogram (MOTSA) of the head. A subtle striping effect can be seen between the individual three-dimensional slabs. Note the excellent spatial resolution, along with good peripheral vessel detail, that is characteristic of this technique.

(e.g., anteroposterior in the case for a straight coronal projection) and the brightest pixel encountered by that ray is displayed in the final image. Any of an infinite range of projections can be created in this fashion and viewed either individually or as a rotating cine loop.

Several characteristics of the MIP algorithm are worthy of note.[5] Because it only displays the brightest pixel along a given axis, it tends to suppress structures of lower signal intensity (e.g., small vessels, vessel loops, or aneurysmal segments). This feature becomes more pronounced as the volume through which the ray is passed becomes larger. Therefore, to adequately assess small vessels and areas of signal loss within vessels, it is important to examine the individual slices and, if necessary, to obtain MIPs on smaller volumes of interest or on fewer slices. Other algorithms that have been applied to angiographic data sets include connectivity algorithms[6,7] and methods designed to maintain three-dimensional perspective[8] in the two-dimensional projections. These methods have some advantages relative to the MIP algorithm, and investigation continues into newer projection methods. Nevertheless, the MIP method, because of its simplicity and rapidity, remains the most widely used projection method in clinical practice.

On TOF slices all vessels flowing into the imaged slices from any direction will be bright, and overlap between arteries and veins may obscure relevant anatomy. This can be overcome by application of presaturation pulses adjacent to the imaged slice to eliminate flow entering from unwanted directions. For example, to adequately visualize the carotid bifurcation, it is necessary to eliminate the jugular veins by superior presaturation. Similarly, when imaging the renal arteries, the inferior vena cava can be eliminated by inferior presaturation.

Phase Contrast MRA

PC angiography takes advantage of the previously discussed phase shifts induced in hydrogen nuclei as they move through magnetic field gradients. In this case, however, the phase shifts are produced by specific *flow-encoding* gradients and are proportional to flow velocity as well as to the amplitude and duration of these gradients (Fig. 16-3). Two approaches have been used to produce images from these phase data. Two sequential flow-encoding gradients of identical magnitude but opposite sign may be applied, with subsequent subtraction of the data sets, which eliminates background signal and sums the signal from moving spins.[9-11] An alternative approach involves application of flow-encoding gradients to yield PC images, fol-

lowed by multiplication of this data pixel by a magnitude or TOF gradient echo image to yield a so-called speed image.[12] The images can be obtained in either the two-dimensional or the three-dimensional mode, just as in TOF MRA.

PC MRA has several potential advantages. It is much less sensitive to saturation effects than TOF MRA, which gives it an advantage in imaging slow flow. For example, in contrast to three-dimensional TOF MRA, it permits imaging of veins as well as arteries. PC MRA is also less affected by the exact orientation of blood vessels to the slice than is TOF MRA. The improved background suppression obtainable with PC MRA has several important advantages: as compared with TOF MRA, thicker slices can be obtained with similar blood vessel contrast since there is no averaging of signal with adjacent stationary tissue. By taking this to the limit, complete projectional angiographic images through the entire body that are exactly comparable with x-ray images can be obtained. Among the capabilities that this makes possible is that of obtaining angiographic images at multiple points of the cardiac cycle.[13]

Another advantage of the improved background suppression available with PC is the ability to reliably suppress the bright signal from clotted blood. Clotted blood in which the hemoglobin has been converted to methemoglobin has a very high signal intensity due to the long T-1 values of methemoglobin. Even the rapid application of radiofrequency pulses in TOF MRA sequences may be inadequate to suppress this signal, which may then appear on the final projections after application of the MIP algorithm. In PC MRA, however, the entire signal comes from the actual motion of hydrogen nuclei, and hematomas are suppressed along with the rest of the stationary tissue.

In PC MRA unwanted vessels can be eliminated by spatial presaturation, just as in TOF MRA. However, the ability to select the flow velocities and directions to be imaged allows elimination of unwanted vessels by appropriate selection of these parameters. Even when, because of their geometry and velocity, unwanted vessels cannot be eliminated, the ability to display flow in opposite directions as shades of black or white may allow one to easily distinguish, for example, arteries from their accompanying veins. Finally, the PC technique is inherently quantitative. While information about flow velocities can be obtained from TOF images by measuring the movement of saturation bands applied within the image,[14] this information is directly obtainable from PC MRA images, since the signal is directly related to flow velocity and the known strength of the flow-encoding gradients. By replacing one spatial dimension with a velocity dimension, a PC technique has been developed in which flow velocities can be tracked over time in a manner comparable with that

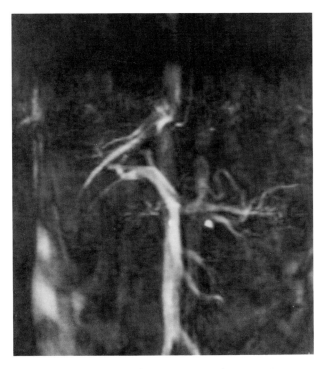

Figure 16-3 Two-dimensional PC MRA of the portal venous system and inferior vena cava. (From Yucel,[47] with permission.)

used in Doppler imaging.[15,16] These techniques have seen limited application to date, but widespread application may be expected as investigation continues in this area.

PC MRA does have several important limitations. One is that it is inherently more time-consuming than TOF MRA because each gradient application encodes flow in only one direction. Therefore, to obtain flow in all three directions, the total acquisition time must be four to six times as long as that for a TOF study, depending on the implementation. This becomes less of a problem, however, if the flow within the vessel of interest is predominantly along one axis.

Another limitation of PC MRA is the necessity to apply flow-encoding gradients of the appropriate amplitude and duration to detect the flow velocity within the vessel of interest. If the gradients are too weak, an inadequate signal will be obtained from slowly moving blood. Conversely, if the gradients are too strong, the signal from rapidly moving blood will alias, which results in loss of signal intensity. Often in cases of pathology, such as proximal occlusion or cardiac dysfunction, the flow rate within a given vessel may not be known, and multiple acquisitions may be necessary to image the vessel of interest.

Flow at Stenoses

One of the primary goals of MRA is to accurately depict areas of stenosis in blood vessels. However, flow at stenoses has several characteristics that make it difficult to image accurately. At the actual site of stenosis there is marked acceleration of flow velocity, resulting in steep velocity gradients along the long and short axes of the blood vessel. For a variable distance beyond the site of stenosis, flow becomes disordered and turbulent, and there may even be areas of flow reversal within eddy currents. These factors contribute to signal loss on MRA at sites of stenosis owing to the presence of an increased range of velocities within each pixel, with resulting intravoxel phase dispersion and cancellation of signal. This tendency for signal loss to occur at sites of stenosis remains the major limitation of MRA. The degree of signal loss is highly dependent on voxel size and TE, with increasing loss of signal as these variables increase.

Black Blood MRA

One proposed solution to the problem of signal loss at sites of stenosis has been black blood angiography.[17] Black blood MRA takes advantage of the tendency for blood to lose signal intensity during MR imaging, as evidenced by the flow voids typically present within vessels on standard MR images. This tendency can be accentuated by the application of presaturation pulses outside the imaged volume. Contrast is provided by the selection of imaging parameters so that signal is present in stationary tissue (i.e., relatively T-1 or proton density-weighted images). Black blood techniques have a theoretical advantage in areas of stenosis in that the natural tendency of turbulent flow to lose signal due to intravoxel phase dispersion promotes, rather than hinders, contrast between blood and stationary tissue. The individual black blood images, once acquired, can be postprocessed in an manner analogous to that used for white blood images, except that a minimum intensity projection algorithm is used. These algorithms are more difficult to apply since bone and air-containing structures also exhibit signal voids on MR imaging and must be excluded from the area of interest to be reconstructed.

CLINICAL APPLICATIONS

Carotid Arteries

Outside of the intracranial circulation, MRA evaluation of the carotid arteries aroused early interest, not least because MR imaging of the brain is already commonly performed for ischemic symptoms, and even a screening examination of the carotids would make a useful adjunct to routine brain MRI. Masaryk and coworkers,[18] using a three-dimensional TOF technique, studied an early group of 22 bifurcations in 15 patients, which were correlated with had x-ray angiographic results. They characterized the internal carotid arteries as normal, mildly, moderately, or severely stenotic or occluded and found complete agreement between MRA and x-ray angiography, except for one case of severe stenosis that was poorly imaged by MRA. They noted a tendency for MRA to slightly overestimate the degree of stenosis. In a follow-up study,[19] the same group performed a blinded comparison of 75 bifurcations in 38 patients. They demonstrated excellent correlation between three-dimensional TOF MRA and x-ray angiography, with correlation coefficients of 0.97 for the left carotid artery and 0.95 for the right. When a cutoff value of 70 percent area stenosis (approximately 55 percent diameter stenosis) was used for the presence of disease, MRA had sensitivities of 100 and 94 percent with specificities of 95 and 93 percent for the left and right carotid arteries, respectively.

The two-dimensional TOF method has also been applied to carotid MRA.[1,20] It has the advantage of being able to cover a large field of view, from the proximal common carotid artery to the carotid siphon, without saturation effects. It is also quite sensitive to slow flow distal to severe stenoses and may be better at distinguishing critical stenosis from occlusion. However, the technique is more susceptible to signal voids at sites of stenosis, especially with longer TEs, and to date has been less successful in accurately delineating carotid stenosis than the three-dimensional techniques (Fig. 16-4).

Edelman and co-workers[17] examined the possibility of using black blood angiography to evaluate the carotid bifurcation. In 13 of 33 diseased carotid vessels the black blood technique was superior to bright blood methods, which tended to overestimate the degree of stenosis, especially severe stenosis. By using a combination of bright blood and black blood MRA, Mattle et al.[21] obtained a sensitivity of 100 percent and specificity of 92 percent in the detection of 70 percent or greater diameter stenosis. In the same study duplex sonography had a sensitivity of 86 percent and specificity of 84 percent. Where duplex sonography and MRA were in agreement, there was 100 percent correlation with the findings of x-ray angiography.

At present MRA appears to be at least as accurate as duplex sonography in the noninvasive evaluation of carotid stenosis. The three-dimensional TOF method has been the most successful. This is accounted for by the small voxel sizes (up to 0.7-mm resolution in all axes) and short TEs obtainable with this method, which tend to diminish the effects of intravoxel phase dispersion and consequent signal loss at stenoses (Fig. 16-5). There remains a slight tendency toward the overestimation of stenosis, but the addition of black blood techniques may help to counteract this effect. Higher spatial resolution and shorter TE techniques are currently under development and can be expected to further improve the accuracy of MRA of the carotid bifurcation. Meanwhile, the combination of duplex sonography and MRA may make routine use of x-ray angiography unnecessary when the former two studies are in agreement.

One area in which MRA has yet to be successfully applied is visualization of the common carotid artery origin. The aortic arch is too deep to be readily accessible to surface coil imaging, although work to develop special surface coils for carotid imaging is in progress. Body coil imaging is limited by lower signal-to-noise ratios, which require thicker slices and therefore result in less accurate imaging than is possible with surface coils. It is possible that some variation of the multislab three-dimensional approach will solve this problem in the not too distant future[22] (Fig. 16-6). MRA is not capable currently of accurately delineating plaque morphology, and x-ray angiography is still necessary

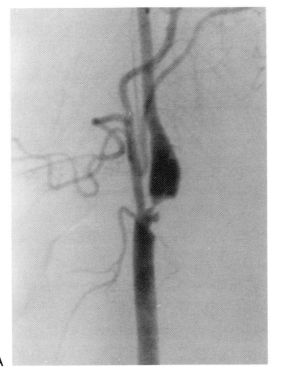
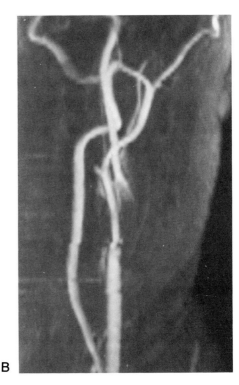

A   B

Figure 16-4 **(A)** Intra-arterial digital angiogram demonstrates severe stenosis of the internal carotid artery origin. **(B)** Corresponding two-dimensional TOF MRA demonstrates large, flame-shaped area of signal void due to turbulence distal to the stenosis. (From Yucel,[47] with permission.)

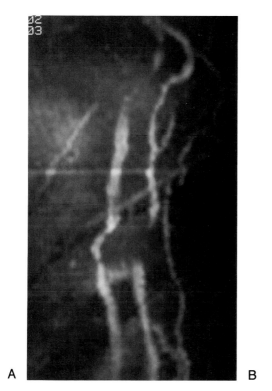
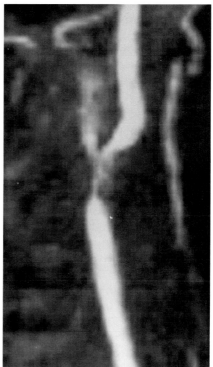

Figure 16-5 (A) Two-dimensional TOF MRA of the carotid demonstrates marked signal void at carotid bifurcation. (B) Three-dimensional multislab (MOTSA) image demonstrates much better delineation of the stenosis at the bifurcation.

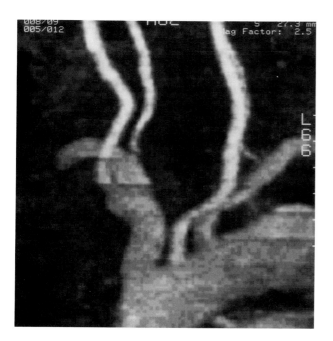

Figure 16-6 MOTSA image of the aortic arch obtained in the body coil.

to establish the presence or absence of plaque ulceration.

Renal Artery

MRA has the potential to be a good screening test for renal artery stenosis. In order to be useful for this application, a test must be able to identify among the population of patients with hypertension or renal insufficiency those with significant (i.e., >50 percent diameter) stenosis. It does not have to give precise information about the degree of stenosis, although it would be ideal if it could do so, since it then could potentially replace x-ray angiography. It is sufficient if it can simply rule in or out the presence of a significant stenosis, so that x-ray angiography could be reserved for the minority of patients with renal artery disease.

Kent and co-workers used two-dimensional TOF MRA to diagnose renal artery stenosis in 37 patients (77 arteries).[23] They obtained 3- to 5-mm coronal and axial slices during breath-holding. Approximately 10 breath-holds were required for each plane, each breath-hold lasting 12 to 16 seconds. The slices were examined individually and also in axial and coronal collapsed images. Of these patients 23 had either unilateral or bilateral renal artery stenosis, which was classified as mild, moderate, severe, or occluded. Agreement with regard to the severity of stenosis was obtained in 91 percent of arteries. With a cutoff of 50 percent diameter stenosis for the presence of significant disease, the sensitivity of MRA was 100 percent and the specificity was 94 percent.

Debatin and co-workers,[24] using a variation of this method to diagnose renal artery stenosis, examined 32 patients by two-dimensional PC MRA. Taking advantage of the improved stationary tissue suppression of PC MRA, they obtained 7-mm slices in the axial and coronal planes, each with flow-encoding in all three directions and with the flow-encoding gradients set to detect mean velocities of 40 cm/s or lower. Each slice took approximately 40 seconds to acquire, so slices were obtained during quiet respiration rather than with breath-holding. The use of both axial and coronal images improved the accuracy of interpretation. For diameter stenosis of more than 50 percent, the overall sensitivity was 91 percent, with a specificity of 98 percent. These workers also obtained TOF MRA images in the coronal plane only, which they did not find as useful as the PC MRA results.

As can be seen from the preceding studies, two-dimensional techniques have been preferred over three-dimensional ones for renal studies by most investigators despite the fact that three-dimensional studies have higher spatial resolution. This is because three-dimensional MR imaging, in general, is more suscepti-

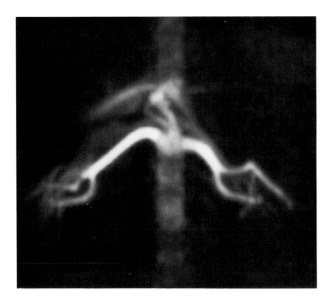

Figure 16-7 Three-dimensional phase contrast angiogram of normal renal arteries. Note the excellent intrarenal vascular detail. (From Yucel,[47] with permission.)

ble to motion-induced artifacts than two-dimensional imaging, and it has been thought that the constant respiratory and bowel motion present in the abdomen would degrade the images. Nevertheless, it has been shown[25] that three-dimensional MRA can give excellent abdominal vascular images. It appears that the motion artifacts, by being averaged over the relatively long three-dimensional acquisition times (10 to 12 minutes for 60 partitions), become nearly imperceptible and do not seriously degrade image quality (Fig. 16-7). Vock and co-workers,[26] using a three-dimensional PC MRA technique to examine the abdominal vessels, were able to detect seven of eight stenotic renal arteries. The potential for improved spatial resolution would certainly encourage the continued investigation of three-dimensional MRA in the evaluation of renal artery stenosis.

Currently MRA performed by either two-dimensional or three-dimensional techniques appears to be a sensitive and specific method for identifying patients at risk for a renovascular cause of hypertension (Figs. 16-8 and 16-9). X-ray angiography remains essential for definitive diagnosis. One group of patients for whom it might be especially useful is those with renal insufficiency suspected to have a renovascular cause. One is especially reluctant to perform renal arteriography on these patients without previously indicated high probability of finding significant disease, which a positive MRA should provide. Conversely, a totally normal bilateral renal MRA would appear to make a renovascular cause for renal failure unlikely. Further investigation into this area is certainly warranted. At present the spatial resolution of MRA is not adequate to evaluate the intrarenal vessels. The majority of patients studied so far have had an atherosclerotic etiology for their renal stenosis, and it is not known whether these results can be extrapolated to patients with fibromuscular dysplasia.

Portal Vein

Portal venous evaluation has been another area in which the applications of MRA has been explored. The portal venous system has been successfully imaged by breath-held two-dimensional TOF MRA[27] as well as by two-dimensional and three-dimensional PC MRA.[25] In a study[26] using three-dimensional PC MRA to examine 13 normal subjects and 10 patients with portal hypertension, 100 percent of patent portal veins were demonstrated by this technique, which was also able to demonstrate more retroperitoneal collaterals than x-ray angiography. The superior mesenteric vein was demonstrated in 92 percent of cases, but the splenic

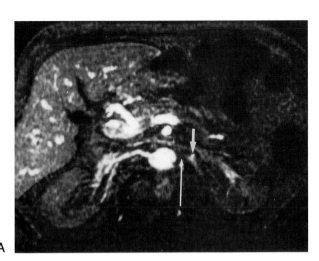

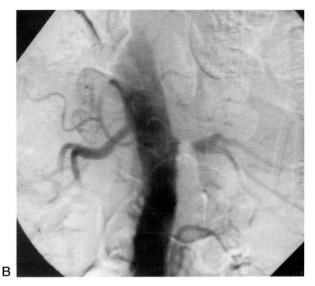

Figure 16-8 (A) Two-dimensional TOF axial collapsed image, demonstrating a patent right renal artery and severe signal void at origin of severely stenotic left renal artery *(long arrow).* Note reconstitution of left renal artery flow signal distally *(short arrow).* **(B)** Corresponding aortogram.

vein was adequately visualized in only 67 percent. In a study of 30 patients being evaluated for liver transplantation,[28] two-dimensional TOF MRA demonstrated patency of the portal vein in 26 of 27 patients and diagnosed portal vein occlusion in all three of the other patients. This study also provided excellent depiction, superior to that obtainable by sonography, of the extent and location of retroperitoneal collateral veins.

The direction and velocity of flow can also be measured in the portal vein by a TOF technique in which the vein is tagged with a saturation band and the movement of this band is observed over time. Measurements of portal vein flow velocity by this method have been found to correlate well with Doppler measurements and to allow detection of flow reversal as well as calculation of volume flow rates.[27-29] Portal vein MRA thus

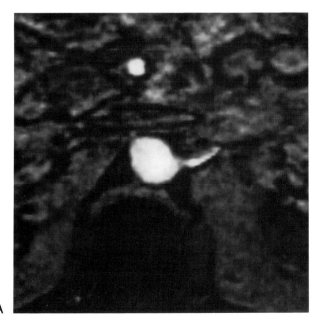

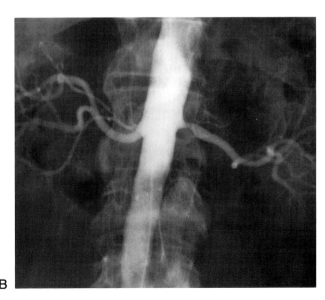

Figure 16-9 (A) Axial MOTSA image showing moderate stenosis at origin of left renal artery. Note excellent correlation without overestimation of degree of stenosis as compared with aortogram **(B)**.

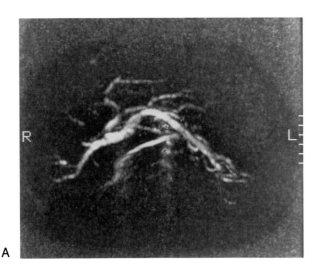
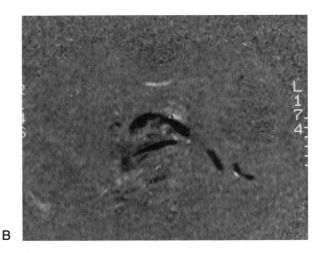

A   B

Figure 16-10 (A) Axial two-dimensional phase contrast angiogram demonstrating patency of the splenic and portal veins. **(B)** Individual image with right-left flow encoding demonstrates hepatopetal flow. On this image flow from left to right is encoded as black, flow from right to left as white.

appears able to fully evaluate the main portal vein for patency and flow direction (Fig. 16-10), as well as to identify retroperitoneal collateral vessels in patients with portal hypertension. It has the advantage over sonography of not being limited by overlying bowel gas or ribs. Angiography can be limited to confirmation of portal vein occlusion, to cases of suspected portal branch vein pathology, and to situations requiring complete evaluation of the splenic or superior mesenteric veins.

Peripheral Vessels

Two-dimensional TOF and PC techniques have been shown to be capable of diagnosing venous thrombosis in the extremities.[30-33] While small series have demonstrated the accuracy of two-dimensional TOF MRA in the diagnosis of proximal deep venous thrombosis (DVT), enthusiasm for MR venography has been diminished by the proven success of compression sonography in the diagnosis of DVT.[34,35] MRA is unlikely to replace sonography in those areas of the body suitable for sonographic evaluation, since it is more expensive and less available than sonography. However, MR venography has a significant role to play in imaging those veins that are poorly or not at all accessible to ultrasound (e.g., the iliac, subclavian, and brachiocephalic veins and the inferior and superior venae cavae). The iliac veins, in particular, are a potential source of serious pulmonary emboli, which cannot be adequately evaluated by sonography, and in patients with a high prior probability of iliac vein or inferior

vena cava thrombosis (i.e., those with leg swelling extending to the hip or a history of pelvic tumor, trauma, or surgery) MR may be used to complement or replace the sonographic evaluation.

Both PC[13,36,37] and TOF[38-40] two-dimensional MRA techniques have been applied to the arterial circulation of the lower extremities. Three-dimensional MRA techniques are not suitable for peripheral artery evaluation because of the large fields of view that must be imaged. TOF MRA has been performed by acquiring sequential axial slices, which are then reprojected into anteroposterior, lateral, and oblique MR angiograms. Venous flow is eliminated by inferior presaturation. The two-dimensional TOF techniques have the advantage of being very sensitive to slow flow distal to occlusions, (Fig. 16-11), which allows visualization of the tibial vessels[39] so that distal runoff can be assessed (Fig. 16-12). One problem with the TOF techniques is that they are relatively time-consuming. A typical examination with an acquisition time of 10 seconds per slice and 3-mm slices would require 20 minutes to cover a 36-cm field of view. This would have to be repeated three times to image from the aortic bifurcation to the calf.

In addition, the highly pulsatile, triphasic flow typical of the normal extremity vessels can produces artifacts in the y-axis of the TOF images. This effect, which is due to the marked variation in flow signal present during the time required for image acquisition, can be reduced by cardiac gating, but this is impractical owing to time constraints. If the y-axis is set in the anteroposterior direction, as is typical, these artifacts are not seen on the straight coronal projections, but they may de-

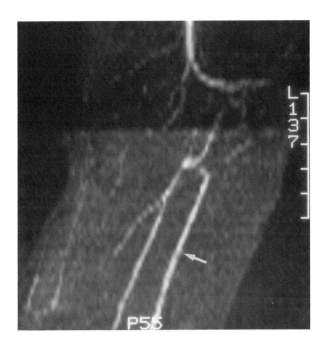

Figure 16-11 Two-dimensional TOF MRA from pediatric patient with traumatic popliteal artery occlusion shows excellent detail of tibial runoff. This study allowed performance of a popliteal-anterior tibial *(arrow)* bypass without angiography. (From Fillmore et al.,[39] with permission.)

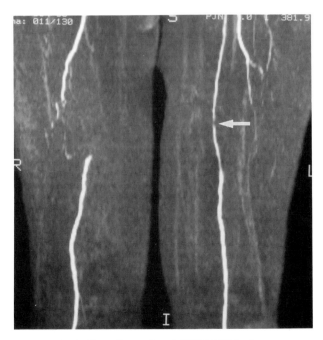

Figure 16-12 Two-dimensional TOF MRA demonstrates long superficial femoral artery occlusion on right with reconstitution of the above-knee popliteal. In contrast, on the left there is a focal superficial femoral artery stenosis *(arrow)*, which would be amendable to percutaneous transluminal angioplasty.

grade image quality on the oblique projections. This is not a problem distal to an occlusive lesion since the flow in these areas assumes a low-resistance pattern, with flow throughout the cardiac cycle resembling that in the carotid arteries. Two-dimensional TOF MRA is also quite sensitive to the orientation of vessels relative to the imaging plane. Therefore, horizontal segments, such as may be present in tortuous iliac arteries, and the deep femoral and anterior tibial artery origins may be relatively poorly visualized. Despite these limitations, TOF MRA has been shown to be an effective modality for visualizing stenoses and occlusions of the peripheral arteries, as well as for visualizing the runoff vessels.[39-41] As mentioned previously, two-dimensional TOF techniques may result in overestimation the degree of stenosis (Fig. 16-13). However, in conjunction with noninvasive pressure measurements, they may provide enough information to obviate x-ray angiography in selected cases.[40,41]

Two-dimensional PC MRA has been tried in an effort to alleviate some of the problems associated with TOF MRA. PC images may be obtained as direct coronal projections (Fig. 16-14). This allows the studies to be gated to the cardiac cycle, eliminating the artifact associated with pulsatile flow. In general, superior-inferior flow encoding is sufficient for arterial visualization, but in selected cases such as tortuous iliacs, all three flow directions may be obtained to compensate for vessel tortuosity. Because the time of the examination is not limited by the field of view selected, PC MRA has an advantage over TOF MRA. With a heart rate of 64 bpm, a study may be obtained in as little as 2 minutes. Additional acquisitions are necessary if additional view angles or flow sensitivities are required, which lengthens the imaging time. PC and TOF MRA must be compared in a prospective fashion before it can be known which method is optimal for lower extremity arterial studies.

CONCLUSIONS

Newly developed ultrafast imaging methods, which either are modifications of standard gradient echo imaging[42] or are based on the echo planar method,[43] allow acquisition of individual slices in less than 1 second. These techniques have been applied to the abdominal[44] and pulmonary[45] vasculature with promising results. Preliminary results have even demonstrated the capability of subsecond imaging to visualize the proximal coronary arteries.[46] Ultrafast MRA holds the promise of being able to "freeze" physiologic and vascular motion. This could dramatically increase the speed with which MRA is performed, as well as extend

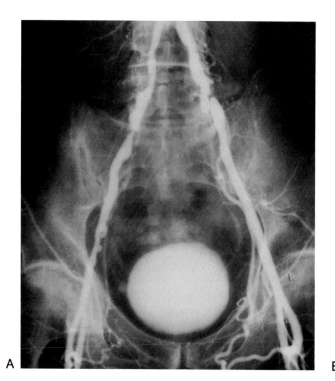

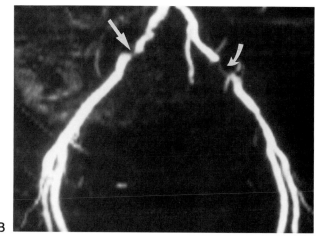

A   B

Figure 16-13 (A) Conventional iliac angiogram. **(B)** Two-dimensional TOF MRA in left posterior oblique equivalent projection only slightly overestimates moderate right common iliac stenosis *(straight arrow)*. The severe left common iliac stenosis results in marked signal loss, with overestimation of the length of the diseased segment. The signal is seen distal to the stenosis *(curved arrow),* indicating the presence of a stenosis rather than an occlusion. (From Potchen et al.[48] with permission.)

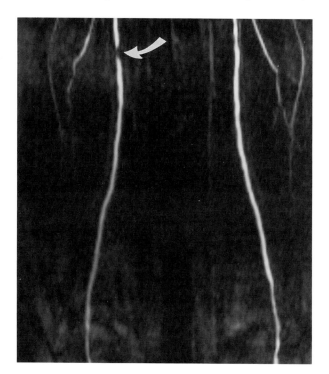

Figure 16-14 Image from cine two-dimensional PC angiogram of the thighs, showing focal stenosis in proximal SFA *(arrow).* (From Yucel,[47] with permission.)

its applicability to areas from which it has heretofore been excluded, such as pulmonary embolism and coronary artery disease. Further studies will be required, however, before these techniques are accepted clinically.

REFERENCES

1. Keller PJ, Drayer BP, Fram EK et al: MR angiography with two-dimensional acquisition and three-dimensional display: work in progress. Radiology 173:527, 1989

2. Ruggieri PM, Laub GA, Masaryk TJ, Modic MT: Intracranial circulation: pulse-sequence considerations in three-dimensional (volume) MR angiography. Radiology 171:785, 1989

3. Schmalbrock P, Yuan C, Chakeres DW et al: Volume MR angiography: methods to achieve very short echo times. Radiology 175:861, 1990

4. Parker DL, Yuan C, Blatter DB: MR angiography by multiple thin slab three-dimensional acquisition. Magn Reson Med 17:434, 1991

5. Anderson CM, Saloner D, Tsuruda JS et al: Artifacts in maximum-intensity-projection display of MR angiograms. AJR 154:623, 1990

6. Cline HE, Dumoulin CL, Lorensen WE et al: Volume

rendering and connectivity algorithms for MR angiography. Magn Reson Med 18:384, 1991

7. Saloner D, Hanson WA, Tsuruda JS et al: Application of a connected-voxel algorithm to MR angiographic data. J Magn Reson Imaging 1:423, 1991

8. Siebert JE, Rosenbaum TL: Projection algorithm imparting a consistent spatial perspective for three-dimensional MR angiography, abstracted. Society of Magnetic Resonance in Medicine, 9th Annual Scientific Meeting, New York, 1990, Program Abstracts, p. 60

9. Dumoulin CL, Hart HR: Magnetic resonance angiography. Radiology 161:717, 1986

10. Dumoulin CL, Souza SP, Hart HR: Rapid scan magnetic resonance angiography. Magn Reson Med 5:238, 1987

11. Dumoulin CL, Souza SP, Walker MF, Wagle W: Three dimensional phase contrast angiography. Magn Reson Med 9:139, 1989

12. Spritzer CE, Pelc NJ, Lee JN et al: Rapid MR imaging of blood flow with a phase-sensitive, limited-flip-angle, gradient recalled pulse sequence: preliminary experience. Radiology 176:255, 1990

13. Steinberg FL, Yucel EK, Dumoulin CL, Souza SP: Peripheral vascular and abdominal applications of MR flow imaging techniques. Magn Reson Med 14:315, 1990

14. Edelman RR, Mattle HP, Kleefield J, Silver MS: Quantification of blood flow with dynamic MR imaging and presaturation bolus tracking. Radiology 171:551, 1989

15. Walker MF, Souza SP, Dumoulin CL: Quantitative flow measurement in phase contrast MR angiography. J Comput Assist Tomogr 12:304, 1989

16. Dumoulin CL, Souza SP, Hardy CJ, Ash SA: Quantitative measurement of blood flow using cylindrically localized Fourier velocity encoding. Magn Reson Med 21:242, 1991

17. Edelman RR, Mattle HP, Wallner B et al: Extracranial carotid arteries: evaluation with "black blood" MR angiography. Radiology 177:45, 1990

18. Masaryk TJ, Modic MT, Ruggieri PM et al: Three-dimensional (volume) gradient-echo imaging of the carotid bifurcation: preliminary clinical experience. Radiology 171:801, 1989

19. Masaryk AM, Ross JS, DiCello MC et al: 3DFT MR angiography of the carotid bifurcation: potential and limitations as a screening examination. Radiology 179:797, 1991

20. Litt AW, Eidelman EM, Pinto RS: Diagnosis of carotid artery stenosis: comparison of 2DFT time-of-flight MR angiography with contrast angiography in 50 patients. AJR 156:611, 1991

21. Mattle HP, Kent KC, Edelman RR et al: Evaluation of the extracranial carotid arteries: correlation of magnetic resonance angiography, duplex ultrasonography, and conventional angiography. J Vasc Surg 13:838, 1991

22. Lewin JS, Laub G, Hausmann R: Three-dimensional time-of-flight MR angiography: applications in the abdomen and thorax. Radiology 179:261, 1991

23. Kent KC, Edelman RR, Kim D et al: Magnetic resonance imaging: a reliable test for the evaluation of proximal atherosclerotic renal arterial stenosis. J Vasc Surg 13:311, 1991

24. Debatin JF, Spritzer CE, Grist TM et al: Imaging of the renal arteries: value of MR angiography. AJR 157:981, 1991

25. Dumoulin CL, Yucel EK, Vock P et al: Two- and three-dimensional phase contrast MR angiography of the abdomen. J Comput Assist Tomogr 14:779, 1990

26. Vock P, Terrier F, Wegmüller H et al: Magnetic resonance angiography of abdominal vessels: early experience using the three-dimensional phase-contrast technique. Br J Radiol 64:10, 1991

27. Edelman RR, Zhao B, Liu C et al: MR angiography and dynamic flow evaluation of portal venous system. AJR 153:755, 1989

28. Finn JP, Edelman RR, Jenkins RL et al: Liver transplantation: MR angiography with surgical validation. Radiology 179:265, 1991

29. Tamada T, Moriyasu F, Ono S et al: Portal blood flow: measurement with MR imaging. Radiology 173:639, 1989

30. Hansen ME, Spritzer CE, Sostman HD: Assessing the patency of mediastinal and thoracic inlet veins: value of MR imaging. AJR 155:1177, 1990

31. Spritzer CE, Sussman SE, Blinder RA et al: Deep venous thrombosis evaluation with limited-flip-angle, gradient-refocussed MR imaging: preliminary experience. Radiology 166:371, 1988

32. Totterman S, Francis CW, Foster TH et al: Diagnosis of femoropopliteal venous thrombosis with MR imaging: a comparison of four MR pulse sequences. AJR 154:175, 1990

33. Erdman WA, Jayson HL, Redman HC et al: Deep venous thrombosis of extremities: role of MR imaging in the diagnosis. Radiology 174:425, 1990

34. White RH, McGahan JP, Daschbach MM, Hartling RP: Diagnosis of deep-vein thrombosis using duplex ultrasound. Ann Intern Med 111:297, 1989

35. Yucel EK, Fisher JS, Egglin TK et al: Isolated calf venous thrombosis: diagnosis with compression US. Radiology 179:443, 1991

36. Lanzer P, Bohning D, Groen J et al: Aortoiliac and femoropopliteal phase-based NMR angiography: a comparison between FLAG and RSE. Magn Reson Med 15:372, 1990

37. Lanzer P, McKibbin W, Bohning D et al: Aortoiliac imaging by projective phase sensitive MR angiography: effects of triggering and timing of data acquisition on image quality. Magn Reson Imaging 8:107, 1990

38. Wendt RE, Nitz W, Morrisett JD, Hedrick TD: A technique for flow-enhanced magnetic resonance angiography of the lower extremities. Magn Reson Imaging 8:723, 1990

39. Fillmore DJ, Yucel EK, Briggs SE et al: MR angiography of vascular grafts in children. AJR 157:1069, 1991

40. Yucel EK, Dumoulin CL, Waltman AC: MR angiography of lower-extremity arterial disease: preliminary experience. J Magn Reson Imaging 2:303, 1992

41. Mulligan SA, Matsuda T, Lanzer P et al: Peripheral arte-

rial occlusive disease: prospective comparison of MR angiography and color duplex US with conventional angiography. Radiology 178:695, 1991

42. Haase A: Snapshot FLASH MRI: application to T1-, T2-, and chemical-shift imaging. Magn Reson Med 13:77, 1990

43. Rzedzian R, Pykett I: Instant images of the human heart using a new, whole-body MR imaging system. AJR 149:245, 1987

44. Haacke EM, Wielopolski PA: High-resolution three-dimensional pulmonary imaging, (abstracted). J Magn Reson Imaging 1:166, 1991

45. Crawley AP, Cohen MS, Yucel EK et al: Single-shot MR imaging: applications to angiography. J Cardiovasc Intervent Radiol 15:32, 1992

46. Edelman RR, Manning WJ, Burstein DB, Paulin S: Coronary arteries: breath-hold MR angiography. Radiology 181:641, 1991

47. Yucel EK: Magnetic resonance angiography. Perspect Vasc Surg 3:35, 1991

48. Potchen EJ, Maacke EM, Siebert JE, Gottschalk A: Magnetic Resonance Angiography: Concepts and Applications. Mosby-Year Book, St. Louis, 1992

Section V

Acute Limb Ischemia

The management of acute extremity ischemia remains a major diagnostic and therapeutic challenge to the vascular surgeon and interventional radiologist. Acute lower-extremity ischemia due to embolic disease continues to cause significant morbidity and mortality despite optimal surgical management. Limb loss rates of 8 to 10 percent and perioperative mortality rates of 10 percent continue to be reported. Maximization of limb salvage while simultaneously minimizing associated morbidity and mortality requires expeditious diagnosis and restoration of perfusion. This may vary from immediate progression to the operating room in the setting of obvious embolic disease to detailed arteriography and preoperative intra-arterial thrombolytic therapy in the setting of intrainguinal graft failure.

In the following chapters we will review the diagnosis and management of various clinical entities responsible for acute extremity ischemia. Acute thromboembolic disease of native vessels continues to be the paradigm of acute extremity ischemia. Differentiation of emboli from native vessel thrombosis can be a difficult but essential factor, as the diagnostic evaluation and approach to treatment may differ greatly. Prompt diagnosis and restoration of perfusion are the main tenets of successful management. The selective application of intra-arterial thrombolytic therapy has added an important diagnostic and therapeutic tool.

Arterial bypass surgery for atherosclerotic occlusive disease is the sine qua non of vascular surgery. Despite significant advances, bypass grafts, whether autogenous or prosthetic, are subject to failure. Generally, graft failure is marked by a recurrence of symptoms that may vary from moderate claudication to profound limb-threatening ischemia. Effective restoration of perfusion and long-term graft patency are the goals of therapy. Long-term secondary graft patencies depend on the successful correction of the lesions responsible for graft failure. Recognition of these lesions depends on an understanding of the various mechanisms of graft failure that are likely to occur at different postoperative intervals. Precise diagnostic studies, including angiography, angioscopy, and duplex scanning contribute to the recognition and repair of these lesions. Management strategies for the failed bypass graft vary with the type of conduit and the cause of graft failure. Understanding and controlling the myointimal hyperplastic reaction, which occurs in response to arterial injury, remains a major challenge of vascular research.

Vascular trauma has become an increasingly common cause of acute extremity ischemia. The diagnostic and therapeutic considerations may vary dramatically, depending on the nature of the injury. For example, a popliteal artery occlusion associated with unstable orthopedic injuries and multisystem blunt injury would pose different challenges than an exsanguinating penetrating injury to the femoral vessels. Iatrogenic vascular trauma to the extremities has become an increasingly common cause of acute ischemia. These injuries often occur in high-risk patients, are generally superimposed on pre-existing atherosclerotic occlusive disease, and may present difficult therapeutic challenges.

Regardless of the mechanism of arterial occlusion or disruption, the subsequent ischemia results in variety of local and systemic effects that threaten both the limb and the patient.

17

Pathophysiology of Acute Extremity Ischemia

Michael Belkin

Fortunately for the vascular surgeon, the lower extremity, as compared with other organs and tissues, is comparatively resistant to the effects of ischemia. Unlike the brain, which suffers infarction after only 4 to 8 minutes of ischemia, or the myocardium, which infarcts after 17 to 20 minutes, the lower extremity may be salvaged after up to 5 to 6 hours of profound ischemia.[1]

Evaluation of the effects of acute ischemia on the extremity is complicated by the fact that the various tissues that comprise the extremity have different susceptibilities to ischemic injury, and manifest the injury in different fashions. Skin and bone are fairly resistant to effects of ischemia and may survive injuries that, by their effect on other tissues, have rendered the limb painful and useless. Nerve is generally the most sensitive tissue in the extremity to the effects of ischemia. Significant morbidity may therefore result from isolated ischemic nerve injury in an otherwise intact limb. Examples of this phenomenon, such as foot drop, due to deep peroneal nerve injury after anterior compartment syndrome, are, unfortunately, well known to the vascular surgeon.

Skeletal muscle is the major structural component of the extremity and, for a variety of reasons, plays a key role in the pathophysiology of extremity ischemia. Skeletal muscle constitutes more than 40 percent of body mass and approximately 75 percent of lower-extremity weight. Although resting skeletal muscle has a relatively slow metabolic rate compared with that of other tissues (e.g., brain, myocardium, and kidney), it is the major metabolic component of the lower extremity, accounting for more than 90 percent of metabolic activity.[2] Skeletal muscle receives 71 percent of the resting lower-extremity blood flow and a larger proportion of the blood flow during reperfusion hyperemia after ischemia.[3] Furthermore, skeletal muscle plays the pivotal role in the numerous local and systemic manifestations of extremity ischemia-reperfusion injury discussed below.

REPERFUSION SYNDROME

The profound systemic effects of revascularization of the lower extremity were described as early as the 1950s by Haimovici[4] (Fig. 17-1). As ischemic skeletal muscle is reperfused, a variety of intracellular ions, structural proteins, enzymes, and other components are released through the damaged sarcolemma into the circulation. The resulting "myonephropathic syndrome," with its associated hemodynamic instability, lactic acidosis, and hyperkalemia, is well recognized by the vascular surgeon.[5,6] Myoglobin released into the circulation is

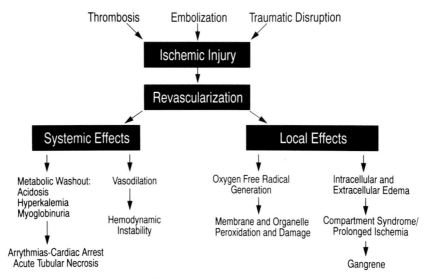

Figure 17-1 Revascularization syndrome. Multiple systemic and local complications of reperfusion of an ischemic extremity.

cleared through the kidneys, resulting in dark red urine (without red blood cells). Myoglobinuria may persist for 2 to 4 days after reperfusion. Acute renal failure may ensue from myoglobin casts, developing in the renal tubules as well as direct toxic effects of myoglobin on the renal tubules.[6] Serum creatine phosphokinase levels may increase dramatically (to > 10,000 units) after reperfusion of ischemic muscle, remaining elevated for days after injury. Similarly, other serum enzyme levels, such as lactate dehydrogenase (LDH_1, LDH_2), serum glutamic-oxaloacetic transaminase (SGOT), and serum glutamic-pyruvic transaminase (SGPT), will also be transiently elevated. Myocardial contractility may become depressed; increased cardiac irritability leading to dysrhythmias may occur.[4] As interventional radiologists have assumed an active therapeutic role in lower-extremity revascularization through the infusion of thrombolytic agents, they have also witnessed these life-threatening complications.[7]

When the lower extremity is subjected to severe ischemia, cellular membrane dysfunction results. In this setting, the reperfusion phase is marked by the development of both intracellular and interstitial edema. Intracellular edema results from membrane damage and failure of membrane-bound ATPase. Interstitial edema results from increased microvascular membrane permeability to ions, water, and proteins.[8,9] This edema may appear within minutes, progressing significantly over the next 24 hours. The extent of edema is dependent on the period of ischemia, the underlying occlusive disease, and the adequacy of revascularization.[10] When muscle edema occurs within the confines of an osseofascial compartment, interstitial pressure

continues to rise. Acute compartment syndrome results as pressure increases beyond capillary perfusion pressure (30 mmHg), and tissue perfusion is impaired. Unless recognized and decompressed, compartment syndromes will lead to prolonged tissue ischemia despite apparent successful revascularization.

Prolongation of the ischemic injury may also occur due to microvascular obstruction to blood flow. Endothelial cell edema may predispose to white blood cell (WBC) and platelet sludging, leading to the so-called no-reflow phenomenon.[11] Similarly, prolonged vascular occlusion can lead to small vessel thrombosis in the muscle and skin, which prevents tissue reperfusion when blood flow is restored to the large vessels.[12] In our laboratory, my associates and I have demonstrated that infusion of urokinase into acutely ischemic skeletal muscle results in increased muscle salvage.[13] These observations are consistent with a significant role for microvascular thrombotic occlusion in the pathophysiology of ischemic injury.

SKELETAL MUSCLE ISCHEMIA-REPERFUSION INJURY

Although our knowledge of the systemic effects of limb revascularization and compartment syndrome is well developed, our understanding of ischemia-reperfusion (IR) injury at the tissue level is only beginning to evolve. The pathophysiology of ischemic injury is complex and involves a variety of factors, including decreased cellular energy charge, inadequate oxygen and substrate delivery, altered ion compartmentalization, and membrane permeability changes. More recently, attention has been focused on "reperfusion injury," (i.e., cellular injury that occurs or is manifested at the time perfusion is restored to ischemic tissue). Most of this injury is believed to be induced by oxygen-derived free radicals, which are formed as oxygen is reintroduced to ischemic tissue.

The relative extent of injury that occurs during the ischemic interval versus the extent that during reperfusion is unclear. Many morphologic and physiologic indicators of injury (e.g., membrane and organelle disruption, cellular and organelle edema, washout of nucleotide precursors) only become manifest as perfusion is restored. It becomes somewhat a semantic argument to discuss whether these injuries represent "reperfusion injury" or simply an overt manifestation of injury initiated during ischemia. Thus, IR injury is best considered a cascade of events that is instigated during the ischemic interval and manifested or intensified during reperfusion.

Perhaps the most important and obvious impact of ischemia on the extremity and skeletal muscle is progressive energy depletion. During profound muscle ischemia, tissue adenosine triphosphate (ATP) levels are initially well maintained at the expense of high-energy creatine phosphate (CP).[14] After approximately 3 hours of ischemia, CP stores are depleted and cellular ATP levels begin to fall linearly, with complete depletion by 7 hours. Muscle subjected to mild ischemic stress (≤ 2.5 hours) demonstrates no necrosis or significant ultrastructural damage and rapidly restores tissue glycogen and high-energy phosphate levels with reperfusion. When muscle is subjected to prolonged ischemic injury (6 to 7 hours), severe ultrastructural injury and extensive necrosis result, preventing the muscle tissue from regenerating glycogen and high-energy phosphates.[14] The inability to restore cellular energy level with reperfusion is due to both damage to metabolic machinery (e.g., mitochondria) and to loss of substrates. During prolonged ischemia, ATP and adenosine diphosphate (ADP) are progressively broken down into lipid-soluble nucleosides and purine bases, which are washed out of the tissue during the initial periods of hyperemic reperfusion. Loss of these nucleosides and purine bases deprives the cell of the substrates necessary to restore ATP levels.[15]

Increased intracellular calcium levels may also contribute to impaired cellular metabolism. At reperfusion, calcium levels increase due to leakage through damaged sarcolemma, through voltage-dependent slow channels, and through sodium-calcium exchange.[16] Increased intracellular calcium may uncouple oxidative phosphorylation, activate cellular proteases, and promote muscle contracture.[17,18]

Thus, during prolonged ischemia, a critical level of energy depletion is reached at which irreversible injury occurs. Less severe ischemia results in minimal or intermediate injury; thus, interventions that optimize the conditions of reperfusion may minimize muscle damage.

The actual mechanisms of reperfusion injury remain controversial. It is generally agreed, however, that oxygen-derived free radicals are generated that damage cellular membranes and intracellular organelles.[8,14,19] Free radicals are highly reactive compounds that result from the univalent reduction of molecular oxygen. The most important free radical species include the superoxide radical (a weak oxidizing agent), hydrogen peroxide, and the extremely reactive hydroxyl radical. These unstable compounds attack the unsaturated bonds of fatty acids within the phospholipid membrane, causing both mechanical and functional derangements.[20]

The precise mechanism of free radical formation in skeletal muscle is somewhat controversial. Figure 17-2 demonstrates an empirically derived explanation for free radical formation, developed from studies of IR in other tissues, such as intestine.[21] This theory holds that during ischemia, high-energy nucleotides are progressively metabolized, until hypoxanthine accumulates in the cell. Simultaneously, progressive ischemia leads to the conversion of xanthine dehydrogenase (XD) to xanthine oxidase (XO) by activation of an intracellular calcium-dependent protease. Reperfusion restores tissue oxygen, and the XO acts on its two substrates, oxygen and hypoxanthine, to form the superoxide radical and NADH. The evidence supporting this theory is indirect and is based largely on the ability of allopurinol (an XO inhibitor) to ameliorate the effects of skeletal muscle IR in several models.[8] Direct measurements of XO activity in skeletal muscle, however, reveal little or no detectable activity compared with that in other tissues.[22] There is also some controversy as to whether the XD-to-XO conversion occurs in skeletal muscle.[23,24] These and other considerations have led researchers to investigate other potential sources of free radicals and mechanisms of IR injury.

The WBC has recently been implicated as an important mediator of skeletal muscle IR injury. Neutrophil infiltration and subsequent activation have been studied extensively in cardiac muscle IR injury, and the mechanisms of injury seem to apply to skeletal muscle as well.[25] Studies from our laboratory and others have demonstrated a protective effect of artificially induced neutropenia against skeletal muscle IR injury.[26,27] Neutrophils are chemotactically attracted to the injured muscle tissue by activated complement factors, leukotrienes, and other factors. Leukocyte infiltration

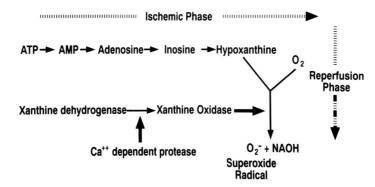

Figure 17-2 Proposed mechanism of free radical generation during reperfusion of ischemic skeletal muscle. During ischemia, xanthine dehydrogenase is converted to xanthine oxidase. During reperfusion, xanthine oxidase converts oxygen and hypoxanthine enzymatically to the superoxide radical and NADH.

into areas of ischemic skeletal muscle has long been recognized; the resulting inflammatory reaction is a fundamental component of the normal response to injury.[28,29] Paradoxically, this intense inflammatory reaction may also contribute to muscle injury through a variety of mechanisms (Fig. 17-3). The activated neutrophil undergoes a complex series of morphologic, metabolic, and functional alterations. In the process of endocytosis, a variety of lysosomal enzymes are released. These enzymes can destroy noncellular tissue (connective tissue components, basement membranes, and proteins), as well as viable and irreversibly injured cellular tissue.[30,31] In addition to lysosomal enzymes, neutrophils have a highly developed mechanism of oxygen-derived free radical formation through an NADPH oxidase on the plasma membrane.[32] Thus, neutrophils may induce the free radical reperfusion injury discussed above. Furthermore, free radicals may be synergistic with lysosomal enzymes in their mechanisms of tissue injury.[31]

The local inflammatory response to ischemic skeletal muscle injury that occurs during reperfusion is ultimately similar to that which occurs elsewhere. We are therefore beginning to recognize the role of the complement cascade, interleukins, and other cytokines. Experimental models of skeletal muscle IR have recently demonstrated activation of the complement cascade, generation of WBC chemotactic peptides (C3a and C5a), and production of interleukin-1 (IL-1).[33,34]

POTENTIAL CLINICAL MODIFICATION OF SKELETAL MUSCLE ISCHEMIA-REPERFUSION INJURY

Although our understanding of the mechanisms of skeletal muscle IR injury is developing, the application of this knowledge to the clinical setting has not yet been

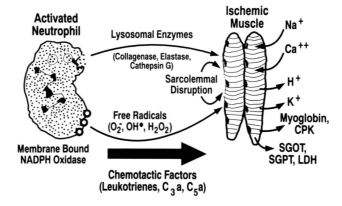

Figure 17-3 Neutrophil-mediated injury in skeletal muscle ischemia-reperfusion injury. Activated neutrophil is attracted to ischemic skeletal muscle by chemotactic factors during reperfusion. It then contributes to local injury through a variety of mechanisms, including free-radical generation and lysosomal enzyme release. CPK, creatinine phosphokinase; SGOT, serum glutamic-oxaloacetic transaminase; SGPT, serum glutamic-pyruvic transaminase; LDH, lactate dehydrogenase.

achieved. Attempts to limit the extent of IR injury by modifying the conditions of reperfusion remain an area of intense investigation.

The infusion of free radical scavengers, such as superoxide dismutase and mannitol, has been useful in mitigating skeletal muscle IR injury in a variety of experimental models.[8,19] The infusion of these agents into an ischemic extremity at reperfusion offers a potential clinical treatment of reperfusion injury. Similarly, the controlled reintroduction of oxygen, by limiting reperfusion hyperemia, has also been useful in animal experiments and may potentially be clinically applicable.[19,35]

Perhaps most interesting is the potential amelioration of reperfusion injury due to activated WBCs. Obviously, artificially induced neutropenia (through radiation or pharmacologic depression), which has been successful in animal experiments, is not a clinical option. Fortunately, there are more elegant and potentially clinically applicable means of decreasing WBC-induced IR injury. The endothelium of ischemic muscle tissue expresses the formation of WBC surface adhesion molecules (endothelial leukocyte adhesion molecules [ELAMs] CD11b/CD18), which are important mediators of WBC sequestration during IR injury. Blockage of these adhesion molecules with monoclonal antibodies has been useful in experimental models and may possibly prove useful in decreasing WBC infiltration and injury.[36]

The development of strategies to decrease IR injury remains hampered by our relative inability to measure the efficacy of treatment in the clinical setting. Unlike in the animal laboratory, muscle cannot be removed en masse to evaluate the extent of injury. Limb salvage and function are of primary importance but are only gross measures of muscle salvage.

The main tenet in decreasing the magnitude of skeletal muscle IR injury remains limiting the ischemic interval to as short a period as possible through expeditious diagnosis and revascularization. Clinical strategies for managing acute extremity ischemia in the setting of native vessel thrombosis, emboli, graft thrombosis, and vascular trauma are detailed in the following chapters.

REFERENCES

1. Abbott WM, Maloney RD, McCabe CC et al: Arterial embolism: a 44 year perspective. Am J Surg 143:460, 1982
2. Ruderman NB, Goodman MN, Berger M et al: Effect of starvation on muscle glucose metabolism: studies with the isolated perfused rat hindquarter. Fed Proc 36:171, 1977
3. Rutherford RB, Valenta J: Extremity blood flow and distribution: the effects of arterial occlusion, sympathectomy and exercise. Surgery 69:332, 1991
4. Haimovici H: Muscular, renal and metabolic complications of acute arterial occlusions: myonephropathic-metabolic syndrome. Surgery 85:461, 1979
5. McCarron Da, Elliot WC, Rose JS et al: Severe mixed metabolic acidosis secondary to rhabdomyolysis. Am J Med 67:905, 1979
6. Rakowski TA, Cerasaro TS: Myoglobinuria. Am Fam Physician 20:129, 1979
7. McNamara TO, Rischer JR: Thrombolysis of peripheral arterial and graft occlusions; improved results using high dose urokinase. AJR 144:769, 1985
8. Korthius RJ, Granger DN, Townsley MI et al: The role of oxygen derived free radicals in ischemia induced increases in canine skeletal muscle vascular permeability. Circ Res 57:599, 1985
9. Wright JG, Valeri CR, Hobson RW: Endothelial permeability to Iodine[125] labeled albumin predicts skeletal muscle injury after ischemia-reperfusion. Curr Surg 45:25, 1987
10. Matsen FE, Krygmire RB: Compartmental syndromes. Surg Gynecol Obstet 147:943, 1978
11. Ernst E, Hammerschmidt DE, Bagge V et al: Leukocytes and the risk of ischemic diseases. JAMA 257:2318, 1987
12. Dunnant JR, Edwards WS: Small vessel occlusion in the extremity after various periods of arterial reperfusion: an experimental study. Surgery 75:240, 1973
13. Belkin M, Valeri R, Hobson RW: Intra-arterial urokinase increases skeletal muscle viability after acute ischemia. J Vasc Surg 9:161, 1989
14. Harris K, Walker PM, Mickle AG et al: Metabolic responses of skeletal muscle to ischemia. Am J Physiol 250:H213, 1986
15. Walker PM, Lindsay T, Liauw S et al: The impact of energy depletion on skeletal muscle. Microcirc Endothelium Lymphatics 5:189, 1989
16. Majed O: The role of reperfusion-induced injury in the pathogenesis of the crush syndrome. N Engl J Med 324:417, 1991
17. Wrogemann K, Pena S: Mitochondrial calcium overload: a general mechanism for cell-necrosis in muscle diseases. Lancet 1:672, 1976
18. Ogilvie RW, Armstrong RB, Baird KE et al: Lesions in the rat soleus muscle following eccentrically biased exercise. Am J Anat 182:335, 1988
19. Walker PM, Lindsay T, Labbe et al: Salvage of skeletal muscle with free radical scavengers. J Vasc Surg 5:68, 1987
20. Freeman BA, Crappo JD: Biology of disease. Free radicals and tissue injury. Lab Invest 47:412, 1982
21. McCord JM: Oxygen derived free radicals in postischemic tissue injury. N Engl J Med 312:159, 1985
22. Wajner M, Harkness RA: Distribution of xanthine dehydrogenase and oxidase activities in human and rabbit tissues. Acta Biochim Biophys Hung 99:79, 1989
23. Roy RS, McCord JM: The pathophysiology of superoxide: roles in inflammation and ischemia. Can J Physiol Pharmacol 60:1346, 1982

24. Smith JK, Carden DL, Sadasivan KK et al: Role of xanthine oxidase in post ischemic microvascular injury in skeletal muscle. Am J Physiol 1993 (in press)

25. Lucchesi BR, Mullane KM: Leukocytes and ischemia induced myocardial injury. Annu Rev Pharmacol Toxicol 26:201, 1986

26. Belkin M, LaMorte WL, Wright J, Hobson RW: The role of leukocytes in the pathophysiology of skeletal muscle ischemic injury. J Vasc Surg 10:14, 1989

27. Korthius RJ, Grisham MB, Granger DN: Leukocyte depletion attenuates vascular injury in post ischemic skeletal muscle. Am J Physiol 254:H823, 1988

28. Dahlback LO, Rais O: Morphologic changes in striated muscle following ischemia. Immediate post ischemic phase. Acta Chir Scand 131:430, 1966

29. Smith JK, Grisham MB, Granger DN et al: Free radical defense mechanisms and neutrophil infiltration in post ischemic skeletal muscle. Am J Physiol 256:H789, 1989

30. Weissman G, Smolen J, Korchak H: Release of inflammatory mediators form stimulated neutrophils. N Engl J Med 303:27, 1980

31. Ward PA, Johnson KJ, Till GO: Oxygen radicals, neutrophils and acute tissue injury. In Taylor AE, Matalon S, Ward PA (eds): Physiology of Oxygen Radicals. American Physiological Society, Bethesda, 1986

32. Babior BA: Oxygen dependent microbial killing by phagocytes. N Engl J Med 298:659, 1978

33. Rubin BB, Smith A, Liauw S et al: Complement activation and white cell sequestration in post ischemic skeletal muscle. An J Physiol 259:H525, 1990

34. Ascer E, Chittur M, Gennaro M et al: Interleukin-1 and thromboxane release after skeletal muscle ischemia and reperfusion. Ann Vasc Surg 6:69, 1992

35. Wright JG, Belkin M, Hobson RW: Hypothermia and controlled reperfusion: two non-pharmacologic methods which diminish ischemia-reperfusion injury in skeletal muscle. Microcirc Endothelium Lymphatics 5:315, 1989

36. Simpson PJ, Todd RF, Fantone JC et al: Reduction of experimental canine myocardial reperfusion injury by a monoclonal antibody (Anti Mo1, Anti CD11b) that inhibits leukocyte adhesion. J Clin Invest 81:624, 1988

18

Basic Pharmacology and Physiology of the Fibrinolytic System

Michael Streiff
William R. Bell

The human fibrinolytic system is a complex system of proteins whose interaction maintains vascular patency without compromising hemostasis. Deficiencies or excesses of any of its components can lead to hemorrhage or thrombosis. During the past two decades, great strides have been made in elucidating the various components of this system and their interactions. Knowledge of this system is essential to all physicians who treat vascular diseases. This chapter reviews the various components of the fibrinolytic system, their interrelationships with each other and with the coagulation cascade, congenital and acquired disorders of the fibrinolytic system, and therapeutic agents that can be used to activate the system.

FIBRINOLYTIC SYSTEM

Plasminogen

The human fibrinolytic system consists of a collection of proteolytic enzymes whose purpose is the dissolution of thrombi. The principal component of this system is plasminogen, which upon activation yields the fibrinolytic enzyme, plasmin. The major site of plasminogen production, as for most other plasma proteins, is the liver.[1,2] The plasma concentration of plasminogen is approximately 20 mg/dl; it has a half-life of approximately 2 days, primarily due to catabolic degradation rather than conversion to plasmin or intravascular consumption.[3,4]

The gene for plasminogen is inherited as two codominant autosomal alleles.[5,6] Several hereditary dysfunctional plasminogen molecules have been described in adults with recurrent thromboembolic disease. The defects in these molecules include abnormal active sites, impaired activator binding, and defective activation.[7-9]

The plasminogen molecule consists of a nonprotease or heavy chain (A-chain) and a serine protease containing a light chain (B-chain) (Fig. 18-1). The heavy chain is composed of an activation peptide (amino acids 1 through 76) and of 5 looped ellipsoid structures known as kringles.[10] These structures are numbered 1 through 5 in sequence, progressing from the amino- to the carboxy-terminus. Each is composed of 80 amino acids

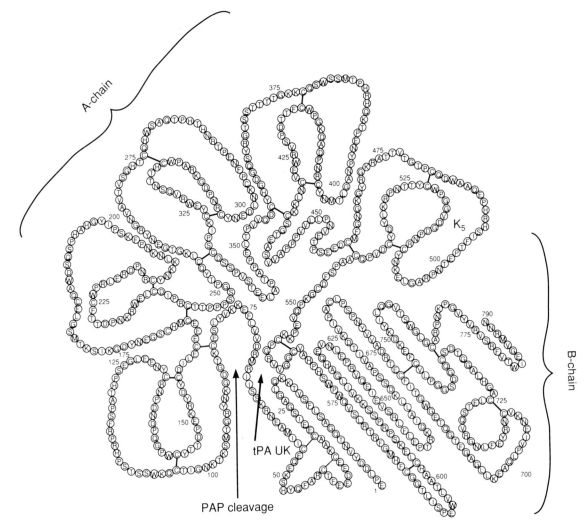

Figure 18-1 Structure of plasminogen. PAP, preactivation peptides; tPA UK, tissue plasminogen activator urokinase. (Modified from Collen and Lijnen,[404] with permission.)

held together by 3 disulfide bonds.[11] These structures are responsible for plasminogen's fibrin binding capability and its interaction with antifibrinolytic agents, such as ε-aminocaproic acid and tranexamic acid.[12] Homologous structures can be found in prothrombin, tissue plasminogen activator (tPA), single-chain urokinase plasminogen activator (scUPA), lipoprotein A, factor XII,[10] vampire bat plasminogen activator, and hepatocyte growth factor.

Using lysine Sepharose column chromatography with ε-aminocaproic acid elution, two different forms of plasminogen have been isolated; native (full-length) glu-plasminogen and partially digested lys-plasminogen.[13-16] Lys-plasminogen is a degradation product resulting from plasmin digestion of glu-plasminogen.[17] The lysine residue at its amino terminus

corresponds to lysine 77 of the parent molecule.[18] The properties of these two molecules differ markedly. Glu-plasminogen exists primarily in a closed conformation with the A-chain in close proximity to the active site of the B-chain. The amino terminal residues of the activation peptide stabilize this conformation. Plasmin digestion releases this segment to produce lys-plasminogen, which exists in an open conformation.[10] This structural change makes lys-plasminogen easier to activate by plasminogen activators (three to ten times as fast by urokinase [UK][19,20] and streptokinase [SK][21]) and increases its binding affinity for fibrin.[18,22,23] In addition, it is probably responsible for the large difference in plasma half-life between lys-plasminogen (0.8 days) and glu-plasminogen (2 days).[24]

Plasminogen Activation

The conversion of plasminogen to plasmin by plasminogen activators is accomplished by the proteolytic cleavage of the arginine 560-valine 561 bond. Two chains are thus formed: the A- (heavy) chain, which comprises the amino-terminus of plasminogen; and the B- (light) chain, which contains the carboxy-terminal active site. The molecular weight of the A- and B-chains is 60,000 and 25,000 daltons, respectively.[25,26]

Three different pathways of plasminogen activation have been proposed on the basis of in vitro studies of native human plasminogen activation. In the absence of any plasmin inhibitors, the activation of glu-plasminogen yields lys-77-plasmin and the so-called preactivation peptides formed by the cleavage of lysine 62-serine 63, arginine 67-methionine 68, or lysine 76-77.[27,28] Wiman and Wallen therefore proposed that activation takes place by a two-step process in which both the release of the preactivation peptides from the amino-terminus of glu-plasminogen and the subsequent cleavage of the arginine 560-valine 561 bond are catalyzed by the activator.[29] Alternatively, Violand and Castellino[30] demonstrated that the presence of the preactivation peptides is not required for plasminogen activation to occur. These investigators proposed that plasmin digestion releases these residues to form lys-77-plasminogen, in which the arginine 560-valine 561 bond is subsequently cleaved by the activator to produce lys-77-plasmin. Finally, Robbins and co-workers[31] showed that when a plasmin inhibitor, such as aprotinin, is present, autodigestion is prevented, and glu-plasmin is the final product. Using a carefully constructed in vitro model of the fibrinolytic system, Rouy and Anglés-Cano[32] recently demonstrated that the latter scheme of plasmin generation is probably the predominant pathway in vivo. These three potential mechanisms are summarized in Figure 18-2.

Plasmin

The B- (light) chain of plasmin contains the proteolytic active site of the molecule, which is formed by three amino acid residues: histidine 602, aspartic acid 645, and serine 740.[33,34] Thrombin, factor Xa, and the pancreatic proteases contain active sites that are homologous in structure and mode of action.[35] Plasmin functions as an endopeptidase with a pH optimum of about 7.[36] It acts specifically as a serine protease, cleaving any synthetic esters and amides of lysine and arginine and peptide bonds having either lysine or arginine on the carboxy side of the molecule.[37]

Fibrin is the principal physiologic substrate of plasmin, although other elements of the coagulation cascade, including factor VIII, factor V, and fibrinogen, are also inactivated by plasmin.[38] Other targets of plasmin include von Willebrand factor, high-molecular-weight kininogen, as well as several components of

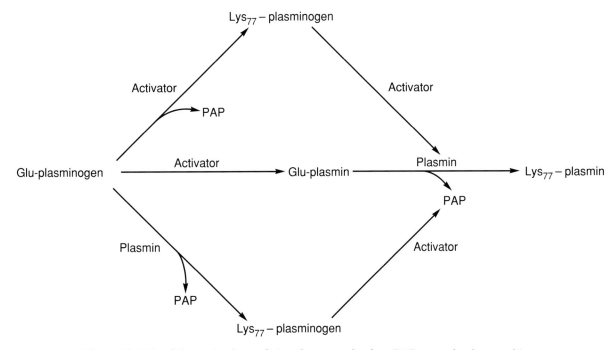

Figure 18-2 Possible mechanisms of plasminogen activation. PAP, preactivation peptides.

basement membranes: fibronectin, collagen, and laminin.[10] Plasmin cleaves fibrin and fibrinogen into a family of fragments known as fibrinogen and fibrin degradation products (FDP-fdp). Fibrinogen degradation products include, in order of decreasing size, fragments X, Y, D, and E[39-42] (Fig. 18-3). Fibrin digestion results in a series of crosslinked fragments, including D-dimers, D₂E complexes, and larger combinations of X and Y[43-50] (Fig. 18-4).

The anticoagulant effects of plasmin result not only from the destruction of fibrin, fibrinogen, and other components of the coagulation cascade, but also from the inhibitory properties of fibrinogen and fibrin degradation products. Fragments Y and D have potent antipolymerizing properties that inhibit the formation of stable fibrin clots.[47] Furthermore, they are no longer able to induce and support platelet aggregation.[48,49]

Plasminogen Activators

Endogenous Activators

Three different systems comprise the endogenous plasminogen activators in humans: the factor XII-dependent pathway, tPA, and scUPA.[50] The presence of the factor XII-dependent pathway was first discovered by Niewiarowski and Prou-Wartelle,[51] who demonstrated that kaolin or glass beads could induce fibrino-lytic activity in the euglobulin fraction of plasma and that factor XII was necessary for this reaction to occur. Subsequently, it has been shown that prekallikrein and high-molecular-weight kininogen are important components of this system.[52,53] Factor XII is thought to induce fibrinolysis through the activation of factor XI and prekallikrein. These substances then directly activate scUPA to two-chain UK, which converts plasminogen into plasmin (Fig. 18-5). High-molecular-weight kininogen acts as a cofactor in the activation of prekallikrein. Activated factor XII also activates plasminogen directly, although much less efficiently than two-chain urokinase. The physiologic significance of these pathways remains unknown.[50]

tPA, a single-chain polypeptide of 527 amino acids and approximately 70,000-dalton molecular weight (Fig. 18-6), is a product of vascular endothelial cells.[54] tPA exists in two forms: a single-chain variety and a two-chain form derived from the former by plasmin hydrolysis of the arginine 275-isoleucine 276 bond.[55-57] The tPA molecule is composed of both a heavy and light chain. The heavy chain contains a fibronectin finger domain, an epidermal growth factor domain, and two kringle domains. The second kringle and the fibronectin finger domain contain fibrin-binding sites that give tPA its fibrin specificity. Researchers have yet to determine the physiologic function of the epidermal growth factor domain.[50]

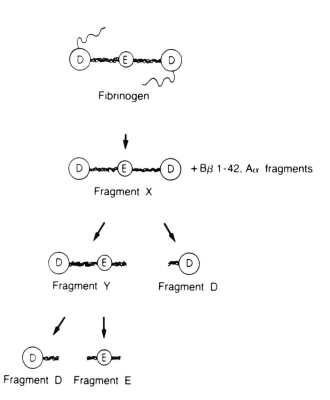

Figure 18-3 Plasmin degradation of fibrinogen. (From Francis and Marder,[41] with permission.)

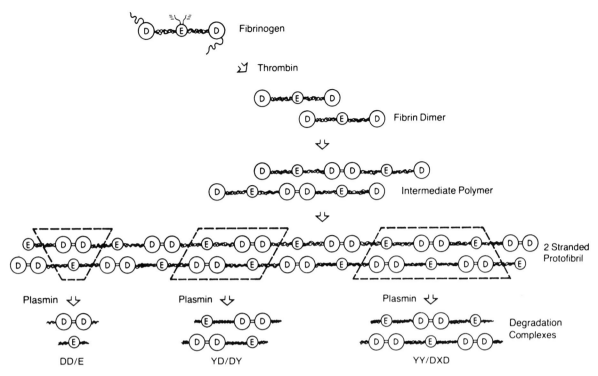

Figure 18-4 Fibrin polymerization and degradation. (From Francis and Marder,[405] with permission.)

The light chain of tPA contains the serine protease active site, which bears considerable homology with trypsin, thrombin, plasmin, and elastase.[54,58] The two-chain variety of tPA activates plasminogen 5 to 10 times as efficiently as the single-chain variety in the absence of fibrin and is also more rapidly inactivated by inhibitors. In the presence of fibrin, however, both forms demonstrate equal efficiency. Conformational changes in the single-chain variety of tPA after fibrin binding are thought to be responsible for its improved enzymatic efficiency.[55,59]

The release of tPA from endothelial cells is triggered by a wide variety of stimuli, including venous stasis, exercise, mental stress, hypoxia, acidosis, thrombin, histamine, bradykinin, and epinephrine. Exogenous agents such as DDAVP also induce tPA release from the endothelium.[50] Others have suggested that the release of tPA may be triggered by a putative hypothalamic hormone, plasminogen activator-releasing hormone (PARH).[60] However, studies in patients who have undergone adenohypophysectomy have failed to document a decrease in DDAVP-induced tPA release.[61] Furthermore, no such hormone has been isolated from bovine pituitary or hypothalamic extracts.[62]

Upon its release, tPA binds to fibrin through its fibronectin finger region and the second kringle and then activates fibrin-bound plasminogen to initiate fibrinolysis. Single-chain tPA is converted to two-chain tPA on the surface of the clot by newly generated plasmin.[56] Critical to the role of tPA as an endogenous plasminogen activator is its fibrin-specificity, which limits systemic plasminogen activation and fibrinogenolysis. In

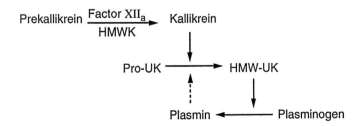

Figure 18-5 Factor XII-dependent fibrinolytic pathway. pro-UK, pro-urokinase; HMWK, high-molecular-weight-kininogen; HMW-UK, high-molecular-weight-urokinase. (From Bachmann,[50] with permission.)

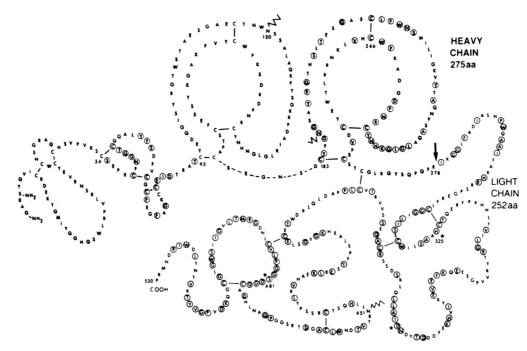

Figure 18-6 Structure of tissue plasminogen activator. *, active site. (From Bachmann,[50] with permission.)

the presence of fibrin, tPA activates one molecule of glu-plasminogen every 5 to 10 seconds. This catalytic efficiency drops to one molecule every 2000 seconds in the absence of fibrin.[50] Changes in the structure of the clot that occur as digestion proceeds increase the concentration of tPA and plasminogen on the surface of the clot, further potentiating thrombolysis.[63,64] Plasminogen activator inhibitors and α_2-antiplasmin also help focus the activity of tPA and plasmin on the surface of the fibrin clot.

Catabolism of tPA occurs mainly in the liver. Its serum half-life is approximately 4 minutes[65,66] (Table 18-1). Several structures on tPA appear to have a role in its clearance from the circulation. Mutants that lack the fibronectin finger domain have been demonstrated to have a longer half-life than does native tPA in an animal model.[67] Glycoprotein side chains such as sialic acid also appear to slow its clearance from the plasma.[68]

The third endogenous plasminogen activator in the human fibrinolytic system is scUPA. The fibrinolytic

Table 18-1 Properties of Thrombolytic Agents

Agent	Source	Molecular Weight (Da)	Type of Agent	Plasma Half-Life (min)	Fibrinolytic Activation	Fibrin Specificity	Antigenicity	Allergic Reactions	Cost
SK	Streptococcal culture	47,400	Bacterial proactivator	23–29	Systemic	Minimal	Yes	Yes	Least expensive
UK	Heterologous mammalian tissue culture	37,000–54,000	tPA	15	Systemic	Minimal	No	No	More expensive
tPA	Heterologous mammalian tissue culture Recombinant bacterial product	70,000	tPA	4	Systemic	Moderate	No	No	Most expensive
APSAC	Streptococcal culture	130,000	Bacterial proactivator	90	Systemic	Minimal	Yes	Yes	More expensive
scUPA	Heterologous mammalian tissue culture Recombinant bacterial product	54,000	tPA	4	Systemic	Moderate	No	No	?

Abbreviations: SK, streptokinase; UK, urokinase; tPA, tissue plasminogen activator; APSAC, anisoylated plasminogen-streptokinase activator complex; scUPA, single-chain urokinase-type plasminogen activator.

activity of urine was first identified in 1946 by Macfarlane and Pilling.[69] Williams later identified this substance as a plasminogen activator in 1951; the next year, Sobel dubbed the responsible enzyme *urokinase*.[70,71] Although evidence for a precursor of UK was first published in 1973,[72] it was not until the early 1980s that several groups isolated and characterized pro-urokinase (pro-UK).[73–77] Subsequently, Pannell and Gurewich and other investigators have demonstrated that pro-UK exhibits intrinsic thrombolytic activity, prompting its current designation, scUPA.[78,79]

scUPA has been isolated from lung and kidney tissue and has also been produced through recombinant technology.[75,80–85] This 411-amino acid molecule has a molecular weight of 54,000 daltons[86] (Fig. 18-7). It consists of three separate domains: an epidermal growth factor domain, a kringle domain, and a serine protease-active site. Unlike tPA, the kringle domain of scUPA lacks a lysine-binding site, which explains its inability to bind to fibrin.[50] Nevertheless, scUPA appears to demonstrate significant fibrin specificity in vivo. Lijnen et al.[79] proposed that a plasma protein that is inactivated by fibrin and competes with plasminogen for binding with scUPA, limits the activity of scUPA to the clot surface. Gurewich and colleagues suggested that conformational changes that occur in glu-plasminogen upon fibrin binding are the critical steps that permit activation by scUPA to occur and account for its fibrin specificity.[87]

Although scUPA possesses minimal intrinsic plasminogen activator capability (approximate 0.4 percent of high-molecular-weight urokinase activity), most of its in vivo thrombolytic potency is mediated by high- and low-molecular-weight urokinase.[87] The current concept of the in vivo activity of scUPA is that after localizing on the clot surface, it activates local plasminogen, which, in addition to digesting fibrin, converts scUPA into high- and low-molecular-weight urokinase. These molecules then mediate the bulk of subsequent fibrinolytic activity (Fig. 18-8).

Recent in vitro studies have demonstrated that scUPA activates a different set of plasminogen molecules than tPA does. scUPA activates plasminogen bound to C-terminal lysine residues, while tPA activates plasminogen bound to internal lysine residues on fibrin.[88] Currently, investigators are attempting to

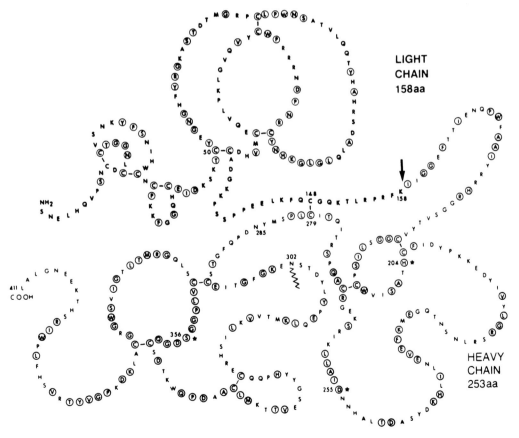

Figure 18-7 Structure of single-chain urokinase-type plasminogen activator. *, active site. (From Bachmann,[50] with permission.)

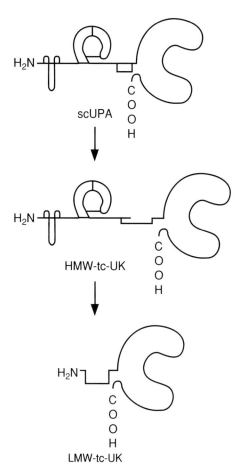

Figure 18-8 Relationship of single-chain urokinase-type plasminogen activator to high- and low-molecular-weight urokinase. scuPA, single-chain urokinase-type plasminogen activator; HMW-tc-UK, high-molecular-weight two-chain urokinase; LMW-tc-UK, low-molecular-weight two-chain urokinase. (From Loscalzo,[406] with permission.)

apply this in vitro synergy to clinical practice in hopes of improving safety, as well as thrombolytic efficiency. The impact of this strategy remains to be seen. Although scuPA has been used in several clinical trials in myocardial infarction, it has yet to establish itself as a force in clinical thrombolysis.[89,90] The plasma half-life of scuPA is approximately 4 minutes, and its plasma concentration is 8 to 10 ng/ml.[91] It is catabolized predominantly in the liver.[92]

In contrast to scuPA, UK is well established as an effective thrombolytic agent for clinical purposes. Depending on the source, urokinase is composed of different proportions of low- and high-molecular-weight forms. Preparations derived primarily from urinary sources contain mostly the high-molecular-weight form (54,000 daltons).[93] Tissue culture preparations

have more low-molecular-weight urokinase.[94] Like scuPA and tPA, UK activates plasminogen directly by cleaving the arginine 560-valine 561 bond. However, unlike these agents, it displays little fibrin specificity. It is cleared by the liver and has a half-life of approximately 15 minutes.[12]

Exogenous Activators

The two exogenous activators in clinical use today are SK and anisoylated plasminogen-streptokinase activator complex (APSAC). Streptokinase was initially discovered in 1933 by Tillett and Garner,[95] who recognized the fibrinolytic properties of an extracellular protein produced by Lancefield group C β-hemolytic streptococci.

A single-chain protein of 415 amino acids with a molecular weight of 47,400 daltons, streptokinase—despite its name—is neither a kinase nor an enzyme. It activates plasminogen in a unique fashion by forming an eqimolar streptokinase-plasminogen complex. Conformational changes in the plasminogen molecule ensue, activating the active center. The complex then proceeds to activate free and complexed plasminogen molecules.[50] The plasmin generated degrades fibrin and fibrinogen as well as free and bound SK molecules releasing a series of SK fragments, ranging from 40,000 to 10,000 daltons,[96,97] all of which retain some degree of activator activity.[98]

Streptokinase interacts with various forms of plasminogen molecule, including glu-plasminogen, lysine-77 plasminogen, valine 442 plasminogen, and the B-chain of plasmin.[99] In vitro studies show that the activity of the activator complex varies with both the size of the streptokinase fragment and the form of plasminogen within the complex.[99-101] The degree of activity is proportional to the size of the SK fragment and inversely proportional to the size of the plasminogen molecule, with the SK B-chain complex having the highest degree of activator activity. Complexes containing glu- and lys-plasminogen retain some degree of fibrin binding because of the intact lysine binding sites on the kringles.[102] This activity is lost in the more digested forms of plasminogen, valine 442 plasminogen and the B-chain of plasmin. Nevertheless, significant fibrinogenolysis results from administration of streptokinase (Fig. 18-9).

Plasmin bound to streptokinase is protected from inhibition by α_2-antiplasmin. The plasmin streptokinase complex is 10^5 times less reactive to α_2-antiplasmin than is plasmin itself.[103] α_2-Macroglobulin, however, does bind to this complex and plays a significant role in the clearance of SK. Antistreptokinase antibodies also appear to play a role. The liver is the major

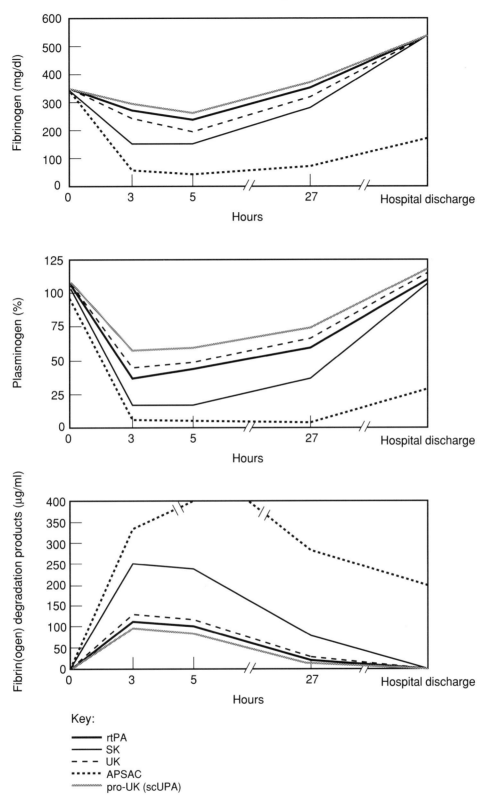

Figure 18-9 Effect of various thrombolytic agents on **(A)** plasma fibrinogen, **(B)** plasminogen, and **(C)** fibrin(ogen) degradation products concentrations. rtPA, recombinant tissue plasminogen activator; SK, streptokinase; UK, urokinase; pro-UK, pro-urokinase; scUPA, single-chain urokinase-type plasminogen activator; APSAC, anisoylated plasminogen-streptokinase activator complex. (From Bell WR: unpublished data.)

organ of catabolism and the half-life of SK in humans is approximately 15 to 30 minutes.[104-106]

Unlike the previously discussed activators, SK is antigenic in humans because of its bacterial origin. As such, it can cause allergic reactions. Furthermore, all individuals have antistreptokinase antibodies in their blood due to previous streptococcal infections in widely varying titers. These antibodies neutralize the effect of the drug, making clinical response unpredictable. Verstraete et al.[107] found that 352,000 U of SK neutralized the antibodies present in 98 percent of patients. However, some patients may require up to 3 million U and others less than 25,000 U to overcome their antistreptokinase antibodies. After exposure to SK, the titer of these antibodies rises rapidly to approximately 100 times their pre-infusion level within 5 to 10 days and persists for up to 6 months.[108]

APSAC is the first synthetic plasminogen activator approved for general clinical use. Although envisioned to be an activator with the efficiency of streptokinase plus a long half-life and improved fibrin specificity, APSAC has been only partially successful in achieving these goals. APSAC consists of a complex of SK and plasminogen with a p-anisoyl group bound reversibly to serine 740 of the plasminogen active site (Fig. 18-10). Its molecular weight is approximately 130,000 daltons. After administration, deacylation of the active site begins to generate active streptokinase-plasmino-gen complexes. Because the kringles of plasminogen are unaffected by the p-anisoyl group, they are free to bind to the surface of the fibrin clot. The gradual deacylation process theoretically allows the complex time to bind to fibrin before activation. Furthermore, the anisoyl group protects the complex from plasmin inhibitors, giving the agent a long half-life. This property simplifies administration (a 2- to 5-minute intravenous bolus) and theoretically should reduce reocclusion.[109] Unfortunately, clinical use has demonstrated that these expectations have been realized only in part. While the agent does have an extremely long half-life (approximately 90 minutes),[109] significant fibrinogenolysis results, as identified in studies performed by us (see Fig. 18-9). The efficacy and frequency of allergic side effects concomitant to APSAC appear to be comparable to streptokinase.[110]

New Developments in Thrombolysis

Current research in thrombolytic therapy is focused on the development of hybrid plasminogen activators, which, it is hoped, will prove safer and more effective than the currently available agents. Several groups have developed genetically engineered mutant tPA molecules that are cleared more slowly than is native tPA.[111-114] Theoretically, these variants should prove more effective and to have reduced rates of reocclusion

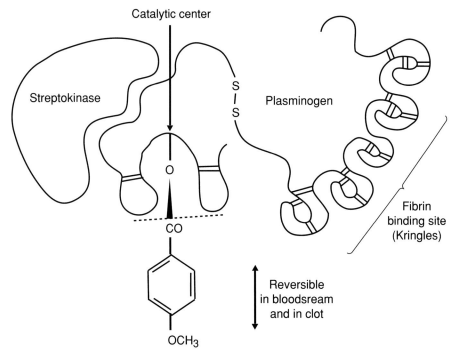

Figure 18-10 Schematic depiction of anisoylated plasminogen-streptokinase activator complex (APSAC). Molecular weight, 131,000 daltons. (From Ferres,[109] with permission.)

compared with native tPA. Others have synthesized tPA mutants resistant to plasminogen activator inhibitor 1 (PAI-1) inactivation[115] (see the section, Plasminogen Activator Inhibitors). However, since doses of tPA currently used easily overwhelm endogenous PAI-1 concentrations, it is doubtful that these congeners will have a significant impact on clinical practice. Likewise, it remains to be seen whether synergistic combinations of agents or newly discovered natural activators (BAT-PA) will make a contribution to therapeutic thrombolysis in the future.[116]

Plasmin Inhibitors

The human body has an extensive system of plasmin and plasminogen activator inhibitors to balance the activity of the fibrinolytic system.

α_2-Antiplasmin

The most important and potent inhibitor of plasmin is α_2-antiplasmin, initially identified in 1976. This single-chain glycoprotein of 452 amino acids has a molecular weight of 67,000 daltons. It belongs to the general class of serine protease inhibitor (serpin), which includes α_1-antitrypsin, inter-α-trypsin inhibitor, antithrombin III, α_2-macroglobulin, and C1 esterase inhibitor.[117,118] The only physiologic role of α_2-antiplasmin appears to be plasmin inhibition.[118] It is synthesized by the liver and has a plasma concentration of 7 mg/dl.[119] Although primarily a plasma protein, small amounts are also found in platelets and are released upon platelet activation by thrombin.[120] Females have higher concentrations than do males. The half-life of α_2-antiplasmin is 2.6 days. When complexed to plasmin, this decreases to 0.5 days.[121]

α_2-Antiplasmin exerts its inhibitory activity on fibrinolysis by forming a 1 : 1 stoichiometric complex with plasmin.[118,122,123] In addition to inhibiting plasmin in the circulation, α_2-antiplasmin inhibits fibrinolysis at the surface of the fibrin clot by interfering competitively with the binding of plasminogen to fibrin and by inactivating plasmin within the substance of the clot.[124-127] α_2-Antiplasmin also inactivates several other components of the coagulation and fibrinolytic cascades, including activated factor XII, factor XI, factor X, thrombin, kallikrein, UK and tPa.[128-131] However, the physiologic importance of these interactions in vivo is likely to be insignificant.

A number of patients have been reported with congenital homozygous α_2-antiplasmin deficiency,[132-137] which appears to be inherited in an autosomal recessive manner. Affected persons have a severe bleeding tendency similar to that of patients with hemophilia A.

Bleeding tends to occur shortly after initial hemostasis, consistent with unrestrained fibrinolysis. In vitro the euglobulin lysis time is markedly shortened. This deficiency can be successfully managed with antifibrinolytic agents, such as ϵ-aminocaproic acid or tranexamic acid.[138]

A number of heterozygotes for α_2-antiplasmin deficiency have also been recognized, with plasma levels ranging from 35 to 71 percent. A few of these cases displayed a mild bleeding tendency.[138]

A number of acquired disorders can result in α_2-antiplasmin deficiency. Liver disease is associated with increased plasmin levels due to impaired production. The half-life of the protein appears to be unchanged.[139-141] By contrast, nephrotic syndrome results in α_2-antiplasmin deficiency due to increased urinary excretion.[142,143] The bleeding tendency associated with amyloidosis has been proposed to be secondary to α_2-antiplasmin deficiency. Avid binding to amyloid fibrils and excess plasminogen activator production have both been suggested as possible causes.[144-146] Striking reductions in α_2-antiplasmin are also seen in disseminated intravascular coagulation (DIC) and thrombolytic therapy as a consequence of accelerated consumption.[147]

α_2-Macroglobulin

The second most important physiologic inhibitor of plasmin is α_2-macroglobulin. Unlike α_2-antiplasmin, α_2-macroglobulin inhibits plasmin selectively. Plasmin retains its fibrinolytic activity but is no longer able to degrade fibrinogen or factor VIII.[148-151] α_2-Macroglobulin has one-tenth the plasmin inhibitory activity of α_2-antiplasmin.[152] While α_2-macroglobulin appears to play a secondary role as a plasmin inhibitor, it has been shown to be the primary inhibitor of plasmin activity when SK is used as a thrombolytic agent.[104] α_2-Macroglobulin also inhibits thrombin, although it is probably only responsible for approximately 25 percent of the thrombin inhibitory activity of plasma, with antithrombin III playing the primary role in this capacity.[153,154] Other proteases inhibited by α_2-macroglobulin include kallikrein, elastase, collagenase, and cathepsin G. Once formed, the protease-α_2-macroglobulin complex is rapidly cleared from circulation by a receptor-mediated mechanism. The liver appears to be the major organ of catabolism.[155]

α_2-Macroglobulin has been found in hepatocytes, endothelial cells, platelets, and white blood cells and may be produced by the monocyte-macrophage system.[156] The plasma concentration of α_2-macroglobulin in adults is approximately 2 mg/ml.[157,158] Children have significantly greater concentrations (2 to 2.5 times normal adult concentrations), and females tend to have 15 percent more than do males.[158]

Elevated levels of α_2-macroglobulin have been reported in a number of disease states, including pulmonary disease, cirrhosis, nephrotic syndrome, and in Down syndrome. Pregnancy and oral contraceptives produce increased serum concentrations as well. Acquired decreases in α_2-macroglobulin have been seen in rheumatoid arthritis and multiple myeloma and during thrombolytic therapy, particularly with streptokinase.[159-161]

α_1-Antitrypsin

α_1-Antitrypsin, whose major purpose is the inhibition of neutrophil elastase, is also a plasmin inhibitor of limited significance, much less even than α_2-macroglobulin.[155,162] It also has minimal inhibitory effects on several components of the coagulation cascade, including thrombin, activated factor XI, and activated factor X.[163,164] Also termed α_1-proteinase inhibitor, it is synthesized in the liver and is distributed widely throughout the body.[162] Its plasma concentration is about 2.5 mg/ml, and its half-life is approximately 1 week. Catabolism occurs in the liver.[128,165] Plasma levels of α_1-proteinase inhibitor are increased during inflammation, neoplasia, pregnancy, and estrogen therapy, indicating that the inhibitor is an acute-phase reactant. In congenital α_1-antitrypsin deficiency, pulmonary and liver damage occur because of the unbridled activity of neutrophil elastase resulting in early emphysema and cirrhosis.[162] Interestingly, cigarette smoke contains oxidants that inactivate the enzyme, producing a local deficiency and gradually leading to emphysematous changes.[166-168] Neither of these deficiency states appears to result in significant disorders of hemostasis.

A number of other plasmin inhibitors have been identified, including C1 inhibitor, a protease that inhibits the activity of C1 (the first component of complement cascade), kallikrein, activated factor XI, activated factor XII, and plasmin. Although its principal physiologic role is the regulation of the complement and kallikrein-kinin systems, it probably plays a minor role in the regulation of fibrinolysis. Still other plasmin inhibitors with limited roles in physiologic plasmin inhibition are antithrombin III, protease nexin, inter-α-trypsin inhibitor, and histidine-rich glycoprotein.[155]

Plasminogen Activator Inhibitors

Inhibition of fibrinolysis also occurs at the level of plasminogen activation. In 1973 Hedner[169] discovered a rapid plasminogen activator inhibitor, which has since been named plasminogen activator inhibitor 1

(PAI-1). The plasma half-life of PAI-1 is 2 hours. Its average plasma concentration is approximately 0.6 U/ml, varying during the day, with its highest concentrations in the morning and lowest in the evening.[170,171] PAI-1 binds tPA or scUPA in a 1:1 molar ratio, preventing the activation of plasminogen. Endothelial cells are the primary source of this protein, although it is also found in platelet α-granules, which release it upon activation.[172,173] Increased levels of PAI-1 have been associated with severe liver disease, pancreatitis, malignancy, deep venous thrombosis, and myocardial infarction. Postoperative patients also exhibit increased levels of PAI-1, as do septic patients. Endotoxin appears to be a potent stimulus for the release of PAI-1 from endothelial cells.[174] Presumably, elevated levels of PAI-1 may predispose to thrombosis, although this suggestion remains to be proved. Protein C has been proposed to serve as a regulator of PAI-1 activity in plasma. While activated protein C does appear to react with and inactivate PAI-1, this reaction is quite slow, and its physiologic significance is unknown.[175]

PAI-2 is another inhibitor of tPA and urokinase-type plasminogen activator. It is present in the placenta and in neutrophils and also circulates in the plasma of pregnant women.[176] PAI-2 has been proposed to play a role in the pathogenesis of eclampsia; however, this suggestion remains to be firmly established.[177] PAI-3 is the most recently described activator inhibitor. This heparin-dependent inhibitor of scUPA is present in urine and plasma; its physiologic significance is unknown.[178]

Most of the proteins that inhibit plasmin also exhibit some inhibitory effect on plasminogen activation. C1 inhibitor is probably the most physiologically important because of its inhibitory effect on kallikrein and activated factor XII. It is responsible for 95 percent of the plasma inhibitory activity of activated factor XII and for 50 percent of the kallikrein plasmin inhibitory activity.[179] Antithrombin III also possesses some inhibitory activity against activated factor XII,[180] while α_2-macroglobulin suppresses kallikrein-mediated fibrinolytic activity.[181] α_2-Antiplasmin displays activity against both kallikrein and activated factor XII. In addition, α_2-antiplasmin, α_2-macroglobulin, α_1-antitrypsin, and antithrombin III all inhibit urokinase.[181]

PHYSIOLOGIC MODEL OF FIBRINOLYSIS IN HUMANS

The body maintains a precise balance between thrombosis and hemorrhage through the complex interaction of the various components of the fibrinolytic system. A highly simplified summary of these events can be described as follows. Vascular injury initiates clot formation via the intrinsic and extrinsic arms of the coagulation cascade, in concert with platelet adhesion and activation. Plasminogen is incorporated into the substance of the clot, as is α_2-antiplasmin, through the thrombin-mediated action of activated factor XIII. tPA is released by endothelial cells in response to high local thrombin concentrations and venous stasis.[182-185] It binds to the fibrin clot and activates the bound plasminogen to plasmin, which digests the fibrin clot. The intrinsically poor plasminogen activator capabilities of tPA in the absence of fibrin, as well as the presence of circulating PAI-1 and α_2-antiplasmin, focus its activity on the surface of the clot. The supply of plasminogen on the clot surface is maintained by the ability of tPA to increase plasminogen binding in a time- and concentration-dependent manner.[186] Since plasmin has both its lysine-binding sites and active site occupied by fibrin, inactivation by α_2-antiplasmin occurs very slowly, as the half-life of plasmin on fibrin is 100 times longer than in its absence.[187] The α_2-antiplasmin crosslinked to fibrin slows fibrinolysis by plasmin, so that adequate endothelial repair can occur before clot lysis. The interaction of these components is depicted in Figure 18-11.

PHYSIOLOGIC AND PATHOLOGIC CHANGES OF THE FIBRINOLYTIC SYSTEM

Variations in fibrinolytic activity occur under a wide range of physiologic circumstances and also in association with certain pathologic conditions. Although fibrinolytic activity has been reported by some to increase with age,[186-189] confirmation by other investigators is lacking.[190,191] The most extensive study of age and fibrinolysis was conducted by Meade and coworkers, who demonstrated a steady decline in fibrinolytic activity in subjects aged 20 to 50, followed by a less prominent increase until age 65.[192] Although no consistent sex differences in fibrinolytic activity have been reported,[190] the decline with age reported by Meade et al.[192] is not as uniform in women, and there is a greater response to exercise in women than in men.[193] Fibrinolytic activity is higher in blacks than in whites,[194] probably due to high levels of plasminogen activator in blacks.[195,196] In addition, fibrinolytic activity seems to decrease with rising social class.[197] Although people with blood group O have slightly higher levels of fibrinolysis than do those with the other blood groups, the differences are not of statistical significance.[198]

The diurnal variation in the level of fibrinolytic activity is lowest in the morning, peaking in the late afternoon and early evening.[199,200] This rise and fall in fibrinolytic activity corresponds to the plasma levels of PAI-1, which is thought to be responsible for this cycle.[174] Venous blood contains slightly higher levels of plasminogen activator, and thus fibrinolytic activity, than does arterial blood.[201] There is no arteriovenous difference, however, in the concentrations of fibrinogen, plasminogen, or α_2-antiplasmin.[202] Elevated temperatures,[203,204] and high altitude[205] also increase fibrinolytic activity.

Exercise has long been associated with increased fibrinolysis.[206,207] This increase is proportional to the intensity and duration of exercise.[208-210] The rise in fibrinolytic activity during exercise is primarily due to the release of tPA from the vascular endothelium.[211] Endothelial trauma, fibrin deposition, increased release of catecholamines and arginine vasopressin, as well as increased body temperature have all been suggested as mediators of this release.[212] Other investigators have suggested that increased blood flow may be responsi-

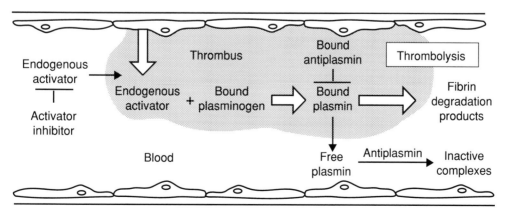

Figure 18-11 Schematic depiction of physiologic fibrinolysis in vivo. (From Francis and Marder,[41] with permission.)

ble. This is supported in a study by Rennie et al.,[213] which demonstrated that the local increase in tPA release induced by exercise could be abolished with arterial occlusion during activity. After exercise, tPA levels fall temporarily, probably as a result of transient endothelial depletion.[214] Reported changes in the plasma levels of plasminogen, fibrinogen,[214] and α_2-antiplasmin[215] are variable, probably reflecting differences in the exercise protocols and laboratory methods used for measurement.

Long-term physical conditioning appears to enhance plasminogen activator release in response to a thrombotic stimulus (venous occlusion) as well as to physical activity.[216] Stratton et al.[216a] demonstrated that six months of physical conditioning increased resting tPA activity and decreased PAI-1 and fibrinogen levels in elderly men. The enhanced fibrinolytic potential and diminished fibrinogen level in the blood associated with conditioning are probably important contributors to the beneficial effect of exercise on the risk of cardiovascular disease.

Dietary habits such as a low-fat diet, onion ingestion, and caffeinated beverages have been associated with reduced fibrinolytic activity.[217-220] By contrast, beer and wine, but not other alcoholic beverages, lower fibrinolytic activity, suggesting that a component unique to beer and wine other than alcohol is responsible.[220,221] Beer also abolishes the diurnal variation in fibrinolytic activity.[222] Obesity lowers fibrinolytic activity by lowering the release of tPA.[192,223-225] The long-term effects of smoking on fibrinolysis are uncertain; both decreased activity and no effect have been reported.[192,226] Anxiety has been shown to increase fibrinolytic activity.[227]

Pregnancy is accompanied by changes in the fibrinolytic system. Fibrinolytic activity steadily declines as pregnancy progresses, while plasminogen and fibrinogen levels rise 50 to 60 percent higher than normal levels.[228,229] These changes rapidly reverse after delivery. Recent research has demonstrated that PAI-1 rises threefold during the second and third trimesters, while PAI-2, the inhibitor of placental origin, rises 25-fold during pregnancy. These changes may be responsible for the decrease in fibrinolytic activity during pregnancy.[230] Kruithof et al.[231] dispute these findings. While they demonstrated increases in PAI-1 and PAI-2 activity in pregnancy, they also found elevated levels of scUPA and tPA. Using a radioactive fibrin-plate method, these workers found no change in total fibrinolytic activity.[230] To date, the controversy remains to be settled. Studies of the fibrinolytic effects of various oral contraceptives indicate that estrogen stimulates fibrinolysis, while progesterone inhibits it.[232,233] Both anabolic steroids[234,235] and intravenous testosterone[236] stimulate fibrinolysis.

Thrombotic and hemorrhagic disorders can result from deficiencies in, or dysfunctional components of, the fibrinolytic system. Thrombosis has been associated with plasminogen deficiency, as well as dysfunctional plasminogen molecules. Several cases of congenital hypoplasminogenemia have been described with antigenic and functional plasminogen levels 30 to 50 percent of normal.[237]

Dysfibrinogenemia and inadequate plasminogen activator levels can also predispose to thrombosis.[238-243] Hemorrhagic disorders can also result from primary imbalances of the fibrinolytic system, such as an excess of plasminogen activator and α_2-antiplasmin deficiency.

DIC is not a primary disease entity, but rather occurs secondary to various pathologic conditions. It involves diffuse derangement of both the coagulation and fibrinolytic systems. Although virtually any pathologic condition can induce DIC, it is most commonly associated with infection,[244] malignant neoplasms,[245,246] liver disease,[247] trauma,[248] snake bites, and obstetric complications such as abruptio placenta,[249] hypertensive toxemia,[250] amniotic fluid embolism,[251] abortion,[252] and postpartum hemolytic uremic syndrome.[253]

The pathophysiologic trigger of DIC is probably the release of thrombotic substances from injured necrotic or neoplastic tissue,[254] which simultaneously activates the coagulation and fibrinolytic systems, causing platelet aggregation.[255] Infectious agents can release substances such as endotoxin, which can result in direct activation of platelets and the coagulation cascade.[256] Alternatively, endotoxin may indirectly activate these systems through endothelial injury. Malignant neoplasms may release thromboplastic substances[245,246] as well as materials that activate the fibrinolytic system.[257,258] In obstetric complications, tissue thromboplastin from the uterus or its contents may be released into the maternal circulation.[259] Acute hypoxia, hypotension, and acidosis resulting from trauma, may also cause release of tissue thromboplastin from injured organs.[260,261] In patients with liver disease, impaired clearance of activated factors and plasminogen activators, as well as decreased synthesis of inhibitors of the coagulation and fibrinolytic system, may contribute to a DIC or hyperfibrinolytic state.[247,262] Recently, Hersch et al.[263] demonstrated that a primary fibrinolytic state may result from acquired deficiencies of PAI-1 and α_2-antiplasmin.

Once the coagulation system is activated, concomitant fibrinolytic activation may occur intrinsically through factor XII or extrinsically through the release of plasminogen activators from endothelium or necrotic or neoplastic tissues. Plasminogen levels in DIC are usually reduced,[264] but plasminogen activator levels are usually normal.[265] As a result of diffuse activation of the coagulation and fibrinolytic systems, many of the components of the coagulation system are either depleted or degraded, or both. Of particular importance are the resultant fibrinogen and FDPs that inhibit the coagulation system by preventing thrombin-induced fibrin formation[266] and platelet aggregation.[48,49]

Although the severity of the clinical presentation of DIC varies greatly from patient to patient, the two major manifestations are a bleeding diathesis and thrombosis. Bleeding is more common and can occur at virtually any site in the body and probably occurs secondary to depletion of coagulation system components, lysis of existing hemostatic plugs, and the anticoagulant effects of fibrin and FDPs. Thrombi and microthrombi can form almost anywhere in the body, causing organ dysfunction.[267]

The diagnosis of DIC can generally be suspected on clinical examination. Although no single laboratory test is pathognomic for DIC,[268] several laboratory studies can help confirm the diagnosis, including an abnormal clotting time, thrombocytopenia, the presence of red blood cell fragments on a peripheral smear, decreased plasma fibrinogen and elevated serum fibrinogen and FDP titers.[269] Recently, enzyme-linked immunosorbent assays (ELISAs) with monoclonal antibodies against crosslinked fragment D of fibrin (D-dimer) have been developed for detecting specifically FDPs. Although these complexes should be very specific markers of ongoing fibrin clot lysis and be elevated in DIC, the specificity of these antibodies has been called into question.[270] Coagulation times (prothrombin time [PTT] and activated partial thromboplastin time [aPTT]) are often prolonged but may be normal; the activated partial thromboplastin time and the thrombin time seem to be more sensitive than the prothrombin time for identifying DIC.[271]

The most important principle in the management of DIC is prompt treatment of the underlying illness. Supportive measures include maintenance of intravascular volume, correction of electrolyte and acid-base disturbances, and avoidance of hypoxia. Transfusions of packed red blood cells and fresh-frozen plasma or cryoprecipitate may be given with caution, but platelet transfusions and individual coagulation factor replacement are of little help. The use of heparin in the treatment of DIC remains controversial. Although initially reported to be of benefit in treatment of DIC,[272] heparin subsequently has been shown to have no effect or worsen the outcome of patients with DIC.[273,274] Similar controversy surrounds the use of antifibrinolytic agents in the treatment of DIC.[275]

Perturbations of the hemostatic system are commonplace in patients with malignant neoplasms. More than 50 percent of patients with primary neoplasms and 95 percent of those with metastatic cancers have some laboratory abnormality of coagulation.[276] The most often recognized abnormalities are elevated fibrin/fibrinogen-split products, thrombocytosis, and elevated fibrinogen levels.[277-279] In 9 to 15 percent of patients, DIC of clinical significance developed, and in 1 to 11 percent, thromboembolic disease developed.[276] Various tumor cell lines have been shown to release membrane components that activate platelets and possess tissue factor-like activity capable of stimulating coagulation.[279-284] Host monocytes appear to respond to cancer cells by synthesizing additional procoagulants.[279,285-288] Devastating coagulopathies, such as Trousseau syndrome, can result.

Malignant cells also appear to possess the capability of synthesizing plasminogen activators. Human ovarian,[289] pancreatic,[290] lung,[291] and breast adenocarcinoma[292] have all been demonstrated to produce urokinase-like plasminogen activators, while brain tumors[293] and melanomas[294] appear to produce tPA. Elevated levels of tissue plasminogen activator and urokinase-type plasminogen activator have also been described in amyloidosis and appear to be responsible for the hemorrhagic diathesis seen in some of these patients. The production of plasminogen activators by tumors also influences their biologic behavior. Human tumor cell lines that secrete urokinase-like plasminogen activator, appear to have greater aggressiveness and metastatic potential than do related lines without this capability. It has been suggested that plasminogen activators enable tumor cells to break through basement membranes and gain access to vascular channels for dissemination. Once in the vasculature, the ability of tumor cells to stimulate platelet aggregation and coagulation allows them to form a protective cocoon of platelets and fibrin which shields them from the immune system.[295,296] In an attempt to interrupt this cycle, various agents that affect the fibrinolytic and coagulation systems have been used in the treatment of cancer, but none has been shown to have a significant impact on survival.

Liver disease is often accompanied by a hemorrhagic diathesis, resulting from a decreased synthesis of coagulation factors by the liver, as well as from increased fibrinolysis.[297-299] Several factors probably play a role in the hyperfibrinolytic state of hepatocellular disease, including decreased hepatic clearance of plasminogen activators and activated coagulation factors,[300,301] increased production of plasminogen activator,[302] and decreased production of fibrinolytic inhibitors, such as α_2-antiplasmin.[301] In contrast to hepatocellular disease, cholestatic liver disease and extrahepatic liver disease are associated with decreased fibrinolytic activity. The reduction in fibrinolysis correlates with the severity of cholestasis. Cholestasis may inhibit fibrinolysis by increasing serum lipids, such as β-lipoprotein and triglycerides, which are known to have antifibrinolytic activity.[303]

Renal disease has been associated with decreased fibrinolytic activity and elevated fibrinogen levels.[304,305] The level of fibrinolysis is not related to the degree of renal excretory function and cannot be improved by hemodialysis.[306] Factors that may contribute to the decreased fibrinolytic activity in renal disease include increased levels of fibrinolytic inhibitors[307] and loss of plasma fibrinolytic proteins due to glomerular injury. Plasminogen is decreased in renal disease[304,306] and can be found excreted in the urine.[308] In nephrotic syndrome, hypoalbuminemia also appears to have a role in suboptimal fibrinolysis.[309]

Fibrin and FDPs are also lost in the urine, the amount and size of the fragments proportional to the degree of proteinuria.[310] Urinary fibrinogen and fibrin degradation products may also result from fibrinolysis of glomerular fibrin deposits that occur in some forms of renal disease.[311] Whether a result of glomerular leakage or of intraglomerular fibrinolysis, the amount of FDP-fdp present in the urine is proportional to the severity of the renal disease.[312]

Atherosclerotic vascular disease, long linked to derangements in lipoprotein metabolism, may also be associated with abnormalities in fibrinolysis. Fibrinogen levels have been found to be significant predictors of cardiovascular disease in several prospective epidemiologic studies, including the Framingham study, the Goteborg study, and the Leigh study.[313-315] Several investigators have demonstrated decreased fibrinolytic activity in the blood of patients with atherosclerosis[316,317] and coronary artery disease.[318-320] Specific fibrinolytic abnormalities in patients with coronary artery disease include impaired diurnal variation of fibrinolysis[321] and reduced fibrinolytic response to venous occlusion,[322] consistent with decreased activator production. Elevated levels of PAI-1 have also been demonstrated in this population. Reduced fibrinolytic activity has also been reported in other atherosclerotic conditions, such as peripheral vascular disease[323] and cerebrovascular disease.[324]

Several risk factors for atherosclerotic vascular disease, including obesity,[223,224] hyperlipoproteinemia,[325] diabetes mellitus,[318,320] and cigarette smoking,[326] have been associated with decreased fibrinolysis. Diabetic patients have both decreased activator levels and increased inhibitor levels.[327] Physical training, while it does increase the fibrinolytic response in diabetic patients, does less so than in control subjects.[328] No correlation has been found between these fibrinolytic abnormalities and the severity of diabetic microvascular

disease.[329] Obesity and hypertriglyceridemia are both associated with elevated PAI-1 levels, while chronic cigarette smoking has been demonstrated to reduce tPA release from endothelial cells in response to DDAVP.[326,330,331]

Defective fibrinolysis has also been associated with recurrent venous thrombosis. Isacson et al.[184] were the first to demonstrate that some patients with recurrent deep venous thrombosis had reduced plasminogen activator stores in their vessel walls. Subsequent studies have shown that as many as 30 to 40 percent of patients with idiopathic recurrent deep venous thrombosis have abnormalities of fibrinolysis.[332-336] In one study, 42 percent of subjects with abnormal fibrinolysis had diminished baseline tPA release, while 26 percent had abnormally high basal PAI-1 activity. Reduced fibrinolytic activity has also been ascribed to women in whom deep venous thrombosis develops while on oral contraceptives.[337,338]

Surgery has long been associated with the development of thromboembolic disease. The increased incidence of DVT in this population has been attributed to temporary increases in PAI-1 that occur during the perioperative period.[339] In several studies of patients undergoing hip operations, elevated preoperative PAI-1 concentrations were associated with postoperative DVT.[340,341] Therapeutically, agents such as ethylestrenol and phenformin, which increase fibrinolytic activity, have been used in patients with defective fibrinolytic systems to prevent deep venous thrombosis.[342] Stanazolol has also been found to increase fibrinolytic activity by decreasing levels of plasminogen activator inhibitor 1.[343]

ANTIFIBRINOLYTIC THERAPY

Therapeutic manipulations of the human fibrinolytic system can be achieved by the administration of antifibrinolytic agents for the treatment of bleeding disorders. Agents available for clinical use include ε-aminocaproic acid ([EACA] or Amicar), trans-p-aminomethylcyclohexane carboxylic acid ([AMCA], or tranexamic acid), and aprotinin, (Trasylol).

ε-Aminocaproic acid and tranexamic acid are effective antifibrinolytic agents because they are lysine analogues. They act by binding to the lysine binding sites of plasminogen and competitively inhibit its interaction with fibrin. Although in vitro these agents render plasminogen more accessible to plasminogen activators by inducing conformational changes in the molecule, they prevent plasminogen from binding to fibrin and degrading it.[344,345-355]

EACA is rapidly absorbed from the gastrointestinal

tract and can thus be administered orally. The drug is excreted by the kidney and has a serum half-life of 1 to 2 hours. After an oral dose, peak serum levels are achieved within 2 hours. About 80 percent of an intravenous dose is cleared by the kidney in 3 hours.[356] The recommended dosage of EACA is 100 mg/kg given orally or intravenously as a loading dose, followed by 0.5 to 1.0 g/h. This regimen maintains plasma concentrations of 13 mg/dl, adequate to inhibit in vivo fibrinolysis.[350,351] EACA is excreted in the urine, where concentrations 75 to 100 times that of plasma levels are achieved. Therefore, much lower doses are required in patients with renal disease or urinary tract bleeding.[356]

Tranexamic acid is 6 to 10 times as potent as EACA; therefore, 10 mg/kg PO every 3 to 4 hours is sufficient to inhibit in vivo fibrinolysis. Like EACA, it has a half-life of approximately 2 hours.[355,357]

Side effects such as nausea, vomiting, diarrhea, abdominal pain, and skin rash have been associated with the use of both agents, although they occur relatively infrequently.[358] Even rarer is rhabdomyolysis with concomitant muscle weakness and myoglobinuria, associated with toxic levels of these medications.[359-362] Thrombosis can also occur but usually only in patients with a predisposing hypercoagulable state. These agents do not induce clot formation but rather prevent normal clot dissolution in the face of generalized pathologic thrombosis.[363,364] EACA has been shown to be teratogenic and is contraindicated in pregnancy.[349]

In contrast to the previous two agents, aprotinin is a serine protease inhibitor derived from bovine parotid gland, pancreas, and lung.[349] Aprotinin inhibits a wide variety of serine proteases other than plasmin, including trypsin, chymotrypsin, and kallikrein.[365,366] It is also a weak anticoagulant.[367] The active site of aprotinin contains lysine.[368] Although aprotinin exerts its antifibrinolytic effect by competitively inhibiting plasminogen activation and noncompetitively inhibiting the action of plasmin on fibrin,[369] its extremely short half-life limits its clinical value as an antifibrinolytic agent.

Antifibrinolytic agents have been employed clinically to treat a number of bleeding conditions, including hyperfibrinolytic states, primary coagulation disorders, and localized imbalances of hemostasis. Primary hyperfibrinolytic states that have been successfully treated with EACA or tranexamic acid include congenital α_2-antiplasmin deficiency,[370] plasminogen activator-secreting tumors,[371] and postoperative bleeding.[349] Several studies in cardiac bypass surgery have demonstrated that EACA as well as aprotinin[372-375] can significantly reduce transfusion requirements and blood loss.[376] These gains were most striking in cases requiring long bypass times and involving cyanotic heart dis-

ease.[372] However, enthusiasm for these agents must be tempered by the occasional reports of disastrous thrombotic consequences in patients who have had unrecognized DIC or in whom large lysis-resistant intrapleural and intrapericardial clots have developed.[353,363,377]

Antifibrinolytic therapy has also been used successfully as an adjunct to coagulation factor replacement in patients with factor deficiencies who undergo surgery. Studies on patients with congenital factor VIII and IX deficiency undergoing dental extraction have shown that the administration of antifibrinolytic agents both improves hemostasis and reduces factor replacement required.[378,379] Since the euglobulin lysis time is unaffected by the administration of antifibrinolytic agents in these patients, it appears that the beneficial effect is a consequence of local, not systemic, inhibition of fibrinolysis. In general, hematuria, especially upper urinary tract bleeding, is not a safe or appropriate indication for antifibrinolytic therapy in this population, unless the bleeding is life-threatening and unmanageable by factor replacement. Several cases of ureteral obstruction by lysis-resistant clots have been reported in this setting.[380-382]

Antifibrinolytic therapy has also been used to control bleeding in patients without factor deficiencies in areas whose inhabitants are susceptible to hyperfibrinolysis. Menorrhagia has been associated with elevated levels of local plasmin activity.[383] Increased plasminogen activator activity has been documented in the secretory phase of the menstrual cycle,[384] in patients with abnormal uterine bleeding,[385] and in those with intrauterine devices (IUDs).[386] Antifibrinolytic therapy has been shown to reduce blood loss significantly in various instances of increased uterine bleeding, including essential menorrhagia,[387] menorrhagia secondary to IUD placement[388] and postoperative bleeding after cervical conization.[389]

The urinary tract is another organ system to which antifibrinolytic therapy has been applied because of the high concentrations of scUPA in these tissues. Although quite successful in managing bleeding associated with prostate surgery as well as rectal biopsy and hematuria due to hemoglobinopathies, antifibrinolytic agents have occasionally resulted in clot-associated urinary tract obstruction.[380,382,390,391] Thus, only severe bleeding resistant to conventional therapy warrants consideration of their use.

Gastrointestinal bleeding also responds to antifibrinolytic therapy. Peptic ulcer disease,[392,393] cirrhosis and its sequelae,[394] and ulcerative colitis[395] have all been associated with local increases in fibrinolysis. Tranexamic acid has been shown to reduce acute upper gastrointestinal bleeding in patients with diffuse gastritis,[396] gastric erosions, gastric ulcers, and esophageal varices.[397] In addition, EACA has been demonstrated to reduce rectal bleeding in patients with ulcerative colitis.[398]

The results of antifibrinolytic therapy in the management of subarachnoid hemorrhage have been less encouraging. Although plasminogen activator activity is normally absent in cerebrospinal fluid (CSF), it can be found in the CSF after subarachnoid hemorrhage.[399] Since EACA and AMCHA both cross the blood-brain barrier, these agents should theoretically reduce the risk of rebleeding, a major contributor to early fatalities after subarachnoid hemorrhage. Unfortunately, although a few controlled studies demonstrated reduced incidence of rebleeding and mortality in the treatment group,[400,401] others have failed to show a mortality benefit, primarily due to an increased incidence of ischemic events.[402,403] The controversy surrounding the use of antifibrinolytic agents for this indication remains unresolved.[404,405]

SUMMARY

The human fibrinolytic system is a complex system of interacting proteins that ensures adequate hemostatic reserves while maintaining vascular patency. Since the 1970s, great strides have been made in understanding and exploiting the various components of this system, primarily by refining and administering fibrinolytic drugs for a wide range of disorders. Many of the applications of fibrinolytic therapy are discussed in the ensuing chapters. It is expected that in the years to come we will become even more adept at manipulating this powerful system to further therapeutic advantage.

ACKNOWLEDGMENTS

This work was supported in part by NIH research grants 36260 and HL 24898 from the National Heart, Lung, and Blood Institute of the National Institutes of Health, Bethesda.

REFERENCES

1. Bohmfalk JF, Fuller GM: Plasminogen is synthesized by primary cultures of rat hepatocytes. Science 209:408, 1980
2. Raum D, Marcus D, Alper CA et al: Synthesis of human plasminogen by the liver. Science 208:1036, 1980
3. Rabiner SF, Goldfine ID, Hart A et al: Radioimmunoassay of human plasminogen and plasmin. J Lab Clin Med 74:265, 1969
4. Collen D, Tytgat G, Claeys H et al: Metabolism of plasminogen in healthy subjects: effects of tranexaminic acid. J Clin Invest 51:1310, 1972
5. Hobart MJ: Genetic polymorphism of human plasminogen. Ann Hum Genet 42:419, 1979
6. Raum D, Marcus D, Alper C: Genetic polymorphism of human plasminogen. Am J Hum Genet 32:681, 1980
7. Miyata T, Iwanaga S, Sakata Y, Aoki N: Plasminogen Tochigi: inactive plasmin resulting from replacement of alanine 600 by threonine in the active site. Proc Natl Acad Sci USA 79:6132, 1982
8. Wohl RC, Summaria L, Robbins KC: Physiological activation of the human fibrinolytic system: isolation and characterization of human plasminogen variants, Chicago I and Chicago II. J Biol Chem 254:9063, 1979
9. Wohl RC, Summaria L, Chediak J et al: Human plasminogen variant Chicago III. Thromb Haemost 48:146, 1982
10. Henkin J, Marcotte P, Yang H: The plasminogen-plasmin system. Prog Cardiovasc Dis 34:135, 1991
11. Magnusson S, Sottrup-Jensen L, Petersen TE et al: Homologous "kringle" structures common to prothrombin and plasminogen. p. 203. In Ribbons DW, Brew K (eds): Proteolysis and Physiological Regulation. Academic Press, San Diego, 1976
12. Collen D, Lijnen HR: The fibrinolytic system in man. CRC Crit Rev Oncol Hematol 4:249, 1990
13. Wallen P, Wiman B: Characterization of human plasminogen I: on the relationship between different molecular forms of plasminogen demonstrated in plasma and found in purified preparations. Biochim Biophys Acta 221:20, 1970
14. Rickli EE, Cuendet PA: Isolation of plasmin-free human plasminogen with N-terminal glutamic acid. Biochim Biophys Acta 250:447, 1971
15. Wallen P, Wiman B: Characterization of human plasminogen. II. Separation and partial characterization of different molecular forms of human plasminogen. Biochim Biophys Acta 257:122, 1972
16. Robbins KC, Summaria L, Elwyn C, Barlow GH: Further studies on the purification and characterization of human plasminogen and plasmin. J Biol Chem 240:541, 1965
17. Claeys H, Molla A, Verstraete M: Conversion of NH$_2$-terminal lysine human plasminogen by plasmin. Thromb Res 3:315, 1973
18. Wiman B, Wallen P: Structural relationship between "glutamic acid" and "lysine" forms of human plasminogen and their interaction with the NH$_2$-terminal activation peptide as studied by affinity chromatography. Eur J Biochem 50:489, 1975
19. Peltz SW, Hardt TA, Mangel WF: Positive regulation of activation of plasminogen by urokinase: differences in Km for (glutamic acid)-plasminogen and lysine-plasminogen and effect of certain alpha, omega-amino acids. Biochemistry 21:2798, 1982
20. Christensen U, Müllertz S: Kinetic studies on the urokinase catalyzed conversion of NH$_2$-terminal lysine

plasminogen to plasmin. Biochim Biophys Acta 480:275, 1977

21. Wohl RC, Summaria L, Arzadon L, Robbins KC: Steady state kinetics of activation of human and bovine plasminogens by streptokinase and its equimolar complexes with various activated forms of human plasminogen. J Biol Chem 253:1402, 1978

22. Thorsen S: Differences in the binding to fibrin of native plasminogen and plasminogen modified by proteolytic degradation. Influence of omega-amino-carboxylic acids. Biochim Biophys Acta 393:55, 1975

23. Rakoczi I, Wiman B, Collen D: On the biological significance of the specific interaction between fibrin, plasminogen and antiplasmin. Biochim Biophys Acta 540:295, 1978

24. Collen D, Verstraete M: Molecular biology of human plasminogen. II. Metabolism in physiological and some pathological conditions in man. Thromb Diath Haemorrh 34:403, 1975

25. Robbins KC, Summaria L, Hsieh B, Shah RJ: The peptide chains of human plasmin. Mechanism of activation of human plasminogen to plasmin. J Biol Chem 242:2333, 1967

26. Summaria L, Hsieh B, Robbins KC: The specific mechanism of activation of human plasminogen to plasmin. J Biol Chem 242:4279, 1967

27. Rickli EE, Otavsky WI: Release of an N-terminal peptide from human plasminogen during activation with urokinase. Biochim Biophys Acta 295:381, 1973

28. Wiman B: Primary structure of peptide released during activation of human plasminogen by urokinase. Eur J Biochem 39:1, 1973

29. Wiman B, Wallen P: Activation of human plasminogen by an insoluble derivative of urokinase. Structural changes of plasminogen in the course of activation to plasmin and demonstration of possible intermediate compound. Eur J Biochem 36:25, 1973

30. Violand BN, Castellino FJ: Mechanisms of the urokinase-catalyzed activation of human plasminogen. J Biol Chem 251:3906, 1976

31. Summaria L, Arzadon L, Bernabe P, Robbins KC: The activation of plasminogen to plasmin by urokinase in the presence of the plasmin inhibitor Trasylol. The preparation of plasmin with the same NH_2-terminal heavy (A) chain sequence as the parent zymogen. J Biol Chem 250:3988, 1975

32. Rouy D, Anglés-Cano E: The mechanism of activation of plasminogen at the fibrin surface by tissue-type plasminogen activator in a plasma milieu in vitro. Role of α_2-antiplasmin. Biochem J 271:51, 1990

33. Groskopf WR, Summaria L, Robbins KC: Studies on the active center of human plasmin. Partial amino acid sequence of a peptide containing the active center serine residue. J Biol Chem 244:3590, 1969

34. Robbins KC, Bernabe P, Arzadon L, Summaria L: The primary structure of human plasminogen II. The histidine loop of human plasmin: light (B) chain active center histidine sequence. J Biol Chem 248:1631, 1973

35. Summaria L, Hsieh B, Groskopf WR et al: The isola-

tion and characterization of the S-carboxyl-methyl B (light) chain derivative of human plasmin. The localization of the active site on the B (light) chain. J Biol Chem 242:5046, 1967

36. Christensen LR, Macleod CM: A proteolytic enzyme of serum: characterization, activation and reaction with inhibitors. J Gen Physiol 28:363, 1975

37. Weinstein MJ, Doolittle RF: Differential specificities of thrombin, plasmin and trypsin with regard to synthetic and natural substrates and inhibitors. Biochim Biophys Acta 258:577, 1972

38. Bick RL: The clinical significance of fibrinogen degradation products. Thromb Haemost 8:302, 1982

39. Ring M, Butman S, Bruck D et al: Fibrin metabolism in patients with acute myocardial infarction during and after treatment with tissue-type plasminogen activator. Thromb Haemost 60:428, 1988

40. Sherman LA, Mossesson MW, Sherry S: Isolation and characterization of the clottable low molecular weight fibrinogen derived by limited plasmin hydrolysis of human fraction I-4. Biochemistry 8:1515, 1969

41. Francis CW, Marder VJ: Physiologic regulation and pathologic disorders of fibrinolysis. p. 358. In Colman RW, Hirsh J, Marder VJ, Salzman EW (eds): Hemostasis and Thrombosis: Basic Principles and Clinical Practice. 2nd Ed. JB Lippincott, Philadelphia, 1987

42. Tockagi T, Doolittle RF: Amino acid sequence studies on plasmin-derived fragments of human fibrinogen: amino-terminal sequences of intermediate and terminal fragments. Biochemistry 14:940, 1975

43. Pizzo SV, Schwartz ML, Hill RL, McKee PA: The effect of plasmin on the subunit structure of human fibrin. J Biol Chem 248:4574, 1973

44. Gaffney PJ, Joe F: The lysis of cross-linked human fibrin by plasmin yields initially a single molecular complex, D-dimer-E. Thromb Res 15:673, 1979

45. Francis CW, Marder VJ, Barlow GH: Plasmic degradation of cross-linked fibrin. Characterization of new macro-molecular soluble complexes and a model of their structure. J Clin Invest 66:1033, 1980

46. Gaffney PJ, Joe F, Mahmoud M: Giant fibrin fragments derived from cross-linked fibrin: structure and clinical implication. Thromb Res 20:647, 1981

47. Marder VJ, Shulman NR, Carroll WR: High molecular weight derivatives of human fibrinogen produced by plasmin. I. Physicochemical and immunological characterization. J Biol Chem 244:2111, 1969

48. Holt JC, Mahmoud M, Gaffney PJ: The ability of fibrinogen fragments to support ADP-induced platelet aggregation. Thromb Res 16:427, 1979

49. Niewiaroski S, Budzynski AZ, Lipinski B: Significance of the intact polypeptide chains of human fibrinogen in ADP-induced platelet aggregation. Blood 49:636, 1977

50. Bachmann F: Plasminogen activators. p. 318. In Colman RW, Hirsh J, Marder VJ, Salzman EW (eds): Hemostasis and Thrombosis: Basic Principles and Clinical Practice. 2nd Ed. JB Lippincott, Philadelphia, 1987

51. Niewiaroski S, Prou-Wartelle O: Rôle du facteur con-

tact (facteur Hageman) dans la fibrinolyse. Thromb Diath Haemorrh 3:593, 1959

52. Saito H, Ratnoff OD, Waldmann R, Abraham JP: Deficiency of a hitherto unrecognized agent, Fitzgerald factor, participating in surface-mediated reactions of clotting, fibrinolysis, generation of kinins and the property of diluted plasma enhancing vascular permeability (PF/DIL). J Clin Invest 55:1082, 1975

53. Weiss AS, Gallin JI, Kaplan AP: Fletcher factor deficiency: a diminished role of Hageman factor activation caused by absence of prekallikrein with abnormality of coagulation, fibrinolysis, chemotactic and kinin generation. J Clin Invest 53:622, 1974

54. Pennica D, Holmes WE, Kohr WJ et al: Cloning and expression of human tissue-type plasminogen activator cDNA in *E. coli.* Nature 301:214, 1983

55. Ranby M, Bergsdorf N, Nilsson T: Enzymatic properties of the one- and two-chain form of tissue plasminogen activator. Thromb Res 27:175, 1982

56. Rijken DC, Hoylaerts M, Collen D: Fibrinolytic properties of one-chain and two-chain human extrinsic (tissue-type) plasminogen activator. J Biol Chem 257:2920, 1982

57. Rijken DC, Groenveld E: Isolation and functional characterization of the heavy and light chains of human tissue-type plasminogen activator. J Biol Chem 261:3098, 1986

58. Strassburger W, Wollmer A, Pitts JE et al: Adaptation of plasminogen activator sequences to known protease structures. FEBS Lett 157:219, 1983

59. Hoylaerts M, Rijken DC, Lijnen HR, Collen D: Kinetics of the activation of plasminogen by human tissue plasminogen activator: role of fibrin. J Biol Chem 257:2912, 1982

60. Cash JD: Control mechanisms of activator release. p. 65. In Davidson JF, Rowan RM, Samama MM, Desnoyers PC (eds): Progress in Chemical Fibrinolysis and Thrombolysis. Vol. 3. Raven Press, New York, 1978

61. Juhan-Vague I, Conte-Devolx B, Aillaud MF et al: Effects of DDAVP and venous occlusion on the release of tissue-type plasminogen activator and von Willebrand factor in patients with pan-hypopituitarism. Thromb Res 33:653, 1984

62. Colucci M, Stassen JM, Salwa J, Collen D: Identification of plasminogen activator releasing activity in the neurohypophysis. Br J Haematol 58:337, 1984

63. Higgins D, Vehar G: Interaction of one-chain tissue plasminogen activator with intact and plasmin-degraded fibrin. Biochemistry 26:7786, 1987

64. Fleury V, Anglés-Cano E: Characterization of the binding of plasminogen to fibrin surfaces: the role of carboxy-terminal lysines. Biochemistry 30:7630, 1991

65. Korninger C, Stassen JM, Collen D: Turnover of human extrinsic (tissue-type) plasminogen activator in rabbits. Thromb Haemost 46:658, 1981

66. Nilsson T, Wallen P, Mellbring G: Turnover of tissue-type plasminogen activator in man, abstracted. Haemostasis 14:90, 1984

67. Larsen GR, Henson R, Blue Y: Variants of human tissue-type plasminogen activator. Fibrin binding, fibrinolytic and fibrinogenolytic characterization of genetic variants lacking the fibronectin finger-like and/or the epidermal growth factor domains. J Biol Chem 263:1023, 1988

68. Beebe DP, Aronson DL: Turnover of t-PA in rabbits: influence of carbohydrate moieties. Thromb Res 51:11, 1988

69. Macfarlane RG, Pilling J: Fibrinolytic activity of normal urine. Nature 159:779, 1947

70. Williams JRB: The fibrinolytic activity of urine. Br J Exp Pathol 32:530, 1951

71. Sobel GW, Mohler SR, Jones NW et al: Urokinase: an activator of plasma profibrinolysin extracted from urine. Am J Physiol 171:768, 1952

72. Bernik MB: Increased plasminogen activator (urokinase) in tissue culture after fibrin deposition. J Clin Invest 52:823, 1973

73. Nielsen LS, Hansen JG, Skriver L et al: Purification of zymogen to plasminogen activator from human glioblastoma cells by affinity chromatography with monoclonal antibody. Biochemistry 21:6410, 1982

74. Sumi H, Kosugi T, Matsuo O, Mihara H: Physicochemical properties of highly purified kidney cultured plasminogen activator (single polypeptide chain urokinase). Acta Haematol Jpn 45:119, 1982

75. Husain S, Gurewich V, Lipinski B: Purification and partial characterization of a single chain high molecular weight form of urokinase from human urine. Arch Biochim Biophys 220:31, 1983

76. Wun TC, Ossowski L, Reich E: A proenzyme form of human urokinase. J Biol Chem 257:7262, 1982

77. Kohno T, Hopper P, Lillquist JS et al: Kidney plasminogen activator: a precursor form of human urokinase with high fibrin affinity. Biotechnology 2:628, 1984

78. Gurewich V, Pannell R, Louie S et al: Effective and fibrin-specific clot lysis by a zymogen precursor form of urokinase (pro-urokinase). A study in vitro and in two animal species. J Clin Invest 73:1731, 1984

79. Lijnen HR, Zamarron C, Blaber M et al: Activation of plasminogen by pro-urokinase. I. Mechanism. J Biol Chem 261:1253, 1986

80. Bernik MB, Oller EP: Plasminogen activator and proactivator (urokinase precursor) in lung cultures. J Am Med Wom Assoc 31:465, 1976

81. Kasai S, Arimura H, Nishida M et al: Proteolytic cleavage of single-chain pro-urokinase induces conformational change which follows activation of the zymogen and reduction of its high affinity for fibrin. J Biol Chem 260:12377, 1985

82. Stump DC, Lijnen HR, Collen D: Purification and characterization of single-chain urokinase-type plasminogen activator from human cell cultures. J Biol Chem 261:1274, 1986

83. Ratzkin B, Lee SG, Schrenk WJ et al: Expression in *Escherichia coli* of biologically active enzyme by a DNA sequence coding for the human plasminogen activator urokinase. Proc Natl Acad Sci USA 78:3313, 1981

84. Nolli ML, Sarubbi E, Corti A et al: Production and characterization of human recombinant single chain urokinase-type plasminogen activator from mouse cells. Fibrinolysis 3:101, 1989

85. Zamarron C, Lijnen HR, Van Hoef B et al: Biological and thrombolytic properties of proenzyme and active forms of human urokinase-I. Fibrinolytic and fibrinogenolytic properties in human plasma in vitro of urokinase obtained from human urine or by recombinant DNA technology. Thromb Haemost 52:19, 1984

86. DeMunk GAW, Rijken DC: Fibrinolytic properties of single chain urokinase-type plasminogen activator (pro-urokinase). Fibrinolysis 4:1, 1990

87. Pannell R, Gurewich V: Pro-urokinase: a study of its stability in plasma and of a mechanism for its selective fibrinolytic effect. Blood 67:1215, 1986

88. Gurewich V: Pro-urokinase: physico-chemical properties and promotion of its fibrinolytic activity by urokinase and by tissue plasminogen activator with which it has a complementary mechanism of action. Semin Thromb Hemost 14:110, 1988

89. Van De Werf F, Nobuhara M, Collen D: Coronary thrombolysis with human single-chain urokinase-type plasminogen activator (pro-urokinase) in patients with acute myocardial infarction. Ann Intern Med 104:345, 1986

90. Meyer J, Bär F, Barth H et al and PRIMI trial study group: randomized double-blind trial of recombinant pro-urokinase against streptokinase in acute myocardial infarction. Lancet 1:863, 1989

91. Huber K, Kirchheimer J, Binder BR: Characterization of a specific anti-human urokinase antibody: development of a sensitive radio-immunoassay for urokinase antigen. J Lab Clin Med 103:684, 1984

92. Collen D, De Cock F, Lijnen HR: Biological and thrombolytic properties of proenzyme and active forms of human urokinase. II. Turnover of natural and recombinant urokinase in rabbits and squirrel monkeys. Thromb Haemost 52:F24, 1984

93. White WF, Barlow GH, Mozen MM: The isolation and characterization of plasminogen activators (urokinase) from human urine. Biochemistry 5:2160, 1966

94. Barlow GH: Urinary and kidney cell plasminogen activator (urokinase). Methods Enzymol 45:239, 1976

95. Tillett WS, Garner RL: The fibrinolytic activity of hemolytic streptococci. J Exp Med 58:485, 1933

96. Brockway WJ, Castellino FJ: A characterization of native streptokinase isolated from a human plasminogen activator complex. Biochemistry 13:2063, 1974

97. Siefring GE, Castellino FJ: Interaction of streptokinase with plasminogen. Isolation and characterization of a streptokinase degradation product. J Biol Chem 251:3913, 1976

98. Chesterman CN, Cederholm-Williams SA, Allington MJ, Sharp AA: The degradation of streptokinase during the production of plasminogen activator. Thromb Res 5:413, 1974

99. Summaria L, Robbins KC: Isolation of a human plasmin-derived functionally active, light (B) chain capable of forming with streptokinase an equimolar light (B) chain-streptokinase complex with plasminogen activator activity. J Biol Chem 251:5810, 1976

100. Markus G, Evers JL, Hobika GH: Activator activities of the human plasminogen-streptokinase complex during its proteolytic conversion to the stable activator complexes. J Biol Chem 251:6495, 1976

101. Robbins KC, Wohl RC, Summaria L: Plasmin and plasminogen activators: kinetics and kinetics of plasminogen activation. Ann NY Acad Sci 370:588, 1981

102. Cederholm-Williams SA: The binding of plasmin-streptokinase complex to fibrin monomer-sepharose. Thromb Res 17:573, 1980

103. Cederholm-Williams SA, De Cock F, Lijnen HR, Collen D: Kinetics of the reactions between streptokinase, plasmin and alpha$_2$-antiplasmin. Eur J Biochem 100:125, 1979

104. Gonias SL, Einarsson M, Pizzo SV: Catabolic pathways for streptokinase, plasmin and streptokinase activator complex in mice: in vivo reaction of plasminogen activator with alpha$_2$-macroglobulin. J Clin Invest 7:412, 1982

105. Pfeifer GW, Doerr F, Brod KH: Zur pharmakokinetik von I^{131} streptokinase un Menschen. Klin Wochenschr 47:482, 1969

106. Robbins KC, Summaria L, Wohl RC, Bell WR: The human plasmin-derived light (B) chain streptokinase complex: a second generation thrombolytic agent. Thromb Haemost 50:787, 1983

107. Verstraete M, Vermylen J, Amery A, Vermylen C: Thrombolytic therapy with streptokinase using a standard dosage scheme. Br Med J 454:5485, 1966

108. Brogden RN, Speight TM, Avery GS: Streptokinase: A review of its clinical pharmacology, mechanism of action and therapeutic uses. Drugs 5:357, 1973

109. Ferres H: Preclinical pharmacological evaluation of anisoylated plasminogen streptokinase activator complex. Drugs, suppl. 3. 3:33, 1987

110. ISIS-3 Collaborative Group: ISIS-3: a randomized comparison of streptokinase vs tissue plasminogen activator vs anistreplase and of aspirin plus heparin vs aspirin alone among 41,299 cases of suspected acute myocardial infarction. Lancet 2:753, 1992

111. Ahern TJ, Morris GE, Barone KM et al: Site-directed mutagenesis in human tissue plasminogen activator. J Biol Chem 265:5540, 1990

112. Burck PJ, Berg DH, Warrick MW et al: Characterization of a modified human tissue plasminogen activator comprising a kringle-2 and a protease domain. J Biol Chem 265:5170, 1990

113. Larsen GR, Timony GA, Horgan PG et al: Protein engineering of novel plasminogen activators with increased thrombolytic potency in rabbits relative to Activase. J Biol Chem 266:8156, 1991

114. Browne MJ, Carey JE, Chapman CG et al: A tissue-type plasminogen activator mutant with prolonged clearance in vivo. J Biol Chem 263:1599, 1988

115. Madison EL, Goldsmith EJ, Gerard RD et al: Serpin-

resistant mutants of human tissue-type plasminogen activator. Nature 339:721, 1989

116. Gardell SJ, Ramjit DR, Stabilito II et al: Effective thrombolysis without marked plasminemia after bolus intravenous administration of vampire bat salivary plasminogen activator in rabbits. Circulation 84:244, 1991

117. Moroi M, Aoki N: Isolation and characterization of alpha$_2$-plasmin inhibitor in human plasma. A novel proteinase inhibitor which inhibits activator-induced clot lysis. J Biol Chem 251:5956, 1976

118. Wiman B, Collen D: Purification and characterization of human antiplasmin, the fast-acting plasmin inhibitor in plasma. Eur J Biochem 78:19, 1977

119. Saito H, Goodnough LT, Knowles BB, Aden DP: Synthesis and secretion of alpha$_2$-plasmin inhibitor by established human liver cell lines. Proc Natl Acad Sci USA 79:5684, 1982

120. Plow EF, Collen D: The presence and release of alpha$_2$-antiplasmin from human platelets. Blood 58:1069, 1981

121. Collen D, Wiman B: Turnover of antiplasmin, the fast-acting plasmin inhibitor of plasma. Blood 53:313, 1979

122. Collen D, De Cock F, Edy J: Identification and some properties of a new fast-reacting plasmin inhibitor in human plasma. Eur J Biochem 69:209, 1976

123. Mullertz S, Clemmensen I: The primary inhibitor of plasmin in human plasma. Biochem J 159:545, 1976

124. Moroi M, Aoki N: Inhibition of plasminogen binding to fibrin by α_2-plasmin inhibitor. Thromb Res 10:851, 1977

125. Aoki N, Moroi M, Tachiya K: Effects of α_2-plasmin inhibitor on fibrin clot lysis. Its comparison with α_2 macroglobulin. Thromb Haemost 39:22, 1978

126. Sakata Y, Aoki N: Crosslinking of α_2-plasmin inhibitor to fibrin by fibrin-stabilizing factor. J Clin Invest 65:290, 1980

127. Sakata Y, Aoki N: Significance of cross linking of α_2-plasmin inhibitor to fibrin in inhibitor of fibrinolysis and in hemostasis. J Clin Invest 69:536, 1982

128. Messmore HL: Natural inhibitors of the coagulation system. Semin Thromb Hemost 8:267, 1982

129. Holmberg L, Lecander I, Astedt B: Binding of urokinase to plasma proteinase inhibitors. Scand J Clin Lab Invest 40:743, 1980

130. Saito H, Goldsmith GH, Moroi M, Aoki N: Inhibitory spectrum of α_2-plasmin inhibitor. Proc Natl Acad Sci USA 76:2013, 1979

131. Korninger C, Collen D: Neutralization of human extrinsic (tissue-type) plasminogen activator in human plasma: no evidence for a specific inhibitor. Thromb Haemost 46:662, 1981

132. Aoki N, Saito H, Kamiya T et al: Congenital deficiency of α_2-plasmin inhibitor associated with severe hemorrhagic tendency. J Clin Invest 63:877, 1979

133. Kluft C, Vellenga E, Brommer EJP: Homozygous α_2 anti-plasmin deficiency. Lancet 2:206, 1979

134. Kluft C, Vellenga E, Brommer EJP, Wijngaards G: A familial hemorrhagic diathesis in a Dutch family: an inherited deficiency of α_2 anti-plasmin. Blood 59:1169, 1982

135. Miles LA, Plow EF, Donnelly KJ, Hougie C et al: A bleeding disorder due to deficiency of α_2 anti-plasmin. Blood 59:1246, 1982

136. Yoshioka A, Kamitsuji H, Takase T et al: Congenital deficiency of α_2-plasmin inhibitor in three sisters. Haemostasis 11:176, 1982

137. Kettle K, Mayne EE: A bleeding disorder due to deficiency of α_2 antiplasmin. J Clin Pathol 38:428, 1985

138. Saito H: α_2-Plasmin inhibitor and its deficiency states. J Lab Clin Med 112:671, 1988

139. Knot EAR, Drijfhout HR, TenCate JW et al: Alpha$_2$ plasmin inhibitor metabolism in patients with liver cirrhosis. J Lab Clin Med 105:353, 1985

140. Aoki N, Yamanaka T: The α_2-plasmin inhibitor levels in liver diseases. Clin Chim Acta 84:99, 1978

141. Teger-Nilsson AC, Gyzander E, Myrwold H et al: Determination of fast-acting plasmin inhibitor (α_2 antiplasmin) in plasma from patients with tendency to thrombosis and increased fibrinolysis. Haemostasis 7:155, 1978

142. Taberner DA, Ralston AJ, Ackril P: Acquired α_2 antiplasmin deficiency in glomerular proteinuria. Br Med J 282:1121, 1981

143. Francis RB, Jr, Sandler RM, Levitan D et al: Reduced α_2 anti-plasmin levels in nephrotic syndrome. Nephron 39:325, 1985

144. Mayer K, Williams EC: Fibrinolysis and acquired α_2-plasmin inhibitor deficiency in amyloidosis. Am J Med 79:394, 1985

145. Clyne LP, Caldwell AB: Acquired α_2 anti-plasmin deficiency secondary to amyloidosis. Thromb Haemost 58:797, 1987

146. Takahashi H, Koike T, Yoshida N et al: Excessive fibrinolysis in suspected amyloidosis: demonstration of plasmin-alpha$_2$ plasmin inhibitor complex and von Willebrand factor fragment in plasma. Am J Hematol 23:153, 1986

147. Aoki N, Moroi M, Matsuda M, Tachiya K: The behavior of α_2-plasmin inhibitor in fibrinolytic states. J Clin Invest 60:361, 1977

148. Ganrot PC: Inhibition of plasmin activity by α_2 macroglobulin. Clin Chim Acta 16:328, 1967

149. Harpel PC, Mosesson MW: Degradation of human fibrinogen by plasma α_2 macroglobulin enzyme complexes. J Clin Invest 52:2175, 1973

150. Veremeenko KN, Kizim AI: Selective action of α_2 macroglobulin-plasmin complex on fibrin. Thromb Res 23:317, 1981

151. Vantera E, Varimo M, Myllyla G: Effect of α_2 macroglobulin-plasmin complexes on factor VIII. Thromb Res 18:247, 1980

152. Aoki N, Moroi M, Tachiya K: Effects of α_2-plasmin inhibitor on fibrin clot lysis. Its comparison with α_2 macroglobulin. Thromb Haemost 39:22, 1978

153. Abildgaard V: Purification of two progressive an-

tithrombins of human plasma. Scand J Clin Lab Invest 19:190, 1967

154. Shapiro SS, Anderson DB: Thrombin inhibition in normal plasma. p. 361. In Lundblad RL, Fenton JW, Mann KG (eds): Chemistry and Biology of Thrombin. Ann Arbor Science, Ann Arbor, MI, 1977

155. Harpel PC: Blood proteolytic enzyme inhibitors: their role in modulating blood coagulation and fibrinolytic enzyme pathways. p. 219. In Colman RW, Hirsh J, Marder VJ, Salzman EW (eds): Hemostasis and Thrombosis: Basic Principles and Clinical Practice. 2nd Ed. JB Lippincott, Philadelphia, 1987

156. Hovi T, Mosher D, Vaheri A: Cultured human monocytes synthesize and secrete α_2 macroglobulin. J Exp Med 145:1580, 1977

157. Wilding P, Adham NF, Mehl JW, Haverback BJ: α_2 Macroglobulin concentration in human serum. Nature 214:1226, 1967

158. Ganrot PC, Schersten B: Serum α_2 macroglobulin concentration and its variation with age and sex. Clin Chim Acta 15:113, 1967

159. James K, Johnson G, Fudenberg HH: The quantitative estimation of α_2 macroglobulin in normal, pathological, and cord sera. Clin Chim Acta 14:207, 1966

160. Housely J: α_2 Macroglobulin levels in disease in man. J Clin Pathol 21:27, 1968

161. Nilehn JE, Ganrot PC: Plasmin, plasmin inhibitors, and degradation products of fibrinogen in human serum during and after intravenous infusion of streptokinase. Scand J Clin Lab Invest 20:113, 1967

162. Morse JO: Alpha$_1$-antitrypsin deficiency. N Engl J Med 299:1045, 1978

163. Gans H, Tan BH: Alpha$_1$-antitrypsin, an inhibitor of thrombin and plasmin. Clin Chim Acta 17:111, 1967

164. Ellis V, Scully M, MacGregor I, Kakkar V: Inhibition of human factor Xa by various plasma protease inhibitors. Biochim Biophys Acta 701:24, 1982

165. Laurell CB, Nosslin B, Jeppson JO: Catabolic rate of alpha$_1$-antitrypsin of Pl type M and Z in man. Clin Sci Mol Med 52:457, 1977

166. Travis J, Salvesen GS: Human plasma proteinase inhibitors. Annu Rev Biochem 52:655, 1983

167. Johnson D, Travis J: Structural evidence for methionine at the reactive site of human alpha-1-proteinase inhibitor. J Biol Chem 253:7142, 1978

168. Matheson NR, Wong PS, Travis J: Enzymatic inactivation of human alpha$_1$-proteinase inhibitor by neutrophil myeloperoxidase. Biochem Biophys Res Commun 88:402, 1979

169. Hedner U: Studies on an inhibitor of plasminogen activation in human serum. Thromb Diath Haemorrh 30:414, 1973

170. Chmielewski J, Ranby M, Wiman B: Evidence for a rapid inhibitor to tissue plasminogen activator in plasma. Thromb Res 31:427, 1983

171. Kluft C, Verheijen JH, Chang GTG et al: Diurnal fluctuations in the activity in blood of the fast-acting tPA inhibitor, abstracted. Haemostasis 14:100, 1984

172. Van Mourik JA, Lawrence DA, Loskutoff DJ: Purification of an inhibitor of plasminogen activator (antiactivator) synthesized by endothelial cells. J Biol Chem 259:14914, 1984

173. Erickson LA, Ginsberg MH, Loskutoff DJ: Detection and partial characterization of an inhibitor of plasminogen activator in human platelets. J Clin Invest 74:1465, 1984

174. Juhan-Vague I, Moerman B, De Cock F et al: Plasma levels of a specific inhibitor of tissue-type plasminogen activator (and urokinase) in normal and pathologic conditions. Thromb Res 33:523, 1984

175. DeFouw NJ, van Hirsbergh VWM, Jong YF et al: The interaction of activated protein C and thrombin with the plasminogen activator inhibitor released from cultured human endothelial cells. Thromb Haemost 57:176, 1987

176. Åstedt B, Lecander I, Ny T: The placental type plasminogen activator inhibitor PAI-2. Fibrinolysis 1:203, 1987

177. Bonnar J, Daly L, Sheppard BL: Changes in the fibrinolytic system during pregnancy. Semin Thromb Hemost 16:221, 1990

178. Stump DC, Taylor FB, Nesheim ME et al: Pathologic fibrinolysis as a cause of clinical bleeding. Semin Thromb Hemost 16:260, 1990

179. Kluft C: Occurrence of C1 inactivator and other proteinase inhibitors in euglobulin fractions and their influence on fibrinolytic activity. Haemostasis 5:136, 1976

180. Rosenberg RD: Mechanism of antithrombin action and the structural basis of heparin's anticoagulant function. p. 353. In Bing DH (ed): The Chemistry and Physiology of the Human Plasma Proteins. Pergamon Press, New York, 1979

181. Harpel PC: Human plasma α_2 macroglobulin: an inhibitor of plasma kallikrein. J Exp Med 132:329, 1970

182. Loskutoff D: Effect of thrombin on the fibrinolytic activity of cultured bovine endothelial cells. J Clin Invest 64:329, 1979

183. Levin EG, Marzec U, Anderson J et al: Thrombin stimulates tissue plasminogen activator release from cultured human endothelial cells. J Clin Invest 74:1988, 1984

184. Isacson S, Nilsson IM: Defective fibrinolysis in blood and vein walls in recurrent "idiopathic" venous thrombosis. Acta Chir Scand 138:313, 1972

185. Kluft C: Studies on the fibrinolytic system in human plasma. Thromb Haemost 41:365, 1979

186. Tran-Thang C, Kruithof EKO, Bachmann F: Tissue-type plasminogen activator increases the binding of glu-plasminogen to clots. J Clin Invest 74:2009, 1984

187. Wiman B, Collen D: Molecular mechanisms of physiological fibrinolysis. Nature 272:549, 1978

188. Hume R: The relationship to age and cerebral vascular accidents of fibrin and fibrinolytic activity. J Clin Pathol 14:167, 1961

189. Swan HT: Fibrinolysis related to age in men. Br J Haematol 9:311, 1963

190. Sawyer DW, Fletcher AP, Alkjaersig N, Sherry S: Studies on the thrombolytic activity of human plasma. J Clin Invest 39:426, 1960

191. Hamilton PJ, Dawson AA, Ogston D, Douglas AS: The effect of age on the fibrinolytic enzyme system. J Clin Pathol 27:326, 1974

192. Meade TW, Chakrabati R, Haines AP et al: Characteristics affecting fibrinolytic activity and plasma fibrinogen concentrations. Br Med J 1:153, 1979

193. Cash JD: Effect of moderate exercise on the fibrinolytic system in normal young men and women. Br Med J 2:502, 1966

194. Walker WR: Fibrinolytic activity of whole blood from South African Banta and white subjects. Am J Clin Nutr 9:461, 1961

195. Ferguson JC, Mackay N, MacNicol GP: Effect of feeding fat on fibrinolysis, stypven time, and platelet aggregation in Africans, Asians and Europeans. J Clin Pathol 23:580, 1970

196. Barr RD, Ouna N, Kendall AG: The blood coagulation and fibrinolytic systems in healthy adult Africans and Europeans—a comparative study. Scot Med J 18:93, 1973

197. Szczeklik A, Dischinger P, Kueppers F et al: Blood fibrinolytic activity, social class and habitual physical activity. II. A study of black and white men in Southern Georgia. J Chron Dis 33:291, 1980

198. Meade TW, North WRS: Population-based distributions of hemostatic variables. Br Med Bull 33:283, 1977

199. Fearnley GR, Balmforth G, Fearnley E: Evidence of a diurnal fibrinolytic rhythm with a simple method of measuring natural fibrinolysis. Clin Sci 16:645, 1957

200. Fornasari PM, Gamba G, Dolci D et al: Circadian rhythms in fibrinolysis. p. 773. In Serneri N, Prentice CRM (eds): Haemostasis and Thrombosis. Academic Press, London, 1979

201. Fearnley GR, Ferguson J: Arteriovenous difference in natural fibrinolysis. Lancet 2:1040, 1957

202. Ogston D, Ogston CM, Bennett NB: Arteriovenous differences in the components of the fibrinolytic enzyme system. Thromb Diath Haemorrh 16:32, 1966

203. Bedrak E, Beer G, Furman KI: Fibrinolytic activity and muscular exercise in heat. J Appl Physiol 19:469, 1964

204. Britton BJ, Hawkey C, Wood WG et al: Adrenergic, coagulation and fibrinolytic responses to heat. Br Med J 4:139, 1974

205. Chochan IS, Singh I, Balakrihshan K: Fibrinolytic activity at high altitude and sodium acetate buffer. Thromb Diath Haemorrh 32:65, 1974

206. Hunter J: Treatise on Blood, Inflammation and Gunshot Wounds. G Nicoll, London, 1794

207. Biggs R, MacFarland RG, Pilling J: Observations on fibrinolysis. Experimental activity produced by exercise or adrenaline. Lancet 1:402, 1947

208. Rosing DR, Brakman P, Redwood DR et al: Blood fibrinolytic activity in man. Diurnal variation and the response to varying intensities of exercise. Circ Res 27:171, 1970

209. Hawkey CM, Britton BJ, Wood WG et al: Changes in blood catecholamine levels and blood coagulation and fibrinolytic activity in response to graded exercise in man. Br J Haematol 29:377, 1975

210. Davis GL, Abilgaard CF, Bernayer EM, Britton M: Fibrinolytic and hemostatic changes during and after maximal exercise in males. J Appl Physiol 40:287, 1976

211. Marsh N, Gaffney P: Some observations on the release of extrinsic and intrinsic plasminogen activators during exercise in man. Haemostasis 9:238, 1980

212. Röcker L, Taenzer M, Drygas WK et al: Effect of prolonged physical exercise on the fibrinolytic system. Eur J Appl Physiol 60:478, 1990

213. Rennie JAN, Bennett B, Ogston D: Effect of local exercise and vessel occlusion on fibrinolytic activity. J Clin Pathol 30:350, 1977

214. Arai M, Yorifuji H, Ikematsu S et al: Influences of strenuous exercise (triathlon) on blood coagulation and fibrinolytic system. Thromb Res 57:465, 1990

215. Ferguson EW, Bernier LL, Banta GR: Effects of exercise and conditioning on clotting and fibrinolytic activity in men. J Appl Physiol 62:1416, 1987

216. Williams RS, Logue EE, Lewis JL et al: Physical conditioning augments the fibrinolytic response to venous occlusion in healthy adults. N Engl J Med 302:987, 1980

216a. Stratton JR, Chandler WL, Schwartz RS et al: Effects of physical conditioning on fibrinolytic variables and fibrinogen in young and old adults. Circulation 83:1692, 1991

217. Lee KT, Kim PN, Keokarn Y, Thomas WA: Geographic pathology of atherosclerosis and thrombosis. Coagulation and clot-lysis phenomena in Koreans on a low-fat diet. J Atheroscler Res 6:203, 1966

218. Menon IS, Kendal RY, Dewar HA, Newall DJ: Effect of onions on blood fibrinolytic activity. Br Med J 3:351, 1968

219. Al Samarrae W, Truswell AS: Short term effect of coffee on blood fibrinolytic activity in healthy adults. Atherosclerosis 26:255, 1977

220. Fearnley GR, Ferguson J, Chakrabati R, Vincent CT: Effect of beer on blood fibrinolytic activity. Lancet 1:184, 1960

221. Nilsson IM, Bjorkman SE, von Studnitz W, Hallen A: Antifibrinolytic activity of certain pectins. Thromb Diath Haemorrh 6:177, 1961

222. Walter E, Birkholz LB, Harenberg J, Weber E: Circadian rhythms of platelet function, fibrinolytic activity of plasma and the influence of reduced food uptake, fat loading and beer drinking on fibrinolytic activity. p. 525. In Serneri N, Prentice CRM (eds): Haemostasis and Thrombosis. Academic Press, London, 1979

223. Ogston D, McAndrew GM: Fibrinolysis in obesity. Lancet 2:1205, 1964

224. Bennett N, Ogston C, McAndrew GM, Ogston D: Stud-

ies on the fibrinolytic enzyme system in obesity. J Clin Pathol 19:241, 1966

225. Almer LO, Janzon L: Low vascular fibrinolytic activity in obesity. Thromb Res 6:171, 1975

226. Janzon L, Nilsson IM: Smoking and fibrinolysis. Circulation 51:1120, 1975

227. Ogston D, McDonald GA, Fullerton HW: The influence of anxiety in tests of blood coagulability and fibrinolytic activity. Lancet 2:521, 1962

228. Bonnar J, McNicol GP, Douglas AS: Fibrinolytic enzyme system and pregnancy. Br Med J 3:387, 1969

229. Biezenski JJ, Moore HC: Fibrinolysis in normal pregnancy. J Clin Pathol 11:306, 1958

230. Wiman B, Csemiczsky L, Marsk L, Robbe H: The fast inhibitor of tissue plasminogen activator in pregnancy. Thromb Haemost 52:124, 1984

231. Kruithof EKO, Tran-Thang C, Gudinchet A et al: Fibrinolysis in pregnancy—a study of plasminogen activator inhibitors. Blood 69:460, 1987

232. Brakman P, Sobrero AJ, Astrupt T: Effects of different systemic contraceptives on blood fibrinolysis. Am J Obstet Gynecol 106:187, 1970

233. Sobrero AJ, Brakman P, Astrupt T: Effects on blood fibrinolysis of an oral contraceptive low in progestin (Ovulen). Am J Obstet Gynecol 110:122, 1971

234. Davidson JF, Lochhead M, McDonald GA, McNicol GP: Fibrinolytic enhancement by stanazol: a double blind trial. Br J Haematol 22:543, 1972

235. Hedner U, Nilsson IM, Isacson S: Effect of ethyloestrenol in the vessel wall. Br Med J 2:729, 1976

236. Fearnley GR, Chakrabati R: Increase of blood fibrinolytic activity by testosterone. Lancet 2:128, 1962

237. Aoki N: Hereditary abnormalities of the fibrinolytic system. p. 264. In Francis JL (ed): Fibrinogen, Fibrin Stabilization and Fibrinolysis. Ellis Horwood, Chichester, UK, 1987

238. Soria J, Soria C, Caen JP: A new type of congenital dysfibrinogenemia with defective fibrin lysis—Dusard syndrome: a possible relation to thrombosis. Br J Haematol 53:575, 1983

239. Beck EA, Charache P, Jackson DP: A new inherited coagulation disorder caused by an abnormal fibrinogen, fibrinogen Baltimore. Nature 208:143, 1983

240. Mondhiry HAB, Bilezikian SB, Nossel HL: Fibrinogen New York, an abnormal fibrinogen associated with thromboembolism: functional evaluation. Blood 45:607, 1975

241. Fuchs G, Egbring R, Havenmann K: Fibrinogen Marburg. A new genetic variant of fibrinogen. Blut 34:107, 1977

242. Sandbjerg-Hansen M, Clemmensen I, Winther D: Fibrinogen Copenhagen, an abnormal fibrinogen with defective polymerization and release of fibrinopeptide A but normal adsorption of plasminogen. Scand J Clin Lab Invest 40:221, 1980

243. Johansson L, Hedner U, Nilsson IM: A family with thromboembolic disease associated with deficient fibrinolytic activity in vessel wall. Acta Med Scand 203:477, 1978

244. Yoshikawa T, Tanaka KR, Guze LB: Infection and disseminated intravascular coagulation. Medicine 50:234, 1971

245. Peck SD, Reiquam CW: Disseminated intravascular coagulation in cancer patients. Supportive evidence. Cancer 31:1114, 1973

246. Sun NCJ, Bowie EJW, Kazmier FJ et al: Blood coagulation studies in patients with cancer. Mayo Clin Proc 49:636, 1974

247. Verstraete M, Vermylen J, Collen D: Intravascular coagulation in liver disease. Annu Rev Med 25:447, 1974

248. Attar S, Boyd D, Layne E et al: Alterations in coagulation and fibrinolytic mechanisms in acute trauma. J Trauma 9:939, 1969

249. Sutton DM: Intravascular coagulation in abruptio placenta. Am J Obstet Gynecol 109:604, 1971

250. Davidson EC, Phillips LL: Coagulation studies in the hypertensive toxemias of pregnancy. Am J Obstet Gynecol 113:905, 1972

251. Bonnar J: Blood coagulation and fibrinolysis in obstetrics. Clin Haematol 2:213, 1973

252. Stim EM: Saline abortion. Obstet Gynecol 40:247, 1972

253. Strauss RG, Alexander RW: Post-partum hemolytic uremic syndrome. Obstet Gynecol 47:169, 1976

254. Hardaway RM, Dixon RS, Foster EF: The effect of hemorrhagic shock on disseminated intravascular coagulation. Ann Surg 184:43, 1976

255. Evensen S, Jeremic M: Platelet and the triggering mechanism of intravascular coagulation. Br J Haematol 19:33, 1970

256. Beller FK: The role of endotoxin in DIC. Thromb Diath Haemorrh, suppl. 36:125, 1969

257. Pitney WR: Disseminated intravascular coagulation. Semin Haematol 8:65, 1971

258. Ossowski L, Quigley JP, Kellerman GM, Reich E: Fibrinolysis associated with oncogenic transformation. J Exp Med 138:1056, 1973

259. Schneider CL: Etiology of fibrinopenia: fibrination defibrination. Ann NY Acad Sci 75:634, 1959

260. Bergentz SE, Nilsson IM: Effect of trauma on coagulation and fibrinolysis in dogs. Acta Chir Scand 122:21, 1961

261. Cafferata HT, Aggeler PM, Robinson AJ, Blaisdell FW: Intravascular coagulation in the surgical patient: its significance and diagnosis. Am J Surg 118:281, 1969

262. MacMahon AG: Disseminated intravascular coagulation in acute alcoholic liver disease. S Afr Med J 47:227, 1973

263. Hersch SL, Kunelis T, Francis RB, Jr: The pathogenesis of accelerated fibrinolysis in liver cirrhosis: a critical role for tissue plasminogen activator inhibitor. Blood 69:1315, 1987

264. Merskey C, Johnson AJ, Kleiner GJ, Wohl H: The defibrination syndrome: clinical features and laboratory diagnosis. Br J Haematol 13:528, 1967

265. Spero JA, Lewis JH, Hasiba U: Disseminated intravascular coagulation. Findings in 346 patients. Thromb Haemost 43:28, 1980
266. Latallo ZS, Budzynski AZ, Lipinski B, Kowalski E: Inhibitors of thrombin and of fibrin polymerization, two activities derived from plasmin-digested fibrinogen. Nature 203:1184, 1964
267. Robboy SJ, Colman RW, Minna JD: Pathology of disseminated intravascular coagulation (DIC): analysis of twenty-six cases. Hum Pathol 3:327, 1972
268. Niewiarowski S, Gurewich V: Laboratory identification of intravascular coagulation. J Lab Clin Med 77:665, 1971
269. Karp JE, Bell WR: Fibrinogen-fibrin degradation products and fibrinolysis following exercise in humans. Am J Physiol 227:1212, 1974
270. Eisenberg PR, Jaffe AS, Stump DC et al: Validity of enzyme-linked immunosorbent assays of cross-linked fibrin degradation products as a measure of clot lysis. Circulation 82:1159, 1990
271. Bell WR: Disseminated intravascular coagulation. Johns Hopkins Med J 146:289, 1980
272. Colman RW, Robboy SJ, Minna JD: Disseminated intravascular coagulation: an approach. Ann J Med 52:679, 1972
273. Green D, Seeler RA, Allen N, Alavi IA: The role of heparin in the management of consumption coagulopathy. Med Clin North Am 56:193, 1972
274. Lasch HG, Heene DH: Heparin therapy of diffuse intravascular coagulation (DIC). Thromb Diath Haemorrh 33:105, 1974
275. Prentice CRM: Basis of antifibrinolytic therapy. J Clin Pathol, suppl. 14. 33:35, 1980
276. Nand S, Messmore H: Hemostasis in malignancy. Am J Hematol 35:45, 1990
277. Davis RB, Theologides A, Kennedy BJ: Comparative studies of blood coagulation and platelet aggregations in patients with cancer and nonmalignant diseases. Ann Intern Med 71:67, 1969
278. Sun NC, McAfee W, Hum GJ et al: Hemostatic abnormality in malignancy. A prospective study of 108 patients. Am J Clin Pathol 71:10, 1979
279. Rickles FR, Edwards RL: Activation of blood coagulation in cancer. Trousseau's syndrome revisited. Blood 62:14, 1983
280. Pearlstein EP, Salk PL, Yogeswaran et al: Correlation between spontaneous metastatic potential, platelet aggregating activity of cell extracts and cell surface siaylation in 10 metastatic variant derivatives of a rat renal sarcoma line. Proc Natl Acad Sci USA 77:4336, 1980
281. Karpatkin S, Pearlstein E: Role of platelets in human tumor cell metastases. Ann Intern Med 95:636, 1981
282. Ewan VA, Edwards LRL, Rickels FR: Induction of tissue factor activity in a monocyte like cell line. J Lab Clin Med 101:401, 1983
283. Garg SK, Niemetz J: Tissue factor activity of normal and leukemic cells. Blood 42:729, 1973
284. Hudig D, Rapaport SI, Bajaj SP: Tissue factor like activity of the human monocyte tumor cell line U-937. Thromb Res 27:321, 1982
285. Edwards RL, Rickels FR, Cronlund M: Abnormalities of blood coagulation in patients with cancer. Mononuclear cell tissue factor generation. J Lab Clin Med 98:917, 1981
286. Morgan D, Edwards RL, Rickels FR: Monocyte procoagulant activity as a peripheral marker of clotting activation in cancer patients. Haemostasis 18:55, 1988
287. Schwartz BS, Edgington TS: Immune complex induced human monocyte procoagulant activity. J Exp Med 154:892, 1981
288. Semararo N: Different expression of procoagulant activity in macrophages associated with experimental and human tumors. Haemostasis 18:47, 1988
289. Astedt B, Holmberg L: Immunological identity of urokinase and ovarian carcinoma plasminogen activator released in tissue culture. Nature 261:595, 1976
290. Wu MC, Adel AY: Comparative studies on urokinase and plasminogen activator from cultured pancreatic carcinoma. Int J Biochem 10:1001, 1979
291. Markus G, Takita H, Cumiolo SM et al: Content and characterization of plasminogen activators in human lung tumors and normal lung tissue. Cancer Res 40:841, 1980
292. Evers JL, Patel J, Madeja JM et al: Plasminogen activator activity and composition in human breast cancer. Cancer Res 42:219, 1982
293. Tucker WS, Kirsch WM, Martinez-Hernandez A, Fink LM: In vitro plasminogen activator activity in human brain tumors. Cancer Res 38:297, 1978
294. Rijken DC, Collen D: Purification and characterization of the plasminogen activator secreted by human melanoma cells in culture. J Biol Chem 256:7035, 1981
295. Sane DC, Pizzo SV, Greenberg CS: Elevated urokinase-type plasminogen activator level and bleeding in amyloidosis: case report and literature review. Am J Hematol 31:53, 1989
296. Kwaan HC, Keer HN: Fibrinolysis and cancer. Semin Thromb Haemost 16:230, 1990
297. Goodpasture EW: Fibrinolysis in chronic hepatic insufficiency. Johns Hopkins Hosp Bull 25:330, 1914
298. DeNicola P, Soardi F: Fibrinolysis in liver diseases. Study of 109 cases by means of the fibrin plate method. Thromb Diath Haemorrh 2:290, 1958
299. Grossi CE, Moreno AH, Rousselot LM: Studies on spontaneous fibrinolytic activity in patients with cirrhosis of the liver and its inhibition by epsilon amino caproic acid. Ann Surg 153:383, 1961
300. Fletcher AP, Biederman O, Moore D et al: Abnormal plasminogen-plasmin system activity (fibrinolysis) in patients with hepatic cirrhosis: its cause and consequences. J Clin Invest 43:681, 1964
301. Tytgat G, Cohen D, deVreker R, Verstraete M: Investigations on the fibrinolytic system in liver cirrhosis. Acta Haematol 40:265, 1968
302. Astrup T, Rasmussen J, Amery A: Fibrinolytic activity of cirrhotic liver. Nature 185:619, 1960

303. Jedrychowski A, Hillenbrand P, Ajdukiewicz AB et al: Fibrinolysis in cholestatic jaundice. Br Med J 1:640, 1973

304. Edward N, Young DPG, MacLeod M: Fibrinolytic activity in plasma and urine in chronic renal disease. J Clin Pathol 17:365, 1964

305. Wardle EN, Menon IS, Rastogi SP: Study of proteins and fibrinolysis in patients with glomerulonephritis. Br Med J 2:260, 1970

306. McNicol GP, Barakat AA, Douglas AS: Plasma fibrinolytic activity in renal disease. Scott Med J 10:189, 1965

307. Larsson SO, Hedner U, Nilsson IM: On coagulation and fibrinolysis in acute renal insufficiency. Acta Med Scand 189:443, 1971

308. Chen HF, Nakabayashi M, Satoh K, Sakamoto S: Studies on the purification and characterization of human urinary plasminogen and plasmin. Thromb Haemost 42:1536, 1980

309. Gandrille S, Aiach M: Albumin concentration influences fibrinolytic activity in plasma and purified systems. Fibrinolysis 4:225, 1990

310. Hall CL, Blainey JD, Gaffney PJ: Origin of urinary fibrin-fibrinogen degradation products in renal glomerular disease. Nephron 23:6, 1979

311. Briggs JD, Prentice CRM, Hutton MM et al: Serum and urine fibrinogen-fibrin related antigen (F.R-antigen) levels in renal disease. Br Med J 4:82, 1972

312. Nilsson IM: Fibrinogen degradation products and renal disease. Scand J Haematol, suppl. 13:357, 1971

313. Shakespeare M, Wolf P: Demonstration of urokinase antigen in blood. Thromb Res 14:825, 1979

314. Wijngaards G, Kluft C, Groenveld E: Demonstration of urokinase-related fibrinolytic activity in human plasma. Br J Haematol 51:165, 1982

315. Wun TC, Schleuning WD, Reich E: Isolation and characterization of urokinase from human plasma. J Biol Chem 257:3276, 1982

316. Naimi S, Goldstein R, Proger S: Studies of coagulation and fibrinolysis of the arterial and venous blood in normal subjects and patients with atherosclerosis. Circulation 27:904, 1963

317. Peabody RA, Tsapogas MJ, Wu KT et al: Altered endogenous fibrinolysis and biochemical factors in atherosclerosis. Arch Surg 109:309, 1974

318. Fearnley GR, Chakrabati R, Avis PRD: Blood fibrinolytic activity in diabetes mellitus and its bearing on ischemic heart disease and obesity. Br Med J 1:921, 1963

319. Chakrabati R, Hocking ED, Fearnley GR et al: Fibrinolytic activity and coronary artery disease. Lancet 1:987, 1968

320. Badawi H, E-Sawi M, Mikhail M et al: Platelet coagulation and fibrinolysis in diabetic and non-diabetic patients with quiescent coronary heart disease. Angiology 21:511, 1970

321. Rosing DR, Redwood DR, Brakman P et al: Impairment of the diurnal fibrinolytic response in man. Effect of age, type IV hyperlipoproteinemia, and coronary artery disease. Circ Res 34:641, 1974

322. Walker ID, Davidson JF, Hutton I, Lawrie TDV: Disordered "fibrinolytic potential" in coronary artery disease. Thromb Res 10:509, 1977

323. Nestel PJ: Fibrinolytic activity of the blood in intermittent claudication. Lancet 2:373, 1959

324. Pilgeram LO: Abnormalities in clotting and thrombolysis as a risk factor for stroke. Thromb Diath Haemorrh 31:245, 1974

325. Andersen P, Arnesen H, Hjermann I: Hyperlipoproteinemia and reduced fibrinolytic activity in healthy coronary high-risk men. Acta Med Scand 209:199, 1981

326. Allen RA, Kluft C, Brommer ETP: Effect of chronic smoking on fibrinolysis. Arteriosclerosis 5:443, 1985

327. Almer LO, Nilsson IM: On fibrinolysis in diabetes mellitus. Acta Med Scand 198:101, 1975

328. Schneider SH, Kim HC, Khachadurian AK, Ruderman NB: Impaired fibrinolytic response to exercise in type II diabetes: effects of exercise and physical training. Metabolism 37:924, 1988

329. Almer LO, Pandolfi M: Fibrinolysis and diabetic retinopathy. Diabetes 25:807, 1976

330. Hamsten A, Wiman B, deFaire U, Blombäck M: Increased plasma levels of a rapid inhibitor of tissue plasminogen activator in young survivors of myocardial infarction. N Engl J Med 313:1557, 1985

331. Mehta J, Mehta P, Lawson D, Saldeen T: Plasma tissue plasminogen activator inhibitor levels in coronary artery disease: correlation with age and serum triglyceride concentrations. J Am Coll Cardiol 9:263, 1987

332. Wiman B, Ljungberg B, Chmielewska J et al: The role of the fibrinolytic system in deep venous thrombosis. J Lab Clin Med 105:267, 1985

333. Nilsson IM, Ljungner H, Tengborn L: Two different mechanisms in patients with venous thrombosis and defective fibrinolysis: low concentration of plasminogen activator or increased concentration of plasminogen activator inhibitor. Br Med J 290:1453,

334. Haggroth L, Mattson C, Felding P, Nilsson IM: Plasminogen activator inhibitors in plasma and platelets from patients with recurrent venous thrombosis and pregnant women. Thromb Res 42:585, 1986

335. Juhan-Vague I, Valadier J, Alessi MC et al: Deficient t-PA release and elevated PA inhibitor levels in patients with spontaneous deep venous thrombosis. Thromb Haemost 57:67, 1987

336. Petaja J: Fibrinolytic response to venous occlusion for 10 and 20 minutes in healthy subjects and in patients with deep vein thrombosis. Thromb Res 56:251, 1989

337. Astedt B, Issacson S, Nilsson IM, Pandolfi M: Thrombosis and oral contraceptives: possible predisposition. Br Med J 4:631, 1973

338. Pizzo SV, Lewis JG, Campbell EE, Dreyer NA: Fibrinolytic response and oral contraceptive-associated thromboembolism. Contraception 23:181, 1981

339. Mellbring G, Dahlgren S, Wiman B: Plasma fibrinolytic activity in patients undergoing major abdominal surgery. Acta Chir Scand 151:109, 1985

340. Paramo JA, Alfaro MJ, Rocha E: Postoperative changes in the plasma levels of tissue-type plasminogen activator and its fast-acting inhibitor-relationship to deep vein thrombosis and influence of prophylaxis. Thromb Haemost 54:713, 1985

341. Eriksson B, Eriksson E, Gryzander E et al: Thrombosis after hip replacement. Relationship to the fibrinolytic system. Acta Orthop Scand 60:159, 1989

342. Nilsson IM, Hedner U, Issacson S: Phenformin and ethylosternol in recurrent venous thrombosis. Acta Med Scand 198:107, 1975

343. Kluft C, Preston EE, Malia RG et al: Stanazolol-induced changes in fibrinolysis and coagulation in healthy adults. Thromb Haemost 51:157, 1984

344. Brockway W, Castellino F: Measurement of the binding of antifibrinolytic amino acids to various plasminogens. Arch Biochem Biophys 151:194, 1972

345. Wallen PL: Activation of plasminogen with urokinase and tissue activator. p. 91. In Paoletti R, Sherry S (eds): Thrombosis and Urokinase. Academic Press, London, 1977

346. Thorsen S, Mullertz S: Rate of activation and electrophoretic mobility of unmodified and partially degraded plasminogen: Effects of 6-aminohexanoic acid and related compounds. Scand J Clin Lab Invest 34:167, 1974

347. Griffin JD, Ellman L: Epsilon-aminocaproic acid (EACA). Semin Thromb Hemost 5:27, 1978

348. Sweeney WM: Aminocaproic acid, an inhibitor of fibrinolysis. Am J Med Sci 249:576, 1965

349. McNicol GP: Disordered fibrinolytic activity and its control. Scott Med J 7:266, 1962

350. McNicol GP, Douglas AS: Epsilon-aminocaproic acid and other inhibitors of fibrinolysis. Br Med Bull 20:233, 1964

351. Niewiarowski S, Wolosowicz N: The in vivo effect of epsilon-aminocaproic acid on human plasma fibrinolytic system. Thromb Diath Haemorrh 15:491, 1966

352. Nilsson IM, Andersson L, Björkman SE: Epsilon-aminocaproic acid (EACA) as a therapeutic agent: based on 5 years clinical experience. Acta Med Scand, suppl. 448:5, 1966

353. Bennett B, Ogston D: Natural and drug-induced inhibition of fibrinolysis. Clin Hematol 2:135, 1973

354. Sherry S, Fletcher AP, Alkjaelsig N et al: Epsilon-aminocaproic acid. "A potent antifibrinolytic agent". Trans Assoc Am Physicians 72:62, 1959

355. Andersson L, Nilsson IM, Nilehn JE et al: Experimental and clinical studies on AMCA, the antifibrinolytically active isomer of p-aminomethyl cyclohexane carboxylic acid. Scand J Haematol 2:230, 1965

356. McNicol GP, Fletcher AP, Alkjaersig N, Sherry S: The absorption, distribution, and excretion of ϵ-aminocaproic acid following oral or intravenous administration to man. J Lab Clin Med 59:15, 1962

357. Okamoto S, Oshiba S, Mihara H et al: Synthetic inhibitors of fibrinolysis: In vitro and in vivo mode of action. Ann NY Acad Sci 146:414, 1968

358. Bergin JJ: The complications of therapy with epsilon-aminocaproic acid. Med Clin North Am 50:1669, 1966

359. Rizza RA, Selonick S, Conley CL: Myoglobinuria following aminocaproic acid administration. JAMA 236:1845, 1976

360. Lane RJM, Mastaglia FL: Drug-induced myopathies in man. Lancet 2:562, 1978

361. Mackay AR, Sang UH, Weinstein PR: Myopathy associated with epsilon-aminocaproic acid (EACA) therapy. J Neurosurg 49:597, 1978

362. Britt CW, Randall RL, Peters BH, Schrochet SS: Rhabdomyolysis during treatment with epsilon-aminocaproic acid. Arch Neurol 37:187, 1980

363. Charytan C, Purtilo D: Glomerular capillary thrombosis and acute renal failure after epsilon-aminocaproic acid therapy. N Engl J Med 280:1102, 1969

364. Gralnick HR, Greipp P: Thrombosis with epsilon aminocaproic acid therapy. Am J Clin Pathol 56:151, 1977

365. Steichele DF, Herschlein HJ: Zur antifibrinolytischen Wirkung des Trypsin-kallikrein inactivators. Med Welt 42:2170, 1961

366. Green NM: Kinetics of the reaction between trypsin and the pancreatic trypsin inhibitor. Biochem J 66:407, 1957

367. Prentice CRM, McNicol GP, Douglas AS: Studies on the anticoagulant action of aprotinin (Trasylol). Thromb Diath Haemorrh 24:265, 1970

368. Chavet J, Acher R: The reactive site of the basic trypsin inhibitor of pancreas. Role of lysine 15. J Biol Chem 242:4274, 1967

369. Dubber AHC, McNicol GP, Uttley D, Douglas AS: In vitro and in vivo studies with Trasylol, an anticoagulant and a fibrinolytic inhibitor. Br J Haematol 14:31, 1968

370. Miura O, Hirosawa S, Kato A, Aoki N: Molecular basis for congenital deficiency of α_2-plasmin inhibitor. J Clin Invest 83:1598, 1989

371. Davidson JF, McNicol GP, Frank GL et al: Plasminogen-activator-producing tumor. Br Med J 1:88, 1969

372. McClure PD, Izsak J: The use of epsilon-amino caproic acid to reduce bleeding during cardiac bypass in children with congenital heart disease. Anesthesiology 40:604, 1974

373. Lambert CJ, Marengo-Rowe AJ, Levenson JE et al: The treatment of postperfusion bleeding using epsilon aminocaproic acid, cryoprecipitate, fresh-frozen plasma and protamine sulfate. Ann Thorac Surg 28:440, 1979

374. Sterns LP, Lillehei CW: Effect of epsilon amino caproic acid upon blood loss following open-heart surgery. An analysis of 340 patients. Can J Surg 10:304, 1967

375. Gralnick HR: Epsilon-aminocaproic acid in preoperative correction of hemostatic defect in cyanotic congenital heart disease. Lancet 2:1204, 1970

376. Bidstrup BP, Royston D, Sapsford RN et al: Reduction in blood loss and blood use after cardiopulmonary bypass with high dose aprotinin. J Thorac Cardiovasc Surg 97:364, 1989

377. Kevy SV, Glickman RM, Bernhard WF et al: The pathogenesis and control of the hemorrhagic defect in open heart surgery. Surg Gynecol Obstet 123:313, 1966

378. Walsh PN, Rizza CR, Matthews JM et al: Epsilon-aminocaproic acid and therapy for dental extraction in hemophilia and Christmas disease: a double-blind controlled trial. Br J Haematol 20:463, 1971

379. Forbes CD, Barr RD, Reid G et al: Tranexamic acid in control of haemorrhage after dental extraction in haemophilia and Christmas disease. Br Med J 2:311, 1972

380. Hilgartner MW: Intrarenal obstruction in haemophilia. Lancet 1:486, 1966

381. Stark SN, White JG, Langer Jr. J, Krivit W: Epsilon aminocaproic acid therapy as a cause of intrarenal obstruction in haematuria in haemophiliacs. Scand J Haematol 2:99, 1965

382. van Itterbeck H, Vermylen J, Verstraete M: High obstruction of urine flow as a complication of the treatment with fibrinolysis inhibitors of haematuria in haemophiliacs. Acta Haematol 39:237, 1968

383. Nilsson IM: Local fibrinolysis as a mechanism for haemorrhage. Thromb Diath Haemorrh 34:623, 1975

384. Albrechtsen OK: The fibrinolytic activity of the human endometrium. Acta Endocrinol 23:297, 1956

385. Rybo G: Clinical and experimental studies on menstrual blood loss. Acta Obstet Gynecol Scand 45:1, 1966

386. Larsson B, Liedholm P, Sjoberg NO, Astedt B: Increased fibrinolytic activity in the endometrium of patients using Copper IUD. Contraception 9:531, 1974

387. Nilsson L, Rybo G: Treatment of menorrhagia with an antifibrinolytic agent, tranexamic acid (AMCA). A double blind investigation. Acta Obstet Gynecol Scand 46:572, 1967

388. Kasonde JM, Bonnar J: Aminocaproic acid and menstrual loss in women using intrauterine devices. Br Med J 4:17, 1975

389. Rybo G, Westerberg H: The effect of tranexamic acid (AMCA) on postoperative bleeding after conization. Acta Obstet Gynecol Scand 51:347, 1972

390. Gobbi F: Use and misuse of aminocaproic acid. Lancet 1:472, 1967

391. McNicol GP, Fletcher AP, Alkjaersig N et al: The use of epsilon aminocaproic acid, a potent inhibitor of fibrinolytic activity in the management of postoperative hematuria. J Urol 86:829, 1961

392. Cox HT, Poller L, Thomson JM: Gastric fibrinolysis. A possible aetiologic link with peptic ulcer. Lancet 2:1300, 1967

393. Low J, Dodds AJ, Biggs JC: Fibrinolytic activity of gastroduodenal secretions—a possible role in upper gastrointestinal hemorrhage. Thromb Res 17:819, 1980

394. Oka K, Tanaka K: Local fibrinolysis of esophagus and stomach as a cause of haemorrhage in liver cirrhosis. Thromb Res 14:837, 1979

395. Kwaan HC, Cocco A, Mendeloff AI: Histologic demonstration of plasminogen activation in rectal biopsies from patients with active ulcerative colitis. J Lab Clin Med 64:877, 1964

396. Biggs JC, Hugh TB, Dobbs AJ: Tranexamic acid and upper gastrointestinal haemorrhage—a double blind trial. Gut 17:729, 1976

397. Cormack F, Jouhar AJ, Chakrabati RR, Fearnley GR: Tranexamic acid in upper gastrointestinal haemorrhage. Lancet 1:1207, 1973

398. Salter RH, Read AE: Epsilon-aminocaproic acid therapy in ulcerative colitis. Gut 11:585, 1970

399. Tovi D, Nilsson IM: Increased fibrinolytic activity and fibrin degradation products after experimental intracerebral hemorrhage. Acta Neurol Scand 48:403, 1972

400. Maurice-Williams RS: Prolonged anti-fibrinolysis: an effective nonsurgical treatment for ruptured intracranial aneurysms. Br Med J 1:945, 1978

401. Chowdhary UM, Carey PC, Hussein MM: Prevention of early recurrence of spontaneous subarachnoid haemorrhage by epsilon-amino caproic acid. Lancet 1:741, 1979

402. van Rossum J, Wintzen AR, Endtz LJ et al: Effect of tranexamic acid on rebleeding after subarachnoid hemorrhage. A double-blind controlled clinical trial. Ann Neurol 2:242, 1977

403. Kaste M, Ramsay M: Tranexamic acid in subarachnoid hemorrhage. A double-blind study. Stroke 10:519, 1979

404. Collen D, Lijnen HR: Molecular and cellular basis of fibrinolysis. p. 1232. In Hoffman R, Benz EJ, Jr, Shattil SJ et al. (eds): Hematology: Basic Principles and Practice. Churchill Livingstone, New York, 1991

405. Francis CW, Marder VJ: Concept of clot lysis. Annu Rev Med 37:187, 1986

406. Loscalzo J: An overview of thrombolytic agents. Chest, suppl. 97:117s, 1990

19

Peripheral Embolization and Thrombosis

William C. Mackey

Primary nontraumatic acute extremity ischemia is caused by either embolism or arterial thrombosis. Prolonged survival of patients with advanced cardiac disease and with significant cardiac dysrhythmias accounts for the increasing incidence of peripheral embolism (23.1 : 100,000 admissions in 1950 to 1964, 50.4 : 100,000 in 1960–1979).[1] Acute arterial thrombosis is at least as common as embolism as a cause of acute extremity ischemia.[2] Prolonged survival of patients with extensive atherosclerotic disease makes peripheral arterial thrombosis an increasingly common clinical presentation.

While the differentiation between embolism and thrombosis is important, patients presenting with embolism and thrombosis are similar in most respects, so that demographic criteria are not useful in distinguishing between these conditions. The mean age of patients presenting with embolization or thrombosis is approximately 65 to 70 years, although patients presenting with aortoiliac "saddle" embolus tend to be younger (mean age 56 in a recent report).[3-6] Men predominate among patients presenting with thrombosis, but in most series of peripheral emboli, women are affected as commonly as men.[3,5,7] Risk factors for atherosclerotic cardiovascular disease are of nearly equal prevalence in patients with embolism and thrombosis.[3]

Peripheral embolism and thrombosis are threatening to both life and limb. In 1978 Blaisdell reviewed 35 series of acute lower-extremity ischemia, published between 1963 and 1977, and found that mortality rates ranged from 15 percent to 48 percent with a mean of approximately 25 percent.[8] Limb salvage rates in these same series ranged from 40 percent to 81 percent.[8]

With improved clinical decision making, pre- and postoperative care, and surgical as well as anesthetic techniques, mortality rates have declined only slightly. In 1984, Dale reported a mortality rate of 7.1 percent in 140 cases of acute ischemia related to embolism or thrombosis.[7] Also in 1984, Cambria and associates from the Massachusetts General Hospital reported mortality rates of 8 percent in 52 cases of thrombosis but 20 percent in 220 case of peripheral embolization.[3] Furthermore, in 1989 Clason et al.[9] from Edinburgh reported a 29.3 percent 30-day mortality in 181 patients undergoing lower-extremity embolectomy. Mortality risk in this series was correlated with increasing age, proximal vascular occlusion, recent myocardial infarction, grade 3 to 4 New York Heart Association functional score, and the presence of preexisting peripheral arterial disease.[9] In a separate report, this same group found that upper-extremity embolization was less likely to result in death (5 percent versus 29 percent) than lower extremity embolization because of less extensive associated cardiopulmonary disease in the former group.[10] In a report by Baxter-Smith et al.[11] from Birmingham, England, mortality was also correlated with duration of symptoms; mortality was 10 percent in patients with symptoms for less than 2 hours and 32 percent in those with symptoms for 5 to 8 hours. A similar correlation was noted in a 1985 series from Copenhagen (18 percent mortality if <6 hours and 33 percent mortality if >48 hours).[12] In general, mortality rates are higher in patients with embolic disease than in those with thrombosis because of the former's more frequent association with acute myocardial infarction or other severe cardiac disease.

While mortality rates have improved very little, especially in patients with emboli, limb salvage rates have improved and are consistently higher in embolic than in thrombotic disease. The underlying peripheral occlusive disease is usually much worse in patients with thrombosis and often renders limb salvage impossible.[3] In separate series by Clason and Tawes of predominantly embolic disease, limb salvage rates of 95 percent were achieved in surviving patients.[4,9] Cambria and Abbott[3] found 85 percent and 67 percent limb salvage rates in patients with embolism and thrombosis, respectively.

While both embolism and thrombosis pose threats to life and limb, the former is more often fatal, and the latter more often results in limb loss. These outcome statistics should guide our approach to the patient with acute limb ischemia secondary to embolism or thrombosis.

PATHOPHYSIOLOGY OF EMBOLISM AND THROMBOSIS

Embolism

The heart is the source of 75 to 90 percent of peripheral emboli.[2,13] Atrial fibrillation is present in approximately 70 percent of patients presenting with embolization, and atrial mural thrombus is the presumed source of the embolus in these patients.[2,3] Rheumatic heart disease, which affected predominantly middle-aged women, was a common cause of atrial fibrillation and subsequent mural thrombus formation but has steadily declined in prevalence since 1950.[14,15] Currently, atherosclerotic heart disease is a much more frequent underlying cause of atrial fibrillation and myocardial infarction, leading to mural thrombi and subsequent embolism. As a result, affected patients are now older and less frequently female.[14,15]

Unfortunately, standard echocardiographic techniques are insensitive in the detection of atrial appendage mural thrombus, so that confirmation of the source of emboli is often not possible.[16] Transesopha-

geal echocardiography and other imaging techniques, such as Indium 111 platelet scintigraphy, iodine 131-fibrinogen scanning, computed tomography (CT), and magnetic resonance imaging (MRI), are significantly more sensitive in the detection of these thrombi.[17-19]

Myocardial infarction, the second most common condition associated with cardioarterial embolization, precedes approximately 24 percent of peripheral embolic events.[2] Left ventricular mural thrombus occurs following 30 percent of acute anterior wall transmural infarcts, but clinically evident embolism occurs in under 5 percent of all acute infarcts.[20,21] Haimovici[14] found that "silent" myocardial infarction was present in 11 percent of patients with peripheral embolization and that embolization may be the presenting symptom of an acute infarction. In patients with embolism and without atrial fibrillation, acute infarction is especially likely, and such patients should be evaluated accordingly.

Acute myocardial infarction, whether or not it is the source of the embolus, is frequently encountered in patients presenting for treatment of acute nontraumatic extremity ischemia. In the Edinburgh series, 11 percent of patients with acute lower-extremity ischemia had suffered an acute infarction within 14 days before their presentation with limb ischemia.[9] In the Copenhagen series, 21 percent of 252 patients presenting with acute embolic ischemia of the legs were under treatment for acute infarction.[12]

Other cardiac diseases may result in peripheral embolization. Although thromboemboli from prosthetic heart valves most frequently involve the cerebral vessels, resulting in stroke, peripheral emboli do occur. The finding of acute extremity ischemia in a patient with a prosthetic heart valve implicates the valve as the source especially if systemic anticoagulation has been inadequate. Components of prosthetic valves may embolize after structural failure of the prosthesis.[22] Disc occluders from tilting disc prostheses may lodge within the aorta parallel to the flow stream and serve as a nidus for later thromboemboli.[22]

Acute and subacute bacterial or fungal endocarditis can result in peripheral embolization. Frequently, such emboli are microemboli and involve distal small vessels, resulting in digital or patchy cutaneous gangrene similar to that seen with atheroembolization, which is discussed below. Moderate sized emboli may lodge in calf or forearm vessels and result in mycotic pseudoaneurysms. Fungal endocarditis, primarily with Candida or Aspergillus, most frequently causes macroemboli resulting in acute peripheral ischemia.[23,24] Intravenous drug abuse and cardiac surgery are the most common factors predisposing to fungal endocarditis and mycotic embolization.[23] Pathologic and microbiologic examination of retrieved emboli is mandatory in patients with suspected mycotic embolization.[23,24]

Rarely, acute extremity ischemia may result from embolization of an atrial myxoma or other intracardiac tumors. Again, pathologic examination of suspicious emboli may provide a potentially life-saving diagnosis.

Emboli of sufficient size to cause acute extremity ischemia may originate from extracardiac sources. The most common extracardiac source for such emboli is the aorta. Atheroembolization from severely ulcerated aortic or peripheral plaques results in the distinctive syndrome of painful blue or purple toes, livido reticularis, and patchy cutaneous gangrene (blue toe syndrome).[25-27] Most frequently, the peripheral pulses are preserved in patients with atheroembolic disease. Frequently the source for such atheroemboli is a severely diseased aorta (Fig. 19-1), and patients may present with atheroemboli after instrumentation of these diseased vessels for angiographic procedures. If the disease extends above the renal and visceral arteries, progressive renal failure and focal intestinal infarction can result. Management of the atheroembolic syndrome involves debridement or amputation of necrotic tissue, exclusion of the source of emboli from the peripheral circulation by arterial replacement or bypass with ligation, and often lumbar sympathectomy.[27]

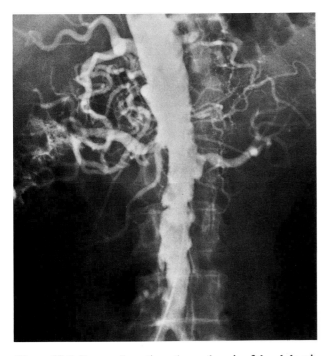

Figure 19-1 Severe ulcerative atherosclerosis of the abdominal aorta is a likely source of atheroemboli to the lower extremities.

Less frequently, mural thrombus from aneurysmal or nonaneurysmal aortas may result in macroembolization and acute peripheral ischemia.[28] Mural thrombus from nonaneurysmal aortas is recognized with increasing frequency to be the source of "cryptogenic" emboli.

Foreign body embolization may be the source of acute ischemia in cases of penetrating trauma.[29,30] The usual presentation includes a small-caliber gunshot wound to the mediastinum or abdomen with tamponade at the cardiac or arterial injury site and bullet migration to the periphery, resulting in acute ischemia or pulse deficit.

Paradoxic embolization is another rare cause of acute peripheral ischemia. Any patient presenting with pulmonary emboli or deep venous thrombosis and associated acute peripheral ischemia should be suspected of having arterial emboli originating in the venous circulation.[31] Many intracardiac defects may predispose to paradoxic embolization, but a patent foramen ovale is by far the most frequently implicated.

Primary or metastatic lung tumors and pulmonary inflammatory lesions may, in rare cases, gain access to the arterial circulation via the pulmonary veins or direct invasion of the left side of the heart. Such tumor emboli are a rare cause of peripheral ischemia.

Despite modern imaging techniques, the source of peripheral embolization will remain inapparent in more than 10 percent of patients presenting with suspected embolization. Some of these suspected cryptogenic emboli may actually represent cases of atypical in situ thrombosis.

Sites of arterial occlusion by peripheral emboli are shown in Table 19-1.[13,14,32] More than 80 percent of extremity embolic events involve the aortic bifurcation or more distal lower extremity vessels, and only 16 percent involve the upper extremities. Emboli to the cerebral, renal, and mesenteric vessels are common but are not included in this table. Emboli tend to lodge at points where the diameter of vessels decreases. Most often this is at branch points such as the aortic bifurcation or the common femoral bifurcation. Alternatively,

Table 19-1 Sites of Extremity Emboli

Location	N	%
Upper extremity	235/1464	16.1
Aortoiliac	372/1464	25.4
Common femoral/profunda femoris	581/1464	39.7
Superficial femoral/popliteal/tibial	276/1464	18.9

(Data from Abbott et al.,[13] Haimovici,[14] and Fogarty et al.[32])

emboli may lodge at points of atherosclerotic stenosis, frequently in the common iliac artery or in the superficial femoral artery at Hunter's canal.

Thrombosis

The superficial femoral artery is the most common site of acute thrombosis. Involvement of the upper extremity is less common. Virtually all nonembolic arterial occlusions are caused by thrombosis within an area of pre-existing atherosclerotic disease. The gradual progression of these stenoses and the concomitant development of collaterals prior to thrombosis may, however, make the acute thrombotic event clinically insignificant. Clinically significant acute thromboses occur when collateral flow is insufficient to maintain adequate distal perfusion. Inadequate collateral flow results when an artery which is not sufficiently stenotic to promote collateral formation suddenly thromboses, or when propagation of thrombus from the inciting point compromises the takeoff or reentry sites for collateral flow. Intraplaque hemorrhage may be one event which causes sudden thrombosis in a previously nonstenotic arterial segment. Popliteal aneurysms are also susceptible to thrombosis and the lack of preformed collaterals in this setting usually results in profound ischemia.

Diabetics and heavy smokers may have inadequate collateral flow because of severe profunda femoris branch disease, inadequate geniculate collaterals, and small vessel disease. In such patients acute thrombosis of even a heavily diseased superficial femoral artery may result in critical ischemia.

The role of hypercoagulability in spontaneous arterial thrombosis remains unclear. Surgical intervention results in abrupt increases in factor VIII levels, in platelet reactivity, and in decreases in antithrombin III levels, so it may be difficult to ascertain whether hypercoagulability is a cause of thrombosis or a result of its treatment.[33] After recovery from the thrombotic event and its treatment, some patients will be found to have hypercoagulable states. The most frequently documented hypercoagulable states in patients undergoing vascular reconstruction are antiphospholipid antibody (lupus-like anticoagulant) syndrome, antithrombin III deficiency, protein C deficiency, and protein S deficiency.[34,35] Heparin-induced platelet activation syndrome should be considered in patients developing arterial or venous thromboses while receiving heparin therapy.[34,35] Spontaneous thrombosis of a normal or minimally diseased artery strongly suggests an underlying hypercoagulable state. Vascular graft thrombosis and iatrogenic and traumatic arterial thrombosis are covered in Chapters 21 and 23, respectively.

Ischemia Following Acute Embolization or Thrombosis

The clinical presentation of patients with embolism or thrombosis depends on the severity of the ischemia and resulting tissue injury. The severity of ischemia is determined by several factors. First, the nature of the precipitating event (embolism versus thrombosis) is important. With embolic disease, the involved vessels are often normal or only mildly diseased, such that the collateral circulation is poorly developed. With thrombotic occlusions, the slowly progressive nature of the atherosclerotic process most often leads to collateral formation and the clinical significance of the thrombosis is, therefore, blunted.

Second, the site of the thrombosis or embolism determines in part the degree of ischemia. An embolus lodging at the common femoral bifurcation may occlude both the superficial femoral and profunda femoris arteries, resulting in more severe ischemia than a smaller embolus lodging at Hunter's canal. Similarly, an embolus that lodges in the axillary artery above the origin of the profunda brachii artery will cause more profound ischemia than a more distal embolus which permits flow through the profunda brachii into the collateral network around the elbow.

Third, proximal and distal propagation of thrombus will influence the degree of ischemia by compromising the takeoff and reentry sites for collaterals. With any arterial occlusion, thrombus will propagate proximally to the next branch point because of stasis within the occluded segment. In addition, thrombus may propagate distally to the point at which collaterals reenter. If flow within the collateral bed is sluggish, or if the collaterals are quite small in relation to the main vessels, the propagating thrombus may obliterate exit and reentry sites and further compromise distal flow.

Fourth, the elapsed time from the embolism or thrombosis to the restoration of flow will in part determine the severity of ischemia-related tissue injury. If the ischemia is absolute, muscle and peripheral nerve infarction will begin within 3 to 4 hours, and significant permanent extremity dysfunction can be expected if flow is not restored within 6 to 12 hours.[33] Absolute ischemia is not commonly encountered in clinical practice because at least some collateral flow usually exists, but recent studies suggest that partial ischemia may cause cellular damage more quickly than absolute ischemia.[36,37]

Fifth, because significant muscle injury occurs as a result of reperfusion, probably because of oxygen free radicals, the degree of muscle injury may be in part determined by the rapidity of reperfusion. Experimentally, muscle injury can be decreased by controlling oxygen delivery by hemodilution during reperfusion.[38] Clinically, patients with chronic superficial femoral occlusions who undergo common femoral embolectomy are less likely than those with patent superficial femorals to develop compartment syndrome and other manifestations of muscle injury.[39]

Other factors may influence the severity of ischemia. Cardiac output may be significantly compromised in the patient with an embolus after myocardial infarction and the associated reflex vasoconstriction may worsen distal perfusion. The use of alpha adrenergic drugs may also compromise acral flow. Venous thrombosis may develop quickly in the ischemic extremity because of immobility and stasis.[8] The subsequent venous hypertension and interstitial edema may further impair tissue oxygenation (for a discussion of the pathophysiology of acute ischemic tissue injury, see Ch. 17).

CLINICAL PRESENTATION AND EVALUATION

The presenting signs and symptoms of acute ischemia include the five "P's": pulselessness, pain, pallor, paresthesias, and paralysis. Pain is present in all cases and is proportional to the severity of the ischemia. Pulselessness is apparent on examination but may be difficult to interpret in the patient with pre-existing occlusive disease. Often examination of the unaffected limbs will offer a clue to the severity of chronic occlusive disease and will permit a more accurate assessment of the significance of pulse deficits. If the pulses in the unaffected limbs are normal and there is no evidence of occlusive disease elsewhere, the absence of pulses in the affected limb is usually highly significant and often related to acute embolism. If, however, there is evidence for severe occlusive disease in the unaffected limb, the examiner should suspect the existence of such disease in the symptomatic limb and consider more carefully the probability of acute thrombosis of diseased vessels. Likewise, pallor must be interpreted in the context of the patients other findings. Pallor is noted in severe acute ischemia when the collateral flow is inadequate. Compensatory cutaneous vasodilatation will cause rubor in more chronic partially compensated ischemia.

Paresthesias suggest sensory nerve dysfunction and progression to numbness will occur if ischemia worsens. Patients presenting with loss of light touch sensation on examination have critical ischemia and require emergent revascularization to avoid long-term neurologic sequelae. Patients with pain but intact sensory and motor examination have less severe ischemia and

may undergo necessary preliminary studies without compromising long-term outcome.

Paralysis after embolism or thrombosis results from motor nerve dysfunction and muscle ischemia. The earliest sign of motor dysfunction in the ischemic foot is sluggish movement when the patient is asked to wiggle the toes. The patient may be able to plantar-flex and dorsiflex the foot and make gross movements of the toes but may be unable to make finer movements. This subtle motor deficit reflects loss of function in the intrinsic muscles of the foot, with preservation of function of the long flexors whose bodies lie within the calf. Paralysis of the muscles in the calf or thigh is ominous.

Useful clinical information can be gained by palpation of the calf muscles. If the calf muscles are soft and nontender, full recovery of function after reperfusion can be anticipated and severe postreperfusion myonephropathic syndrome and compartment syndromes are unlikely. Tenderness of the calf muscle suggests that significant ischemic injury has occurred and that reperfusion may well be followed by myonephropathic and compartment syndromes. Rigidity of the calf muscles (rigor mortis), when accompanied by other signs of severe acute ischemia, suggests that at least significant portions of the muscle are infarcted, so that reperfusion will not result in complete functional recovery. In addition, reperfusion in these patients will be accompanied by severe myonephropathic syndrome and compartment syndromes. Such patients are often best treated by heparin administration and expeditious primary amputation in order to avoid the potentially life-threatening complications of reperfusion.

Careful history and physical examination, along with simple Doppler assessment, usually will permit accurate localization of the site of arterial occlusion in acute ischemia. Bilateral acute lower-extremity ischemia associated with absence of both femoral pulses is diagnostic of aortic bifurcation saddle embolus. Often, cutaneous mottling or cyanosis extending above the groin creases and occasionally to the umbilicus is noted. In cases of embolization to the common femoral artery bifurcation, the femoral pulse is often preserved but takes on an obstructed quality. Continuous wave Doppler may reveal the "drumbeat" sound characteristic of distal obstruction. Preservation of a normal femoral pulse and Doppler signal in the presence of acute ischemia suggests more distal localization, usually to the popliteal artery, either above the knee at Hunter's canal or, more commonly, at the popliteal trifurcation. In the latter case the popliteal pulse will be preserved. More distal emboli, those traveling to tibial vessels are most often clinically inapparent, unless they occur in the setting of severe associated occlusive disease, such that the site of embolism lies in the sole remaining patent vessel, or unless they occur in association with more proximal thromboembolic disease.

Similar clinical localization of the embolus is often possible in cases of upper-extremity embolization. Absence of the axillary artery pulse suggests occlusion at, or just beyond, the thoracic outlet and is most often associated with profound ischemia. Presence of the axillary pulse and absence of the brachial pulse in the antecubital area suggests occlusion in the mid-brachial region. In this case, preservation of flow in the profunda brachii system usually lessens the degree of ischemia. In thin patients, precise localization of the occlusion is possible by palpation of the exact point of loss of pulsation. More distal emboli are characterized by the presence of the brachial pulse in the antecubital fossa. In this setting, ischemia may be severe if there is involvement of both the radial and ulnar arteries and significant distal clot propagation.

Occasionally, peripheral emboli will result in subacute ischemia or in a subtle worsening of chronic symptoms. In a series from Wisconsin, 22 patients presented 2 to 30 days after the onset of symptoms.[40] On the basis of clinical evaluation, these patients were thought to have chronic ischemia or acute exacerbation of chronic ischemia due to thrombosis. Arteriography, however, revealed intraluminal filling defects suggestive of emboli; 19 of these patients were treated successfully with embolectomy alone. This series demonstrated that (1) emboli can occasionally present a more subtle clinical syndrome, (2) simple embolectomy can be successful even after a prolonged delay, and (3) the clinical status of the limb is a more reliable guide to viability and ease of treatment than is elapsed time between event and presentation.[40]

History and physical examination are not only sufficient for assessment of limb viability and for localization of the occlusion—they may permit assessment of etiology as well. Among clinical findings, atrial fibrillation, which occurred in 74 percent of patients with embolism and in 4 percent of patients with thrombosis in one recent series, is of most discriminative value in differentiating between these conditions.[3] Because peripheral atherosclerosis predisposes to thrombosis, it is surprising that only 40 percent of patients with acute arterial thrombosis in this series had a history of intermittent claudication.[3] In another series, however, 86 percent of patients judged to have thrombosis gave a history of claudication.[5] Therefore, a history of claudication or other evidence of chronic ischemia of the affected limb, especially in the absence of atrial fibrillation or recent myocardial infarction, is most often associated with a thrombotic etiology.

In most cases of acute ischemia secondary to embolism, history and physical examination alone are sufficient to make an appropriate diagnosis. Laboratory testing, therefore, can be used sparingly and only to establish that surgical intervention can be carried out safely. In light of the frequent association between embolism and acute myocardial infarction, a 12-lead electrocardiogram (ECG) should be obtained preoperatively. In cases associated with recent-onset atrial fibrillation, a chest radiograph and arterial blood gas should be helpful in ruling out pulmonary embolism or other mechanical causes of this arrhythmia. Routine coagulation studies and platelet count will be helpful preoperatively. A urinalysis might reveal hematuria and lead to increased suspicion of associated renal artery embolization.

In suspected embolic disease, preoperative arteriography is rarely indicated. If peripheral embolization is associated with abdominal or flank pain, biplanar aortography should be considered, to rule out associated mesenteric or renal emboli. Patients with an atypical presentation for embolic disease may undergo arteriography for suspected thrombosis. Typical arteriograms obtained in patients with embolization are seen in (Figures 19-2 to 19-5). Aortic saddle embolus (Fig. 19-2) and embolus to the proximal superficial femoral artery (Fig. 19-3) are characterized in these films by discrete intraluminal filling defects, lack of collateral flow, poor distal flow, and lack of atherosclerotic disease in adjacent arterial segments. Emboli to the superficial femoral and profunda femoris arteries (Fig. 19-4) and to the infrageniculate popliteal artery (Fig. 19-5) are here characterized by abrupt arterial cutoff, poor distal flow, and again, absence of atherosclerosis.

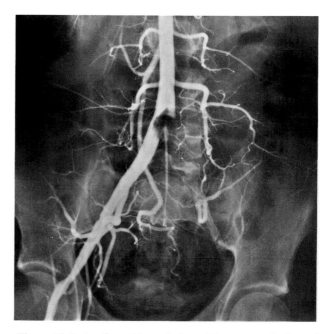

Figure 19-2 Aortic saddle embolus with acute occlusion of the left iliac artery and near occlusion of the right iliac artery.

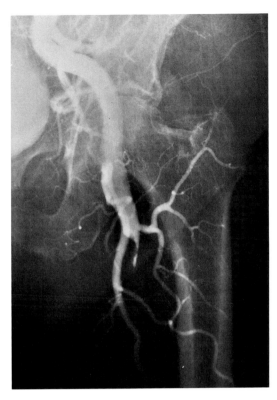

Figure 19-3 Acute embolus to the left superficial femoral artery origin with preservation of profunda femoris flow.

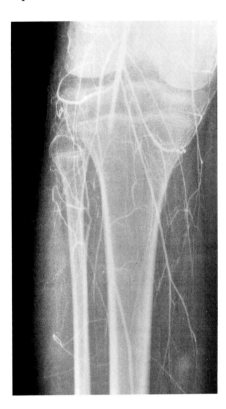

Figure 19-5 Acute embolic occlusion of the infrageniculate popliteal artery.

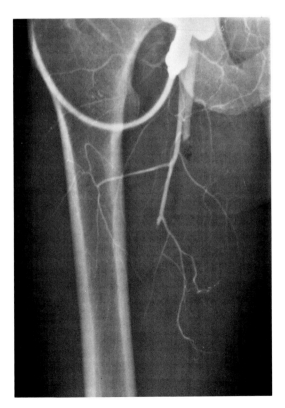

Figure 19-4 Emboli to the right superficial femoral and profunda femoris arteries with abrupt cutoff of flow in both arteries.

Because the management of patients with thrombotic acute ischemia often requires complex and lengthy arterial reconstruction, a more detailed preoperative assessment is desirable, if the condition of the limb permits. Because of the preexisting collateral bed, the severity of ischemia in patients with thrombosis is often less than that seen in patients with embolization and permits a period for medical evaluation and arteriography. Heparin is administered at presentation, and necessary evaluations conducted expeditiously. Arteriography (Figs. 19-6 and 19-7) is almost always indicated in these patients, in order to define the optimal form of reconstruction. Arteriograms typical for thrombosis of atherosclerotic vessels are shown in Figures 19-6A,B and 19-7A. In Figure 19-6A, the abrupt iliac cutoff is consistent with embolization or thrombosis, but the abundant collateral supply reconstituting the common femoral (Fig. 19-6B) suggests a slowly progressive atherosclerotic stenosis eventuating in thrombosis. In Figure 19-7A, the significant atherosclerosis of the more proximal superficial femoral artery suggests a thrombotic etiology. In this patient, the absence of atrial fibrillation or a recent myocardial infarction further supported this diagnosis. With the advent of thrombolytic therapy, arteriography and intra-arterial thrombolysis might permit exact identification

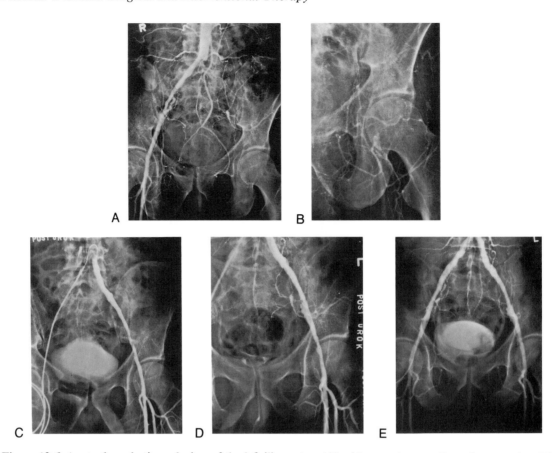

Figure 19-6 Acute thrombotic occlusion of the left iliac artery **(A)** with prominent collaterals suggesting **(B)** progressive atherosclerosis as the etiology. Treatment with thrombolytic agent restored patency uncovering **(C)** external iliac stenosis, which was treated with **(D)** balloon angioplasty. **(E)** Patency maintained at 16 months. See text for discussion.

of the cause of thrombosis and expeditious treatment with balloon angioplasty or local surgical intervention.

In many patients, the differential diagnosis of embolism and thrombosis will not be clear cut. Often in such patients the degree of ischemia allows time for arteriography which usually renders a definitive diagnosis and allows optimal treatment planning. If the ischemia is severe, however, immediate operative intervention is indicated despite the diagnostic uncertainty.

TREATMENT

Initial treatment should be based on history and physical examination data. An algorithm for the management of acute nontraumatic limb ischemia is shown in Figure 19-8. Virtually all patients presenting with acute nontraumatic limb ischemia should receive intravenous heparin at the time of presentation. Initially, limb salvageability and likely etiology must be assessed. If the limb is not salvageable, expeditious amputation

should be undertaken in order to avoid systemic toxicity from muscle breakdown. If the limb is salvageable and embolism is suspected, the patient should be prepared for the operating room as quickly as possible. Brachial and femoral embolectomies can be conducted under local anesthesia and intravenous sedation, but axillary block or spinal may provide better anesthesia and, therefore, a less stressful procedure for the patient. If popliteal exploration is anticipated, spinal, epidural, or general anesthesia are necessary. The entire affected extremity should be sterilely prepped to permit assessment of distal perfusion after embolectomy and prior to wound closure, to provide an appropriate field, if more extensive reconstruction becomes necessary, and to facilitate the harvest of autogenous vein, if needed.

Most upper-extremity embolectomies are carried out through a longitudinal incision at or just above the antecubital area. Rarely, it will be necessary to extend the incision distally in order to identify the origins of the radial and ulnar arteries in order to guide the

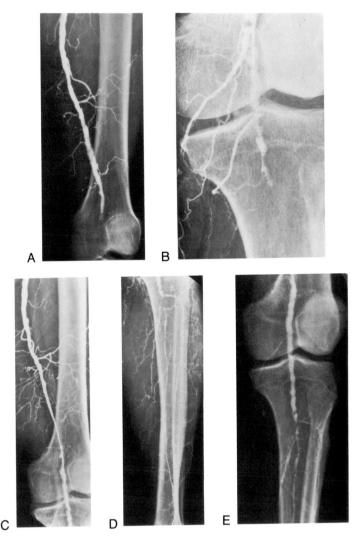

Figure 19-7 **(A)** Acute thrombotic occlusion of popliteal artery. **(B)** Early recanalization after bolus of thrombolytic agent. Progressive recanalization after **(C)** 6 hours and **(D)** 19 hours of thrombolytic infusion. **(E)** Continued patency at 14 months despite severe underlying atherosclerosis. See text for discussion.

thrombectomy catheter selectively into each distal artery. In exposing the brachial artery, care must be taken to avoid injury to the adjacent median nerve. Because the brachial artery is usually free from atherosclerosis, a transverse arteriotomy is appropriate for embolectomy. Embolectomy catheters (#2 or #3) are passed distally after arterial control is achieved with vessel loops. It is usually unnecessary to pass catheters beyond the flexor crease at the wrist. Passage into the small vessels of the hand with subsequent overzealous balloon inflation may result in arterial rupture or pseudoaneurysm formation in the hand. Once all retrievable clot is removed the catheter (#3 or #4) is passed proximally as far as the subclavian. Removal of proximal clot should be followed by return of pulsatile flow at the

arteriotomy, and catheter passage should be repeated until no additional clot can be extracted. In the rare instance in which adequate inflow cannot be restored, the patient should be closed and taken for immediate angiography for better delineation of the cause of proximal obstruction. After embolectomy and arteriotomy closure, the distal perfusion should be assessed before removal of the patient from the operating room. Return of a palpable pulse in the radial artery at the wrist and return of a normal Doppler signal in the palmar arch is evidence for an adequate embolectomy. If the radial pulse does not return or the palmar arch Doppler signal is absent, damped, or monophasic, operative arteriography should be carried out and residual embolus or thrombus removed as necessary. Rarely, in cases of

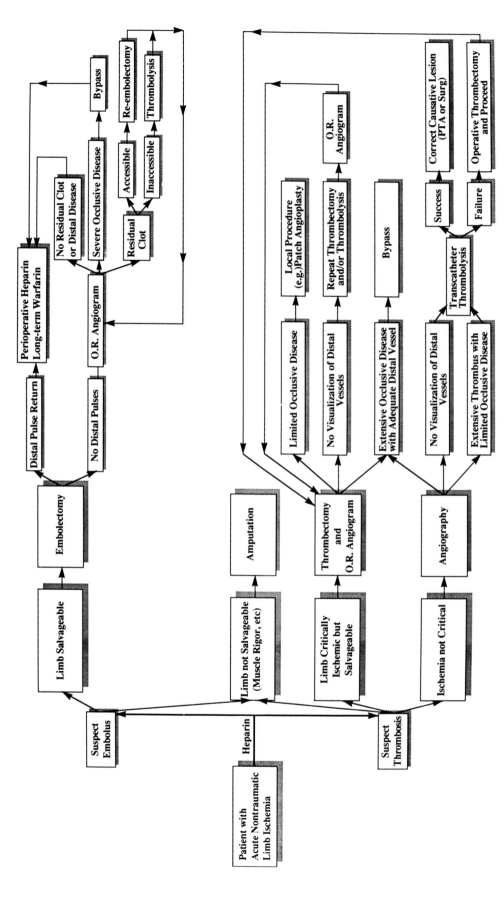

Figure 19-8 Algorithm for the management of acute nontraumatic limb ischemia. See text for discussion.

upper-extremity embolism, intraoperative thrombolysis with urokinase (50,000 to 250,000 units intra-arterial) will be necessary to clear residual surgically inaccessible thrombus.[41-45]

Embolism to the lower extremity is handled similarly. If the femoral pulse is absent or suggests occlusion at the femoral bifurcation, a longitudinal groin incision is used. If significant atherosclerosis is present in the common femoral artery, a longitudinal arteriotomy is advisable for adequate exposure of the lumen, to permit local endarterectomy, if necessary. Longitudinal arteriotomy, especially in a heavily diseased artery may necessitate patch closure. Transverse arteriotomy is simpler in a normal or minimally diseased artery.

If physical examination suggests more distal embolization, and especially if the popliteal pulse is preserved, a below-knee popliteal exposure is indicated.[46] As in the common femoral artery, significant disease in this artery may necessitate longitudinal arteriotomy and patch closure. Endarterectomy in the below-knee popliteal or more distal vessels should be avoided. In the setting of a palpable popliteal pulse, below-knee popliteal exposure will permit ready exposure and selective catheterization of the peroneal and tibial arteries.

Embolectomy catheters (#2 or #3 for tibial vessels, #3 or #4 for SFA, #3 for profunda, and #4 or #5 for iliac) are passed distally first and then proximally. Inadequate restoration of inflow is, as in the upper extremity, an indication for immediate arteriography, if possible, or immediate inflow reconstruction, if necessary. After arteriotomy closure, and before wound closure, the distal perfusion is assessed. If ankle pulses are present and the foot becomes hyperemic, no further evaluation is indicated in the operating room. If distal pulses do not return, or if the foot remains ischemic in appearance, operative angiography is indicated. If no residual clot is noted, and if the distal occlusive disease does not jeopardize continued limb viability, the procedure may be terminated. If surgically accessible residual thrombus is noted, repeat passage of the catheter into the affected vessel is indicated. Direct cut-down over a tibial vessel at the ankle may be necessary to clear residual tibial or pedal artery thrombus.[47] Meticulous closure of such distal arteriotomies, including liberal use of vein patching, is necessary to avoid iatrogenic distal occlusions.

Surgically inaccessible residual thrombus is treated with intra-arterial thrombolytic therapy (50,000 to 250,000 units urokinase), followed by repeat arteriography and retreatment, if necessary. The efficacy and safety of intraoperative thrombolysis have been well documented.[41-45]

Patients treated for embolism should undergo assessment of the source of embolization, and virtually all patients should be treated with postoperative heparin and long-term warfarin. With anticoagulation, the incidence of early recurrent embolization is 9 percent; without anticoagulation, it is 31 percent.[48] With long-term warfarin anticoagulation, the 5-year incidence of recurrent embolization is 22 percent; without anticoagulation, it is 38 percent.[1]

If spontaneous thrombosis is suspected to be the etiology of the acute ischemia, the management algorithm is more complex (Fig. 19-8). Heparin is administered at presentation. As with embolization, nonviable limbs should be amputated expeditiously, to avoid the complications of muscle necrosis. If the limb is judged to be critically ischemic but salvageable, immediate operative thrombectomy and operative angiography are indicated. If the post-thrombectomy operative arteriogram reveals extensive occlusive disease with adequate distal vessels, a distal bypass is carried out. If the distal vasculature is not visualized, a more distal thrombectomy is carried out, and intraoperative thrombolytic therapy is employed if extensive distal or small vessel thrombosis is encountered. If the operative arteriogram reveals only a well-localized arterial lesion responsible for the thrombosis, a local procedure such as endarterectomy with patch angioplasty or short segment bypass may be appropriate.

If thrombosis is suspected, but the degree of ischemia is not immediately limb-threatening, angiography should be carried out in the angiography suite. This usually results in more detailed delineation of the inflow and of the distal anatomy, especially if techniques such as reactive hyperemia or balloon occlusion angiography are used to enhance distal visualization. If the angiogram reveals extensive disease with good distal anatomy, distal bypass is carried out at a time determined by the status of the limb. If there is poor visualization of the distal vessels or if extensive thrombus is visualized, transcatheter thrombolytic therapy is carried out (for the protocols used, see Ch. 20). Successful thrombolysis will uncover the anatomy responsible for the thrombosis. Definitive correction of this causative anatomic lesion by surgical reconstruction or percutaneous angioplasty is a prerequisite for a successful outcome in most cases.[49-51] Urokinase is currently preferred over streptokinase in transcatheter thrombolytic therapy because of superior efficacy and safety.[52] Early experience with recombinant human tissue-type plasminogen activator (tPA) is also promising.[53]

Illustrative examples of transcatheter thrombolytic therapy are given in Figures 19-6 and 19-7. In Figure 19-6A, and B, common iliac thrombosis is suggested. After 6 hours of thrombolytic therapy, recanalization of the iliac is apparent (Fig. 19-6C), and a significant external iliac stenosis is uncovered. Angioplasty of this lesion was successful (Fig. 19-6D), and follow-up angiography 16 months later (Fig. 19-6E) reveals a satisfactory long-term result.

Figure 19-7A shows an arteriogram with acute popliteal occlusion. No runoff vessels were visualized. This patient had medical risk factors believed to preclude surgery. After 2 hours of thrombolytic therapy, early popliteal recanalization is apparent (Fig. 19-7B); after 6 hours (Fig. 19-7C), recanalization has progressed, revealing severe underlying popliteal atherosclerosis and occlusion of the tibial vessel origins. By 19 hours (Fig. 19-7D), recanalization is complete, and the limb has returned to its baseline condition. Follow-up angiography 14 months later (Fig. 19-6E) revealed continued patency of the left popliteal despite severe occlusive disease.

If thrombolysis in the angiography suite is unsuccessful and the reconstructibility of the limb remains uncertain, duplex imaging of the distal vessels may be carried out in an effort to find a patent potential recipient vessel in the distal calf or foot.[54] Operative thrombectomy via a below knee popliteal approach followed by operative angiography is another means of establishing reconstructibility after failed thrombolysis. A patent distal vessel can usually be identified using one of these approaches. Outcome in this setting will be determined by the quality of the recipient vessel, the quality of the vein conduit, and the extent of distal small vessel thrombosis. The latter factor may be favorably influenced by the use of intraoperative thrombolytic agents. Despite all aggressive attempts at limb salvage, up to 33 percent of patients presenting with thrombotic limb ischemia will require amputation either as a primary procedure or after failed salvage attempts.[3,7]

The contraindications to thrombolytic therapy should be carefully considered before choosing this option. Hemorrhagic complications of thrombolysis, especially intracranial hemorrhage, can be devastating; such complications may be minimized by careful patient selection and adherence to well-defined thrombolytic protocols (see Ch. 20) that limit dose and length of infusion.

All patients undergoing revascularization of an acutely ischemic limb are at risk of the postreperfusion myonephropathic syndrome. Haimovici[55,56] first brought attention to, and later fully described, the salient features of this syndrome, which occurs to a clinically significant degree in 7.5 to 15 percent of patients undergoing revascularization for acute ischemia. Acutely, washout of potassium and hydrogen ion from the ischemic limb can result in myocardial depression or dysrhythmias, or both. The anesthesiologist should anticipate this possibility and treat the patient with bi-carbonate and/or calcium just prior to reperfusion. Myoglobin and other products of skeletal muscle breakdown can precipitate within the kidney and result in acute renal failure. Maintenance of a brisk diuresis and alkalinization will prevent renal shutdown in most cases. Severe swelling within the calf or even thigh can result in secondary muscle or nerve injury, venous compression and further edema, and arterial compression with secondary ischemia. After reperfusion, the extremity should be assessed immediately, and at regular intervals, for evolving compartment syndromes. The indications for and technique of fasciotomy are covered in the chapter on traumatic limb ischemia. Almost 9 percent of patients undergoing emergent revascularization for embolic or thrombotic limb ischemia will require fasciotomy.[2]

Because of the severe morbidity associated with reperfusion syndrome and the high mortality associated with the treatment of embolic disease, Blaisdell et al.[8] have advocated the use of high-dose heparin (2000 to 4000 U/h after an initial bolus of 10,000 to 20,000 units) in the management of virtually all patients with thromboemblic disease, except those requiring immediate amputation. With this approach and the selective use of later surgical thromboembolectomy or bypass, Blaisdell achieved a limb-salvage rate of 84 percent in patients with heparin treatment and a mortality rate of 7.5 percent. Although most surgeons now prefer early surgical revascularization in combination with heparin anticoagulation, Blaisdell's conservative approach may be useful in the patient at very high mortality risk.

Finally, the approach to the patient with acute limb ischemia of either embolic or thrombotic etiology should be tempered by the patients medical condition and risk factors. Patients moribund after massive myocardial infarction should undergo conservative therapy with heparin and the least invasive operation possible when clinically stable. Loss of limb is certainly preferable to loss of life. In addition, patients severely disabled after a major stroke or disabled by other chronic medical illness who will derive little benefit from limb salvage should undergo primary amputation if revascularization is complex or risky.

Associated cardiac disease is the major determinant of mortality risk in patients with embolism or thrombosis. Mortality risk is greater in patients with emboli (> 10 percent) than in patients with thrombosis (5 percent). In high-risk patients with emboli, greater attention to associated cardiac disease and more frequent use of conservative therapy or delayed surgical therapy might decrease mortality, though probably with a corresponding increase in limb loss. In patients with thrombosis, surgical mortality may be reduced further only by cardiac screening with stress testing and subsequent selective coronary revascularization, which is applicable only to patients with less severe ischemia. Cardiac mortality risk (approximately 5 percent) in patients with thrombosis, therefore, may have reached an irreducible minimum, and efforts should be directed at improving limb-salvage rates through aggressive revascularization, even complex definitive reconstruction in the acute setting. Experienced judgement is essential in determining the optimal timing and type of intervention in these patients.

SUMMARY

Patients with acute embolic or thrombotic limb ischemia require prompt intervention in order to provide limb salvage and to avoid the systemic toxicity associated with muscle necrosis. Unlike patients with traumatic limb ischemia, those with thrombosis or embolization are most often old and infirm with a variety of significant medical problems which complicate surgical decision making and management. Initial assessment of these patients must include a rapid assessment of the degree of ischemia, the potential for salvage of a functional limb, the probable etiology, the site of occlusion, and the confounding medical problems. Treatment plans and contingency plans are based on this clinical assessment (see Fig. 19-8). With careful attention to the fundamentals of diagnosis and management reviewed in this chapter, limb salvage rates should exceed 95 percent for patients with emboli and 75 percent for patients with thrombosis, while mortality rates should be less than 10 percent for both groups.

REFERENCES

1. Elliot JP, Hageman JH, Szilagyi DE et al: Arterial embolization: problems of source, multiplicity, recurrence, and delayed treatment. Surgery 88:833, 1980
2. Mills JL, Porter JM: Basic data related to clinical decision making in acute limb ischemia. Ann Vasc Surg 5:96, 1991
3. Cambria RP, Abbott WM: Acute arterial thrombosis of the lower extremity: its natural history contrasted with arterial embolism. Arch Surg 119:784, 1984
4. Tawes RL, Harris EJ, Brown WH et al: Arterial thromboembolism: a 20 year perspective. Arch Surg 120:595, 1985
5. McPhail NV, Fratesi SJ, Barber GG et al: Management of acute thromboembolic limb ischemia. Surgery 93:381, 1983
6. Busuttil RW, Keehn G, Milliken J et al: Aortic saddle embolus: a twenty year experience. Ann Surg 197:698, 1983
7. Dale WA: Differential management of acute peripheral arterial ischemia. J Vasc Surg 1:269, 1984
8. Blaisdell FW, Steele M, Allen RE: Management of acute lower extremity arterial ischemia due to embolism and thrombosis. Surgery 84:822, 1978
9. Clason AE, Stonebridge PA, Duncan AJ et al: Morbidity and mortality in acute lower limb ischemia: a 5 Year Review. Eur J Vasc Surg 3:339, 1989
10. Stonebridge PA, Clason AE, Duncan AJ et al: Acute ischemia of the upper limb compared with acute lower limb ischemia: a 5 year review. Br J Surg 76:515, 1989
11. Baxter-Smith D, Ashton F, Slaney G: Peripheral arterial embolism: a 20 year review. J Cardiovasc Surg 29:453, 1988
12. Bugge M, Jelnes R, Arendrup H et al: Arterial embolism of the legs: a follow-up study of 252 patients. Ann Chir Gynaecol 74:137, 1985
13. Abbott WM, Maloney RD, McCabe CC et al: Arterial embolism: a 44 year perspective. Am J Surg 143:460, 1982
14. Haimovici H: Peripheral arterial embolism: a study of 330 unselected cases of embolism of the extremities. Angiology 1:20, 1950
15. Haimovici H, Moss CM, Veith FJ: Arterial embolectomy revisited. Surgery 78:409, 1875
16. Shrestha NK, Moreno FL, Narcisco FV et al: Two dimensional echocardiographic diagnosis of left atrial thrombus in rheumatic heart disease: a clinicopathologic study. Circulation 67:341, 1983
17. Wakefield TW: Noninvasive methods of diagnosing cardiac sources for macroemboli. p. 604. In Ernst CB, Stanley JC (eds): Current Therapy in Vascular Surgery. 2nd Ed. BC Decker, Philadelphia, 1991
18. Cujec B, Polasek P, Voll C, Shuaib A: Transesophageal echocardiography in the detection of potential cardiac sources of embolism in stroke patients. Stroke 122:727, 1991
19. Lee RJ, Bartzokis T, Tiong-Keat Y et al: Enhanced detection of intracardiac sources of cerebral emboli by transesophageal echocardiography. Stroke 122:734, 1991
20. Asinger RW, Mikell FL, Elsperger J et al: Incidence of left ventricular thrombosis after acute transmural myocardial infarction. Serial evaluation by two dimensional echocardiography. N Engl J Med 305:297, 1981
21. Keating EC, Gross SA, Schlamowitz RA: Mural thrombi in myocardial infarctions. Am J Med 74:989, 1983
22. Schwarz TH, Coffin LH, Pilcher DB: Renal failure after embolization of a prosthetic mitral valve disc and review of systemic disc embolization. J Vasc Surg 2:697, 1985
23. Vo NM, Russell JC, Becker DR: Mycotic emboli of the peripheral vessels; analysis of 44 cases. Surgery 90:541, 1981
24. Swensson EE, Willman VL, Peterson GJ: Acute aortic occlusion from aspergillosis in a healthy patient with survival. J Vasc Surg 4:187, 1986
25. Wingo JP, Nix ML, Greenfield LJ et al: The blue toe syndrome: hemodynamics and therapeutic correlates of outcome. J Vasc Surg 3:475, 1986

26. Fisher DF, Clagett GP, Brigham RA et al: Dilemmas in dealing with the blue toe syndrome: aortic versus peripheral source. Am J Surg 148:836, 1984

27. Kaufman JL, Stark K, Brolin RE et al: Disseminated atheroembolism from extensive degenerative atherosclerosis of the aorta. Surgery 102:63, 1987

28. Machleder HI, Takiff H, Lois JF et al: Aortic mural thrombus: an occult source of arterial thromboembolism. J Vasc Surg 4:473, 1986

29. Michelassi F, Pietrabissa A, Ferrari M et al: Bullett emboli to the systemic and venous circulation. Surgery 107:239, 1990

30. Shannon JJ, Vo NM, Stanton PE et al: Peripheral arterial missile embolization: A case report and 22 year literature review. J Vasc Surg 5:773, 1987

31. Langdon TJ, Bandyk DF, Olinger GN et al: Multiple paradoxical emboli. J Vasc Surg 4:284, 1986

32. Fogarty TJ, Daily PO, Shumway NE et al: Experience with balloon catheter technique for arterial embolectomy. Am J Surg 122:231, 1971

33. McDaniel MD, Pearce WH, Yao JST et al: Sequential changes in coagulation and platelet function following femorotibial bypass. J Vasc Surg 1:261, 1984

34. Eldrup-Jorgensen J, Flanigan P, Brace L et al: Hypercoagulable states and lower limb ischemia in young adults. J Vasc Surg 9:334, 1989

35. Donaldson MC, Weinberg DS, Belkin M et al: Screening for hypercoagulable states in vascular surgical practice. A preliminary study. J Vasc Surg 11:825, 1990

36. Malan E, Tattoni G. Physio- and anatopathology of acute ischemia of the extremities. J Cardiovasc Surg 4:2, 1963

37. Perry MO, Fantini G. Ischemia: Profile of an enemy. Reperfusion injury of skeletal muscle. J Vasc Surg 6:231, 1987

38. Walker PM, Lindsay TF, Libbe R et al: Salvage of skeletal muscle with free radical scavengers. J Vasc Surg 5:68, 1987

39. Matsen FF, Krygmire RB: Compartmental syndromes. Surg Gynecol Obstet 147:943, 1978

40. Jarrett F, Dacumos GC, Crummy AB et al: Late appearance of arterial emboli: diagnosis and management. Surgery 86:898, 1979

41. Norem RF, Short DH, Kerstein MD: Role of intraoperative fibrinolytic therapy in acute arterial occlusion. Surg Gynecol Obstet 167:87, 1988

42. Garcia R, Saroyan RM, Senkowsky J et al: Intraoperative intraarterial urokinase infusion as an adjunct to Fogarty catheter embolectomy in acute arterial occlusion. Surg Gynecol Obstet 171:201, 1990

43. Quinones-Baldrich WJ, Zierler RE, Hiatt JC: Intraoperative fibrinolytic therapy: an adjunct to catheter thromboembolectomy. J Vasc Surg 2:319, 1985

44. Parent FN, Bernhard VM, Pabst TS et al: Fibrinolytic treatment of residual thrombus after catheter embolectomy for severe lower limb ischemia. J Vasc Surg 9:153, 1989

45. Cohen LH, Kaplan M, Bernhard VM: Intraoperative streptokinase. Arch Surg 121:708, 1986

46. Abbott WM, McCabe C, Maloney RD et al: Embolism of the popliteal artery. Surg Gynecol Obstet 159:533, 1984

47. Youkey JR, Clagett GP, Cabelloni S et al: Thromboembolectomy of arteries explored at the ankle. Ann Surg 199:367, 1984

48. Green RM, DeWeese JA, Rob CG: Arterial embolectomy before and after the Fogarty catheter. Surgery 77:24, 1975

49. Ferguson LJ, Faris I, Robertson A et al: Intraarterial streptokinase therapy to relieve acute limb ischemia. J Vasc Surg 4:205, 1986

50. Hallett JW, Yrizzarry JM, Greenwood LH: Regional low dosage thrombolytic therapy for peripheral arterial occlusions. Surg Gynecol Obstet 156:148, 1983

51. Berni GA, Bandyk DF, Zierler E et al: Streptokinase treatment of acute arterial occlusion. Ann Surg 198:185, 1983

52. Belkin M, Belkin B, Bucknam CA et al: Intra-arterial thrombolytic therapy: efficacy of streptokinase vs. urokinase. Arch Surg 121:769, 1986

53. Graor RA, Risius B, Young JR et al: Peripheral and bypass graft thrombolysis with recombinant human tissue-type plasminogen activator. J Vasc Surg 3:115, 1986

54. Collier PE: Limb salvage surgery without arteriography: is it possible? Presented at the Fourth Annual Meeting of the Eastern Vascular Society, Boston, May 1990

55. Haimovici H: Arterial embolism with acute massive ischemic myopathy and myoglobinuria: evaluation of a hitherto unreported syndrome with a report of two cases. Surgery 47:739, 1960

56. Haimovici H: Muscular, renal, and metabolic complications of acute arterial occlusions: myonephropathic–metabolic syndrome. Surgery 85:461, 1979

20

Thrombolysis Treatment for Acute Lower Limb Ischemia

Thomas O. McNamara

Acute lower limb ischemia (ALLI) continues to be a very difficult clinical problem that endangers both life and limb. In this chapter I propose a major change in the treatment of ALLI, specifically, the use of percutaneous intra-arterial thrombolysis (PIAT) as the initial treatment for ALLI in limbs that continue to have at least partial neurosensory function, plus angiographic findings of patent collateral and distal vessels. This may seem revolutionary to some, but in our view it is merely evolutionary. To put this proposal into proper perspective and to explain the theoretical basis for this approach, the evolving body of knowledge regarding ALLI is reviewed.

HISTORY

Conservative management of ALLI resulted in many limbs lost to amputation or in disability due to ischemic neuropathy, rest pain, or severe claudication. Surgical intervention was pursued to improve on these unsatisfactory outcomes, with direct embolectomy first performed in 1911 by Labey.[1] Subsequently, a range of methods of indirect clot extraction were developed to minimize the extent of the surgical procedure and to retrieve distal thrombus. Retrograde flushing, described in 1930, was an attempt to force distal clot proximally to facilitate removal.[2] A less invasive modi-

fication, described in 1951,[3] was the use of rubberized bandages to accomplish retrograde milking of distal clot to allow removal from a proximal arteriotomy. In 1960 Shaw described a corkscrew type wire to remove clot distal to the arteriotomy.[4] In 1961, Oeconomus reported the successful use of a special vein stripper with an olive-shaped head for the removal of a clot distant from the arteriotomy.[5] All these techniques have been superseded by indirect embolectomy/thrombectomy using the Fogarty technique and balloon-tipped catheter for clot extraction, introduced in 1963 and found superior to the other indirect methods and devices.[6]

The Fogarty procedure offers many advantages over direct embolectomy/thrombectomy. These include the ability to reach either proximally to the aortoiliac junction or distally to the pedal vessels after introduction of the device into the common femoral artery. Surgical access is relatively easy, requiring only dissection through soft tissue and limited exposure. The catheter manipulations are limited, straightforward, and rapidly accomplished. Thus, the procedure can be performed rather quickly, often under local anesthesia. Theoretically, the combination of these features would be expected to be associated with less surgical "stress" to the patient, reduced anesthesia risk, less postoperative morbidity, and both lower operative and in-hospital mortality than with direct embolectomy.

The combination of these theoretical advantages and the excellent results described in the initial reports resulted in the use of this procedure with increasing frequency for ALLI.[7,8] The rapid acceptance and general enthusiasm for the Fogarty procedure is exemplified by Thompson's description of it, in 1974, as the "single most important advance in the management of embolism in the last decade."[9] As a result of this enthusiasm, utilization expanded to include patients with ischemia of longer duration, those with more tissue at risk, and those with more extensive peripheral and coronary artery disease.

Although most early reports on the use of the Fogarty procedure for ALLI endorsed its expanded applications, some began to note higher than expected mortality and amputation rates. In 1966, Blaisdell et al.[10] noted a 7.3 percent mortality rate in patients undergoing emergency thromboembolectomy for ALLI versus 1.5 percent for similar occlusions treated with elective reconstruction. Although deaths were initially ascribed to congestive heart failure, myocardial infarction, or pneumonia, retrospective review of clinical and pathologic findings demonstrated a great similarity to patients dying after emergency surgery for ruptured abdominal aortic aneurysm. Both groups appeared to have massive pulmonary damage due to microemboli from the lower limbs. Blaisdell and colleagues judged that this accounted for hypoxia, tachypnea, elevated central pressure, the appearance of congestive heart failure, and cardiorespiratory death. Microemboli were found in the venous effluent from lower extremities during operations for ALLI and in most of the lungs, during autopsy examinations. For the most part, the microemboli consisted of platelet-fibrin aggregates, which were assumed to have been formed on the venous side of the capillary circulation and flooded the lungs during the initial washout phase after successful surgery and restoration of flow. These findings were reproduced in a dog model in which the aorta was cross-clamped and the collateral flow to the lower extremities interrupted for several hours. After release of the clamp, the initial venous effluent from the lower extremities demonstrated a high concentration of platelet-fibrin emboli. Subsequent lung biopsies showed microemboli in the pulmonary arterioles "identical to those found in [their] clinical material."[11]

Microemboli were judged to be the cause of the pathologically observed pulmonary perivascular edema, hemorrhage, and atelectasis. Blaisdell's group reasoned that serotonin release from the platelets and histamine release from pulmonary macrophages would occur and cause both vaso- and bronchoconstriction, leading to arteriovenous shunting, atelectasis, arterial desaturation, increased pulmonary vascular resistance, subse-

quent reduction in cardiac output, and, ultimately, cardiopulmonary failure.[10] The lower incidence of this phenomenon after elective procedures for chronic lower-extremity arterial occlusions was attributed to the presence of well-developed collaterals that provided adequate blood supply to the distal tissues, whereas the collaterals in ALLI were either occluded or inadequately developed, resulting in significant distal ischemia with anoxia, progressive acidosis, and slow flow. This was equated to "local shock." Other investigators had previously shown that clotting in capillaries and venules accompanies shock[12–15] and that clotting on the venous side of the capillary is potentiated by the usually lower pH, which would be exaggerated in ALLI.[16] This was substantiated by the frequent finding of gross clot in the leg veins associated with ALLI and by the occasional observation of pulmonary embolism after successful arterial embolectomy.[17]

Blaisdell and co-workers had noted a 53 percent incidence of this cardiopulmonary failure syndrome after emergency surgery for ruptured abdominal aortic aneurysm, during the course of this study.[10] They believed that the larger amount of tissue made ischemic by the required aortic cross-clamping would effect a greater degree of "local shock," with a greater amount of microemboli flooding the lungs after restoration of flow. They suggested that the aortic cross-clamping would be akin to an acute thromboembolic aortic occlusion. Occlusion at this level was associated with the greatest mortality in the ALLI patients. They reasoned that the mechanism of death was probably the same in both groups of patients.[10] They also reasoned that these platelet-fibrin aggregates and venous thrombi would not form in the presence of adequate heparinization. In 1969 a review of the results of embolectomy for ALLI demonstrated that the mortality was chiefly in patients with obstruction of the iliac or common femoral arteries, particularly if, on physical examination, the ischemic demarcation was found to be at or above the knee.[18] In this group, the mortality rate was 81 percent. By contrast, mortality was uncommon in patients with upper-extremity or below-knee occlusions. This finding supported the concept that the larger the region involved with "local shock," the greater the potential insult to the lungs from platelet-fibrin microemboli and venous clot after restoration of flow. Similar findings regarding increased risk of mortality with more proximal occlusions had also been observed during the era of direct embolectomy, but a pathophysiologic explanation had not previously been offered.[19] Blaisdell and co-workers supported their pathophysiologic explanation by the demonstration of pulmonary microemboli in 56 percent of autopsies performed after thromboembolectomy for ALLI.[18] They therefore recommended routine venous thrombectomy and arteriovenous irrigation to reduce the risk of gross and microscopic pulmonary embolism after restoration of flow, observing, however, that this treatment did not consistently prevent pulmonary complications. They again also recommended heparinization before, during, and after the procedure, reasoning that it would limit the secondary development of arterial and venous thrombus, as well as platelet-fibrin aggregates, thereby reducing the risk of micro- and macroembolization. They believed that such heparinization would also reduce the risk of prompt reocclusion due to thrombosis in the damaged vascular bed after successful use of the Fogarty balloon-tipped catheter.

The use of heparinization to reduce the risk of reocclusion after embolectomy had also been advised during the era of direct embolectomy, but it was routinely discontinued during the first 48 hours postsurgery due to "prohibitive morbidity."[19] The lesser amount of surgery associated with the Fogarty procedure/device could be expected to be associated with less postoperative bleeding during uninterrupted heparinization, but initial reports were unfavorable. In 1967 Darling et al.[20] stated that the risks associated with the use of heparin outweighed its benefit during the early postoperative period. However, in 1972 Holm and Schersten[21] presented very strong evidence in favor of the use of full therapeutic doses of heparin during the entire perioperative period, when treating ALLI with the Fogarty procedure. They reported a 4.5 percent mortality and 4.5 percent amputation rate in those patients treated uninterruptedly with "adequate anticoagulation" versus a 25.6 percent mortality rate and a 22.2 percent amputation rate in those not adequately treated. They defined "adequate anticoagulation" as heparinization beginning before and maintained for 1 week after thromboembolectomy (minimum heparin dose 5000 units every 6 hours), plus 3 months of "antiprothrombin therapy." Although they did note a higher incidence of wound complications (i.e., bleeding and infection) in the patients treated "adequately," none had been serious. They observed that most deaths after thromboembolectomy for ALLI were clot related, including myocardial infarction, pulmonary embolism, and cerebral embolism. Continuous "adequate anticoagulation" could, they believed, be expected to reduce the likelihood of such thrombus-induced pathology.

Blaisdell and co-workers subsequently demonstrated the presence of ischemic metabolites in the venous efflux from ischemic limbs, which could damage the lungs.[22] In an elegant experiment, they demonstrated the production of multiple sites of pulmonary hemorrhage in both lungs of a dog after prolonged ischemia of the lower limbs despite lack of direct exposure of

one lung to this blood. Obviously, microemboli were not the only by-product of ALLI capable of causing pulmonary damage, but more pulmonary injury was observed in their presence, indicating that they were an independent pathologic factor. Pulmonary damage was prevented when the venous efflux was routed through the liver, possibly due to both the filtering of embolic debris and the detoxification of ischemic metabolites by the liver. Others had shown that the liver is capable of removing activated clotting factors, fibrin, and some vasoactive substances, such as thromboplastin, adenosine diphosphate (ADP), histamine, serotonin, fibrinopeptides, and kinins from the circulation.[23-27] Blaisdell and co-workers postulated that the platelet-fibrin aggregates might be the source of some of these substances and that the ischemia produced the others, but the nature of the substances and the mechanism of pulmonary injury were not clear. Subsequent investigation into both acute coronary and peripheral arterial ischemia by others has validated their observations and answered some of the questions raised by their postulates.

We now know that a fresh clot is continually undergoing breakdown by fibrinolysis, as well as reformation by clot-bound thrombin-induced accretion. Thus, the pooled or sludging blood in the ischemic area may contain proteolytic fragments of fibrin(ogen), such as $B\beta1$-42, which have been shown to increase vascular permeability.[28] Also, platelets contain and can release thromboxane A_2, a prostanoid that causes endothelial cell microfilaments to become disassembled, reducing junctional membrane apposition and increasing permeability.[29] Monocytes can release interleukin, and lymphocytes can release leukotriene. Experimentally, both produce leakage of albumin through the arteriolar walls.[30-32] Other leukocytic factors, such as tumor necrosis factor, platelet-activating factor,[33] and interferons, have similar effects on vascular permeability.[30,32,34] It is noteworthy that large numbers of leukocytes and lymphocytes are observed between severely ischemic or necrotic muscle bundles.[35] Freischlag et al[36] have elegantly demonstrated that white blood cells in acutely ischemic tissue appear to release these substances.

The sudden flushing into the circulation of a highly concentrated bolus of such substances after thromboembolectomy might be expected to cause marked pulmonary vascular leak with thickening of the walls of the precapillary arterioles and intra-alveolar hemorrhage, as was seen in the human and animal autopsy findings reported by Blaisdell and co-workers. Serotonin, which they originally suggested to be causative agent, may actually promote capillary integrity instead.[37-39]

Additional mechanisms by which the ischemia-induced release of intracellular substances can cause death or severe morbidity were noted by Haimovici in 1970.[35] He reported four cases of hyperkalemia and myoglobinuric nephrosis complicating ALLI after successful thromboembolectomy. Each patient had a large volume of severely ischemic tissue ". . . the level of ischemic manifestations exceeded the usual level seen in the common forms of an acute arterial occlusion." He judged that the increased severity of ischemia resulted from the proximal level of the occlusion plus significant loss or ineffectiveness of collateral flow.

Haimovici likened this phenomenon associated with the treatment of massive, severe ALLI to the experimental crush syndrome,[40] in which the reestablishment of blood flow to previously compressed and ischemic limbs results in myoglobinuria, hyperkalemia, and frequently, renal insufficiency. Muscle necrosis appears to be required for myoglobinuria to induce acute tubular necrosis (ATN).[41] The observation that myoglobinuria and ATN could follow thromboembolectomy for ALLI had been independently reported in 1969 by Winninger.[42]

In 1969, Fogarty and colleagues[43] reported on the biochemical analysis of the venous efflux from limbs made temporarily ischemic during cardiopulmonary bypass and in patients treated with embolectomy for iliac or common femoral emboli. They found severe venous hypoxia, moderate hypercarbia, and mild lowering of pH in the venous efflux of the legs made temporarily ischemic, whereas venous hypoxia and hypercarbia in patients with emboli were more profound, presumably due to more complete occlusion of the collaterals and the longer duration of the ischemia. This finding confirmed earlier animal work performed by Provan et al.,[44] who demonstrated hypotension, a drop in systemic pH, hypercarbia, and venous hypoxia after unclamping of the aorta (and the major collateral channels) after 30 minutes of total ischemia. Fogarty and co-workers[43] documented that an abrupt fall in systemic venous pH and marked elevation of serum potassium promptly followed restoration of flow via embolectomy and postulated that cardiac arrhythmias may have caused the reported sudden deaths and near-deaths immediately after thromboembolectomy for ALLI. They also noted elevated creatine phosphokinase (CPK) levels in both the venous efflux and the systemic circulation of the patients with acute arterial emboli, a finding consistent with Haimovici's observation that muscle necrosis occurs with prolonged, complete arterial occlusions.[35]

In 1978, Blaisdell et al.[45] published a landmark article in which he challenged the efficacy of emergency thromboembolectomy for ALLI. This article reviewed the results of 3345 patients who had undergone emergency/urgent balloon-catheter clot extraction surgery for the treatment of ALLI, with a cumulative mortality rate of approximately 25 percent while approximately 30 percent of the survivors required amputation. These results prompted Blaisdell's group to propose an algorithm in which patients received massive doses of heparin, rather than emergency surgery, and were then treated medically in preparation for either subsequent reconstructive/restorative surgery, if their limbs improved over several days, or to undergo primary amputation if they did not. These investigators reported a substantially lower mortality rate without an attendant higher amputation rate with this approach; they postulated that the reduction in mortality was partly due to better preparation of these patients for the "stress" of surgery. Many of the deaths reported with emergent revascularization were attributed to pulmonary microembolization by platelet-fibrin aggregates.[11,22] It was postulated that, with marked heparinization, these were less likely to form, and that they were likely to clear, due to endogenous fibrinolysis, during a 72-hour (or longer) course of heparinization. Thus, initial heparin treatment and delayed surgery should reduce the risk of pulmonary microemboli.[45] Blaisdell and coworkers differed from their predecessors by (1) suggesting doses of heparin of up to 4000 U/h, and (2) delaying surgery to avoid the risk of wound bleeding and to provide time for endogenous fibrinolysis to clear distal small vessel thrombus. This approach would obviate the risk of microembolization and, possibly, macroembolization of lungs and provide an open distal vascular bed with low outflow resistance.

Others reported results confirming Blaisdell's observations, with mortality rates of 15 to 22 percent after emergency thromboembolectomy for ALLI, amputation rates of 3 to 25 percent in the survivors, and even higher mortality rates with aortoiliac or aortic bifurcation occlusions.[46–53] These studies confirmed the earlier observation by Blaisdell and others that the risks were much higher than after elective revascularization surgery on chronically ischemic limbs (1 to 2 percent)[10,54] or for amputation (3 to 4 percent) without initial attempts at reperfusion.[46,55]

In 1982, Abbott et al.[56] published their review of the results of conservative versus surgical management of acute upper and lower limb ischemia at the Massachusetts General Hospital over a 44-year period (1937 to 1981). They noted that during 1937 to 1964, only 23 percent of patients with emboli had been treated surgically, whereas during 1964 to 1981, after the introduction of the Fogarty device, 88 percent had undergone embolectomy. Throughout the 44-year period, the limb salvage rate after surgical treatment in 498 patients was 89 percent, versus 77 percent in the 235 patients treated conservatively. Abbott et al. also noted that surgical limb salvage rates after the introduction of the Fogarty device/procedure were not significantly improved: 83 percent after versus 82 percent prior. Despite theoretical predictions that this form of surgery for ALLI would dramatically reduce risk, the mortality rate decreased only 5 percent, from 24 percent to 19 percent.

Fogarty embolectomy did lower the mortality associated with surgical treatment of arm emboli (from 21 percent to 6 percent), while the mortality rate after the same treatment for lower extremities remained at about 20 percent. No explanation was offered. Possibly the Fogarty device is most efficacious when used to extract clot from an otherwise normal vascular tree, such as the arteries in the upper extremities, which are more likely to be free of atherosclerosis than those in the lower extremity.

These reports prompted some, including Fogarty, to suggest that the best application of emergency clot removal was for use in relatively normal vessels occluded with an acute embolus that might also have an associated secondary distal thrombus. It was advised that the use of the device/procedure for thrombectomy and "blind endarterectomy" in an atherosclerotic vessel might be successful but should be expected to be associated with more complications, including perforation, dissection, arterial rupture, plaque avulsion, intimal damage, and retention of broken catheter part.[45,57,58]

McPhail et al.[59] reported improved results by performing emergency clot extraction surgery only on embolic occlusions and using Blaisdell's approach of heparinization and delayed surgery for thrombotic occlusions. Emergent embolectomy was accompanied by 8.7 percent mortality and 7.5 percent amputation rates versus 12 percent mortality and 22 percent amputation rates for the thrombotic occlusions. Fogarty[60] suggested that differentiation of embolic versus thrombotic occlusions based on a history of atrial fibrillation, prior claudication, and physical findings would be accurate in 85 percent of cases.

However, Blaisdell and others have countered that such clinical differentiation is very difficult.[45] Cambria and Abbott[61] stated that atrial fibrillation is the only reliable clinical predictor of an embolic etiology.

One of the few analyses of the accuracy of clinically diagnosing an embolic etiology for ALLI was published in 1986 by Jivegård et al.[62] While attempting to use the approach of emergency clot extraction only for those patients with the clinical diagnosis of embolic occlusions, they reported a misdiagnosis based on operative findings in 29 percent in 122 patients. They confirmed the previously reported poor prognosis after emergency

thrombectomies in patients with unsuspected underlying atherosclerosis and spontaneous in situ thrombosis as the etiology of ALLI, in whom they experienced a 50 percent surgical failure rate versus 13 percent for embolic occlusions. One-half the surgical failures in the thrombotic group involved the development of gangrene, with many patients dying of sepsis, versus only 14 percent of cases of gangrene in the failed embolic group. The thrombotic occlusion group experienced a 30-day mortality rate of 27 percent and a 50 percent amputation rate, as opposed to the 25 percent mortality rate and a 6 percent amputation rate in those correctly diagnosed as having an embolic occlusion.

In 1986 Jivegård et al.[62] reviewed the surgical literature of 1978 to 1984, including reports of 2495 cases of ALLI treated with emergency thromboembolectomy, with a cumulative 30-day mortality rate of 18 percent and an amputation rate of 16 percent in the survivors. This report bolstered the view of those who believed that the results reported by Blaisdell et al. reflected outmoded surgical and postoperative treatment. Jivegård et al.[62] also proposed that the results could be further improved by delaying surgery so that the operator would be one who could perform reconstructive surgery if the simpler thromboembolectomy approach failed.

In 1982, Field et al.[63] reported their experience with 61 patients with ALLI who underwent thromboembolectomy an average of 37 hours after the onset of symptoms. In 18 patients (30 percent), restorative surgery attempts failed, which led immediately to reconstructive surgical attempts. They cited a 14 percent mortality rate and a 12 percent amputation rate after the use of thromboembolectomy, versus 0 percent and 12 percent in those 18 patients treated with additional reconstructive surgery. It was stressed that there was no increase in the incidence of either mortality or amputation by the addition of reconstructive surgery.

There has been a trend toward reconstructive surgery in patients with thrombotic disease instead of emboli. A recent report by Yeager et al.[64] included results of surgical management of 74 patients with ALLI with reconstructive procedures in 84 percent and simple thrombectomy or embolectomy in only 12 percent. Only six (8 percent) of their occlusions were judged to be due to emboli. This more aggressive approach was associated with a 30-day mortality rate of 15 percent (8 percent due to myocardial infarction, 7 percent due to cancer) and major amputation rate of 30 percent.

Timing of surgery has also been controversial; in contrast to Blaisdell's recommendation against immediate surgery, most investigators have stressed the importance of operating as early as possible for ALLI. Consistently, the reports of direct embolectomy demonstrated a marked increase in amputations with increasing time between the onset of symptoms and surgical treatment. In 1933, Pearse[65] reported on a series of 282 cases collected from the literature; when embolectomy was performed within 10 hours, the limb was saved in 40 percent of these cases; after 10 to 15 hours, in only 16 percent; and after 30 hours, in none. Similar statistics were reported by others.[66-69] Linton[70] demonstrated in 1941 that this phenomenon was due to persistent occlusion by distal thrombus despite successful embolectomy. He also demonstrated "spasm" in the vessels distal to the embolus and postulated that, with time, this vasoconstriction would promote secondary thrombosis, which would be difficult to clear with direct embolectomy. He suggested empirically that 6 hours was the grace period.

Mortality rates were found to parallel these results. Using direct embolectomy, Sterling et al.[19] in 1963, noted increasing mortality with increasing delay between the onset of symptoms and surgery, ranging from 19 percent after 0 to 6 hours to 67 percent after 24 hours or more. Despite the theoretical ability of the Fogarty procedure/device to extract the secondary distal thrombus thought to account for the failures of "late" embolectomy, the same association between duration of ischemia and morbidity and mortality was noted with catheter thromboembolectomy.[56-71]

Several studies have noted that duration of symptoms alone should not be used as a criterion to exclude patients from thromboembolectomy (direct or indirect),[19,56,71] and Field et al.,[63] Fogarty,[72] Spencer and Eisman[73] all cite excellent results after delayed embolectomy for occlusions up to 90 days in duration. Jivegård et al.[74] found that thromboembolectomies performed in the time period of 13 to 24 hours after the onset of ALLI carried the greatest risk of mortality (48 percent), a threefold greater risk than when surgery was performed within 3 hours or beyond 72 hours after the onset of ischemia. This may be due to the effect of endogenous fibrinolysis on peripheral microemboli.

Information regarding the extent of arterial occlusion, including the presence and quality of collateral flow and the degree of patency of distal vessels, might be expected to provide valuable prognostic and decision-making information in the presence of ALLI. Simply put, the more completely the clotting process has occluded blood flow, the more likely and rapid the development of lethal biochemical and coagulation products, as evidenced by studies of complete vascular occlusion and limb reimplantation.[75-77] This had been recognized by early investigators, who speculated that their success with late embolectomies was due to adequate collateral flow despite the presence of pain, pallor, and decreased sensorimotor function.[19,43,56,72,73]

Arteriography would have been expected to clarify the issue and aid in treatment planning; however, it was invariably not performed because of concern that the attendant delay would prejudice a good surgical outcome.

Haimovici et al.[78] were among the first (1975) to recommend preoperative arteriography for the patient with ALLI, as part of treatment planning and as an aid to prognosis due to recognition of the significance of atherosclerotic disease. This confirmed the experience of Freund et al.,[79] who had reported a 52 percent mortality in ALLI patients with underlying atherosclerosis versus 18 percent in those without. To date the best results for limb salvage are with embolectomy, reported by Fogarty[73] to be 95 percent, but still associated with a substantial mortality (16 percent).

Major risk factors associated with even higher mortality rates include advanced age (32 percent mortality in octogenarians),[80] recent myocardial infarction (RMI) (within 2 weeks) of 40 to 100 percent,[71,74,80] and irreversible ischemia (46 to 73 percent).[64,71] This led Jivegård, in 1986, to state that "acute limb ischemia threatens the limb of the young but the life of the old."[74] This is of note in that most patients who present with ALLI are elderly and frequently have extensive underlying cardiovascular disease. Many are also debilitated due either to advanced age or to underlying malignancy.[64]

This brief historical review explains the rationale for exploring the potential benefits of PIAT as the initial therapy for selected patients with ALLI. Initially, use of this therapy was limited to patients at high risk of surgery (elderly, debilitated, RMI, significant cardiac disease), when surgery could not be performed promptly or in an effort to identify the underlying flow-limiting lesion in occluded bypass grafts for optimal preoperative treatment planning. Initial results were satisfactory, and led to an expansion of indications. We now use PIAT as the initial treatment for virtually all patients with ALLI who present without anesthesia and paralysis.[81]

Table 20-1 Clinical Classification of Degree of Acute Lower Limb Ischemia

Class	Clinical Classification	Sensorimotor Function	Pedal Doppler Signal — Artery/Vein
I	Viable	Intact	+/+
II	Threatened	Impaired	−/+
III	Irreversible	Absent	−/−

Table 20-2 Correlation Between Angiographic Pattern and Clinical Degrees of Ischemia

Angiographic Vessel Category	Clinical Classification of Ischemia	Angiographic Pattern			
		Occluded Segments	Inflow	Collaterals	Distal Vessels Seen to Be Patent
I	Viable	Single	Normal	Patent	Yes
II	Threatened	Tandem	Normal	Patent	Yes
		Single	Stenotic	Patent	Yes
		Single	Normal	Stenotic	Yes
III	Irreversible (profound)	Multiple	Normal	Patent	No
		Multiple	Normal	Occluded	No[a]

[a] In this instance, the inability to visualize the distal vessels may not mean that they are occluded.

RESULTS OF PIAT

The first 72 consecutive cases treated with PIAT demonstrated a positive thrombolysis outcome in 85 percent, with an additional 5 percent treated successfully with surgery after either failure of thrombolysis or reocclusion within 30 days. This yielded a total limb salvage of 90 percent at 30 days. The 30-day mortality rate was 1.6 percent (1 in 63 patients), and the amputation rate was 8.3 percent (6 in 72 limbs). Arteriography before PIAT demonstrated a strong correlation between the angiographic pattern of vascular occlusion(s) and the clinical degree of ischemia,[82] as described by the Ad Hoc Committee on Reporting Standards of the Society for Vascular Surgery/North American Chapter and the International Society for Cardiovascular Surgery.[83] An abbreviated version is shown in Table 20-1. The correlation between angiographic patterns and clinical degree of ischemia is shown in Table 20-2. The angiographic pattern also correlated very strongly with the outcome of PIAT, as shown in Table 20-3. Illustrations of the angiographic patterns are shown in Figures 20-1 to 20.3. The illustrations depict the multiple variations within an angiographic category that affect similar sensorimotor impairment and have a nearly equivalent likelihood of success with PIAT.

Unlike the case with surgical treatment,[19,22] the level of occlusion was not a strong predictor of outcome from PIAT for ALLI.[81,82] Proximal arterial occlusions (iliac and common femoral) yielded a 6 percent mortality and 6 percent amputation rate versus 0 percent mortality and 8 percent amputation for the 25 distal arterial occlusions. The 14 suprainguinal grafts yielded 0 percent mortality and 7 percent amputation rate versus a 0 percent mortality and 13 percent amputation rate for the 16 infrainguinal grafts. These results suggest that the greatest risk of mortality is with proximal arterial occlusions (6 percent) and of amputation with infrainguinal bypass graft thromboses (13 percent).

The angiographic demonstration of single versus tandem (or more) segments of occlusion was a far better predictor of outcome than location alone (Table 20-3). Consistently, treatment of single segment occlusions yielded better results than tandem occlusions. In arterial occlusions, PIAT yielded 100 percent success with single versus 79 percent with tandem segment occlusions; in bypass graft occlusions the respective results were 91 percent and 74 percent.[81]

The six amputations were all in patients who had at least tandem lesions. They were performed after unsuccessful attempts at both PIAT and surgery, unless the risk/benefit ratio for surgery was considered too

Table 20-3 Correlation Between Outcome of PIAT and Initial Angiographic Pattern

Pattern	No.	% Positive Thrombolysis Outcome	% Amputation	% Mortality
I	13	100	0	0
II	51	85	7.8	0
III	8	63	25	16

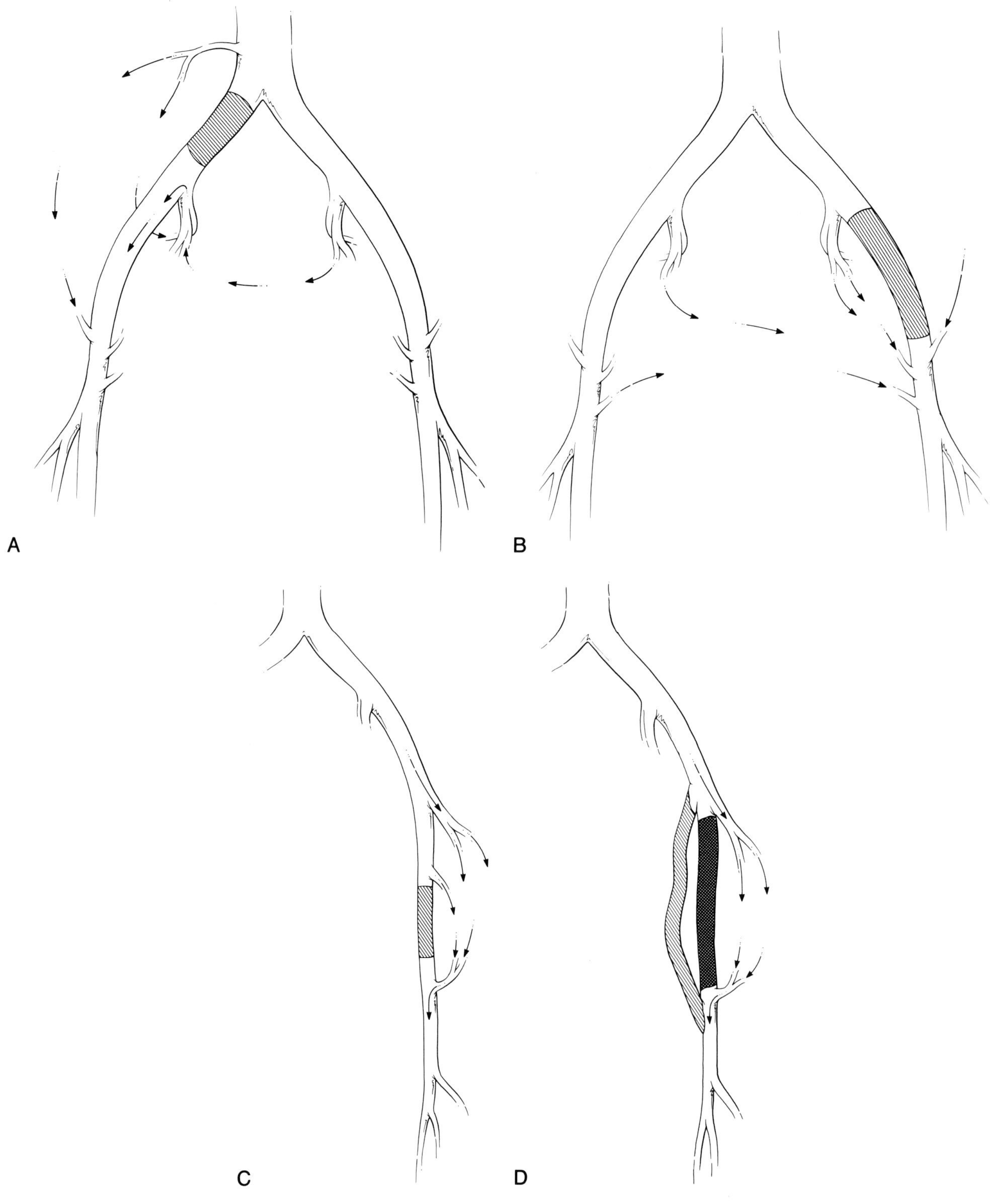

Figure 20-1 Category I with single segment occlusion, patent collaterals, and distal vessels. **(A)** Common iliac occlusion. **(B)** External iliac occlusion. **(C)** Superficial femoral artery (SFA) occlusions, but patent popliteal and distal segments. **(D)** Femoropopliteal above-knee (AK) bypass graft occlusion, but patent popliteal and distal segments. *(Figure continues.)*

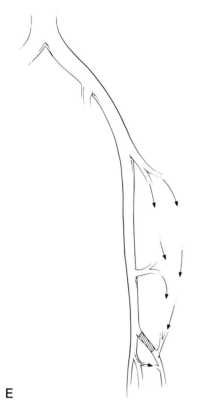

E

Figure 20-1E *(Continued).* **(E)** Occlusion of proximal segment of only one trifurcation artery and patent distal portion.

poor to justify surgery (one case). The amputations were all in patients with thrombotic occlusions. Amputations resulted in 2 of 8 patients (25 percent) who presented with class III (irreversible) ischemia, in 4 of 51 (7.8 percent) of patients in class II, and none in patients with class I ischemia (viable).

As has been the experience with surgery, the commonest cause of failure of PIAT was inadequate runoff. The distal runoff bed was more often severely compromised in patients with occluded bypass grafts than in those with a native artery occlusion. Progressive atherosclerotic obliteration of the distal runoff bed may more often be the cause of graft occlusions, whereas the native artery occludes at the site of the worst disease with the distal runoff bed not as consistently diseased/occluded.

The single death occurred in a patient who presented with irreversible clinical ischemia and a category III angiographic pattern. Reperfusion of a cadaveric extremity resulted in hyperkalemia and lactic acidosis, adult respiratory distress syndrome (ARDS), and ATN associated with myoglobinuria. Thus, the systemic complications of reperfusion of a large mass of severely ischemic or necrotic muscle previously described with

surgery can also occur after thrombolysis, although this occurred surprisingly infrequently in our series. It is possible that thrombolytic therapy directly clears or diminishes the lethal coagulation and metabolic by-products of ischemia.

PIAT for ALLI offers the advantage of dissolving the platelet-fibrin aggregates and venous thromboses described by Blaisdell and co-workers[10,11,22,45] and others,[17] potentially reducing the risk of pulmonary and cardiac complications these cause. This should reduce the likelihood of death after reperfusion due to cardiopulmonary insufficiency. Since thrombolysis accomplishes restoration of flow gradually rather than suddenly, this may reduce the likelihood of serious hyperkalemia and its attendant complications. In surgical series hyperkalemia follows the abrupt flushing of the highly concentrated ischemic limb blood into the circulation and then clears.[43] PIAT may allow a more gradual release of potassium and other anaerobic metabolites of ischemia, which is better tolerated physiologically.

In the past, surgeons have relied either solely or primarily on the physical findings to make the assessment of salvageability. They have used findings of "early rigor," "stiff joints," and "extreme tenderness of the muscles"[35] and the extension of skin discoloration to the thigh[22,45] as manifestations of the degree of ischemia and extent of vascular occlusion. They have also used the operative finding of backbleeding following thromboembolectomy[62,70] to provide information relative to the adequacy of collateral flow and patency of the distal vessels. The validity of these criteria is limited by their subjectivity, allowing for significant differences of opinion between examiners, unlike the more objective demonstration of the vascular occlusive pattern by angiography. Furthermore, Spencer and Eisman demonstrated the patency of the small distal vessels despite the physical findings of mottling, paralysis, and anesthesia.[73] In our view, the most accurate method of establishing the mass of ischemic muscle and the likelihood of rapid progression to necrosis is the combination of the physical examination findings of ischemia and the angiographic pattern (Table 20-4). They usually match and enable the interventional radiologist and vascular surgeon to confirm one another's independent assessment.

Nonagreement also provides critical information. For example, angiographic demonstration of complete occlusion of both the main and collateral channels (angiographic category III) (Fig. 20-3A), despite the physical findings of ischemia in the threatened (class II) group, would lead us to avoid PIAT, as these patients may rapidly progress to the irreversible class. Reliance on angiographic findings mandates excellent angio-

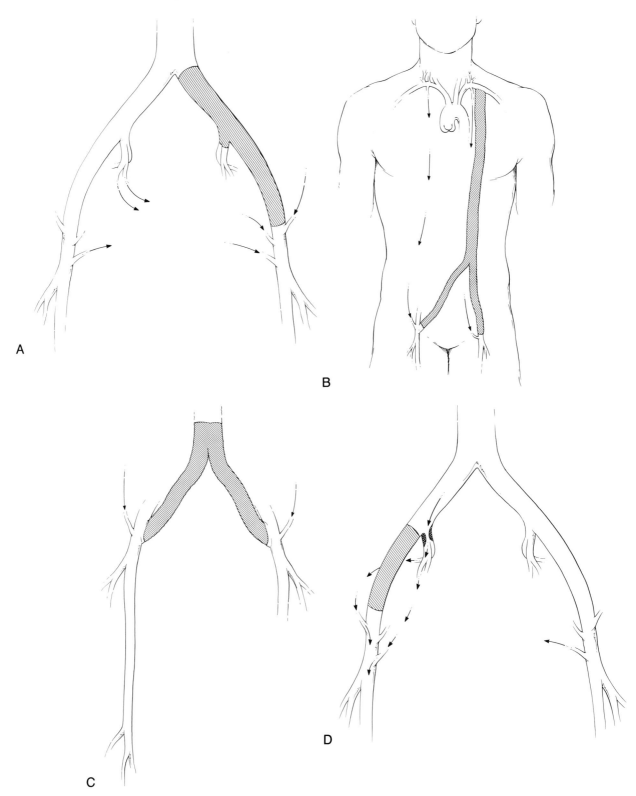

Figure 20-2 Category II with tandem or parallel segments of occlusion versus single-segment occlusion plus a tandem or parallel stenosis. **(A)** Occlusion of common, external, and origin of internal iliac arteries. **(B)** Occlusion of axillobifemoral graft. **(C)** Occlusion of aortobifemoral graft. **(D)** Occlusion of external iliac plus stenosis of (collateral) internal iliac artery. *(Figure continues.)*

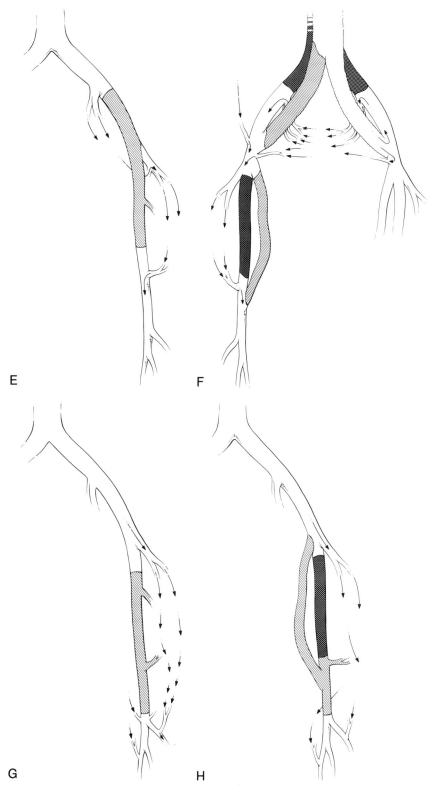

Figure 20-2E *(Continued).* **(E)** Occlusion of contiguous aortofemoral segments: external iliac, common femoral, and proximal superficial femoral artery (SFA). **(F)** Occlusion of separated iliofemoral segments: aortofemoral graft limb plus ipsilateral femoropopliteal (above-knee [AK]) graft. **(G)** Contiguous femoropopliteal segments: SFA plus popliteal. **(H)** Contiguous graft plus artery segments: femoropopliteal (AK) graft plus popliteal artery. *(Figure continues.)*

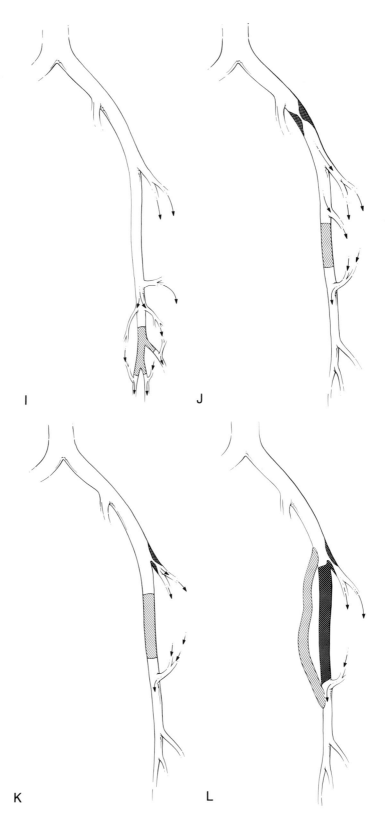

Figure 20-2I *(Continued).* **(I)** Parallel segmental occlusions: proximal portion of all of the trifurcation arteries. **(J)** Inflow stenosis plus single segment occlusion. **(K)** Parallel (collateral) stenosis plus single segment arterial occlusion. **(L)** Parallel (collateral) stenosis plus single segment graft occlusion.

Table 20-4 Correlation Between Categories of Ischemia and Time Required to Re-establish Flow and Status after 30 Days

Angiographic Category/ Clinical Description	Re-establishment of Flow on Angiography[a] (h)	Mean Time For Complete Clot Lysis (h)	Results at 30 Days (%)		
			Patent	Death	Amputation
I/Viable	2.5	10	100	0	0
II/Threatened	4.0	18	85	0	8.0
III/Irreversible	10.0	25	63	12.5	25.0

[a] Repeat angiography performed at 2, 4, 8 to 18, and 24 to 36 hours after onset of infusion.

graphic technique to avoid underestimation of collateral and distal perfusion. A false impression of occlusion of the distal vessels (category III) can be seen in any situation in which tandem occlusions of two or more segments are present, such that the collateral flow is quite slow (occlusions of superficial femoral + popliteal + proximal trifurcation) (Fig. 20-4). This can usually be clarified by prolonged filming and the use of digital subtraction arteriography (DSA). Occlusion of

the proximal portion of collateral channels can yield a false impression of occlusion of the distal vessels beyond a main channel segmental occlusion (Fig. 20-5). Advancement of a catheter through these occlusions, followed by small injections of contrast material, will clarify distal patency. We would perform PIAT if they are patent and sensory function remains.

We would also recommend PIAT in the occasional patient who presents with clinically irreversible ische-

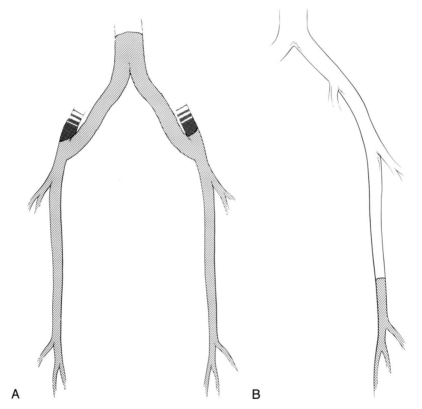

Figure 20-3 Category III patterns consisting of occlusion of tandem (or more) segments plus lack of filling of either collaterals or distal vessels. **(A)** Occlusion of multiple contiguous segments plus occlusion of collateral and distal (trifurcation) arteries. **(B)** Tandem and parallel occlusions of distal superficial femoral artery (SFA), popliteal, and trifurcation arteries without distal reconstitution (nonsegmental).

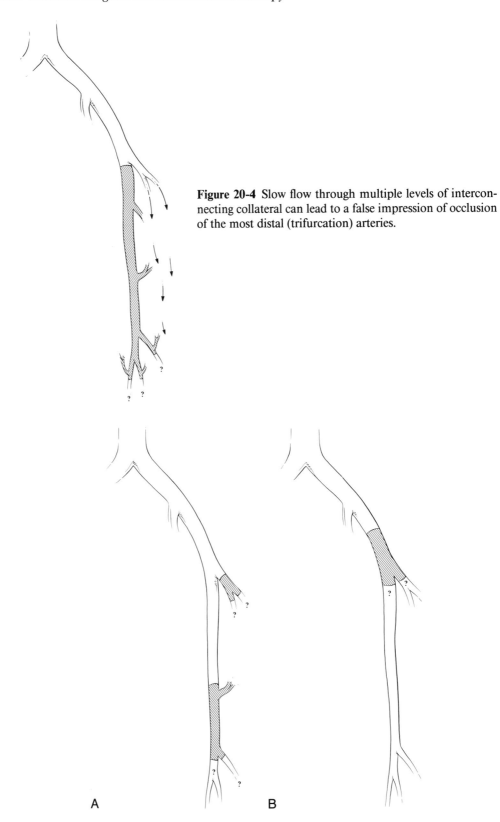

Figure 20-4 Slow flow through multiple levels of interconnecting collateral can lead to a false impression of occlusion of the most distal (trifurcation) arteries.

A   B

Figure 20-5 Occlusion of proximal portion of collateral channel obscures segmental nature of main channel occlusion, giving false impression of category III pattern. **(A)** Segmental occlusions of profunda femoris plus contiguous segments of distal superficial femoral artery (SFA) and popliteal artery. **(B)** Contiguous tandem occlusions of external iliac, common femoral, and origins of profunda femoris and SFA (parallel channels).

mia, but with angiographically patent collateral and distal vessels (category I or II). When these patients present within a few hours of the onset of their occlusion, they invariably have return of sensorimotor function with institution of heparinization and PIAT. The severity of ischemic signs may be due to reflex initial spasm of the distal vessels.[45,70]

The risks of systemic reperfusion and death are minimal in the absence of prolonged total occlusion of blood supply to a large muscle mass. More proximal occlusions, with incontrovertible angiographic evidence of loss of collateral and distal vessels (Fig. 20-3A), are at greater risk than more complete distal vessel occlusions (Fig. 20-3B). Complete occlusion of the profunda femoris distal to contiguous tandem iliofemoral occlusions puts the patient at considerable risk from reperfusion despite the rare instance of continued patency of the SFA (Fig. 20-6). We would have the greatest apprehension in utilizing PIAT for ALLI in patients in whom the thigh musculature is clearly ischemic due to the large muscle mass affected. We have not treated aortic bifurcation occlusions because of the concern that there would be insufficient collateral flow to prevent the thigh and buttock musculature from undergoing necrosis (Fig. 20-3A). Our experience matches that of Stallone et al.,[18] in that we believe the

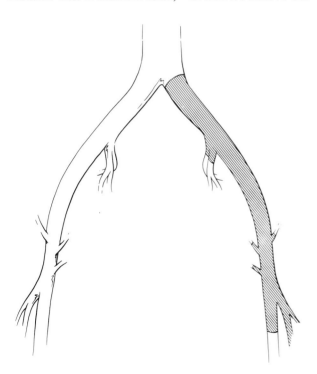

Figure 20-6 Contiguous tandem segmental occlusions of the iliofemoral arteries plus complete (nonsegmental) occlusion of the profunda femoris. Despite the rare patency of the superficial femoral artery (SFA), considerable muscle mass is at risk of necrosis due to occlusion of the profunda femoris.

risk of life-threatening reperfusion complications is minimal if the ischemia is limited to the arm or to below the knee, where the reperfusion injury is a local one.

Ischemic injury to the endothelial cell promotes extravasation of fluid through the vessel wall after restoration of flow. This causes swelling of the muscle compartment with associated increase in subfascial pressure from normal values of 0 to 5 mmHg to as much as 40 mmHg.[84] This can result in compression of the capillaries with reocclusion and then necrosis of muscle due to both ischemia and pressure, the so-called compartment syndrome.[85,86] Fasciotomy is an effective method of treatment, but should be performed prior to loss of pulses or the development of marked swelling and tenderness.[87] Loss of the ability to dorsiflex the foot requires consideration of prompt fasciotomy. Although this complication most often occurs after completion of lysis, thrombolysis can be continued during and after fasciotomy.

We noted three instances of compartment syndrome (4 percent) in our series of 72 infusions. Two were detected early and responded well to prompt fasciotomy. The other was detected late, did not have a fasciotomy, and developed a foot drop.[81]

The low incidence of compartment syndrome may have been due to the protective effect of the gradual reperfusion inherent in current PIAT methods. There is animal and clinical evidence that the slow restoration of flow over a period of hours may significantly reduce the risk of severe swelling that occurs following sudden restoration of flow at normal arterial pressure in reperfusion of ischemic skeletal and cardiac muscle.[88-91] Reperfusion at half the normal pressure has prevented such swelling in Beyerdorf's rat hindlimb model.[88] Beyerdorf et al. demonstrated that after 4 hours of total ischemia, the musculature experienced complete recovery of contractile function with only minimal increase in leg volume, when gentle reperfusion pressure of 50 mmHg and a modified substrate-enriched, hyperosmotic, alkalotic, low Ca^{2+} reperfusate were used. By contrast, uncontrolled reperfusion at 100 mmHg with Krebs-Henseleit solution resulted in severe reperfusion injury: massive edema, increased leg volume, and no contractile function after electrical stimulation. Similar findings have been noted in an ischemic cardiac muscle animal model by Buckberg and co-workers.[89-91] Although current PIAT regimens do not use a markedly altered reperfusate fluid, as used in these models, there are several similarities. One is the supply of glucose, which may help initiate anaerobic energy production at the start of reperfusion. Hypoxia stimulates glucose uptake in skeletal muscle.[92-94] The ischemic tolerance of skeletal muscle is improved by an increase in carbohydrate metabolism induced by glucose-enriched perfusion solutions.[95,96] In addition, PIAT duplicates the gentle and slow reperfusion of this regimen, as well as normothermia, to optimize the rate of cellular repair.

Myopathic-nephrotic-metabolic syndrome requires a massive volume of necrotic muscle[35,47] and results in renal tubular necrosis due to myoglobin precipitation. It is akin to the crush syndrome.[40,41] Haimovici's original description matches the clinical and angiographic patterns we term irreversible or category III.[35] These patients had excruciating pain with any attempt to mobilize the extremity, a much more proximal level of ischemia than usual, and marked "rigidity of the extremity" or "stiffness of the joints." Massive swelling of the extremity occurred within 12 to 24 hours of successful embolectomy, which was initially thought to be due to excessive venous thrombosis. However, postmortem examination demonstrated absence of venous clot and the presence of pale swollen muscle, presumably due to increased vascular permeability after the severe ischemia. Lymphocytes and leukocytes were seen to have infiltrated the spaces between the muscle bundles.[35] These findings and Freischlag's animal work support the concept that ischemic white blood cells release substances that promote vascular permeability.[36] The extensive occlusion required to produce this severe ischemia is uncommon (Fig. 20-3A) and should be treated with emergency surgery and intraoperative thrombolysis. Urinary alkalinization and expectant management of hyperkalemia, acidosis, arrhythmias, and hypotension are required.

We found myoglobin in the urine of a few of our patients, but in none of these cases did renal insufficiency develop. We do not try to alkalinize the urine during our PIAT infusions, but we do recommend sufficient hydration to maintain a minimum urine output of 50 ml/h.

Significant puncture site bleeding occurred in 2 of our 72 infusions (2.8 percent). We did not find the fibrinogen levels to be predictive of the likelihood of bleeding, but we did find levels below 100 mg/dl to be associated with more difficulty in controlling bleeding, if it occurred.

The risk of hemorrhagic stroke during PIAT for ALLI is difficult to determine because of the small size of reported series. We did not experience any in our series of 72 cases.[81] In our overall experience with almost 900 urokinase (UK) infusions, we have had only one instance of hemorrhagic stroke (nonfatal, full recovery) (McNamara TO, unpublished data, UCLA Medical Center). In a similarly large experience with UK infusions, for venous and arterial occlusions, Graor reports an incidence of approximately 0.1 percent (Graor RA, personal communication, 1992).

In the GISSI-2 study of more than 20,000 patients treated with thrombolysis for acute coronary occlusions with either recombinant tissue plasminogen activator (rtPA) or streptokinase (SK), an overall risk of stroke of 1.14 percent was found. Of these, 0.36 percent had hemorrhagic strokes, 0.48 percent ischemic strokes, and 0.30 percent strokes of undefined cause. Hemorrhagic stroke was significantly more frequent in patients with a diastolic blood pressure of 110 mmHg.

The doses of thrombolytic agent used for PIAT for ALLI are well below those used for coronary occlusions and may explain the lower incidence of stroke. Another potential explanation is that UK may be less likely to induce intracranial hemorrhage as it is less fibrin-specific than rtPA. Also, it has been demonstrated to cause less bleeding during PIAT for peripheral occlusions than SK.[97-102] This may relate to less disruption of the coagulation system with UK.[103] Current data suggest a trend of less bleeding with UK than rtPA for PIAT.[104]

In our series, embolic occlusions were more successfully treated than thrombotic occlusions, 94 percent versus 82 percent patency at 30 days despite earlier concerns that emboli could be more resistant to lysis, since they may be partly organized. Edwards[105] has reported that cardiac mural thrombi larger than 5 mm are rarely organized, regardless of their age. The likelihood that thrombolysis might promote detachment of residual intracardiac clot and result in cerebral embolization and death is unknown. To date, the largest experience with the use of thrombolysis in the face of intracardiac clot has been reported by Kremer et al.[106] In 1986 these investigators reported their experience in 16 patients with known intracardiac clot due to RMI treated with thrombolysis to clear the intracardiac clot. In 10 of 16 patients, this was successful when UK was administered at a dosage of 60,000 IU/h with concomitant intravenous heparinization. No instances of embolization were noted during those 2- to 8-day treatment periods, including three patients who had come to medical attention because of peripheral embolization. We do not interpret this experience to mean that repeat embolization cannot occur during this type of treatment, but it would seem to indicate that this complication is not a common accompaniment. Only two of the 16 embolic occlusions in our series had residual intracardiac clot on an echocardiogram; neither had repeat embolization during PIAT. The definitive therapy for embolic occlusions is PIAT. When the embolus is cleared, the patient's peripheral vascular tree does not require further treatment, unlike in patients with underlying atherosclerotic flow-limiting lesions for which further treatment is necessary to prevent reocclusion. The relatively less diseased state of the peripheral vascular tree in patients with embolic occlusions may explain why our success rate in treating embolic occlusions with PIAT was higher than for thrombotic occlusions.

While the presence of intracardiac mural thrombus in the left ventricle puts patients at higher risk of stroke, especially during the first 2 weeks after a myocardial infarction, patients with RMI represent a small percentage of patients presenting with ALLI (8 percent in our series).[81] We routinely obtain a transthoracic echocardiogram to search for residual intracardiac clot in patients with an embolic etiology for ALLI, but we do not obtain a transesophageal echocardiogram, nor do we delay the onset of the PIAT while awaiting the performance or interpretation of the echocardiogram.

In our experience, the embolic occlusions that involve the upper extremities are easily treated with PIAT, although upper-extremity embolectomy also yields very good results. We currently favor an initial trial at PIAT, based on our perception that it carries less morbidity than does embolectomy. If, after a few hours of PIAT, the occlusion proves resistant to thrombolysis, embolectomy can be performed only with mild prolongation of the duration of ischemia.

Spontaneous thromboses of native arteries and bypass grafts allow stabilization and better medical evaluation in both groups. Surgery, if needed, can be done on a more elective basis. In most instances, PIAT will serve to resolve the occlusion and permit optimal arteriographic definition of the underlying flow-limiting lesion(s). Although arteriography can be performed in the operating room after thrombectomy, it is more optimally performed in angiographic suites after PIAT, since this setting provides for more complete evaluation of inflow and outflow vessels. In addition, thrombolysis provides an opportunity to use the various endovascular techniques to treat the underlying flow-limiting lesion.

Furthermore, the use of PIAT addresses the group of patients for whom the use of a Fogarty device/procedure has had the poorest results, specifically, patients with spontaneous in situ arterial occlusions who have had the lowest incidences of limb salvage and the highest incidences of mortality,[45,57,59,61-63] possibly because removing the clot with the Fogarty balloon will not clear the underlying flow-limiting lesion.

As previously noted, some address these problems by performing primary reconstruction rather than thrombectomy,[64] but this approach has not received uniform endorsement. There remains the concern that the more extensive procedure may be associated with a higher mortality rate, unless it is performed on a delayed basis after stabilization of the patient. Published reports of reconstructive surgery for ALLI have not shown higher mortality and amputation rates than thrombectomy, but the rates have been substantial (15 percent and 30 percent, respectively).[64] In our experience, PIAT for

thrombotic ALLI has yielded better results than have those reported with the use of either restorative (thrombectomy) or reconstructive surgery. In a retrospective review of our initial 56 thrombotic occlusions, we demonstrated a 30-day patency of 82 percent, mortality of 1.8 percent, and amputation rate of 10.7 percent. The 30-day patency rate was higher after PIAT of native arterial occlusions (88 percent) as opposed to graft occlusions (80 percent).[81] (For a discussion of the role of PIAT in ALLI due to graft occlusion, see Ch. 22.) At times a combined lytic and surgical approach is warranted. PIAT for proximal occlusions may be of value to improve inflow before an infrainguinal reconstruction. Direct comparisons of the results of PIAT with surgery, which would optimally be done with a prospective randomized study, are not yet available.

In surgical series, advanced age[74,80] and or RMI[64,71,74,80] have had an adverse impact on the risk of mortality associated with treatment of ALLI. We have not noted this correlation with PIAT.[81] Our series included five patients with RMI and 20 patients 75 years of age or older, none of whom experienced myocardial infarction or death. This could be explained on the basis of less stress with PIAT than with surgery and attendant anesthesia. An additional factor could be the decrease in serum fibrinogen levels associated with PIAT, as it has been demonstrated to have a strong correlation with the incidence of myocardial infarctions.[107] Some have gone so far as to suggest that it represents an independent risk factor that perhaps should be modified by lowering in those patients who are at a higher than normal risk of myocardial infarction. Thus, PIAT may prove particularly efficacious for the elderly and those with RMI.

TECHNIQUE

The technique of PIAT during treatment of ALLI is less controversial than patient selection, but the approach is still evolving. Currently, UK is widely preferred as the thrombolytic agent for such infusions based on multiple studies confirming a higher incidence of lysis, in less time and with fewer complications than with SK.[97-102] UK is also regarded as preferable to SK, in that it is a direct plasminogen activator, yielding a more predictable response.

A review of results reported in eight series using SK for ALLI in 60 patients yields a success rate of 53 percent in 42 hours, with an 11.25 percent incidence of significant bleeding,[108-115] versus 85 percent success, in 18 hours, with a 2.8 percent incidence of significant bleeding when using UK.[81] There is not sufficient information at this time regarding the use of rtPA. Regimens for rtPA that yield faster lysis may do so only with a somewhat higher incidence of bleeding.[104] We and others have found UK to cause less bleeding than SK[97-103] and have therefore been reluctant to use rtPA, as it has not been found to have a better bleeding profile than SK.

The dose of UK is probably more controversial than the question of which agent to use. We use an initial dose rate of 4000 IU/min, until flow has been reestablished. This is coupled with either advancement of the end-hole catheter at 2-hour intervals or the use of a coaxial or multisidehole system, such that virtually all of the occlusion is bathed with drug from the outset of the infusion. In the latter instance, the catheter does not need to be advanced, and re-examination for the purposes of altering the dose can be performed at 4-hour intervals. In most instances, flow is re-established by 4 hours. The dose is then reduced to 1000 to 2000 IU/min, to clear up the small amount of residual clot.[97,102,116]

The angiographic patterns of occlusion are predictive of both ultimate outcome and the time required to obtain reestablishment of antegrade flow (see Tables 20-3 and 20-4). With single segment occlusions (category I), we have angiographically demonstrated restoration of flow in 2 hours; tandem lesions (category II) have antegrade flow at 4 hours. Occlusion of the distal vessels (category III) required a mean infusion of 10 hours to reestablish antegrade flow throughout the entirety of the original occlusions[82] and until the distal most vessels have flow through them.

Once flow has been re-established, infusion is continued from just within the origin of the vessel/graft; this minimizes flow limitation and the risk of pericatheter thrombus. A lower dose of 1000 U/min is used until there has been complete clot lysis, generally from 4 to 12 hours. The slower lysis during this phase may result from antegrade flow, limiting the interaction of drug with clot.[123] Infusion should be continued to ensure that all residual clot is lysed before presuming that residual filling defects represent a fixed anatomical lesion. It can be very difficult to differentiate residual thrombus from a fixed stenosis after only a few hours of infusion. Empirically and experimentally, it has been noted that the last bits of clot clear slowly. The premature performance of angioplasty can result in distal embolization.

Although we use 4000 IU/min to re-establish flow in patients with threatened (class II) or irreversible (class III) ischemia, those with an intact sensorimotor examination (viable—class I) can be treated with a lower dose of 1000 IU/min. This degree of ischemia does not demand rapid re-establishment of flow. On occasion we have used doses of 6000 and 8000 U/min and have noted that this has effected lysis more quickly, but with

a much more rapid fall in serum fibrinogen and more instances of significant bleeding. Although this experience is limited, we do not currently use these higher dosages routinely.

We favor uniform use of concomitant heparinization based on the surgical experience that patients treated with systemic heparinization as part of their treatment of ALLI, have both lower amputation and mortality rates.[21,45,56] Furthermore, heparinization may reduce the probability of distal propagation of clot in major vessels of thrombus in small branch vessels. Extensive experience with fibrinolysis for acute myocardial infarction has demonstrated a lower incidence of reocclusion and death in patients treated conjunctively with aspirin and heparin during fibrinolytic infusions.[124-129] This may extrapolate to a lower incidence of both myocardial infarctions and peripheral reocclusions during and after the fibrinolytic treatment of ALLI if concomitant heparinization is performed.

Continued anticoagulation is not necessary if PIAT and subsequent PTA have provided sufficiently brisk blood flow. Systemic anticoagulation is continued in those patients with residual flow-limiting lesions until operative repair can be performed. In those instances, we usually leave a vascular sheath in place to prevent puncture site bleeding.

Surgery can be performed immediately after the cessation of PIAT. In our experience, the dosages of UK that we have used for PIAT (1000 to 4000 IU/min) have not disrupted the coagulation system to such a degree that significant bleeding has been encountered during operations performed within a few hours of PIAT.[81,104]

CONCLUSIONS

The proposition that PIAT has a role as the initial treatment for ALLI represents a major change in treatment. The introduction of the Fogarty device/procedure in 1963 led to its adoption as the most favored method of treating ALLI, despite considerable controversy over higher than expected morbidity, mortality, and amputation rates. Much of the controversy stems from the lack of uniformity in classifying the degree of clinical ischemia and the angiographic findings. Without a uniform classification, efforts to sort out the appropriate role for each form of therapy are doomed to failure because of the inadvertent blending together of different degrees of ischemia and extent of vascular occlusion.

There is a persistent belief that only a narrow window of opportunity of 6 to 8 hours is available to the surgeon in which to perform thromboembolectomy or reconstructive surgery based primarily on animal work done by Dunant and Edwards in 1963.[75] Their demonstration of the detection of spontaneous thrombosis of distal muscular and skin vessels as early as 8 hours after occlusion of the femoral arteries has been used to justify the emergency performance of thromboembolectomy because of fear of "no reflow," despite successful removal of clot from the major arteries. Omitted from this interpretation of that experiment is that small vessel thrombosis was never seen unless *both* the femoral artery and *all* the collaterals were occluded. Furthermore, the process was only beginning at 8 hours and required 24 hours for progressive obliteration of the entire small vessel bed.

In most patients with ALLI who have open collaterals supplying angiographically visible vessels distal to the occlusion, our experience indicates that the time limit of 6 hours does not pertain. It is more reliable to select patients for thrombolysis on the basis of the combination of their sensorimotor examination and their angiographic pattern than simply on the duration of symptoms.

Just as the indiscriminate use of emergency surgery for all instances of ALLI is inappropriate, we believe that PIAT should not be used indiscriminately in this clinical setting. Treatment should be individualized. The technique, dose of thrombolytic agent, time between catheter manipulations, and extent of concomitant heparinization should be based on the patient's degree of clinical ischemia and pattern of vascular occlusion.[116] The most efficacious combination of those variables will be determined only with the consistent use of agreed-on classifications of the different degrees of clinical ischemia and the reporting of the pattern of the underlying extent of vascular occlusion.[82,129]

ALLI remains a serious threat for both life and limb, despite almost a century of evolving treatment methods. The Fogarty procedure/device is a marvelous advance, but it is far from a panacea. It would appear to be most efficacious at removing embolic occlusions from relatively normal arteries between the origin of the iliacs and the origin of the trifurcation vessels. However, an increasing preponderance of acute occlusions are due to spontaneous in situ thrombosis superimposed on atherosclerosis, the patient group in which the results with balloon-catheter clot extraction are the least promising and in which this mode of treatment is associated with the highest mortality. In our experience, PIAT does well in this group of occlusions.[81]

PIAT offers the potential for relatively rapid, but not sudden, removal of all clot without trauma to the vessel and with a low mortality rate. It may yield a lower amputation rate. The apparent reduction in mortality in the elderly and those with RMI may make it most efficacious in those decidedly high-risk groups. Although controversial, the use of PIAT for embolic occlusions offers the potential for definitive therapy of the occlusion without the need for either subsequent PTA or surgery. In both thrombotic and embolic occlusions, PIAT extends the potential of endovascular therapy. Although the ultimate role and method of thrombolysis in ALLI have not been established, this modality offers considerable promise for a disease process that has remained difficult to treat.

Other regimens include 4000 IU/min after deposition of loading dose through the clot (lacing) before beginning the continuous infusion,[117] or continuous infusion with a higher dosage of 6000 IU/min (Graor RA, personal communication, 1992). The pulse spray technique uses 10,000 IU/min delivered with frequent, small bursts through special catheters[118,119] or larger volume boluses every few minutes via an end-hole catheter (Yamada R, personal communication, 1992). Advocates of pulse spray argue that lysis is hastened by better dispersion of drug through the clot and by the mechanical disruption of clot caused by the jet effect. Still others use continuous infusions of 1000 to 1500 IU/min to avoid a systemic fibrinolytic effect.[117] All investigators report approximately the same incidences of success, with the higher doses yielding earlier re-establishment of flow. Definitive comparisons between the various techniques are currently lacking. In general, those who use the lower doses perform fewer repeat angiograms and make catheter adjustments after longer time intervals than do those who use higher doses.

It is not surprising that virtually any dose of thrombolytic agent delivered directly into a fresh clot would effect fibrinolysis. It is my view that although higher doses will effect lysis more quickly, this must be coupled with infusion delivery techniques or systems that enable the higher dose of drug to maintain contact with the clot throughout the period of higher dose infusion, or else the higher dose will not yield faster lysis.[116] This impression is based upon extensive clinical experience plus numerous in vitro and in vivo animal experiments that demonstrate progressively faster lysis with higher doses of both UK and rtPA (Becker G, personal communication).[120-123] Accepting that as a premise, the question then becomes what is the best dose and technique to use. Adequate studies are not available to answer this question.

REFERENCES

1. Labey G, cited by Mosny M, Dumont MJ: Embolie fémorale au cours d'un rétrécissment mitral pur artériotomie. Guérison Bull Acad Med (Paris) 66:358, 1911

2. Lerman J, Miller FR, Lund CC: Arterial embolism and embolectomy. JAMA 94:1128, 1930

3. Keeley JL, Rooney JA: Retrograde milking; an adjunct in embolectomy. Ann Surg 184:1022, 1951

4. Shaw RS: A method for the removal of the adherent distal thrombus. Surg Gynecol Obstet 110:255, 1960

5. Oeconomos N: L'embolectomie retrograde; technique simplifié et résultats. J Chir pear 81:185, 1961

6. Fogarty TJ, Cranley JJ, Krause RJ et al: A method for extraction of arterial emboli and thrombi. Surg Gynecol Obstet 116:241, 1963

7. Fogarty TJ: Catheter technique for arterial embolectomy. J Cardiovasc Surg 8:22, 1967

8. Fogarty TJ, Dailey PO, Shumway NE, Krippaehne H: Experience with balloon catheter technique for arterial embolectomy. Am J Surg 122:231, 1971

9. Thompson JE: Acute peripheral arterial occlusions. N Engl J Med 290:950, 1974

10. Blaisdell FW, Lim RC, Amberg JR et al: Pulmonary microembolism. Arch Surg 93:776, 1966

11. Lim RC, Choy SH, Blaisdell FW et al: Massive pulmonary microembolism in regional shock. Surg Forum 27:14, 1966

12. Hardaway RM: Syndromes of Disseminated Intravascular Coagulation. p. 43. Charles C Thomas, Springfield, IL, 1966

13. McKay DG: Disseminated Intravascular Coagulation. p. 103. Harper & Row, New York, 1965

14. Hardaway RM, Chun B, Rutherford RB: Coagulation in shock in various species, including man. Acta Chir Scand 130:157, 1965

15. Robb HJ: The role of microembolism in the production of irreversible shock. Ann Surg 158:685, 1963

16. Hardaway RM, Brewster WR, Jr, Elovitz MJ: The influence of vasoconstriction and acidosis on disseminated intravascular coagulation. Surgery 59:804, 1966

17. Jackson BB: Venous aspiration as an adjunct in the management of late arterial embolectomy. Surgery 57:358, 1965

18. Stallone RJ, Blaisdell FW, Cafferata HT, Levin SM: Analysis of morbidity and mortality from arterial embolectomy. Surgery 65:207, 1969

19. Sterling GR, Morris KN, Officer Brown CJ, Barnett AJ: Arterial embolectomy. Med J Aust 2:255, 1963

20. Darling C, Austen WG, Linton R: Arterial embolism. Surg Gynecol Obstet 124:106, 1967

21. Holm J, Scherstén T: Anticoagulant treatment during and after embolectomy. Acta Chir Scand 138:683, 1972

22. Stallone J, Lim C, Blaisdell FW: Pathogenesis of pulmonary changes following ischemia of the lower extremities. Ann Thorac Surg 7:539, 1969

23. Deykin D: The role of the liver in serum-induced hypercoagulability. J Clin Invest 45:256, 1966

24. Gans H: Preservation of vascular patency as a function of reticuloendothelial clearance. Surgery 60:1216, 1966

25. Prose PH, Lee L, Balk SD: Electron microscopic study of the phagocytic fibrin-cleaning mechanism. Am J Pathol 47:403, 1965

26. Spaet TH: Studies on the in vivo behavior of blood coagulation product I in rats. Thromb Diath Haemorrh 8:276, 1962

27. Thomas DP, Bane JR: 5-Hydroxytryptamine in the circulation of the dog. Nature 216:335, 1967

28. Cierniewski CS, Poniatowski J, Urbanczyk J: The peptide of $B\beta1$-42 which increases microvascular permeability is released by plasmin during cleavage of fragment Y of fibrinogen. Biochim Biophys Acta 884:594, 1986

29. Golino P, Ashton JH, McNatt J et al: Simultaneous administration of thromboxane A_2-serotonin S_2-receptor antagonists markedly enhances thrombolysis and prevents or delays reocclusion after tissue-type plasminogen activator in a canine model of coronary thrombosis. Circulation 79:911, 1989

30. Martin S, Maruta K, Burkart V et al: IFN-gamma increase vascular permeability. Immunology 64:301, 1988

31. Bjork J, Headqvist P, Arfors KE: Increase in vascular permeability induced by leukotriene B_4 and the role of polymorphonuclear leukocytes. Inflammation 6:189, 1986

32. Royall JA, Berkow RL, Beckman JS et al: Tumor necrosis factor and interleukin 1 increase vascular endothelial permeability. Am J Physiol 257:L399, 1989

33. Garcia JGN, Azghani A, Caloahan KS, Johnson AR: Effect of platelet activating factor on leukocyte-endothelial cell interactions. Thromb Res 51:83, 1988

34. Rudd MA, George D, Amarante P et al: The temporal effects of thrombolytic agents on platelets function in vivo and the modulation of prostaglandins. Circ Res 67:1175, 1990

35. Haimovici H: Arterial embolism, myoglobinuria and renal tubular necrosis. Arch Surg 100:639, 1970

36. Freischlag J, Hanna D: Superoxide anion release (O_2^-) after ischemia and reperfusion. J Surg Res 50:565, 1991

37. Sweetman HE, Shepro D, Hechtman HB: Inhibition of thrombocytopenic petechiae by exogenous serotonin administration. Haemostasis 10:65, 1981

38. Shepro D, Wells SL, Hechtman HB: Vasoactive agonists prevent erythrocyte extravasation in thrombocytopenic hamsters. Thromb Res 35:421, 1984

39. Shepro D, Hechtman HB: Endothelial serotonin uptake and mediation of prostanoid secretion and stress fiber formation. Fed Proc 44:2616, 1985

40. Snyder DB, Campbell GS: Humoral effects of experimental crush syndrome. Surgery 47:217, 1960

41. Montagni CA, Simeone FA: Observations of the liberation and elimination of myohemoglobin and of hemoglobin at the release of muscle ischemia. Surgery 34:169, 1953

42. Winninger A: Consequences generales de la revascularisation après ischémie aigue des membres. Presse Med 77:1319, 1969

43. Fisher RD, Fogarty TJ, Morrow AG: Clinical and biochemical observations of the effect of transient femoral artery occlusion in man. Surgery 68:323, 1970

44. Provan JL, Frankel GJ, Austen WG: Metabolic and

hemodynamic changes after temporary aortic occlusion in dogs. Surg Gynecol Obstet 123:544, 1966

45. Blaisdell FW, Steele M, Allen RE: Management of acute lower extremity arterial ischemia due to embolism and thrombosis. Surgery 84:822, 1978

46. Eriksson J, Holmberg JT: Analysis of factors affecting limb salvage and mortality after embolectomy. Acta Chir Scand 143:237, 1977

47. Haimovici H: Myopathic-nephrotic-metabolic syndrome associated with massive acute arterial occlusions. J Cardiovasc Surg (Torino) 14:589, 1973

48. Abbott WM, McCabe C, Maloney RD, Wirthlin RS: Embolism of the popliteal artery. Surg Gynecol Obstet 159:533, 1984

49. Volmar J: Rekonstruktive Chirurgie der Arterien. p. 263. Thieme, Stuttgart, 1982

50. Balas P, Bonatsos G, Xeromeritis N et al: Early surgical results on acute arterial occlusions of the extremities. J Cardiovasc Surg (Torino) 26:262, 1985

51. Larcan A, Mathieu P, Hellmer J, Fieve G: Severe metabolic changes following delayed revascularization: Legrain-Cormier syndrome. J Cardiovasc Surg (Torino) 14:609, 1973

52. Littoy FN, Baker WH: Acute aortic occlusion—a multi-faceted catastrophe. J Vasc Surg 4:211, 1986

53. Baetz W, Brückner R: Symptomatik und therapie der aortenbifurkationsembolie. Chirurgie 56:166, 1985

54. Couch NP, Wheeler HB, Hyatt DF et al: Factors influencing limb survival after femoropopliteal reconstruction. Arch Surg 95:163, 1967

55. Bodily KC, Burgess EM: Contralateral limb and patient survival after leg amputation. Am J Surg 146:280, 1983

56. Abbott WM, Maloney RD, McCabe CC et al: Arterial embolism: a 44 year perspective. Am J Surg 143:460, 1982

57. Gordon D, Fogarty TJ: Peripheral arterial embolism. p. 449. In Rutherford RB (ed): Vascular Surgery. 2nd Ed. WB Saunders, Philadelphia, 1984

58. Fogarty TJ: Complications of arterial embolectomy. p. 95. In Beebe HG (ed): Complications in Vascular Surgery. Vol. 4. JB Lippincott, Philadelphia, 1973

59. McPhail MV, Fratesi SJ, Barber GG, Scobie TK: Management of acute thromboembolic limb ischemia. Surgery 93:381, 1983

60. Fogarty TJ: Management of arterial emboli. Surg Clin North Am 59:749, 1979

61. Cambria RP, Abbott WM: Acute arterial thrombosis of the lower extremity. Arch Surg 119:784, 1984

62. Jivegård L, Holm J, Scherstén T: The outcome in arterial thrombosis misdiagnosed as arterial embolism. Acta Chir Scand 152:251, 1986

63. Field T, Littoy FN, Baker WH: Immediate and long-term outcome of acute arterial occlusion of the extremities: the effect of added vascular reconstruction. Arch Surg 117:1156, 1982

64. Yeager RA, Moneta GL, Taylor LM et al: Surgical management of severe acute lower extremity ischemia. J Vasc Surg 15:385, 1992

65. Pearse HE, Jr: Embolectomy for arterial embolism of the extremities. Ann Surg 98:17, 1933

66. Danzis M: Arterial embolectomy. Ann Surg 98:249, 1933

67. Key E: Embolectomy in circulatory disturbances in the extremities. Surg Gynecol Obstet 36:309, 1923

68. Petitpierre M: Ueber embolektomie der extremitäte narterien. Dtsch Z Chir 210:184, 1928

69. Dschanelidze JJ: Embolektomie. Arch Klin Chir 149:55, 1927

70. Linton RR: Peripheral arterial embolism: a discussion of the post-embolic vascular changes and their relation to the restoration of circulation in peripheral embolism. N Engl J Med 224:189, 1941

71. Gregg RO, Chamberlain BE, Myers JK, Tyler DB: Embolectomy or heparin therapy for arterial emboli? Surgery 93:377, 1983

72. Fogarty TJ: Sudden arterial occlusion: surgical aspects. Cardiovasc Clin 3:173, 1971

73. Spencer FC, Eisman B: Delayed arterial embolectomy—a new concept. Surgery 55:64, 1964

74. Jivegård L, Holm J, Scherstén T: Acute limb ischemia due to arterial embolism or thrombosis: influence of limb ischemia vs. pre-existing cardiac disease on postoperative mortality rate. J Cardiovasc Surg 29:32, 1988

75. Dunant JH, Edwards WS: Small vessel occlusion in the extremity after various periods of arterial obstruction: an experimental study. Surgery 73:240, 1973

76. Mehl RL, Paul HA, Shorey W et al: Treatment of "toxemia" after extremity replantation. Arch Surg 89:871, 1964

77. Malette WG, Armstrong RG, Criscuolo D: A second mechanism in hypotension following release of abdominal aortic clamps. Surg Forum 14:292, 1964

78. Haimovici H, Moss CM, Veith FJ: Arterial embolectomy revisited. Surgery 78:409, 1975

79. Freund U, Romanoff H, Flomen Y: Mortality rate following lower limb embolectomy: causative factors. Surgery 77:201, 1975

80. Allermand H, Westergaard-Nielsen J, Nielsen OS: Lower limb embolectomy in old age. J Cardiovasc Surg 27:440, 1986

81. McNamara TO, Bomberger RA, Merchant RF: Intra-arterial urokinase as the initial therapy for acutely ischemic lower limbs. Circulation, suppl I. 83:I-106, 1991

82. McNamara TO: The correlation of the initial arteriographic pattern with clinical degree of ischemia and outcome in acute lower limb ischemia. Presented at the 75th Annual Meeting of the Radiological Society of North America, Dec. 1989, Chicago

83. Rutherford RB, Flanigan DP, Gupta SK et al: Suggested standards for reports dealing with lower extremity ischemia. J Vasc Surg 4:80, 1986

84. Schmidt-Neuerburg KP: Diagnose und differential-diagnose des kompartmentsyndroms. Langenbecks Arch Chir 358:221, 1982

85. Herman BE, Wallace HW, Gadboys HL, Litwak RS: Anterior curral syndrome as a complication of cardio-

pulmonary bypass. J Thoras Cardiovasc Surg 52:755, 1966

86. Lanz, Folgezastånde des kompartmensyndroms an den unteren extremitåten. Langenbecks Arch Chir 358:237, 1982

87. Rosato FE, Barker CF, Roberts B, Danielson GK: Subcutaneous fasciotomy—description of a new technique and instrument. Surgery 59:383, 1966

88. Beyersdorf F, Matheis G, Krüger S et al: Avoiding reperfusion injury after limb revascularization: experimental observations and recommendations for clinical application. J Vasc Surg 9:757, 1989

89. Rosencranz ER, Buckberg GD: Myocardial protection during surgical coronary reperfusion. J Am Coll Cardiol I:1235, 1983

90. Buckberg GD: Studies of controlled reperfusion after ischemia. I. When is cardiac muscle damaged irreversibly? J Thorac Cardiovasc Surg 92:483, 1986

91. Allen BS, Okamoto F, Buckberg GD: Studies of controlled reperfusion after ischemia. XV. Immediate functional recovery after six hours of regional ischemia by careful control of conditions of reperfusion and composition of reperfusate. J Thorac Cardiovasc Surg 92:621, 1986

92. Dietze G, Wicklmayer M, Mayer L: Evidence for a participation of the Kallikrein-Kinin system in the regulation of muscle metabolism during hypoxia. Hoppe-Seylers Z Physiol Chem 358:633, 1977

93. Randle PJ, Smith GH: Regulation of glucose uptake by muscle. The effect of insulin, anaerobiosis, and cell poisons on the uptake of glucose and release of potassium by isolated rat diaphragm. Biochem J 70:490, 1958

94. Newsholme EA, Randle PJ: Regulation of glucose uptake by muscle. V. Effects of anoxia, insulin, adrenalin, and prolonged starving on concentrations of hexosphosphates and isolated rat diaphragm and perfused isolated hearts. Biochem J 80:655, 1961

95. Falholt K, Falholt W: Metabolism in ischemic muscle before and after treatment with glucose-insulin-potassium infusions. Acta Med Scand, suppl. 687:77, 1984

96. Idström JP, Rennie MJ, Scherstén T, Bylund-Fellenius AC: Membrane transport in relation to net uptake of glucose in the perfused rat hind limb. Stimulatory effect of insulin, hypoxia, and contractile activity. Biochem J 233:131, 1986

97. McNamara TO, Fischer JR: Thrombolysis of peripheral arterial and graft occlusions: improved results using high-dose urokinase. AJR 144:769, 1985

98. Belkin M, Belkin B, Bucknam CA et al: Intraarterial fibrinolytic therapy: efficacy of streptokinase vs. urokinase. Arch Surg 121:679, 1986

99. Gardiner GA, Loktun W, Kandarpa K et al: Thrombolysis of occluded femoropopliteal grafts. AJR 147:621, 1986

100. van Breda A, Katzen BT, Deutsch AS: Urokinase versus streptokinase in local thrombolysis. Radiology 165:109, 1987

101. Bell WR: Update on urokinase and streptokinase: a comparison of their efficacy and safety. Hosp Formul 23:230, 1988

102. McNamara TO: Technique and results of "higher-dose" infusion. Cardiovasc Intervent Radiol 11:548, 1988

103. Tennant SN, Dixon J, Venable TC et al: Intracoronary thrombolysis in patients with acute myocardial infarction: comparison of the efficacy of urokinase with streptokinase. Circulation 69:756, 1984

104. Meyerovitz MF, Goldhaber SZ, Reagan K et al: Recombinant tissue-type plasminogen activator versus urokinase in peripheral arterial and graft occlusions: a randomized trial. Radiology 175:75, 1990

105. Edwards WD: Aneurysms and mural thrombi of the left ventricle. Mayo Clin Proc 56:129, 1981

106. Kremer P, Fiebig R, Tilsner V et al: Lysis of left ventricular thrombi with urokinase. Circulation 72:112, 1985

107. Wilhelmsen L, Svärdsudd K, Korsan-Bengsten K, Larsson B, Welin L, Tibblin G. Fibrinogen as a risk factor for stroke and myocardial infarction. N Engl J Med 311:501, 1984

108. Fong H, Downs A, Lye C, Morrow I: Low-dose streptokinase infusion therapy of peripheral arterial occlusions and occluded vein grafts. Can J Surg 29:259, 1986

109. Kakkasseril JS, Cranley JJ, Arbaugh JJ et al: Efficacy of low-dose streptokinase in acute arterial occlusion and graft thrombosis. Arch Surg 120:427, 1985

110. Seeger JM, Flynn TC, Quintessenza JA: Intraarterial streptokinase in the treatment of acute arterial emboli. Surg Gyn Obstet 164:303, 1987

111. Battey PM, Fulenwider JT, Smith RB III et al: Intraarterial thrombolysis for acute limb ischemia: a three year experience. South Med J 80:479, 1987

112. Berni GA, Bandyk DF, Zierler RE et al: Streptokinase treatment of acute arterial occlusion. Ann Surg 198:185, 1983

113. Rush DS, Gewertz BL, Lu CT et al: Selective infusion of streptokinase for arterial thrombosis. Surgery 93:828, 1983

114. Hargrove WC III, Barker CF, Berkowitz HD et al: Treatment of acute peripheral arterial and graft thromboses with low-dose streptokinase. Surgery 92:981, 1982

115. Taylor LM, Jr, Porter JM, Baur GM et al: Intraarterial streptokinase infusion for acute popliteal and tibial artery occlusion. Am J Surg 147:583, 1984

116. McNamara TO, Gardner K: Coaxial system improves thrombolysis of ischemia. Diagn Imaging 8:122, 1991

117. Sullivan KL, Gardiner GA, Shapiro MJ, Levin D: Acceleration of thrombolysis with a high-dose transthrombus bolus technique. Radiology 173:805, 1989

118. Valji K, Roberts AC, Davis GB, Bookstein JJ: Pulsed-spray thrombolysis of arterial and bypass graft occlusions. AJR 156:617, 1991

119. Mewissen MW, Minor PL, Beyer GA, Lipchik EO: Symptomatic native arterial occlusions: early experience with "over-the-wire" thrombolysis. JVIR 1:43, 1990

120. Collen D, Stassen JM, Verstraete M: Thrombolysis with human extrinsic (tissue-type) plasminogen activator in rabbits with experimental jugular vein thrombosis: effect of molecular form and dose of activator, age of the thrombus, and route of administration. J Clin Invest 71:368, 1983

121. Korninger C, Matsuo O, Suy R et al: Thrombolysis with human extrinsic (tissue-type) plasminogen activator in dogs with femoral vein thrombosis. J Clin Invest 69:573, 1982

122. Matsuo O, Rijken DC, Collen D: Comparison of the relative fibrinogenolytic, fibrinolytic, and thrombolytic properties of tissue plasminogen activator and urokinase in vitro. Thromb Haemost 45:225, 1981

123. Walker JE, Flook V, Ogston D: An artificial circulation for the study of thrombolysis. Acta Hematol 69:41, 1983

124. ISIS-2 Study Group: Randomized trial of intravenous streptokinase, oral aspirin, both, or neither among 17,187 cases of suspected myocardial infarction: ISIS-2. Lancet 2:349, 1988

125. The Scati Group: Randomized controlled trial of subcutaneous calcium-heparin in acute myocardial infarction. Lancet 2:182, 1989

126. Bleich SD, Schumacher RR, Cooke DH et al: Effect of heparin on coronary arterial patency after thrombolysis with tissue plasminogen activator in acute myocardial infarction. Am J Cardiol 66:1412, 1990

127. Hsia J, Hamilton WP, Kleiman NS et al: A comparison between heparin and low-dose aspirin as adjunctive therapy with tissue plasminogen activator for acute myocardial infarction. N Engl J Med 323:1433, 1990

128. Sobel BE, Hirsch J: Principles and practice of coronary thrombolysis and conjunctive treatment. Am J Cardiol 68:382, 1991

129. de Bono DP, Simoons ML, Tijssen J et al, for the European Cooperative Study Group: Early intravenous heparin improves coronary patency in thrombolysis with recombinant tissue-type plasminogen activator. Br Heart J 67:122, 1992

21

Acute Limb Ischemia Resulting from Graft Failure

Harold J. Welch
Michael Belkin

Graft failure may result from a variety of etiologies and requires the surgeon and interventional radiologist to combine their skills, judgment, and experience to provide the best outcome for the patient. As surgical techniques advance and indications for surgery broaden, there will be more patients at risk of graft occlusion. The saying that "an ounce of prevention is worth a pound of cure" is well taken for vascular grafts, in that it is well documented that revision of a failing graft results in higher patency rates than thrombectomy of an occluded graft.[1] Close, frequent follow-up of all grafts to the lower extremity, with physical examination and noninvasive studies, may provide evidence that a graft is in jeopardy. Despite even the most rigorous postoperative surveillance, grafts may fail unexpectedly. This will usually result with recrudescence of ischemic symptoms and often limb-threatening ischemia, mandating urgent intervention. The many types of bypass grafts and graft materials have generated a myriad of opinions and techniques on how to re-establish flow when they occlude.

DIAGNOSIS

Graft thrombosis may manifest in a number of ways. Early failure usually results in acute ischemia, with a cold, mottled, pulseless extremity, often worse than the preoperative state. Physical examination and Doppler assessment by an experienced examiner are usually all that are necessary to confirm the diagnosis. Failure of a graft in the late postoperative period may manifest with a wide spectrum of symptoms, ranging from negligible to limb-threatening ischemia. Gradual graft failure, for example, from vein valve fibrosis, may allow for the development of extensive collateral flow. Thus, the patient may present with the mild symptoms of claudication, coolness, mild pain, or the formation of new superficial ischemic ulcers. Acute late failure will usually produce limb-threatening ischemia, which requires prompt recognition. Patient recognition of the signs and symptoms of graft failure is an important tool in the post-operative surveillance protocol. Patients are instructed to seek immediate attention if symptoms of graft occlusion occur. Early intervention to restore flow in occluded grafts has been shown to be more successful than later attempts.[2-4]

Diminution of pulses, decreased Doppler signals and ankle-brachial index, and pulsed volume waveforms are usually diagnostic of the failing graft. Duplex scan examination is often helpful, and in those cases in which urgent invasive therapy is unnecessary, may be the test of choice. Arteriography is indicated to determine the optimal management strategy for those patients with recurrent ischemia for which intervention will eventually be required. In addition to its diagnostic value, it may allow for potential therapeutic intervention with thrombolytic drugs and percutaneous transluminal angioplasty (PTA).

ETIOLOGY

The etiology of graft occlusion characteristically varies with the interval from operation to thrombosis (Fig. 21-1.) Occlusions that occur within the first 30 days of surgery are generally attributable to errors of operative technique (i.e., judgmental or technical errors). These include graft kinking or twisting, clamp injuries, anastomotic defects, inadequate flushing of clots from the graft, use of inadequate venous conduit, and intimal flaps. In some cases, early graft thrombosis may be due to graft surface thrombogenicity or hypercoagulable states. Other early graft failures may be due to low flow states from inadequate inflow or outflow. Grafts that fail from 30 days to 2 years postoperatively characteristically do so as a result of neointimal hyperplastic lesions. Healing of the arterial lumen after reconstruction (whether it be endarterectomy, valve lysis, or bypass anastomosis) is a normal response to injury. A hyperplastic response is responsible for 19 to 55 percent of intermediate graft failures,[5,6] although these lesions may be responsible for even later failures.[1,5,7] This may occur at either anastomosis with vein or synthetic grafts, and anywhere along the length of autogenous vein grafts. The hyperplastic lesions are white, firm, and fibrotic on gross inspection, usually appearing within 6 months of surgery (Fig. 21-2).

From experimental work on animal models, much has been learned about the vascular hyperplastic response, though many questions remain unanswered. It appears that intimal hyperlasia is dependent on smooth muscle cell proliferation and migration, and matrix deposition, which is regulated by a number of both stimulatory and inhibitory factors from the blood, leukocytes, and vascular wall cells. The process is explained in detail in Chapter 3, and synopsized in Figure 21-3.

Thrombosis of an anastomotic aneurysm can also lead to intermediate and late graft failure. Failure of grafts beyond 2 years is characteristically due to the progression of distal atherosclerotic disease, which limits outflow and ultimately leads to graft occlusion.

Aortofemoral Grafts

Aortofemoral graft limb occlusion may affect up to 15 to 30 percent of patients if followed up to 10 years after surgery,[8–12] with early thrombosis (< 30 days) accounting for 18 to 28 percent of overall graft failure in reported series.[2,13] The most common interval for aortic graft failure is within the range of 24 to 36 months. This is usually due to fibrointimal hyperlasia at or just distal to the femoral anastomosis, typically in the profunda femoris orifice. Graft infection, although rarely leading to occlusion, does usually require removal of the graft, and can be considered to be a cause of graft failure. Fortunately, it is rare, occurring in about 1 to 2

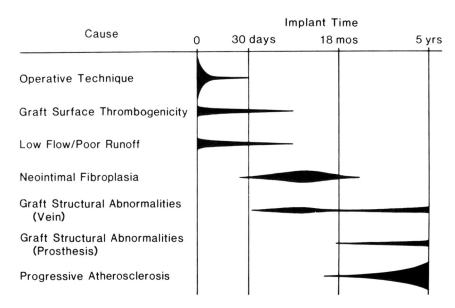

Figure 21-1 Etiology of graft failure temporally related to graft insertion. (From Rutherford,[71] with permission.)

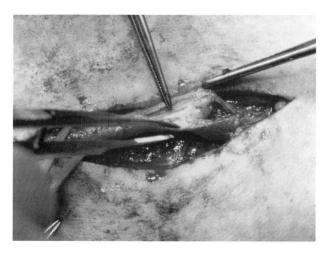

Figure 21-2 Intimal hyperplastic lesion at valve site in a reversed saphenous vein femoropopliteal bypass.

percent of published series.[14-16] Graft infection may become manifest at any time after implantation, but most occur within 2 to 5 years after implantation.[17] Mortality rates for this formidable complication range from 25 percent to 75 percent and amputations occur in approximately 30 percent of patients.[14-16,18-22]

Axillofemoral Grafts

Extra-anatomic bypass grafts, usually placed in the high-risk patient, may occlude for a number of reasons. Unrecognized inflow problems may contribute to early occlusions. For this reason, Calligaro et al.[23] recommend arteriography of the subclavian and axillary arteries to avoid originating a graft distal to a severe stenosis. Others believe that physical examination and blood pressure measurements are the only necessary confirmation of adequate inflow.[24] A triphasic brachial Doppler signal, which we rely on, also indicates normal inflow.

Proper configuration of the graft is felt to be essential in maintaining high patency rates. O'Donnell and co-workers[25] and others[26-28] advocate the "common hood" for the femorofemoral limb (Fig. 21-4A). Not only does this eliminate a low flow segment of the graft, as is the case with other configurations, such as the "lazy S," but it allows for thrombectomy of both limbs through one graftotomy (Fig. 21-4B). The axillary artery anastomosis should be performed as close to the chest wall as possible, generally in the segment of artery between the pectoralis minor muscle tendon and the clavicle. This will limit traction on the anastomosis caused by movement of the arm, thereby preventing kinking or disruption of the anastomosis, leading to bleeding or pseudoaneurysm formation. In addition, the axillofemoral tunnel should follow a gentle curve, in the mid-axillary line to just medial to the anterior iliac spine, and the graft pulled relatively taut through the tunnel, so as to prevent kinking when the patient sits up (Fig. 21-5).

Graft compression is widely thought to be a major factor in axillofemoral graft failure. Although this may have been a factor prior to externally supported grafts, several recent studies have shown excellent patency rates with externally supported grafts.[26,29] We recently demonstrated that external graft compression did not change graft flow velocity as measured by Duplex scanning, nor did it effect the ankle-brachial indices.[30] Additionally, in our laboratory, we found externally supported ePTFE grafts to be five times more resistant to an external compressive force compared to thin-walled ePTFE or knitted Dacron (Welch HJ, Pontoriero M, Xhang X, O'Donnell TF: unpublished data). A possible explanation for the observation that these grafts occlude during sleep is a decrease in cardiac output and graft flow. A review of the literature does not support any significant difference in patency rates between PTFE and Dacron in axillofemoral grafts.[25]

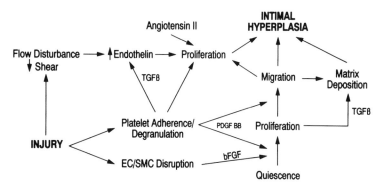

Figure 21-3 Factors contributing to intimal hyperplasia.

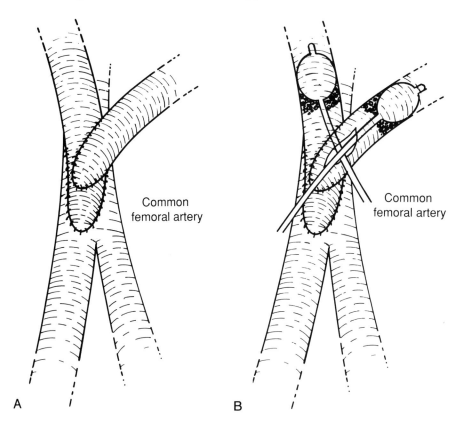

Figure 21-4 **(A)** Preferred configuration of the axillobifemoral graft in the groin. There is no "isolated" low-flow segment of the graft and blood flow hemodynamics do not cause decreased pressures in the contralateral leg. **(B)** Common hood allows for thrombectomy of both limbs of the graft through one graftotomy.

Infrainguinal Grafts

Polytetrafluoroethylene Grafts

Although it is well documented that ePTFE grafts have lower patency rates for infrainguinal bypass than autogenous saphenous vein (ASV), they generally remain the graft material of choice when vein is not available. Patency rates for ePTFE and ASV grafts to the popliteal artery are comparable for approximately $2\frac{1}{2}$ years, after which the ePTFE grafts showed decreased patency. At 4 years, ASV grafts had a 68 percent patency rate, while the ePTFE grafts only a 38 percent patency rate, a statistically significant difference. This difference was most pronounced in the below-knee grafts.[31] Bypass patency to the infrapopliteal vessels is significantly improved using autogenous vein, which has a 49 percent 4-year patency rate compared with a 12 percent patency rate with PTFE grafts.[31]

Early failure (< 1 month) accounts for approximately 25 percent of ePTFE graft failures. While mechanical problems of the graft itself are rare, kinking or tunneling problems may occur. Like all prosthetic conduits, thrombogenicity is increased in low-flow states,[32] which may be present with restricted runoff or congestive heart failure. Veith et al.[33] could not find a cause of graft thrombosis in 41 percent of their early ePTFE failures. Late failure is due to intimal hyperplasia (19 to 21 percent), progression of distal disease (37 to 64 percent), inflow disease (12 to 17 percent), and technical or unknown causes (31 percent).[6,34] Unexplained graft failure should prompt screening for hypercoagulability. Many vascular surgeons will place patients on warfarin after restoring patency to a previously thrombosed prosthetic graft.

Vein Grafts

Early occlusions account for 3 to 16 percent of vein graft failures.[35-39] Those that remain open beyond the perioperative period have a 3-year patency rate of 74 to 80 percent and a 5-year cumulative patency rate of 62 to 82 percent. As delineated in Figure 21-1, a technical cause of early vein graft failure may range from 14 to 100 percent.[35-40] Particular to in situ vein grafts are retained valves and valvulotome injuries. Retained

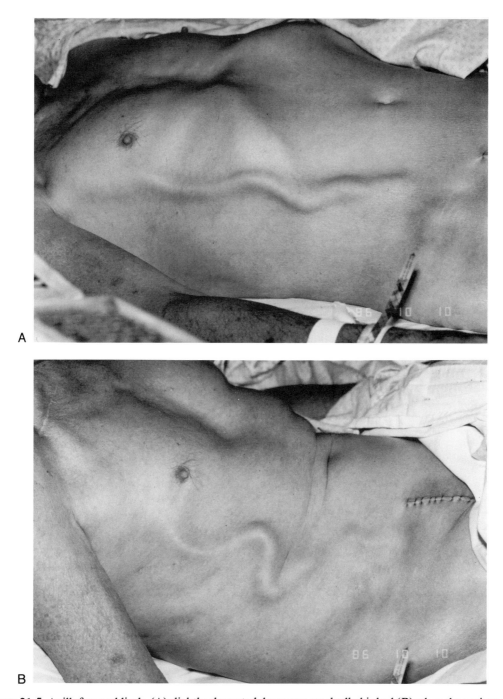

Figure 21-5 Axillofemoral limb, (**A**) slightly elongated, becomes markedly kinked (**B**) when the patient sits up. (Courtesy of Anthony Whittemore, M.D.)

valves accounted for 31 percent of early graft failure at our institution.[41] Donaldson et al.[42] reported a 4 percent incidence of retained valve leaflets and an 11 percent incidence of valvulotome injury leading to in situ graft failure. As with other grafts, the predominant cause of intermediate failure is myointimal hyperplasia, either at the anastomosis, or at valve sites. Figure 21-6 is a scanning electron micrograph of a typically tattered valve leaflet disrupted with a valvulotome, which when repaired and thickened during the healing process, can result in a stricture. Leather et al.[43] noted that postoperative stenotic lesions occurred in their in situ venous bypasses primarily at valve sites. We also found the majority (54 percent) of intermediate and

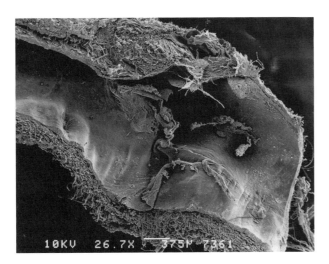

Figure 21-6 Scanning electron micrograph of a dog greater saphenous vein valve disrupted with a Mills valvulotome.

late in situ graft failures were secondary to intrinsic graft lesions.[5] In Bandyk's series, 52 percent of their failing grafts were found to have problems involving the in situ conduit,[37] and Whittemore et al reported that the most probable cause of vein graft failure was due to lesions within the graft.[1] Stept et al.[40] found that three of eight early vein graft failures were due to mid-graft valves, with intimal flaps at the anastomoses also responsible for three of eight failures. Beyond 2 years after surgery, progressive atherosclerosis in the distal outflow tract is responsible for most vein graft failures.

MANAGEMENT

The approach to the failed graft must be a flexible one. The patient with minimal symptoms and absence of tissue loss may require no further intervention.[44] Occasional patients who are deemed nonreconstructable may tolerate relative ischemia for several years before amputation is eventually necessary.[5] The asymptomatic patient with graft failure, however, is uncommon. Most patients whose graft has failed have recurrence of their ischemic symptoms and will require aggressive intervention. Arteriography should be performed to delineate the potential cause of the failure, and to delineate outflow vessels for possible reconstruction. Balloon occlusion arteriography, where inflow to the leg is occluded by a balloon catheter, followed by contrast injection distal to the balloon, is used extensively at our institution with excellent results.

Rarely, the patient will present with a critically ischemic, threatened limb and should be taken directly to the operating room. Arteriography and thrombolytic therapy would only prolong the ischemia time to the leg and decrease the chance for a successful outcome. Optimal surgical management of the ischemic limb is controversial. While most surgeons and patients would opt for an aggressive attempt at limb salvage with revascularization, others believe that amputation and early prosthetic rehabilitation will provide the best outcome for the patient.[45] Many factors enter the decision-making process, including the likelihood of successful revascularization, the potential for rehabilitation, the ambulatory status of the patient, and the anticipated life expectancy of the patient.

Early failure of any graft is almost always the result of a technical error and is best corrected in the operating room. The proximal and distal anastomoses are exposed; thrombectomy of the graft, and native vessels if necessary, is performed. Intraoperative angioscopy or arteriography is then done to identify and evaluate the cause of the graft failure, if it is not otherwise readily apparent. Graft failure beyond 30 days may result from several factors; the approach to revascularization varies with each type of graft.

Aortofemoral Grafts

Occlusion of an aortofemoral graft limb, or rarely the entire graft, presents a myriad of management options to the surgeon. Observation, thrombectomy, extra-anatomic reconstruction, graft replacement, and thrombolytic therapy are all potential choices, after thorough appraisal of the clinical situation. Variables entering into the decision-making process include the degree of limb ischemia, the associated medical risk factors, the experience of the surgeon or the interventional radiologist or both, and the presumed cause of the graft occlusion. All these factors indicate that there is no uniform procedure to reestablish graft flow; each case must be approached on its own merits.

Unless the patient's limb is acutely threatened from critical ischemia, biplanar arteriography is extremely helpful in the management of aortic graft thrombosis. If only one limb of the graft is occluded, arteriography can be performed through the contralateral groin. Direct graft puncture can be safely done with minimal complications. If there are no femoral pulses, the axillary, brachial, or translumbar approach can be used, depending on the radiologist's preference and experience. Arteriography is useful in evaluating the proximal anastomosis for thrombus, kinks, pseudoaneurysm, or progressive atherosclerotic disease. The aorta above the anastomosis should be visualized as a potential inflow source. Outflow vessels should be sought, but may not be seen if there is little collateral flow.

In most instances of unilateral limb occlusion, graft limb thrombectomy will be successful. Thrombectomy of the graft limb has been shown to be effective in both early and late occlusions.[3,46,47] Using the previous incision, the native femoral vessels and the hood of the graft are exposed and controlled. After heparinization, a longitudinal incision is made in the hood of the graft, and balloon thrombectomy catheters are passed proximally in the graft. Thrombus is usually retrieved, and good inflow reestablished after several passes. There may be pseudointima or organized thrombus adherent to the wall of the graft which continue to impede inflow. In this circumstance, loop endarterectomy strippers may be used in conjunction with balloon catheters as described by Ernst and Daugherty.[48] This technique has proved very effective at removing the endothelialized plug and maintaining long-term patency[46] (Fig. 21-7). The new wire thrombectomy catheters, designed to remove adherent clots, may also prove to useful in this situation.

Most late occlusions are associated with outflow problems, primarily progression of disease at the profunda orifice. Thrombectomy combined with profundaplasty has been used with excellent success, and is considered the procedure of choice by many.[3,46,47] Bernhard et al.[3] had an early 97 percent graft patency following thrombectomy, while Brewster et al.[47] reported 100 percent success with early occlusions and 95 percent success with late limb occlusions. Thrombectomy is a low risk procedure that can be used on repeated occasions if necessary.

Extra-anatomic grafting is an alternative method of providing inflow to an ischemic leg after aortofemoral graft failure. The simplest method is a femorofemoral crossover graft. Provided there is normal inflow on the donor side, the proximal anastomosis can be made over the graft hood, the common femoral artery, or over the profunda orifice if necessary to improve the outflow on the donor side. Generally a 6-mm or 8-mm ringed ePTFE graft is used for the bypass, and the tunnel is

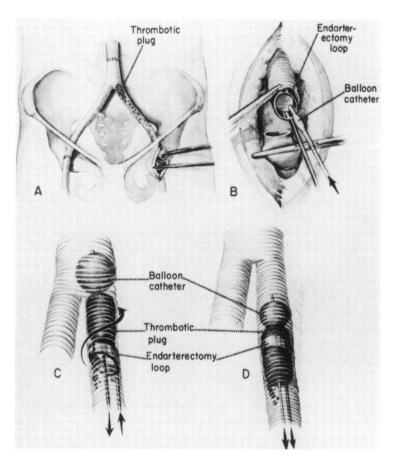

Figure 21-7 Technique of removing a thrombotic plug from an occluded aortofemoral graft limb. **(A)** Occluded graft limb is transected. **(B)** Loop endarterectomy stripper with balloon catheter inserted through loop is introduced up the transected occluded limb. **(C)** Balloon catheter snugged down as loop stripper clears the adherent thrombotic plug. Vector arrows indicate direction of manipulation. **(D)** The catheter, loop stripper, and thrombotic plug are removed as one. (From Ernst and Daugherty,[48] with permission.)

made with blunt finger dissection, so the graft will lie in a gentle inverted U, coursing superior to the pubic bone. The recipient anastomosis is determined according to the outflow. If the superficial femoral artery is patent, then the anastomosis is placed on the distal common femoral artery. If the superficial femoral artery is diseased, the anastomosis should be directed down the proximal profunda. When infection is present in the groin, the SFA or profunda must be approached through clean noninfected tissue planes. Femorofemoral bypass for aortobifemoral graft failure has a high early patency rate and acceptable late patency rates.[13,49]

Axillofemoral bypass is rarely indicated for unilateral aortofemoral graft limb failure; however, an axillobifemoral bypass is an acceptable option for complete graft failure. This procedure has been shown to have good patency rates and is appropriate in the high-risk patient.

For the patient who has occluded the entire aortic graft and who is a good surgical risk, replacement of the entire graft is often the favored option. Aortic inflow will provide the best long-term patency. If there is enough of a cuff of infrarenal aorta, the proximal anastomosis can be performed at this level. If not, an excellent alternative is the usually nonatherosclerotic descending thoracic aorta,[50-52] or supraceliac aorta.[53] In some instances, the native infrarenal aorta will have thrombosed above a low-lying proximal anastomosis up to the level of the renal arteries. When this occurs, suprarenal aortic control can be achieved and thrombectomy of the native infrarenal aorta performed. If the redo proximal anastomosis is done at the infrarenal aorta, a portion of the previous graft will need to be resected to allow the new graft to lay properly. Because of possible scarring of the ureters to the graft, care and judgement must be exercised in attempting to remove the femoral limbs of the graft. If there is any question, the limbs of the old graft should be left in place and the new graft limbs tunneled alongside them.

Thrombolytic therapy for aortobifemoral graft occlusion has not had widespread use. Transgraft hemorrhage, resulting from lysis of fibrin ingrowth during thrombolytic therapy, has been reported through knitted Dacron and PTFE grafts,[54-57] but is usually not significant. Most workers recommend against using lysis on these grafts if they occlude with several months of initial placement to decrease the likelihood of significant bleeding. McNamara et al.[58] recently reported on the use of intra-arterial urokinase for acutely ischemic lower limbs. They were able to successfully restore patency in 10 of 11 occluded Dacron aortobifemoral grafts, (presumably all unilateral occlusions), without significant transgraft bleeding.[58] Despite the reported success, most aortofemoral graft occlusions will need surgical correction for the cause of the failure, and thus routine use of thrombolytic therapy in this situation is not advocated. (For a detailed discussion of thrombolytic therapy, see Chs. 20 and 22.)

When outflow restriction is the primary cause of aortofemoral graft failure, as is usually the case with late occlusions, several options are available to restore adequate outflow. Profundaplasty, as previously discussed, is the most common and often the most direct method. Profundaplasty is achieved by several possible techniques. If the limb of the aortofemoral graft is anastomosed to the common femoral artery, the orifice of the profunda may be patched open. Saphenous vein, Dacron, PTFE, or an endarterectomized segment of occluded superficial femoral artery may be used for the patch. Conversely, the limb of the graft may be extended down the proximal profunda femoris artery, or a bypass to a more distal undiseased segment of PFA may be used (Fig. 21-8). When these simpler techniques do not optimize outflow, a bypass to the popliteal or tibial vessels may be necessary. Brewster and associates found that the addition of a distal bypass was necessary in 26 percent of initial reoperations for graft limb failure and in 53 percent of tertiary or greater procedures for occluded graft limbs.[2]

Infrainguinal Grafts

Vein Grafts

Vein graft failure during the perioperative period mandates a return to the operating room to correct the technical problem that is generally responsible for graft occlusion. The distal anastomosis should be exposed first, and a longitudinal arteriotomy made in the hood of the graft. This incision permits removal of local thrombus and direct inspection of the distal anastomosis. A balloon catheter (usually #3 or #4) is passed retrograde up the graft and the thrombus is gently extracted. Two or three passes are generally required to extract all the thrombus and restore arterial inflow. Often, thrombus extends into the distal arterial tree requiring distal thrombectomy with a #2 or #3 balloon catheter. If excellent inflow cannot be restored, further attempts at thrombectomy through an incision in the proximal vein graft hood must be undertaken. Incising the graft hood will allow inspection and evaluation of the proximal anastomosis. Upon successful thrombectomy, completion arteriography may identify a retained valve cusp, large arteriovenous fistula, valvulotome injury or twist in the graft, in addition to visualization of the distal arterial tree. Alternatively, visualization of the graft with the angioscope will often

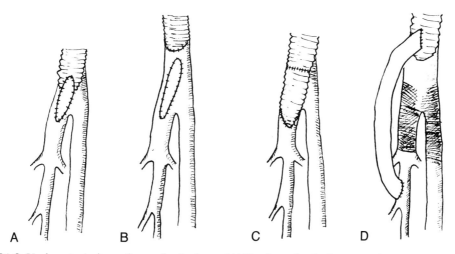

Figure 21-8 Various techniques for profundaplasty. **(A)** Patch profundaplasty crossing graft-artery anastomosis if graft onlay onto distal common femoral artery. **(B)** Patch of profunda femoris origin. Patch material can be vein, prosthetic, or endarterectomized superficial femoral artery. **(C)** Extension of graft onto profunda femoris. **(D)** Jump bypass from original graft to mid-profunda if profunda origin is occluded.

delineate subtle defects not visualized by arteriography. Embolization of plaque or platelet aggregates to distal vessels may have occluded outflow leading to graft thrombosis. If the small vessels of the distal arterial tree are occluded beyond the limits of the balloon catheter, intraoperative thrombolytic therapy may be used. There is no single clearly defined protocol for employing intraoperative thrombolytic infusion. Our protocol uses 250,000 units of urokinase reconstituted in 30 ml of normal saline; 10 ml is infused into the distal vessels, and inflow is occluded. After 10 to 15 minutes, inflow is restored to flush the distal vessels. This sequence is repeated twice more. Lack of improvement on the postlytic therapy angiogram has been shown to portend future graft rethrombosis and thus may require additional or alternative outflow procedures.[59]

As previously discussed, vein graft failure during the intermediate postoperative period is most often secondary to an intrinsic graft lesion. The defect must be identified in order to be corrected. The two options available to initially restore patency are thrombolysis and balloon thrombectomy. Balloon catheter thrombectomy of occluded grafts followed by vein patch has been shown by Whittemore et al.[1] to have a low 19 percent patency rate at 5 years, compared with a 86 percent 5-year cumulative patency rate for those failing grafts repaired with vein patch prior to occlusion. Several authors believe the endothelial trauma from the balloon stimulates intimal hyperplasia leading to subsequent graft failure.[60,61] (For a discussion of the role of thrombolysis in the management of occluded grafts, see Ch. 22.) It is important to note that thrombolytic

agents offer several theoretical advantages over the balloon catheter. Foremost is the lack of mechanical endothelial trauma produced by the balloon. If the clot is completely lysed, the follow-up arteriogram may identify the cause of the occlusion. If the cause of the graft failure is identified, this will enable more precise surgical or radiologic intervention. The thrombolytic agent may also leave less residual thrombus in the graft than balloon thrombectomy, and can also clear thrombus from distal runoff arteries. Lastly, in patients who have medical contraindications to surgery, thrombolytic therapy may permit for nonsurgical treatment.

Despite these theoretical advantages, thrombolytic therapy is most often a temporizing measure. When vein graft lesions are identified with thrombolytic therapy, and then subsequently treated, the long-term results are disappointing. Belkin et al.[4] showed there was a high rethrombosis rate, with patency rates of only 37 percent and 23 percent at 1 and 3 years, respectively. Similarly, Graor et al.[62] had an 18 percent patency rate at 1 year with thrombolysis. While early reports of balloon angioplasty for vein graft defects were encouraging, long-term follow-up of such treatment has been disappointing. Whittemore et al.[1] found only an 18 percent 4-year patency rate after PTA of 54 lesions in 30 patients. They did find a higher 3-year patency rate for grafts requiring a single PTA (59 percent patency) compared with those that required repeated dilatation (6 percent patency). Vein grafts initially treated with thrombolytic therapy and then with PTA had only an 11 percent 3-year patency, although this was not statistically different from those grafts whose lesions were angioplastied prior to graft occlusion (29 percent patency).[63] Others have noted better long-term results, however[64] (see Ch. 22).

Depending on the nature of the defect responsible for thrombosis, a variety of surgical interventions may be employed to revise the vein graft. These include patch angioplasty of a vein graft stenosis or anastomotic stenosis, a jump graft extension beyond the distal obstruction, a new bypass graft, or a profundaplasty. The options are dependent on several factors: the availability of vein, the patient's medical condition and life expectancy, and the experience of the surgeon. Bandyk et al.[65] reported the most success when the lesion was excised and treated with autologous tissue; a small number of grafts treated with PTA had high restenosis rates. If a *failing* graft is identified before thrombosis, high (85 percent) 5-year patency rates can often be achieved with simple vein patch angioplasty,[1] although others have had limited success with this option.[65] However, when actual thrombosis of the graft occurs, the long-term patency of the simpler procedures is disappointing. Secondary revascularization for infrainguinal graft failure also shows clear differences in conduit patency rates. Brewster et al.[44] reported a 5-year patency rate of 63 percent with autogenous veins and 18 percent with a variety of prosthetic devices. Green et al.[66] used prosthetic grafts for their new bypasses after failed grafts and had only a 22 percent patency rate at 4 years, no better than treatment by thrombectomy and angioplasty. Conversely, Edwards et al.[67] used autogenous reversed vein and achieved excellent 5-year primary and secondary patencies of 57 percent and 71 percent, respectively. Yang et al.[68] used PTFE in 73 secondary procedures for failed infrainguinal bypasses and

achieved a 55 percent secondary patency rate at 4 years, although these secondary grafts required aggressive follow-up and frequent reintervention. Bartlett et al.[69] investigated an aggressive surgical approach to failed infrainguinal bypasses. Most (87 percent) of their reoperative bypasses were done using PTFE and they achieved a 37 percent cumulative patency rate at 5 years.[69] Therefore, when a infrainguinal vein graft fails, and there is sufficient outflow, the optimal management is the insertion of an entirely new graft, preferably with autogenous vein.[4,44,66,67] Figure 21-9 shows patency results after intervention for failed vein grafts in selected series.

Our approach to vein graft failure beyond the perioperative period is outlined in the algorithm depicted in Figure 21-10. Very rarely have we been unable to identify usable autologous vein and thus resort to prosthetics only as a last option for secondary or tertiary reoperations.

Polytetrafluoroethylene Grafts

Direct operative intervention, with thrombectomy and revision, has been the most common approach in the management of failed PTFE infrainguinal grafts, although thrombolytic therapy has been employed by some authors. The rational for surgical thrombectomy is that the defect is usually at an anastomosis (most often the distal) and rarely (if ever) in the graft itself. In addition, the graft is not subject to mechanical damage by thrombectomy as may occur with a vein graft. Early failure requires a return to the operating room to correct the technical problem. If no discernible cause can be found, the patient should be screened for a

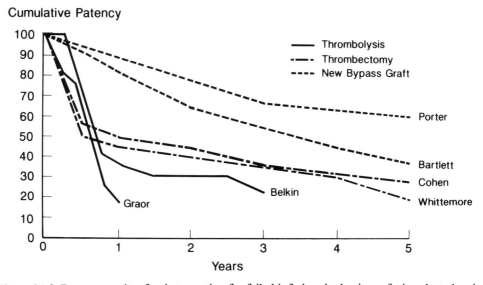

Figure 21-9 Patency results after intervention for failed infrainguinal vein grafts in selected series.

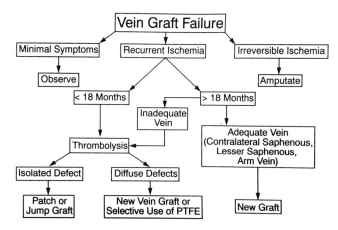

Figure 21-10 Treatment algorithm for failed infrainguinal vein grafts.

hypercoagulable state. Late graft failure can be treated with thrombectomy or thrombolytic therapy. We have had success with the use of urokinase in opening these grafts.[71] Most patients, however, will subsequently require surgical revision of the graft, usually at the distal anastomosis (Fig. 21-11). Ascer et al.[34] showed that treatment by patch angioplasty yields acceptable (52 percent at 3 years) long-term patency rates only in the femoral above-knee popliteal bypasses. In the femoral below-knee popliteal, or femoral distal bypass, graft salvage resulted in poor (13 to 15 percent) 3-year patency rates. New grafts to a more distal outflow site had 3-year patency rates of 39 to 48 percent.[34] Thus, when a below-knee PTFE graft fails, the optimal therapy is the insertion of a completely new bypass, preferably with vein, to a more distal outflow artery.

Extra-anatomic Grafts

As with other grafts, extraanatomic grafts that fail within the perioperative period must be returned to the operating room for correction of the likely technical problem. Like other prosthetic grafts, intimal hyperplasia at the anastomoses must be corrected by patch angioplasty, graft extension, or an entirely new graft. New inflow (e.g., contralateral axillary artery, supraceliac, or descending thoracic aorta) or outflow (e.g., profunda, popliteal) sources may be used, particularly if the indications for revascularization have changed. For instance, if an axillofemoral graft that was initially placed for treatment of an infected aortic graft subsequently fails, it may in turn be replaced by a thoracic aorta to femoral bypass, provided the patient is a good surgical risk. Because extra-anatomic grafts are often the last option when revascularization is necessary, failure of these grafts will frequently lead to amputation.

SUMMARY

Arterial grafts fail for a variety of reasons that are usually identifiable and temporally related to graft insertion. Technical mistakes, intimal hyperplasia, and progressive atherosclerosis are the most common mechanisms responsible for graft thrombosis. Throm-

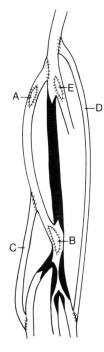

Figure 21-11 Available options for treatment of failed infrainguinal bypass graft. **(A)** Patch angioplasty of graft stenosis. **(B)** Patch angioplasty of outflow stenosis at distal anastomosis. **(C)** Jump graft to patent distal artery beyond occlusive disease in native vessels. **(D)** Entirely new bypass graft. **(E)** Profundaplasty to increase collateral flow if new bypass not feasible. (From Bernhard,[72] with permission.)

bolytic therapy has made great strides during the past decade but should be viewed as an adjunctive measure to restore graft patency, since almost all graft failures will need some type of further intervention. Thrombectomy, angioplasty, graft extension, and new bypasses remain the primary procedures for restoring blood flow to the ischemic limb. Until intimal hyperplasia and atherosclerosis can be controlled, careful follow-up and timely intervention are the best method of prolonging graft patency.

REFERENCES

1. Whittemore AD, Clowes AW, Couch NA, Mannick JA: Secondary femoropopliteal reconstruction. Ann Surg 193:35, 1981
2. Brewster DC, Meier GH III, Darling RC et al: Reoperation for aortofemoral graft limb occlusion: optimal methods and long-term results. J Vasc Surg 5:363, 1987
3. Bernhard VM, Ray LI, Towne JB: The reoperation of choice for aortofemoral graft occlusion. Surgery 82:867, 1977
4. Belkin M, Donaldson MC, Whittemore AD et al: Observations on the use of thrompolytic agents for thrombotic occlusion of infrainguinal vein grafts. J Vasc Surg 11:289, 1990
5. Nitzberg R, Coleman JA, Belkin M et al: The management of intermediate and late in situ saphenous vein bypass occlusions. Presented at the Eastern Vascular Society, May 1990, Boston
6. O'Donnell TF, Mackey WC, McCullough JL et al: Correlation of operative findings with angiographic and noninvasive hemodynamic factors associated with failure of polytetrafluoroethylene grafts. J Vasc Surg 1:136, 1984
7. Szilagyi DE, Elliot JP, Hageman JH et al: Biologic fate of autogenous vein implants as arterial substitutes: clinical, angiographic, and histopathologic observations in femero-popliteal operations for athersclerosis. Ann Surg 178:232, 1973
8. Crawford ES, Bomberger RA, Glaeser DH et al: Aorto-iliac occlusive disease: factors influencing survival and function following reconstructive operation over a 25-year period. Surgery 90:1055, 1981
9. Szilagyi DE, Elliot JP, Jr, Smith RF et al: A thirty-year survey of the reconstructive surgical treatment of aorto-iliac occlusive disease. J Vasc Surg 3:421, 1986
10. Malone JM, Moore WS, Goldstone J: The natural history of bilateral aortofemoral bypass grafts for ischemia of the lower extremities. Arch Surg 110:1300, 1975
11. Mulcare RJ, Royster TS, Lynn RA, Conners RB: Long-term results of operative therapy for aortoiliac disease. Arch Surg 113:601, 1978
12. Nevelsteen A, Suy R, Daenen W et al: Aortofemoral grafting: factors influencing late results. Surgery 88:642, 1980
13. LeGrand DR, Vermillion BD, Hayes JP, Evans WE: Management of the occluded aortofemoral graft limb. Surgery 93:818, 1983
14. O'Hara PJ, Hertzer NR, Beven EG, et al: Surgical management of infected abdominal aortic grafts: review of a 25-year experience. JVS 3:725, 1986
15. Goldstone J, Moore WS: Infection in vascular prosthesis: clinical manifestations and surgical management. Am J Surg 128:225, 1974
16. Jamieson GG, DeWeese JA, Rob CG: Infected arterial grafts. Ann Surg 181:850, 1975
17. Reilly LM, Stoney RJ, Goldstone J et al: Improved management of aortic graft infection: the influence of operation sequence and staging. J Vasc Surg 5:421, 1987
18. Lorentzen JE, Nielsen OM, Arendrup H et al: Vascular graft infection: an analysis of sixty-two graft infections in 2411 consecutively implanted synthetic vascular grafts. Surgery 98:81, 1985
19. Bunt TJ: Synthetic vascular graft infections. I. Graft infections. Surgery 93:733, 1983
20. Szilagyi DE, Smith RF, Elliott JP, Vradecic MP: Infection in arterial reconstruction with synthetic grafts. Ann Surg 176:321, 1972
21. Daugherty SH, Simmons RL: Infection in bionic man; the pathology on infections in prosthetic devices. Part 2. Curr Probl Surg 19:281, 1982
22. Reilly LM, Altman H, Lusby RJ et al: Late results following surgical management of vascular graft infection. J Vasc Surg 1:36, 1984
23. Calligaro KD, Ascer E, Veith FJ et al: Unsuspected inflow disease in candidates for axillofemoral bypass operations: a prospective study. J Vasc Surg 11:832, 1990
24. Taylor LM, Hamre D, Moneta GL et al: Axillobifemoral bypass. In Veith FJ (ed): Current Critical Problems in Vascular Surgery. Vol. 3. Quality Medical Publishing, St. Louis, 1991
25. Nitzberg RS, Welch HJ, O'Donnell TF et al: The influence of graft material on patency of axillofemoral grafts. p. 270. In Veith FJ (ed): Current Critical Problems in Vascular Surgery. Vol 3. Quality Medical Publishing, St. Louis, 1991
26. Harris EJ, Taylor LM, McConnell DB et al: Clinical results of axillobifemoral bypass using externally supported polytetrafluoroethylene. J Vasc Surg 12:416, 1990
27. Ray LI, O'Connor JB, Davis CC et al: Axillofemoral bypass: a critical reappraisal of its role in the management of aortoiliac occlusive disease. Am J Surg 138:117, 1979
28. Ward RE, Holcroft JW, Conti S, Blaisdell FW: New concepts in the use of axillofemoral bypass grafts. Arch Surg 118:573, 1983
29. Nitzberg RS, Prendiville E, O'Donnell TF et al: Does graft material and the status of outflow influence the patency of axillofemoral bypass? Presented at the Southern Association for Vascular Surgery, Jan. 24–27, 1989, Acopulco, Mexico
30. Welch HJ, Heggerick P, McLaughlin R et al: Duplex assessment of external compression of axillobifemoral

grafts. Presented at the Society of Vascular Technology, June 1991, Boston
31. Veith FJ, Gupta SK, Ascer E et al: Six-year prospective multicenter randomized comparison of autologous saphenous vein and expanded polytetrafluoroethylene grafts in infrainguinal arterial reconstructions. J Vasc Surg 3:104, 1986
32. Eldrup-Jorgensen J, Mackey WC, Connolly RJ et al: Evaluation of arterial prostheses in a baboon ex-vivo shunt: the effect of graft material and flow on platelet deposition. Am J Surg 150:185, 1985
33. Veith FJ, Gupta S, Daly V et al: Management of early and late thrombosis of the expanded polytetrafluoroethylene femoral popliteal bypass grafts: favorable prognosis with appropriate reoperation. Surgery 87:581, 1980
34. Ascer E, Collier P, Gupta SK, Veith FJ: Reoperation for polytetrafluoroethylene bypass failure: the importance of distal outflow site and operative technique in determining outcome. J Vasc Surg 5:298, 1987
35. Leather RP, Shah DM, Karmody AM: Infrapopliteal artery bypass for limb salvage: increased patency and utilization of the saphenous vein used in situ. Surgery 90:1000, 1981
36. Gruss JD, Bartels D, Vargas H et al: Arterial reconstruction for distal disease of the lower extremities by the in situ vein graft technique. J Cardiovasc Surg 23:231, 1982
37. Bandyk DF, Kalbrick HW, Stewart GW, Towne JB: Durability of the in situ saphenous vein bypass: a comparison of primary and secondary patency. J Vasc Surg 5:256, 1987
38. Donaldson MC: Lessons from initial experience with the in situ saphenous vein graft. Arch Surg 119:766, 1984
39. Dunton RF, Donovan TJ, Drezner AD et al: Early experience with in situ saphenous vein grafts for severe ischemia of the lower extremity. Surg Gynecol Obstet 158:472, 1984
40. Stept LL, Flinn WR, McCarthy WJ et al: Technical defects as a cause of early graft failure after femorodistal bypass. Arch Surg 122:599, 1987
41. Shoenfeld NA, O'Donnell TF, Bush HL et al: The management of early in situ saphenous vein bypass occlusions. Arch Surg 122:871, 1987
42. Donaldson MC, Mannick JA, Whittemore AD: Causes of primary graft failure after in-situ saphenous vein bypass. Presented at the Thirty-ninth Scientific Meeting of the ISCVS, June 1991, Boston
43. Leather RP, Shah DM, Corson JD, Karmody AM: Instrumental evolution of the valve incisions method of in situ saphenous vein bypass. J Vasc Surg 1:113, 1984
44. Brewster DC, LaSalle AJ, Robison JG et al: Femoropopliteal graft failures. Clinical consequences and success of secondary reconstructions. Arch Surg 118:1043, 1983
45. Stoney RJ: Ultimate salvage for the patient with limb-threatening ischemia. Am J Surg 136:228, 1978
46. Hyde GL, McCready RA, Schwartz RW et al: Durability of thrombectomy of occluded aortofemoral graft limbs. Surgery 94:748, 1983
47. Brewster DC, Meier GH III, Darling RC et al: Reoperation for aortofemoral graft limb occlusion: optimal methods and long term results. J Vasc Surg 5:363, 1987
48. Ernst CD, Daugherty ME: Removal of a thrombotic plug from an occluded limb of an aortofemoral graft. Arch Surg 113:301, 1978
49. Frisch N, Bour P, Berg P et al: Long-term results of thrombectomy for late occlusions of aortofemoral bypass. Ann Vasc Surg 5:16, 1991
50. Rosenfeld JC, Savarese RP, DeLaurentis DA: Distal thoracic aorta to femoral artery bypass; a surgical alternative. J Vasc Surg 2:747, 1985
51. McCarthy WJ, Rubin JR, Flinn WR et al: Descending thoracic aorta-to-femoral artery bypass. Arch Surg 121:681, 1986
52. Schultz RD, Sterpetti AV, Feldhaus RJ: Thoracic aorta as source of inflow in reoperation for occluded aortoiliac reconstruction. Surgery 100:635, 1986
53. Canepa CS, Schubart PJ, Taylor LM, Porter JM: Supraceliac aortofemoral bypass. Surgery 101:323, 1987
54. Rabe FE, Becker GJ, Richmond BD et al: Contrast extravasation through Dacron grafts: a sequela of low dose streptokinase therapy. AJR 138:917, 1982
55. Rosner NH, Dous PE: Contrast extravasation through Dacron grafts: a sequela of low dose streptokinase therapy. AJR 148:668, 1984
56. van Breda A, Robison JC, Feldman L et al: Local thrombolysis in the treatment of arterial graft occlusions. J Vasc Surg 1:103, 1984
57. Perler B, Kinnison M, Halden W: Transgraft hemorrhage: a serious complication of low dose thrombolytic therapy. J Vasc Surg 3:936, 1986
58. McNamara TO, Bomberger RA, Merchant RF: Intra-arterial urokinase as the initial therapy for acutely ischemic lower limbs. Circulation, [Suppl. I.] 83:I-106, 1991
59. Quinones-Baldrich WJ, Ziomek S, Henderson T et al: Intraoperative fibrinolytic therapy: experimental evaluation. J Vasc Surg 4:229, 1986
60. Dobrin PB: Mechanisms and prevention of arterial injuries caused by balloon embolectomy. Surgery 106:457, 1989
61. Bowles CR, Olcott C, Pakter RL et al: Diffuse arterial narrowing as a result of intimal proliferation: a delayed complication of embolectomy with the Fogarty balloon catheter. J Vasc Surg 7:487, 1988
62. Graor RA, Risius B, Young JR et al: Thrombolysis of peripheral arterial bypass grafts: surgical thrombectomy compared with thrombolysis. A preliminary report. J Vasc Surg 7:347, 1988
63. Whittemore AD, Donaldson MC, Polak JF, Mannick JA: Limitations of balloon angioplasty for vein graft stenosis. J Vasc Surg 14:340, 1991
64. Sullivan KL, Gardiner GA, Jr, Kandarpa K et al: Efficacy of thrombolysis in infrainguinal bypass grafts. Circulation, Suppl. I. 83:I99, 1991
65. Bandyk DF, Bergamini TM, Towne JB et al: Durability of vein graft revision: the outcome of secondary procedures. J Vasc Surg 13:200, 1991
66. Green RM, Ouriel K, Ricotta JJ, DeWeese JA: Revision

of failed infrainguinal bypass graft: principles of management. Surgery 100:646, 1986

67. Edwards JE, Taylor LM, Porter JM: Treatment of failed lower extremity bypass with new autogenous vein bypass grafting. J Vasc Surg 11:136, 1990

68. Yang PM, Wengerter KR, Veith FJ et al: Value and limitations of secondary femoropopliteal bypasses with polytetrafluoroethylene. J Vasc Surg 14:292, 1991

69. Bartlett ST, Olinde AJ, Flinn WR et al: The reoperative potential of infrainguinal bypass: long term limb and patient survival. J Vasc Surg 5:170, 1987

70. O'Donnell TF, Coleman JC, Sentissi J et al: Comparison of direct intra-arterial streptokinase infusion to urokinase infusion in the management of failed infrainguinal ePTFE grafts. p. 80. In Veith FJ (ed): Current Critical Problems in Vascular Surgery. Vol. 3. Quality Medical Publishing, St. Louis, 1989

71. Rutherford RB: The prevention and management of graft thrombosis. p. 496. In Kempczinski RF (ed): The Ischemic Leg. Year Book Medical Publishers, Chicago, 1985

72. Bernhard VM: Late vascular graft thrombosis. p. 198. In Bernhard VM, Towne JB (eds): Complications in Vascular Surgery. 2nd Ed. Harcourt Brace Jovanovich, Orlando, FL, 1985

22

Thrombolysis of Acute Occlusions of Infrainguinal Grafts

Kevin L. Sullivan

Geoffrey A. Gardiner, Jr.

Detection and correction of flow-limiting lesions prior to graft thrombosis represent the best strategy for maintaining graft patency[1-3] (see Ch. 21). When this approach fails, a choice must be made between thrombectomy, thrombolysis, and graft replacement. The poor long-term patency following thrombectomy and local surgical revision has led investigators to examine the potential of intraarterial thrombolysis.[2-4] It was hoped that this technique would improve long-term patency compared with thrombectomy by lysing peripheral thrombus inaccessible to thombectomy catheters, and also by producing less trauma to the occluded artery and graft. To assess the degree to which thrombolysis has succeeded in the management of occluded grafts and determine the role it should play, three factors must be considered: the initial success rate, the complication rate, and the long-term patency. Since the time necessary to complete thrombolysis may be an important clinical factor in some cases, the duration of infusion must also be considered.

INITIAL SUCCESS

Success rates are dependent on the criteria used to define success. Initial outcome of lytic therapy for thrombosed grafts can be divided into technical and clinical success. Technical success, defined as complete or near-complete resolution of thrombus within the occluded graft, is not necessarily associated with restored antegrade blood flow or improved clinical status. Using this definition, initial success of graft thrombolysis is achieved in 74 to 88 percent of cases.[5-8]

Clinical success, defined as complete resolution of thrombus resulting in restoration of antegrade blood flow and resolution of ischemic symptoms, has resulted in initial success rates of 66 to 88 percent.[5-8] This definition includes any additional surgical or interventional procedures required for correction of an associated flow-limiting lesion but does not include surgical thrombectomy of the graft or distal vessels. In general, clinical success will occur less often than will technical success. However, neither of these definitions account for patients who improve clinically despite residual thrombus, or those for whom subsequent surgical management was made easier. Using this more liberal approach, overall success rates may be higher because of partial graft recanalization or improved runoff. Graor achieved a 97 percent success rate when success was defined as clot lysis resulting in a return to preocclusive symptoms, an increase in the ankle:brachial index greater than 0.25, or a reduction in the magnitude of the operative procedure required.[9]

A number of factors appear to influence the initial success rate. Techniques employed for regional thrombology of thrombosed grafts are one important factor. In general, these techniques are similar to those for occluded native arteries. One exception is the need to locate the graft origin. The proximal segment of the graft can often be visualized on angiography, but sometimes multiple views are necessary to detect a more subtle irregularity in the vessel wall representing the graft origin (Fig. 22-1A). With this anatomic knowledge, it is generally possible to direct a guidewire and catheter into the graft. Direct infusion of plasminogen activator into the graft is necessary for efficient thrombolysis, and minimal activation of the systemic fibrinolytic system.

The choice of plasminogen activator apparently plays a role in determining initial success. Primary success has been reported in 27 to 72 percent of grafts using streptokinase (SK), compared with 66 to 97 percent of grafts using urokinase (UK) or recombinant tissue plasminogen activator (tPA).[8-15] The lower success rate with SK is probably due in part to inactivation by antistreptococcal antibodies, and early termination of infusions because of bleeding complications.[14]

Graft material also appears to influence initial success. Most investigators have noted higher success rates with prosthetic grafts compared to autologous vein grafts.[5,8] The higher success rate with prosthetic grafts may be related to the different modes of failure for vein and prosthetic materials. Vein grafts are more likely to have a flow-limiting lesion identified as the cause of thrombosis, and such lesions can contribute to failure of the procedure.[8] These include diffuse wall thickening, anastomotic stenoses, or stenoses from valve hypertrophy or clamp injuries. Grafts with diffuse wall thickening cannot be salvaged. Focal high-grade stenoses may prevent selective catheterization of the graft, or impair antegrade flow, leading to acute rethrombosis before completion of lysis and repair of the stenosis.

While the data on graft thrombolysis are predominantly from experience with infrainguinal grafts, there is limited evidence that graft location influences success. Experience with aortofemoral grafts suggests that a higher level of success can be expected here. McNamara and Bomberger[12] achieved a 91 percent success rate in aortobifemoral grafts, compared with 68 percent success in infrainguinal grafts. Durham et al.[5] reported a success rate of 88 percent for suprainguinal compared with 59 percent for infrainguinal grafts.

The duration of graft occlusion is another factor that may have a role in initial success. However, this is a difficult variable to assess, since most patients present acutely because limb viability depends on graft patency. Therefore, few chronically occluded grafts are lysed. For this same reason, occlusion age is generally not an important issue in graft thrombolysis.

The rate at which plasminogen activator has been infused has not been demonstrated to be a determinant of success. In a randomized comparison of two different infusion rates which span the range of rates commonly used in clinical practice (50,000 versus 250,000 units of urokinase/h), Cragg et al.[6] found no difference in the initial success.

Failure of graft thrombolysis can be attributed to a number of causes. Discontinuation of infusion due to a complication related to lytic therapy is one of the most frequent. The risk of acute rethrombosis exists as long as the catheter remains in a vessel with little or no blood flow. Pericatheter thrombosis was reduced from 35 percent to 11.8 percent in one study when adequate anticoagulation with heparin was employed.[15] Atherosclerotic or neointimal hyperplastic lesions causing complete or near-complete luminal occlusion occasionally preclude passage of a guidewire or catheter into a graft, preventing delivery of plasminogen activator to the occluding thrombus. Uncommonly, a patient with a chronically occluded graft will present with symptoms of acute ischemia from progression of disease elsewhere, leading to failure of graft lysis due to occlusion age. Rarely does failure of lytic therapy interfere with successful surgical replacement or revision of the graft.

COMPLICATIONS

Complications remain a major concern in graft thrombolysis. Bleeding is the most common complication, but other complications such as distal embolization, sepsis, and reperfusion syndrome are well-recognized risks. Major complications, defined as an event leading to unanticipated surgery, bleeding requiring transfusion, or an event prolonging hospitalization, occur in 13 to 30 percent of graft thrombolysis procedures.[5,8,11,14]

Major bleeding complications have been reported in 7 to 17 percent of graft thrombolysis procedures.[5,7,8,10]

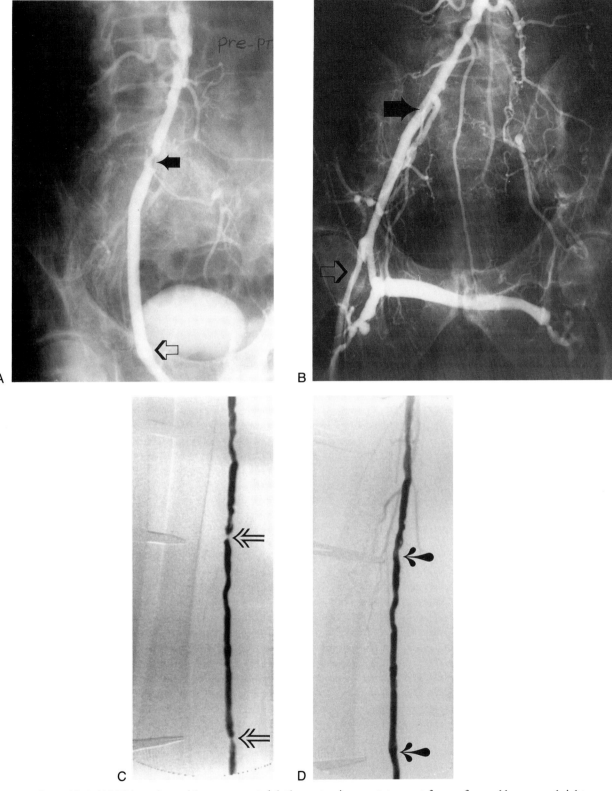

Figure 22-1 **(A)** This patient with acute-onset right leg rest pain was status post-femorofemoral bypass and right femoropopliteal autologous vein bypass. Physical examination suggested an occluded femoropopliteal graft. Angiography revealed an occluded femoropopliteal graft, and a right external iliac artery stenosis *(solid arrow)*. Note the slight bulge in the common femoral artery *(open arrow)*, which represents the origin of the femoropopliteal graft. **(B)** Angioplasty eliminated the external iliac artery stenosis *(solid arrow)*. The femoropopliteal graft *(open arrow)* was successfully thrombolysed. Two focal stenoses in the femoropopliteal graft *(open arrows)* **(C)** were successfully dilated with balloon angioplasty *(markers)* **(D)**.

The large majority of these occur locally at the arterial puncture site or in the extremity being perfused. Hemorrhage in these locations can generally be detected and controlled quickly. Intracranial bleeding, the most feared complication of lytic therapy, was reported in 0.5 percent of procedures in a compilation of 1787 cases of regional thrombolysis for native artery and graft thrombosis.[16] Bleeding from an anastomosis is a common problem in recently placed grafts, occuring in approximately one-third of grafts lysed when they are less than 1 month old.[8] Transgraft extravasation has been demonstrated through both Dacron and polytetrafluoroethylene (PTFE) and is not limited to new grafts.[17-20] This is rarely a significant problem, although life-threatening bleeds of this type have been reported.

Distal embolization can produce increased ischemia during thrombolytic infusions. However, this is almost always transient, resolving with continued infusion. It may be necessary to advance the infusion catheter into the distal vessel for direct bolus injection or infusion of the thrombolytic agent to resolve this problem. Although amputation as a result of distal embolization has been reported, it appears to be rare.

Several factors have been identified which may influence the complication rate. Total complications probably rise with the duration of the thrombolytic infusion.[21] This may be related to the increasing likelihood of developing a systemic lytic state, leading to bleeding complications. Also, prolonged catheterization can lead to sepsis. Finally, contrast-induced renal failure can result from repeated angiograms during a short time interval. The choice of plasminogen activator may influence the bleeding complication rate, with urokinase producing fewer major bleeds than streptokinase or tPA.[9] Unfortunately, hematological parameters measuring the presence of a lytic state, such as fibrinogen levels, do not seem useful in predicting hemorrhagic complications.[22,23]

Careful patient selection remains the most important factor in minimizing the chance of a major complication. In addition to standard exclusion criteria used for all forms of lytic therapy, a recently placed graft is a relative contraindication to thrombolysis. The combination of poor long-term patency and high bleeding complication rates argue against lysing such grafts in most cases.[8] These grafts generally require surgical revision, since early failure will probably be due to a defective anastomosis, or poor choice of distal anastomotic site. Transgraft extravasation above the inguinal ligament is a relative contraindication to further thrombolysis since bleeding in this location is difficult to monitor and control.

DURATION OF INFUSION

Infusion duration is an important factor, since time to restored flow may have a role in determining the choice of therapy in an ischemic limb. Antegrade flow is usually restored within several hours of initiating thrombolysis, and ischemic symptoms may improve when this occurs. However, the course of thrombolytic procedures is quite variable. Often, there are short segments of thrombus more resistant to thrombolysis, which may require prolonged infusion before resolution occurs. Distal embolization during the course of infusion may also retard resolution of ischemia. Largely because of these factors, complete lysis generally requires 12 to 24 hours of infusion with current methods. Therefore, thrombolysis should be limited to those patients who can tolerate at least several hours of ischemia.

Many of the innovations in this field have been directed toward accelerating thrombolysis. Techniques for increasing the lysis rate have the common theme of rapid introduction of the plasminogen activator into thrombus, thereby activating intrathrombic plasminogen. Contradictory results have been reported on the value of an initial intrathrombic bolus in accelerating thrombolysis.[6,21] The pulse-spray technique, in which highly concentrated urokinase is forcefully injected into thrombus, has achieved average lysis times as short as 1 hour in grafts.[24,25] If further experience confirms these early results, it would support the hypothesis that activation of intrathrombic plasminogen accelerates thrombolysis.

LONG-TERM PATENCY

Long-term patency is a major factor in evaluating the role of thrombolysis in the management of occluded grafts. To date, only several small studies have analyzed long-term patency following graft thrombolysis, and therefore the conclusions at this point are tentative.

Most of the important determinants of long-term graft patency are unrelated to the thrombolysis procedure itself. Factors known to affect primary graft patency, such as graft material and status of runoff vessels, can be expected to influence significantly the durability of secondary graft patency following thrombolysis. These and other patient selection factors probably account for the variations in reported results after successful lytic procedures.

The 1-year patency of infrainguinal vein and prosthetic grafts after successful recanalization using regional thrombolysis ranges from 28 percent to 56 percent using life-table analysis. At 3 years, patencies as low as 0 percent and as high as 42.4 percent have been reported.[5,8,26] A number of factors have been identified that appear to influence long-term patency. The most important of these is detection and correction of the lesion(s) thought to be responsible for graft thrombosis (Fig. 22-1). Such lesions have been found in approximately half of all successful procedures, but seem to be more frequent in vein grafts.[5,8,26] A 1-year patency of 89 percent was found in those grafts with a corrected flow-limiting lesion, compared with 23 percent in grafts without such a lesion.[8] This difference persisted at 2 years, with 79 percent as compared with 10 percent patency. At 6 months, McNamara and Bomberger[12] found an 80 percent patency rate in grafts with repaired flow-limiting lesions, compared with 7 percent patency in grafts without such lesions corrected. Many patients with detectable lesions as a cause of graft thrombosis require limited surgical procedures. Some lesions will be amenable to transluminal angioplasty or other interventional technique. Recanalized grafts without an identified cause for graft occlusion may benefit from long-term anticoagulation.

Graft material may influence long-term patency. In at least one study, the successfully recanalized vein grafts seem to have better long-term patency than that of prosthetic grafts, 69 percent versus 29 percent at 2 years.[8] However, in another series limited to vein grafts, a 37 percent 1-year and 23 percent 2-year patency was achieved.[26] Yet another investigator failed to demonstrate any significant difference in long-term patency based on graft materials.[5] The reason for this widely disparate experience is uncertain.

Graft location has not been consistently demonstrated to effect long-term patency. Most studies have documented no significant difference between suprainguinal and infrainguinal long-term graft patency.[5,27] However, McNamara and Bomberger[12] found that suprainguinal grafts had better long-term patency than infrainguinal grafts. No difference in patency between popliteal and infrapopliteal vein bypass was found by Belkin et al.[26] Graft age at the time of thrombosis may affect long-term patency, with a trend toward improved long-patency with increasing graft age.[8]

concern during any thrombolytic procedure, do not represent an unacceptable risk in properly selected patients. The duration of infusion does contribute to patient discomfort but is tolerable unless the severity of ischemia will lead to tissue necrosis during the time necessary to complete thrombolysis. The optimal dose and delivery of the thrombolytic agent remains ill-defined. Data on long-term patency, and relative efficacy of lysis versus other salvage techniques are limited and contradictory. For this reason, definitive statements regarding the role of regional thrombolysis in patients with occluded grafts are premature.

At the current time, factors that influence the decision of when to utilize thrombolysis include the degree of limb ischemia, the availability of vein for graft replacement, and contraindications to thrombolysis or surgery. Certain groups of patients would seem most likely to benefit from thrombolysis. In those with thrombosed outflow vessels distal to an occluded graft, thrombolysis is probably the best approach, if the outflow vessels must be recanalized. Very poor long-term graft patency after thrombectomy of distal runoff vessels has been achieved under these circumstances.[3] For thrombosed vein grafts below the knee, thrombolysis should probably be used to salvage the graft if replacement with autologous vein is not possible.

The ability of thrombolysis to uncover the cause of graft failure may be its greatest value. Correction of a flow-limiting lesion by surgery or angioplasty has resulted in excellent long-term patency. Such lesions are found in about one-half of occluded grafts, but their presence is seldom known before thrombolysis. As a result, this cannot be used to select patients for thrombolysis. If newer techniques currently under development can consistently recanalize grafts in several hours with a low complication rate, the routine use of thrombolysis to detect the cause of graft failure may become more acceptable and may lead to better planned therapeutic procedures. Until such time, the optimal therapy for a patient with an occluded peripheral bypass graft should include consideration of both surgical and interventional options, individualized to the specific clinical situation.

CURRENT ROLE
OF THROMBOLYSIS

Although there is considerable clinical experience and accumulated information in the field of graft thrombolysis, some important unresolved questions remain. Initial success of graft thrombolysis has been high with both urokinase and tPA. Complications, a

REFERENCES

1. Bandyk DF, Bergamini TM, Towne JB et al: Durability of vein graft revision: The outcome of secondary procedures. J Vasc Surg 13:200, 1991
2. Whittemore AD, Clowes AW, Couch NP et al: Secondary femoropopliteal reconstruction. Ann Surg 193:35, 1981
3. Green RM, Ouriel K, Ricotta JJ et al: Revision of failed

infrainguinal bypass graft: principles of management. Surgery 100:646, 1986

4. Brewster DC, LaSalle AJ, Robison JG et al: Femoropopliteal graft failures. Clinical consequences and success of secondary reconstructions. Arch Surg 118:1043, 1983

5. Durham JD, Geller SC, Abbott WM et al: Regional infusion of urokinase into occluded lower-extremity bypass grafts:long-term clinical results. Radiology 172:83, 1989

6. Cragg AH, Smith TP, Corson JD et al: Two urokinase dose regimens in native arterial and graft occlusions: initial results of a prospective randomized clinical trial. Radiology 178:681, 1991

7. Seabrook GR, Mewissen MW, Schmitt DD et al: Percutaneous intraarterial thrombolysis in the treatment of thrombosis of lower extremity arterial reconstructions. J Vasc Surg 13:646, 1991

8. Sullivan KL, Gardiner GA, Jr, Kandarpa K et al: Efficacy of thrombolysis in infrainguinal bypass grafts. Circulation, suppl. I. 83:I-99, 1991

9. Graor RA, Olin J, Bartholomew JR et al: Efficacy and safety of intraarterial local infusion of streptokinase, urokinase, or tissue plasminogen activator for peripheral arterial occlusion: a retrospective review. J Vasc Med Biol 2:310, 1990

10. van Breda A, Robison JC, Feldman L et al: Local thrombolysis in the treatment of arterial graft occlusions. J Vasc Surg 1:103, 1984

11. LeBolt SA, Tisnado J, Shao-Ru C: Treatment of peripheral arterial obstruction with streptokinase: results in arterial vs graft occlusions. AJR 151:589, 1988

12. McNamara TO, Bomberger RA: Factors affecting initial and 6 month patency rates after intraarterial thrombolysis with high dose urokinase. Am J Surg 152:709, 1986

13. Gardiner GA, Jr, Koltun W, Kandarpa K et al: Thrombolysis of occluded femoropopliteal grafts. AJR 147:621, 1986

14. van Breda A, Katzen BT, Deutsch AS: Urokinase versus streptokinase in local thrombolysis. Radiology 165:109, 1987

15. Becker GJ, Rabe FE, Richmond BD et al: Low-dose fibrinolytic therapy. Radiology 148:663, 1983

16. Gardiner GA, Jr, Sullivan KL: Complications of regional thrombolytic therapy. p. 87. In Kadir S (ed): Current Practice of Interventional Radiology. BC Decker, Philadelphia, 1991

17. Perler BA, Kinnison M, Halden WJ: Transgraft hemorrhage: a serious complication of low-dose thrombolytic therapy. J Vasc Surg 3:936, 1986

18. Rabe FE, Becker GJ, Richmond BD et al: Contrast extravasation through Dacron grafts: a sequela of low-dose streptokinase therapy. AJR 138:917, 1982

19. Becker GJ, Holden RW, Rabe FE: Contrast extravasation from a Gore-Tex graft: a complication of thrombolytic therapy. AJR 142:573, 1984

20. Rosner NH, Doris PE: Contrast extravasation through a Gore-Tex graft: a sequela of low-dose streptokinase therapy. AJR 143:633, 1984

21. Sullivan KL, Gardiner GA, Jr, Shapiro MJ et al: Acceleration of thrombolysis with a high-dose transthrombus bolus technique. Radiology 173:805, 1989

22. Graor RA, Risius B, Young FR et al: Low-dose streptokinase for selective thrombolysis: systemic effects and complications. Radiology 152:35, 1984

23. Mori KW, Bookstein JJ, Heeney DJ et al: Selective streptokinase infusion: clinical and laboratory correlates. Radiology 148:677, 1983

24. Kandarpa K, Drinker PA, Singer SJ et al: Forceful pulsatile local infusion of enzyme accelerates thrombolysis: in vivo evaluation of a new delivery system. Radiology 168:739, 1988

25. Valji K, Roberts AC, Davis GB et al: Pulsed-spray thrombolysis of arterial and bypass graft occlusions. AJR 156:617, 1991

26. Belkin M, Donaldson MC, Whittemore AD et al: Observations on the use of thrombolytic agents for thrombotic occlusion of infrainguinal vein grafts. J Vasc Surg 11:289, 1990

27. Gardiner GA, Jr, Harrington DP, Koltun W et al: Salvage of occluded arterial bypass grafts by means of thrombolysis. J Vasc Surg 9:426, 1989

23

Acute Ischemia: Upper- and Lower-Extremity Trauma

Mark C. Goldberg
Thomas F. O'Donnell, Jr.

And from the purple fountain Brutus
  drew
The murd'rous knife, and, as it left
  the place,
Her blood, in poor revenge, held it
  in chase

This passage from Shakespeare's *The Rape of Lucrece* (line 1734) describes a colorful scene involving cardiovascular trauma. Most of our knowledge concerning vascular trauma originates with the care of wounded soldiers. Ligation of bleeding vessels was the treatment of choice until the conclusion of World War II.[1] It was during this war that the concepts of lateral repair and end-to-end anastomosis were developed.[2] Antibiotic prophylaxis and advances in the techniques of vascular surgery occurred during the Korean War. Anesthesia advanced at this time and allowed for more technically difficult procedures with lower morbidity. Amputation rates after lower-extremity trauma fell from 49.6 percent during World War II[1] to 13 percent during the Korean conflict.[3] Prompt transportation, effective resuscitation, antibiotics, arteriography, and improvements in operative technique are responsible for the improvement now seen in the treatment of lower-extremity trauma.

ETIOLOGY

Vascular injuries can be the result of penetrating or blunt trauma, drug abuse, or an iatrogenic diagnostic/therapeutic procedure. Obviously, the military experience is biased toward penetrating trauma (94 percent).[3] In most cities, the majority of injuries are sustained by gunshot or stab wounds. Interestingly, Mattox and DeBakey and co-workers[4] established a correlation between the mechanism of penetrating cardiovascular injuries to the economy. An increase in gunshot wounds was observed during times of prosperity. Conversely, stab wounds equaled or exceeded the incidence of gunshot wounds during those periods corresponding to economic decline. However, in some countries, and in rural America, blunt vascular injuries resulting from motor vehicle accidents play a larger role. A significant number of patients are subjected to a vascular injury as a result of a diagnostic or therapeutic procedure. This includes angiographic, orthopaedic,[5] urologic,[6] as well as other surgery-related vascular injuries. Even MAST trousers (Military Anti-Shock Trousers) have been observed to cause an injury ultimately requiring a fasciotomy.[7]

399

MECHANISM

Projectiles can produce injury either by direct trauma or by way of a blast effect. The blast effect plays a more substantial role in high-velocity injuries seen primarily in a military context. Blunt trauma produces injuries through direct energy transfer to the vessel, compression, crushing forces, traction from bone displacement, or direct injuries relating to bone fragments.

The kinetic energy released into the tissue resulting from a ballistic missile equals mass times velocity squared, divided by two times the gravity ($KE = mV^2/2g$). Obviously, small increases in the velocity will result in tremendous increases in the kinetic energy imparted to the tissues. Generally, military missiles can generate a velocity over 2000 ft/s and are classified as high velocity.[8] Civilian missiles do not obtain velocities greater than 1600 ft/s, and most handguns generate velocities below 1000 ft/s.

Blunt trauma injuries that do not result in disruption of all three layers of an artery can precipitate damage to the intima. The result of this intimal disruption can range from simply a flow disturbance to thrombosis at the site of injury and beyond. In cases in which the injury results in partial or complete disruption, a hematoma will form and, if contained, a false aneurysm may result. Injury to the intima may led to thrombosis, distal arterial emboli, and ultimately, profound limb ischemia. Vessel spasm frequently occurs after injuries to surrounding tissues or to the vessel itself. Spasm rarely results in significant lower extremity ischemia. However, it bespeaks the potential for an occult arterial lesion later manifested in another form.

The risk of a nonreconstructable arterial injury to the lower extremity is greatest with blunt and high-velocity missiles.[9] This risk is related to the associated tissue damage. This is best illustrated by the high amputation rate with fractures or dislocations (26 percent) as compared with a rate of 0.6 percent in extremities without skeletal trauma.[10]

LOCATION

Cardiovascular trauma presents predominantly in the extremities (Tables 23-1 and 23-2). This may, in part, be attributed to the higher immediate mortality of vascular trunk injuries and to the proximity of extremity arteries and veins to the surface. Sites of injury most apt to result in limb loss are the popliteal artery, tibial vessels, and brachial artery.

Table 23-1 Distribution of Arterial Injuries in a Series of 665 Patients

Site of Injury	No.
Extremity	501
Aorta	31
Visceral	37
Cervical	96

(From Perry,[11] with permission.)

DIAGNOSIS

Priorities

The rules of general body trauma also apply to the patient with an acutely ischemic extremity resulting from an injury. The golden rules consist of the ABCs of trauma care (airway, breathing, circulation). One must first protect the airway and cervical spine before attempting management of all other injuries. The second priority is to rule out problems of the cardiovascular system. This pertains to injuries contributing to decreased cardiac output including tension pneumothorax and pericardial tamponade. The third priority is to maintain circulatory stability. Sources of hemorrhage and initial fluid resuscitation should be controlled. Large-bore intravenous lines should be established in nontraumatized extremities. A minimum of two 16-gauge lines is recommended. Lactated Ringer's solution is an appropriate fluid for initial resuscitation.

History

The evaluation begins with determination of the agent and circumstances surrounding the injury. Ambrose Paré is credited with first proposing to analyze the

Table 23-2 Distribution of Vascular Injuries in a Series of 4459 Patients

Site of Injury	%
Abdomen	35
Extremity	34
Lower	19
Upper	15
Cardiac/arch	14
Cervical	12

(From Mattox et al.,[4] with permission.)

trajectory of the missile. He would instruct the patient to assume the body position at the time of the injury. The awareness of mechanism, trajectory, and anatomy can often help, especially in cases of an occult vascular injury. A history of sensory and/or motor loss should be elicited. Obviously, questions pertaining to past medical history, including cardiac disease and current medications, are important. Equally important is eliciting a history of the last meal eaten as well as allergies.

Physical Examination

Trauma-induced lower-extremity arterial injuries present primarily with hemorrhage and/or distal ischemic symptoms. Hemorrhage is often easily controlled with external compression. A trauma patient with arterial bleeding, an expanding/pulsatile mass, distal ischemia, or diminished pulses is considered to have a vascular injury until proved otherwise. Pulsatile bleeding or the combination of distal ischemia and diminished pulses are pathognomonic for an arterial injury.[12] The difficulty lies in detecting the occult injury and having an index of suspicion for initiating further diagnostic studies. One can attempt to predict the possibility of an arterial injury by assessing the trajectory of the penetrating weapon based on the location of the entrance and exit wounds. It should be noted, however, that the presence of a pulse does not rule out a vascular injury. If the index of suspicion is high, one should proceed with further evaluation of the vascular system. Signs of vascular injury with an intact pulse can include a thrill, bruit, hematoma formation, loss of blood through an open wound, and sensory loss in the distribution of a nerve closely associated with the artery. Other important observations include diminished capillary refill time, color of the extremity, temperature, and a full motor and sensory examination.

Clearly, the observation of associated injuries plays a significant role in focusing on the physical examination. A history of a fracture or dislocation should raise the index of suspicion for an arterial injury. This is particularly important with a posterior dislocation of the knee.

In a study of 70 civilian trauma victims submitted for physical examination, arteriography, and, if indicated, surgical intervention, the most reliable clinical sign of underlying arterial injury was a diminished or absent pulse (83.3 percent).[13] This has been confirmed by other investigators.[14] Diminished pulses without signs of distal ischemia, however, do not constitute absolute evidence for an arterial injury. Associated hypotension may diminish the validity of this physical finding. On the other hand, the finding of a palpable distal pulse does not rule out an arterial injury.[13,15–18]

Arteriogram

The most appropriate method for evaluation of the trauma patient with a potential vascular injury has undergone significant changes during the past 10 years. Routine surgical exploration of all wounds in proximity to major vessels, even in the absence of arterial compromise, was advocated during the 1960's and 1970's.[17,19,20] This approach arose from an effort to minimize missed vascular injuries and to avoid diagnostic delays that might compromise a vascular reconstruction. More recently, however, this was questioned with the finding of a negative exploration in 57 to 88 percent of patients.[12,21] Furthermore, a negative exploration results in a morbity rate ranging from 5 to 31 percent[21,22] and a prolonged hospital stay, if there are no other associated injuries.

Arteriography can reduce the number of unnecessary surgical explorations in patients with equivocal signs of vascular trauma. The false-positive rate ranges from zero to 4 percent.[13,15,21,23] More important, however, is the false-negative rate, which ranges from 0 to 1.8 percent.[13,15,24,25] More recently, routine arteriography of patients without clear signs of vascular injuries has also been questioned.

Indications for Arteriogram

An obvious arterial injury in an unstable and hypotensive patient should be explored immediately in the operating room. In general patients, with an obvious injury above the knee without evidence of atherosclerosis can be explored without obtaining a preoperative arteriogram. Arteriography, however, can provide a road map that is particularly helpful in the atherosclerotic patient. It can also clarify situations in which the diagnosis is in question. Ultimately, sound judgment is crucial in defining the need for an arteriogram versus the immediate need for surgical exploration.

The most reliable clinical sign of an arterial injury is an abnormal pulse examination.[13] There are vessels, however, that cannot be palpated, such as the profunda femoris artery. In addition, there are situations in which the absence of pulses does not help during the evaluation of a trauma victim. Arteriography may be most helpful in evaluating the patient with peripheral vascular atherosclerosis displaying signs of distal ischemia.

The most controversial indication for an arteriogram is proximity of a penetrating object to a major vessel.

Several studies have demonstrate a low diagnostic yield of arterial injuries, using proximity as the exclusive criterion for arteriography.[13,26] Thus, proximity alone is not sufficient to determine the need for exploration or arteriography. Rather, it should raise the possibility in conjunction with other signs and symptoms. We have found that close clinical observation, supplemented with noninvasive arterial pressure and imaging studies, has decreased the need for arteriography in this setting. This policy has also been adopted by Anderson and associates, who prospectively examined penetrating trauma to the extremities.[27] Randomly selected patients with gunshots to the extremities (n = 23) were studied using B-mode ultrasound, segmental Doppler pressure measurements, and arteriography. The sensitivity and specificity of B-mode ultrasound were 83 percent and 100 percent, respectively. Doppler segmental pressures (67 percent sensitive) did not improve on the sensitivity or the specificity of B-mode ultrasound. The drawback to B-mode ultrasound is that it is a technician-dependent study that requires each vascular laboratory to determine its own accuracy. These findings have been substantiated by Bynoe and associates with an observed 95 percent specificity, 99 percent sensitivity, and a 98 percent accuracy of duplex ultrasound.[28]

Blunt lower-extremity trauma is associated with an incidence of vascular injuries approaching as high as 40 percent.[29] Angiograms, either preoperatively or intraoperatively, are recommended to detect the stretch injury to the popliteal artery associated with knee fractures and posterior dislocations.[30] It has also been recommended to evaluate the axillary artery after shoulder dislocations[31] and the brachial artery after supracondylar fractures.[32]

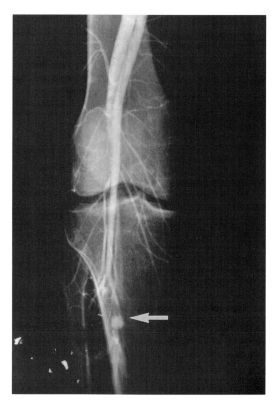

Figure 23-1 A pseudoaneurysm *(arrow)* and an arteriovenous fistula, resulting from a gunshot wound to the lower leg.

Radiographic signs of arterial trauma include the findings of extravasation, obstruction/narrowing, arterial wall contour irregularity/intimal flaps, false aneurysms, and early venous filling/arteriovenous fistula (Fig. 23-1).[18,32] Extravasation of contrast material is the most common finding in penetrating trauma and is best seen using several projections. One of the greatest

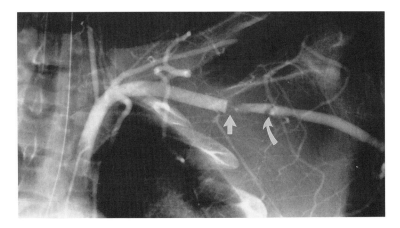

Figure 23-2 Stretch injury to the axillary artery in a young man, the result of a motorcycle accident. A filling defect is present in the proximal axillary artery *(arrow)*, and an intimal defect is demonstrated several centimeters distally *(arrow)*.

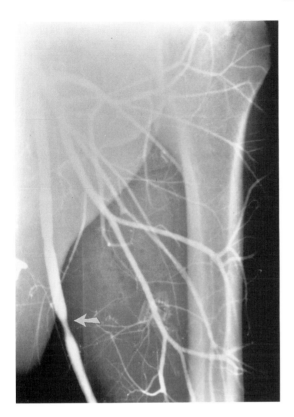

Figure 23-3 Focal vasospasm of the superficial femoral artery *(arrow)*, resulting from a gunshot wound to the thigh.

errors in interpreting angiograms, in trauma, includes evaluation based on a single projection film.[32] Delayed films have been suggested as the best method for delineating subtle signs of extravasation.[33]

The second most common finding is arterial occlusion (Fig. 23-2), seen in 22 percent of patients undergoing arteriograms to exclude vascular injuries.[32] It often occurs in combination with extravasation, extrinsic

compression, and luminal narrowing. Mechanisms for occlusion range from intimal defects that result in thrombosis to transmural disruption of the vessel.

Luminal narrowing is a difficult finding to interpret (Fig. 23-3). The differential diagnosis includes transient spasm, intramural hematoma, compression by an extraluminal structure, intraluminal thrombus, an intimal flap, and atheromatous plaque. Differentiation of the causes may be difficult. Fortunately, most of the causes of narrowing are associated with another sign of arterial injury. In a review of 1200 angiograms obtained to rule out vascular trauma, only 14 vessels demonstrated luminal narrowing as the sole sign of vascular injury.[32]

An intraluminal flap may appear as a radiolucent defect (Fig. 23-4). The disruption of the intima may take on several manifestations, such as a short horizontal lucent line or a long spiraling linear lesion. Intimal flaps are often associated with arterial spasm[32] and can result in thrombosis. Intraluminal thrombus presents as either a complete or partial occlusion. Intraluminal thrombus without occlusion can present with a central defect or with a filling defect along the arterial wall. In the latter situation, it appears as a luminal narrowing.

Angiography, on occasion, can also be used to obtain proximal control with the placement of a balloon catheter. Intraluminal control of vessels has been reported in selected situations.[34-36] Belkin and associates described two patients who underwent preoperative arteriography during which the injured vessel was identified.[35] Before transfer to the operating room, a balloon catheter, placed proximal to the injury, established preoperative proximal control and simplified the procedure. The value of this approach is reserved for situations in which the patient can be safely transported to the angiography suites without endangering life or limb.

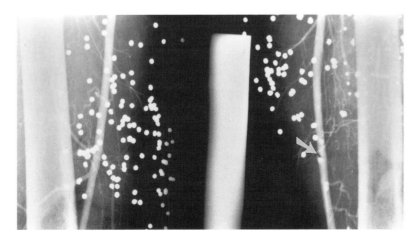

Figure 23-4 Intimal flap in the superficial femoral artery *(arrow)* of a young man, resulting from a shotgun injury.

Intraoperative Arteriography

Intraoperative arteriography may be necessary in those patients requiring immediate intraoperative control in whom when additional anatomic information is necessary for revascularization. Its limitations preclude its routine substitution for properly performed higher-quality diagnostic angiography. The techniques for arteriography must be modified to obtain the best possible film with only a single exposure. A film cassette is wrapped in a sterile plastic bag and positioned directly beneath the extremity. The cassette and the limb should be positioned close together to enhance resolution and decrease the magnification. The patient should be positioned to minimize the projection of vessels over opaque structures, such as heavy bones. For the arteries of the thigh and popliteal region, an anterioposterior projection is most useful. The vessels of the calf are best seen with a slight internal rotation of the foot, which will minimize the overlap of the three tibial vessel. The distal tibial arteries and vessels in the foot are often best seen with external rotation and plantar flexion. Vessels of the upper extremity are best demonstrated with the palm up to provide the least overlap of the radial, ulnar and interosseous arteries. A C-arm image intensifier with a video recorder has the advantage of providing anatomic information quickly.

GENERAL PRINCIPLES OF MANAGEMENT

Early recognition of an arterial injury is mandatory. The failure to identify signs and symptoms of ischemia remains the most important immediate limiting factor to limb salvage.[10,37-51] During transport to the operating room, direct pressure over the bleeding wound will adequately control most bleeding. General anesthesia is the preferred method in the setting of trauma. Positioning of the patient is determined by the type of injury, the types of associated injuries, the possible need for autogenous vein from the contralateral extremity, and the ability to access the distal pulses intraoperatively. With proximal injuries of the upper or lower extremity, one should be prepared to gain access within the chest or abdomen, respectively. In the extremity, longitudinal incisions are made over the vessels. Proximal and distal control should be obtained before entering a hematoma or suspected area of injury. The vessels are encircled with tapes or a loop. If hemorrhage is present and proximal control is incomplete, one can in some instances apply digital pressure to control the

bleeding while the dissection is completed. The injured artery is identified and the extent of damage assessed. Examination should also rule out associated damage to veins, nerves, soft tissue and bony structures. The edges of the vessel should be debrided. One may be reluctant to debride the vessel adequately. Leaving some portion of damaged vessel, however, may result in thrombosis of the repair or in late pseudoaneurysm formation. Thrombus may often be present proximal and distal to an injury, and balloon catheter thrombectomy may be required for restoration of flow. Local application of heparin, if necessary, is indicated at this time, as many patients may have contraindications to systemic heparin.

It is crucial to obtain coverage of exposed vessels after a vascular repair. Some investigators have stated that insufficient tissue coverage of traumatized vessels and repairs may be an indication for primary amputation.[52] In some instances, extra-anatomic bypass can be performed to avoid devitalized tissue wounds. This is rarely an option, and consultation with a plastic surgeon may be fruitful. Intraoperative management must keep in mind the final method of wound closure to preserve the vascular supply to important muscle groups, which may be a source of coverage.[53-55] Alternative methods include the use of porcine skin[56] and transplantation of omentum.[57,58] Others have advised early second-look operations to assess the extent of soft tissue and muscle necrosis.[59]

Vasospasm as a result of trauma, particularly in younger patients, can compromise attempts at revascularization. Tolazoline is a α-adrenergic blocker that has a direct effect on smooth muscle cells. Intra-arterial use of tolazoline has been reported to decrease vascular spasm.[60] Peck et al. reported 15 trauma patients who, despite successful vascular reconstruction, persisted in significant vasospasm and ischemia. Tolazoline in combination with heparin was administered continuously into the femoral artery. Ischemia was reversed in 87 percent of patients, with a limb salvage rate of 67 percent.

TYPES OF REPAIR: PRIMARY VERSUS INTERPOSITION GRAFTS

The mechanism and extent of injury in association with the requirement for debridement of the vessel determine the method of repair (Table 23-3). Lateral repairs are the simplest and are usually performed for minor lacerations and iatrogenic arterial injuries. A vein patch angioplasty may be sufficient if debride-

Table 23-3 Methods for Repair of Vessels

Primary
    Lateral
    Patch angioplasty
    End-to-end anastomosis

Interposition graft
    Autogenous
    Synthetic

ment has compromised the diameter of the lumen, but an interposition graft is not required. In this situation, one may use a small vein present in the wound. It is important not to compromise the venous drainage of the injured extremity. If there is any question regarding the venous system, it is preferable to harvest vein from an uninjured limb. End-to-end anastomosis or interposition grafts are often required for more extensive injuries. Published reports vary in regard to the techniques required for arterial repair. Drapanas and associates[16] reported 70 percent of arterial repairs using primary techniques and only 16 percent using an interposition graft. The success of revascularization is not affected by the specific technique employed,[11,17] but anastomotic tension is the most common cause of failure.[17]

Prosthetic grafts have proved useful (1) if inadequate veins are present, (2) if significant wound contamination is observed, and (3) to reduce operative time. Feliciano and associates[61] have one of the largest experiences with polytetrafluoroethylene (PTFE) grafts in the setting of vascular trauma. In 1985, these workers published a series of 206 patients treated for arterial injuries with 236 PTFE grafts.[61] Most injuries encountered in this series were in the upper (39 percent) and lower (46 percent) extremities, and most of the interposition grafts were to the superficial femoral and brachial artery. Interposition grafts of the brachial artery with 4-mm PTFE were associated with a high immediate and late failure rate. Its use in the lower extremity was limited by a slightly lower long-term patency rate, as compared with saphenous vein. PTFE grafts were not associated with graft infections in trauma wounds except for those exposed or in proximity to osteomyelitis. Exposed PTFE was more easily managed in Feliciano's experience but was associated with delayed blowout, occlusion, and infection if coverage was delayed too long. Several other papers have been published supporting the notion that PTFE is useful in the trauma setting, particularly in contaminated wounds.[62,63] Most surgeons, however, exclusively use autogenous grafts.

SPECIFIC AREAS OF ARTERIAL INJURY

Lower Extremity

Femoral, Profunda, and Superficial Artery

Femoral, profunda, and superficial arterial injuries most commonly result from penetrating trauma.[64] The superficial artery is injured four times as frequently as the common femoral artery.[17,65] The incidence of profunda femoris injuries is incompletely documented in most series but appears almost to equal the frequency of common femoral arterial injures.[17] Several reports have noted that femoral vein injuries are associated with 50 percent of arterial injuries in this region.[2,3] Signs of distal ischemia indicate the need for immediate reconstruction. As a general rule, above-knee injuries producing signs of distal ischemia do not require a preoperative arteriogram. The first few centimeters of the profunda femoris should be reconstructed in a conventional method. Distal profunda femoris arterial injuries are best managed by simple ligation.

Surgical exposure in the groin may require proximal exposure and control of the common or external iliac artery. Table 23-4 summarizes the indications for an extraperitoneal approach to the iliac artery. The patient is placed in a supine position, and a roll may be placed under the buttocks. A skin incision is made 2 to 3 cm above and parallel to the inguinal ligament. The aponeuroses of the external oblique, internal oblique, and transversus muscles are also incised parallel to the inguinal ligament. The transversalis fascia is divided, and the properitoneal fat and viscera are retracted medially. The common, external, and internal iliac arteries are now visualized. Exposure of the groin vessels uses a standard longitudinal femoral incision. The inguinal ligament may be divided for control of the distal external iliac artery. The profunda is usually a single vessel but occasionally has a double origin.

Popliteal Artery

The most serious and complicated lower-extremity injury facing a vascular surgeon involves the popliteal artery. The risk of amputation with ligation of the pop-

Table 23-4 Indications for an Extraperitoneal Approach to the Iliac Artery

Hematoma extending to the inguinal ligament
Bleeding from groin wound requiring external compression for control
Previous groin surgery and immediate proximal control required

liteal artery is 73 percent in the DeBakey-Simeone series.[1] Despite improved techniques, civilian popliteal injuries resulted in a high amputation rate relative to other vascular injuries. Only 10 percent of all vascular injuries involve the popliteal artery, but 65 percent of amputations after trauma are associated with a popliteal fossa injury.[45] In general, higher amputation rates are seen with blunt trauma than with penetrating injuries to the popliteal space.[16,40,51,66,67] Thus, injuries in this region represent a complex problem, due in part to the relative lack of collateral vessels for both the popliteal artery and vein.

Factors that have an impact on salvage of the extremity include the mechanism of the injury, ischemic interval, age, degree of atherosclerosis, and associated soft tissue, nerve, bone, and venous injuries. The major obstacles to lower-extremity salvage with popliteal arterial injuries are the extent of soft tissue injury and the delay of treatment, which can result in the thrombosis of distal tibial vessels and muscle necrosis. In the Tulane group's experience, a delay in treatment correlated positively with the amputation rate (5.7 hours versus 3.1 hours).[51] The Albany group reports that, although they had no amputations, significant neuromuscular impairment resulted from delay of surgical intervention.[66]

Once the diagnosis of a popliteal arterial injury is made, the patient should be heparinized if no contraindications are present (Tables 23-5). The probability of an arterial contusion and thrombosis is significant with popliteal injuries. Intravenous heparin should be given at systemic doses to prevent clot formation and propagation into the distal vessels as well as the collaterals and muscular branches. During a 20-year period, Wagner et al.[42] reported on 99 patients treated for blunt popliteal injuries. The amputation rate early on in the series was 15 percent, but this dropped to 6 percent toward the end of the series. Despite a 15.8-hour mean ischemic interval, the improvement seen was attributed to the routine preoperative use of systemic heparin and to an increased number of primary repairs.

The vascular injury should be addressed first and should take precedence over operative stabilization of fractures if limb-threatening ischemia is present. Depending on the extent of ischemia, initial stabilization

Table 23-5 Indications for Arteriogram to Exclude Blunt Popliteal Arterial Injury

Knee dislocation
Fractures adjacent to the popliteal fossa
Orthopaedic procedure following trauma that will require a tourniquet
Crush injuries to the popliteal fossa

of skeletal injuries may be preferable in selected situations. The key to a successful outcome is the early reversal of significant tissue ischemia. This will greatly decrease the risk of permanent neurologic disability, myonecrosis and, ultimately, amputation. If a compartment syndrome is suspected, it is best to perform a fasciotomy early on to improve the collateral flow to the ischemic distal extremity.

Exposure of the popliteal artery is best approached using a standard medial incision. It allows the surgeon to extend the incision to include the distal superficial artery, as well as the tibial vessels. Distal exposure of the below knee popliteal artery is obtained by continuing the skin incision distally along the medial aspect of the leg. A posterior approach is discouraged. It is confined to the popliteal space and is suboptimal for surgical exposure in the setting of trauma.

In those patients with combined popliteal artery and vein injuries, we generally repair the vein after restoration of the arterial system. During the Vietnam War, Rich[3] reported the importance of venous repairs. This has been confirmed in the civilian experience.[40,51,68,69] The possibility of a compartment syndrome should again be addressed at the completion of the arterial repair. An intraoperative arteriogram should be used to ensure technical adequacy as well as to assess for any evidence of thrombus or unrecognized distal injuries. Any technical errors or arterial or vein graft defects must be addressed at this time.

Once skeletal stabilization has been achieved, the vascular repair should be reinspected and assessed using a Doppler. Soft tissues are now debrided and it is important to obtain adequate coverage of exposed nerves and blood vessels. If fasciotomies have been performed, significant edema and swelling will preclude complete coverage of these structures. It may be necessary to mobilize viable muscle to cover vessels and nerves. Open wounds should be kept moist to prevent tissue desiccation (Table 23-6).

Tibial Vessels

Arterial injuries of the tibial vessels are relatively infrequent and accounted for only 9.3 percent of all arterial lower-extremity injuries in the Mattox-DeBakey series.[4] Results in a civilian population with blunt trauma and shotgun injuries appear to parallel the wartime experience with primary amputation rates of 17 percent and 33 percent respectively.[70] Blunt and shotgun trauma accounted for 90 percent of three-vessel injuries.

The critical factors involved in the care of these injuries includes a high index of suspicion, a short interval before surgical intervention, and the application of

Table 23-6 Popliteal Arterial Injury: Summary of Management

Preoperative
  Arteriogram
  Perioperative systemic heparin (if isolated injury)
  Perioperative antibiotics

Intraoperative
  Adequate vascular exposure
  Arterial debridement
  Thrombectomy of proximal and distal arteries
  Local application of heparin, if systemic heparin contraindicated
  Vascular repair without tension
  Repair of associated venous injury
  Completion angiogram
  Fasciotomy, if indicated
  Immobilization of fractures
  Soft tissue debridement
  Soft tissue coverage

Postoperative
  Postoperative leg elevation
  Wound care

sound surgical judgment and technique in the operating room. If two or more vessels are injured, at least one should be repaired. In patients who have one occluded artery and no bleeding or ischemia, vascular exploration is not required. A single-vessel injury requiring exploration for bleeding may be ligated. Ligation of a single tibial vessel carries a minimal risk of an ensuing amputation.[70-72] This does not apply to the tibioperoneal trunk which is functionally two vessels.

The proper surgical management of the arterial injury is best dictated by those observations made at exploration. A medial incision is positioned slightly below the knee to expose the below-knee popliteal artery, the common tibioperoneal trunk, and the peroneal and posterior tibial arteries. On occasion, it is possible to expose the anterior tibial artery through this incision. The anterior tibial artery is best exposed along the anterolateral aspect of the leg. The peroneal artery may be exposed though a medial incision along the upper two-thirds of the leg. It then takes a lateral course and becomes intimately associated with the fibula. We prefer to expose the distal one-third of the peroneal artery, using a lateral approach with resection of the fibula.

The extent of the injury, limited mobility of the tibial arteries, and the small size often limit the clinical value of a lateral arterial repair. Debridement of nonviable vessel wall often renders a gap that must be bridged by a vein interposition graft. Techniques involved in exploration of tibial artery trauma is similar in principle to the popliteal artery wound. Systemic or local heparin is

useful to prevent distal thrombosis if the situation allows for its application. Gentle balloon thrombectomy with a 2 or 3 French catheter proximally and distally may be required. Small-vessel techniques using surgical loops, 7-0 suture, and spatulation of the anastomosis are required. A completion arteriogram is important to evaluate the anastomosis and the distal outflow. Repair of small fragile tibial veins is difficult, and ligation is usually the only option. Fasciotomy is often indicated. Other adjunctive measures may include soft tissue debridement, musculocutaneous flaps, and intra-arterial infusion of a vasodilator.

Upper Extremity

Upper-extremity vascular trauma is defined as an injury sustained distal to the lateral border of the first rib and extending to the fingers. This includes the subclavian, axillary, brachial, radial, and ulnar arteries. Adjacent structures include the accompanying veins and nerves. A knowledge of the anatomy, including the rich collateral system of the upper extremity, will aid the vascular surgeon in the management of these injuries. The presenting symptoms of the patient are dependent on the location of the injury relative to the collateral network.

Upper-extremity trauma is often a complex and challenging problem. Before World War II, arterial ligation was the surgical procedure of choice with an amputation rate that exceeded 40 percent.[1] As in the case of lower-extremity trauma, subsequent wars contributed to the refinements in vascular technique and modern civilian upper-extremity salvage rates ranging from 96 to 100 percent (Table 23-7). Despite successful restoration of the vascular system, concomitant nerve and musculoskeletal injuries often compromise the functional results.

Subclavian and Axillary Arteries

Owing to the protective coverage of the clavicle, most injuries to these vessels results from penetrating trauma. Gunshot wounds are the most common mechanism.[73,75,77] On physical examination, 30 to 50 percent of patients will have pulses present. Therefore, the presence of pulses does not rule out a vascular injury.[74-76]

Proximal control requires control of the subclavian artery. Exposure of the proximal left subclavian artery can be accomplished using a high left anterolateral thorocotomy. The proximal right subclavian artery is displayed through a median sternotomy. The second and third portions of both the right and left subclavian artery may be approached via a resection of the clavi-

Table 23-7   Amputation and Disability Rates Secondary to Upper-
Extremity Trauma

Investigators	Amputation Rate		Neurologic Deficit	
	Primary (%)	Secondary (%)	Moderate (%)	Major (%)
Hardin et al.[73]	2	4	23	23
Sitzmann and Ernst[74]	0	0	N/A	7 (upper)
				21 (lower)
Occutt et al.[75]	0	0	10	16
Borman et al.[76]	0	1.5	34	17
Myers et al.[77]	0	0	N/A	17

cle. The right subclavian, as compared to the left, rises slightly higher into the supraclavicular fossa. The second portion of the subclavian artery is exposed by dividing the scalene muscle. The third portion is the most superficial and is easily identified during this dissection. A median sternotomy may be combined with a clavicular resection ("open book" incision), if further exposure is required. The morbidity associated with resection of the clavicle is minimal and does not result in significant alteration in the motion of the shoulder.

Exposure of the axillary artery is accomplished using a skin incision 1 cm below the midportion of the clavicle and continued laterally along the deltopectoral grove. The pectoralis major muscle fibers are split. The pectoralis minor muscle and tendon are divided. The cephalic vein lies in the deltopectoral grove and should be preserved. The artery lies lateral to the vein, and the brachial plexus surrounds both structures.

Ideally, the arterial injury should be repaired primarily. This is not often possible. An interposition saphenous vein or synthetic graft can be used.[78] Limb salvage in situations of penetrating injuries is usually good. This may be, to some extent, secondary to the rich collateral system of both the arterial and venous systems. If the subclavian or axillary vein is injured it may be repaired with a lateral venorrhaphy. Otherwise, it is safe to ligate either vein. The long-term morbidity is determined by any associated neurologic trauma to the brachial plexus. If a neurologic deficit is observed in the acute postoperative period, it may be prudent to re-explore the wound, since an expanding hematoma may be responsible for compression of the brachial plexus. Evacuation of a hematoma under these circumstances carries a good prognosis for recovery of function over the course of several months.

Avulsion injuries at the shoulder are among the most difficult problems that can face a surgeon. Typically, the patient sustains an injury to the shoulder while riding a motorcycle. A shear force can result in a mangled extremity with injuries to the axillary and brachial arteries as well as the brachial plexus. In combination with significant soft tissue loss and a brachial plexus injury, the prognosis is poor. In cases with uncertainty concerning the brachial plexus, an aggressive effort at salvage should be attempted.

Brachial Artery

The brachial artery is one of the most frequently injured vessels in civilian, military, iatrogenic, and drug abuse situations.[3,11,17,79-81] Arterial injuries are commonly seen with fractures and dislocations at the elbow. Volkmann's contracture is the consequence of an untreated compartment syndrome, with its ensuing ischemia. It often results from an untreated supracondylar fracture of the humerus. The brachial artery is exposed, using a skin incision along the medial border of the biceps grove. Care should be taken during the dissection, given the close proximity of the median nerve to the brachial artery. On occasion, a high bifurcation can occur above the elbow. The brachial artery can often be repaired laterally or mobilized for a primary end-to-end anastomosis.

FASCIOTOMY

Indications

A compartment syndrome may follow penetrating or blunt trauma. It can also occur either before or after revascularization. The indications for a fasciotomy are not as well defined as those for revascularization. When preformed at the appropriate juncture, however, fasciotomy, can help prevent ongoing limb ischemia. Bardenheuer[82] first described the procedure to prevent

dinal curvilinear incision begun overlying and above the elbow along the course of the brachial artery. The incision is continued in a gentle arching pattern initially, laterally, then medially, and ending in the central portion of the wrist. The incision may be continued into the central portion of the palm with a slightly lateral sweep. Attention should be directed toward identifying and releasing the fascia of the lacertus fibrosus, the proximal edge of the pronator teres, the superficial flexor muscles, and the carpal tunnel.[83] On occasion, a fasciotomy of the hand compartments may also be required.

PRIMARY AMPUTATION

Indications

Delayed amputations result in increased morbidity to the patient and increased hospital costs.[84] While limb salvage is an admirable goal for any surgeon, it is important to make an initial assessment of the extent of injuries. The goal is to salvage a functional extremity. It is possible to execute a successful revascularization, only later to find that the extremity is insensate and nonfunctional. The frequency of primary amputations in the literature is not a reliable indicator of successful outcome. Many secondary amputations are performed later in the course of care, as a result of disabling associated injuries. Determining clearly defined criteria for primary amputation of an extremity is complex (Table 23-9).

The proximity of nerves, bone, and vessels can result in complex injuries requiring difficult decisions. Large forces are often necessary to produce concomitant neurovascular, skeletal, and soft tissue injuries. These types of injuries, in civilian experiences, often result from blunt trauma.[41,85-87] Severe peripheral nerve deficits are perhaps the most significant limiting factor in the reconstruction of a limb. Peacock and Proctor[87] reported in 1977 that the absence of a nerve injury is ultimately the most important determinant of a successful limb reconstruction. A clean nerve transection

Table 23-9 Factors Responsible for Limiting Rehabilitation of an Extremity

Prolonged ischemia
Late recognition of a vascular injury
Nerve injury
Extensive skeletal and soft tissue injuries
Compartment syndrome—untreated
Concomitant venous injury—untreated

that can be primarily repaired is rare and, even in those cases, the functional results are suboptimal.[87,88] Thus, the finding of a significant neurologic deficit in a limb indicates a poor prognosis for a functional result. The difficulty is that the patients often present unconscious or in an altered state due to drugs or alcohol. An attempt to salvage a denervated devascularized extremity with devastating skeletal and soft tissue loss is ill-advised. It is particularly prudent to consider the option of amputation in the setting of extensive lower-extremity trauma, concomitant trauma to other areas of the body, and hypotension. Obviously, there is a fine line between a limb that can be reconstructed with function and a nonsalvageable extremity. As one considers all the possible situations that may present in an ischemic lower extremity in the trauma setting, it is difficult to establish clearly defined criteria for primary amputation. If there is any doubt it is best to err on the side of revascularization.

VASCULAR INJURIES RELATED TO DRUG ABUSE

Drug abuse is seen in all walks of life, and the complications are increasingly being recognized. The ingenuity of drug abusers has given rise to an unlimited variety of injury sites. Even reports of repeated intracardiac injections have been published.[81] Because the drug abuser requires access to vascular structures to achieve a "rush," the vascular surgeon is seeing a greater number of injuries related to this epidemic problem.

The vascular surgeon must be aware of the different drugs injected, as well as the methods used for injection. Heroin is the most commonly abused drug of injection. Other drugs of abuse include cocaine, barbiturates, and amphetamines. Outside of the well-known systemic effects of these drugs, inadvertent direct arterial injection can result in limb-threatening ischemia. The most common arteries involved at presentation are the brachial and femoral arteries. A hyperemic flush is initially observed, followed by ischemic symptoms. The symptoms and physical signs include the absence of pulses, loss of sensation, cyanosis, edema, and ultimately gangrene. The extremity ischemia occurs by way of several mechanisms, including vasospasm, intimal damage, and thrombosis from mechanical trauma (e.g., intimal flaps, arteriovenous fistulas), infection, chemical arteritis as well as foreign-body reactions and particulate emboli. The final outcome is determined by the type of drug, its concentration, the method of injection, and the time delay until initiation of treatment. The actual incidence of arterial injections is unknown. Those patients who do present are the worst cases, or simply drug abusers who are concerned enough to seek medical attention.

Mechanism for Extremity Ischemia

Early work in the 1940s focused on the vasospatic response as a result of intra-arterial injection of thiopental[89] and barbiturates.[90] In 1959, Kinmonth and Shepherd[91] published a study which dismissed vasoconstriction as the direct cause of distal ischemia and gangrene. Using a rabbit model, 5 percent thiopental was injected into the femoral artery. The vasospasm lasted only 30 seconds, and no tissue loss was observed. This was substantiated several years later by Engler et al.,[92] who also attempted to induce gangrene with intra-arterial injections of several drugs (dextroamphetamine sulfate, promazine hydrochloride, ether, and sulfobromophthalein sodium). In these early experiments, femoral arterial injections did not induce gangrene. It was with the temporary proximal occlusion of the femoral artery that tissue necrosis was observed. It was concluded that the drug must be transported undiluted in a highly irritating bolus. Vasospasm would appear to increase the duration of exposure, and the effect of vasoconstriction is not a direct cause of necrosis. Thus, vasospasm may be important in increasing the duration of exposure of the endothelium to highly irritating cytotoxic drugs.[81] A chemical endarteritis can result from some of these drugs, ultimately resulting in thrombosis of the vessel. Necrotizing angitis, a potentially lethal syndrome, has been associated with drug abuse.[93] The histologic pattern is indistinguishable from periarteritis nodosa.

Obstruction of the vessel can also occur as a result of foreign bodies and crystallization of some drugs. During the preparation of drugs, talc, cornstarch, and other fillers may be introduced before intravenous injection. Wright[93a] demonstrated that intra-arterial injection of a suspension of cornstarch and talc could reduce arterial flow in the femoral artery using a primate animal model. A second mechanism for obstruction is due to crystallization of some drugs. Drugs are occasionally prepared in an aqueous, alkaline solution. If the pH were suddenly decreased without dilution, precipitation could occur with crystal formation. It has been suggested that crystal formation during an intra-arterial injection could result in an intimal injury and thrombosis.[94] Furthermore, the crystal formation could mechanically obstruct the lumen of arterioles. Thrombosis of an artery may also be induced by mechanical trauma. Depending on the skill of a particular addict, an intimal flap or perivascular injection may lead to a thombogenic surface.

Compression of a limb may initiate muscle ischemia and result in a compartment syndrome.[95-97] Measurement of intracompartmental pressures is a useful method for establishing the diagnosis in unconscious patients with a suspected compartment syndrome. If the patient is conscious, the diagnosis can usually be made on clinical grounds.

Management

The management of drug-induced vascular injuries has been disappointing. In part, this may relate to the late presentation of patients at an irreversible point. It is clear that, like other diseases, the treatment begins with a thorough history and physical examination. Noninvasive arterial studies are useful to help establish the diagnosis as well as to develop a base of reference. The patient should be resuscitated vigorously to prevent hemoconcentration and the extremity elevated to reduce edema formation. Arteriography should be reserved for those cases suspected of large-vessel disease. Experimental and clinical data support the use of sympathectomy in an attempt to increase tissue perfusion and reduce tissue loss.[90,91] Because thrombosis plays a significant role in this complex problem, anticoagulation with systemic heparin has uniformly been recommended. Prophylactic antibiotics and tetanus prophylaxis are also strongly encouraged. The possibility of a compartment syndrome should lower the threshold for a fasciotomy. Steroids have been advocated by some authorities.[98] The management of ischemic extremities induced by intra-arterial injection of drugs is reviewed in Figure 23-7.

IATROGENIC INJURIES

Diagnostic and therapeutic interventional methods have increased over the last decade. As the number and sophistication of invasive procedures have increased, so too have the number and types of iatrogenic injuries. The vascular system is at particularly high risk of an iatrogenic injury. These injuries are often underemphasized in the surgical literature. In fact, many vascular trauma reports fail to discuss inatrogenic vascular injures.[16,17,65,99-102]

Operations for iatrogenic vascular injuries constitute 10 to 29 percent of all civilian vascular trauma.[103] Many believe that most series underestimate the true incidence of iatrogenic arterial injuries. Arterial complications are more common (90 percent) than venous injuries (10 percent).[104] The experience at the Walter Reed Army Hospital with iatrogenic vascular trauma is reviewed in Table 23-10.

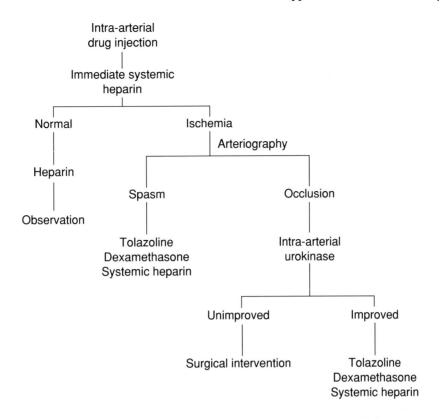

Figure 23-7 Suggested algorithm for treatment of intra-arterial drug injection.

In the Walter Reed experience, the femoral artery is the most commonly injured vessel, followed by the brachial artery[104,105] (Table 23-11). Early correction is essential. As a general rule, there is no place for expectant management of acute limb-threatening ischemia. Vascular consultation should be obtained immediately, if vascular injuries are suspected. Prompt recognition and intervention, if required, is probably the most important factor. A delay in surgical intervention was attributed by the Walter Reed vascular group to be the responsible factor in six of eight permanent functional disabilities and in three of four amputations.[105] Obviously, other important factors include the use of anticoagulation, proper surgical exposure, familiarity with the anatomy, and the use of appropriate techniques for vascular repair. These issues are covered separately in this chapter.

The following sections address the most common types of iatrogenic vascular complications.

Angiography

Angiography has remained the most important diagnostic modality to demonstrate graphically the location and extent of vascular disease. In 1953, Seldinger[106] published his technique for percutaneous vascular catheterization which has formed the basis for

Table 23-10 Walter Reed Army Hospital Experience: Iatrogenic Vascular Injuries

Source of Injury	%
Cardiac catheterization	30
Angiography	30
Surgical complications	30
Miscellaneous procedures	10

(Data from Rich et al.[104] and Youkey et al.[105])

Table 23-11 Walter Reed Army Hospital Experience: Distribution of Iatrogenic Vascular Injuries

Site of Injury	%
Femoral artery	42
Brachial artery	17
Axillary artery	14
Iliac artery	11
Aorta	4

(Data from Rich et al.[104] and Youkey et al.[105])

angiographic access. Angiography has become widely available, nearly every general and tertiary care hospital has these facilities. Because of the large number of procedures performed in the world, iatrogenic vascular injuries are increasingly recognized and reported in the literature. A national survey of hospitals in the United States was conducted by Hessel and associates[107] to determine the incidence of angiographically related injuries. The incidence of vascular complications was dependent on the site of cannulation. The transfemoral technique is the most common approach and has a 1.7 percent incidence of complications. The translumbar technique originally described by Dos Santos[107a] in 1929 and the transaxillary approach had a 2.9 percent and 3.3 percent incidence, respectively. Thirty deaths were reported out of 118,591 angiographic procedures.

The techniques of vessel cannulation, large sheaths, and use of a guidewire are most commonly responsible for vascular complications. The injuries most frequently encountered include vessel perforation with hemorrhage, thrombosis, embolism, pseudoaneurysm formation, and arteriovenous fistula. The axillary/brachial arterial approach has the highest rate of complications. This is related in part to the relatively small size of the vessel compared to the catheter, particularly in children.[108] Hemorrhagic injuries have been observed, resulting in brachial plexus compression injuries.[109] Venous angiography can cause endothelial damage and result in venous thrombosis.[110,111]

On numerous occasions, the history of medicine has recorded serendipitous and fortuitous discoveries as a result of technical misadventure. An example was the discovery of percutaneous transluminal angioplasty (PTA). It was the accidental placement of a catheter retrograde through an occluded iliac artery in 1963 that led Dotter to carry out the first transluminal dilatation in January 1964.[112,113] Subsequent requirements by Porstmann, Zeitler, van Andel, Staple, and Grüntzig led to the development of the modern technique of PTA. PTA and other endovascular therapeutic techniques, including atherectomy and vascular stenting, are finding increased utilization in the treatment of vascular disease, due in part to acceptable results and lower costs relative to surgical revascularization. As with all interventions for vascular disease, though, complications can occur. Complication rates of 2 to 25 percent have been reported for PTA. In a review of the literature, Weibull et al.[114] looked at the complication rates of 2043 PTAs. The overall complication rate was 8.6 percent. Vascular complications that did not require surgery consisted of groin hematoma (2.0 percent), guidewire perforation of the vessel (0.25 percent), subintimal dissection (0.75 percent), and arteriovenous fistula (0.25 percent). Vascular compli-

cations requiring surgical intervention included distal embolization (2.0 percent), vessel thrombosis (1.8 percent), groin hematoma (0.25 percent), retroperitoneal hemorrhage (0.1 percent), pseudoaneurysm (0.1 percent), and intimal injury (0.1 percent). As with many reviews of the literature, the incidence of complications was inversely related to the interventionist's experience. (For a more comprehensive discussion of the complications of interventional procedures and their management, see Ch. 86.)

Cardiology

The advent of cardiac intervention, including fibrinolytic therapy, angioplasty, and valvuloplasty, has led to a corresponding increase in iatrogenic vascular injuries. Patients with congestive heart failure, female gender, smaller weight, and smaller body surface area are at increased risk of a vascular complication.[115] Procedures associated with the greatest risk of a vascular complication include PTA and valvuloplasty.[115] This is related in part to the larger sheaths required for interventional procedures.

In the Coronary Artery Surgery Study (CASS), 7551 coronary angiograms were reviewed for complications.[116] Arterial embolization, thrombosis, and dissection occurred more frequently with the transbrachial route (2.85 percent) than with the transfemoral route (0.45 percent). The brachial artery approach is particularly risky for women, with a relative risk of 11.6, as compared with men.[117] The brachial artery often has excellent collaterals and, in a few cases, observation of a brachial artery thrombosis has been acceptable.[118] We do not recommend this approach, as it can result in hand ischemia and fatigue. Exploration of the brachial artery, thrombectomy, and vein patch angioplasty are simple procedures that should be preformed at diagnosis.

Intra-aortic Balloon Counterpulsation

The insertion and use of intra-aortic balloon counterpulsation (IABP) are often associated with vascular injuries in extremely sick patients. These injuries occur frequently and have been observed in 8 to 36 percent of patients with IABP.[103,119,120] In Perler's experience, the vascular complications consisted of ischemic extremities (4.5 percent), arterial injury (2.5 percent), and hemorrhage (0.9 percent). Lower-extremity ischemia was due to either thromboemboli dislodged during insertion and/or operation of the pump or to obstruction of the arterial lumen by the large balloon catheter and sheath.

Local injuries are managed most often with simple repairs. Arterial dissection of the iliac artery and the aorta, however, can be devastating with five of six patients dying in one series.[120] Several factors are important in the prevention of these injuries. Care must be given to examine the insertion site for the presence of arterial disease. Selection of the appropriate balloon size is also important. During insertion, care must be taken to avoid forcing the catheter. If it does not pass easily or an ischemic extremity results after the insertion, the balloon catheter should be removed and, if necessary, inserted at another site. An ischemic extremity that does not improve with the removal of a catheter should be explored. Diagnostic angiography can help identify the cause of ischemia and limit the required repair. If the patient is dependent on an IABP and no other sites are available, a cross-femoral bypass below the catheter is an acceptable solution.

Vascular Injuries During Surgical Procedures

Surgical intervention carries the risk of intraoperative and postoperative complications. These complications are not exclusively the domain of one surgical speciality but should be considered by all physicians practicing the art and science of surgery. The more common iatrogenic vascular surgical complications merit review.

Femoral artery and vein injuries can occur during inguinal hernia repairs.[104,105,121] Classically, this occurs with the transition sutures placed during a Cooper ligament repair. Vascular injuries have been reported with tumor resections and placement of chemotherapy and hyperalimentation catheters.[122] In Myers's series, four mechanisms for vascular injuries were identified. These mechanisms consisted of direct trauma to a vascular structure, long-term presence of an indwelling catheter, local tumor invasion, and radiation necrosis.[122]

Laparoscopy is a commonly performed diagnostic and therapeutic procedure. During insertion of the laparoscope, the proximity of the aorta, vena cava, and iliac arteries and veins places these structures at increased risk of injury. In one series, a vascular complication was attributed to a constellation of factors, including a thin abdominal wall in a young woman with lumbar lordosis.[123] Peritoneal dialysis trocars have been reported to result in iliac and aortic arterial injury.[124,125] The angle of insertion of the trocar is critical and has been emphasized in the literature.[123,126] The

needle must be inserted at a 45-degree angle to the abdominal wall.

Arterial and venous injuries after orthopaedic procedures are unusual despite the close association of vascular to bony structures. Orthopaedic procedures resulting in vascular injuries have included lumbar laminectomy,[5] total hip replacement,[5,127,128] open reduction and internal fixation in the lower extremity,[5] closed reduction of humeral fracture,[5] and hip flexion contracture release.[5] Vascular surgical intervention can range from intraoperative consultation for uncontrolled bleeding to postoperative limb-threatening ischemia. Some reports have documented pseudoaneurysm formation resulting from unsuspected trauma at hip replacement surgery.[129,130] Thrombobosis of the distal superficial femoral and popliteal artery may result from the application of a pneumatic tourniquet. This device has also caused dislodgement of atheromatous plaque and blunt injuries due to compression of the vessel against a bony structure. Arthroscopic procedures can result in both blunt and penetrating injuries to the popliteal artery. The extensive manipulation of the limb during an orthopaedic procedure can result in stretch injuries to the superficial femoral and popliteal arteries. Patients with prior vascular procedures are at risk as demonstrated by a report of patient with a femoral-to-popliteal PTFE bypass, which thrombosed at the conclusion of a limb-shortening procedure for a comminuted supracondylar femur fracture.[131]

Retroperitoneal dissections have been associated with both arterial and venous injuries.[105] In Youkey's series, injuries were observed in urologic, general surgical, and gynecologic procedures. Factors contributing to these injuries are related to the proximity of the vessels, the disruption of anatomic planes by the tumor, and the radical nature of the surgery. Venous injuries are more common than arterial iatrogenic injuries during the course of a retropertoneal dissection.[6] Veins are difficult to appreciate by palpation and are therefore easily damaged. Venous injuries are often difficult to control. The principle of venous trauma is to obtain proximal and distal control without extending the injury; the closure should not compromise the lumen. Not all venous injuries result in bleeding; thrombosis resulting from trauma is underreported in the literature. Acute deep venous thrombosis can result in phlegmasia cerulea dolens.

Arterial thrombosis or distal embolization may occur as a result of blunt trauma or unrecognized compression. These events may be initiated by an event as simple as placement of a retractor blade. Without systemic anticoagulation, local thrombosis can occur and propagate distally. Discovery of the ischemic extremity may be delayed until the postoperative period. Time is of the essence and intervention critical to reverse the ischemia. Atheroemboli are often a more serious threat to limb viability than thrombosis since emboli may lodge in the digital vessels or the plantar arch, a location, not amenable to mechanical embolectomy. Lumbar sympathectomy may enhance the microcirculation in the skin overlying the endangered foot or digits.

PEDIATRIC INJURIES

Many principles established for adult vascular trauma are not directly applicable to the pediatric population. Pediatric vascular trauma poses new problems that often must be approached with a variety of different considerations. This is complicated by less well-defined principles and guidelines concerning vascular trauma in children. Most surgeons often have relatively limited experience with pediatric vascular trauma. On the other hand, it is not a rare event.[132-142] In the Johns Hopkin's series, pediatric vascular trauma increased over the 10-year period of the review, and 25 percent of reported cases were seen during the last year.[138]

Because of the small size of their vessels, these patients present a technical challenge. Even the simple act of mobilizing the femoral artery has been shown to result in thrombosis requiring a thrombectomy in a 3-year-old.[143] Arteries in children under 3 years of age are particularly susceptible to vasospasm. Because of these observations and the relative infrequency of tissue loss and limb-threatening ischemia, some surgeons have advocated a conservative approach to iatrogenic injuries.[133,136] Opponents to this approach site case reports of limb shortening that have been observed in growing children with arterial insufficiency of an extremity.[132,133,135,136,138]

The mechanisms and etiology of vascular trauma are similar to those in adults, except for distribution, which varies with age. Certainly, iatrogenic injuries are the most common mechanism (86 percent) in newborns and children under 2 years of age.[138] In a review of the Johns Hopkins Hospital 10-year experience (1965–1975), Shaker and associates[138] reported on 118 children under the age of 15 with vascular injuries. The extremities were the most commonly reported site of injury. Iatrogenic injuries comprised 58 percent of all

Table 23-12 Distribution of Iatrogenic Pediatric Vascular Injuries

Location	%
Femoral	66
Brachial	27

Table 23-13 Distribution of Penetrating Pediatric Vascular Injuries

Location	%
Subclavian	13.6
Vertebral	4.5
Carotid	4.5
Radial	36
Femoral	18
Popliteal	13.6

cases reported and 59 percent of iatrogenic injuries occurred in children under 4 years of age. By contrast, only 42 percent were penetrating injuries in children under 4 years of age. Penetrating vascular injuries predominate in children over 6 years of age (63 percent). When major vascular injuries do occur, they are similar to the adult experience in location and indications for surgery. In a review of 233 children with major trauma, 5 percent were vascular injuries and all required surgical intervention[144] (Tables 23-12 and 23-13).

Vascular injuries with impending tissue loss require surgical intervention. Nonoperative management in these situations, regardless of age, has no role. The main controversy concerns the care of nonischemic, iatrogenic vascular injuries. Children with iatrogenic vascular injuries have excellent collaterals and are often able to avoid tissue loss.[133,135,138,145] Despite the rarity of acute symptomatic limb ischemia, reports have focused on the long-term consequences of nonoperative management. Particular attention has been directed at limb growth retardation. This was first observed by Harris and associates[146] in a child who underwent a Blalock-Taussing procedure. Since then there are numerous reports documenting the occurrence of limb shortening in children after nonoperative management of an iatrogenic injury, although the incidence of limb shortening in a control group is not established. Taylor and associates[133] were concerned with this issue. In their careful retrospective review, it was found that limb shortening develops in children with iatrogenic catheter-related injuries at the same incidence as a similar cohort group. These investigators concluded that children under the age of 5 may be observed for clinical symptoms. In the absence of symptoms, surgical intervention does not appear to be warranted.

REFERENCES

1. DeBakey M, Simeone F: Battle injuries of the arteries in World War II: an analysis of 2,471 cases. Ann Surg 123:534, 1946

2. Rich N: Vascular trauma. Surg Clin North Am 53:1367, 1973
3. Rich N, Baugh J, Hughes C: Acute arterial injuries in Vietnam: 1000 cases. J Trauma 10:359, 1970
4. Mattox KL, Feliciano DV, Burch J et al: Five thousand seven hundred sixty cardiovascular injuries in 4459 patients. Epidemiologic evolution 1958 to 1987. Ann Surg 209:698, 1989
5. Freischlag JA, Sise M, Quinones BWJ et al: Vascular complications associated with orthopedic procedures. Surg Gynecol Obstet 169:147, 1989
6. Hertzer NR: Vascular problems in urologic patients. Urol Clin North Am 12:493, 1985
7. Brotman S, Browner BD, Cox EF: MAS trousers improperly applied causing a compartment syndrome in lower-extremity trauma. J Trauma 22:598, 1982
8. Wilson J: Shotgun ballistics and shotgun injuries. West J Med 129:149, 1978
9. Seller J, Richardson J: Amputation after extremity injury. Am J Surg 152:260, 1986
10. Shah P, Ito K, Clauss R: Is limb loss avoidable in civilian vascular injuries? Am J Surg 154:202, 1987
11. Perry M: Vascular injuries. p. 177. In Shires G (ed): Principles of Trauma Care. McGraw-Hill, New York, 1985
12. Spencer A: The reliability of signs of peripheral vascular injury. Surg Gynecol Obstet 114:490, 1962
13. Tohmeh AG, Perler BA: Angiography in the evaluation of proximal arterial injury. Surg Gynecol Obstet 170:117, 1990
14. Menzoian J, Doyle J, Cantelmo N: A comprehensive approach to extremity vascular trauma. Arch Surg 120:801, 1985
15. Smith RE, Elliott JD, Hageman JH: Acute penetrating arterial injuries of the neck and limbs. Arch Surg 109:198, 1974
16. Drapanas T, Hewitt R, Weichert R: Civilian vascular injuries: a critical appariasal of three decades of management. Ann Surg 172:351, 1970
17. Perry M, Thal E, Shires G: Management of arterial injuries. Ann Surg 173:403, 1971
18. Saletta J, Freeark R: The partially severed artery. Arch Surg 97:198, 1968
19. Patman D, Foulos E, Shires G: The management of civilian arterial injuries. Surg Gynecol Obstet 118:725, 1964
20. Dillard B, Nelson D, Norman H: Review of 85 major arterial injuries. Surg 63:391, 1968
21. Sirinek K, Levine B, Gaskill H III, Root V: Reassessment of the role of routine operative exploration in vascular trauma. J Trauma 21:339, 1981
22. Getzen L, Bellinger S, Kendall L: Should all neck, axillary, groin, or popliteal wounds be explored for possible vascular or visceral injuries? J Trauma 12:906, 1972
23. Chakravarty M: Utilization of angiography in trauma. Radiol Clin North Am 24:383, 1986
24. Sirinek K, Gaskill H III, Dittman W, Levine B: Exclusion angiography for patients with possible injuries of the extremity: a better use of trauma center resources. Surgery 94:598, 1983
25. McDonald EJ, Goodman P, Winestock M: The clinical indications for arteriography in trauma to the extremity. Radiology 116:45, 1975
26. McCorkell S, Harley S, Morishima M, Cummings D: Indications for angiography in extremity trauma. AJR 145:1245, 1985
27. Anderson R, Hobson RI, Lee B et al: Reduced dependency on arteriography for penetrating extremity trauma: influence of wound location and noninvasive vascular studies. J Trauma 30:1059, 1990
28. Bynoe R, Miles W, Bell R et al: Noninvasive diagnosis of vascular trauma by duplex ultrasonography. J Vasc Surg 14:346, 1991
29. Shields L, Mohinder M, Cave D: Complete dislocation of the knee: experience at the Massachusetts General Hospital. J Trauma 9:192, 1969
30. O'Donnell TJ, Brewster D, Darling R et al: Arterial injuries associated with fractures and/or disruption of the knee. J Trauma 17:775, 1977
31. Barrata J, Lim V, Mastromonaco E, Edilon E: Axillary artery disruption secondary to anterior dislocation of the shoulder. J Trauma 23:1009, 1983
32. Sclafani SJ, Cooper R, Shaftan GW et al: Arterial trauma: diagnostic and therapeutic angiography. Radiology 161:165, 1986
33. Sampson R, Pasternak B: Traumatic arterial spasm: rarity or nonentity. J Trauma 20:607, 1980
34. Cohen I, Chretien P: Control of hemorrhage from the internal jugular vein by a balloon catheter. Surg Gynecol Obstet 132:791, 1973
35. Belkin M, Dunton R, Crombie HDJ, Lowe R: Preoperative percutaneous intraluminal balloon catheter control of major arterial hemorrhage. J Trauma 28:548, 1988
36. McCaughan J, Young J: Intra-arterial occlusion in vascular surgery. Ann Surg 171:695, 1970
37. Sher MH: Principles in the management of arterial injuries associated with fracture/dislocations. Ann Surg 182:630, 1975
38. Miller H, Welch C: Quantitative studies on the time factor in arterial injuries. Ann Surg 130:428, 1949
39. Bongard FS, White GH, Klein SR: Management strategy of complex extremity injuries. Am J Surg 158:151, 1989
40. Weimann S, San NM, Sandbichler P et al: Civilian popliteal artery trauma. J Cardiovasc Surg (Torino) 28:145, 1987
41. Weaver FA, Rosenthal RE, Waterhouse G, Adkins RB: Combined skeletal and vascular injuries of the lower extremities. Am Surg 50:189, 1984
42. Wagner W, Calkins E, Weaver F et al: Blunt popliteal arterial trauma: one hundred consecutive injuries. J Vasc Surg 7:736, 1988
43. Snyder WH III, Watkins WL, Whiddon LL, Bone GE: Civilian popliteal artery trauma: an eleven year experience with 83 injuries. Surgery 85:101, 1979
44. Peck JJ, Eastman AB, Bergan JJ et al: Popliteal vascular

trauma. A community experience. Arch Surg 125:1339, 1990

45. Daughterty M, Sachatello C, Ernst C: Improved treatment of popliteal arterial injuries. Arch Surg 113:1317, 1978

46. Fabian TC, Turkleson ML, Connelly TL, Stone HH: Injury to the popliteal artery. Am J Surg 143:225, 1982

47. Gnanadev DA, Fandrich BL: Popliteal artery trauma: update and recent advances in management. Ann Vasc Surg 2:332, 1988

48. Howe HRJ, Poole GVJ, Hansen KJ et al: Salvage of lower extremities following combined orthopedic and vascular trauma. A predictive salvage index. Am Surg 53:205, 1987

49. Jaggers R, Feliciano D, Mattox K et al: Injury to popliteal vessels. Arch Surg 117:657, 1982

50. Krige JE, Spence RA: Popliteal artery trauma: a high risk injury. Br J Surg 74:91, 1987

51. Armstrong K, Sfeir R, Rice J, Kerstein M: Popliteal vascular injuries and war: are Beirut and New Orleans similar? J Trauma 28:836, 1988

52. Cohen A, Baldwin J, Grant R: Problems in the management of battlefield vascular injuries. Am J Surg 118:526, 1969

53. Ger R: The coverage of vascular repairs by muscle transposition. J Trauma 16:974, 1976

54. Rodgers CM, Ketch LL: Management of associated soft-tissue injury. Surg Clin North Am 68:823, 1988

55. Swartz WM, Jones NF: Soft tissue coverage of the lower extremity. Curr Probl Surg 22:1, 1985

56. Ledgerwood A, Lucas C: Biological dressings sfor exposed vascular grafts: a reasonable alternative. J Trauma 16:974, 1975

57. Goldsmith HS, Beattie EJJ: Protection of vascular prostheses following radical inguinal excisions. Surg Clin North Am 49:413, 1969

58. Watkins RM, Thomas JM: The role of greater omentum in reconstructing skin and soft tissue defects of the groin and axilla. Br J Surg 72:925, 1985

59. Lange RH, Bach AW, Hansen STJ, Johansen KH: Open tibial fractures with associated vascular injuries: prognosis for limb salvage. J Trauma 25:203, 1985

60. Peck JJ, Fitzgibbons TJ, Gaspar MR: Devastating distal arterial trauma and continuous intraarterial infusion of tolazoline. Am J Surg 145:562, 1983

61. Feliciano DV, Mattox KL, Graham JM, Bitondo CG: Five-year experience with PTFE grafts in vascular wounds. J Trauma 25:71, 1985

62. Shah P, Katsuki I, Clauss R et al: Expanded microporous polytrtrafluroethylene (PTFE) grafts in contaminated wounds: experimental and clinical study. J Trauma 23:1030, 1983

63. Vaughan GD, Mattox KL, Feliciano DV et al: Surgical experience with expanded polytetrafluoroethylene (PTFE) as a replacement graft for traumatized vessels. J Trauma 19:403, 1979

64. Kelly G, Eiseman B: Civilian vascular injuries. J Trauma 15:507, 1975

65. Reynolds RR, McDowell HA, Diethelm AG: The sur-

gical treatment of arterial injuries in the civilian population. Ann Surg 189:700, 1979

66. Shah DM, Naraynsingh V, Leather RP et al: Advances in the management of acute popliteal vascular blunt injuries. J Trauma 25:793, 1985

67. Orcutt MB, Levine BA, Root HD, Sirinek KR: The continuing challenge of popliteal vascular injuries. Am J Surg 146:758, 1983

68. Feliciano DV, Herskowitz K, OGorman RB et al: Management of vascular injuries in the lower extremities. J Trauma 28:319, 1988

69. Ashworth EM, Dalsing MC, Glover JL, Reilly MK: Lower extremity vascular trauma: a comprehensive, aggressive approach. J Trauma 28:329, 1988

70. Keeley SB, Snyder WH III, Weigelt JA: Arterial injuries below the knee: fifty-one patients with 82 injuries. J Trauma 23:285, 1983

71. McNutt R, Seabrook GR, Schmitt DD et al: Blunt tibial artery trauma: predicting the irretrievable extremity. J Trauma 29:1624, 1989

72. Yeager RA, Hobson RW II, Lynch TG et al: Popliteal and infrapopliteal arterial injuries. Differential management and amputation rates. Am Surg 50:155, 1984

73. Hardin WJ, O'Connell R, Adinolfi M, Kerstein M: Traumatic arterial injuries of the upper extremity: determinants of disability. Am J Surg 150:266, 1985

74. Sitzmann J, Ernst C: Management of arm arterial injuries. Surgery 96:895, 1984

75. Orcutt MB, Levine BA, Gaskill HV, Sirinek KR: Civilian vascular trauma of the upper extremity. J Trauma 26:63, 1986

76. Borman K, Snyder W, Weigelt J: Civilian arterial trauma of the upper extremity. Am J Surg 148:796, 1984

77. Myers SI, Harward TR, Maher DP et al: Complex upper extremity vascular trauma in an urban population. J Vasc Surg 12:305, 1990

78. Graham J, Feliciano D, Mattox K et al: Management of subclavian vascular injuries. J Trauma 20:539, 1980

79. Alix E, Bogumill G, Wright C: Intra-arterial injection of abused drugs. Cardiovasc Res 9:266, 1975

80. Benitez PR, Newell MA: Vascular trauma in drug abuse: patterns of injury. Ann Vasc Surg 1:175, 1986

81. Ryan J, Hooper J, Jabaley M: Drug injection injuries of the hands and forearms in addicts. Plast Reconstr Surg 53:445, 1974

82. Bardenheuer L: Die Entstehung und Behandlung der ischämischen Muskelkowtmktur und Gangrän. Dtsch Z Chir 108:44, 1911

83. Mubarak S, Hargens A: Acute compartment syndromes. Surg Clin North Am 63:539, 1983

84. Bondurant FJ, Cotler HB, Buckle R et al: The medical and economic impact of severely injured lower extremities. J Trauma 28:1270, 1988

85. Odland MD, Gisbert VL, Gustilo RB et al: Combined orthopedic and vascular injury in the lower extremities: indications for amputation. Surgery 108:660, 1990

86. Ransom K, Shatney C, Soderstom C, Cowley R: Man-

agement of arterial injuries in blunt trauma of the extremity. Surg Gynecol Obstet 153:241, 1981

87. Peacock J, Proctor H: Factors limiting extremity function following vascular injury. J Trauma 17:532, 1977

88. Visser P, Hermerck A, Pierce G et al: Prognosis of nerve injuries incurred during acute trauma to peripheral arteries. Am J Surg 134:226, 1980

89. VanderPost C: Report of case of mistaken injection of pentothal sodium into an aberrant ulnar artery. S Afr Med J 16:182, 1942

90. Cohen S: Accidental intra-arterial injection of drugs. Lancet 2:311, 1948

91. Kinmonth J, Shepherd R: Accidental injection of thiopentone into arteries. Studies of pathology and treatment. Br Med J 2:914, 1959

92. Engler H, Freeman R, Kanavage C et al: Production of gangrenous extremities by intra-arterial injections. Am Surg 30:602, 1964

93. Citron B, Halpern M, McCarron M et al: Necrotizing angiitis associated with drug abuse. N Engl J Med 283:1003, 1970

93a. Wright AE, Douglas SR: An experimental investigation of the role of the blood fluids in connection with phacocytosis. Proc Roy Soc (Lond) 72:357, 1903–1904

94. Brown S, Lyons S, Sundee J: A study of some factors leading to intravascular thrombosis. Br J Anaesth 40:13, 1968

95. Kaufer H, Spengler DM, Noyes FR, Louis DS: Orthopaedic implications of the drug subculture. J Trauma 14:853, 1974

96. Dolich B, Aiache A: Drug-induced coma: a case of crush syndrome and ischemic contracture. J Trauma 13:223, 1973

97. Owen C, Mubarka S, Hargens A et al: Intramuscular pressures with limb compression: clarification of the pathogenesis of the drug-induced muscle-compartment syndrome. N Engl J Med 30:1169, 1979

98. Buckspan G, Franklin J, Novak G et al: Studies of etiology and potential treatment. J Surg Res 24:294, 1978

99. Frykberg ER, Vines FS, Alexander RH: The natural history of clinically occult arterial injuries: a prospective evaluation. J Trauma 29:577, 1989

100. Frykberg ER, Crump JM, Dennis JW et al: Nonoperative observation of clinically occult arterial injuries: a prospective evaluation. Surgery 109:85, 1991

101. Cikrit D, Dalsing M, Bryant B et al: An experience with upper-extremity vascular trauma. Am J Surg 160:229, 1990

102. Borman KR, Jones GH, Snyder WH III: A decade of lower extremity venous trauma: patency and outcome. Am J Surg 154:608, 1987

103. Orcutt MB, Levine BA, Gaskill HV III, Sirinek KR: Iatrogenic vascular injuries. A reducible problem. Arch Surg 120:384, 1985

104. Rich N, Hobson R, Fedde C: Vascular trauma secondary to diagnostic and therapeutic procedures. Arch Surg 128:715, 1974

105. Youkey JR, Clagett GP, Rich NM et al: Vascular trauma secondary to diagnostic and therapeutic proce-

dures: 1974 through 1982. A comparative review. Am J Surg 146:788, 1983

106. Seldinger S: Catheter replacement of needle in percutaneous arteriography: new technique. Acta Radiol (Stockh) 39:368, 1953

107. Hessel S, Adams D, Abrams H: Complications of angiography. Radiology 138:273, 1981

107a. Dos Santos R, Lamas A, Pereira-Caldas J: Arteriografia da aorta e dos vasos abdominais. Med Contemp 47:53, 1929

108. Franklin E, Girod A, Sequeira F et al: Femoral artery spasm in children: catheter size is the principle cause. AJR 138:295, 1982

109. Menzoian J, Corson J, Bush H, LoGerfo F: Management of the upper extremity with absent pulses following cardiac catheterization. Am J Surg 135:484, 1978

110. Laerum F, Laake K: Phlegmasia coerulea dolens after pelvic phlebography with meglumine metrizoate. Eur J Radiol 1:117, 1981

111. Laerum F: Injurious effects of contrast media on human vascular endothelium. Invest Radiol, suppl. 1. 20:PS98, 1985

112. Dotter C, Judkins M: Transluminal treatment of arteriosclerotic obstruction: description of a new technic and a preliminary report of its application. Circulation 30:654, 1974

113. Dotter C: Transluminal angioplasty: a long view. Radiology 135:561, 1980

114. Weibull H, Berqvist D, Jonsson K et al: Complications after percutaneous transuminal angioplasty in the iliac, femoral, and popliteal arteries. J Vasc Surg 5:681, 1987

115. McCann R, Schwartz L, Pieper K: Vascular complications of cardiac catheterization. J Vasc Surg 14:375, 1991

116. Davis K, Kennedy J, Kemp H et al: Complications of coronary angiography from the collaborative study of coronary artery surgery (CASS). Circulation 59:1105, 1979

117. Harris J: Coronary angiography and its complications, the search for risk factors. Arch Intern Med 144:337, 1984

118. Gallen J, Wiss D, Cantelmo N, Menzoian J: Traumatic pseudoaneurysm of the axillary artery: report of three cases and review of literature. J Trauma 24:350, 1984

119. Alpert J, Bhaktan E, Gielchinsky I et al: Vascular complications of intra-aortic balloon pumping. Arch Surg 111:1190, 1976

120. Perler B, McCabe C, Abbott W et al: Vascular complications of intra-aortic balloon counterpulsation. Arch Surg 118:957, 1983

121. Natali J, Benhamou AC: Iatrogenic vascular injuries. A review of 125 cases (excluding angiographic injuries). J Cardiovasc Surg (Torino) 20:169, 1979

122. Myers S, Harward T, Putman J, Frazier O: Vascular trauma as a result of therapeutic procedures for the treatment of malignancy. J Vasc Surg 14:314, 1991

123. McDonald PT, Rich NM, Collins GJJ et al: Vascular

trauma secondary to diagnostic and therapeutic procedures: laparoscopy. Am J Surg 135:651, 1978

124. Day R, White R: Peritoneal dialysis in children; review of 8 years experience. Arch Dis Child 52:56, 1977

125. Sanchez CA, Fernandez FW, Alarcon ZA et al: [Puncture of a great vessel: an uncommon complication of peritoneal dialysis.] Rev Clin Esp 134:583, 1974

126. Palmer R: Safety in laparoscopy. J Reprod Med 13:1, 1974

127. Zahrani H, Cuschieri R: Vascular complications after total knee replacement. J Cardiovasc Surg 30:951, 1989

128. Matos MH, Amstutz HC, Machleder HI: Ischemia of the lower extremity after total hip replacement. J Bone Joint Surg 61A:24, 1979

129. Kroese A, Robertson H, Gorniosky M: Traumatic aneurysm of the common femoral artery after hip endoprosthesis: a case report. Acta Orthop Scand 46:119, 1975

130. Dorr L, Conaty J, Kohl R, Harvey J: False aneurysm of the femoral artery following total hip surgery. J Bone Joint Surg 56A:1059, 1974

131. Ellenhorn JI, Fowl RJ, Akers DL, Kempczinski RF: Femur fracture with limb shortening causing occlusion of a polytetrafluoroethylene femoral popliteal graft. J Vasc Surg 12:558, 1990

132. Bassett F, Lincoln C, King T, Canent R: Inequality in the size of the lower extremities following cardiac catheterization. South Med J 61:1013, 1968

133. Taylor L, Troutman R, Feliciano P, Menashe V et al: Late complications after femoral artery catheterization in children less than five years of age. J Vasc Surg 11:297, 1990

134. Barlow B, Niemirska M, Gandhi R: Ten years' experience with pediatric gunshot wounds. J Pediatr Surg 17:927, 1982

135. Klein M, Coran A, Whitehouse W et al: Management of iatrogenic arterial injuries in injuries in infants and children. J Pediatr Surg 17:933, 1982

136. Smith C, Green R: Pediatric vascular injuries. Surgery 90:20, 1981

137. Wolf Y, Reyna T, Schropp K, Harmel R: Arterial trauma of the upper extremity in children. J Trauma 30:903, 1990

138. Shaker I, White J, Signer R et al: Special problems of vascular injuries in children. J Trauma 16:863, 1976

139. Rothrock SG, Howard RM: Delayed brachial artery occlusion owing to a dog bite of the upper extremity. Pediatr Emerg Care 6:293, 1990

140. Reed MK, Lowry PA, Myers SI: Successful repair of pediatric popliteal artery trauma. Am J Surg 160:287, 1990

141. Myers SI, Reed MK, Black CT et al: Noniatrogenic pediatric vascular trauma. J Vasc Surg 10:258, 1989

142. Holcomb GW III, Meacham PW, Dean RH: Penetrating popliteal artery injuries in children. J Pediatr Surg 23:859, 1988

143. Cahill J, Talbert J, Otteson O et al: Arterial complications following cardiac catheterization in infants and children. J Pediatr Surg 2:134, 1967

144. Breaux CWJ, Smith G, Georgeson KE: The first two years' experience with major trauma at a pediatric trauma center. J Trauma 30:37, 1990

145. Salerno F, Collins O, Redmond D: External iliac artery occlusion in a newborn infant. Surgery 67:863, 1970

146. Harris A, Segel N, Bishop J: Blalock-Taussig anastomosis for tetralogy of fallot. A ten to fifteen year follow-up. Br Heart J 26:266, 1964

Section VI

Chronic Arterial Disease

The management of chronic occlusive arterial disease dominates the clinical efforts of most practitioners treating patients with vascular disease. The disciplines of vascular surgery and interventional radiology have both made great strides in this arena since the advent of bypass surgery, which preceded by a decade the description of angioplasty by Charles Dotter. Since these pioneering efforts, there has been considerable elucidation of the indications, techniques, pathophysiology and results of both surgical and interventional techniques. This progress has improved the lifestyle and salvaged the limbs of many patients suffering from chronic occlusive disease. Nevertheless, the treatment of vascular disease is overwhelmingly palliative. Atherosclerosis, the underlying pathology of the majority of patients, is a systemic disease process that may be manifest in only one vascular bed but may be a silent cause of co-morbidity when more aggressive treatment is considered. Furthermore, vascular disease is often inexorably progressive, albeit slowly. These attitudes should help place enthusiasm for aggressive intervention in the appropriate perspective.

Over the last several decades, indications for specific therapeutic approaches have evolved and are now widely accepted. Short segment iliac artery stenoses are ideally treated by angioplasty; long segment infrainguinal occlusions are optimally treated, when appropriate indications are met, with bypass grafting. Between these two relatively clear extremes, there are instances where selection of appropriate treatment involves careful consideration of a wide range of variables including the expected outcome, potential risks, and reasonable alternatives; selection of a treatment option

for any patient requires consideration of all these factors with input from the appropriate specialists and the informed patient. At times, there will be disagreement as to the best treatment option. This diversity of opinions indicates the evolving state of vascular intervention. It is the goal of the authors of the following chapters to try to help put the treatment options into appropriate perspective. Ongoing trials comparing some of the newer treatment options will help to clarify their role in the optimum treatment for patients with chronic occlusive vascular disease. Continued cooperative efforts between surgeons and interventionalists, adoption of uniform terminology and classification and a commitment to careful, long-term follow-up of all interventions will improve our abilities to provide the best treatment to these patients.

Many of the considerations relevant to treatment of chronic vascular disease are discussed within the following sections; however, it is important for the clinician treating these patients to consider all options in each patient, giving foremost consideration to conservative management. A concerted effort toward disease prevention, including stronger emphasis on the dangers of tobacco abuse, sedentary lifestyle, and poor dietary habits is a responsibility that physicians all share. Furthermore, at times the most important decision made in the care of patients with chronic occlusive vascular disease is the decision not to intervene. Commitment to the long-term care of these patients mandates incorporation of conservative management techniques that are vital to successful management of all patients. This, appropriately, is emphasized in each of the ensuing chapters.

The following chapters will review the current status of surgical and interventional management of chronic occlusive vascular disease. It is fitting that this section be as well represented in this text as will be apparent from the ensuing chapters, since it is in the treatment of chronic occlusive disease that the surgical and interventional approaches best complement each other. In these difficult management problems, both the surgical and interventional approaches contribute greatly; indeed, this is the area of closest cooperation between our disciplines. We hope that the contributions in this section serve to further this cooperation and understanding.

24

Clinical Evaluation of Occlusive Peripheral Vascular Disease

B. Clay Parker   Dennis F. Bandyk

Joseph L. Mills   Arina van Breda

Atherosclerotic femoropopliteal occlusive disease may be clinically silent; approximately 10 percent of patients with demonstrable arterial occlusive disease do not claudicate.[1] Most patients come to evaluation because of a range of clinical symptoms including intermittent claudication, ischemic rest pain, ischemic ulceration, tissue necrosis or gangrene, and "blue toe syndrome." These clinical presentations are often well defined and diagnosis may be made on the basis of an adequate history and physical examination. In a significant number of patients, the diagnosis may be less certain. In these patients, noninvasive vascular testing can provide supplemental and confirmatory information essential to treatment planning and patient management. Objective and quantifiable data about the severity of vascular disease is invaluable in proper management. Knowledge of the presentation, evaluation, and natural history of vascular disease is required of all physicians participating in care of these patients. This clinical assessment must be undertaken prior to invasive evaluation and determination of treatment.

HISTORY

The majority (70 percent) of patients presenting for evaluation of peripheral vascular disease have claudication; a smaller number (approximately 25 to 30 per-

cent) have a threatened limb at initial evaluation with ischemic ulcers, rest pain, or gangrene.[1-4] The prevalence of occlusive peripheral vascular disease increases with age, occurring in 3 percent of patients less than 60 years old and in more than 20 percent of the population over 75 years old.[5] Of those patients less than 40 years old at presentation, more than one-half have aortoiliac disease only, while those patients over 40 years old are more likely to have femoropopliteal disease. Multisegment disease occurs in over 20 percent of all patients with intermittent claudication, regardless of age at presentation. Long-term studies of patients with vascular disease have emphasized the relative stability of symptoms and the benefit of conservative management. Only about 25 percent of patients with claudication are likely to have significant progression of symptoms.[2,3,6,7] The majority of patients (60 percent) will have stabilization of symptoms and about 15 percent will improve.[7] The likelihood of amputation in all patients is approximately 5 to 6 percent over 10 years, but is higher in smokers and especially in diabetics, where the likelihood of amputation is 20 percent or more in long-term follow-up.[5]

Intermittent claudication is defined as muscle pain induced by exercise and relieved by rest. The pain is typically produced by the same level of exercise, and usually resolves rapidly with cessation of exercise and without change in position.[8] Onset may be earlier if the patient walks uphill or at a more rapid pace. The pain characteristically develops in the calf muscles in patients with isolated superficial femoral artery (SFA) disease but may be in the thigh or buttocks in patients with aortoiliac disease. Foot claudication can be a presenting symptom in patients with Buerger's disease.[9] Patients will occasionally describe leg fatigue, numbness, or heaviness, rather than pain or cramping. Vasculogenic claudication must be differentiated from neurogenic or pseudoclaudication, which results from spinal stenosis. Neurogenic claudication often has a variable or unpredictable onset and may require a change in position for relief. Patients with purely neurogenic claudication have normal peripheral pulses. However, the two conditions can coexist; evaluation with exercise testing can be extremely useful in differentiating these conditions.[10]

Ischemic rest pain occurs when the resting limb blood flow is insufficient to meet the basal metabolic demands of the extremity. It characteristically develops in the forefoot and is aggravated by elevation and relieved by dependency; it often occurs when the patient goes to bed at night. The loss of gravitational pressure in the supine position is insignificant in patients with normal lower extremity blood flow, but can be critical in patients with marginal limb pressures at rest. Patients will seek relief by sleeping upright, standing and shaking the foot, or paradoxically, by getting out of bed and walking. All these maneuvers restore the beneficial effect of gravity on circulation to the foot.[11]

Ischemic ulcers usually occur on the distal toes but can also occur on the malleoli or on the shins. They may result from minor traumatic skin breaks which fail to heal because of inadequate basal circulation. Ischemic ulcers are characterized by "punched out" borders and a lack of surrounding erythema unless there is superimposed infection. The clinical course is prolonged and the ulcers are characteristically difficult or slow to heal.[12] Ischemic ulcers should be distinguished from neuropathic ulcers, which occur at sites of pressure in patients with abnormal neurologic (sensory) function.[13]

Gangrene develops when ischemia is sufficiently severe to result in tissue necrosis. This process generally begins in the digits and distalmost aspect of the extremities.

An occasional patient with lower extremity vascular disease will present with "blue toe syndrome." The sudden onset of painful, "blue toe(s)" in the presence of palpable pedal pulses should lead the clinician to suspect this entity. It is caused by atheromatous digital embolization from an ulcerated atherosclerotic lesion, and is generally considered an indication for intervention. It may also be superimposed on a more typical history of claudication or rest pain.

The abrupt onset of pain, numbness, paresthesia, coolness, or inability to move the lower leg and/or foot may be indicative of acute lower extremity ischemia related either to an embolic phenomenon or thrombosis of a previously stenotic vessel or thrombosis of a lower extremity aneurysm (e.g., popliteal aneurysm thrombosis); lower extremity bypass graft thrombosis may present in a similar fashion. Careful questioning of patients with acute and severe symptoms may reveal a prior history of milder symptoms indicating underlying vascular disease, which may alter treatment and options (i.e., thrombolysis rather than thrombectomy).

An adequate history specifically seeking symptoms of the various manifestations of atherosclerotic occlusive disease listed above will serve to direct the physical examination. While gathering historical information, the presence of significant risk factors for the development of atherosclerotic disease should be sought. The dominant risk factors are age, male sex, cigarette smoking, diabetes mellitus, obesity, hyperlipidemia, hypertension, and family history of atherosclerotic vascular disease. Coronary artery disease frequently accompanies peripheral vascular disease and its presence should be questioned.[5] The incidence of death due to coronary disease is two to five times greater in claudicants than the general population.[5] Coronary disease accounts for 30 to 70 percent of deaths in patients with obstructive peripheral vascular disease.[5] Significant coronary disease (greater than 70 percent stenosis in at least one coronary artery) is present in as many as 57 percent of such patients.[5] A history of angina, myocardial infarction, congestive heart failure, and previous coronary artery bypass should be specifically sought. A detailed discussion of the management of associated coronary artery disease is beyond the scope of this chapter, but the presence of clinically significant coronary disease may certainly alter patient selection for intervention and choice of intervention. Previous harvesting of the ipsilateral saphenous vein for aortocoronary bypass grafting may similarly alter clinical decision making. Cerebrovascular manifestations of atherosclerotic disease are likewise associated with peripheral vascular disease.[5] The history should include an interrogation regarding previous vascular interventions, surgical or percutaneous, and determination of current medications, especially propranolol[14] and nicotine patches,[8] which may exacerbate symptoms.

PHYSICAL EXAMINATION

A thorough physical examination should include pulse examination and auscultation for carotid, abdominal, and femoral bruits. The abdomen should be carefully palpated for the presence of an abdominal aortic aneurysm (AAA). Brachial pressures should be obtained bilaterally, as the atherosclerosis process can involve the subclavian artery origins and result in an artificially lowered reading; a difference of 20 mmHg between the two arms is significant. Inspection of the legs and feet may reveal trophic changes of thin, shiny pretibial skin, loss of hair from the lower legs and feet, and thick brittle nails, indicative of chronic peripheral vascular insufficiency. A stark white appearance of the foot with collapsed foot veins or a pale, mottled-appearing foot are signs of acute, profound arterial insufficiency. Conversely, a red foot which deepens in intensity upon placing the foot in a dependent position (dependent rubor) or becomes pale upon elevation correlates with fairly severe chronic arterial insufficiency. Focal areas of discoloration, especially bluish or reddish discoloration of one or more toes, may be a sign of microemboli from a stenotic or ulcerated plaque in the more proximal vasculature; frankly blue or purple painful digits are likely to represent "blue toe syndrome."[15]

Inspection of the foot also includes a search for skin breakdown or ulceration. The feet should be carefully examined for the presence of calluses and other cutaneous lesions. The spaces between each of the toes should be specifically examined. Areas over bony prominences, such as the metatarsal heads in diabetic patients, are particularly prone to the development of ulcers. The heel should also be carefully examined for breakdown in the integrity of the integumentary system. Evidence of venous disease, including thickened or indurated skin around the lower leg/ankle, brownish discoloration of the skin, ulcers about the malleolus, or superficial varicosities should also be noted, as this can be an associated factor or the primary cause of the lower extremity complaints. Palpation of the lower extremities establishes a subjective determination of warmth or coolness of the legs, making note of the ambient temperature of the examination room. In extremely ischemic patients with rest pain, light touch can severely exacerbate the discomfort. Pulses should be sought, particularly at the femoral, popliteal, dorsalis pedis, and posterior tibial levels. All peripheral pulses should be palpated, and judged to be absent, diminished, normal, or hyperactive.[15] Although the dorsalis pedis pulse may be absent in up to 12 percent of normal subjects, absence of the posterior tibial pulse is a strong clinical sign of peripheral vascular disease.[16] Capillary refill can be evaluated by application of pressure to the toenail and/or toe and rapidly releasing after observation for the normal, pink color to return (normal = about 1 second). Another simple bedside test that can be incorporated into the physical examination is a postural elevation/dependency examination, which can also give supportive information about the

presence of peripheral vascular disease. With the patient supine, the examiner elevates and supports the legs at a 65-degree angle with the knees straight. The patient exercises the feet and/or toes by dorsiflexion and plantar flexion. In the presence of arterial insufficiency, the involved extremity will become pale and the veins of the foot will collapse. At this point, the patient should be moved to a sitting position, with the feet in a dependent position; the time for the foot to resume a normal color and the time required for the foot veins to redistend should be noted. Normally, the color should return within 10 seconds and the veins fill within 15 seconds. In moderate ischemia, 25 to 30 seconds may pass before color and venous distention return; when the times are longer than 30 to 40 seconds, severe ischemia is indicated.[15] Proprioception and light touch sensory testing are important in patients with acute arterial insufficiency as loss of any of these is a sign of limb-threatening ischemia, as well as in diabetics with suspected peripheral vascular disease since diabetic neuropathy may be a contributing or complicating factor in peripheral vascular disease. Muscle strength should be assessed on an ongoing basis in patients with acute, severe ischemia, as this may be another sign of impending irreversible ischemia.

NONINVASIVE VASCULAR TESTING

While history and physical examination will establish the diagnosis of vascular disease in the majority of patients with advanced disease, patients with milder disease may prove more difficult to evaluate. Both false-positive and false-negative diagnoses may result from reliance on historical and physical examination only.[17] To objectively and accurately establish the etiology of extremity complaints and, more significantly, to quantify the severity of disease, noninvasive testing is essential.

Quantification of severity is one of the major benefits of noninvasive testing. As is evident elsewhere in this text, published results of treatment of vascular disease are often difficult to assess due to the varied and at times subjective parameters used for patient selection and to define success. Classification of vascular patients by the historical and noninvasive criteria as proposed by the Society of Vascular Surgery and modified by Rutherford has been accepted by the surgical and interventional communities[18] (Table 24-1). Use of this classification is of value in accurately assessing and describing vascular status, and provides a common basis for definition of clinical status.

Noninvasive testing can identify patients with nonvascular etiology of complaints and can alert the clini-

Table 24-1 Clinical Categories of Limb Ischemia

Acute Limb Ischemia

Category	Description	Capillary Return	Muscle Weakness	Sensory Loss	Doppler Signals	
					Arterial	Venous
Viable	Not immediately threatened	Intact	None	None	Audible AP more than 30 mmHg	Audible
Threatened	Salvageable if promptly treated	Intact, slow	Mild, partial	Mild, incomplete	Inaudible	Audible
Irreversible	Major tissue loss, amputation required regardless of treatment	Absent (marbling)	Profound, paralysis (rigor)	Profound, anesthetic	Inaudible	Inaudible

Chronic Limb Ischemia

Grade	Category	Clinical Description	Objective Criteria
	0	Asymptomatic, no hemodynamically significant occlusive disease	Normal results of treadmill[a]/stress test
I	1	Mild claudication	Treadmill exercise completed, postexercise AP is greater than 50 mmHg but more than 25 mmHg less than normal
	2	Moderate claudication	Symptoms between those of categories 1 and 3
	3	Severe claudication	Treadmill exercise cannot be completed, postexercise AP is less than 50 mmHg
II	4	Ischemic rest pain	Resting AP of 40 mmHg or less, flat or barely pulsatile ankle or metatarsal plethysmographic tracing, toe pressure less than 30 mmHg
III	5	Minor tissue loss, nonhealing ulcer, focal gangrene with diffuse pedal ischemia	Resting AP of 60 mmHg or less, ankle or metatarsal plethysmographic tracing flat or barely pulsatile, toe pressure less than 40 mmHg
	6	Major tissue loss, extending above transmetatarsal level, functional foot no longer salvageable	Same as for category 5

Abbreviation: AP, ankle pressure.
[a] Five minutes at 2 mph on a 12-degree incline.
(From Rutherford and Becker,[18] with permission.)

cian to those patients in whom symptoms are multifactorial in origin. This determination is critical in decision making, such as in the patient with coexistent vascular disease and neuropathy. Noninvasive studies can be used as a baseline for clinical follow-up in the large majority of patients with claudication who are treated nonoperatively to accurately measure progression or document stabilization of disease. In those patients who undergo surgical or percutaneous intervention, postoperative studies can be compared with those obtained prior to intervention to document the patency and hemodynamic success of the reconstruction, to identify a failing or failed intervention, and to determine long term efficacy. Noninvasive testing techniques are described in greater detail in Chapters 13 and 14; their application in the assessment of peripheral vascular disease is briefly highlighted here.

Blood Pressure Measurement

Blood pressure measurement in the extremities of a patient with known or suspected peripheral vascular disease is the most basic aspect of noninvasive testing. Using a simple sphygmomanometer and hand-held Doppler, bilateral brachial pressures as well as bilateral ankle pressures (measuring both dorsalis pedis and posterior tibial pressures) quickly and easily allows one to determine the ankle-brachial index (ABI). This quick and easily reproducible test can give significant objective evidence regarding the degree of impairment of perfusion of a particular limb. The ankle-brachial index should normally be 0.95 or greater. Though there is some individual variability, generally patients with ABIs in the 0.5 to 0.9 range have complaints of claudication, whereas patients with ABIs less than 0.5 are likely to have rest pain or nonhealing ulcers. Likewise, an absolute ankle pressure of less than 50 mmHg is indicative of severe ischemia.[18,19]

Segmental blood pressure measurements adds some anatomic specificity. Measurements are made with a series of blood pressure cuffs at the thigh, calf, and ankle levels. The stronger of the dorsalis pedis and posterior tibial Doppler signals at the ankle level is monitored as the cuffs are sequentially inflated and deflated to determine the systolic pressure at each level along the limb. A drop in pressure of 20 to 30 mmHg between segments is a significant drop, indicative of a significant stenosis between the two locations that the measurements are taken. Likewise, a 20-mmHg difference in pressure at the same level between the two lower extremities suggests significant occlusive disease.[20] Due to the relatively larger circumference of the upper thigh, relative to the lower thigh, calf and ankle levels, a mismatch can occur between the thigh size and the cuff size. This will result in artificially elevated upper thigh pressures. Some vascular laboratories accept this thigh-cuff size discrepancy and look for a 20- to 30-mmHg higher thigh pressure than brachial pressure as a normal finding (no significant occlusive disease in the aorto-iliac segment). Other labs correct for this discrepancy by using relatively larger cuffs at the upper thigh levels, with the normal upper thigh pressures being recorded nearly equivalent to the brachial pressure. Obviously the interpreter of the noninvasive examination must be familiar with this aspect of a particular laboratory's testing technique to avoid a potential pitfall.

A well-known pitfall of lower extremity blood pressure measurements is artifactually elevated ankle pressures (and hence ABIs) in patients with noncompressible vessels. The most common etiology of this is Monckeberg's medial sclerosis, found in patients with diabetes mellitus. The great toe pressure measurement — either as an absolute value or indexed to the brachial pressure (the great toe-brachial index) — can be used in such cases, as the digital arteries are less likely to be noncompressible. A normal great toe-brachial index is 0.6 or greater; absolute toe pressures of 30 mmHg or greater are typically required for healing.[19]

Doppler Waveform Analysis

Directional Doppler waveform analysis is an additional source of information about the presence or ab-

sence of occlusive vascular disease (see Ch. 13).[20] While a degraded waveform may be due to proximal occlusive disease, probe malalignment relative to the arterial flow, superimposed venous flow signal, patient motion, and arterial wall or plaque calcification are but a few possible causes of artifactually degraded Doppler waveforms. It is imperative, therefore, to incorporate the Doppler waveform analysis with other aspects of noninvasive testing.

Plethysmography

Segmental limb plethysmography, also known as volume pulse recordings, pulse volume recordings, or PVRs, is a reproducible noninvasive test that has the advantage of allowing a global assessment of segmental perfusion regardless the route of delivery of blood to a given segment (native vessel versus collateral flow versus bypass graft). This unique characteristic makes it a useful modality in the evaluation of limb perfusion. Degradation of the plethysmographic curve implies impairment of perfusion of a given segment due to obstructive disease proximal to that segment.

Segmental plethysmographic recordings are especially useful in diabetic patients, as the recordings are not affected by noncompressible vessels (as are segmental limb pressure measurements) and the test avoids many of the previously described pitfalls involved with directional doppler waveform recordings.[21] Transmetatarsal waveforms are routinely available to evaluate distal disease. A potential source of error in interpretation of segmental plethysmographic waveform is isolated profunda femoris disease. In this clinical situation, the patient will complain of thigh claudication, which might suggest aortoiliac segmental disease. The thigh plethysmographic recordings will be degraded, again, possibly implicating aortoiliac disease. The presence of a triphasic Doppler signal at the common femoral artery level or a normal high thigh pressure measurement would be the needed clues that the true disease is not in the aortoiliac region. This potential pitfall illustrates the necessity of integration of presenting symptoms with several different modes of noninvasive vascular testing.

Photoplethysmography (PPG) is a means of determining perfusion at the cutaneous level.[21] Evaluation of the cutaneous perfusion of the feet and toes is particularly useful in patients with nonhealing wounds in helping to establish the vascular component of the delayed healing as well as the response to therapy. PPGs are also useful in evaluating patients with suspected very distal vascular occlusive disease.

Exercise Testing

While resting noninvasive tests are adequate in patients with characteristic symptoms and moderate or advanced disease, patients with atypical or exertional symptoms only will require a more complete evaluation. In these patients, exercise testing is vitally important to ensure accurate diagnosis. It allows the clinician to observe, record, and correlate the patient's symptoms while reproducing the physiologic state that leads to these symptoms. Exercise testing should be performed on all patients with normal or near-normal resting studies and in those patients with abnormal resting studies where there is a question or possibility of nonvascular causes contributing to the symptoms.

The standard exercise treadmill test is performed on a 12-degree grade at 1.7 to 2 mph until the patient is forced to stop. These parameters may be adjusted based on the presenting symptoms and the patient's overall condition. After the exercise, repeat ankle and brachial blood pressure measurements are recorded, followed by repeat ankle plethysmographic recordings. The normal response is a postexercise ankle systolic pressure greater than 80 percent of the pre-exercise value as well as maintenance of good plethysmographic waveform morphology, although with augmented amplitude when compared with pre-exercise data. Significant reductions in ankle pressures and/or degradation of the plethysmographic recordings which correlate with the development of leg pain objectively document a vasculogenic cause. Patients with pure neurogenic claudication will not demonstrate an exercise-induced reduction in ABI.[22] Again, careful correlation of the results of exercise testing and the patient's symptoms is mandatory to avoid errors in diagnosis. Patients who develop claudication during exercise testing must be questioned as to whether their typical symptoms are the same as those induced on the treadmill.

An alternative to exercise testing is the reaction hyperemia testing, using a 4-minute thigh occlusion cuff, followed by measurement of ankle blood pressure. Normally, the postocclusion ankle pressure should be greater than 80 percent of the preocclusion value.[23]

Color-Flow Doppler

Recent interest has developed in mapping the lower extremity arterial tree with color-flow Doppler imaging. The main value of this technique is that it can differentiate stenotic arterial segments from complete occlusions. By using the criteria of an increased flow velocity of 100 percent in an area of stenosis relative to the flow velocity in an immediately proximal arterial segment, and loss of the reversed component of the normally triphasic Doppler waveform, a hemodynam-

ically significant focal stenosis in the femoropopliteal segment of the leg can be determined with good specificity, sensitivity, and accuracy.[24] Likewise, areas of long segment arterial occlusion in the femoropopliteal segments are typically easily diagnosed. This anatomic information is particularly useful in selecting patients (prior to angiography) who will be suitable candidates for transluminal revascularization techniques (i.e., patients with focal areas of hemodynamically significant stenosis or short segmental occlusions).[25] Patients with long segment occlusions or long segment severe stenosis can then be stratified into those who, due to severity of symptoms (i.e., lifestyle limiting claudication, rest pain, or potential tissue loss) will require bypass surgery, and those with claudication that is less severely limiting who may be treated with risk factor modification and exercise. A second area in which duplex imaging is useful is evaluation of common femoral and popliteal aneurysms and pseudoaneurysms.[26] Some have recommended that patients undergoing carotid or peripheral studies also be examined to determine occult AAAs. The reasons for instituting such a screening program are the high occurrence of AAAs in patients with carotid, coronary, and peripheral vascular disease; the relative insensitivity of the abdominal physical examination for detection of abdominal aortic aneurysms; and the marked disparity in morbidity and mortality rates (as well as cost) comparing elective versus emergency repair of abdominal aortic aneurysms.[27-33]

An additional aspect of peripheral vascular disease testing that is well served by duplex imaging is surveillance of lower extremity bypass grafts. Determination of velocities within a bypass graft allows earlier detection of impending graft failure (typically when the velocities are less than 45 cm/sec) and thus elective repair or revision before thrombosis.[34]

While duplex imaging does provide unique information with both anatomic information and flow disturbance information within a given focal area of stenosis, there are limitations to this modality that preclude its use as a solitary modality in the evaluation of occlusive atherosclerotic peripheral vascular disease. Vessel wall calcification or plaque calcification results in a large acoustic impedance mismatch between the surrounding soft tissues (including flowing blood) and the area of calcification. This impedance mismatch results in reflection of a large percentage of the incident sound waves both for imaging and for velocity interrogations, resulting in acoustical shadowing. Thus in a heavily calcified plaque, the data required for determination of a significant stenosis may, in fact, not be obtainable.[35] Imaging of the distal abdominal aorta and iliac segments is at best difficult with duplex techniques. Depth of the vessels (especially in obese patients), overlying bowel gas (again, resulting in acoustical shadowing), and vessel tortuosity (resulting in varying Doppler angles relative to the transducer face) may all contribute to degradation of duplex imaging of the pelvic vessels.[36] While analysis of various Doppler waveform parameters at the more easily obtainable common femoral artery level, including spectral analyses and pulsatility indices, have been used to infer presence or absence of occlusive aortoiliac segment disease, results of these methods have been poor.[37] Imaging of the infrapopliteal arterial runoff vessels is also limited due to small vessel size, lower flow velocities in this segment, and arterial plaque calcifications. Within the femoropopliteal segment, the previously mentioned duplex criteria are very good at grading a given focal stenosis, although the utility of this modality in multifocal, sequential stenoses is less clear.[38] Finally, though most importantly, the greatest limitation of duplex scanning is its lack of the important physiologic information regarding the overall perfusion of the limb or a given segment of the limb. The central issue of the adequacy of compensation for a given stenosis by collateral blood flow is not addressed by duplex. This aspect of patient evaluation, however, is of critical importance when initially evaluating peripheral vascular disease patients, when following the patients on conservative therapy, and when following patients who have undergone revascularization procedures.

Color-flow imaging is expensive and should not be used for routine screening. It may be useful in selecting patients who are candidates for balloon angioplasty prior to angiography.[25] We firmly believe, however, that color duplex technology should not be routinely used to identify focal lesions for nonsurgical treatment in patients whose symptoms are not severe enough to warrant any intervention.

Magnetic Resonance Imaging

Magnetic resonance imaging (MRI) has been applied to the heart and vascular system since the early discovery of the absence of signal from rapidly flowing arterial blood. This flow void can in certain cases result in excellent contrast with the adjacent soft tissue structures, resulting in generally good anatomic detail. Multiplanar imaging and reconstruction capabilities added to the interest in applying this modality to the vascular tree.[39] Acquired vascular disorders (specifically, aortic dissections and AAAs) have been delineated with this modality.[40,41] More recently images of the isolated blood vessels of a given region of the body can be generated by computer-assisted manipulation of the MR acquired information. In addition to its applications in the carotid and intracranial circulation, this MR angiography (MRA) has been used to address occlusive

atherosclerotic disease of the lower extremities. The angiographic images generated by this modality, in light of the noninvasive nature of the technique and lack of patient exposure to intravascular contrast material, has prompted use of MRA in patients with contrast allergy or medically tenuous patients with encouraging initial results.[42-44] Evaluation of infrapopliteal runoff vessels in patients with severe proximal occlusive vascular disease by MRA has more recently been described.[44] However, MRA suffers from the same limitation of duplex imaging as a sole method of studying vascular disease; that is, the lack of physiologic correlation. Determination of the hemodynamic consequence of a stenosis or occlusion must be independently determined; furthermore, the cost of the examination, motion degradation, acquisition time, flow-related artifacts, and lack of interventional capability with MRA limit its current usefulness.

A potential future application of magnetic resonance technology in the evaluation of patients with occlusive peripheral vascular disease is the use of nuclear magnetic resonance spectroscopy in studying noninvasively the biochemical effects of muscle ischemia.[45,46]

CONCLUSION

Optimum care of the patient with peripheral vascular disease is predicated on accurate clinical assessment, including history; physical examination; and noninvasive testing, when appropriate. These data must be integrated by the physician to insure accurate diagnosis and appropriate therapy. While the history and physical examination alone may be diagnostic in patients with advanced disease, those patients with less severe disease at presentation may be diagnostic dilemmas. Noninvasive testing provides objective and quantifiable assessment of the presence as well as the severity of vascular disease. It allows distinction between vascular and nonvascular causes of extremity symptoms, thereby facilitating appropriate patient selection for more invasive assessment and for therapy. This assessment must be physiologic, since the prevalence of asymptomatic or mildly symptomatic vascular disease in the aging population could lead to overtreatment if anatomic criteria only were used for treatment selection. This is to be avoided by all practitioners treating these patients, given the frequently benign course of the peripheral component of vascular disease and the accelerated morbidity and mortality due to the coronary and cerebrovascular components that frequently coexist. Accurate, standardized description of the severity of vascular disease, using a widely accepted classification such as the SVS criteria, is mandatory in the evaluation of outcomes and to ensure consistency in reporting. Finally, ongoing clinical assessment is important to the long-term management of these patients. Objective evaluation of progression of disease and documentation of the benefits of surgical or interventional therapies can be obtained by noninvasive testing.

REFERENCES

1. McDaniel MD, Cronenwett JL: Basic data related to the natural history of intermittent claudication. Ann Vasc Surg 3:273, 1989
2. Glagov S, Weisenberg E, Zarins CK et al: Compensatory enlargement of human atherosclerotic coronary arteries. N Engl J Med 316:1371, 1987
3. Zarins CK, Weisenberg E, Kolettis G et al: Differential enlargement of artery segments in response to enlarging atherosclerotic plaques. J Vasc Surg 7:386, 1988
4. Hertzer NR: The natural history of peripheral vascular disease: implications for its management. Circulation 83 (suppl I):I12, 1991
5. Vogt MT, Wolfson SK, Kuller LH: Lower extremity arterial disease and the aging process: a review. J Clin Epidemiol 45:529, 1992
6. Imparato AM, Kim GE, Davidson T, Crowley JG: Intermittent claudication: its natural course. Surgery 78:795, 1975
7. Cronenwett JL, Warner KG, Zelenock GB et al: Intermittent claudication: current results of nonoperative management. Arch Surg 119:430, 1989
8. Criado E, Ramadan F, Keagy B et al: Intermittent claudication. Surg Gynecol Obstet 173:163, 1991
9. Treiman RL: Peripheral vascular disease in diabetic patients: evaluation and treatment. Mt Sinai J Med 54:241, 1987
10. Gordreau JJ, Creasy JK, Flanigan P et al: Rational approach to the differentiation of vascular and neurogenic claudication. Surgery 84:749, 1978
11. Ritz G, Friedman S, Osbourne A: Diabetes and peripheral vascular disease. Clin Podiatr Med Surg 9:125, 1992
12. Friedman SA: The diagnosis and medical management of vascular ulcers. Clin Dermatol 8:30, 1990
13. Edmonds ME: The diabetic foot: pathophysiology and treatment. Clin Endocrino Metab 15:889, 1986
14. Roberts DH, Tsao Y, McGloughlin GA et al: Placebo controlled comparison of captopril, atenold, labetolol, and pindolal in hypertension complicated by intermittent claudication. Lancet 2:650, 1987
15. Nelson JP: The vascular history and physical examination. Clin Podiatr Med Surg 9:1, 1992
16. Spittell JA: Diagnosis and management of occlusive peripheral vascular disease. Curr Probl Cardiol 15:1, 1990
17. Marinelli MR, Beach KW, Glass MJ et al: Noninvasive testing vs clinical evaluation of arterial disease: a prospective study. JAMA 241:2031, 1979
18. Rutherford RB, Becker GJ: Standards for evaluating and reporting the results of surgical and percutaneous therapy for peripheral arterial disease. J Vasc Intervent Radiol 2:169, 1991
19. Barnes RW, Thornhill B, Nix L et al: Predictions of amputation wound healing: role of doppler ultrasound and digital photoplethysmography. Arch Surg 116:80, 1981
20. Baker JD: The vascular laboratory. p. 205. In Moore WS (ed): Vascular Surgery—A Comprehensive Review. Grune & Stratton, Orlando, FL, 1986
21. Barnes RW: Noninvasive diagnostic assessment of peripheral vascular disease. Circulation (suppl I) 83:I20, 1991
22. Carter SA: Response of ankle systolic pressure to leg exercise in mild or questionable arterial disease. New Engl J Med 287:578, 1972
23. Fronek A, Johansen K, Dilley RB et al: Ultrasonographically monitored post-occlusive reactive hyperemia in the diagnosis of peripheral arterial occlusive disease. Circulation 48:149, 1973
24. Strandness DE: Duplex scanning for diagnosis of peripheral arterial disease. Herz 13:372, 1988
25. Edwards JM, Coldwell DM, Goldman ML et al: The role of duplex scanning in the selection of patients for transluminal angioplasty. J Vasc Surg 13:69, 1990
26. Coughlin BF, Paushter DM: Peripheral pseudoaneurysms: evaluation with duplex ultrasound. Radiology 168:339, 1988
27. Brown DW, Hollier LH, Pairoleno PC et al: Abominal aortic aneurysm and coronary artery disease. Arch Surg 116:1484, 1981
28. Galland RB, Simmons MJ, Torric EPH: Prevalence of abominal aortic aneurysm in patients with occlusive peripheral vascular disease. Br J Surg 78:1259, 1991
29. Graham M, Chan A: Ultrasound screening for clinically occult abdominal aortic aneurys. Can Med Assoc J 138:627, 1988
30. Twomey A, Twomey E, Wilkins RA et al: Unrecognized aneurysmal disease in male hypertensive patients. Int Angiol 5:269, 1986
31. Allardice JT, Allwright GJ, Wofinler JMC, Wyatt AP: High prevalence of abdominal aortic aneurysm in men with peripheral vascular disease: screening by ultrasonography. Br J Surg 75:240, 1988
32. Shapiro OM, Pasik S, Wasserman JP et al: Ultrasound screening for abdominal aortic aneurysms in patients with atherosclerotic peripheral vascular disease. J Cardiovasc Surg 31:170, 1990
33. Berridge DC, Griffith CDM, Anan SS et al: Screening for clinically unsuspected abdominal aortic aneurysm in patients with peripheral vascular disease. Eur J Vasc Surg 3:421, 1989
34. Bandyk DF: Postoperative surveillance of femorodistal grafts: the application of echo-doppler (duplex) ultrasonic scanning. p. 59. In Bergan JJ, Yao JST (eds): Reoperative Arterial Surgery. Grune & Stratton, Orlando, FL, 1986
35. Strandness DE: The use of ultrasound in the evaluation of peripheral vascular disease. Progr Cardiovasc Dis 20:403, 1978
36. Kholer TR, Nicholls SC, Zierler RE et al: Assessment of

pressure gradients by Doppler ultrasound: experimental and clinical observations. J Vasc Surg 6:460, 469, 1987

37. Moneta GL, Strandness DE: Peripheral arterial duplex scanning. J Clin Ultrasound 15:645, 1987
38. Rosenfield K, Kelly SM, Fields CD et al: Noninvasive assessment of peripheral vascular disease by color flow Doppler/two dimensional ultrasound. Am J Cardiol 64:247, 1989
39. Weeden VJ, Menli RA, Edelman RR et al: Projective imaging of pulsatile flow with magnetic resonance. Science 230:946, 1985
40. Dinsmore RE, Liberthson RR, Wiener GL et al: Magnetic resonance imaging of thoracic aortic aneurysms: comparison with other imaging methods. AJR 146:309, 1986
41. Lee JKT, Ling D, Heiken JP et al: Magnetic resonance imaging of abdominal aortic aneurysms. AJR 143:1197, 1984

42. Menli RA, Wedam VJ, Geller SE et al: MR gated subtraction angiography: evaluation of lower extremities. Radiology 159:411, 1986
43. Yucel EK, Dumoulin CL, Waltman AC: MR angiography of lower extremity arterial disease: preliminary experience. JMRI 2:303-309, 1992
44. Owen RS, Carpenter JP, Baum RA et al: Magnetic resonance imaging of angiographically occult runoff vessels in peripheral arterial occlusive disease. New Engl J Med 326:1577,
45. Zatima MA, Berkowitz HD, Gross GM et al: 31P nuclear magnetic resonance spectroscopy: noninvasive biochemical analysis of the ischemic extremity. J Vasc Surg 3:411, 1988
46. Hands LJ, Sharif MH, Payne GS et al: Muscle ischemia in peripheral vascular disease studied by 31P-magnetic resonance spectroscopy. Eur J Vasc Surg 4:637, 1990

25

Percutaneous Intervention for Aortoiliac Disease

Kenneth S. Rholl
Arina van Breda

When Dotter first considered the possibility of percutaneous treatment of atheromatous obstruction in arteries in 1963,[1] few could have envisioned the tremendous impact and growth of this technique over the next three decades. In 1964, using coaxial polyethylene catheters, Dotter successfully restored perfusion in the leg of an elderly woman who had refused amputation, reversing the gangrenous changes that had begun.[2] However, the first reports of successful restoration of blood flow by percutaneous technique were met with little enthusiasm in either the surgical or radiologic communities. Dotter recalled an early requisition for arteriography reading, "Visualize, but do not try to fix!".[3] The use of coaxial polyethylene catheters required large arteriotomies and limited the lumen achieved; despite this, Dotter correctly predicted the expansion of percutaneous vascular dilatation techniques to multiple organ systems. The introduction of the double lumen balloon catheter by Grüntzig in 1974[4] revolutionized the field, allowing more complete dilatation of larger arteries while maintaining a smaller arteriotomy site. With this development came the ability to successfully treat aortoiliac disease. During the ensuing two decades, numerous studies documented the efficacy of aortoiliac angioplasty, both in terms of primary technical and clinical success as well as the longevity of the result.[5-61] Since Grüntzig's important advance, other techniques and devices have expanded the application of percutaneous vascular intervention; notable among these are lytic therapy and stents. Yet other technologies, such as atherectomy and lasers, have undergone scrutiny for possible utility in the vascular system but elude a well defined role. While the utility of these newer procedures is still under investigation, percutaneous transluminal angioplasty (PTA) remains the cornerstone of percutaneous treatment of atherosclerotic vascular disease.

PATIENT EVALUATION

While the clinical evaluation of peripheral vascular disease is covered in detail elsewhere in this book, a brief review of the evaluation of patients for aortoiliac intervention is in order. Patients with aortoiliac disease may present with intermittent claudication of the calves, although symptoms frequently include the thighs, hips, and buttocks. The severity and duration of symptoms and the degree of limitation should be noted. Impotence in men may also be a presenting or accompanying complaint. The constellation of all of these symptoms, including impotence, may indicate distal aortic occlusion or the "Leriche syndrome." If the onset of occlusive disease is acute, with limited collateralization, the ischemic symptoms may be more severe and may include rest pain or tissue loss. A unique clinical presentation of aortic occlusive disease is the "small aorta" syndrome or focal atherosclerotic stenosis of the lower abdominal aorta. This typically occurs in younger women (40 to 50 years old) with a history of cigarette use.[62] The younger age and female predilection, a deviation from the classic clinical profile of atherosclerotic disease, often leads to delay in diagnosis at times with profound consequences (Fig. 25-1).

Aortoiliac lesions may result in distal embolic events causing the "blue toe syndrome," in which embolization results in focal painful areas of bluish discoloration of the digits.[63,64] The patient may recall multiple episodes of these painful symptoms involving the digits of one or both feet. Stenotic disease may or may not be present; therefore, there may not always be a history of claudication accompanying these symptoms.

Examination of the patient with aortoiliac disease frequently, but not invariably, reveals decreased femoral pulses. Although the pulses may be intact at rest, they may decrease dramatically with exercise as outflow demand increases. Auscultation may reveal the presence of a bruit over the aortoiliac segment. Physical evidence of distal embolization should also be sought.

In addition to the history and physical examination, a formal noninvasive vascular examination identifying sites of involvement and estimating severity can be indispensable in documenting indications for the procedure, establishing a vascular baseline, and planning the procedure to follow.

TECHNIQUES

A complete description of the technique of aortoiliac angioplasty is beyond the scope of this chapter. Several key points warrant mention, however. Patients who are

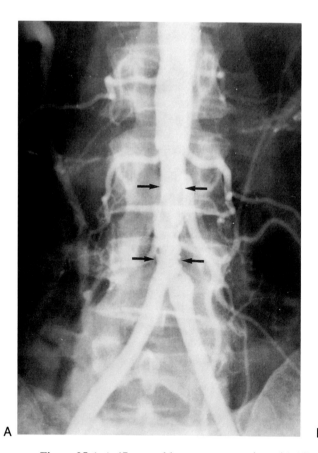
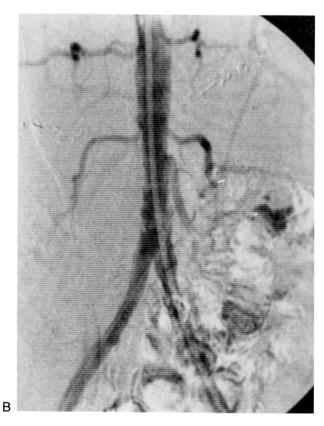

A

B

Figure 25-1 A 47-year-old woman presenting with bilateral hip and thigh claudication. **(A)** Diagnostic aortogram demonstrating a "hypoplastic" distal aorta with focal atherosclerotic disease involving the aortic bifurcation *(arrows)*. A 25-mm trans-stenotic resting gradient was present, increasing to 40 mmHg following intra-arterial nitroglycerine administration. **(B)** Following PTA of the distal aorta and its bifurcation no residual gradients were present with resolution of the patient's symptoms.

candidates for aortoiliac intervention should undergo complete diagnostic angiography. When iliac arterial disease is suspected, a contralateral femoral approach to the diagnostic angiographic study is preferred to minimize the possibility of inadvertent occlusion of the affected iliac vessel by passage of the diagnostic catheter through a tight stenosis. The diagnostic study allows careful planning of the proposed intervention and should include evaluation of the abdominal aorta, the iliac vessels, and the runoff of both lower extremities. The abdominal aorta should be studies for not only stenotic disease, but also the presence of aneurysm formation. Loss of the lumbar arteries, even in the presence of normal caliber of the aortic lumen, should raise suspicion of an aneurysm. In the case of suspected embolic disease, the entire aorta may be studied for evidence of a lesion likely to produce emboli. Pelvic imaging should include multiple oblique projections to identify eccentric lesions and to evaluate the region of the common iliac artery bifurcations. Similarly, if not included in the oblique pelvic views, ipsilateral oblique views of the common femoral artery bifurcations are useful in analyzing the origins of both the superficial and deep femoral arteries. Finally, arteriography of the lower extremities is performed to assess the runoff vessels. Continued refinements in digital vascular imaging have allowed more complete study of the arterial system with improved patient comfort and often reduced contrast load.

Intra-arterial pressure measurements should be obtained as part of the routine diagnostic arteriographic procedure when there is clinical suspicion or angiographic evidence of significant aortoiliac disease. A resting peak systolic pressure gradient greater than 10 to 15 mmHg is hemodynamically significant. In the absence of a resting gradient, as may be seen in patients with only exertional symptoms, intra-arterial administration of vasodilators such as nitroglycerine 100 to 200 μg or Priscoline 25 μg may reveal a hemodynamically significant lesion. The vasodilation caused by these agents in the distal vascular beds simulates the increased blood flow demand seen with exercise. Generally, a peak systolic gradient of greater than 15 to 20 mmHg or 15 percent indicates that the lesion is flow limiting. In patients in whom a mild-to-moderate stenosis is identified, the presence or absence of a gradient can help establish the significance of the lesion. When no specific lesion is identified angiographically, the intra-arterial pressure measurements may occasionally reveal a significant underlying stenosis (Fig. 25-2). Finally, repeating these measurements following treatment of the vessel documents the success of the procedure and identifies any residual stenosis. While generally very accurate, there are times when intra-arterial pressure measurements may be misleading. Specifically, the presence of a gradient is dependent on unobstructed outflow. Without outflow, a gradient may be absent despite even a severe stenosis. This consideration is important in treatment of multilevel disease, where a combined approach such as iliac PTA and subsequent femoropopliteal bypass for revascularization is being considered. Since patency of the distal graft is dependent on adequate inflow, underestimation of the significance of a lesion by relying solely on the hemodynamic data or angiographic appearance alone can compromise the clinical result.

Preprocedural administration of antiplatelet agents (primarily aspirin) and intraprocedural use of heparin are routine in many institutions, although the value of these are unconfirmed. Most authors suggest the intraoperative use of vasodilators such as nitrates and calcium channel blocking agents to minimize vasospasm.[5,14,20,30,37,65-67] Patients should be encouraged to refrain from smoking or use of transdermal nicotine prior to the procedure.

A retrograde approach is preferred for routine iliac angioplasty, but PTA has been successfully performed from the contralateral approach (i.e., over the aortic bifurcation) without a significant increase in complications[68,69] (Fig. 25-3). An axillary or brachial approach is rarely necessary for intervention in the aortoiliac vessels and should be avoided because of decreased control over the guidewire and catheter and, more importantly, a greater risk of complications, especially those related to the puncture site.

Lesions involving the origins of the common iliac arteries may require the use of simultaneous bilateral retrograde balloon catheters extending into the distal abdominal aorta — the "kissing balloon" technique.[45,46,48-50,53-55] Aortic lesions may also require this technique to obtain adequate lumen size. (Fig. 25-4) The successful use of as many as three balloons has been described to obtain sufficient diameters for dilatation in the abdominal aorta.[43,45,48-51,54-56,70] Care must be taken to avoid significant oversizing of the balloon, as this can lead to dissection or rupture.

Thrombolysis has been used successfully in the treatment of occluded arteries and grafts.[71-81] The occluded segment is traversed with a catheter-guidewire combination with placement of an infusion system within the thrombosed vessel. By eliminating the thrombus, the underlying stenotic lesion can be identified and subsequent appropriate treatment administered. Techniques of thrombolysis are described in Chapter 20.

Balloon expandable stents have recently become available in the United States for placement in iliac arteries. The Palmaz stent (Johnson & Johnson) is

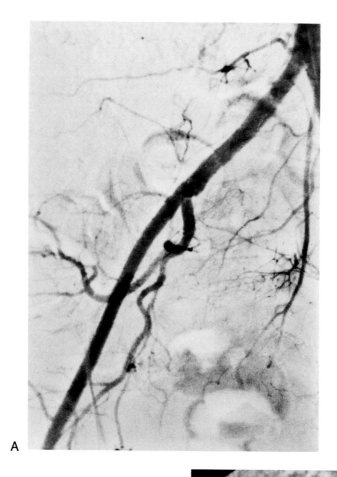

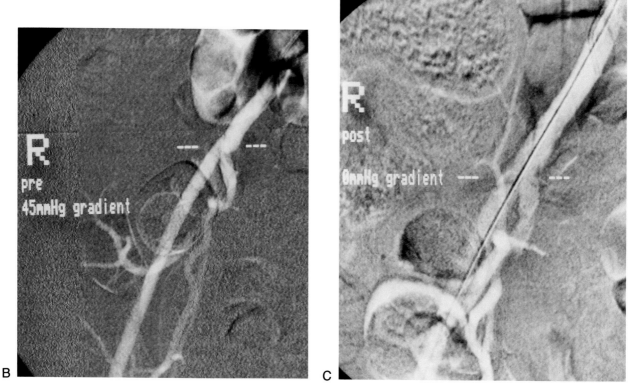

Figure 25-2 A 52-year old woman who presented with right calf and thigh claudication. **(A)** Diagnostic arteriography revealed no obvious high-grade stenosis. **(B)** Intra-arterial pressure measurements, however, revealed a 45-mm gradient across the origin of the right external iliac artery. **(C)** Following PTA, repeat intra-arterial pressure measurements revealed no residual gradient. The patient subsequently became asymptomatic.

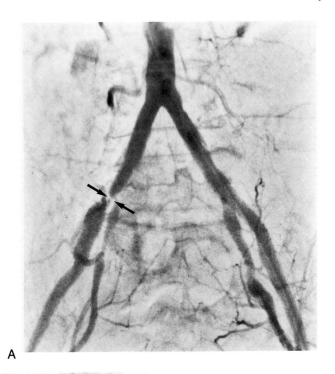

A

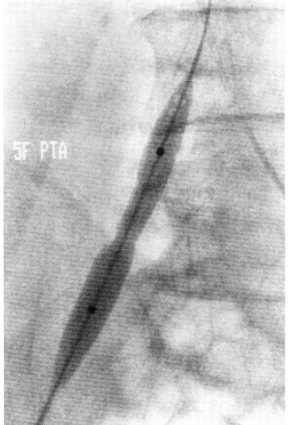

B

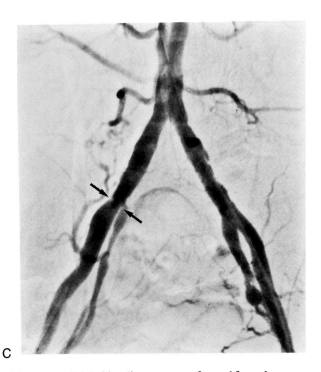

C

Figure 25-3 **(A)** Diagnostic arteriography in this patient with suspected right iliac disease was performed from the contralateral femoral artery. This approach allowed complete diagnostic assessment and avoided possible occlusion of the severe right external iliac stenosis *(arrows)* by the diagnostic catheter. **(B)** Following the diagnostic study, ipsilateral PTA was performed. **(C)** Post-PTA angiogram demonstrated an excellent result *(arrows)*.

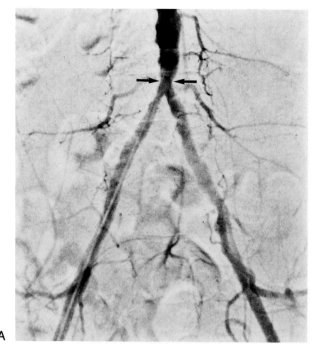

A

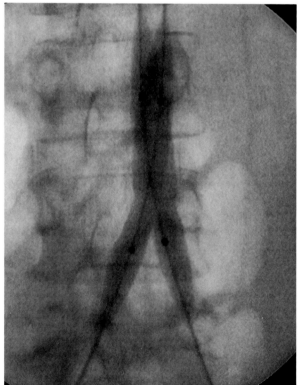

B

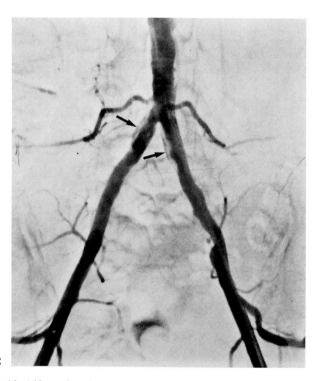

C

Figure 25-4 **(A)** A concentric stenosis of the distal aorta and its bifurcation *(arrows)* was identified in this patient with symptoms of bilateral lower extremity claudication. **(B)** Dilatation was performed using the "kissing balloon" technique with simultaneous inflation of bilateral balloons. **(C)** Following dilatation, repeat study revealed a good angiographic result. Small intimal cracks *(arrows)* are present in both common iliac arteries; these are of no significance in the absence of hemodynamic gradients.

mounted on an angioplasty balloon catheter, which is then used to deploy the stent in the offending region of the vessel. These stents have been used quite successfully for lesions that respond poorly to PTA, including eccentric calcified lesions, lesions with significant elastic recoil, and dissections in which the dissecting flap continues to obstruct the flow of blood[82-89] (Fig. 25-5). Because these stents are rigid, an ipsilateral approach is generally necessary. The relatively large size of the device and delivery sheath make its use in smaller diseased vessels problematic. Smaller rigid stents and flexible self-expanding stents, while not yet approved for use in the vascular system, may prove useful in these circumstances.

The use of directional atherectomy has also been described in the iliac arteries.[30,90-92] Theoretically, by removing the offending atheroma rather than using balloon dilatation, elastic recoil is eliminated. In addition, the smoother lumen following atherectomy may provide less stimulus for thrombus formation and result in less turbulent flow, reducing the likelihood of restenosis. (Fig. 25-6) These potential advantages, however, have not been demonstrated in large clinical series. In addition, the working diameter of the available Simpson Atherectomy Device (Devices for Vascular Intervention, Inc., Temecula, CA) limits its usefulness in the iliac arteries. The largest Simpson peripheral atherectomy device provides a maximum working diameter of only 7.7 mm. The newer over-the-wire atherectomy device has a slightly larger working diameter of 9.7 mm. Both devices require an 11 French introducer sheath, again limiting the utility of the technique and likely resulting in a higher rate of puncture site complications. One potential use of atherectomy involves its use in the removal of obstructing intimal flaps following PTA.[93] In the iliac arteries, however, stents have largely become the treatment of choice for obstructing intimal flaps.[83,87]

PATIENT SELECTION

Over the last decade, despite considerable early resistance, balloon angioplasty has become the treatment of choice for the focal, symptomatic iliac stenosis.[6,11,13,21,26,36,65,94-96] Surgical reconstruction remains the treatment of choice for bilateral long segment severe stenotic or occlusive disease, where there is severe restriction of flow to the lower extremities.[11,15,65,94,96-99] Many patients, however, do not fall neatly into these categories, but rather represent a spectrum of clinical and angiographic presentations. The decision to proceed with intervention should be based on several factors. Foremost among these is consideration of the severity of symptoms. Mild symptoms often do not require any intervention other than an exercise program with follow-up. Only patients in whom a conscientious program of exercise fails to achieve sufficient palliation should undergo further therapy. Patients with more severe symptoms at presentation may require more prompt intervention. Classifications of acute and chronic ischemia[100,101] proposed by Rutherford et al. and adopted by the Society of Vascular Surgery (SVS) and the Society of Cardiovascular and Interventional Radiology (SCVIR) are useful in evaluating the clinical effects of ischemia.

Second, the overall health of the patient must be considered. Is the patient a candidate for percutaneous and/or surgical intervention? The risks of intervention must be weighed against the possible benefits. Although percutaneous intervention is generally less stressful, the unusual complication may force surgical intervention and its increased risks.

Third, the morphology of the disease should be appraised. Guidelines for PTA of arteries including the aorta and iliac arteries have been developed by SCVIR[94] (Table 25-1), (Fig. 25-7 and 25-8). Lesions are classified by their morphologic characteristics, including length and severity of occlusive changes, as well as the presence of concomitant disease such as aneurysm formation and embolic events. Recommendations for therapy for various categories are outlined depending on the clinical situation and expected results. The best results with angioplasty are obtained in short, focal stenoses in arteries of larger diameter. Longer stenoses, occlusions, and smaller vessels are less desirable lesions for PTA. It follows, then, that aortoiliac stenotic disease is most ideally suited to angioplasty. However, within the spectrum of aortoiliac disease a range of treatment options will exist. These criteria are meant to serve as guidelines rather than steadfast rules; the entire clinical picture must be taken into account before a therapeutic course is decided upon.

The most common indication for aortoiliac intervention is lifestyle limiting claudication, SVS grades 2B and C. These are patients whose affected limb is not threatened but who are unable to ambulate sufficiently to maintain their desired lifestyle. For a given vascular lesion, the degree of limitation will vary widely between an active, athletic patient and the sedentary person. Patients with appropriate symptoms and a suitable lesion for percutaneous treatment (in the absence of contraindications) should be considered candidates for intervention, but only after an adequate trial of conservative management including graded exercise, abstinence from tobacco use, and weight loss.[102,103]

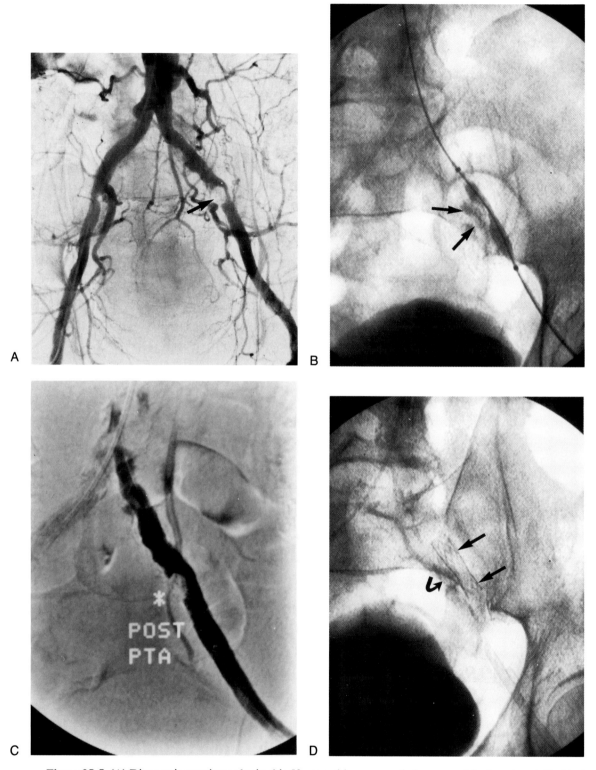

Figure 25-5 **(A)** Diagnostic arteriography in this 59-year-old man revealed an eccentric densely calcified lesion near the left common iliac bifurcation *(arrow)*. The left hypogastric artery was occluded, filling from collateral pathways. **(B)** PTA was performed from a retrograde approach, displacing the calcified lesion *(arrows)* medially. **(C)** Post-PTA digital imaging revealed significant elastic recoil and residual stenosis. **(D)** A Palmaz intravascular stent *(arrows)* was deployed with an 8-mm balloon. The calcified lesion *(curved arrow)* is seen medial to the stent. *(Figure continues.)*

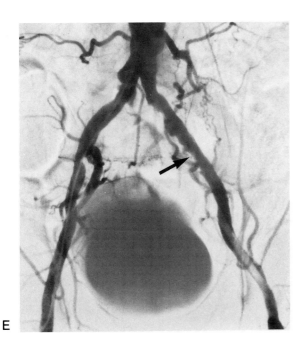

E

Figure 25-5 *(Continued.)* **(E)** Following stent deployment, no significant residual stenosis or gradients were present at the site *(arrow).*

More severe disease may result in resting symptoms and tissue loss (SVS grades 3 and 4). In these patients, there is little place for conservative management when intervention is plausible. Lesions suitable for percutaneous treatment should definitely be considered for intervention. Lesions in these patients may be less than ideal for percutaneous therapy (i.e., longer stenoses, occlusions and multilevel and/or diffuse disease). However, many of these patients are also less than ideal candidates for surgical revascularization. Since the morbidity and mortality of percutaneous therapy are significantly lower than that associated with surgery, and since failure of percutaneous therapy generally does not preclude a surgical option,[11,12,40,61,66,104] a trial of percutaneous therapy may be warranted.

Occlusive disease in the aortoiliac region was once the domain of the surgeon alone. More recently, percutaneous intervention has begun to make inroads in the treatment of segmental occlusions of these vessels. Direct recanalization and angioplasty has been used but was limited by a significant incidence of complications, including embolism and reocclusion.[105–111] Thrombolysis has been used to convert longer segments of occluded vessel to short stenoses. Theoretically, this may improve both the immediate complication rate by re-

moval of much of the offending thrombus prior to PTA, as well as the long-term results by converting the lesion to a more favorable category. Thrombolytic therapy has allowed interventional treatment of patients who might otherwise not have been candidates for nonsurgical therapy, and therefore has become an important adjunctive technique in management of iliac artery disease. More recently, primary stenting is being evaluated as a means of treating patients with iliac occlusions. While initial results look promising, long-term results are not yet available.[88,112–114]

Although lesions causing distal emboli were once thought to represent a relative contraindication to percutaneous therapy, they have been successfully treated with PTA and other percutaneous techniques without significant additional embolization[64,115,116]: there is no evidence that these patients should not be considered candidates for PTA. We have found that rather than ulcerative lesions, many patients presenting with "blue toe syndrome" have high grade stenotic lesions without angiographic evidence of ulceration as a source of their emboli (Fig. 25-9). These may be associated with thrombus and, if so, a trial of thrombolytic therapy may be warranted. These patients respond extremely well to PTA of these lesions, which both eliminates the embolic episodes, and increases perfusion to the distal extremities. PTA in this group often obviates the need for surgical bypass.

Multilevel disease may be an indication for a combined percutaneous and surgical approach.[117–131] Iliac PTA improves inflow prior to a femoropopliteal or femorodistal bypass and has been used successfully in numerous studies. Iliac PTA may also be used in the face of a contralateral iliac occlusion in patients not candidates for an aortofemoral or aortoiliac bypass to allow a femoro-femoral crossover graft to be placed (Fig. 25-10).

Impotence may also be an indication for percutaneous intervention in aortoiliac disease.[45,58,132–134] Aortic and/or bilateral common iliac or hypogastric artery lesions are potential contributors to impotence when there is evidence of arterial insufficiency; these proximal vessel lesions respond well to PTA. More distal, or small vessel disease, is less likely to have long-term patency postangioplasty. A steal phenomenon in a case of external iliac artery disease has also been reported as a cause of impotence.[133] As impotence has many potential causes, a noninvasive examination of penile arterial blood flow may be useful in determining whether arterial insufficiency is in fact present.

Hypertension secondary to aortoiliac disease proximal to a renal transplant has also been reported as an unusual indication for aortoiliac intervention.[135]

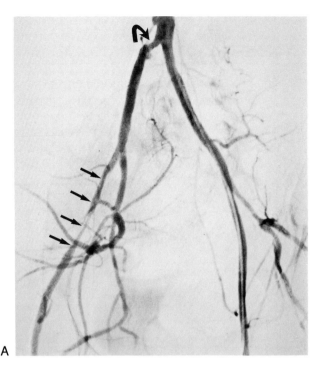

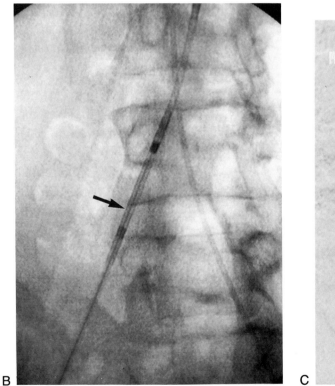

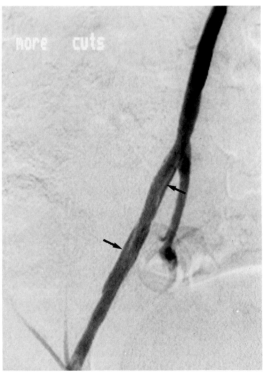

Figure 25-6 A 41-year-old woman with right lower extremity claudication. **(A)** Diagnostic angiography revealed a long fusiform stenosis of the right external iliac artery *(arrows)*. A moderate common iliac artery stenosis *(curved arrow)* was also present on the right. **(B)** As the external iliac lesion was suboptimal for PTA, atherectomy was performed with the Simpson atherectomy device *(arrow)*. **(C)** Following atherectomy, there is marked improvement in the lumen caliber. The nonobstructing intimal crack *(arrows)* was felt secondary to overinflation of the atherectomy balloon. The patient has done well at 1 year follow-up.

Table 25-1 SCVIR Guidelines for Iliac PTA

Category	Description	Guidelines
1	Stenoses <3 cm, concentric, noncalcified	PTA treatment of choice
2	Stenoses 3–5 cm, concentric, noncalcified Stenoses <3 cm, eccentric, calcified	Well suited for PTA. Includes lesions followed by distal bypass
3	Stenoses 5–10 cm Chronic occlusions <5 cm	Amenable to PTA. Moderate chance of success versus surgery. PTA may be performed in patients with high surgical risk or lack of surgical material
4	Stenoses >10 cm Chronic occlusions >5 cm, after thrombolysis Extensive bilateral disease Stenoses associated with aneurysms or other lesions requiring surgery	PTA has limited role. Low technical success. Poor long-term benefit. PTA only when no surgical options or in very hgh-risk patients

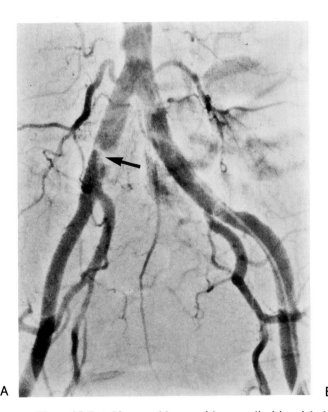
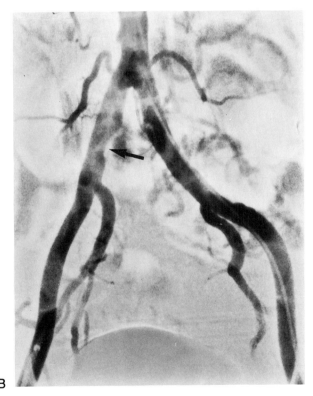

Figure 25-7 A 58-year-old man with severe limiting right lower extremity claudication. **(A)** Diagnostic arteriography revealed focal short eccentric stenosis of the right common iliac artery, SCVIR lesion category 2. **(B)** The lesion responded well to angioplasty with only minimal eccentric residual narrowing *(arrow)* and no residual hemodynamic pressure gradient, the residual narrowing was felt to be insignificant. The patient continues to do well 3 years post-PTA.

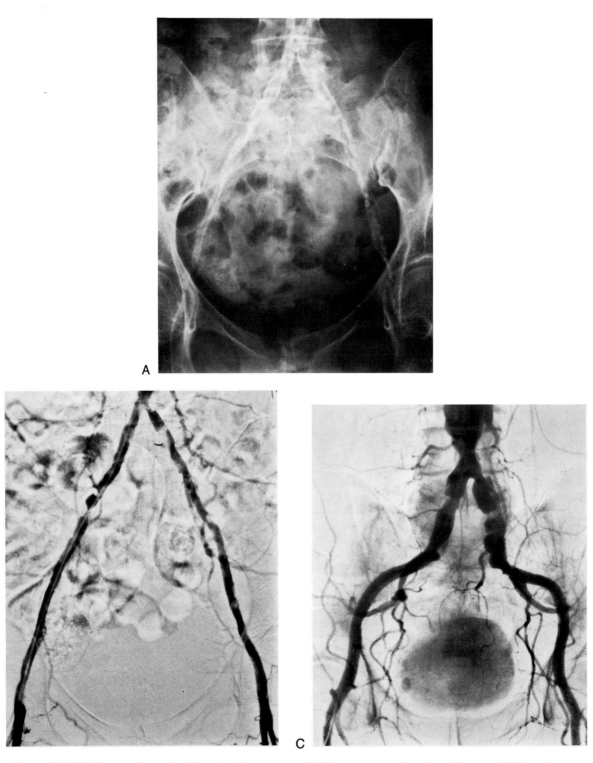

Figure 25-8 (**A**) Scout radiograph of the pelvis demonstrated diffuse severe calcification of the aortic bifurcation and iliac vessels. (**B**) Subsequent subtraction angiography confirmed extensive bilateral disease, SCVIR lesion category 4. (**C**) Category 4 disease is also demonstrated in this patient with distal aortic and bilateral common iliac artery stenoses, which are also associated with aortic and iliac aneurysmal disease.

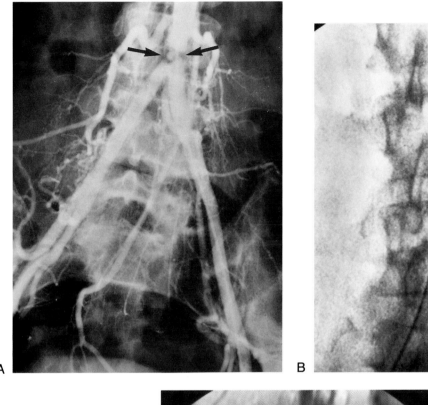

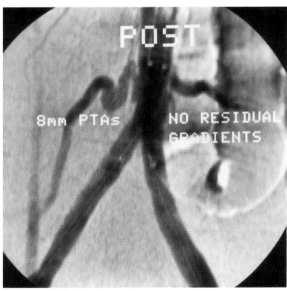

Figure 25-9 (**A**) A 62-year-old woman presented with multiple episodes of blue toe syndrome occurring in both feet. The diagnostic arteriogram revealed a severe concentric stenosis in the distal abdominal aorta *(arrows)*. (**B**) PTA of the distal aortic lesion was performed using bilateral 8-mm balloons. (**C**) Following PTA, there is excellent morphologic result with no residual hemodynamic pressure gradient. At 4-year follow-up, the patient is asymptomatic with no further embolic episodes.

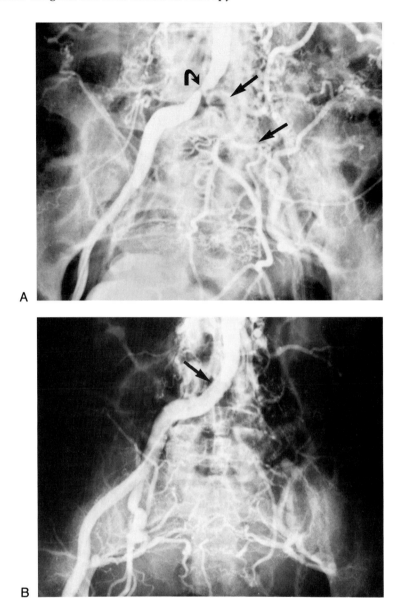

Figure 25-10 A 61-year-old man with significant coronary artery disease and nonhealing ulcer of the left foot. **(A)** Diagnostic arteriography revealed occlusion of the left common iliac artery *(arrows)* with focal high grade stenosis of the right common iliac artery *(curved arrow)*. **(B)** PTA of the right common iliac artery lesion was performed with complete obliteration of the stenosis *(arrow)*. A femorofemoral crossover graft was subsequently placed with eventual healing of the left foot ulceration.

CONTRAINDICATIONS

Few absolute contraindications to percutaneous aortoiliac intervention exist, as these procedures generally have a very low morbidity and mortality. The patient with severe, acute, limb-threatening ischemia who would best be treated by surgical intervention may represent such a contraindication; however, even this contraindication is becoming relative rather than absolute (see Ch. 20). Other contraindications to percutaneous

intervention in aortoiliac disease are relative to the situation at hand. Clinical contraindications include coagulopathies, severe medical disease, and the uncooperative patient. Contraindications regarding the disease process itself include lack of safe vascular access; involvement of the vessel by aneurysmal disease; involvement of the vessel by extensive exophytic plaque with a high risk of embolization; diffuse severe stenotic disease; and lesions with low likelihood of success, which are better treated by surgical bypass. Occlusions, once felt to represent a contraindication to percutaneous intervention due to a possibly higher risk of embolization, are now successfully treated by a variety of nonsurgical techniques including thrombolysis and stenting as noted above. Occlusions, therefore, no longer represent a contraindication to interventional therapy.

When contemplating any intervention, percutaneous or surgical, the potential risks and benefits to the patient must be considered. As the morbidity and mortality associated with percutaneous intervention is less than that associated with surgery,[61,66,95,104,136] the indications for percutaneous intervention extend beyond the more conservative indications for surgery. Moderate claudication not sufficiently improved with conservative management may not be an indication for surgical bypass, but might be appropriately treated by PTA. Similarly, the medical contraindications to surgical bypass do not always apply to percutaneous intervention. Patients with significant coronary or pulmonary disease in whom anesthetic risk is prohibitive can often safely undergo iliac PTA.

RESULTS

When evaluating the efficacy of aortoiliac interventions, several factors should be taken into consideration. Certainly the long-term durability of any revascularization procedure is a prime consideration; one can evaluate this in terms of primary and secondary patency rates (those patent following additional intervention), as well as clinical results. Morbidity and mortality associated with these procedures must be included in any assessment. In addition, with ever increasing concern over the escalating costs of health care, the direct and indirect costs of these interventions cannot be ignored. Significant cost advantages of PTA over surgical reconstruction in appropriate patients have been shown, largely resulting from shorter hospitalization, avoidance of general anesthesia, and decreased costs of procedural rooms and fees.[59,60]

Angioplasty

Iliac Artery PTA

Early reports suggested an extremely high patency rate for iliac artery PTA, approaching 90 percent at 5 years.[6,7,13,41] Subsequent investigators have reported a wide variety of "patency" rates ranging from 30 to 90 percent at 5 years. Review of the literature suggests the actual long-term durability of iliac artery PTA to be much better than the most pessimistic reports, though

perhaps not as good as first thought.[5-42,95,96,117-122,124-127,131,137-141] Table 25-2 summarizes the data from a large number of series reporting on a total of over 6000 procedures. Primary success (although not always precisely defined in the same fashion) is approximately 92 percent. Combining multiple series, patency rates at 1, 3, and 5 years are reasonable estimated at 91, 80, and 72 percent, respectively.

The wide variation on reported results stems from numerous differences in evaluation and reporting techniques, as well as from likely differences in patient populations. Standardization of reports has not been consistent. First, patency may be expressed in terms of procedures attempted or successful procedures. Many authors have felt justified in reporting long-term patency as a percentage of initial technical successes, since attempted PTA rarely resulted in worsening of the patient's vascular status, nor removed him or her from candidacy for surgical therapy.[96,142] A technically unsuccessful angioplasty does not have the same consequences or implications as a failed surgical procedure. Second, primary and secondary patency rates are not always strictly defined in reports of long-term success. Third, the determination of "patency" can be difficult at best, and misleading at worst. Techniques and definitions of patency vary between studies. Simple ankle-brachial indices, a frequently used modality, may not adequately assess the PTA site itself. Continued improvement in clinical symptomatology, while important, may not in fact indicate the status of the PTA site. Although a recurrence of symptoms and/or a decrease in the ankle-brachial index may represent recurrence of disease at the prior site of intervention, it may also result from progression of disease remote to the PTA site (Fig. 25-11). Imaging with hemodynamic measurements at the prior PTA site will often reveal continued patency even though recurrence is suspected.[27] Fourth, as with surgical bypass, the characteristics of the patient population in each series can have a profound effect on

Table 25-2 Cumulative Iliac PTA Patency Data[a,b]

Time	Mean (%)	Range (%)
Primary success	92.3	73–100
1 Year	91.0	63–100
3 Years	80.0	58–95
5 Years	72.0	32–92

[a] n = 6564.

[b] The follow-up period for each individual series was variable, not all series had follow-up to 5 years.

(Data from references, 5–42, 95, 96, 117–122, 124–127, 130, 131, 137–141.)

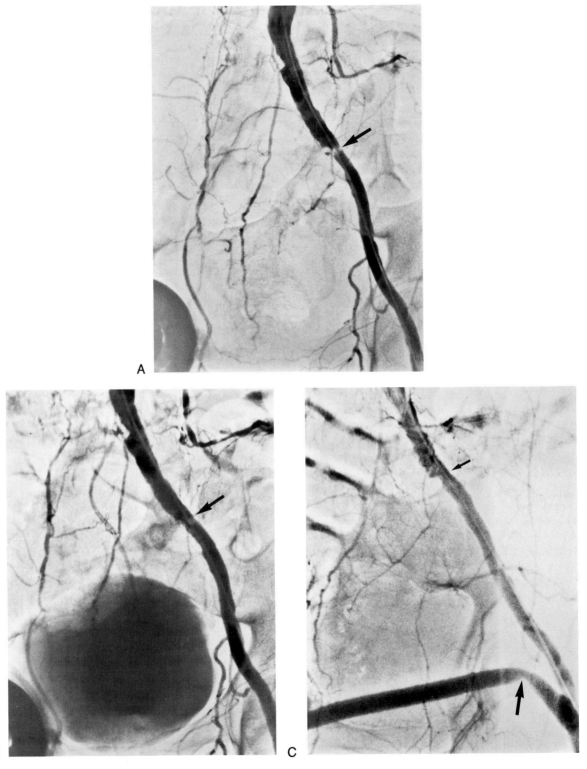

Figure 25-11 (A) Severe focal concentric stenosis at the origin of the left external iliac artery *(arrow)* with occlusion of the left hypogastric artery was demonstrated in this patient with a chronic right iliac occlusion. **(B)** Successful PTA *(arrow)* was performed prior to subsequent femorofemoral crossover graft placement. **(C)** When recurrent right lower extremity symptoms occurred, despite a clinically patent graft, recurrent stenosis of the left iliac PTA site was suspected. Angiography with hemodynamic pressure measurements, however, demonstrated the angioplasty site to be widely patent *(small arrow)*. A stenosis of the graft itself was instead demonstrated *(large arrow)*. Translesion gradients confirmed this to be hemodynamically significant.

clinical outcome and long term success. Several authors have studies factors that may influence the outcome of PTA, particularly long-term patencies[11,15,29,34-36,39] (Table 25-3). Many of these factors are interrelated: the effects of each are difficult to separately analyze. For instance, patients referred for limb salvage will generally have more severe disease with poor runoff. Stokes et al.[35] demonstrated no difference between patients with and without diabetes if the severity of their disease was accounted for. Similarly, Spence et al.[11] did not find a significant difference in outcome in diabetic patients when only iliac lesions were considered. Despite this lack of specific correlation, these factors can be used to aid in prediction of outcome for patients being considered for PTA. Interestingly, there is little available data to support the generally held tenet that patients who continue to smoke will have a poorer long-term patency rate than those who do not.

The overall success rates with iliac artery PTA listed in Table 25-2 compare quite well with those reported with aortoiliac reconstruction listed in Table 25-4. Five- and 10-year patency rates of 80 to 90 percent and 70 to 75 percent are derived from multiple series.[98,130,143] Wilson et al.,[95] in a prospective, randomized trial, found no significant difference in long-term durability when comparing PTA with surgery once an initial increased failure rate of PTA was accounted for; those patients failing PTA underwent surgical reconstruction without increased morbidity and mortality over surgery alone.

It should be noted that technical failures of PTA rarely result in changes in vascular status or are the cause of significant morbidity.[95,96,137,142] Johnston et al.[96] reported only 3.8 percent of failed iliac PTAs resulted in worsening of the patient's clinical grade. Similarly, late failure of iliac angioplasty generally results in reversion to the initial presenting symptoms, and sec-

Table 25-3 Factors Influencing PTA Outcome

Predictive Factor	Better	Worse
Indication	Claudication	Limb salvage
Site	Proximal	Distal
Runoff	Intact	Diseased
Severity	Short	Long
	Stenosis	Occlusion
	Concentric	Eccentric
	Noncalcified	Calcified
Diabetes	Absent	Present

(Data from references 11, 15, 29, 34, 35, 36, 39.)

Table 25-4 Cumulative Aortoiliac Reconstruction Patency Data[a]

Time	Mean (%)	Range (%)
Primary success	98	80-100
5 Years	80-90	68-96
10 Years	70-75	62-86

[a] The follow-up period for individual series was variable.
(Data from references 98, 130, 143.)

ondary patency with repeat angioplasty can be accomplished without an increase in morbidity or mortality and with the same expected results as the primary angioplasty.[142] These results must be compared with results with surgical failures. Although in general the reported patency rates for surgical bypass are slightly higher than for PTA, the morbidity and mortality associated with aortoiliac reconstruction is not insignificant, with perioperative mortality rates estimated at 2 to 5 percent.[130,143] Furthermore, failure of a bypass procedure can have devastating consequences. Crawford et al.[144] reported a 12 percent mortality rate for patients undergoing "redo" surgery for failed aortoiliac reconstructions.[144] Finally, when evaluating the long-term durability of these procedures and weighing therapeutic options, one must consider the life expectancy of this group of patients. The natural history of patients with vascular disease demonstrates significant mortality in these patients, approaching 20 to 30 percent at 5 years and 50 to 60 percent at 10 years.[98,143]

Aortic PTA

While iliac artery PTA has been evaluated in many series, much less information is available regarding aortic PTA. Aortic occlusive disease, however, has been successfully treated with PTA techniques in a number of series,[43-58,145] which are summarized in Table 25-5 and Figure 25-12. Primary success rates

Table 25-5 Cumulative Aortic PTA Patency Data[a]

Time	Mean (%)	Range (%)
Primary success	95	83-100
1 Year	98	83-100
3 Years	87	83-96
5 Years	80	70-92

[a] The follow-up period for each individual series was variable; not all series had follow-up to 5 years.
(Data from references: 43-58, 145.)

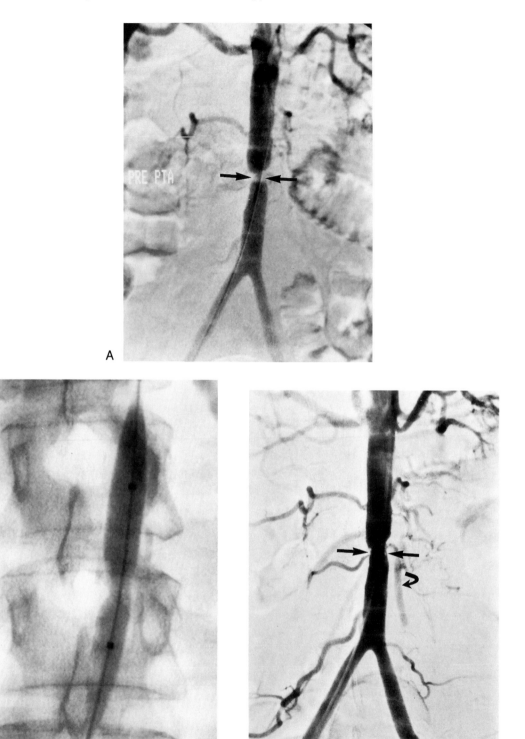

Figure 25-12 **(A)** A focal severe concentric stenosis *(arrows)* of the infrarenal abdominal aorta was demonstrated in this patient presenting with bilateral buttock, thigh, and calf claudication. The inferior mesenteric artery was not visualized. **(B & C)** Balloon dilatation of the stenosis was performed with marked improvement in lumen caliber *(arrows)* and resolution of the trans-stenotic gradient. Minimal filling of the inferior mesenteric artery was noted *(curved arrow)*. Follow-up noninvasive study at 3 years revealed normal ankle-brachial indices with no return of symptoms.

averaged 95 percent with 1-, 3-, and 5-year patency rates of 93, 87, and 80 percent, respectively. Our experience with 12 patients who underwent PTA of the infrarenal aorta also resulted in excellent long-term durability, demonstrating a 92 percent patency rate with an average followup of 5.2 years (range 0.6 to 9.8 years).[145] As might be expected, these results are quite similar to iliac artery angioplasty, as both deal with treatment of larger vessels. In addition, the aortic bifurcation is a common site of occlusive disease extending into the common iliac artery origins. Treatment of these lesions has met with good success, frequently employing the "kissing balloon" technique to simultaneously dilate the aorta and both iliac artery origins.[43,45,46,48,49,50,53-55] The results are comparable to those of aortic bypass surgery, but with lower morbidity and mortality. Embolization from the seemingly exophytic plaque frequently seen in the aorta has been reported in less than 1 percent of reported cases.[43-58]

Thrombolysis

Thrombolytic therapy of acute limb ischemia is discussed in detail in Chapter 20. In this setting, McNamara[79,146] has reported excellent results with thrombolysis, even in the face of severe ischemia. In situations where there was acute ischemia but the extremity remained viable (SVS acute ischemia category 1), a success rate of 100 percent was noted. When the limb became threatened, a success rate of 84 percent was reported. Finally, even in those patients with acute profound or irreversible ischemia (SVS acute ischemia category 2), 60 percent had a positive outcome. Primary PTA is generally not indicated, as embolization of the acute thrombus distally may further compromise the vascular status. The SCVIR guidelines[94] therefore recommend thrombolysis of acute occlusions prior to attempted PTA if the percutaneous option is chosen (Table 25-1).

Thrombolysis of subacute and chronic occlusions, although somewhat more time-consuming and cumbersome than primary PTA and/or stent placement, may reduce the risk of embolization[105] and poorer results[106-111] when PTA is attempted without lysis. Furthermore, by converting an occlusion to a stenosis, the long-term durability may be improved to that of the underlying stenotic disease (Figs. 25-13 and 25-14). Deeter et al.[147] reported the results of thrombolysis in 19 iliac artery occlusions including 11 chronic occlusions (range 1 month to 6 years). The primary success rate for complete revascularization of the occluded segments was 89 percent with 85 of these remaining patent

at a mean follow-up of 1 year. Minor embolization occurred in 5 percent with no episodes of clinically significant emboli. Importantly, failure of the procedure did not worsen the vascular status of any patient nor preclude that patient from possible surgical alternatives. Overall successful lysis can be obtained in 75 to 80 percent of patients in whom lysis of iliac occlusions is undertaken.[71-79,147]

With appropriate patient selection, thrombolysis can be a safe and useful adjunct to angioplasty or surgery in patients with both acute and chronic iliac artery occlusive disease. Current trials of primary stent placement in chronic occlusive disease should help clarify the relative roles of thrombolysis and stents in these patients.

Intravascular Stents

Many of the failures of PTA procedures, particularly in the immediate periprocedural period, have occurred in vessels in which there was an initial suboptimal result. When significant elastic recoil is encountered, there is immediate partial restenosis of the vessel at the PTA site when the balloon is deflated. This frequently occurs with more densely calcified lesions, which may be eccentric. Furthermore, extensive dissection of the vessel following PTA may result in partial or complete obstruction to flow. Suboptimal PTA results not only account for immediate failures, but also may lead to an increase in delayed failure of PTA with more rapid recurrence of the stenosis. Intra-arterial measurements made both prior to and following PTA are extremely useful as an adjunct to post-PTA angiography, further defining the hemodynamic result of the procedure. In cases where angiographic and hemodynamic evaluation suggest that the response to PTA is suboptimal, intravascular stenting has proven valuable in providing improved short- and long-term outcomes[82-89,113,148-156] (Fig. 25-15).

Although intravascular stenting is still in its infancy, the iliac artery has been the site of the majority of peripheral intravascular stent placements. The Palmaz stent (Johnson & Johnson, Warren, NJ) was the first stent widely available and is the stent with the greatest clinical experience thus far. Palmaz recently reported the results of a multicenter trial investigating the use of the Palmaz stent in iliac arteries.[82] Clinical success was 99 percent initially, 91 percent at 1 year and 84 percent at 2 years. At 43 months, clinical success dropped to 69 percent, although angiographic patency was found in 92 percent (Fig. 25-16). This highlights the difficulty in determining the durability of the procedure. Many of the patients who had recurrent symptoms did not ex-

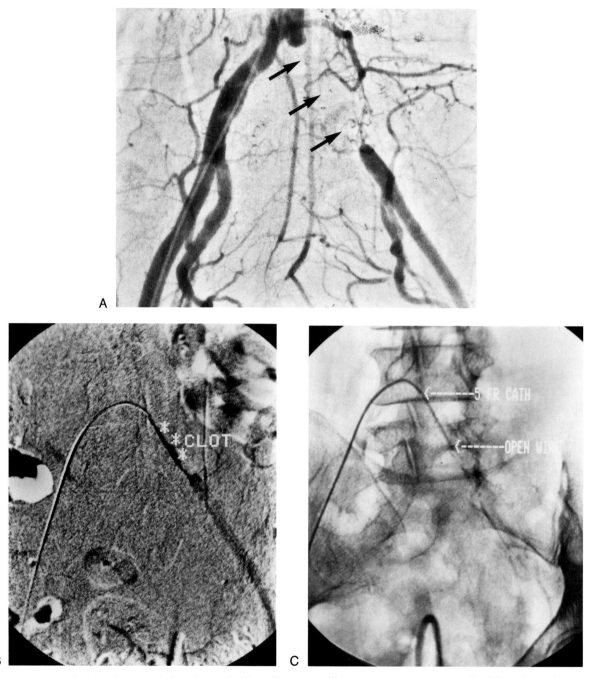

Figure 25-13 (A) A 6-cm occlusion *(arrows)* of the left common iliac artery was demonstrated in this patient with limiting left thigh and calf claudication. **(B)** The occluded segment was recanalized from a contralateral approach. Injection of the catheter demonstrated thrombus within the occluded segment. **(C)** Urokinase infusion was performed through a coaxial catheter and infusion wire at 100,000 units/hr. *(Figure continues.)*

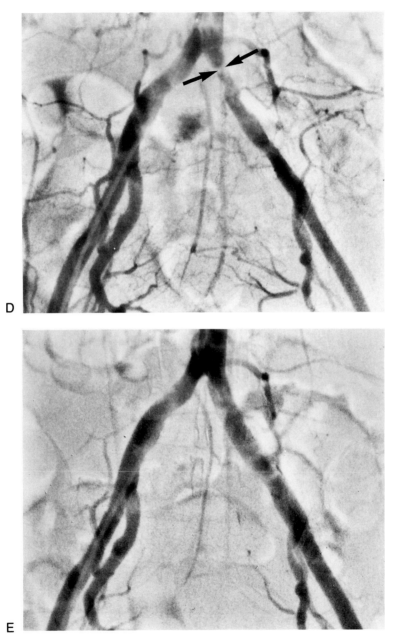

Figure 25-13 *(Continued.)* **(D)** After 12 hours of infusion, lysis of the thrombus had occurred revealing underlying concentric focal stenosis *(arrows)*. **(E)** Following PTA, there is restoration of a normal caliber lumen and brisk flow into the left extremity.

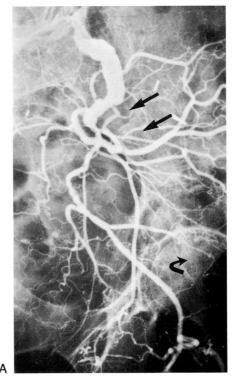

A

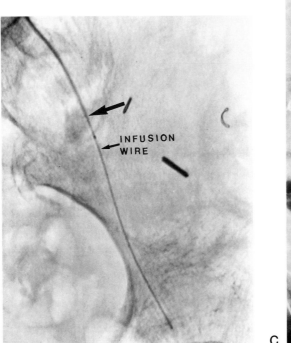

B

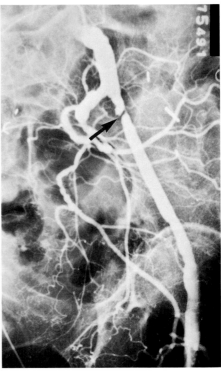

C

Figure 25-14 A 56-year-old woman with abrupt worsening of claudication, 3 months prior to presentation in the noninvasive laboratory. **(A)** Angiography performed following noninvasive studies confirmed left external iliac artery occlusion. *(arrows)* The abrupt onset of the patient's symptoms 3 months prior suggests the occlusion was chronic. Faint opacification of the common femoral artery *(curved arrows)* was noted. **(B)** A coaxial infusion system was placed from a contralateral approach with an infusion wire *(small arrow)* being positioned throughout the occlusion. The 5 French catheter *(large arrow)* was positioned at the proximal aspect of the occlusion. **(C)** Following overnight low dose urokinase infusion, there was complete lysis of the thrombus revealing a severe eccentric left external iliac artery stenosis *(arrow)*. *(Figure continues.)*

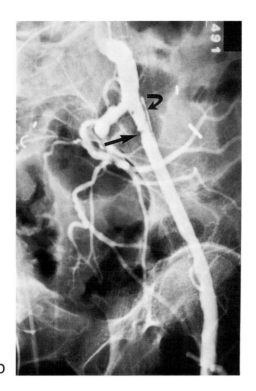

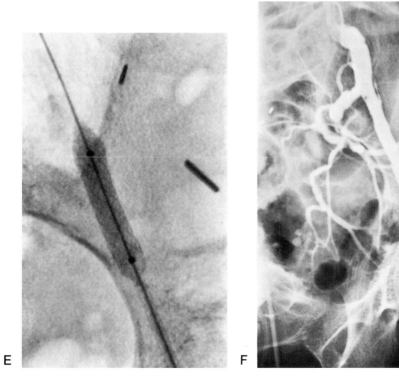

Figure 25-14 *(Continued.)* **(D)** From a retrograde approach, PTA of the external iliac artery lesion was performed resulting in marked improvement in the lumen. A small dissection *(curved arrow)* and moderate residual stenosis *(large arrow)* were, however, present. A residual gradient of 20 mmHg following intra-arterial nitroglycerine administration was measured. **(E)** A Palmaz intravascular stent was deployed at the angioplasty site. **(F)** Repeat evaluation demonstrated complete resolution of stenosis and trans-stenotic gradient.

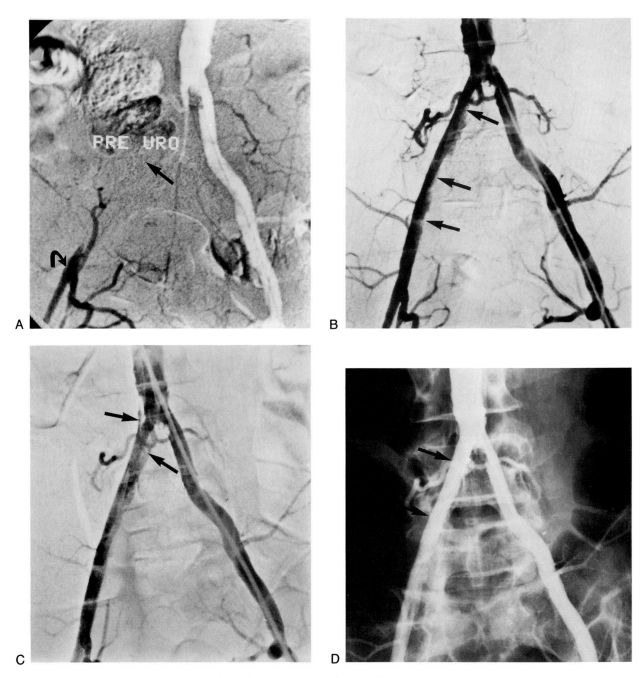

Figure 25-15 A patient presenting with a 6-month history of severe right lower extremity claudication. **(A)** Complete occlusion of the right common iliac artery *(arrow)* with reconstitution of the external iliac artery *(curved arrow)* was present. **(B)** Following thrombolytic infusion, there is restoration of antegrade flow through the common iliac artery. Eccentric stenosis of the common iliac artery *(arrows)* was present over a long segment. **(C)** Following PTA, there is some improvement in the lumen, however, extensive intimal flaps *(arrows)* were present in the proximal common iliac artery with a significant residual gradient. **(D)** Two Palmaz intravascular stents *(arrows)* were deployed in the common iliac artery with good morphologic result and resolution of the residual pressure gradient.

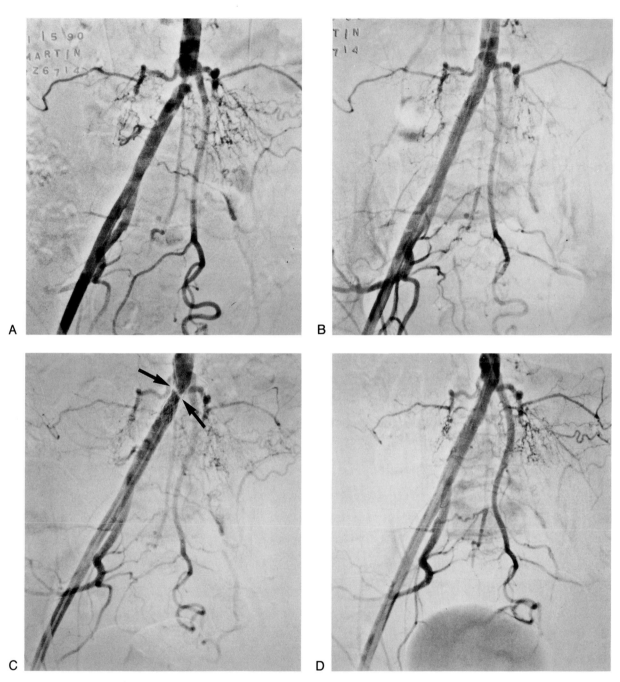

Figure 25-16 A patient with bilateral lower extremity claudication left greater than right. **(A)** Severe concentric stenosis of the origin of the right common iliac artery and a chronic left iliac artery occlusion were demonstrated. **(B)** PTA and stent placement were performed in the right common iliac artery prior to planned femorofemoral crossover graft. Both extremities improved so that the patient was no longer limited and the graft not necessary, presumably due to transpelvic collaterals. **(C)** One year following treatment, however, the patient returned with identical symptoms. Repeat angiography revealed recurrent stenosis within the Palmaz stent *(arrows)*. **(D)** Repeat dilatation was performed without difficulty, again providing relief in both lower extremities.

perience failure within the stented portion of the vessel, but rather underwent progression of disease remote to the site. Richter et al.[15] recently reported the updated results of a randomized trial comparing PTA and primary stent placement in iliac arteries in 247 patients. Initial success rates were 98 percent with stent placement and 91 percent with PTA. Cumulative 5-year patency rates determined angiographically were 93.6 percent for stent placement and 64.6 percent for the PTA group. Their study suggests that overall, long-term patency of treated iliac lesions may be significantly improved if stents are placed primarily. It is not entirely clear whether there is a definable subset of patients and/or lesions in whom stent placement may or may not be beneficial. For instance, 13 of 19 recurrent stenoses following PTA occurred in external iliac arteries, suggesting these arteries may respond less well to PTA than common iliac arteries.

The Wallstent (Schneider) has also been used with some frequency in the iliac arteries.[113,114,148,149,152,153,155,156] Advantages include a smaller, more flexible delivery device, the self-expanding nature of the stent, and the inherent flexibility of the stent, which may be more appropriate for tortuous vessels (Fig. 25-17). Initial reports outlining use of the Wallstent in the iliac arteries are extremely encouraging. Primary technical success is reported to be 99 percent (n = 170).[152,155,156] Long-term patency rates, though limited in number, averaged 95 percent at 1 year (n = approximately 120) and 88 percent at 2 years (n = approximately 60).

Occasional reports have surfaced regarding the use of stents in the infrarenal abdominal aorta and its bifurcation.[148-151] Generally, these have been used in smaller-caliber aortas. The maximum optimal diameter for the clinically available Palmaz stent is 12 mm while the currently available Wallstent is limited to 10 mm in diameter. Although the Palmaz stent can be expanded beyond 12 mm, the length of the stent becomes quite short and the ratio of surface area covered by the struts of the stent increases. Alterations in current designs may allow treatment of larger vessels with these devices.

The use of stents for primary recanalization of occluded iliac arteries deserves some mention here. Primary PTA of occluded vessels has resulted in lower patency rates and higher rates of complications, specifically distal embolization.[105-111] Investigators have reported increased success with primary use of intravascular stents during recanalizations.[88,112,113,152] Cumulative patency rates for stented occlusions are similar to that seen in stenotic disease if the technical failures related to recanalization are excluded in one series reported by Vorwerk et al.[152] Embolization did

occur in 4.7 percent, although this was usually treated successfully by either percutaneous or surgical techniques. Rees[112] described a secondary patency rate of 100 percent with follow-up of 1 to 14 months and an embolization rate of 16.7 percent.[112] The role of stents in the primary treatment of iliac artery occlusions remains unclear, with larger series and long-term results needed. Thrombolysis, though somewhat more cumbersome, may reduce the risk of embolization while converting occlusive disease to stenotic disease.

Atherectomy

Results from iliac artery atherectomy to date have not been significantly different from standard balloon angioplasty.[30,90-92] Primary technical success averaged 85 percent, although the definition of success varied widely. Three-year patency ranged from 57 to 84 percent, not clearly improving over standard PTA. Furthermore, investigators have generally limited the use of atherectomy to focal lesions, selecting a group of patients expected to have better outcomes, both short- and long-term. There was a significant increase in the number of complications encountered with atherectomy, largely related to the arteriotomy site. Puncture site hematomas were noted in up to 24 percent. This is hardly surprising when one considers the large arteriotomy necessary for these devices. Cost of the devices to the patient is estimated to be in the range of $600 to $1000 versus $200 for a PTA catheter. In addition, the costs of increased procedure time are generally passed through to the patient. At this time, there would appear to be little evidence to support the use of atherectomy in the iliac arteries.

COMPLICATIONS

Although the long-term durability of aortoiliac reconstructive surgery may surpass that of aortoiliac PTA, the marked difference in morbidity and mortality when comparing the two revascularization techniques has led to the general acceptance of PTA as the initial treatment of choice for many patients suffering from aortoiliac disease. Table 25-6 summarizes available literature reporting the complication rates for patients undergoing aortoiliac PTA.[6-13,15-17,19-26,30-32,35-37,39-41,65-67,96,104,125,126,136,158,159] The overall complication rate for all aortoiliac PTA where complications were reported was 8.1 percent. Major complications occurred in only 2.7 percent, with only 1.2 percent requiring surgical intervention. The mortality rate attributable to PTA was 0.2 percent, about one-tenth that

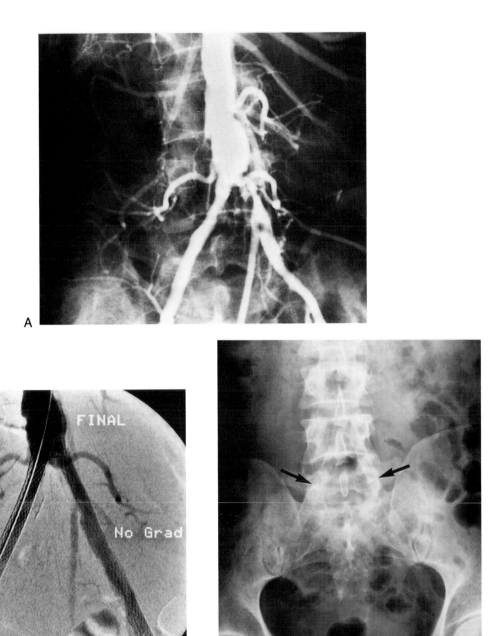

Figure 25-17 (A) Diffuse common iliac artery disease was present in this patient, who was not an operative candidate. **(B)** Following PTA, bilateral Wallstents were deployed, recreating the aortic bifurcation. Minimal residual gradient was present on the right with no residual gradient being present on the left. **(C)** A KUB 3 months later demonstrated stability in the position of the Wallstents *(arrows).*

Table 25-6   Complication Rates for Aortoiliac
PTA[a]

Complication	Rate (%)
Mortality	0.2
Limb loss	0.1
Arterial rupture	0.2
Occlusion (acute)	1.9
Embolization	1.6
Hematoma	2.9
Pseudoaneurysm/arteriovenous fistula	0.5
Renal dysfunction	0.7
Severity	
Major complications	2.7
Major complications requiring surgery	1.2
Minor complications	5.4
Overall complication rate	8.1

[a] n = 6620 procedures.
(Data from references 6–13, 15–17, 19–26, 30–32, 35–37, 39–41, 65–67, 96, 104, 125, 126, 136, 139, 158.)

generally assessed to surgical reconstruction. As the coexistence of coronary artery disease is significant in these patients, it is no surprise that myocardial infarction accounted for many of these mortalities. Arterial rupture at the site of PTA occurred in 0.3 percent. Although conservative management has been suggested,[159] rupture is generally an indication for emergency surgery. Reinflation of the balloon at the site of rupture will tamponade any hemorrhage until surgery can be performed (Fig. 25-18). Acute arterial occlusion was reported in 1.9 percent. Etiologies include primary thrombosis, dissection and vasospasm. Vasodilator administration, antiocoagulation, and repeat dilatation will frequently result in a patent lumen. A local thrombolytic infusion may be necessary if there is significant thrombus formation. Recently, stents have been used with good success to salvage these complications.[87,88] Clearly, many of the infrequent complications of angioplasty can be managed by adjunctive interventional techniques and do not require surgery.

Minor complications were noted in 5.4 percent. The majority of minor complications involved hematomas at the arterial access site. Minor complications generally required minimal if any additional treatment. This review is comparable to those of Becker, Gardiner, and Casarella.[65,67,134] The slightly higher rates noted by these authors is in part related to their inclusion of PTA at sites other than the aortoiliac segment. Generally, there is agreement that aortoiliac PTA carries a lower complication rate than do more distal lower and upper extremity procedures and those dealing with visceral vessels.

Difficulty in determining the exact rate of complications for aortoiliac PTA is to be expected as there are no standards for the reporting of complications. While a small puncture site hematoma may represent a complication to one author, another may consider it an expected consequence of the procedure. Similar difficulty is encountered when comparing the complication rates of PTA to those of surgical reconstruction of the aortoiliac segment. Blood loss such as occurs routinely with surgical procedures would be considered a major complication were it to occur during PTA. Much of the expected postoperative course of patients undergoing surgical reconstruction would and should be considered unacceptable for PTA. Reports suggesting that the complication rates for the two procedures are similar generally are not holding the two techniques to similar standards.[158] Careful review of the literature leaves little doubt as to the markedly increased safety of PTA over surgical techniques.

CONCLUSIONS

Iliac artery PTA has gained widespread acceptance in both the surgical and medical disciplines, and as such, has become one of the most commonly performed procedures for peripheral vascular disease. A high rate of technical and clinical success combined with a low complication rate have largely been responsible for this acceptance. Iliac PTA has not only been used as a primary modality of restoring perfusion to the lower extremities, but also has been found valuable in optimizing inflow prior to infra-inguinal bypass procedures. Excellent patient tolerance and extremely short recovery periods have allowed patients to return rapidly to normal daily activity. Finally, significant savings, in terms of not only the treatment costs, but also the savings associated with a decreased recovery time, can be realized with these procedures when compared to their surgical alternatives.

The safety margin of PTA has led many to expand its indications beyond those for the corresponding surgical procedures. As previously noted, moderate claudication would generally not be an indication for surgical intervention. However, failing conservative therapy, PTA may well be appropriate. In addition, this same safety margin exists should the occlusive disease recur or progress to another site. Recurrence at an angioplasty site is usually not limb-threatening and redilatation is frequently a simple procedure carrying no additional risk. A graft failure, on the other hand, may be catastrophic, often presenting with an acutely threatened limb.

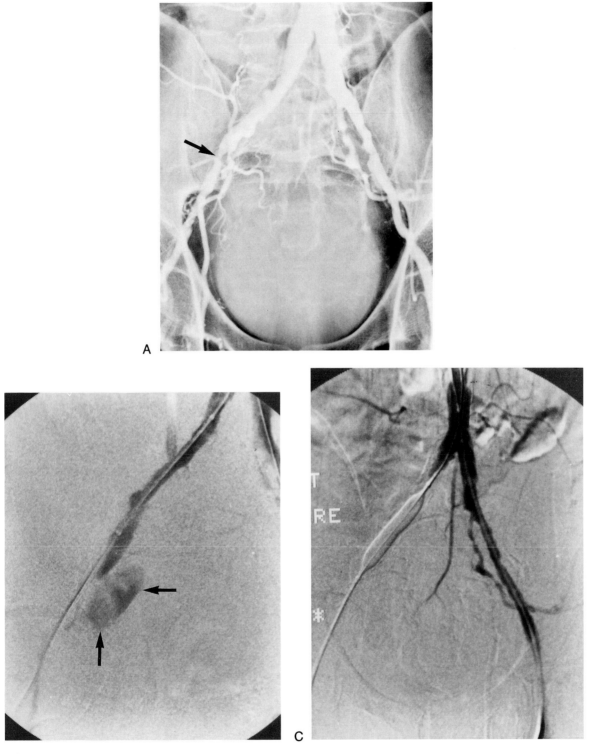

Figure 25-18 A 71-year-old man with severe coronary artery disease presented with nonhealing ulceration of the right lower extremity. **(A)** Despite diffuse disease, a focal gradient in the proximal right external iliac artery *(arrow)* was demonstrated by intra-arterial pressure measurements. As the patient was felt to represent a high surgical risk, balloon dilatation limited to this area was attempted. **(B)** Following dilatation, the patient experienced severe pelvic pain. Digital imaging revealed extravasation of contrast from the dilatation site indicating vascular rupture. **(C)** Reinflation of the angioplasty balloon resulted in tamponade of the rupture site allowing emergency surgical repair.

Although aortoiliac reconstructive surgery has somewhat better long-term durability than PTA, new technologies may improve the short- and long-term results of percutaneous therapy. Thrombolysis has been used to convert occlusive disease to stenotic disease, more readily treated by PTA. Intravascular stents, still in their infancy, have been demonstrated to be beneficial both in salvage of the suboptimal PTA result and in prolongation of patency. Continued refinements in technology may further expand the indications and success of percutaneous treatment of aortoiliac disease.

REFERENCES

1. Dotter CT: Cardiac catheterization and angiographic technics of the future. Cesk Radiol XIX:217, 1965
2. Dotter CT, Judkins MP: Transluminal treatment of arteriosclerotic obstruction: description of a new technic and a preliminary report of its application. Circulation 30:654, 1964
3. Dotter CT: Transluminal angioplasty: a long view. Radiology 135:561, 1980
4. Grüntzig A: Die perkutane rekavalisation chrovischer artelieller verschlusse (Dotter-Privzip) mit einem nemen doppellumingen dilatationskatheter. Rofo 124:80, 1976
5. Katzen BT: Percutaneous transluminal angioplasty for arterial disease of the lower extremities. AJR 142:23, 1984
6. van Andel GJ, van Erp WF, Krepel VM, Breslau PJ: Percutaneous transluminal dilatation of the iliac artery: long term results. Radiology 156:321, 1985
7. Kadir S, White RI, Kaufman SL et al: Long-term results of aortoiliac angioplasty. Surgery 94:10, 1982
8. Freiman DB, Spence R, Gatenby R et al: Transluminal angioplasty of the iliac and femoral arteries: follow-up results without anticoagulation. Radiology 141:347, 1981
9. Tegtmeyer CJ, Hartwell GD, Selby JB et al: Results and complications of angioplasty in aortoiliac disease. Circulation 83 (suppl I)I-53, 1991
10. Katzen BT, Chang J, Knox WG: Percutaneous transluminal angioplasty with the Grüntzig balloon catheter: a review of 70 cases. Arch Surg 114:1389, 1979
11. Spence RK, Freiman DB, Gatenby R et al: Long-term results of transluminal angioplasty of the iliac and femoral arteries. Arch Surg 116:1377, 1981
12. Mosley JG, Gulati SM, Raphael M, Marstron A: The role of percutaneous transluminal angioplasty for atherosclerotic disease of the lower extremities. Ann Coll R Surg Engl 67:83, 1985
13. van Andel GJ: Transluminal iliac angioplasty: long term results. Radiology 135:607, 1980
14. Katzen BT, van Breda A: Transluminal angioplasty of the iliac arteries. Sem Intervent Radiol 2 (suppl):196, 1985
15. Johnston KW, Rae M, Hogg-Johnston SA et al: 5-year results of a prospective study of percutaneous transluminal angioplasty. Ann Surg 206:403, 1987
16. Colapinto RF, Harries-Jones EP, Johnston KW: Percutaneous transluminal dilatation and recanalization in the treatment of peripheral vascular disease. Radiology 135:583, 1980
17. Kumpe DA, Kempczinski RF: Percutaneous transluminal angioplasty in the selected management of proximal arterial occlusive disease of the lower extremities: a preliminary report. Surgery 87:488, 1980
18. van Andel GJ: Long-term results of iliac and femoral angioplasty. Ann Radiol 24:365, 1981
19. Waltman AC, Greenfield AJ, Novelline RA et al: Transluminal angioplasty of the iliac and femoropopliteal arteries. Arch Surg 117:1218, 1982
20. Grüntzig A, Kumpe DA: Technique of percutaneous transluminal angioplasty with the Grüntzig balloon catheter. AJR 132:547, 1979
21. Glover JL, Bendick PJ, Dilley RS et al: Efficacy of balloon catheter dilatation for lower extremity atherosclerosis. Surgery 91:560, 1982
22. Zeitler E, Richter EI, Roth FJ, Schoop W: Results of percutaneous transluminal angioplasty. Radiology 146:57, 1983
23. Korogi Y, Takahashi M, Bussada H et al: Percutaneous transluminal angioplasty of the iliofemoropopliteal arteries: initial and long-term results. Radiat Med 5:68, 1987
24. In der Maur GAP, de Boo T, Boeve J et al: Angioplasty of the iliac and femoral arteries: initial and long-term results in short stenotic lesions. Eur J Radiol 11:163, 1990
25. Lancashire MJR, Torrie EPH, Galland RB: Percutaneous angioplasty in a district general hospital: impact and implications. JR Coll Surg Edinb 37:183, 1992
26. Blankensteijn JD, van Broonhoven TJ, Lampmann L: Role of percutaneous transluminal angioplasty in aortoiliac reconstruction. J Cardiovasc Surg 27:466, 1986
27. Thorvinger B, Norgren L, Albrechtsson. Patency after iliac and femoro-popliteal angioplasty. Acta Radiol 33:29, 1992
28. Lynch RD: Percutaneous transluminal angioplasty (PTA) and the community hospital: experience with 126 cases. J Am Osteopath Assoc 81:155, 1981
29. Wilson SE, Sheppard B: Results of percutaneous transluminal angioplasty for peripheral vascular occlusive disease. Ann Vasc Surg 4:94, 1990
30. Kotb MM, Kadir S, Bennett JD, Beam CA: Aortoiliac angioplasty: is there a need for other types of percutaneous intervention? J Vasc Intervent Radiol:67, 1992
31. Waltman AC: Percutaneous transluminal angioplasty of the iliac and deep femoral arteries. p. 273. In Athanasoulis C(ed): Interventional Radiology, WB Saunders, Philadelphia, 1982
32. Simonetti G, Urigo F: Percutaneous transluminal angioplasty of the iliac arteries. p. 610 In Interventional Radiology, Dondelinger RF, Rossi P, Kurdziel JC, S Wallace (eds): Thieme Medical Publishers, New York, NY, 1990

33. Olbert F, Karnel F: Angioplasty of iliac artery stenoses. p. 295. In Current Practice of Interventional Radiology. Kadir S (ed): BC Decker, Philadelphia, 1991

34. Davies AH, Cole SE, Magee TR et al: The effect of diabetes mellitus on the outcome of angioplasty for lower limb ischemia. Diabetic Med 9:480, 1992

35. Stokes KR, Strunk HM, Campbell DR et al: Five-year results of iliac and femoropopliteal angioplasty in diabetic patients. Radiology 174:977, 1990

36. Johnston KW: Factors that influence the outcome of aortoiliac and femoropopliteal percutaneous transluminal angioplasty. Endovasc Surg 72:843, 1992

37. Tyagi S, Malhotra A, Khalilullah M: Percutaneous transluminal angioplasty for ischaemic arterial disease of the lower extremities. Indian Heart J 42:419, 1990

38. Borozan PG, Schuler JJ, Spigos DG, Flanigan DP: Long-term hemodynamic evaluation of lower extremity percutaneous transluminal angioplasty. J Vasc Surg 2:785, 1985

39. Graor RA, Young JR, McCandless M et al: Percutaneous transluminal angioplasty: review of iliac and femoral dilatations at the Cleveland Clinic. Cleve Clin Q 51:149, 1984

40. Gallino A, Mahler F, Probst P, Nachbur B: Percutaneous transluminal angioplasty of the arteries of the lower limbs: a 5 year follow-up. Circulation 70:619, 1984

41. Motarjeme A, Keifer JW, Zuska AJ: Percutaneous transluminal angioplasty of the iliac arteries: 66 experiences. AJR 135:937, 1980

42. Waltman AC: Percutaneous transluminal angioplasty: iliac and deep femoral arteries. AJR 135:921, 1980

43. Morag B, Garnick A, Bass A et al: Percutaneous transluminal aortic angioplasty: early and late results. Cardiovasc Intervent Radiol 16:37, 1993

44. Grollman JH, Del Vicario M, Mittal AK: Percutaneous transluminal abdominal aortic angioplasty. AJR 134:1053, 1980

45. Tegtmeyer CJ, Kellum CD, Kron IL, Mentzer RM. Percutaneous transluminal angioplasty in the region of the aortic bifurcation. Radiology 157:661, 1985

46. Arbona GL, van Aman ME, Smead WL: Percutaneous transluminal angioplasty of the abdominal aortic bifurcation. Southern Med J 76:22, 1983

47. Tadavarthy AK, Sullivan WA, Nicoloff D et al: Aorta balloon angioplasty: 9 year follow-up. Radiology 170:1039, 1989

48. Belli AM, Hemingway AP, Cumberland DC, Welsh CL. Percutaneous transluminal angioplasty of the distal abdominal aorta. Eur J Vasc Surg 3:449, 1989

49. Morag B, Rubinstein Z, Kessler A et al: Percutaneous transluminal angioplasty of the distal abdominal aorta and its bifurcation. Cardiovasc Intervent Radiol 10:129, 1987

50. Odurny A, Colapinto RF, Sniderman KW, Johnston KW: Percutaneous transluminal angioplasty of abdominal aortic stenoses. Cardiovasc Intervent Radiol 12:1, 1989

51. Heeney D, Bookstein J, Daniels E et al: Transluminal angioplasty of the abdominal aorta. Radiology 148:81, 1983

52. Mitchell SE, Kadir S, Kaufman SL et al: Percutaneous angioplasty of aortic graft stenoses. Radiology 149:439, 1983

53. Tegtmeyer CJ, Wellons HA, Thompson RN: Balloon dilation of the abdominal aorta. JAMA 244:2636, 1980

54. Velasquez G, Castaneda-Zuniga W, Formanek A et al: Nonsurgical aortoplasty in Leriche syndrome. Radiology 134:359, 1980

55. Yakes WF, Kumpe DA, Brown SB et al: Percutaneous transluminal aortic angioplasty: techniques and results. Radiology 172:965, 1989

56. Charlebois N, Saint-Georges G, Hudon G: Percutaneous transluminal angioplasty of the lower abdominal aorta. AJR 146:369, 1986

57. Selby JB, Tegtmeyer CJ: Angioplasty of abdominal aortic stenoses. In Kadir S (ed): Current Practice in Interventional Radiology, BC Decker, Philadelphia, 1991

58. Ravimandalam K, Rao VRK, Kumar S et al. Obstruction of the infrarenal portion of the abdominal aorta: results of treatment with balloon angioplasty. AJR 156:1257, 1991

59. Jeans WD, Danton RM, Baird RN, Horrocks M: A comparison of the costs of vascular surgery and balloon dilatation in lower limb ischaemic disease. Br J Radiol 59:453, 1986

60. Kinnison ML, White RI, Bowers WP, Dunlap ED. Cost incentives for peripheral angioplasty. AJR 145:1241, 1985

61. Stanson AW: A perspective of percutaneous transluminal angioplasty (editorial). Clin Vasc Dis

62. Cronenwett J, Davis J, Gooch J et al: Aortoiliac occlusive disease in women. Surgery 88:775, 1980

63. Karmody AM, Powers SR, Monaco VJ, Leather RP: Blue toe syndrome: an indication for limb salvage surgery. Arch Surg 111:1263, 1976

64. Brewer ML, Kinnison ML, Perler BA, White RI: Blue toe syndrome: treatment with anticoagulants and delayed percutaneous transluminal angioplasty. Radiology 166:31, 1988

65. Becker GJ: Noncoronary angioplasty. Radiology 170:921, 1989

66. Gardiner GA, Meyerovitz MF, Stokes KR et al: Complications of transluminal angioplasty. Radiology 159:201, 1986

67. Casarella WR: Noncoronary angioplasty. Current Probl Cardiol 11:138, 1986

68. Kashdan BJ, Trost DW, Jagust MB et al: Retrograde approach for contralateral iliac and infrainguinal percutaneous transluminal angioplasty: experience in 100 patients. J Vasc Intervent Radiol 3:515, 1992

69. Bachman DM, Casarella WJ, Sos TA: Percutaneous iliofemoral angioplasty via the contralateral femoral artery. Radiology 130:617, 1979

70. Kumpe DA: Percutaneous dilatation of an abdominal aortic stenosis. Radiology 141:536, 1981

71. Dotter CT, Rosch J, Seaman AJ: Selective clot lysis with low dose streptokinase. Radiology 111:31, 1974

72. Becker GJ, Rabe FE, Richmond BD et al: Low dose

fibrinolytic therapy: results and new concepts. Radiology 148:663, 1983

73. Katzen BT, van Breda A: Low dose streptokinase in the treatment of arterial occlusions. AJR 136:1171, 1981

74. Hess H, Ingrisch H, Mietaschk A, Rath H: Local low dose thrombolytic therapy of peripheral arterial occlusions. N Engl J Med 307:1627, 1982

75. McNamara TO, Fischer JR: Thrombolysis of peripheral arterial and graft occlusions: improved results using high dose urokinase. AJR 144:769, 1985

76. McNamara TO, Bomberger RA: Factors affecting initial and 6 month patency rates after intraarterial thrombolysis with high dose urokinase. Am J Surg 152:709, 1986

77. van Breda A, Katzen BT, Deutsch AS: Urokinase versus streptokinase in local thrombolysis. Radiology 165:109, 1987

78. Auster M, Kadir S, Mitchell SE et al: Iliac artery occlusion: management with intrathrombus streptokinase infusion and angioplasty. Radiology 153:385, 1984

79. McNamara TO: Thrombolysis as an alternative initial therapy for the acutely ischemia lower limb. Semin Vasc Surg 5:89, 1992

80. Mingoli A, Dimarzo L, Sciacca V et al: Thrombolysis of graft occlusion using high dose urokinase. An alternative to surgical treatment. Ital J Surg Sci 19:79, 1989

81. Bookstein JJ, Valji K: Pulse-spray pharmacomechanical thrombolysis. Cardiovasc Intervent Radiol 15:228, 1992

82. Palmaz JC, Laborde JC, Rivera FJ et al: Stenting of the iliac arteries with the Palmaz stent: experience from a multicenter trial. Cardiovasc Intervent Radiol 15:291, 1992

83. Becker GJ: Intravascular stents: general principles and status of lower extremity arterial applications. Circulation 83(suppl I):I-122, 1991

84. Palmaz JC, Garcia OJ, Schatz RA et al: Placement of balloon-expandable intraluminal stents in iliac arteries: first 171 procedures. Radiology 174:969, 1990

85. Cikrit DF, Becker GJ, Dalsing MC et al: Early experience with the Palmaz expandable intraluminal stent in iliac artery stenosis. Ann Vasc Surg 5:150, 1991

86. Bonn J, Gardiner GA, Shapiro MJ et al: Palmaz vascular stent: initial clinical experience. Radiology 174:741, 1990

87. Becker GJ, Palmaz JC, Res CR et al: Angioplasty-induced dissections in human iliac arteries: management with Palmaz balloon-expandable intraluminal stents. Radiology 176:31, 1990

88. Gunther RW, Vorwerk D, Antonucci F et al: Iliac artery stenosis or obstruction after unsuccessful balloon angioplasty: treatment with a self-expandable stent. AJR 156:389, 1991

89. Palmaz JC. Balloon-expandable intravascular stent. AJR 150:1263, 1988

90. Kim D, Gianturco LE, Porter DH et al: Peripheral directional atherectomy: 4-year experience. Radiology 183:773, 1992

91. Clugston RA, Eisenhauer AC, Matthews RV: Atherec-

tomy of the distal aorta using a "kissing-balloon" technique for the treatment of blue toe syndrome. AJR 159:125, 1992

92. Hinohara T, Selmon MR, Robertson GC et al: Directional atherectomy: new approaches for treatment of obstructive coronary and peripheral vascular disease. Circulation 81(suppl IV):IV-79, 1991

93. Maynar M, Reyes R, Cabera V et al: Percutaneous atherectomy as an alternative treatment for post-angioplasty obstructive intimal flaps. Radiology 170:1029, 1989

94. Guidelines for Percutaneous Transluminal Angioplasty. Standards of Practice Committee of the Society of Cardiovascular and Interventional Radiology. Radiology 177:619, 1990

95. Wilson SE, Wolf GL, Cross AP: Percutaneous transluminal angioplasty versus operation for peripheral arteriosclerosis. J Vasc Surg 9:1, 1989

96. Johnston KW, Colapinto RF, Baird RJ: Transluminal dilation—an alternative? Arch Surg 117:1604, 1982

97. Hallett JW: Trends in revascularization of the lower extremity. Mayo Clin Proc 61:369, 1986

98. Brothers TE, Greenfield LJ: Long-term results of aortoiliac reconstruction. J Vasc Intervent Radiol 1:49, 1990

99. Whittemore AD, Mannick JA: The ischemic leg. Adv Surg 15:293, 1981

100. Rutherford RB, Flanigan DP, Gupta SK et al: Suggested standards for reports dealing with lower extremity ischemia. J Vasc Surg 4:80, 1986

101. Rutherford RB, Becker GJ: Standards for evaluating and reporting the results of surgical and percutaneous therapy for peripheral arterial disease. J Vasc Intervent Radiol 2:169, 1991

102. McAllister FF: The rate of patients with intermittent claudication managed nonoperatively. Am J Surg 132:593, 1976

103. Ekroth R, Dahllof AG, Gundevall B et al: Physical training of patients with intermittent claudication: indications, methods, and results. Surgery 84:640, 1978

104. Armstrong MWJ, Torrie EPH, Galland RB: Consequences of immediate failure of percutaneous transluminal angioplasty. Ann R Coll Surg Engl 74:265, 1992

105. Ring EJ, Freiman DB, McLean GK, Schwarz W: Percutaneous recanalization of common iliac artery occlusions: an unacceptable complication rate? AJR 139:587, 1982

106. Colapinto RF, Stronell RD, Johnston WK: Transluminal angioplasty of complete iliac obstructions. AJR 146:859, 1986

107. Simonetti S, Rossi G, Passariello R et al: PTA in external iliac artery occlusion. Eur J Radiol 1:184, 1981

108. Daniell SJN, Dacie JE, Lumley JSP: Is percutaneous transluminal angioplasty for common iliac occlusion a safe procedure? J Vasc Intervent Radiol 2:89, 1987

109. Ginsburg R, Thorpe P, Bowles CR et al: Pull-through approach to percutaneous angioplasty of totally occluded common iliac arteries. Radiology 172:111, 1989

110. Pilla TJ, Peterson GJ, Tantana S et al: Percutaneous

recanalization of iliac artery occlusions: an alternative to surgery in the high risk patient. AJR 143:313, 1984

111. Graziani L: Percutaneous recanalization of total iliac and femoro-popliteal artery occlusions. Eur J Radiol 7:91, 1987

112. Rees CR, Palmaz JC, Garcia O et al: Angioplasty and stenting of completing occluded iliac arteries. Radiology 172:953, 1989

113. Gunther RW, Vorwerk D, Bohndorf K et al: Iliac and femoral artery stenoses and occlusions: treatment with intravascular stents. Radiology 172:725, 1989

114. Vorwerk D, Guenther RW: Mechanical revascularization of occluded iliac arteries with use of self-expandable endoprosthesis. Radiology 175:411, 1990

115. Dolmatch BL, Rholl KS, Moskowitz LB et al: Blue toe syndrome: treatment with percutaneous atherectomy. Radiology 172:799, 1989

116. Kumpe DA, Zwerdzinger S, Griffin DJ: Blue digit syndrome: treatment with percutaneous transluminal angioplasty. Radiology 166:37, 1988

117. Weber G, Kiss T: Intraoperative balloon angioplasty. Eur J Vasc Surg 3:153, 1989

118. Wilms G, Nevelsteen A, Baert A, Suy R: Intraoperative angioplasty. Cardiovasc Intervent Radiol 10:8, 1987

119. Al-Salman M, Doyle DL, Hsiang YN et al: Intraoperative balloon angioplasty: a surgical approach. Can Society for Vascular Surgery 35:265, 1992

120. Spoelstra H, Nevelsteen A, Wilms G and Suy R: Balloon angioplasty combined with vascular surgery Eur J Vasc Surg 3:381, 1989

121. Griffith CDM, Harrison JD, Gregson RHS et al: Transluminal iliac angioplasty with distal bypass surgery in patients with critical limb ischaemia. JR Coll Surg Edinb 34:253, 1989

122. Zeitler E, Raithel D, Gailer H et al: PTA combined with surgical vascular operations in iliac and femoral obstruction. Ann Radiol 30:142, 1987

123. Olbert F, Weidinger P, Schlegl A et al: Combined transluminal percutaneous dilation and surgical reconstruction of the iliac, femoral and popliteal arteries. Ann Radiol 24:369, 1981

124. Wilson SE, White GH, Wolf G, Cross AP: Proximal percutaneous balloon angioplasty and distal bypass for multilevel arterial occlusion. Ann Vasc Surg 4:351, 1990

125. Walker PJ, Harris JP, May J: Combined percutaneous transluminal angioplasty and extraanatomic bypass for symptomatic unilateral iliac artery occlusion with contralateral iliac artery stenosis. Ann Vasc Surg 5:209, 1991

126. Brewster DC, Cambria RP, Darling RC et al: Long-term results of combined iliac balloon angioplasty and distal surgical revascularization. Ann Surg 210:324, 1989

127. Kadir S, Smith GW, White RI et al: Percutaneous transluminal angioplasty as an adjunct to the surgical management of peripheral vascular disease. Ann Surg 195:786, 1982

128. Motarjeme A, Keifer JW, Zuska AJ: Percutaneous transluminal angioplasty as a complement to surgery. Radiology 141:341, 1981

129. Corey CJ, Bush HL, Widrich WC, Nabseth DC: Combined operative angiodilation and arterial reconstruction for limb salvage. Arch Surg 118:1289, 1983

130. Bunt TJ: Aortic reconstruction vs extra-anatomic bypass and angioplasty. Arch Surg 121:1166, 1986

131. Peterkin GA, Belkin M, Cantelmo NL et al: Combined transluminal angioplasty and infrainguinal reconstruction in multilevel atherosclerotic disease. J Surg 160:277, 1990

132. Castaneda-Zuniga WR, Smith A, Kaye K et al: Transluminal angioplasty for treatment of vasculogenic impotence. AJR 139:371, 1962

133. Van Unnik JG, Marsman JWP: Impotence due to the external iliac steal syndrome treated by percutaneous transluminal angioplasty. J Urol 131:544, 1984

134. Becker GJ, Rowe DM, Holden RW et al: Percutaneous transluminal angioplasty for vasculogenic impotence. Indiana Med 79:256, 1986

135. Weigele JB: Iliac artery stenosis causing renal allograft-mediated hypertension: angiographic diagnosis and treatment. AJR 157:513, 1991

136. Belli AM, Cumberland DC, Knox AM et al: The complication rate of percutaneous peripheral balloon angioplasty. Clin Radiol 41:380, 1990

137. Clement C, Costa-Foru B, Vernon P Nicaise H: Transluminal angioplasty performed by the surgeon in lower limb arterial occlusive disease: one hundred fifty cases. Ann Vasc Surg 4:519, 1990

138. Harris RW, Dulawa LB, Andros G et al: Percutaneous transluminal angioplasty of the lower extremities by the vascular surgeon. Ann Vasc Surg 5:345, 1991

139. Cole SEA, Baird RN, Horrocks M, Jeans WD: The role of balloon angioplasty in the management of lower limb ischaemia. J Vasc Surg 1:61, 1987

140. Glover JL, Bendick PJ, Dilley RS et al: Balloon catheter dilation for limb salvage. Arch Surg 118:557, 1983

141. Kwasnik EM, Siouffi SY, Jay ME, Khuri SF: Comparative results of angioplasty and aortofemoral bypass in patients with symptomatic iliac disease. Arch Surg 122:288, 1987

142. Samson RH, Sprayregen S, Veith FJ et al: Management of angioplasty complications, unsuccessful procedures and early and late failures. Ann Surg 199:234, 1984

143. Brewster DC: Clinical and anatomical considerations for surgery in aortoiliac disease and results of surgical treatment. Circulation 83(suppl I): I-42, 1991

144. Crawford ES, Manning LG, Kelly TF: "Redo" surgery after operations for aneurysm and occlusion of the abdominal aorta. Surgery 81:41, 1977

145. Hallisey M, Meranze S, Parker BC et al: Percutaneous transluminal angioplasty of the abdominal aorta, abstracted. Society of Cardiovascular and Interventional Radiology, Annual Meeting, New Orleans, LA, 1993.

146. McNamara TO: Thrombolytic therapy for iliac artery occlusions. p. 301. In Kadir S (ed): Current Practice of Interventional Radiology, BC Decker, Philadelphia, 1991

147. Deeter W, Meranze S, Rholl K, et al: Thrombolytic therapy in iliac artery occlusive disease, abstracted. Society of Cardiovascular and Interventional Radiology, Annual Meeting, Washington, DC, 1991.

148. El Ashmaoui A, Do DD, Triller J et al: Angioplasty of the terminal aorta: follow-up of 20 patients treated by PTA or PTA with stents. Eur J Radiol 13:113, 1991

149. Vorwerk D, Gunther RW, Bohndorf K, Keulers P: Stent placement for failed angioplasty of aortic stenoses: report of two cases. Cardiovasc Intervent Radiol 14:316, 1991

150. Palmaz JC, Encamacion CE, Garcia OJ et al: Aortic bifurcation stenosis: treatment with intravascular stents. J Vasc Intervent Radiol 2:319, 1991

151. Kuffer G, Spengel F, Steckmeier B: Percutaneous reconstruction of the aortic bifurcation with Palmaz stents: case reports. Cardiovasc Intervent Radiol 14:170, 1991

152. Vorwerk D, Gunther RW: Stent placement in iliac arterial lesions: three years of clinical experience with the wallstent. Cardiovasc Intervent Radiol 15:285, 1992

153. Rousseau H, Joffre F, Raillat C et al: Iliac artery endoprosthesis: radiologic and histologic findings after 2 years. AJR 153:1075, 1989

154. Long AL, Page PE, Raynaud AC et al: Percutaneous iliac artery stent: angiographic long-term followup. Radiology 180:771, 1991

155. Zollikofer CL, Antonucci F, Pfyffer M et al: Arterial stent placement with use of the wallstent: midterm results of clinical experience. Radiology 179:449, 1991

156. Raillat C, Rousseau H, Joffre F, Roux D: Treatment of iliac artery stenoses with the wallstent endoprosthesis. AJR 154:613, 1990

157. Richter G, Roeren T, Brado M, Noeldge G: Further update of the randomized trial: iliac stent placement versus PTA—morphology, clinical success rates, and failure analysis, abstracted. Society of Cardiovascular and Interventional Radiology, Annual Meeting, New Orleans, LA, 1993

158. Weibull H, Bergqvist D, Jonsson K et al: Complications after percutaneous transluminal angioplasty in the iliac, femoral, and popliteal. J Vasc Surg 5:681, 1987

159. Joseph N, Levy E, Lipman S: Angioplasty-related iliac artery rupture: treatment by temporary balloon occlusion. Cardiovasc Intervent Radiol 10:276, 1987

26

Surgical Management of Aortoiliac Occlusive Disease

John D. Horowitz
Joseph R. Durham

Since the mid-nineteenth century descriptions of atherosclerotic occlusive disease by Cruvheiler and Charcot, involvement of the aortoiliac segment has remained a well-recognized cause of severe disabling claudication, tissue ischemia, and limb loss.[1-3] The modern concept of "segmental" arterial obstruction as the cause of lower limb ischemia was postulated by these vascular pioneers on the basis of history, physical examination, and postmortem dissection.[4] The subsequent development of contrast arteriography revolutionized patient evaluation by providing an anatomic framework for surgical intervention, a diagnostic algorithm still practiced today.[5] Despite accurate clinical and anatomic diagnosis, for years it was technically impossible to apply direct surgical reconstruction to correct the pathophysiologic derangements of aortoiliac occlusive or aneurysmal disease. When Leriche[6] described aortitis terminalis during the 1920s, the only surgical interventions offered were lumbar sympathectomy and amputation. During the subsequent 40 years, the discovery of heparin, the development of durable and biocompatible vascular prostheses, the refinement of vascular surgical technique, and advances in perioperative care succeeded in making aortoiliac revascularization a safe and effective undertaking.

The spectrum of symptomatic aortoiliac occlusive disease mandates that intervention be tailored to each patient. Since a number of surgical and endovascular options exist, treatment strategy must address the anatomic pattern of disease, severity of limb ischemia, and be tempered by a risk/benefit assessment of procedure durability and morbidity relative to concomitant medical conditions. The development of sophisticated endovascular techniques has permitted treatment of focal lesions by a less invasive approach, an option that should be considered in every patient. Safe, successful correction of aortoiliac arterial insufficiency requires an understanding of the anatomic patterns of atherosclerotic disease, clinical manifestations, natural history, relevant pathophysiology, and expected outcome after endovascular angioplasty or direct surgical repair/bypass.

DISEASE PATTERNS AND PRESENTING SIGNS

Aortoiliac atherosclerotic occlusive disease occurs in distinct anatomic and manifests characteristic clinical symptoms/signs[7-10] (Table 26-1). The majority (approximately 70 percent) of patients with severe lower limb ischemia due primarily to aortoiliac atherosclero-

Table 26-1 Patterns of Aortoiliac Occlusive Disease

Type	Pattern
Above inguinal ligament (30%)	
I	Distal aorta and common iliac
II	Distal aorta, common iliac, external iliac, common femoral
Multisegment disease (70%)	
III	Segmental involvement of aorta and iliac system combined with superficial femoral and/or tibial disease

sis also demonstrate multilevel occlusive lesions (type III) with involvement of infrainguinal arteries (common femoral, superficial femoral, popliteal, and tibial). In only one-third of patients is the occlusive process limited to vessels (infrarenal aorta, common and external iliac arteries) above the inguinal ligament (type II). Focal disease limited to the aortic bifurcation (type I) is the least common disease pattern (10 percent of patients). In all the disease patterns, the juxtarenal segment of the abdominal aorta is typically least involved with atherosclerosis. Even in instances of infrarenal aortic occlusion, the aorta immediately distal to the renal arteries will manifest only retrograde thrombotic occlusion and minimal atherosclerotic plaque. Plaque development is always more extensive on posterior walls, a feature that can compromise collateral compensation through the lumbar and median sacral arteries.

Terminal Aorta and Iliac Artery Disease

Patients with segmental type I disease are typically younger (under 60 years of age) and fervent cigarette smokers (more than 2 packs/day). Compared with the cohort with multisegment (type III) disease, the incidence of hypertension and diabetes mellitus is lower, but serum lipid abnormalities (cholesterol, triglycerides, low levels of high-density lipoproteins) are common. The sex distribution fails to show the male predominance generally associated with vascular disease; women account for approximately one-half of patients. Epidemiologically, affected women have commonly experienced premature menopause secondary to hysterectomy or radiation therapy and loss of the protective effect of estrogen against the development of atherosclerosis.[11-13] Hypoplasia of the aortoiliac segment has also been described as predisposing factor.[14-17] Several investigators have characterized a sub-

set of women with symptomatic aortoiliac disease whose aortic diameter was smaller than average. A suprarenal aorta diameter of 19 mm or less and infrarenal aorta diameter of 13 mm or less was judged consistent with "hypoplasia." Using these criteria, approximately one-fourth of women who were candidates for aortoiliac revascularization demonstrated hypoplasia of the aortoiliac *and* infrainguinal vessels. The etiology of this entity may involve overfusion of the fetal double aortae, as there is a single large distal lumbar artery in many of these patients, in contrast to expected paired lumbar arteries. The "classic" presentation would involve a woman under 50 years of age, short in stature, with a history of heavy tobacco use, and an abnormal lipid profile. Atherosclerotic disease is limited to the distal aorta, less commonly to the iliacs, and with sparing of the superficial femoral arteries. The young age of presentation in these women may be the consequence of moderate plaque development in small-caliber vessels resulting in a hemodynamically significant lesion.

The Leriche syndrome, thrombo-obliteration of the terminal aorta, represents a distinct patient population with localized aortoiliac disease. Impotence is a classically associated complaint. Occlusion of the common iliac arteries or terminal aorta leads to retrograde thrombus propagation to the next large uninvolved artery orifice, typically the inferior mesenteric or renal arteries. Approximately 10 percent of candidates for surgical intervention will present with infrarenal aortic occlusion. Lumen encroachment at or above the renal arteries can complicate presenting signs and management if disease severity is sufficient to produce renovascular hypertension and/or ischemic nephropathy as a result of blood flow compromise or atheroembolism to the renal parenchyma. In autopsy studies, Leriche observed that patients with terminal aortic thrombo-obliteration have a short infrarenal aorta and a high iliac bifurcation with an acute takeoff angle (38 degrees); he postulated that these anatomic variations create turbulent flow and a propensity for atherogenesis.[18,19] These early observations stimulated investigations that continue today regarding the role of hemodynamics and shear stress on atherosclerotic plaque development.

Patients with occlusive disease limited to the aortoiliac segment (types I and II) usually present with claudication of buttock, hip, thigh, and calf musculature. Muscle weakness with walking is a common complaint. Collateral compensation includes both visceral (inferior mesenteric artery, superior hemorrhoidal, meandering mesenteric artery) and parietal (inferior epigastric artery, intercostal and lumbar arteries, hypogastric and gluteal arteries) routes. Collateral flow reenters at the level of the circumflex iliac, common femoral, and profunda femoris arteries. Patients rarely present with critical limb ischemia (dependent rubor, pallor on elevation, and tissue loss), except in the case of atheromatous embolism, a process of plaque degeneration with accumulation and dislodgement of thrombus, platelet aggregations, or atherosclerotic debris into the distal terminal circulation.

Patients with type III or combined aortoiliac and infrainguinal occlusive disease are usually older by a decade; have a higher incidence of diabetes, hypertension, associated cardiac and cerebrovascular disease; and are usually men (6:1 male predominance). Short-distance (<50 m) claudication or advanced limb ischemia are prevalent complaints. Patients with multilevel disease constitute up to two-thirds of patients selected for a surgical approach, with operation often undertaken for limb salvage, rather than disabling claudication. Of note, aortoiliac reconstruction/bypass is usually sufficient to relieve critical ischemia, although claudication will persist due to infrainguinal disease (i.e., superficial femoral artery occlusion).

Unilateral Iliac Artery Disease

Hemodynamically significant unilateral iliac artery disease can cause significant limb ischemia and, in the presence of femoropopliteal occlusive disease, can lead to critical limb ischemia. Iatrogenic artery trauma associated with diagnostic angiography, percutaneous transluminal angioplasty (PTA), or intra-aortic balloon pumps may be a cause of unilateral iliac artery disease (Fig. 26-1). In instances of atherosclerosis obliterans, the left common iliac artery is more commonly involved, a finding attributed to the more acute angle of origin, as compared with the right side.[20] Unilateral iliac disease is equally divided between men and women.[21] The role of variation in the aortic bifurcation anatomy as regards the development of atherosclerosis remains speculative.

Disease progression in the aortoiliac segment is unpredictable. Unilateral iliac artery disease may not progress to bilateral disease. When surveillance of the contralateral asymptomatic iliac artery of patients with symptomatic unilateral iliac disease has been performed, disease progression assessed by symptomatology, pulse examination, and angiographic evaluation developed in 15 to 40 percent of patients, depending on the diagnostic method.[22-24] The lowest rates of disease progression were reported when objective physiologic (aorta to femoral artery systolic pressure gradient) assessment of hemodynamic significance was used. Kikta and colleagues[25] have shown that angiographic abnormalities, if not hemodynamically significant by

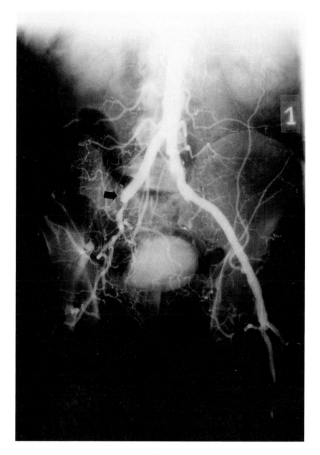

Figure 26-1 Right external iliac artery occlusion after cardiac catheterization 1 year previously. Note reconstitution of the distal external iliac artery and common femoral artery. The left side is relatively free of significant disease.

femoral artery systolic pressure measurement with papaverine administration, rarely become a cause of inflow failure for distal grafts.[25] Furthermore, late failure of crossover femorofemoral grafts is usually secondary to outflow disease, not from progression of inflow disease,[4] a clinical and experimental observation attributed to a protective effect of the increased flow in the donor artery after femorofemoral bypass.[26-29]

DIAGNOSTIC CONSIDERATIONS

Clinical diagnosis of aortoiliac arterial insufficiency is usually straightforward and is based on the location of symptoms and peripheral pulse examination. Proximal limb muscle weakness, progressive intermittent claudication of the buttock and thigh, and, in males, penile erectile dysfunction, are typical presenting symptoms. With type II multilevel disease, symptoms are not localized, and limb ischemia may be advanced at presentation with complaints of ischemic rest pain, foot paresthesia, or tissue loss. An absent or diminished femoral pulse is the hallmark physical finding of aortoiliac occlusive disease. A weak femoral pulse can be present despite iliac occlusion, if collateral development is extensive. A bruit transmitted from the iliac or femoral vessels indicates turbulent blood flow produced by a proximal stenosis.

Aortography with lower limb arterial runoff imaging is an important component of patient evaluation before intervention but is rarely used for solely diagnostic purposes. Arterial imaging by arteriography is used to characterize the extent and nature of the disease, the morphology of plaque and areas of stenosis and to identify concomitant involvement of the celiac, mesenteric, renal, or hypogastric vasculature—features that have implications for patient management.

Femoral pulse palpation and grading cannot accurately assess the hemodynamic significance of an anatomically abnormal aortoiliac arterial segment. This caveat is especially pertinent after prior groin procedures, in obese patients, and in instances of extensive femoral artery calcification.[30-34] Arteriography, considered the "gold standard" of predicting hemodynamic significance, often under- or overestimates severity and extent of atherosclerotic aortoiliac disease.[31-34] Since plaque development is on the posterior wall of the vessels, accurate diagnosis requires imaging in multiple planes.[35] Successful management of aortoiliac disease requires precise determination of which lesions are both hemodynamically significant and responsible for limb ischemic symptomatology.

The correlation of clinical symptoms to segmental limb pressures is widely accepted,[36] but noninvasive pressure measurements for the aortoiliac segment are often inaccurate. Thigh cuff pressure measurements have been used to determine thigh pressure indices[37] and thigh/ankle indices,[38] in an attempt to assess both inflow and outflow at the femoral level, respectively. These measurements can be quite inaccurate in the large patient or in those with distal segmental disease. The overall accuracy for both wide and narrow cuffs appears to be poor compared with intra-arterial pressure measurements.[39] Studies have shown that 55 percent of patients with angiographically proven aortoiliac stenosis had normal proximal thigh indices, while 31 percent of those with superficial femoral artery occlusion in the absence of proximal disease had a falsely elevated thigh pressure index.[40] A more recent study, however, has shown that for isolated segmental proximal disease only, cuff pressure measurements may approach 90 to 95 percent sensitivity and specificity but, in the face of tandem disease distally, sensitivity and specificity still drop to the 50 percent range.[41]

Several investigators have attempted to use femoral artery waveform analysis to assess the hemodynamic significance of inflow aortoiliac lesions. Proximal damping quotient,[42] pulse rise time,[43] waveform and pulsatility index,[44] and, more recently, waveform transformation analysis[45] have all been derived from the femoral artery waveform to predict the significance of inflow lesions with variable success. In a prospective analysis, Thiele et al.[46] used the femoral pulsatility index (FPI) calculated from the femoral waveform amplitude in select patients and found that they could achieve 94 percent accuracy. In 38 percent of patients, however, FPI was not feasible, and invasive pressure readings were required.[46] In a similar study, Flanigan et al.[47] compared FPI with intra-arterial measurements; they found only 62 percent sensitivity and determined 69 percent specificity by algorithm. They concluded that FPI was not accurate enough to determine hemodynamic significance for aortoiliac lesions. By calculating the mean power frequency index from digital signal processing of aortic and femoral waveform spectra, Sawchuk et al.[45] used a computer-derived technique to assess critical and subcritical stenoses of the aortoiliac segment. While they have shown this technique to compare favorably with intra-arterial measurements with and without papaverine-induced reactive changes, their technique is not widely available, nor is it generally applicable. Isotope transit time from the aorta to the femoral region has been investigated as a means of assessing the reduction in flow caused by stenotic lesions but remains experimental and is of unproven benefit.[21]

The duplex ultrasound scanner has the ability to detect flow abnormalities and, when combined with real-time B-mode imaging, can provide valuable anatomic information. Hershey and co-workers[48] reported extensive experience with this technique and concluded that it remains a valuable tool in the initial assessment of hemodynamic significance in aortoiliac disease. A normal noninvasive study of the aorta and iliac arteries that included both Doppler and hemodynamic measurements excluded significant occlusive disease, obviating the need for angiography except to evaluate distal disease. Difficulties with this technique include extreme operator variability, a requisite fasting state for 12 hours before the study, and impaired or absent visualization in the obese patient or in those with limited visualization due to bowel gas. As a result, duplex scanning has not replaced arteriography for the routine preoperative assessment.

Invasive measurement of femoral artery pressure (FAP) remains the most reliable and universally applicable method of assessing the hemodynamic significance of aortoiliac lesions. First described by Brener et al.,[49] FAP measurement has been the "gold standard" against which other diagnostic modalities have been judged. FAP measurement is a straightforward assessment of flow dynamics obtained at angiography by measuring pressures from the catheter as it traverses the stenotic lesion. A drop of 5 mmHg in peak systolic pressure measured by pull-through technique, or a drop of 10 to 15 percent in femoral artery pressure in response to vasodilator injection, constitutes a positive study and implies that the inflow lesion is hemodynamically significant. Flanigan et al.[50] reported that several subcritical stenoses in series can produce a significant reduction in distal flow detectable by FAP measurement alone. Brewster et al.[30] used FAP measurements to predict the success of proximal reconstruction alone in patients with multisegment disease. Of 51 patients with a positive FAP test, 96 percent resolved their indications for surgery with proximal revascularization alone. Of seven patients with a negative FAP, 57 percent failed to improve with proximal revascularization alone and went onto require distal bypass later. For the present time, FAP before and after vasodilator injection remains the single best method of assessing the true hemodynamic significance of an anatomic lesion in the aortoiliac segment.

THERAPEUTIC STRATEGIES

Medical Management

Nonoperative treatment of aortoiliac insufficiency is appropriate for patients with tolerable levels of claudication or those patients with such advanced co-morbid illness that surgical intervention is considered too risky. For those patients with preocclusive subcritical atherosclerosis, the treatment should focus on preventing disease progression and stimulating the formation of collateral circulation. By altering vascular risk factors, such as cigarette smoking, hypertension, hyperlipidemia, diabetes, and exercise tolerance, patients can increase their level of activity and their claudication distance.[51-54]

Pharmacotherapy for chronic lower-extremity ischemia has been attempted for years with variable results. The benefit of circulation-enhancing drugs, such as hemorrheologic agents, vasodilators, prostaglandins, and calcium channel blockers, is being tested. Pentoxifylline (Trental) seems to be the only medication shown by multicenter double-blind placebo-controlled trial to enhance treadmill walking distance in patients with claudication.[55] Actual symptom reduction in daily life seems to be of less obvious benefit.[56] By altering blood viscosity and the rheology of the red blood cell, pentoxifylline enhances perfusion through

capillary beds and collateral circulation pathways and may thus benefit patients with unreconstructable small vessel disease and ischemic ulceration.[57] It is unclear whether pentoxifylline alters the natural disease course of these patients in their need for later extremity revascularization. Claudicants as a group are known to eventually succumb to co-morbid illness and only ten to twelve percent will later go on to develop limb-threatening ischemia over 10-year follow-up periods. In this setting, it is difficult to assess the long-term benefit of pharmacotherapy with pentoxifylline in preventing the tissue effects of chronic lower-extremity ischemia.

Indications for Surgical Management

The least controversial group of patients requiring surgical treatment of aortoiliac occlusive disease includes those with limb-threatening ischemia. Patients with rest pain, nonhealing infection, ulceration, or gangrene will progress rapidly to require major amputation, if revascularization is not achieved. Every effort should be made to assess and to optimize their medical status and to attempt revascularization.

Claudication from aortoiliac insufficiency can be extremely debilitating yet needs to be assessed in light of the patient's operative risks and the anatomy of the disease. Successful management of disabling claudication should be undertaken with consideration of the anatomic, extra-anatomic, and endovascular reconstruction techniques available so as to select the appropriate procedure with an acceptable risk to the appropriate patient. The inactive elderly patient with advanced infrainguinal disease that will probably progress should not be offered surgical revascularization for claudication alone. Patients with isolated aortoiliac disease respond extremely well to revascularization and maintain close to a 90 to 95 percent patency rate at 5 years. They are usually younger healthier patients who are trying to live a more active life-style, and their disease may not progress to involve infrainguinal arterial segments as well. The threshold for surgical intervention in this setting is usually lower.

Patients with distal atheroembolism should be managed surgically. Any type of plaque is subject to degeneration and can shower cholesterol, calcium and thrombotic debris to the distal circulation.[58] The "shaggy aorta," described by Kazmier,[59] is lined with ulcerated, irregular, and diffuse plaque and seems to be particularly susceptible to embolization. Emboli can lodge in the microvasculature of the foot and give rise to the classic "blue toe syndrome." Ischemia of the legs can become limb threatening if the ongoing embolic process is not interrupted. Renal and visceral embolization can give rise to renal failure, hypertension, bleeding, segmental bowel infarction, and pancreatitis.[45,60] In the Mayo Clinic experience of 52 patients with peripheral embolic symptoms, 85 percent were managed surgically. The mortality associated with medical management was significant, as recurrent embolization was common and led to relentless tissue infarction. Mortality of surgical correction by exclusion bypass and sympathectomy was only 4.3 percent, with a 75 percent 5-year survival and only one instance of recurrent embolization.[61] Foremost in the surgical correction of this problem is aortic exclusion with bypass or removal of the embolic source by endarterectomy. The role of anticoagulation remains controversial in this setting, as it may have a permissive effect on embolization by interfering with the organization of the native plaque.[62]

Vasculogenic impotence is a common cause of organic failure of erectile function and may be amenable to surgical correction. Arterial perfusion can be assessed by Doppler examination and peak systolic pressure measurement. The penile/brachial index of less than 0.75 is usually indicative of penile arterial insufficiency. Pulse volume recording of the penile arterial waveform can also reveal flow abnormalities.[63] Arteriography is mandatory to evaluate the level and extent of vascular occlusion. Once all psychogenic and neurogenic causes of sexual dysfunction are ruled out, revascularization of the hypogastric circulation is often successful in restoring erectile function.[35] On occasion, microvascular reconstruction of the pudendal or penile arteries may be necessary to regain erectile function.

Surgical Options

When Leriche described "aortitis terminalis" in 1923, he recommended amelioration of the obstructive problem by direct reconstruction of the pathology itself. It took 25 years for aortoiliac endarterectomy and almost 30 years for prosthetic bypass graft replacement to become a reality. Currently aortofemoral bypass (AFB) remains the procedure of choice in more than 90 percent of patients with symptomatic disease of the aortoiliac segment. Primary patency rates approach 95 percent for localized disease and remains as high as 85 percent for multisegment disease at 5 years. The previously high attendant mortality has been lowered to 3 to 5 percent in most series.[64-68] Patients with localized aortoiliac disease are usually younger and healthier and have little distal outflow disease. They should be offered aortofemoral bypass as the surgical procedure of choice. Most patients with aortoiliac embolic disease require AFB, since aortic exclusion is the main component of treating these patients. Aortoiliac hypoplasia

should also be treated with AFB for the above reasons and because it provides the best inflow to an already diminished vascular system. Despite such positive results, some controversy exists as to whether the higher patency rates of aortofemoral bypass should be pursued at the expense of an increased morbidity and mortality when compared to the results of less stressful, but less durable, angioplasty and extra-anatomic procedures such as femorofemoral or axillofemoral bypasses.

Bunt[69] and Couch et al.[70] have described protocols whereby they classified patients according to the extent of their co-morbid illness. They found that by reserving the more stressful and potentially complex aortobifemoral reconstruction for those patients with only class I and II concomitant medical illness they could reduce perioperative and postoperative morbidity and mortality greatly. Class III and IV patients were offered extra-anatomic bypass and/or PTA.

Controversy still exists whether the technique of proximal anastomosis in aortic reconstruction for occlusive disease should be an end-to-end or an end-to-side reconstruction. All patients with aneurysmal disease, atheroembolism, or aortic occlusion to the level of the renal arteries should be treated with an end-to-end anastomosis. Preference for end-to-end anastomosis is based on the following principles: (1) it is more physiologic with respect to less turbulent antegrade flow[71]; (2) it will not create competitive flow with distal circulation; (3) the graft does not protrude anteriorly and may be less likely to create an aortoduodenal fistula[72]; (4) the distal aorta does not require manipulation before vascular clamping, and the incidence of intraoperative atheroembolism may be less; and (5) late graft occlusion seems to be greater with the end-to-side anastomosis.[73-75] Advocates of end-to-side reconstruction believe that (1) the operation is easier to perform; (2) antegrade flow is preserved to the inferior mesenteric artery, the lumbar arteries, and the hypogastric circulation, with less chance of bowel ischemia and erectile dysfunction; (3) it provides preservation of flow in the case of total graft occlusion; and (4) less dissection of the distal aorta is required with less chance of creating neurogenic sexual dysfunction. Pierce et al.[76] reported better patency rates with the end-to-end configuration at the expense of a 14 percent higher incidence of new-onset impotence. Dunn et al.[72] found no difference in patency rates, yet did acknowledge a higher incidence of aortoduodenal fistula and new onset impotence with the end-to-side graft.

Aortoiliac Endarterectomy

Although bypass grafting has become the procedure of choice for diffuse or severe aortoiliac disease, there remains some role for endarterectomy in the treatment of localized aortoiliac occlusive disease (Fig. 26-2). The procedure can be performed in a contaminated field because no prosthetic is required. Moreover, antegrade flow to the hypogastric circulation is preserved. Endarterectomy should not be performed in any patient with aneurysmal changes of the distal aorta or common iliac arteries nor in any patient with total occlusion of the infrarenal aorta. The extent of iliac plaque should stop 1 to 2 cm short of the iliac bifurcation, as it has been shown that external iliac endarterectomy has a high incidence of early thrombosis and late failure secondary to recurrent stenosis. The 5-year patency of aortoiliac endarterectomy has been reported to be 94 percent if limited to the aorta and common iliacs only. External iliac endarterectomy decreases the patency to 79.6 percent at 5 years.[75]

Unilateral Iliac Surgical Intervention

Surgical options for unilateral iliac artery disease include unilateral aortofemoral bypass, iliofemoral bypass, femorofemoral bypass, iliac endarterectomy, and

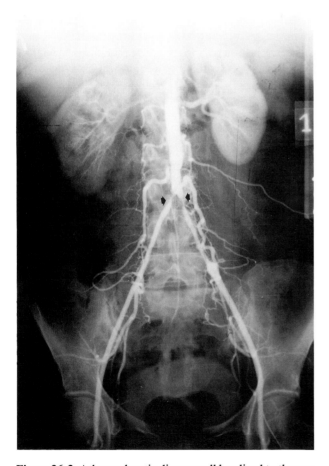

Figure 26-2 Atherosclerotic disease well localized to the aortic bifurcation and the origins of both common iliac arteries. The distal iliac arterial tree is normal bilaterally.

axillofemoral bypass procedures. As previously mentioned, in highly selected patients, endarterectomy has some distinct advantages over bypass. It has been shown to have similar patency rates at 5 years, if one terminates the endarterectomy site above the iliac bifurcation.[77] For bypass techniques, it remains unknown whether the contralateral uninvolved side requires concomitant revascularization. Proponents of unilateral aortofemoral or iliofemoral bypass propose similar patency rates for limb salvage and claudication as compared with aortofemoral bypass, but with less morbidity and little evidence to suggest that the contralateral side will ever need revascularization. These procedures do require a disease-free distal aorta. Aortofemoral and iliofemoral grafts are performed through "renal transplant incisions" in the lower abdominal wall and are usually well tolerated even in the obese patient. These grafts have prograde flow and are shorter, more protected, and probably have better inflow than femorofemoral grafts or axillofemoral grafts. Excellent long-term patency rates with minimal morbidity and mortality have been demonstrated by Kalman et al.[78] and Couch et al.,[79] if outflow was adequate. These investigators recommend that if outflow is compromised, a femorofemoral bypass should be added to the axillofemoral graft and anastomosed to the contralateral uninvolved side; similarly, an extension of the axillofemoral or femorofemoral graft to the popliteal artery of the affected side will enhance flow through the axillofemoral graft component. Such technical modifications not only boost blood flow to the ischemic limb but also increase flow through the main body of the graft, with resultant improvement in patency rates.

Until recently, crossover femorofemoral bypass grafting was reserved for the high-risk patient with iliac artery disease who could not safely tolerate an aortic reconstruction. This form of extra-anatomic bypass is relatively easy to perform, avoids the hemodynamic stress of direct aortic surgery, and does not require an abdominal operation. Superficial femoral artery (SFA) patency is an important consideration for the long-term success of extra-anatomic bypass as compared with AFB. Occlusion of the superficial femoral artery decreases the long-term 5-year patency rates.[49,80] Success of crossover grafting also depends on a relatively disease-free distal aorta and donor iliac artery. Atherosclerotic disease in the contralateral donor iliac system can often be successfully ameliorated by percutaneous transluminal angioplasty.[69,81] Opponents of the femorofemoral bypass technique claim that the nonanatomic route of blood flow, the precarious suprapubic subcutaneous position of the graft, manipulation of the uninvolved side, and the possibility of hemodynamic steal from the uninvolved contralateral side detract from the appeal of crossover grafting. However, there is little evidence that progression of disease in the donor iliac artery is accelerated, nor does the asymptomatic side become symptomatic. Graft failure is rarely due to progression of disease in the donor iliac artery but is more commonly secondary to progression of outflow disease or to stenosis of the distal femoral anastomosis. Graft revisions usually can use the same donor artery for inflow. Contemporary externally supported grafts have increased the patency of these bypasses, as compared with results previously quoted in the literature. Several investigators propose that femorofemoral crossover grafting not only be reserved for patients with prohibitive co-morbidities but that it also be used in even low-risk patients as the initial attempt at revascularization.[49,82-84]

Axillofemoral reconstruction remains an option for patients with aortoiliac occlusive disease who cannot tolerate the cardiopulmonary stress of direct aortic reconstruction. The axillary artery ipsilateral to the poorest arterial outflow is chosen for inflow because it will yield higher flow in the crossover segment. Normal pressures in the donor axillary artery must be ascertained before operation. The 5-year primary patency rates range from 50 to 75 percent, and secondary patency rates from 45 to 85 percent, depending on the series reviewed. Graft failure is usually unrelated to intimal changes in the graft but rather secondary to low flow and thrombosis.[85] With externally supported polytetrafluoroethylene (PTFE) grafts, long-term patency may even be greater than previously reported and more liberal use in the low-risk patient may be warranted. The use of any surgical revascularization should be tempered by the results and availability of endovascular techniques (see Ch. 25).

Surgical Management of Multisegment Disease

In patients with significant disease present in both the aortoiliac and infrainguinal segments, standard practice has been to proceed with the proximal revascularization first and assess the clinical improvement postoperatively. Nearly 80 to 90 percent of patients with multisegment disease will resolve their indications for surgery without requiring distal revascularization. Some patients will remain unimproved after proximal reconstruction alone, but this is difficult to predict preoperatively. If symptoms persist or tissue healing has not improved after the inflow procedure, distal revascularization can be done in a staged fashion. This approach avoids the excess morbidity of a combined initial procedure and does not compromise eventual outcome by waiting. The presence of tissue loss in the foot or a poorly developed profunda to popliteal collateral system would favor immediate distal revascularization combined with the inflow procedure. Staged procedures invoke the following risks: (1) a second operative procedure with additive anesthetic risks, (2) progression of disease in an already threatened limb, and (3) reoperative exploration of the femoral region. The timing of procedures for patients with multisegment disease should be tempered by these considerations.

Success of staged reconstruction rests on accurate assessment of individual contributions of each level to the overall hemodynamic compromise. Patients with abnormal FAP studies with vasodilator challenge who undergo distal revascularization alone without correction of the inflow disease have poor short-term graft patency.[30,46,86] Conversely, the patency of proximal reconstruction only is diminished in those patients with severe outflow disease. The patency of aortofemoral bypass in patients with superficial femoral artery occlusion can be as low as 65 percent if no outflow procedure is performed,[87] and can be significantly improved with the addition of a profundaplasty or an infrainguinal bypass procedure. Preoperative evaluation of profunda collateralization by calculating the profunda collateral index and thigh pressure index will be helpful as a measure of the adequacy of arterial outflow. Bone et al.[37] and Brewster et al.[88] showed that these values can correlate with the success of proximal reconstruction alone.

Intraoperative inspection of the caliber of the profunda orifice can often predict the adequacy of collateralization. If a No. 8 Fogarty embolectomy catheter can pass 20 cm, it is likely that profunda collaterals are adequate. Darling et al. found a 91 percent 5-year patency rate in those aortofemoral bypass grafts that had profunda preservation and only a 70 percent 5-year patency rate in those cases in which little consideration was given to profunda preservation.[8] In the patient with combined inflow and outflow disease, the distal anastomosis of the inflow procedure must be placed over the profunda orifice and serve as an inflow source and patch angioplasty.

The management of multisegment disease has been greatly affected by percutaneous balloon angioplasty of inflow lesions in the iliac system. Brewster et al.[88] reported a series of 75 patients with iliac lesions amenable to angioplasty and distal occlusive disease requiring revascularization. The iliac lesions particularly well suited for PTA were short-segment common iliac stenoses. These were hemodynamically significant lesions that would not provide normal inflow upon which to base a distal bypass graft. Distal revascularization was based on iliac artery PTA, resulting in primary and secondary patency rates of 76 percent and 88 percent, respectively, at 5 years. In grafts that failed, the sites of previous iliac PTA were still patent and considered to be adequate inflow for later revisions. Thus, for suitable iliac lesions, PTA can be used to provide inflow for more distal revascularization. This will be particularly useful in the high-risk patient with concomitant cardiac or cerebrovascular disease who would then need only to undergo a single infrainguinal procedure. The role of angioplasty is discussed at greater length in Chapters 25 and 27.

Complications in Aortoiliac Occlusive Disease

The surgical correction of aortoiliac occlusive disease can incur a high morbidity and mortality. The immediate morbidities may include myocardial ischemia with infarction or dysrhythmia, bleeding, renal failure, hindgut ischemia, and/or atheroembolism. Late complications may include graft infection, aortointestinal fistula, and/or sexual dysfunction. The immediate mortality related to cardiopulmonary disease and other comorbidities should be maintained in the range of 3 to 5 percent for elective procedure. Any algorithm for surgical versus endovascular management must objectively consider the potential morbidities of each modality. However, an in-depth discussion of each of these entities is beyond the scope and intent of this chapter.

Complications of endovascular management, while less physiologically profound, can nevertheless be quite devastating. Balloon catheters can cause arterial rupture, intimal injury with distal dissection, and/or distal embolization. Endovascular complications usually require surgical correction, thereby incurring the risks of emergency operative intervention.

An understanding of the potential complications of all surgical procedures as well as the endovascular techniques designed to complement them is essential to be able to choose a successful treatment plan. While the potential complications of aortic replacement may be a greater risk at the outset, the procedure is considered the most definitive operation with the most durable long-term outcome and in a young, low-risk patient may be more advantageous than iliac angioplasty. However, in other cases, the reverse may be true. Only when the risks and potential benefits of each intervention are known can a true risk/benefit ratio be calculated and a course of action tailored to the individual patient.

SUMMARY

Chronic occlusive disease of the aortoiliac segment is one of the most common and debilitating forms of atherosclerosis. Successful management of these patients requires a balance of surgical risk against the outcome of nonoperative and endovascular measures. An understanding of the various arterial disease patterns, of the hemodynamic significance of arterial stenoses, and of the natural history of arterial disease is crucial to matching the appropriate procedure to the patient. Aortic surgery often invokes tremendous physiologic stress that may be minimized by extra-anatomic bypass or by iliac PTA in properly selected patients. The combined use of endovascular and open surgical techniques can be extremely effective in treating disease involving the aortoiliac segment. Nowhere do endovascular techniques combine so well with operative revascularization as in the aortoiliac segment. Continued close interaction between the interventional radiologist and the vascular surgeon will ensure the selection of the safest, most durable procedure in the treatment of the broad spectrum of disease patterns involving the aortoiliac segment of the arterial tree.

REFERENCES

1. Cruvheilier J: Senile gangrene. p. 1. In: Anatomie Pathologique du Corps Humain. Sect. 27. (Maladies des Arteres. Paris, 1835–1842
2. Von Rokitansky C: A Manual of Pathologic Anatomy. Vol 4. Translated by GE Day. The Sydenham Society, 1849, p. 261
3. Virchow R: Cellular Pathology. Translated by F Chance. Robert M. DeWitt, New York, 1860, p. 394
4. Charcot J-M: Obstruction artérielle et claudication intermittente dans le cheval et dans l'homme. Mem Soc Biol 1:225, 1858
5. Leriche R: Des obliterations artérielles hautes (obliteration de la termination de l'aorte) comme causes des insuffisances circulatoires des membres inférieurs. Bull Mem Soc Chir (Paris) 49:1404, 1923
6. Leriche R: Des obliterations artérielles hautes (obliteration de la termination de l'aorte) comme causes des insuffisances circulatoires des membres inferieurs. Bull Mem Soc Chir (Paris) 49:1404, 1923
7. DeBakey ME, Lawrie GM, Glaeser DH: Patterns of atherosclerosis and their surgical significance. Ann Surg 210:115, 1985
8. Darling RC, Brewster DC, Hallett JW Jr et al: Aortoiliac reconstruction. Surg Clin North Am 59:565, 1979
9. Bergan JJ: Variations of the Leriche syndrome. p. 149. In Bergan JJ, Yao JST (eds): Aortic Surgery. WB Saunders, Philadelphia, 1989

10. Brewster DC: Direct reconstruction for aortoiliac disease. p. 667. In Rutherford RB (ed): Vascular Surgery. 3rd Ed. WB Saunders, Philadelphia, 1989
11. Cronenwett JL, Davis JT Jr, Gooch JB et al: Aortoiliac occlusive disease in women. Surgery 88:775, 1980
12. Weiss NS: Premature menopause and aortoiliac occlusive disease. J Chron Dis 25:133, 1972
13. VanVroonhoven TJMV: Intermittent claudication in premenopausal women: A correlation with the long-term use of oral contraceptives? J Cardiovasc Surg 18:291, 1977
14. Greenhalgh RM: Small aorta syndrome. p. 183. In Bergan JJ, Yao JST (eds): Surgery of the Aorta and Its Branches. Grune & Stratton, New York, 1979
15. DeLaurentis DA: Small aorta syndrome. p. 168. In Brewster DC (ed): Common Problems in Vascular Surgery. Year Book Medical Publishers, Chicago, 1989
16. DeLaurentis DA, Freidman P, Wolferth CC et al: Atherosclerosis and the hypoplastic aortoiliac system. Surgery 83:27, 1978
17. DeLaurentis DA: Aortoiliac hypoplasia. p. 156. In Ernst CB, Stanley JC (eds): Current Therapy in Vascular Surgery. BC Decker, Burlington, Ontario, Canada, 1987
18. Leriche R, Morel A: The syndrome of thrombotic obliteration of the aortic bifurcation. Ann Surg 127:193, 1948
19. Sharp WV, Donovan DL, Teague PC et al: Aortic occlusive disease: a function of vessel bifurcation angle. Surgery 91:680, 1982
20. Shah PM, Tsapogus MJ, Scarton HA et al: Predilection of occlusive disease for the left iliac artery. J Cardiovasc Surg 17:420, 1976
21. Hurlow RA, Chandler ST, Hardman J, Strachan CJL: The noninvasive assessment of aorto-iliac disease: a comparison of dynamic isotope angiology with thigh/brachial pressure index. Surgery 84:278, 1978
22. Dawson JM, Raphael MJ: Serial aortography in the study of peripheral vascular disease — a clinical-radiological study. Br J Radiol 41:333, 1968
23. Kuthan F, Burkhalter A, Baitsch R et al: Development of occlusive arterial disease in lower limbs. Arch Surg 103:545, 1971
24. Chilvers AS, Thomas ML, Browse NL: The progression of arteriosclerosis: a radiological study. Circulation 50:402, 1974
25. Kitka MJ, Flanigan DP, Bishara RA et al: Long-term follow-up of patients having infrainguinal bypass performed below stenotic but hemodynamically normal aortoiliac vessels. J Vasc Surg 5:319, 1987
26. Dick LS, Brief DK, Alpert JA et al: A 12-year experience with femorofemoral crossover grafts. Arch Surg 115:1359, 1980
27. Brief DK, Brener BJ, Alpert J, Parsonnet V: Crossover femorofemoral grafts followed up five years or more. Arch Surg 110:1294, 1975
28. Sumner DS, Strandness DE: The hemodynamics of the femorofemoral shunt. Surg Gynecol Obstet 134:692, 1972
29. Williams LR, Flanigan DP: Alterations in femoral artery hemodynamics associated with femoropopliteal bypass. J Surg Res 26:97, 1971
30. Brewster DC, Waltman AC, O'Hara PJ, Darling RC: Femoral artery pressure measurement during aortography. Circulation (suppl 1):120, 1979
31. Moore WS, Hall AD: Unrecognized aorto-iliac stenosis: a physiologic approach to the diagnosis. Arch Surg 103:633, 1971
32. Brener BJ, Raines JK, Darling RC, Austen WG: Measurement of systolic femoral artery pressure during reactive hyperemia: an estimate of aorto-iliac disease. Circulation 49, 50:(suppl II):II-259, 1974
33. Weismann RE, Upson JF: Intraarterial pressure studies in patients with arterial insufficiency of lower extremities. Ann Surg 157:501, 1963
34. Lorentsen E, Hoel BL, Hol R: Evaluation of the functional importance of atherosclerotic obliterations in the aorto-iliac artery by pressure/flow measurements. Acta Med Scand 191:399, 1972
35. Flanigan DP, Sobinsky KR, Schuler JJ et al: Internal iliac artery revascularization in the treatment of vasculogenic impotence. Arch Surg 120:271, 1985
36. Carter SA: Clinical measurement of systolic pressures in limbs with arterial occlusive disease. JAMA 207:1869, 1969
37. Bone GE, Hayes AC, Slaymaker EE, Barnes RW: Value of segmental limb blood pressure cuffs in the hemodynamic assessment of aortoiliac occlusive disease. Surgery 92:16, 1976
38. Kempczinski RF: The role of noninvasive testing in the evaluation of extremity arterial insufficiency. p. 229. In Kempczinski RF, Yao JST (eds): Practical Noninvasive Vascular Diagnosis. 2nd Ed. Year Book Medical Publishers, Chicago, 1987
39. Flanigan DP, Gray B, Schuler JJ et al: Utility of wide and narrow blood pressure cuffs in the hemodynamic assessment of aortoiliac occlusive disease. Surgery 92:16, 1982
40. Brener BJ, Tiro AC, Alpert J et al: Three techniques for assessing iliac artery stenosis: external femoral artery compression, segmental thigh pressures and intraarterial femoral pressures. In Diethrich ED (ed): Noninvasive Cardiovascular Diagnosis. 2nd Ed. University Park Press, Baltimore, 1981
41. Lynch TG, Hobson RW, Wright CB et al: Interpretation of Doppler segmental pressures in peripheral vascular occlusive disease. Arch Surg 119:465, 1984
42. Waters KJ, Chamberlain J, McNeil IF: The significance of aortoiliac atherosclerosis as assessed by Doppler ultrasound. Surgery 134:338, 1977
43. Fronek A, Johansen KH, Dilley RB et al: Noninvasive physiologic tests in the diagnosis and characterization of peripheral arterial occlusive disease. Am J Surg 126:205, 1973
44. Johnston KW, Taraschuk I: Validation of the role of pulsatility index in quantitation of the severity of peripheral arterial occlusive disease. Am J Surg 131:295, 1976
45. Sawchuck AP, Flanigan DP, Tober JC et al: A rapid, accurate, noninvasive technique for diagnosing critical and subcritical stenoses in aortoiliac arteries. J Vasc Surg 12:158, 1990
46. Thiele BL, Bandyk DF, Zierler RE, Strandness E, Jr: A

systematic approach to the assessment of aortoiliac disease. Arch Surg 118:477, 1983

47. Flanigan DP, Colling JT, Schwartz JA et al: Hemodynamic and arteriographic evaluation of femoral pulsatility index. J Surg Res 32:234, 1982

48. Langsfield M, Nepute J, Hershey F et al: The use of deep duplex scanning to predict hemodynamically significant aortoiliac stenoses. J Vasc Surg 7:395, 1988

49. Brener BJ, Cross F, Brief DK et al: Comparison of aortofemoral and femorofemoral bypass for iliac artery occlusive disease. p. 255. In Veith FJ (ed): Current Critical Problems in Vascular Surgery. Quality Medical Publishers, St. Louis, 1990

50. Flanigan DP, Tullis JP, Streeter VL et al: Multiple subcritical arterial stenoses: Effect of poststenotic pressure and flow. Ann Surg 186:663, 1977

51. Imparato AM, Kim GE, Davidson T et al: Intermittent claudication: its natural course. Surgery 78:795, 1975

52. Cronenwett JL, Warner KG, Zeleneck GB et al: Intermittent claudication: current results of nonoperative management. Arch Surg 119:430, 1984

53. Skinner JS, Strandness DE, Jr: Exercise and intermittent claudication. ii. Effect of physical training. Circulation 36:23, 1967

54. McAllister FF: The fate of patients with intermittent claudication managed nonoperatively. Am J Surg 132:593, 1976

55. Porter JM, Cutler BS, Lee BY et al: Pentoxifylline efficacy in the treatment of intermittent claudication: multicenter controlled double blind trial objective assessment of chronic occlusive arterial disease patients. Am Heart J 104:66, 1982

56. Green RM, McNamara JM: The effect of pentoxifylline on patients with intermittent claudication. J Vasc Surg 7:356, 1988

57. Strano A, Davi G, Avellone G et al: Double-blind, crossover study of the clinical efficacy and hemorrheologic effects of pentoxifylline in patients with occlusive arterial disease of the lower limbs. Angiology 35:459, 1984

58. Gore I, Collins DP: Spontaneous atheromatous embolization: Review of the literature and a report of 16 additional cases. Am J Clin Pathol 33:416, 1960

59. Kazmier FJ: Shaggy aorta syndrome and disseminated atheromatous embolization. p. 189. In Bergan JJ, Yao JST (eds): Aortic Surgery. WB Saunders, Philadelphia, 1989

60. Carvajal JA, Anderson WR, Weiss L et al: Atheroembolism: an etiologic factor in renal insufficiency, gastrointestinal hemorrhages, and peripheral vascular disease. Arch Intern Med 119:593, 1967

61. Kaufman JL, Stark K, Brolin RE: Disseminated atheroembolism from extensive degenerative atherosclerosis of the aorta. Surgery 162:63, 1987

62. Bruns FJ, Segel DP, Adler S: Control of cholesterol embolization by discontinuation of anticoagulant therapy. Am J Med Sci 265:105, 1978

63. Stauffer D, DePalma RG: A comparison of penile-brachial index (PBI) and penile pulse volume recordings (PVR). Bruit 17:29, 1983

64. Martinez BD, Hertzer NR, Beven EG: Influence of distal arterial occlusive disease in prognosis following aortobifemoral bypass. Surgery 88:795, 1980

65. Nevelsteen A, Suy R, Daenen W et al: Aortofemoral grafting: factors influencing late results. Surgery 88:642, 1980

66. Crawford ES, Bomberger RA, Glaeser DH et al: Aortoiliac occlusive disease: factors influencing survival and function following reconstructive operation over a twenty-five year period. Surgery 90:1055, 1981

67. Szilagyi DE, Elliott JP, Jr, Smith RF et al: A thirty year survey of the reconstructive surgical treatment of aortoiliac occlusive disease. J Vasc Surg 3:421, 1986

68. Ouriel K: Long-term results of abdominal aortic reconstruction. p. 175. In Bergan JJ, Yao JST (eds): Aortic Surgery. WB Saunders, Philadelphia, 1989

69. Bunt TJ: Aortic reconstruction vs extra-anatomic bypass and angioplasty: thoughts on evolving a protocol for selection. Arch Surg 121:1166, 1986

70. Couch NP, Clowes AW, Whittemore AD et al: The iliac-origin graft: a useful alternative for iliac occlusive disease. Surgery 97:83, 1985

71. LoGerfo FW, Sancrant T, Teel T et al: Boundary layer separation in models of side-to-end arterial anastomosis. Arch Surg 114:1369, 1979

72. Dunn DA, Downs AR, Lye CR: Aortoiliac reconstruction for occlusive disease: comparison of end-to-end and end-to-side proximal anastomoses. Can J Surg 25:382, 1982

73. Brewster DC, Darling RC: Optimal methods of aortoiliac reconstruction. Surgery 84:739, 1978

74. Mulcas RJ, Royster TS, Lynn RA, Conners RB: Long-term results of operative therapy for aortoiliac disease. Arch Surg 113:601, 1978

75. Gaylis H: Aortoiliac bypass grafting: end-to-end or end-to-side anastomosis? S Afr J Surg 11:45, 1973

76. Pierce GE, Turrentine M, Stringfield S et al: Evaluation of end-to-side v. end-to-end proximal anastomosis in aortobifemoral bypass. Arch Surg 117:1580, 1982

77. Szilagyi DE, Smith RF, Whitney DG et al: The durability of aortoiliac endarterectomy. Arch Surg 89:827, 1964

78. Kalman PG, Hosang M, Johnston KW et al: Unilateral iliac disease: the role of iliofemoral bypass. J Vasc Surg 6:139, 1987

79. Couch NP, Clowes AW, Whittemore AD et al: The iliac-origin arterial graft: A useful alternative for iliac occlusive disease. Surgery 97:83, 1985

80. Piotrowski JJ, Pearce WH, Whitehill T et al: Aortobifemoral bypass: the operation of choice for unilateral iliac occlusion? J Vasc Surg 8:211, 1988

81. Brewster DC, Cambria RP, Darling RC et al: Long-term results of combined iliac balloon angioplasty and distal surgical revascularization. Ann Surg 210:324, 1989

82. Dick LS, Brief DK, Alpert JA et al: A 12-year experience with femorofemoral crossover grafts. Arch Surg 115:1359, 1980

83. Brener BJ: Unilateral iliac artery occlusion. p. 157. In Brewster DC (ed): Common Problems in Vascular Surgery. Year Book Medical Publishers, Chicago, 1989

84. Lamerton AJ, Nicolaides AN, Eastcott: The femoro-

femoral graft: hemodynamic improvement and patency rate. Arch Surg 120:1274, 1985

85. Johnson WC: Axillofemoral bypass for aortoiliac occlusive disease. p. 416. In Ernst CB, Stanley JC (eds): Current Therapy in Vascular Surgery. 2nd Ed. BC Decker, Philadelphia, 1991

86. Baird RJ: Multilevel occlusive disease. p. 143. In Brewster DC (ed): Common Problems in Vascular Surgery. Year Book Medical Publishers, Chicago, 1989

87. Harris PL, Cave Bigley DJ, McSweeney L: Aortofemoral bypass and the role of concomitant femorodistal reconstruction. Br J Surg 72:317, 1985

88. Brewster DC, Perler BA, Robison JG et al: Aortofemoral graft for multilevel occlusive disease. Arch Surg 177:1597, 1982

27

Femoropopliteal Disease

Mark W. Mewissen

The reported results of femoropopliteal percutaneous transluminal angioplasty (PTA) vary widely, making assessment of its role in management of vascular disease problematic. The reasons for this disparity are multiple and include use of different patient populations, dissimilar indications for intervention, lack of PTA reporting standards, and failure to account for the technically imperfect PTA.[1,2] Recently a variety of "new devices" such as lasers, atherectomy catheters, and metallic stents have been developed as an alternative to balloon PTA in an attempt to find better methods of treating progressive occlusive disease. Because these new devices have not yet been fully evaluated, balloon PTA remains the "gold standard" against which they should be compared in appropriate clinical trials. Balloon PTA is safe, is less invasive than surgery, and has demonstrated long-term hemodynamic benefit in selected patients, although it has not shown the long-term durability of autologous vein bypass. For these reasons balloon PTA plays an important role in the treatment of femoropopliteal occlusive disease and should be performed for specific morphologic and clinical indications.

INDICATIONS

Indications for PTA in the femoropopliteal segment include intermittent claudication, ischemic rest pain, ischemic ulceration, and gangrene. These indications are similar to those for infrainguinal bypass grafting,

but because PTA is relatively safer than surgery, patients with less severe degree of claudication and greater comorbidity (such as cardiorespiratory disease and critical ischemia) are also considered candidates for percutaneous endovascular intervention. Noninvasive studies, including resting ankle-brachial indices (ABIs), segmental limb blood pressures, and toe pressure measurements should be obtained routinely prior to intervention. These indirect noninvasive hemodynamic tests correlate well with the severity of ischemic symptoms, but they do not differentiate short stenotic from long occlusive lesions nor do they provide accurate measurements in diabetic patients with calcified, incompressible arteries. For these reasons, angiography remains a mandatory part of the assessment of patients being considered for intervention. Angiography allows detection, localization, and quantification of arterial occlusive disease, but because it is invasive and expensive, it should only be performed in patients who have been appropriately screened for an intervention; it is not suitable for routine screening or follow-up examinations. Color duplex scanning, a direct noninvasive imaging technique, has recently been used to differentiate arterial stenoses from occlusions and it can grade the severity of flow-limiting lesions by peak systolic velocity (PSV) measurements with an accuracy comparable with that of angiography.[3,4]

Most patients with intermittent claudication do not require intervention unless their ischemic symptoms are incapacitating. A program of cigarette smoking cessation, progressive walking exercise, and control of risk factors is highly successful in improving or stabilizing symptoms in most patients.[5,6] Only patients with severe, disabling claudication who fail conservative management and those with limb-threatening ischemia should be considered candidates for intervention.

In the femoropopliteal arterial segment, technical success and durability of PTA strongly correlate with lesion morphology.[7-10] A 5-year cumulative patency rate of 75 percent can be expected for short (smaller than 2 cm) focal stenoses, but the 1-year cumulative patency rate for occlusions longer than 3 cm is significantly lower.[8] Reported 6-month cumulative patency rates have been 86.8 percent for stenoses shorter than 7 cm and 23.1 percent for those longer than 7 cm,[9] and in general balloon PTA of lesions shorter than 5 cm is more durable than PTA of longer than 10-cm.[10]

In 1990 the Standards of Practice Committee of the Society of Cardiovascular and Interventional Radiol-ogy proposed guidelines derived from variables known to affect success and patency rates of PTA.[11] Each type of vascular lesion is classified into four categories (Fig. 27-1 and Table 27-1). Typically, category 1 lesions (short, focal stenoses or occlusions) are most suitable for an endovascular procedure, and PTA should be the initial mode of therapy. Such treatment results in a high technical success rate and can yield clinical results similar to those following bypass grafting. Category 2 and 3 lesions are amenable to PTA, but such treatment does not yield durable long-term patency results that compare favorably with those of bypass grafting. Category 4 lesions (long-segment occlusions or long, diffuse stenoses), are best treated with infrainguinal arterial reconstruction. In general, PTA of category 3 and 4 lesions carries a lower technical success rate and poorer long-term patency. PTA of such lesions has a limited role and should only be considered in patients with con-

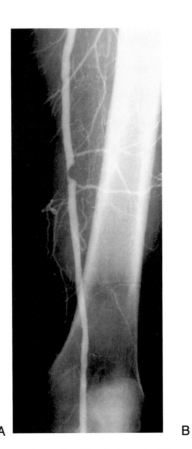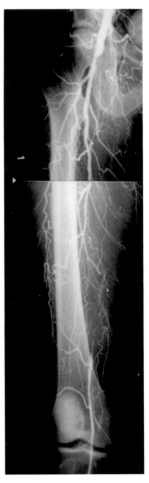

Figure 27-1 **(A)** Angiogram shows short focal stenosis of the superficial femoral artery (SFA) in a patient with calf claudication, ideally suited for PTA. **(B)** Angiogram shows complete occlusion of the SFA in a patient with critical ischemia, best suited for bypass grafting.

Table 27-1 Lesion Categories for Angioplasty From the Society of Cardiovascular and Interventional Radiology

Lesion Categories	Lesion Morphology	Expected Outcome
Category 1	Less than 3-cm single stenosis or occlusion not involving origin of SFA or PA trifurcation	High technical and clinical success PTA is procedure of choice
Category 2	3- to 10-cm single stenosis or occlusion, not involving the distal PA <3-cm calcified stenosis <3-cm multiple stenoses or occlusions No continuous distal runoff	Well suited for PTA Significant improvement in symptoms, pulses, or pressure gradients
Category 3	3- to 10-cm single lesion involving the distal PA Multiple 3- to 5-cm calcified focal lesions Single > 10-cm stenosis or occlusion	High early failure rate Bypass grafting is procedure of choice Attempt only if patient is high risk for revascularization if lacking of suitable bypass material
Category 4	Complete SFA/PA occlusion	PTA has very limited role PTA should only be attempted if surgery alternative is not an option

Abbreviations: SFA, superficial femoral artery; PA, popliteal artery, PTA, percutaneous transluminal angioplasty.
(From Standards of Practice Committee of the SCVIR,[11] with permission.)

comitant cardiorespiratory disease and critical ischemia, in patients with nonreconstructible anatomy, or in the absence of suitable bypass material.[11]

In some patients long-segment occlusions can be treated with thrombolytic therapy prior to PTA. These patients may describe an acute exacerbation or worsening of claudication or may present with an acutely cold foot. Recent experience with catheter-directed thrombolytic therapy has shown that many complicated (i.e., involving both thrombus and plaque) long-segment occlusions in the femoropopliteal arterial segment may be converted to short stenotic lesions, which are readily treated with PTA[12-15] (Fig. 27-2). Although this approach is more complicated, in selected patients it obviates the need of surgical grafting and therefore preserves the native artery (Fig. 27-3). Ulcerated atherosclerotic lesions in the femoropopliteal segment may be associated with distal embolization of atheromatous debris to the digital arteries, the so-called blue toe syndrome.[16] This syndrome has been successfully managed with balloon angioplasty,[17,18] and there is no evidence that these patients should not be treated by percutaneous techniques. Indeed, the same morphologic criteria should apply in considering angioplasty of these lesions.

At present there are no data to identify the most appropriate lesions for alternative revascularization techniques such as atherectomy, laser-assisted angioplasty, or stents which in large part is due to the paucity of well controlled clinical trials that allow an accurate determination of the utility of such techniques. Some may never have any significant role in the treatment of femoropopliteal disease; others may become useful adjuncts. As clinical experience with each new device grows, the spectrum of lesions for which it is appropriate should become better defined.

Initially, lasers were heralded as a technique that would allow treatment of those lesions not amenable to standard balloon PTA, (i.e., long-segment stenoses or occlusions or diffuse disease). A wide variety of laser systems have been used to treat vascular disease, each consisting of a laser power source, a delivery system, and a targeting system (lens, catheter, and shielding) to avoid damage to nondiseased tissue. Each system has featured unique advantages and claimed superiority in its effect on atherosclerotic plaque. In most systems the primary effect of the laser energy on the vessel is a thermal one, causing heating of the tissue; even in those systems designed to be "cool" lasers, some thermal injury appeared to occur.[19,20] Although most early laser systems have been abandoned, other systems are in investigational stages.

Atherectomy is a technique whereby elements of the vessel wall are mechanically removed by cutting or are

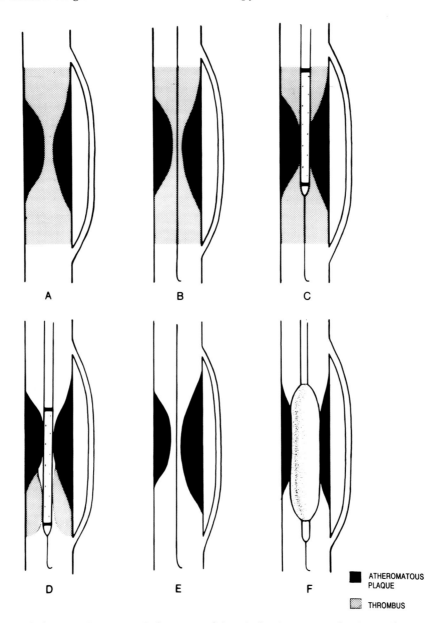

Figure 27-2 Technique used to revascularize an arterial occlusion by means of catheter-directed thrombolysis. **(A)** Complex arterial occlusion consisting of thrombus superimposed on an atheromatous plaque. **(B)** Occlusion crossed with a 0.035-inch guidewire. **(C)** A 5 French multiple side-hole catheter is advanced over the wire into the arterial occlusion to initiate thrombolysis. **(D)** Thrombolysis by further distal advancement of the catheter. **(E)** Complete thrombolysis; note guidewire left across the unmasked stenosis. **(F)** PTA of the uncovered stenosis.

pulverized and abraded with either downstream embolization or suction removal. A number of devices are available or are undergoing evaluation.[21-25] The rationale behind these devices is that the patency rate after intervention would be improved owing to a reduction in the restenosis. Mechanisms proposed for this anticipated result include decreased activation of medial smooth muscle cells and decreased bulk of residual atheroma. Although appealing concepts, there has

been relatively little in the way of documentation of either of these effects. Atherectomy devices have in common that the effective diameter (lumen size) achieved is limited in relation to the size of the device, which makes their percutaneous use in larger vessels above the inguinal ligament difficult. Most such devices are therefore limited to infrainguinal applications, and in many cases supplemental balloon PTA is needed to provide reasonable lumen sizes. Some, such

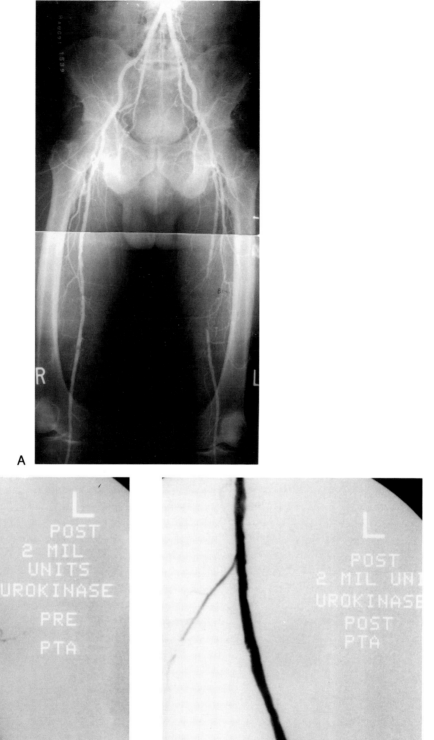

Figure 27-3 (**A**) Bilateral lower extremity runoff angiogram reveals an 8-cm segmental occlusion of the left distal superficial femoral artery (SFA) in a claudicator with acute onset of resting pain (ABI 0.4). (**B**) Angiogram following intrathrombotic delivery of 2 million units of urokinase identifies patent recanalized SFA with uncovered focal stenosis *(arrowheads)*. (ABI 0.95). (**C**) Angiographic success following PTA.

as the Simpson Atherocath device (Peripheral Systems Group, Redwood City, CA), use a balloon attached to the atherectomy device itself to allow the cutter to be applied to the vessel wall in an asymmetric fashion, so that rotating the device to circumferentially cut plaque allows it to achieve a lumen wider than the device itself (directional atherectomy). Rotational atherectomy uses devices that nonselectively affect the vessel wall, circumferentially removing plaque, and yet other devices abrade the vessel wall with high-speed drills. For most of these devices very little in the way of intermediate or long-term follow-up has been reported.

As with lasers, there is a paucity of well documented prospective comparative trials that would allow one to determine appropriate indications for the use of any or all of the atherectomy devices. Given the increased cost and possible increased risk (due to larger device size and greater entry site trauma) associated with the use of atherectomy devices, routine substitution of these devices for balloon PTA is unwarranted in the absence of evidence of improved patency. Nonetheless, there are circumstances in which directional atherectomy may be useful; these include the presence of focal, weblike lesions that prove resistant to balloon dilatation or of large obstructing flaps after standard balloon PTA.[26] Atherectomy is not useful for calcified lesions.

TECHNICAL CONSIDERATIONS

Lower extremity angiography is a preliminary step to every planned endovascular procedure, whether surgical or interventional, and it should be approached as not only a diagnostic study but also a potential percutaneous therapeutic procedure. A thorough knowledge of the patient's ischemic symptoms, physical examination findings, and noninvasive test results will allow the angiographer to determine the arteriographic access site (right or left groin, antegrade or retrograde) and to adjust the angiogram according to each clinical circumstance. In general, the puncture site should be at the common femoral artery contralateral to the more ischemic limb so that the options of antegrade or retrograde puncture on the symptomatic side remain open. Initial detailed angiographic evaluation of the runoff in multiple oblique projections is obtained by both screen-film and digital subtraction techniques. Complete opacification of the runoff vessels is of paramount importance because in situ bypasses to subtrifucation vessels have become routine revascularization procedures. Furthermore, the status of the distal runoff has been shown to predict and correlate with the patency rate of PTA.[27,28]

Balloon PTA in the femoropopliteal arterial segment is usually performed via antegrade puncture of the ipsilateral common femoral artery, although lesions in the proximal superficial femoral artery (SFA) are best approached from the contralateral groin. Careful documentation of the result is an important step in angioplasty. It is generally accepted that technical success is reached if less than 30 percent residual stenosis is present at the PTA site by angiography and distal embolization has not occurred. The presence of a split caused by focal intimal dissection is an expected angiographic finding, although it does not correlate with PTA durability[29] (Figs. 27-4 to 27-6). With directional atherectomy, correct sizing of the catheter as well as multiple circumferential passes of the cutter blade are important because excessive residual stenosis at the treated site increases the risk of early restenosis and clinical failure (Fig. 27-7).

Heparin for anticoagulation is administered as a bolus (5000 units) during endovascular procedures to prevent thrombosis during balloon inflation. After femoral PTA, full anticoagulation is usually continued for 12 to 24 hours to maintain the partial thromboplastin time (PTT) at 2 to 2.5 times normal. Vasodilators such as nifedipine (10 mg sublingually) and intra-arterial nitroglycerin (50 to 100 μg boluses) are routinely administered during the procedure because vasoconstriction may contribute to early occlusion. Oral platelet aggregation inhibitors may also be used, although there is no evidence to support a beneficial effect. Nevertheless, most interventionalists do routinely have their patients start taking aspirin. Technical failures occur in approximately 10 to 15 percent of PTA procedures[10,30,31] and result from failed arterial access, unsuccessful or extraluminal passage of the guidewire through the lesion, failure to dilate the arterial site, or premature termination of the intervention due to a complication.

The technical failure rate is directly related to the features of the lesion treated[11] and is higher for occlusions (17 to 22 percent) than for stenoses (4 to 7 percent). There is controversy as to whether the status of runoff vessels affects long-term patency.[10,30–32] Recent advances in catheter and guidewire technology, frequent use of intra-arterial vasodilators, and "road mapping" capabilities all contribute to greater ease of performance and improved technical success of endovascular procedures.[33]

RESULTS

Meaningful comparison of PTA results with those of alternative forms of therapy remains difficult because not all PTA studies have adhered to rigid reporting

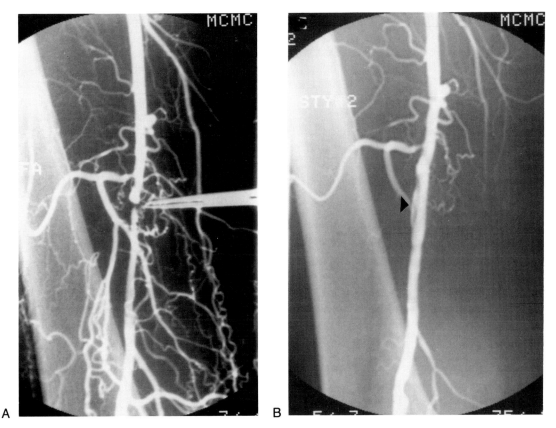

Figure 27-4 **(A)** Angiogram of right SFA shows short focal stenosis. **(B)** Post-PTA angiogram shows "split" at the PTA site *(arrowhead)*.

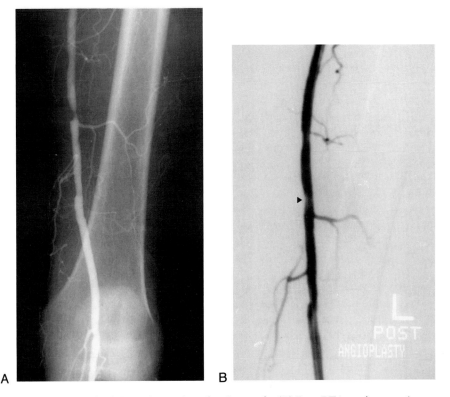

Figure 27-5 **(A)** Angiogram of left SFA shows short focal stenosis. **(B)** Post-PTA angiogram shows no "split" at the PTA site *(arrowhead)*.

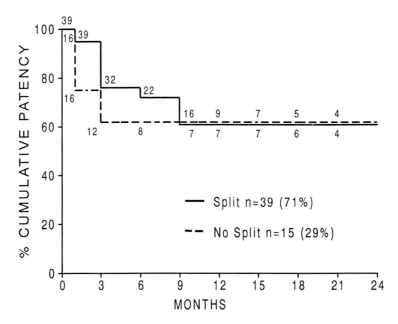

Figure 27-6 Life-table analysis of duration of clinical and hemodynamic success in 55 limbs after successful PTA in the femoropopliteal artery with presence of a split *(solid lines)* or absence *(broken line)* of a split at the PTA site by angiography. (From Mewissen et al.,[29] with permission.)

standards recommended for peripheral arterial reconstruction.[34] Only a few reports have used the life-table method for estimation of successful outcome by objective hemodynamic criteria,[10,29–32,35] and some have included analysis of patients only after successful PTA, omitting technical and early clinical failures (Table 27-2). Such omissions can account for a substantial number of poor results.[34]

The early failure rate of PTA, defined as technical failures plus technical success without clinical improvement at 1 month after treatment, correlates with the status of the distal runoff and the level of ischemia.[30,31,35] Milford et al.[31] showed a 48 percent early failure rate in 27 patients who underwent PTA for limb salvage, whereas this rate was 9 percent in a report by Hewes et al.,[30] in which the majority (70 percent) of the patients were claudicants. Other factors that affect the early failure rate include early restenosis at the PTA site (due to elastic recoil, spasm, or dissection) and early progression of disease in an area remote from the treated site.[7]

It is important to include early failures because they have considerable prognostic implications. Jeans et al.[35] reported that 39 percent of patients with early PTA failures received a bypass graft, 24 percent eventually underwent amputation of the affected limb and the 5-year mortality rate among these patients was twice that in the successful PTA group. It is important to recall that the morbidity of an attempted angioplasty is

not the same as that of a failed surgical procedure; furthermore, failed PTA rarely precludes subsequent surgery.[28] Late failure of PTA results from restenosis at the treated arterial site (myointimal hyperplasia), progression of atherosclerosis remote from the treated site, or a combination of both effects. Restenosis at the PTA site does not appear to preclude redilatation, and a repeat PTA carries the identical prognosis as the initial PTA.[10]

When lesions (stenoses and occlusions) and early failures are included, the 5-year cumulative patency rate is about 40 percent.[10,32,35] With exclusion of early failures, patency rates have been 81 percent at 1 year, 63 percent at 2 years, 61 percent at 3 and 4 years, and 58 percent at 5 years according to a 1991 report.[10]

In a retrospective reanalysis of 254 femoropopliteal angioplasties, Johnston[32] analyzed variables for their impact on long-term patency. Overall, the success of angioplasty was 35.7 percent at 6 years. For stenoses with good runoff, success rate was 53 percent at 5 years, versus 31 percent for stenoses with poor runoff; for occlusions with good runoff, the success rate was 36 percent at 5 years versus 16 percent for occlusions with poor runoff. This analysis included initial technical failures and defined success as clinical improvement combined with improved objective vascular laboratory findings. The mortality rate in this series was 0.4 percent with significant complications in 6.6 percent of patients; these included emergency surgery in 1.2 per-

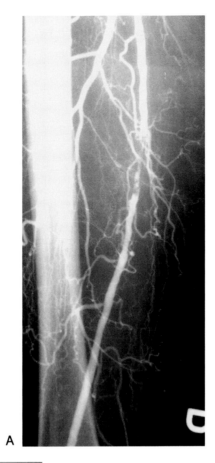

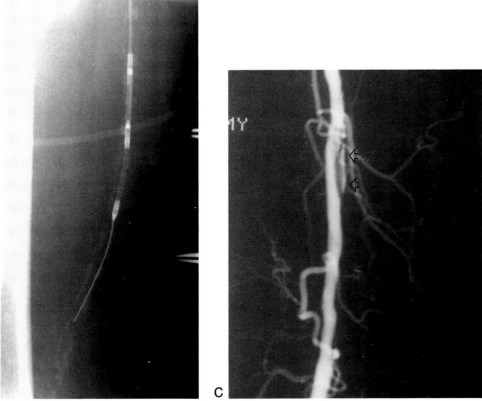

Figure 27-7 (A) Angiogram of right SFA shows lobulated, eccentric plaque ideally suited for atherectomy procedure. **(B)** Simpson Atherocath during atherectomy. **(C)** Angiogram following atherectomy shows technical success. Note "split" at the treated site due to balloon inflation of the device *(arrows)*.

Table 27-2   Early and Late Results of Femoropopliteal Balloon PTA

Authors	No. of PTAs	Level of Ischemia (%) C	LS	Early Failures Technical	Clinical	Total	Cumulative Patency (yr) 1	2	3	4	5	Mortality (30 days)
Jeans[35]	190	51	49			57%					41	3%
Capek[10]	217	74	26	10%		19% at hosp D/C	81^a	63^a	61^a	61^a	58^a	1.3%
Milford[31]	27	7	93	16%		48	47	47				7%
							64^a	64^a				
Hewes[30]	137	70	30	16%	9%	34%	81^a	81^a	61^a	61^a		
							82_o^a	77_o^a	61_o^a	68_o^a		
Johnston[32]	254	80.3	19.7	4%		11% at 1 mo.	63%	53%	51%	44%	38%	0.4%

Abbreviations: PTA, percutaneous transluminal angioplasty; C, claudication; D/C, discharge; LS, limb salvage; s, stenosis; o, occlusion.
[a] Excluding early failures.

cent, transfusion in 1.6 percent, and delayed hospital discharge in 3.2 percent. This study confirms findings of others that patients with less extensive disease (stenoses versus occlusions, good runoff versus poor outflow) do better with angioplasty.

Hemodynamic improvement, as documented by Doppler-derived pressure measurements, is an excellent predictor of subsequent clinical success and limb salvage even in patients with poor runoff, critical ischemia, or diabetes.[30,31,36] Even in limbs with improved Doppler-derived pressure measurement, flow hemodynamics at the treated arterial site significantly affects

PTA durability. Using duplex scanning, Mewissen et al.[29] in 1991 showed that the presence of a greater than 50 percent diameter residual stenosis can be masked by angiography and is predictive of clinical deterioration and PTA failure, whereas normalization of flow correlated with PTA durability[29] (Fig. 27-8).

Using the Simpson Atherocath, Graor and Whitlow[37] reported a 30-day patency rate of 100 percent for simple lesions (less than 5 cm) and 93 percent for complex lesions (more than 5 cm) in 112 patients with SFA stenosis or occlusion. After a mean follow-up period of 12 months, the patency rates were 93 percent and 86

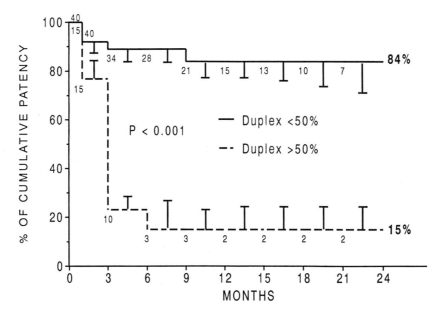

Figure 27-8 Life-table analysis of duration of clinical and hemodynamic success in 55 limbs after successful PTA in the femoropopliteal artery with presence of a less than 50 percent diameter-reducing stenosis *(solid line)* or a greater than 50 percent diameter-reducing residual stenosis *(broken line)* by duplex velocity criteria. (From Mewissen et al.,[29] with permission.)

percent for simple and complex lesions, respectively. In this study follow-up beyond 1 year was not reported. Subsequently, Katzen et al. treated 207 femoropopliteal arteries with the Simpson device. Patency was 69 percent at 1 year and 37 percent at 2 years.[38] Similarly poor long-term patency was reported by Dorros et al., who observed restenosis in 53 percent of patients on angiographic follow-up after a mean time of 5 months.[21] Limited studies suggesting better long-term results with directional atherectomy than with standard balloon angioplasty,[39] bias patient selection to those with short focal stenoses, in whom the best long-term patency for balloon angioplasty is also expected.

Results with other atherectomy devices are limited, frequently including only short-term technical success and little in the way of long-term studies. One high-speed drill (Auth Rotoblator, Heart Technology Inc., Bellevue, WA) has had technical success rates of 89 to 92 percent,[22,40] but with a 2-year patency in one small series of only 12 percent and a high incidence of complications. There is no evidence that atherectomy has in any way improved the results of treatment of femoropopliteal segment disease over standard balloon angioplasty except in limited applications, including resection of obstructing flaps after angioplasty.[26]

The results of laser-assisted balloon angioplasty in the femoropopliteal arterial segment have not been encouraging and are at best similar to those obtained after balloon angioplasty alone, when early failures are excluded (70 and 57 percent at 1 and 3 years).[41,42] At worst, the patency with lasers is considerably worse than that with balloon angioplasty,[43] and several prospective trials have failed to demonstrate improved efficacy of lasers over standard balloon angioplasty.[44-46] The technique carries a high technical failure rate, most commonly due to unsuccessful vessel recanalization and a high incidence of vessel perforation.[20,43,47] The view that lasers can ablate atherosclerotic plaque and therefore improve long-term patency has not been proved to date. Therefore, there are at present no indications for which laser angioplasty appears appropriate.[19]

Intravascular metallic stents have been used in the femoropopliteal segment but to a lesser extent than in the iliac arteries. While stents can moderate the elastic recoil that accounts for early (and immediate) restenosis after angioplasty and can be used to treat obstructing flaps after angioplasty, their usefulness in preventing intimal hyperplasia and preventing long-term restenosis has been very limited in the infrainguinal region. Several relatively small studies have documented the feasibility of placing a variety of vascular stents, including balloon-expandable and self-expanding stents, in the femoral arteries.[48-51] on the basis of this limited experience, the restenosis or reocclusion rate with stents in the femoropopliteal segment is as high as 50 percent. This appears to be related to the relatively smaller size of the femoral arteries as compared with the iliac arteries. The potential impact of anticoagulation on this high rate of restenosis and reocclusion has yet to be determined. At present, intravascular stents should be considered of limited applicability in the femoropopliteal segment.

COMPLICATIONS

The overall incidence of complications related to balloon PTA varies between 5 and 7 percent.[28,52] The majority are benign, not requiring surgical intervention; they include hematoma formation at the PTA site (5 to 10 percent), acute thrombosis at the PTA site (1 to 2 percent), distal embolization (2 percent), vessel perforation (1 percent), guidewire dissection (1 percent) and renal failure (2 percent). Groin hematomas account for most complications associated with directional atherectomy procedures; this is related to larger sheath sizes, and the rigidity of the devices.

Serious complications associated with angioplasty or atherectomy occur in less than 5 percent of cases. If an operation is required for either complications or failure of angioplasty, it can be done safely with satisfactory results, and usually the same operation would have been required had PTA not been performed.[28]

The reported mortality rate directly related to PTA in most series is low (less than 1 percent).[7] However, if PTA is to be compared with other forms of therapy, the mortality rate within 30 days of its performance should be included. Weibull et al.[53] applied criteria used in surgical series to report morbidity and mortality after PTA and found them to be similar to those of surgery. In the recent literature only a few reports have adhered to such standards (Table 27-2). Prospective evaluations are underway, which should address the limitations of prior reports on the usefulness of angioplasty.

SUMMARY

PTA has a definite role in the treatment of patients with femoropopliteal atherosclerotic vascular disease. The greatest utility of this technique appears to be in those patients with relatively short segment, focal disease. Patency rates in appropriately selected patients are comparable with those achieved with synthetic bypass material. While autologous vein bypass remains the most durable intervention for femoropopliteal disease, the lower morbidity of percutaneous intervention has increased the use of angioplasty in many patients.

REFERENCES

1. Flanigan DP, Shuler JJ, Spigos G, Lim LT: Anatomic and hemodynamic evaluation of percutaneous transluminal balloon angioplasty. Surg Gynecol Obstet 154:181, 1982

2. Walden R, Siegel Y, Rubinstein ZJ et al: Percutaneous transluminal angioplasty: a suggested method for analysis of clinical, arteriographic, and hemodynamic factors affecting the results of treatment. J Vasc Surg 3:583, 1986

3. Foley DW: Color Doppler Flow Imaging. Andover Medical Publishers, Andover, MA, 1991

4. Kohler TR, Nance DR, Cramer MM et al: Duplex scanning for diagnosis of aortoiliac and femoropopliteal disease: a prospective study. Circulation 76:1074, 1987

5. Feinberg RL, Gregory RT, Wheeler JR et al: The ischemic window: a method for the objective quantification of the training effect in exercise therapy for intermittent claudication. J Vasc Surg 16:244, 1992

6. Criado E, Ramadan F, Keagy BA, Johnson G: Intermittent claudication. Surg Gynecol Obstet 173:163, 1991

7. Becker GJ, Katzen BT, Dake MD: Noncoronary angioplasty. Radiology 170:921, 1989

8. Krepel VM, van Andel GJ, van Erp WFM et al: Percutaneous transluminal angioplasty of the femoropopliteal artery: initial and long term results. Radiology 156:325, 1985

9. Murray RR Jr, Hewes RC, White RI Jr et al: Long segment femoropopliteal stenoses: is angioplasty a boon or a bust? Radiology 162:473, 1987

10. Capek P, McLean GK, Berkowitz HD: Femoropopliteal angioplasty: factors influencing long-term success. Circulation (suppl. I) 83:I-70, 1991

11. Standards of Practice Committee of the Society of Cardiovascular and Interventional Radiology: Guidelines for percutaneous transluminal angioplasty. Radiology 177:619, 1990

12. Lammer J, Pilger E, Neumayer K et al: Intraarterial thrombolysis: long-term results. Radiology 161:159, 1986

13. Hess H, Mietaschk A, Bruckl R: Peripheral arterial occlusions: a 6-year experience with low-dose thrombolytic therapy. Radiology 163:753, 1987

14. McNamara TO, Fisher JR: Thrombolysis of peripheral arterial and graft occlusions: improved results using high dose urokinase. AJR 144:769, 1985

15. Mewissen MW, Minor PL, Beyer GA, Lipchik EO: Symptomatic native arterial occlusions: early experience with "over-the-wire" thrombolysis. J Vasc Intervent Radiol 1:43, 1990

16. Karmody AM, Powers SR, Monaco VJ, Leather RP: "Blue toe" syndrome. Arch Surg 111:1263, 1976

17. Kumpe DA, Zwerdlinger S, Griffin DJ: Blue digit syndrome: treatment with percutaneous transluminal angioplasty. Radiology 166:37, 1988

18. Brewer ML, Kinnison ML, Perler BA, White RI Jr: Blue toe syndrome: treatment with anticoagulants and delayed percutaneous transluminal angioplasty. Radiology 166:31, 1988

19. Van Breda A: Laser angioplasty. Radiol Clin North Am 27:1217, 1989

20. Cragg AH, Gardiner GA, Smith TP: Vascular applications of laser. Radiology 172:925, 1989

21. Dorros G, Lyer S, Lewin R et al: Angiographic follow-up and clinical outcome of 126 patients after percutaneous directional atherectomy for occlusive peripheral vascular disease. Cathet Cardiovasc Diagn 22:79, 1991

22. Ahn SS, et al. Intraoperative peripheral rotary atherectomy: early and late clinical results. Ann Vasc Surg 6:272, 1992

23. Vallbracht C, Liermann DD, Prignitz I et al: Low-speed rotational angioplasty in chronic peripheral artery occlusion: experience in 83 patients. Radiology 172:327, 1989

24. Triller J, Do DD, Maddern G, Mahler F: Femoropopliteal artery occlusion: clinical experience with the Kensey catheter. Radiology 182:257, 1992

25. Atheroma curettage: an idea whose time may come as several devices begin trials. JAMA 261 (4):498, 1989

26. Maynar M, Reyes R, Cabrera V et al: Percutaneous atherectomy as an alternative treatment for post-angioplasty obstructive intimal flaps. Radiology 170:1029, 1989

27. Rooke TW, Stanson AW, Johnson CM et al: Percutaneous transluminal angioplasty in the lower extremities: a 5-year experience. Mayo Clin Proc 62:85, 1987

28. Samson RH, Sprayregen S, Veith FJ et al: Management of angioplasty complications, unsuccessful procedures and early and late failures. Ann Surg 199:234, 1984

29. Mewissen MW, Kinney EV, Bandyk DF et al: The role of duplex scanning versus angiography in predicting outcome after balloon angioplasty in the femoropopliteal artery. J Vasc Surg 15:860, 1992

30. Hewes RC, White RI Jr, Murray RR et al: Long term results of superficial femoral artery angioplasty. AJR 146:1025, 1986

31. Milford MA, Weaver FA, Lundell CJ, Yellin AE: Femoropopliteal percutaneous transluminal angioplasty for limb salvage. J Vasc Surg 8:292, 1988

32. Johnston KW: Femoral and popliteal arteries: reanalysis of results of balloon angioplasty. Radiology 1992; 183:767-771

33. Darcy MD: Reanalyzing the reanalysis of femoropopliteal angioplasty. Radiology 183:621, 1992

34. Rutherford RB, Flanigan DP, Gupta SK, et al: Suggested standards for reports dealing with lower extremity ischemia. J Vasc Surg 4:80, 1986

35. Jeans WD, Armstrong S, Cole SEA et al: Fate of patients undergoing transluminal angioplasty for lower limb ischemia. Radiology 177:559, 1990

36. Spence R, Freiman D, Gatenby R et al: Long-term re-

28

Surgical Management of Femoropopliteal Occlusive Disease

Joseph L. Mills
Dennis F. Bandyk

The superficial femoral artery (SFA) is the infrainguinal vessel most commonly involved with arteriosclerotic occlusive disease. Hemodynamically significant lesions usually develop in the distal superficial femoral artery at the adductor hiatus. It has been suggested that the adductor magnus tendon at this location prevents the normal compensatory arterial dilatation which occurs at other anatomic sites in response to the progressive development of atherosclerotic plaque.[1] Such compensatory arterial enlargement has been shown to occur in human coronary arteries,[2,3] as well as in the thoracic and abdominal aorta[4] where, unlike the SFA, local anatomic factors do not similarly restrict this adaptive response. Such SFA stenoses usually develop gradually over long periods of time, but flow may eventually be reduced below the thrombotic threshold velocity and cause the SFA to undergo short segment thrombosis. Flow to the popliteal artery is usually maintained by collaterals from the deep femoral artery. Clot will propagate proximally to the level of the first major collateral, often up to the bifurcation of the common femoral artery.

Isolated superficial femoral artery stenosis or segmental occlusion usually manifests clinically as intermittent claudication in the calf muscles. Claudication occurs because a hemodynamically significant arterial lesion prevents the normal exercise-induced increase in lower-extremity blood flow, resulting in insufficient blood flow to meet the metabolic demands of the exercising muscle.

The great majority of patients with claudication caused by isolated superficial femoral artery disease are appropriately treated *nonoperatively*. This conservative approach is based primarily on the relatively benign nature of the condition, as well as the long-term clinical outcome of noninterventional treatment. Conservative, nonoperative therapy for claudication traditionally includes cessation of smoking, a regular exercise program (usually daily walking), weight loss for obese patients, and appropriate management of associated diseases and risk factors (hypertension, diabetes, and coronary artery disease). Approximately 75 percent of patients with claudication will stabilize or improve with conservative management alone; only 25 percent will ever require operation, and only 4 to 5 percent will require major limb amputation.[5-7] The

5-year mortality for claudicants, however, is 20 to 30 percent,[5] usually as a result of associated coronary artery disease. These basic natural history statistics thoroughly support an initial nonoperative approach to most cases of mild to moderate claudication. Intervention is reserved for selected patients with severely disabling symptoms, for those with progressive symptoms after a reasonable trial of conservative treatment, and for those in whom ischemic pain at rest, ischemic ulceration, or tissue loss develops. The latter conditions rarely occur with isolated superficial femoral artery disease, and usually signal the development of progressive atherosclerotic disease in the aorto-iliac segment, the common femoral artery or profunda femoral orifice, or in the infrageniculate outflow vessels.

Femoropopliteal bypass using autogenous saphenous vein is the standard procedure for the surgical management of femoropopliteal occlusive disease. The operation was first performed by Kunlin in 1949,[8] and remains the most durable form of treatment for this condition. The following discussion examines the clinical presentation, patient evaluation, indications for operation, results of surgery, and recommendations for appropriate postoperative follow-up for patients with femoropopliteal occlusive disease.

INDICATIONS AND CONTRAINDICATIONS FOR SURGERY

Limb salvage is the major indication for femoropopliteal bypass surgery. In most reported clinical series, 70 to 90 percent of patients undergoing infrainguinal bypass surgery suffer from ischemic rest pain, ischemic ulceration, or gangrene.[9-12] Patients with blue toe syndrome are also generally considered operative candidates for removal or bypass with exclusion of the atherosclerotic lesion which is the source of distal atheroembolization. Disabling or life-style limiting claudication is a relative indication for surgery; such patients account for no more than 20 to 25 percent of patients undergoing infrainguinal bypass. We generally reserve operation in claudicants for patients who are severely limited (i.e., those with less than one block claudication). These patients generally have an ankle/brachial index (ABI) of less than 0.5 at rest and a post-exercise ankle pressure of less than 50 mmHg.[13]

Nearly all functional ambulatory patients with threatened limb loss are candidates for infrainguinal bypass. The major exception is in patients who are institutionalized, nonambulatory, and severely neurologically impaired. Limb salvage is of no benefit in such cases, and above-knee primary amputation should be performed. Recent reports also suggest that in diabetic patients with end-stage renal disease on dialysis and large gangrenous or nonhealing ulcers of the foot, particularly with advanced heel necrosis, the likelihood of complete healing even in the presence of a patent bypass is poor.[14,15] In addition, the 3- to 5-year survival in such patients approaches zero.[15] Primary amputation may be a better option in such patients, particularly if a difficult reconstructive procedure with modified vein conduits, followed by multiple debridements and a free flap, would be required for soft tissue coverage.

Excepting the above-mentioned circumstances, there are few other absolute contraindications to infrainguinal bypass surgery for limb salvage. Patients with critical limb ischemia who are denied revascularization unavoidably face major limb amputation. Ouriel and associates recently reported that in comparable groups of high-risk patients, primary amputation resulted in higher mortality, longer hospital stay, and lower long-term survival than revascularization.[16] The cost issue has also been carefully examined, and the cost of primary amputation equals or exceeds that of revascularization.[17] Major improvements in anesthetic technique and perioperative management have made limb salvage surgery a viable option even in patients with severe coronary artery disease and associated multiple medical conditions.

Mortality rates from modern series of infrainguinal vein grafts for limb salvage are nearly all below 4 percent,[9,10,12,18,19] with selected centers reporting rates of only 1.4 to 2 percent.[18,20] Functional patients who are ambulatory should rarely be denied the potential and real benefits of limb revascularization. This aggressive approach to limb salvage is one of the major advances in vascular surgery over the past two decades.

SURGICAL APPROACHES AND CHOICE OF CONDUIT

Hemodynamically significant inflow disease should be corrected before attempting femoropopliteal bypass surgery. In claudicants, normalization of inflow to a widely patent profunda femoris artery may markedly improve or completely relieve symptoms. Isolated inflow stenoses, particularly focal common iliac stenoses, are often amenable to percutaneous transluminal angioplasty. The hemodynamic significance of iliac artery stenoses should be determined by pullback pressures with and without vasodilators at diagnostic angiography. Hemodynamically significant lesions should be addressed prior to distal reconstruction, although we occasionally accept small gradients (< 10 to 15 mmHg at rest; < 30 mmHg after administration of

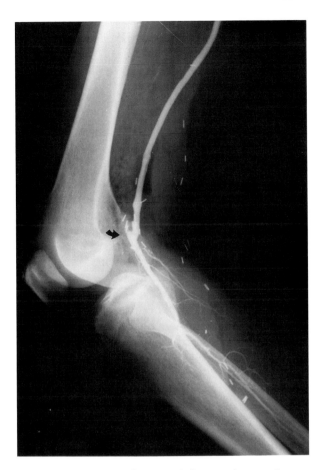

Figure 28-1 Intraoperative completion arteriogram demonstrates satisfactory anastomosis of reversed vein graft to above-knee popliteal artery *(arrow)*. Despite atherosclerotic disease in the distal popliteal artery and single-vessel runoff, this graft remained patent for over 5 years.

30 mg of intra-arterial papaverine) in elderly patients requiring femorodistal bypass for limb salvage.

Femoropopliteal bypass is the procedure of choice in patients requiring operation for severe claudication or limb salvage if the popliteal artery reconstitutes above or below the knee and is in continuity with at least one of the three infrageniculate vessels (Fig. 28-1). If the above-knee popliteal artery is of good quality and widely patent distally, we would choose this artery as an outflow site. Modern results, including our own series, however, indicate that below-knee femoropopliteal bypasses are more durable than above-knee bypasses when autogenous vein conduits are used.[21-23] We preferentially bypass to a good below-knee popliteal artery rather than a mild to moderately diseased above-knee popliteal artery, if adequate autogenous vein is available. Prosthetic conduits should be avoided, except when an above-knee bypass is required and adequate autogenous vein is unavailable in either leg.

An all-autogenous policy for all below-knee and infrapopliteal bypasses has been adopted by many major vascular centers.[9-12,20] The results of prosthetic bypass to the arteries below the knee are poor. A meticulous and thorough search for vein in all four extremities with splicing of suitable segments will usually result in a conduit of sufficient length to perform a bypass. In descending order of preference, the vein conduits of choice are ipsilateral greater saphenous vein, contralateral greater saphenous vein, lesser saphenous vein, cephalic vein, and basilic vein. Because of the great variability in lower-extremity venous anatomy, a significant number of patients will have duplicated venous systems. If such a system is noted at a primary operation, this should be indicated in the operative note. If repeat operation is later required, such information can be extremely valuable. Preoperative venous duplex scanning is sometimes useful in identifying potentially usable vein segments in patients with extensive prior surgery. The results of operation with spliced vein, arm vein, and vein other than the greater saphenous are not equivalent to those in which good-quality greater saphenous vein is present, but they are far better than the use of prosthetic.

Bypass to an isolated or blind popliteal segment is useful for patients with ischemic rest pain or severe claudication. In patients with tissue necrosis, if adequate vein length is available, we prefer bypass to a good-quality patent tibial artery rather than to a blind-segment popliteal vessel. Restoration of pulsatile flow to the foot will most reliably result in healing.

Bypass vein grafts to the infrapopliteal arteries are nearly always reserved for patients with limb salvage indications. Modern reported series of such grafts now show a 5-year patency rate equivalent to that of vein grafts to the popliteal artery.[9,10,20,23] This improvement in modern patency rates for infrapopliteal bypass has been variously attributed to the use of the in situ conduit, as well as to improvements in technique such as loop magnification, use of fine suture, careful vein graft preparation and handling, and mandatory, objective, intraoperative graft assessment with completion arteriography and duplex scanning.

The factor having the greatest influence on patency after infrainguinal vein grafting is the quality of the conduit used (Table 28-1). Patency rates with good ipsilateral greater saphenous vein, both in the reversed and in the in situ configurations, exceed those obtained with alternate or modified conduits. Primary patency rates of 80 to 85 percent at 5 years for infrainguinal bypass grafts using ipsilateral greater saphenous vein have been reported from multiple centers.[9-12,20] Comparable patency rates fall to 60 to 70 percent when alternate vein sources are required, such as lesser sa-

Table 28-1 Factors Affecting Patency After Infrainguinal Arterial Reconstruction

Factor	5-Year Patency (%)	References
Vein quality		
Good-quality ipsilateral greater saphenous vein		
Popliteal bypass	85	9, 18
Infrapopliteal bypass	80	9
Modified greater saphenous vein, lesser saphenous vein	65	9, 18
Arm vein, infrapopliteal bypass	53	47
Repeat operation (after failed bypass)		
With vein conduit	57	42
With polytetrafluoroethylene conduit	31 (2-year)	42, 43
End-stage renal disease (on dialysis)		
Diabetics with end-stage renal disease	22	15

phenous vein, spliced vein segments, and arm vein.[18,20,24-26] Nevertheless, the results of below-knee and infrapopliteal bypass with autogenous vein of any configuration are far superior to those obtained with prosthetic. For this reason, we continue to recommend an all-autogenous policy for such reconstructions. A patient and meticulous search for vein will usually result in a conduit of sufficient length. In addition, sites of origin distal to the common femoral artery can be used for inflow without compromising long-term graft patency. The presence of nonhemodynamically significant stenosis in the superficial femoral artery has not been shown to adversely effect patency of distal origin grafts.[27] The profunda femoris artery can also be used as an inflow site, particularly in repeat operations in which vein length may be a problem.[28]

Prospective randomized studies have demonstrated no significant difference in patency between in situ and reversed vein grafts.[19,29,30] Preliminary data suggest a possible advantage with the in situ conduit for long bypass grafts originating from the groin and extending to the ankle or foot, especially if vein caliber is small (<3 mm).[31] Nevertheless, excellent results with multiple techniques, including in situ vein, nonreversed vein, and reversed vein, have been reported. A summary of recent patency data based on outflow site and type of conduit[32] is presented in Table 28-2. Table 28-3 summarizes the results of available prospective trials of

PTFE versus vein and reversed vein versus in situ vein for femoropopliteal and infrapopliteal arterial reconstruction.

If the in situ technique is used, careful and precise valvulotomy is required. Thorough assessment of the entire graft for the adequacy of valvulotomy is mandatory. Intraoperative graft assessment with pulsed Doppler spectral analysis and color-flow duplex imaging have documented residual competent valve cusps in 5 percent and anastomotic stenoses in 6 percent of in situ vein grafts.[33] Identification and correction of these lesions at the initial operation should optimize graft patency. The flow pattern detected by pulsed Doppler spectral analysis is also of prognostic significance after distal lower-extremity bypass. In patients operated on for critical limb ischemia, a hyperemic pattern with antegrade flow throughout the pulse cycle should be present, as well as a peak systolic velocity in excess of 40 cm/s.[34] If a low-flow graft is present and no focal correctable lesions are identifiable by careful assessment with color-flow scanning or arteriography, consideration should be given to addition of a sequential bypass to a more distal target artery or relocation of the distal anastomosis to an alternate target artery to augment outflow. Completion arteriography is also an excellent technique to exclude anastomotic or vein conduit stenoses; 7 to 10 percent of grafts will have a significant defect identified on routine completion arteriography which requires correction.[35] With mandatory intraoperative graft assessment, the early failure

Table 28-2 Patency Rates of Infrainguinal Bypass Surgery

Site of Distal Anastomosis and Type of Conduit	Patency (%)	
	3-Year Primary (Secondary)	4-Year Primary (Secondary)
Above-knee popliteal		
Saphenous vein	73	69
Polytetrafluoroethylene (PTFE)	66	60
Below-knee popliteal		
Reversed saphenous vein	78	77
In situ vein bypass	73 (86)	68 (81)
PTFE	44	40
Infrapopliteal arteries		
Reversed saphenous vein	66 (78)	62 (76)
In situ vein bypass	74 (84)	68 (81)
PTFE	32	21

Table 28-3 Results of Prospective Trials of Infrainguinal Arterial Reconstruction

Type of Graft	Patency (%)[a]		
	Vein	PTFE	p Value
Vein versus prosthetic			
Veith et al.[22] (n = 845 grafts)			
AK popliteal	61	38	>0.025 (NS)
BK popliteal	76	54	<0.05[b]
Infrapopliteal	49	12	<0.001[b]
Veterans Administration Cooperative Study Group 141[19] (n = 596 grafts)			
BK popliteal	76	64	0.08
Infrapopliteal	73	30	0.001[b]

	Patency (%)[a]		
	RVG	In Situ	p Value
In situ versus reversed vein			
Watelet et al.[30] (n = 100 grafts)			
AK/BK popliteal	88	71	NS
Harris et al.[29] (n = 215 grafts)			
AK/BK popliteal	77	68	NS
Veterans Administration Cooperative Study Group 141[19] (n = 461 grafts)			
BK popliteal	75	78	NS
Infrapopliteal	67	76	NS
Wengerter et al.[31] (n = 125 grafts)			
Overall	67	69	NS
<3-mm veins	37	61	NS

Abbreviations: PTFE, polytetrafluorethylene; NS, not significant; AK, above-knee; BK, below-knee; RVG, reversed vein grafts.

[a] Veith et al.,[22] values at 48 months; Veterans Administration Cooperative Study Group 141[10] values at 24 months; Watelet et al.,[30] values at 36 months; Harris et al.,[29] values at 36 months; Wengerter et al.,[31] values at 30 months.

[b] Denotes statistically significant difference.

rate after infrainguinal vein bypass has been reduced to 3 to 5 percent.[10,11,35] Early graft failure occurs almost exclusively in the more difficult infrapopliteal reconstructions; 30-day failure rates for popliteal reconstructions with vein conduits should be less than 2 to 3 percent.

Compulsive graft surveillance after infrainguinal re-construction is mandatory. The intermediate postoperative interval (3 to 18 months) is the critical time frame during which intrinsic graft lesions develop that can threaten graft patency. Serial duplex graft surveillance now permits detection of these lesions prior to graft occlusion. In 10 to 20 percent of vein grafts, intrinsic graft lesions will develop during this postoperative interval.[10,36,37] The most common lesions are focal, intimal hyperplastic stenoses in the juxta-anastomotic vein graft or fibrotic midgraft valvular stenoses.[23,37] Hemodynamically significant stenoses associated with peak systolic graft velocities of greater than 180 cm/s, or a reduction in ABI exceeding 0.2 should be repaired. Although some of these lesions are amenable to percutaneous balloon angioplasty, the most durable results are obtained when the lesion is excised or replaced.[38] The superficial location of in situ conduits renders postoperative duplex imaging of the entire graft easier and makes focal repair simpler. However, deeply tunnelled reversed vein grafts can also be imaged and focal stenoses identified and repaired. The five-year patency of "failing" grafts after repair of focal graft stenosis exceeds 80 percent, comparable to the extended patency of an unrevised graft.[38-40] This stands in marked contrast to the 26 to 50 percent patency rates reported after thrombectomy or thrombolysis and revision of a failed vein graft.[41] Detection and treatment of graft stenosis before graft occlusion represent a major advance in the management of patients after infrainguinal reconstruction.

The patency rates following reoperation for infrainguinal graft occlusion are significantly less than for primary operations. When reoperation is required, autogenous vein is the conduit of choice. Alternate and spliced vein conduits are frequently necessary; consideration should be given to using a site of origin distal to the common femoral artery if required to permit the use of a completely autogenous conduit. The 5-year patency of reoperation with vein conduits is 55 to 60 percent.[42] When PTFE conduits are used in patients requiring reoperative infrainguinal revascularization, the 2-year patency is less than 30 percent.[43] The addition of a distal arteriovenous (AV) fistula in such cases may extend PTFE graft patency, but convincing long-term data with this technique are lacking.[44,45]

It is critical that all reports of infrainguinal revascularization procedures rigidly adhere to the recommendations of the Ad Hoc Committee on Reporting Standards in Arterial Bypass Surgery of the Joint Vascular Societies.[46] The use of these standards is essential to permit comparison of alternative techniques, whether they be surgical series of vein or prosthetic bypass, or interventional procedures such percutaneous balloon angioplasty, laser-assisted angioplasty, and stenting.

SUMMARY

The natural history of claudication caused by isolated femoropopliteal artery occlusive disease is benign; 75 percent of such patients can be effectively treated with conservative nonoperative management. Ischemic rest pain and tissue necrosis usually develop only in the presence of multilevel occlusive disease; aortoiliac disease, progressive disease of the common femoral and profunda femoral orifice, or infrageniculate occlusive disease in combination with femoropopliteal occlusive disease usually exists in such patients. Bypass with good-quality saphenous vein remains the most durable procedure for patients requiring intervention for femoropopliteal occlusive disease.

REFERENCES

1. Blair JM, Glagov S, Zarins CK: Mechanism of superficial femoral artery adductor canal stenosis. Surg Forum 41:359, 1990
2. Glagov S, Weisenberg E, Zarins CK et al: Compensatory enlargement of human atherosclerotic coronary arteries. N Engl J Med 316:1371, 1987
3. Zarins CK, Weisenberg E, Kolettis G et al: Differential enlargement of artery segments in response to enlarging atherosclerotic plaques. J Vasc Surg 7:386, 1988
4. Zarins CK, Xu C, Glagov S: Atherosclerotic enlargement of the human abdominal aorta. Presented at the Midwestern Vascular Surgery Society, Sept 11, 1992
5. McDaniel MD, Cronenwett JL: Basic data related to the natural history of intermittent claudication. Ann Vasc Surg 3:273, 1989
6. Imparato AM, Kim G-E, Davidson T, Crowley JG: Intermittent claudication: its natural course. Surgery 78:795, 1975
7. Cronenwett JL, Warner KG, Zelenock GB et al: Intermittent claudication; current results of nonoperative management. Arch Surg 119:430, 1989
8. Kunlin J: Le traitement de l'artérite oblitérante par la greffe veineuse. Arch Mal Coeur 42:371, 1949
9. Taylor LM, Jr, Phinney ES, Porter JM: Present status of reversed vein bypass for lower extremity revascularization. J Vasc Surg 3:288, 1986
10. Bandyk DF, Kaebnick HW, Stewart GW, Towne JB: Durability of the in situ saphenous vein arterial bypass: a comparison of primary and secondary patency. J Vasc Surg 5:256, 1987
11. Leather RP, Shah DM, Chang BB, Kaufman JL: Resurrection of the in situ saphenous vein bypass 1000 cases later. Ann Surg 208:435, 1988
12. Mills JL, Taylor SM: Results of infrainguinal revascularization with reversed vein conduits: a modern control series. Ann Vasc Surg 5:156, 1991
13. Rutherford RB: Standards for evaluating results of interventional therapy for peripheral vascular disease. Circulation, suppl. I. 83:6, 1991
14. Edwards JM, Taylor LM, Jr, Porter JM: Limb salvage in end-stage renal disease (ESRD). Arch Surg 123:1164, 1988
15. Whittemore AD, Donaldson MC, Mannick JA: Infrainguinal reconstruction for patients with chronic renal insufficiency. J Vasc Surg 17:32, 1993
16. Ouriel K, Fiore WM, Geary JE: Limb-threatening ischemia in the medically compromised patient: amputation or revascularization. Surgery 104:667, 1988
17. Gupta SK, Veith FJ, Ascer E et al: Cost factors in limb-threatening ischaemia due to infrainguinal arteriosclerosis. Eur J Vasc Surg 2:151, 1988
18. Taylor LM, Jr, Porter JM: Clinical and anatomic considerations for surgery in femoropopliteal disease and the results of surgery. Circulation, suppl. I. 83:63, 1991
19. Veterans Administration Cooperative Study Group 141: Comparative evaluation of prosthetic, reversed, and in situ vein bypass in distal popliteal and tibial-peroneal revascularization. Arch Surg 123:434, 1988
20. Mannick JA, Whittemore AD, Donaldson MC: Clinical and anatomic considerations for surgery in tibial disease and the results of surgery. Circulation, suppl. I. 83:81, 1991
21. Brewster DC, LaSalle AJ, Darling RC: Comparison of above-knee and below-knee anastomosis in femoropopliteal bypass grafts. Arch Surg 116:1013, 1981
22. Veith FJ, Gupta SK, Ascer E et al: Six-year prospective multicenter randomized comparison of autologous saphenous vein and expanded polytetrafluoroethylene grafts in infrainguinal arterial reconstructions. J Vasc Surg 3:104, 1986
23. Mills JL, Fujitani RM, Taylor SM: The characteristics and anatomic distribution of lesions that cause reversed vein graft failure: a five-year prospective study. J Vasc Surg 17:195, 1993
24. Chang BB, Paty PSK, Shah DM, Leather RP: The lesser saphenous vein: an underappreciated source of autogenous vein. J Vasc Surg 15:152, 1992
25. Weaver FA, Barlow CR, Edwards WH et al: The lesser saphenous vein: autogenous tissue for lower extremity revascularization. J Vasc Surg 5:687, 1987
26. Harris RW, Andros G, Dulawa LB et al: Successful long-term limb salvage using cephalic vein bypass grafts. Ann Surg 200:785, 1984
27. Veith FJ, Gupta SK, Samson RH et al: Superficial femoral and popliteal arteries as inflow sites for distal bypasses. Surgery 90:980, 1981
28. Stabile BE, Wilson SE: The profunda femoris-popliteal artery bypass. Arch Surg 112:913, 1977
29. Harris PL, How TV, Jones DR: Prospectively randomized clinical trial to compare in situ and reversed saphenous vein grafts for femoropopliteal bypass. Br J Surg 74:252, 1987
30. Watelet J, Cheysson E, Poels D et al: In situ versus reversed saphenous vein for femoropopliteal bypass: a prospective randomized study of 100 cases. Ann Vasc Surg 1:441, 1986

31. Wengerter KR, Veith FJ, Gupta SK: Prospective randomized multicenter comparison of in situ and reversed vein infrapopliteal bypasses. J Vasc Surg 13:189, 1991

32. Dalman RL, Taylor LM, Jr: Basic data related to infrainguinal revascularization procedures. Ann Vasc Surg 4:309, 1990

33. Bandyk DF, Jorgensen RA, Towne JB: Intraoperative assessment of in-situ saphenous vein arterial grafts using pulsed Doppler spectral analysis. Arch Surg 121:292, 1982

34. Bandyk DF, Kaebnick HW, Bergamini TM et al: Hemodynamics of in situ saphenous vein arterial bypass. Arch Surg 123:477, 1988

35. Mills JL, Fujitani RM, Taylor SM: Contribution of routine intraoperative completion arteriography to early infrainguinal bypass patency. Am J Surg 164:506, 1992

36. Mills JL, Harris EJ, Taylor LM, Jr et al: The importance of routine surveillance of distal bypass grafts with duplex scanning: a study of 379 reversed vein grafts. J Vasc Surg 12:379, 1990

37. Berkowitz HD, Fox AD, Deaton DH: Reversed vein graft stenosis: early diagnosis and management. J Vasc Surg 15:130, 1992

38. Bandyk DF, Bergamini TM, Towne JB et al: Durability of vein graft revision: the outcome of secondary procedures. J Vasc Surg 13:200, 1991

39. Green RM, McNamara J, Ouriel K, DeWeese JA: Comparison of infrainguinal graft surveillance techniques. J Vasc Surg 11:207, 1990

40. Whittemore AD, Clowes AW, Couch NP, Mannick JA: Secondary femoropopliteal reconstruction. Ann Surg 193:35, 1981

41. Belkin M, Donaldson MC, Whittemore AD et al: Observations on the use of thrombolytic agents for thrombotic occlusion of infrainguinal vein grafts. J Vasc Surg 11:289, 1990

42. Edwards JM, Taylor LM, Jr, Porter JM: Treatment of failed lower extremity bypass with new autogenous vein bypass. J Vasc Surg 11:132, 1990

43. Dennis JW, Littooy FN, Greisler HP, Baker WH: Secondary vascular procedures with polytetrafluoroethylene grafts for lower extremity ischemia in a male veteran population. J Vasc Surg 8:137, 1988

44. Dardik H, Sussman B, Ibrahim IM et al: Distal arteriovenous fistula as an adjunct to maintaining arterial and graft patency for limb salvage. Surgery 94:478, 1983

45. Jacobs MJHM, Gregoric ID, Reul GJ: Prosthetic graft placement and creation of a distal arteriovenous fistula for secondary vascular reconstruction in patients with severe limb ischemia. J Vasc Surg 15:612, 1992

46. Ad Hoc Committee on Reporting Standards, SVS/ISCVS: Suggested standards for reports dealing with lower extremity ischemia. J Vasc Surg 4:80, 1986

47. Andros G, Harris RW, Salles-Cunha SX et al: Arm veins for arterial revascularization of the leg: arteriographic and clinical observations. J Vasc Surg 4:416, 1986

29

Interventional Management of Tibial and Peroneal Disease

Donald E. Schwarten

The first report of infrapopliteal angioplasty for chronic lower limb ischemia appeared in 1964 when Dotter and Judkins described three cases of tibial-peroneal trunk angioplasty as a part of their classic description of percutaneous angioplasty.[1] Subsequent reports in the early 1980s described techniques and results achieved with large-caliber catheters designed primarily for use in more proximal inflow vessels.[2-4]. These relatively large balloon and nonballoon catheters caused unacceptable sheer force damage to the smaller-caliber infrapopliteal arteries. While these series were of some interest, and at the time offered benefits for patients who were less than optimal surgical candidates, technological progress has relegated the series to historical interest only.

Much of the current literature pertinent to tibial and peroneal angioplasty not only reflects the advances in catheter technology that were spurred largely by the desire to successfully treat the coronary arteries percutaneously, but also reflects significant advances in understanding the pathophysiology of atherosclerosis and angioplasty as well as the pharmacology of atherogenesis, anticoagulation, vasospasm, and restenosis. Only four years after Gruntzig and Hopff's original description in 1974 of the coaxial balloon dilatation catheter,[5] Gruntzig described a percutanous angioplastic procedure suitable for use in the coronary arteries,[6] and eight years after this report, the use of "coronary" angio-

plasty systems in the treatment of infrapopliteal atherosclerosis was presented. Currently numerous reports are available that describe more or less standard techniques and equipment for the performance of tibial and peroneal angioplasty, the primary technical success rates that can be achieved, and the long-term benefit rates that accrue.[8-14]

The numerous publications regarding tibial and peroneal angioplasty would suggest that this procedure has become rather widely accepted and that it is routinely employed in the management of patients with chronic lower limb ischemia. However, I believe that in most communities even patients who would appear on the basis of both clinical and anatomic criteria to be ideal candidates for tibial or peroneal anioplasty are more often treated surgically. There are, no doubt, numerous reasons for this, but perhaps not the least important are the real and perceived deficiencies in much of the earlier literature on tibial and peroneal angioplasty. The Society of Cardiovascular and Interventional Radiology has adopted a modified version of the standards for classifying lower extremity ischemia that were proposed by Rutherford and colleagues[15,16] and adhered to in some of the later literature on infrapopliteal angioplasty; this may have a considerable impact on the use of tibial and peroneal angioplasty in appropriate clinical and anatomic settings (Tables 29-1 and 29-2).

Table 29-1 Clinical Categories of Chronic Limb Ischemia

Grade	Category	Clinical Description	Objective Criteria
	0	Asymptomatic, no hemodynamically significant occlusive disease	Normal results of treadmill[a] stress test
1	1	Mild claudication	Treadmill exercise completed; postexercise AP >50 mmHg but >25 mmHg below normal
	2	Moderate claudication	Symptoms between those of categories 1 and 3
	3	Severe claudication	Treadmill exercise cannot be completed; postexercise AP <50 mmHg
2	4	Ischemic rest pain	Resting AP 40 mmHg or less; flat or barely pulsatile ankle or metatarsal plethysmographic tracing; toe pressure <30 mmHg
3	5	Minor tissue loss, nonhealing ulcer, focal gangrene with diffuse pedal ischemia	Resting AP 60 mmHg or less; ankle or metatarsal plethysmographic tracing flat or barely pulsatile; toe pressure <40 mmHg
	6	Major tissue loss, extending above transmetatarsal level, functional foot no longer salvageable	Same as for category 5

Abbreviations: AP, ankle pressure.
[a] Five minutes at 2 mph on a 12-degree incline.
(From Rutherford and Becker,[15] with permission.)

PATIENT SELECTION

In recognition of the increased risks of tibial and peroneal angioplasty relative to iliac and femoropopliteal angioplasty, as well as the need for somewhat enhanced skill levels when performing tibial and peroneal angioplasty, almost all authors have reserved this procedure for patients with ischemic rest pain or more advanced ischemic changes (grades 2 and 3, categories 4 through 6). Recent publications recognizing the increased safety associated with low-profile angioplasty systems have suggested expanding selection criteria to include patients with incapacitating intermittent claudication (grade 1, category 3).[14] Horvath et al. have pointed out that, particularly in patients with proximal disease that is treated by percutaneous methods, the likelihood of long-term benefit is enhanced as the runoff status is improved.[12] The finding that long-term patency for any revascularization procedure for chronic lower extremity ischemia is better with optimum runoff is based on analyses of unaltered native vessel status, and it may be premature to conclude that angioplasty to enhance runoff will necessarily result in improved long-term patency rates for more proximal

Table 29-2 Clinical Categories of Acute Limb Ischemia

Category	Description	Capillary Return	Muscle Weakness	Sensory Loss	Doppler Signals	
					Arterial	Venous
Viable	Not immediately threatened	Intact	None	None	Audible AP >30 mmHg	Audible
Threatened	Salvageable if promptly treated	Intact, slow	Mild, partial	Mild, incomplete	Inaudible	Audible
Irreversible	Major tissue loss, amputation required regardless of treatment	Absent (marbling)	Profound, paralysis (rigor)	Profound, anesthetic	Inaudible	Inaudible

Abbreviations: AP, ankle pressure.
(From Rutherford and Becker,[15] with permission.)

interventions. Therefore, for a variety of reasons it would seem in most cases appropriate to reserve angioplasty below the tibioperoneal trunk for patients with rest pain and minor or major tissue loss.

Most patients, except diabetics, with rest pain or more advanced ischemic changes have multilevel disease. It is distinctly unusual for atherosclerotic occlusive disease to be confined to the infrapopliteal arterial vasculature. For the purposes of this discussion, we will assume (1) that either there is no hemodynamically significant proximal disease or such disease has been managed percutaneously or surgically, recently or remotely; and (2) that the necessary indices to relieve rest pain or permit healing have not been achieved and distal intervention is therefore necessary.

Percutaneous transluminal angioplasty enjoys the highest technical success rates and long-term patency rates when short focal concentric atherosclerotic lesions are treated.[17,18] With increasing length of atherosclerotic disease by virtue of either multiple stenoses or long segment occlusions, both the immediate and long-term benefits of balloon angioplasty suffer. Therefore percutaneous angioplasty for limb salvage should ideally be reserved for patients with relatively focal disease. This selection criterion obviously creates a dilemma: patients at greatest risk from operative intervention are likely to have the most advanced peripheral disease and would apparently stand to benefit the most from the least invasive therapy, but, unfortunately, with more extensive disease they are less likely to achieve optimum results from angioplasty. Nevertheless, while ideally angioplasty should be reserved for patients with relatively focal disease, it should be considered when there are compelling reasons to avoid surgical intervention (e.g., the presence of coronary and/or cerebral vascular comorbidity or the lack of suitable conduit). Angioplasty may provide sufficient benefit to permit the affected limb to heal, which may be all that is required.

Under no circumstances should patients with grade 1, category 3 (severe claudication) with extensive infrapopliteal disease be considered candidates for percutaneous intervention.

We have somewhat arbitrarily defined *relatively focal disease* as fewer than four or five stenoses or a less than 6 cm long occlusion in a single tibial or peroneal artery.[13] It is our philosophy that all patients who meet these anatomic criteria and have a clinical indication for revascularization should be treated with percutaneous transluminal angioplasty. Only a minority of patients satisfy these criteria; at our institution approximately 80 percent of patients with tibial disease undergo distal bypass graft surgery for the appropriate clinical indications.[19]

TECHNICAL ASPECTS

Prior to angioplasty, all patients receive the appropriate clinical and noninvasive examinations by a vascular surgeon and an interventionalist. Subsequent diagnostic arteriography is performed from the contralateral approach whenever possible.

If the diagnostic study was obtained more than 24 hours prior to the angioplasty, preangioplasty images must be obtained to ensure that no fresh thrombus has formed in the interval and that it is therefore safe to proceed with angioplasty without prior thrombolysis.

The angioplasty itself is performed from an ipsilateral antegrade approach. Although it is technically possible to perform below-knee angioplasty from the contralateral approach, an ipsilateral antegrade approach is the most desirable, as it facilitates catheter and guidewire control.

MEDICATION

Whenever possible, patients undergoing distal angioplasty should be pretreated with salicylates. During the angioplasty procedure the patient should receive anticoagulation treatment with parenteral heparin, an initial bolus being followed by a maintenance infusion as needed to maintain an activated clotting time of about 200 seconds and a partial thromboplastin time of 2.5 times the control value. If following a successful procedure the runoff is subjectively assessed as brisk, cessation of heparin therapy may be considered. However, if runoff appears to be slow or if persistent vasospasm has been an ongoing problem during the procedure, it may be appropriate to maintain systemic heparin therapy for as long as 72 hours. Some authors advocate continued heparin therapy for all patients for up to 72 hours postangioplasty and subsequent administration of warfarin prior to discharge.[14]

Surprisingly, even densely calcified atherosclerotic tibial and peroneal arteries can respond to catheter and guidewire manipulations with severe vasospasm. For this reason most authors [8-13] advocate routine use of 10 to 20 mg of oral nifedipine as a premedication, although in a recent report the routine use of preprocedure calcium channel blockers was omitted.[14]

Most interventionalists appear to rely on small intraarterial boluses of nitroglycerin to overcome catheter- or guidewire-induced vasospasm; 100-μg boluses of nitroglycerin given via the catheter or sheath are apparently most widely used. A more persistent effect from nitroglycerin can be achieved by use of transdermal patches.

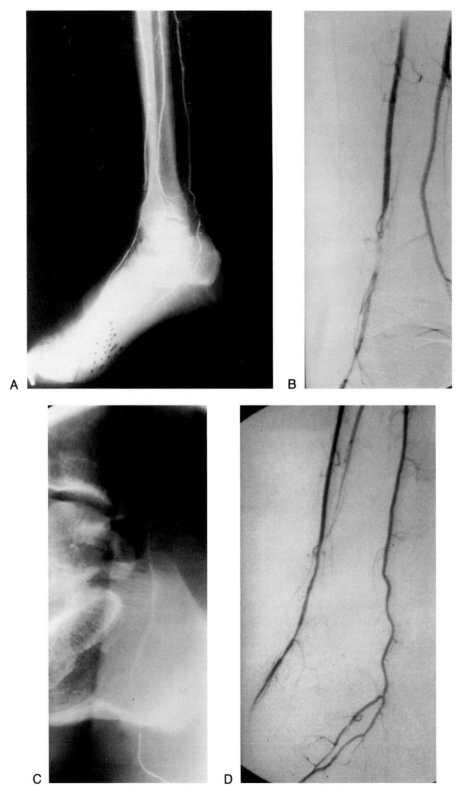

Figure 29-1 **(A)** Stenoses of the dorsalis pedis artery, posterior tibial artery, and mediolateral plantar artery bifurcation. Note swelling of forefoot secondary to infection. **(B)** Close-up of digital subtraction angiogram of dorsalis pedis stenosis. **(C)** Close-up of guidewire in posterior tibial artery. **(D)** Following angioplasty of dorsalis pedis and posterior tibial arteries.

Persistent vasospasm in face of adequate doses of intra-arterial nitroglycerin may be successfully treated with papaverine (60 mg) or, when not contraindicated by pre-existing bradyarrhythmias or congestive heart failure, small incremental doses (1 mg) of intra-arterial verapamil.

TECHNIQUE AND INSTRUMENTATION

When performing angioplasty from the level of the tibial peroneal trunk to the midcalf for most tibial and peroneal arteries, 3.5 to 4.5 French catheters designed to be used with 0.018-inch guidewires are adequate. However, angioplasty in the distal third of the calf or in the foot requires 2.5 to 3.3 French catheters and 0.010- to 0.014-inch guidewires. These smaller systems are more sophisticated, more delicate, and therefore more costly, but they are invaluable in the dorsalis pedis artery, the posterior tibial artery, the extreme distal peroneal artery, and the medial and lateral plantar arteries (Fig. 29-1).

As with any angioplastic procedure, careful technique is mandatory. Optimal imaging equipment and

documentation with angiography of the result of intervention are critical in tibial angioplasty (Fig. 29-2).

Atherosclerosis tends to occur at arterial bifurcations, and there is a risk that angioplasty at a bifurcation may result in occlusion in one of the branch vessels. To minimize this risk when lesions are at or close to bifurcations, two guidewires are placed through the sheath across the bifurcation lesion and into distal branch vessels. Angioplasty is performed over one of the wires, and a low-volume digital arteriogram is obtained to ensure patency of both branch vessels. If one vessel is compromised, angioplasty over the appropriate wire can be performed to restore luminal patency of the compromised vessel origin (Fig. 29-3).

Angioplasty Through Grafts

Aggressive graft surveillance programs frequently permit the detection of intragraft or perianastomotic lesions before graft thrombosis can develop, allowing intervention prior to graft failure.[20] If abnormal velocities are detected, duplex imaging of the graft may allow localization of the pathology, so that a "complete" arteriogram is unnecessary and antegrade puncture of the

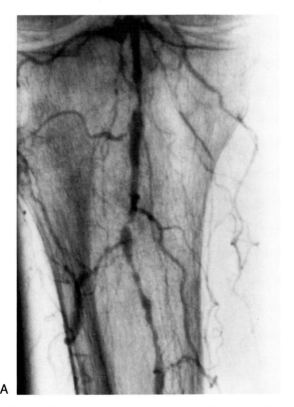
A

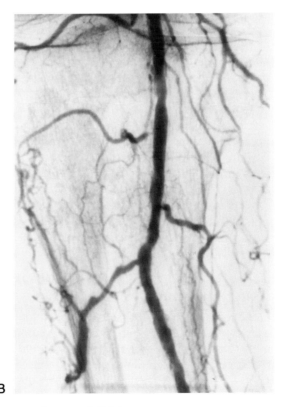
B

Figure 29-2 (A) Preocclusive stenosis of distal popliteal artery and peroneal tibial trunk. **(B)** Following angioplasty of popliteal and tibial arteries.

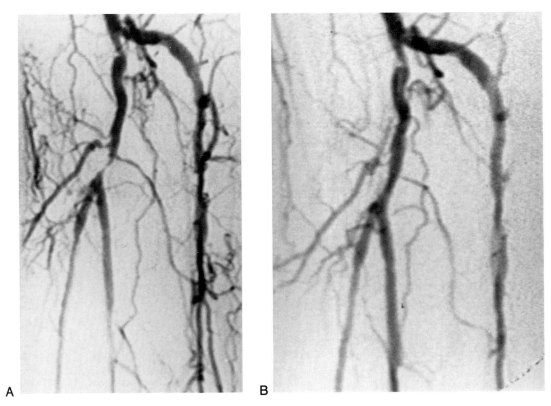

Figure 29-3 (A) Stenosis at bifurcation of tibial and peroneal trunk. **(B)** Following angioplasty after guidewire placement in both branches.

ipsilateral common femoral artery or proximal graft may be done directly. An arteriogram of the affected graft and its runoff may be followed immediately by percutaneous intervention. (The management of a failed graft is addressed elsewhere.) Tibial bypasses are also amenable to interventional salvage. If the pathology is within the vein graft or on the side of the anastomosis and surgical intervention is not planned, my colleagues and I favor directional atherectomy in these instances. If, however, the pathology is in the native artery distal to the distal anastomosis, we believe balloon angioplasty is the percutaneous treatment of choice (Fig. 29-4).

Alternative Techniques

In an extensive review of the vascular applications of laser therapy, Cragg et al.[21] concluded that use of laser technology in peripheral vascular disease should be considered experimental until there are adequate clinical studies to confirm its efficacy. To date there are no clinical studies—prospective, randomized, or otherwise—that confirm the efficacy of laser therapy in peripheral vascular disease.

There have been suggestions that atherectomy devices or drills may enhance the outcome of percutaneous therapy for tibial and peroneal disease. We have not found directional atherectomy to be of value.[22] Ahn (personal communication) found that use of high-speed directional atherectomy in the tibial and peroneal arteries produces dismal 1- to 2-year patency rates: in patients who had an initially technically acceptable angiographic result, patency rates of 20 percent at 1 year and 10 percent at 2 years were found.

One area of potential benefit that will likely be significantly expanded is a combined surgical and interventional approach to the management of patients with extensive infrainguinal disease,[23] especially those requiring a prosthetic conduit. The combined skills of the vascular surgeon and interventional radiologist to maintain an above-knee bypass with the aid of intraoperative balloon angioplasty of outflow vessels has been shown to yield good results.[24] This, in fact, is the essence of management of the patient with tibial and peroneal occlusive disease and the threatened limb. Surgical and percutaneous options are not necessarily competitive; each has its appropriate place in the management of these patients, and in many cases vascular

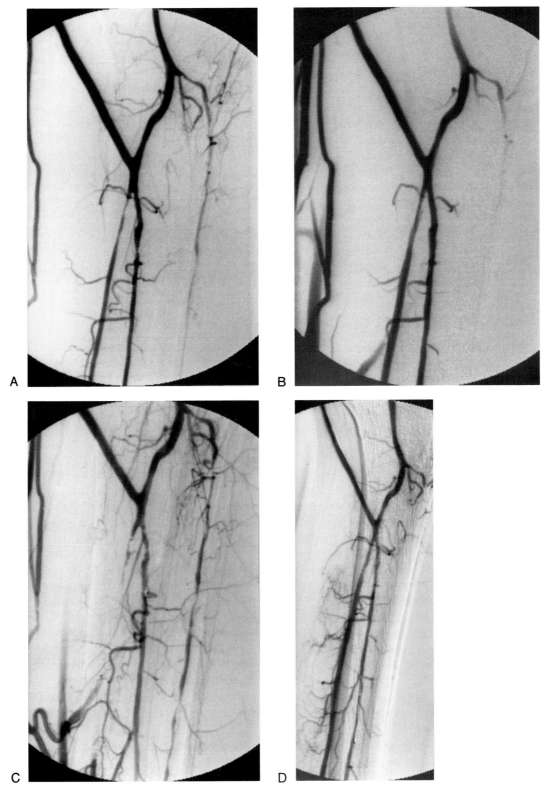

Figure 29-4 (A) Native posterior tibial and peroneal stenosis after in situ graft. **(B)** Immediately following angioplasty of both stenoses. **(C)** 30 minutes after angioplasty, thrombus in posterior tibial artery. **(D)** After treatment with intra-arterial urokinase, patency is restored.

surgery and vascular interventional radiology are adjunctive.

RESULTS

In a retrospective study of 57 procedures in 53 patients, Bakal et al.[10] clearly defined the differences between balloon angioplasty and catheter angioplasty for tibial and peroneal disease. They achieved an 86 percent primary technical success rate with the balloon method, whereas a technical success rate of only 29 percent was achieved by the older method of tibial and peroneal angioplasty using one or a series of tapered catheters. They furthermore documented the benefit of continuous outflow, which when present was associated with a 97 percent clinical benefit rate, in contrast to a 36 percent clinical benefit rate when absent.

There are relatively few reports on the long-term results of tibial angioplasty. Horvath and co-workers[12] achieved cumulative patency rates by life table analysis of 79.8 percent at 1 year and 75.3 percent at 2 years. In reviewing their results with distal angioplasty in a series of 168 patients, Bull and co-workers[14] found a cumulative clinical success rate at 2 years of 83 percent in patients with a single stenosis and a 67 percent clinical success rate in multilevel disease. Their cumulative patency rate at 2 years was 55 percent when lytic therapy had been employed, 52 percent for segmental occlusions, and only 27 percent for anastomotic stenoses. The mean follow-up period was 26.1 months. They concluded that statistically significant factors in predicting long-term patency include (1) a single patent tibial artery, (2) anastomotic stenoses, and (3) acute ischemia. Life table analysis of limb salvage in their series revealed that 20 percent of patients had undergone major amputation, the highest rate of limb loss being observed in patients with failing grafts (27 percent). They furthermore found that the post-treatment ankle-brachial index (ABI) seemed to predict lasting benefit. This would appear to support the conclusion of Bakal et al. that establishment of continuous outflow is important to long-term patency.

In a previous report of my own experience with 96 patients, primary anatomic success (defined as a residual stenosis of less than 30 percent) was achieved in all tibial vessels exhibiting only stenotic disease and in 87 percent of totally occluded vessels, with an overall technical success rate of 97 percent.[13] Prior to angioplasty, the average ABI was 0.27; following tibial or peroneal angioplasty, it was 0.62. At 2 years 81 percent of these patients who were available for follow-up had viable, pain-free extremities, although the average ABI had decreased slightly to 0.57. To date, a randomized prospective trial of surgery versus angioplasty of tibial artery disease has not been undertaken.

The reported complications associated with percutaneous management of tibial and peroneal disease vary widely. In our series only two groin hematomas required other than conservative managment, and in two angioplasties thromboses developed during the procedure and were successfully managed with thrombolysis.[13] Bakal et al.[14] reported one death and one cerebrovascular accident[10]; Horvath et al.[12] reported an overall major complication rate of 4 percent and a minor complication rate of 26.4 percent. These "minor" complications included vessel occlusion and transient renal failure. Bull et al.[14] reported that three of their 168 consecutive patients died following periprocedural complications.

CONCLUSIONS

There is sufficient support in the current literature to suggest that when state-of-the-art techniques are employed good results can be anticipated from percutaneous angioplasty of tibial and peroneal arteries in selected patients with clinical grade 2 or 3 chronic lower limb ischemia. Furthermore, there is evidence that percutaneous angioplasty may be appropriate in the rare patient with isolated tibioperoneal trunk or proximal tibial artery disease with grade I, category 3, chronic limb ischemia. It is also clear that patient selection based largely on angiographic anatomy is the key to success for tibial and peroneal angioplasty and that the majority of patients with rest pain or tissue loss will not fit the ideal angiographic anatomic model for which tibial and peroneal angioplasty gives optimum results. Most patients will be better served with operative intervention because of the extensive nature of their disease. While it is difficult for reasons previously outlined to compare the results of surgical intervention for tibial and peroneal disease with those reported for angioplasty, it is well known that patients with infrainguinal peripheral vascular disease treated surgically may have a periprocedural (30-day) mortality associated with infrainguinal reconstruction of 2 to 6 percent.[25] Furthermore, the fact that the 5-year survival of patients undergoing infrainguinal surgical reconstruction is only 48 percent would seem to dictate use of the least invasive procedure that provides acceptable clinical results in the management of tibial and peroneal occlusive disease. Given these limitations, angioplasty should be the procedure of choice in anatomically suitable patients; it may also be the best option for certain patients with less than optimal angiographic anatomy.

REFERENCES

1. Dotter CT, Judkins MP: Transluminal treatment of arteriosclerotic obstruction: description of a new technique and a preliminary report of its application. Circulation 30:654, 1964

2. Greenfield AJ: Femoral, popliteal and tibial angioplasty. AJR 135:927, 1980

3. Sprayragen S, Sniderman KW, Sos TA et al: Popliteal artery branches: percutaneous transluminal angioplasty. AJR 135:945, 1980

4. Tamura W, Sniderman KW, Beinart C, Sos TA: Percutaneous transluminal angioplasty of the popliteal artery and its branches. Radiology 143:645, 1982

5. Gruntzig A, Hopff H: Perkutane Rekanalisation chronisch arteriellen Verschlusse mit einem neuen Dilatationskatheter: Modifikations der Dotter-Technik. Dtsch Med Wochenschr 99:2502, 1974

6. Gruntzig AR: Transluminal dilatation of coronary artery stenosis (left). Lancet 1:263, 1978

7. Schwarten DE: Extracardiac uses for the "steerable" coronary balloon angioplasty systems. Ann Radiol 29(2):120, 1986

8. Schwarten DE, Cutcliff WC: Arterial occlusive disease below the knee: treatment with percutaneous transluminal angioplasty performed with low-profile catheters and steerable guidewires. Radiology 169:71, 1988

9. Brown KT, Shoenberg NY, Moore ED, Saddekni S: Percutaneous transluminal angioplasty of the infrapopliteal vessels: preliminary results and technical considerations. Radiology 169:75, 1988

10. Bakal CW, Sprayragen S, Scheinbaum K et al: Percutaneous transluminal angioplasty of the infrapopliteal arteries. AJR 154:171, 1990

11. Jeans DJ, Armstrong S, Cole SEA et al: Fate of patients undergoing transluminal angioplasty for lower limb ischemia. Radiology 177:559, 1990

12. Horvath W, Oertl M, Haidinger D: Percutaneous transluminal angioplasty of crural arteries. Radiology 177:565, 1990

13. Schwarten DE: Clinical and anatomical considerations for non-operative therapy in tibial disease and the results of angioplasty. Circulation suppl. T 83:T-86, 1991

14. Bull PG, Mendel H, Hold M et al: Distal popliteal and tibioperoneal transluminal angioplasty; long term follow-up. J Vasc Intervent Radiol 3:45, 1992

15. Rutherford RB, Becker GJ: Standards for evaluating and reporting the results of surgical and percutaneous therapy for peripheral arterial disease. J Vasc Intervent Radiol 2:169, 1991

16. Rutherford RB, Flanigan DP, Gupta SV et al: Suggested standards for reports dealing with the lower extremity ischemia. Prepared by Ad Hoc Committee on Reporting Standards, Society for Vascular Surgery, North American Chapter, International Society for Cardiovascular Surgery. J Vasc Surg 4:80, 1986

17. Capek P, McLean G, Berkowitz H: Femoropopliteal angioplasty: factors influencing long term success. Circulation, suppl. T 83:T-70, 1991

18. Johnston KW, Rae M, Hogg-Johnston SA et al: Five year results of a prospective study of percutaneous transluminal angioplasty. Ann Surg 206:403, 1987

19. Schwarten DE: The role of percutaneous intervention in limb salvage. Second Annual Pacific Northwest Vascular Symposium, Seattle, Sept. 1991

20. Bandyk DF, Cato RF, Towne JB: A flow velocity predicts failure of femoropopliteal and femorotibial grafts. Surgery 98:799, 1985

21. Cragg AH, Gardiner GA, Smith TP: Vascular applications of laser. Radiology 172:925, 1989

22. Schwarten DE: Percutaneous peripheral atherectomy. Presented at Radiology/91, Society of Cardiovascular and Interventional Radiology, University of Minnesota, Minneapolis, Oct. 14, 1991

23. Michel JS: Review of femorodigital bypass procedure in view of a mathematical model. Br J Surg 152:4, 1989

24. Olbert F, Weidingers P, Schlegl A et al: Combined transluminal percutaneous dilatation and surgical reconstruction of the iliac, femoral and popliteal arteries. Ann Radiol 24:369, 1981

25. Veith FJ, Gupta SK, Samson RH et al: Progress in limb salvage by reconstructive arterial surgery combined with new or improved adjunctive procedures. Ann Surg 194:386, 1981

30

Bypass Operations to the Infrapopliteal Arteries and Their Terminal Branches

Enrico Ascer

Mark Gennaro

The origin of modern limb salvage surgery can be attributed to Jean Kunlin, who in a landmark publication in 1949 described his clinical experience with a new type of arterial reconstruction to avert a major amputation in patients with severe occlusive disease of the superficial femoral artery.[1] The efficacy and durability of femoropopliteal bypasses using reversed saphenous vein was confirmed by other investigators and has since become the procedure of choice over lumbar sympathectomy and endarterectomy.[2-5] Encouraged by these reports, Morris and his colleagues[6] and McCaughan[7] were the first surgeons to extend this type of operation to include the major branches of the popliteal artery. Although these authors used synthetic as well as homograft conduits for their infrapopliteal bypasses, the superiority of autogenous vein for arterial reconstructions of these smaller arteries has been well established.

Almost four decades after Kunlin's contribution, we had the opportunity to further extend his original concept by constructing bypasses to the plantar arteries and other branches of the tibial arteries. This aggressive approach allowed us to offer limb salvage surgery to patients presenting with very advanced atherosclerotic disease in whom the only usable outflow tract was one of the branches of the tibial arteries.[8]

In the present chapter we focus primarily on the long-term results of infrapopliteal bypass operations in terms of graft patency and limb salvage. In addition, we discuss several factors that could be associated with the outcome of these bypasses, including inflow and outflow sources, reversed versus in situ vein techniques, and type of graft material. Last, we report on some of the available adjunctive techniques that could potentially enhance patency rates for synthetic grafts placed in the infrapopliteal position.

GENERAL CONSIDERATIONS

Distribution of Atherosclerotic Disease

Although the extent, degree, and location of atherosclerotic disease are subject to great individual variation, certain general patterns of involvement have been identified.[9] In a study of 321 angiograms of patients with peripheral vascular disease, infrapopliteal arteries alone were found to be involved in approximately 27 percent. In this group diabetic patients had occlusion of two and three arteries about twice as often as did nondiabetics (68.9 percent versus 35 percent). Conversely,

511

nondiabetics had single artery occlusion in 65 percent of cases, while only 31.1 percent of diabetics had only one infrapopliteal artery occluded. Reflecting the generalized nature of the disease, atherosclerotic lesions ranging from intimal plaques to significant stenoses involving more proximal parts of the arterial tree were present in 62.5 percent of nondiabetic and 95.4 percent of diabetic patients. In diabetic patients, 40 percent of these proximal lesions were located in the femoropopliteal segments. Patients with ischemic limbs can have multisegmental disease involving both supra and infrainguinal segments; but in the majority (63 percent) of patients with multilevel disease, it is entirely below the inguinal ligament.[10]

Indications for Surgery

Critical ischemia is the principal indication for reconstructions to the infrapopliteal arteries. The majority (65 to 70 percent) of patients have tissue loss as the presenting problem, and ischemic rest pain accounts for the remainder.[11,12] We believe that symptoms limited to intermittent claudication do not constitute an indication for small vessel bypass.

Perioperative Evaluation

A major source of morbidity in patients undergoing distal bypass is cardiac disease, with the incidence of perioperative myocardial infarction varying from 2.6 to 5.4 percent. The mortality rate ranges from 1.3 to 7.6.[13-17] Advances in preoperative cardiac assessment have included liberal use of dipyridamole-thallium scanning to unmask significant coronary artery disease in patients who are unable to perform a treadmill stress test. Although the results of this test should not be used as a sole criterion for cardiac catheterization, coronary angioplasty, or coronary bypass operations prior to the lower limb revascularization, multiple defects on thallium scan have, in general, led us to pursue coronary angiography and proceed with cardiac revascularization. Invasive perioperative monitoring routinely includes use of a pulmonary artery catheter and a radial arterial line for continuous blood pressure measurement.

The cornerstone of preoperative evaluation of the ischemic limb remains angiography, although recently duplex scanning and magnetic resonance imaging (MRI) of the peripheral vascular system have been reported as potential alternatives.[18-20] In our experience angiography can demonstrate a patent distal artery in over 95 percent of patients despite multisegmental dis-

ease. Selective catheterization, delayed filming, injection of intra-arterial vasodilators, and digital subtraction angiography can identify suitable target arteries for distal bypass.[21,22]

CHOICE OF INFLOW

Successful distal vascular reconstruction requires selection of an adequate arterial inflow source. This necessitates optimal biplanar angiographic visualization of all proximal inflow arteries, noting in particular the bifurcation of the common iliac and femoral arteries for stenoses not evident in only one view. The hemodynamics of potentially significant stenoses should be documented by intra-arterial pressure measurements, with liberal use of vasodilators. If a significant pressure gradient is measured above the contemplated bypass inflow site, prebypass angioplasty is an accepted alternative to lengthening of the graft. For example, a significant stenosis in the external iliac artery may be better treated by angioplasty, followed by the distal bypass.[22] At times, significant stenoses may be corrected by the graft angioplasty technique[23] (i.e., placing the hood of the anastomosis over the stenotic segment and thereby restoring normal luminal diameter). For example, a stenotic lesion in the common femoral artery which would otherwise require a more proximal anastomosis to the iliac artery, can be used as the inflow source with this technique, thereby averting a suprainguinal approach.

Common Femoral Artery

Although frequently used, the common femoral artery is not invariably considered the inflow site of choice for infrapopliteal revascularizations. However, ease of dissection and the relatively large caliber of the vessel facilitate its use. Despite the artery's predilection for involvement with varying degrees of atherosclerosis and the potential for infection during groin dissection, the common femoral artery can usually provide durable inflow for bypasses to arteries distal to the popliteal.

Superficial Femoral and Popliteal Arteries

Infrapopliteal bypass with inflow originating from vessels distal to the common femoral artery has historically been viewed with skepticism, since it was believed that progression of atherosclerotic occlusive disease would ultimately compromise inflow and result in graft failure. Nevertheless, this view has not been confirmed. In fact, there are several advantages associated with the use of more distal arteries as inflow sites; these include increased vein utilization, the option to discard imperfect vein segments, avoidance of a scarred or infected groin, fewer complications from vein harvest wounds, and the option to preserve the ipsilateral common femoral artery as an inflow source in case of graft failure.[24] More importantly, the long-term patency of these bypasses does not seem to be adversely affected by proximal disease progression.

Veith and co-workers[25] reported a 58 percent 5-year primary patency for bypasses to infrapopliteal arteries originating from the superficial femoral and popliteal arteries; this was not significantly different from the 50 percent patency achieved with bypasses originating from the common femoral artery. Moreover, operative mortality was not different between the two groups. Disease progression compromising inflow and possibly causing graft thrombosis occurred in only 3 percent of graft failures (1 of 32). Others have also noted acceptable results and no significant difference in long-term patency between grafts originating from the superficial versus the common femoral arteries performed by either the reversed vein[26] or in situ[27] technique. In another study, a proximal stenosis of 20 percent or more in the superficial femoral artery was found to be predictive of decreased long-term (6-year) graft patency for bypasses originating from the distal superficial femoral or popliteal arteries.[28]

One-year primary patency rates ranging from 79 to 97 percent have been reported for bypasses originating from the popliteal artery,[25,28–31] with extended patency at 4 years ranging from 61 to 82 percent[25,28,29] and limb salvage rates at 3 years varying from 67 to 82 percent.[28,29,31] The patency of the pedal arch has been found not to affect extended patency by some authors,[30] while others have noted the severity of the runoff disease to be predictive of long-term patency.[28] Distal bypasses originating from the superficial and popliteal arteries are an acceptable and even desirable alternative to more proximally located bypass grafts and can yield excellent patency and limb salvage results.

Deep Femoral Artery

Leather and colleagues[27] reported that patency results of bypasses originating from the deep femoral artery were equivalent to those using the common femoral artery as an inflow site. Other authors have reported acceptable results even when the distal two-thirds of the deep femoral artery was used as an inflow source for infrapopliteal bypass.[32]

Tibial Arteries

Successful experience with very distal inflow sites for infrapopliteal bypasses were reported in 1985 by Veith and co-workers,[33] who found that 11 of 14 patients (79 percent) maintained a patent graft and functional limb 6 to 50 months postoperatively after undergoing tibiotibial bypass for limb salvage. Our group subsequently reported 24 short tibiotibial vein bypasses, which resulted in a 2-year patency rate of 86 percent.[24] These short vein bypasses had significantly better patency rates than longer femorodistal tibial bypasses (Fig. 30-1). These reports demonstrate the benefit of short vein bypasses even in cases of severely compromised outflow.

Other Donor Arteries

In patients with previously operated or infected groins and extensive atherosclerotic disease of more distal arteries, which precludes their use as an inflow source, the external iliac artery can be used for inflow.[34] We have preferentially used this vessel as the inflow source in 38 cases in which a previously dissected groin relegated the common, proximal superficial, or deep femoral artery to a tertiary choice. Six of nine infrapopliteal bypasses were patent an average of 12 months postoperatively.

CHOICE OF OUTFLOW

Ideally, the choice of outflow artery usually is dictated by the angiographic appearance of the least diseased artery and by local factors such as ulceration or infection. While preoperative angiography will delineate the distal arterial anatomy in most cases, occasionally it will inadequately demonstrate the distal circulation, which makes proper planning of the distal anastomosis uncertain. In these situations intraoperative arteriography may offer better visualization of arteries suitable for bypass.[14] Imparato et al.[35] indicated in 1973 that when the distal arterial vessels are optimally demonstrated, the angiographic criteria initially believed to contribute to graft patency include an intact pedal arch with connections to the distal tibioperoneal arteries. In contrast, others have more recently demonstrated acceptable patency of distal bypass to arteries with restricted runoff and absent pedal arches.[24,33,36] In addition to the angiographic findings, the clinical presentation must be taken into account. For those patients with extensive soft tissue gangrene of the foot to the metatarsal level, while bypass to a proximal "blind"

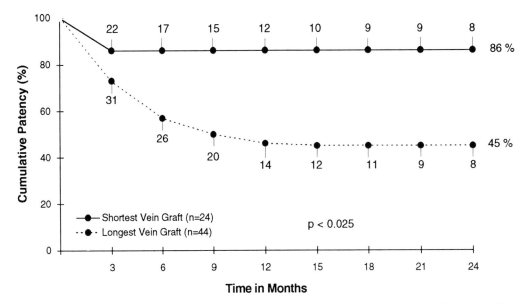

Figure 30-1 Cumulative life table primary patency rates for the 44 longest vein bypasses (i.e., those from the common femoral to the distal third of the infrapopliteal arteries) and for the 24 shortest vein bypasses (tibiotibial). The number of patients at risk is shown at 3-month intervals (p < .025). (From Ascer et al.,[24] with permission.)

popliteal segment can have acceptable long-term patency,[37,38] the distal anastomosis should be constructed to the most distal, least diseased-appearing segment that brings pulsatile flow to the ischemic tissues directly instead of via collaterals.

Tibial/Peroneal Artery

Several reports have demonstrated statistically equivalent patency rates with use of reversed vein or in situ techniques to bypass to any one of the three infrapopliteal arteries.[26,27,39,40] Furthermore, the length of the vein bypass does not appear to affect patency, at least for grafts performed by the in situ method. Leather et al.[27] reported no significant difference in 5-year patency between grafts whose distal anastomosis was within 10 cm of the malleolus and those with more proximally located distal anastomoses (71 versus 74 percent). However, prosthetic grafts anastomosed to more distally located arteries have been noted to have significantly reduced patency rates as compared with those having proximally located anastomoses (25 versus 48 percent).[41]

Paramalleolar and Pedal Arteries

Several reports of paramalleolar and foot bypasses have cited successful results in situations formerly offering little hope of limb preservation.[8,15,16,36,42] Most of these patients are elderly (>65 years), diabetic, and smokers. Coronary artery disease is prevalent. Primary patency rates at 2 years ranged from approximately 67 to 90 percent,[8,15,16,36] and 5-year secondary patency rates varied from 42 to 81 percent.[15,16,36] Statistically insignificant differences in long-term patency with use of the in situ technique resulted from bypasses originating from either the common, superficial, or deep femoral arteries.[36] Similarly, no difference in patency based on the site of distal anastomosis to any of the three tibial arteries was noted. The patency of bypasses to the ankle or foot originating from the popliteal artery was not affected by the technique of bypass, whether in situ or reversed vein.[16] However, prosthetic bypasses can be expected to fail early and result in amputation rates of more than 60 percent by 2 years.[16,42]

Plantar/Tarsal Arteries

Infrequently, patients with limb-threatening ischemia will have all major infrapopliteal arteries occluded as determined by adequate preoperative angiography. Rather than resorting to an amputation, we have attempted bypasses to patent branches of the tibial arteries in the foot, such as the tarsal and plantar arteries. We have achieved an 81 percent 2-year patency rate in 20 bypasses to these branches using reversed saphenous vein[8] (Fig. 30-2); Limb salvage at 2 years was 85 percent. These results underscore the value of this extended approach to limb salvage in situations where major amputations were previously thought to be indicated.

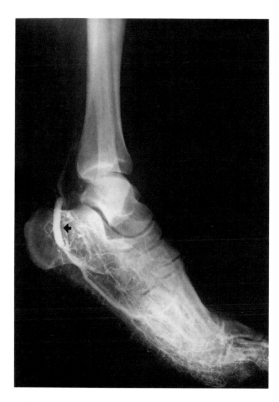

Figure 30-2 Completion angiogram of a very short vein bypass originating from the distal portion of the posterior tibial artery to the lateral plantar artery. Following this procedure, the patient's rest pain subsided, and the ischemic ulcers on his second and third toes healed within a few days.

CHOICE OF CONDUIT

Autologous Vein

Autologous vein used in the reversed position initially was adopted as the conduit and technique of choice for performing infrapopliteal bypasses, since prosthetic conduits were generally associated with poor results. The vein most often used for infrapopliteal bypass procedures was and remains the greater saphenous vein (GSV). In several recent reports by centers committed to using autologous vein for popliteal and infrapopliteal bypass by either the in situ or reversed vein technique, the availability of suitable ipsilateral GSV (usually defined as nondiseased, distensible, and having a diameter ≥ 2.5 to 3.0 mm) ranged from 55 to 96 percent.[11,27,43–46] Saphenous vein utilization rates can be higher with use of the in situ technique and have been reported at approximately 90 to 95 percent.[27,47,48] However, although GSV utilization appears modest in studies in which the reversed vein technique was used, total vein utilization in three studies ranged from 83 percent[49] to approximately 93 percent.[11,50] Frequent

reasons for the unavailability or unacceptability of the GSV are prior removal, inadequate length, and diseased or small segment.

Venous characteristics thought to improve graft patency rates (and therefore limb salvage rates) include the presence and preservation of endothelium, with its elaboration of vasodilatory and antithrombotic biochemical mediators[51,52]; arteriovenous compliance matching[49,50]; and favorable hemodynamic factors.[47,48] Regardless of the exact mechanism, infrapopliteal bypasses with autologous vein result in clearly superior patency compared with bypasses performed with prosthetics. While this issue of which conduit provides optimal patency in distal bypass has been conclusively answered, questions remain regarding the optimal technique (reversed versus in situ) for performing these distal bypasses. However, despite the limitations of comparing varying series from different institutions, and despite the lack of universal adherence to recommended reporting standards,[53] certain generalizations can be made.

Reversed Vein Grafts

Table 30-1 lists the results of several recent studies of infrapopliteal bypass using reversed autogenous vein, most using primarily saphenous vein. Early patency rates (<3 months) varied from approximately 84 to 100 percent,[40,43,54,55] with early failure resulting most often from technical factors such as errors in construction of the anastomoses, use of an inadequate vein, or selection of an inappropriate distal outflow vessel.[56] The greatest proportion of grafts destined to fail did so during the first year. Primary patency rates at 2 years varied from 52 to 76 percent.[41,43,44,55,57]; long-term (5-year) primary patency rates ranged from 35 to 69 percent[40,43,54–56]; and secondary patency rates ranged from 70 to 77 percent[43,56] at 5 years. Limb salvage rates at 5 years varied from 28 to 86 percent.[12,40,54–56]

In Situ Vein Grafts

Although the first report of the in situ technique was published in 1962 by Hall,[58] 17 years elapsed before Leather and colleagues[59] reported their excellent results with the technique and its subsequent popularity. Technical refinements and modifications and the resulting favorable experience with the method eventually led to controversy regarding which technique of lower extremity revascularization, reversed GSV or in situ, provided superior results. Several prospective randomized studies comparing the in situ and reversed saphenous vein techniques were instituted to address this debate, and the results of these and other series of in situ bypasses are listed in Table 30-2.

Table 30-1   Reversed Vein Results

Authors	Year	No. of Bypasses	Patency (%)[a]					Limb Salvage (%)[a]				
			1 yr	2 yr	3 yr	4 yr	5 yr	1 yr	2 yr	3 yr	4 yr	5 yr
Buchbinder et al.[107]	1981	8	63	63								
Hobson et al.[54]	1985	50	62		45		42	70	53	47	47	47
Dalsing et al.[40]	1985	22	65		65		65	70		60		28
LoGerfo[108]	1985	78			71							
Veith et al.[12]	1986	106	64	59	55	49		79	75	71	57	
Rafferty et al.[57]	1987	98	64		43		29	67		59		48
Berkowitz & Greenstein[56]	1987	102	64		57		47	90	90	90	86	86
Fogle et al.[60]	1987	86	65	62	62							
Ascer et al.[24]	1988	237			54		37					
VA study[41]	1988	85	77	67					79			
Rutherford et al.[55]	1988	22	75	75	63							
Taylor et al.[43]	1990	243	81	76	72	69	69					
Wengerter et al.[11]	1991	62	64		61					87		
Mills & Taylor[44]	1991	49	87	74	74							

[a] Some values are approximations based on graphs within the reports.

Early (1-month) patency rates of in situ distal bypass range from 89 to 97 percent.[27,41,45,55,60,61] Early graft failures result from retained valves, anastomotic stenosis, arteriovenous fistulae, small vein diameter (<2 mm), unrecognized coagulopathy, or unexplained reasons.[27,61] Intraoperative evaluation of the bypass with pulsed Doppler spectral analysis can detect abnormalities and lead to improved short- and long-term patencies.[27,46,61] Intraoperative modification of the bypass (ligation of arteriovenous fistula or ablation of residual valve) did not significantly affect primary patency.[46] Primary patency rates at 1 year varied from 64 to 87 percent[11,41,46,55,60]; a 5-year primary patency rate of 73 percent has been reported.[27] Secondary patency rates are higher than primary patency rates and increase to 80 percent at 5 years.[62]

Various factors have been examined for their effect on graft patency. In contrast to reversed vein grafting to infrapopliteal vessels,[11] small vein diameter (<3 mm) has been found not to adversely affect long-term patency.[27,46] The enhanced patency with small diameter veins may be responsible for the greater vein utilization rates. Certain events that may occur during the initial procedure have been found to reduce long-term patency; these include intraoperative graft modification (either correction of an inadequate vein or technical failure of an adequate vein) or reconstruction of a diseased inflow artery (by endarterectomy, vein or pros-

Table 30-2   In Situ Vein Results

Authors	Year	No. of Bypasses	Patency (%)[a]					Limb Salvage (%)[a]				
			1 yr	2 yr	3 yr	4 yr	5 yr	1 yr	2 yr	3 yr	4 yr	5 yr
Buchbinder et al.[107]	1981	22		96								
Carney et al.[45]	1985	31	85	72	72							
Fogle et al.[60]	1987	65	87		87							
Bandyk et al.[61]	1987	124	74	66	63							
VA study[41]	1988	171	83	76					82			
Rutherford et al.[55]	1988	50	88	88	88							
Leather et al.[27b]	1988	608					73					
Wengerter et al.[11]	1991	62	64	58					76			
Mannick et al.[62b]	1991	?	82	80	80	80	80					81
Bergamini et al.[46]	1991	246	75	66	63	63				92		

[a] Some values are approximations based on graphs within the reports.
[b] Values represent secondary patency.

thetic patch angioplasty, or interposition graft). Post-operatively, failure to revise a graft before thrombosis resulted in significantly reduced long-term patency.[46] Not surprisingly, therefore, most causes of graft failure were secondary to defects intrinsic to the graft itself.[63] Finally, prolonged experience with the technique overcame a learning curve and yielded improved results.[46,63] Reported limb salvage rates at 2 and 5 years are 82 percent[41] and 81 percent,[62] respectively.

Arm Vein and Lesser Saphenous Vein Grafts

Other sources of vein, such as arm and lesser saphenous veins, can be used for infrapopliteal bypass when the GSV is not available. Early reports using arm veins, alone or in combination with other veins or graft materials, reported acceptable patency rates ranging from 71 to 84 percent at 1 year to approximately 58 to 63 percent at 3 years.[64-66] Later reports have cited 1-year primary and secondary patency rates for infrapopliteal bypass using arm veins of 63 and 79 percent, respectively.[67] In Taylor et al.'s series,[43] the primary patency for all grafts using "venovenostomy" and "alternate vein sources" was significantly inferior to that of bypasses with GSV, while secondary patency rates were not statistically different at 5 years. Thus, although the primary patency rates achieved with arm veins may be inferior to those with the GSV as a conduit, acceptable secondary patency can result from their use.

The lesser saphenous vein can provide acceptable patency rates for infrapopliteal bypass when the GSV is unavailable. The 3-year patency rates approximate 55 to 60 percent, but results are worse when composite autogenous grafts are required.[68,69]

Prosthetic Grafts

Patients with limb-threatening ischemia in whom autologous conduit is inadequate, diseased, or absent must necessarily undergo revascularization with prosthetic conduit. Fortunately, these circumstances are relatively infrequent, and in groups committed to using entirely autologous tissue for lower extremity vascular reconstructions, only 5 to 16 percent of bypasses will be performed with prosthetic graft material.[10,27,43,62] This percentage will probably increase as the burgeoning elderly population with peripheral vascular disease requires reoperation for limb salvage. Table 30-3 shows the results of several recent reports of infrapopliteal bypass performed with prosthetic conduit.

Polytetrafluoroethylene Grafts

More than 90 percent of patients receiving prosthetic conduit for infrapopliteal bypass have limb-threatening ischemia, and many have had a prior ipsilateral vascular reconstruction. In several reports, initial early (1-month) patency rates ranged from 33 to 78 percent,[55,68,70] and 2-year primary patency rates varied from 11 to 54 percent.[12,13,41,54,55,70-74] Primary patency rates at 5 years ranged from 12 to 50 percent[54,71,73]; however, only one study reported late primary patency rates higher than 37 percent.[71] Secondary patency rates of 73 percent at 1 year, 27 percent at 3 years, and 7 percent at 5 years have been reported.[74] We have reported 37 percent secondary patency at 4 years[75] and attribute our improved results to an aggressive approach to salvage occluded PTFE grafts by performing a totally new bypass rather than thrombectomy, angioplasty, or extension.[76] Limb salvage rates at 1 year have

Table 30-3   Prosthetic Grafts

Authors	Year	No. of Bypasses	Patency (%)[a]					Limb Salvage (%)[a]				
			1 yr	2 yr	3 yr	4 yr	5 yr	1 yr	2 yr	3 yr	4 yr	5 yr
Bergan et al.[72]	1982	58	48	24	19							
Yeager et al.[70]	1982	33	14	11								
Christenson et al.[71]	1985	54	56	54	52	50	50		59			57
Hobson et al.[54]	1985	41	21	12	12	12	12	20	20	20	15	15
Veith et al.[12]	1986	98	45	33	29	12		75	64	61	61	
VA study[41]	1988	68	38	30					58			
Rutherford et al.[55]	1988	14	25	25	17							
Flinn et al.[13]	1988	75	58	45	37	37						
Whittemore et al.[73]	1989	21	28	12	12	12	12	38	28	14	14	14
Londrey et al.[74b]	1991	33	73	38	27	7	7	63	38	26	7	7

[a] Some values are approximations based on graphs within the reports.
[b] Values represent secondary patency.

varied from 25 to 75 percent,[12,54,73,74] and 5-year limb salvage rates ranging from 7 to 57 percent have been reported.[54,71,73,74] Thus, PTFE grafts clearly have reduced early and late patency rates in the infrapopliteal position as compared with autogenous bypass. However, in those patients without an autologous conduit who are faced with limb-threatening ischemia, prosthetic reconstruction can achieve worthwhile patency results and obviate the need for major amputation.

Human Umbilical Vein Grafts

Experience with human umbilical vein (HUV) graft for lower extremity bypass procedures is less extensive than that with PTFE. However, Table 30-4 contains the results of a considerable number of infrapopliteal bypasses.[52,77-79] In one report patency rates for tibial and peroneal artery bypass at 1 and 5 years were approximately 58 and 32 percent respectively.[79] Limb salvage at 2 years was approximately 80 percent in the tibial bypass group and 65 percent after peroneal bypass; limb salvage at 5 years decreased to approximately 70 and 55 percent for tibial and peroneal artery bypasses, respectively. Similar results have been reported by some,[78] while others[55,77] have noted markedly lower primary patency rates of 7 to 9 percent at 2 years. Graft dilatation and aneurysmal degeneration occurred in 21 and 36 percent of grafts, respectively at 5 years, but only 6 percent required surgical intervention.[79] Other authors have found much higher aneurysmal changes (57 percent) at approximately 5 years and recommend that HUV be used sparingly, with careful follow-up evaluation by duplex scanning to ascertain aneurysmal degeneration.[80] New manufacturing modifications aimed at correcting this problem may reduce the incidence of graft dilatation, thereby improving long-term results.

Composite Grafts

Bypass grafts constructed of prosthetic material and vein composites have been used when an adequate length of vein for the entire extent of the bypass is unavailable. Some surgeons are unwilling to use a full-length prosthetic graft in such cases, believing that better compliance matching between artery and vein at the distal anastomosis will lead to decreased intimal hyperplasia and improved patency. The 1-year primary patency rates reported for composite grafts to infrapopliteal vessels (almost exclusively for limb salvage) range from 35 to 70 percent[74,81-85]; 2-year patency rates vary from 48 to 59 percent[74,82]; and 5- to 7-year patencies range from 28 to 30 percent.[74,85] One recent retrospective study comparing autogenous, prosthetic, and composite grafts for infrapopliteal revascularization reaffirmed the clear superiority of vein for maintaining long-term patency.[74] Although composite graft patency was approximately fourfold greater (28 versus 7 percent) than the patency of prosthetic grafts, the difference was not significant. Limb salvage rates for composite grafts varied from 62 to 43.5 percent at 1 and 2 years, respectively.[81] Thus, despite the acceptable limb salvage achieved with composite grafts as compared with infrapopliteal bypass using PTFE entirely,[12,41] no obvious superiority is evident to support the preferential use of one over the other.

Other Grafts

The importance of the venous endothelium in maintaining patency in adverse, low-flow situations has led to attempts to improve upon the poor results achieved with prosthetics by using cryopreserved homologous vein[86,87] and endothelial cell-lined conduit[88-92] as an alternative. Although holding promise, the preliminary results have not led to unanimous endorsement or conversely, to the abandonment of the clinically available prosthetic materials. Until the results of further clinical investigations evaluating long-term patency and limb salvage are available, more general use of these conduits will be limited.

ADJUNCTIVE TECHNIQUES

Alteration of the clotting properties of blood by pharmacologic manipulation with a variety of drugs

Table 30-4 Human Umbilical Vein Grafts

Authors	Year	No. of Bypasses	Patency (%)[a]					Limb Salvage (%)[a]				
			1 yr	2 yr	3 yr	4 yr	5 yr	1 yr	2 yr	3 yr	4 yr	5 yr
Klimach & Charlesworth[77]	1983	112	28	9								
Nevelsteen et al.[78]	1986	65	72	45	41	41	41	69	62	55	55	55
Dardik et al.[79]	1988	181	58	51	43	37	32					

[a] Some values are approximations based on graphs within the reports.

has been used to improve patency in disadvantaged circumstances. Raising the thrombotic threshold of blood may prevent graft closure even in situations of low flow. In addition, pharmacologic modification of the platelet-prosthetic interaction may inhibit the fibrous hyperplastic response, preventing anastomotic or graft stenosis and improving patency. A second method for maintaining flow in situations of limited runoff is to lower the hemodynamic resistance of the outflow circuit by creation of an arteriovenous fistula.

Anticoagulation/Antiplatelet Therapy

Reports evaluating postoperative anticoagulation or antiplatelet treatments are not in agreement regarding their efficacy in prolonging graft patency. Green et al.[93] noted significantly improved 1-year patency rates in above-knee femoropopliteal bypasses with PTFE in patients receiving either aspirin (100 percent) or aspirin and dipyridamole (100 percent) versus control subjects (50 percent). Patients treated with aspirin alone after below-knee bypass had an improved 1-year patency as compared with the other two groups, although the difference was not statistically significant. In another study Flinn et al.[13] treated patients undergoing infrapopliteal bypass with PTFE with coumadin anticoagulation and reported improved 2- and 4-year patencies of 45 and 37 percent, respectively, as compared with other reports in the literature.[12,41] Others have also noted enhanced patency rates in patients undergoing either autologous or prosthetic femoropopliteal bypass who were treated with coumadin or antiplatelet therapy.[94-97] However, at least two prospective, double-blind randomized trials have failed to demonstrate a significant effect of antiplatelet therapy in improving patency rates in prosthetic or venous grafts.[98,99] Therefore, any potential benefit in terms of increased patency must be weighed against the potential risk of increased perioperative bleeding. In one study, this occurred in more than 13 percent of patients.[13] In dependable, compliant patients without significant risk factors for bleeding, anticoagulation may improve long-term patency.

Distal Arteriovenous Fistula

Although vein grafts to small arteries can remain patent despite minimal flow rates, prosthetic grafts, with their inherent thrombogenicity, require higher flow rates to maintain patency. This problem is further compounded when prosthetic bypasses to infrapopliteal arteries require distal anastomoses to disadvantaged, high-resistance outflow tracts, reducing flow

through the graft. Physiologic conversion of these high-resistance systems to a low-resistance arterial circuit by construction of an arteriovenous fistula has been performed in this clinical setting to improve patency.

In 1980 Ibrahim et al.[100] of Dardik's group began to use adjunctive distal arteriovenous (AV) fistulae in an attempt to enhance patency results of glutaraldehyde-tanned HUV grafts inserted below the popliteal artery. These fistulae were constructed by joining the common wall of the opened adjacent artery and vein and then suturing the graft end-to-side to the resulting common ostium. Although their initial experience was limited to patients with disadvantaged outflow tracts, they subsequently liberalized their indications to include all non-autogenous vein bypasses. In 1991, Dardik et al.[101] published a 10-year experience with adjunctive AV fistulae in 210 cases, demonstrating 2-year graft patency rates that varied from 18 percent for bypasses constructed during the first 4 years of the study to 44 percent for those performed in the last 3 years. Harris and Campbell[102] also encouraged the use of AV fistulae by reporting a 47 percent 1-year graft patency in high-risk reconstructions. Moreover, Hinshaw and co-authors[103] published good results with this technique; in a relatively short follow-up of 4 to 24 months, only 6 (16 percent) of their 37 grafts became occluded, and the limb salvage rate was 75 percent. Conversely, Sommoggy et al. of Snyder's group found a high rate of 8-month fistula failure (70 percent) and limb loss (37 percent) in 30 common ostium arteriovenous fistulas constructed in 27 patients. In addition, they reported excessive limb edema in 27 percent of their patients, and serous wound healing problems in 12 percent.

The distal superficial venous system can also be used as an additional outflow site for high-risk paramalleolar bypasses. Our experience with this technique has been obtained with 12 patients who presented with a very limited distal runoff and in whom no autogenous vein or vein segments of sufficient length for bypass grafting were available. In addition, neither a common ostium nor a remote AV fistula would have been feasible in these patients because of the small size of the veins accompanying the arterial outflow segment. Adjunctive AV fistulae were constructed with the GSV in 9 patients and with the lesser saphenous vein in 3 patients (Fig. 30-3). Nine patients have had a patent graft and fistula for over 1 year, and two have had a patent graft without venous outflow for over 1 year. Three patients have had patent grafts and fistulae for over 2 years.

At present we limit the construction of complementary arteriovenous fistulae, utilizing either superficial or deep veins, to patients in whom (1) a prosthetic bypass to an infrapopliteal artery has failed; (2) severely restricted runoff is demonstrated by adequate arteriography; (3) a paramalleolar prosthetic reconstruction is required; or (4) chronic anticoagulation is contraindicated or not advisable. Nevertheless, we recognize that these indications are based on personal bias and we await the outcome of properly controlled studies to prove the value and identify the exact role of complementary arteriovenous fistulae for treating patients who are facing the threat of a major amputation and in whom a more standard revascularization procedure is not feasible.

sufficient, prosthetic grafts can be used, with clearly reduced patency but acceptable short-term limb salvage. Adjunctive methods such as anticoagulation may extend patency after revascularization with prosthetics. Adjunctive AV fistulae can be created to improve patency although more extensive long-term results are needed to confirm the role of this technique. Sound judgment, meticulous operative technique, and conscientious and aggressive postoperative surveillance are mandatory to achieve excellent results in this group of patients with difficult vascular problems.

CONCLUSIONS

Bypass to branches of the popliteal and tibial arteries routinely can be performed for limb preservation. Autologous vein conduits provide superior and durable patency results as compared with prosthetic grafts. The in situ technique may confer some advantage over the reversed vein technique for long bypasses to distally located outflow tracts. When autologous conduit is in-

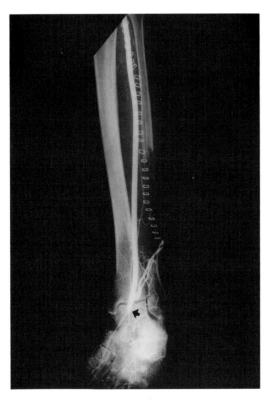

Figure 30-3 Angiogram depicting a polytetrafluoroethylene (PTFE) bypass from the distal portion of an external iliac artery to the dorsalis pedis artery with an adjunctive AV fistula. The lesser saphenous vein was turned down and anastomosed to the dorsalis pedis artery after ablation of the distal vein valves. The distal end of a PTFE graft *(arrow)* was inserted onto the hood of the arteriovenous anastomosis.

REFERENCES

1. Kunlin J: Le traitment de l'artérite obliterante par la greffe veineuse. Arch Mal Coeur 42:371, 1949
2. Julian OC, Dye WS, Olwin JH, Jordan PH: Direct surgery of arteriosclerosis. Ann Surg 136:459, 1952
3. Pratt GH, Krahl E: Surgical therapy for the occluded artery. Am J Surg 87:722, 1954
4. Shaw RS, Wheelock F: Blood vessel grafts in the treatment of chronic occlusive disease in the femoral artery. Surgery 37:94, 1955
5. Dye WS, Grove WJ, Olwin JH, Julian OC: Two and four year behavior of vein grafts in the lower extremities. Arch Surg 72:164, 1956
6. Morris GC, DeBakey ME, Cooley DA, Crawford ES: Arterial bypass below the knee. Surg Gynecol Obstet 108:321, 1956
7. McCaughan JJ: Successful arterial grafts to the anterior tibial, posterior tibial (below the peroneal) and peroneal arteries. Angiology 12:91, 1961
8. Ascer E, Veith FJ, Gupta SK: Bypasses to plantar arteries and other tibial branches: an extended approach to limb salvage. J Vasc Surg 8:434, 1988
9. Haimovici H: Patterns of arteriosclerotic lesions of the lower extremity. Arch Surg 95:918, 1967
10. Veith FJ, Gupta SK, Wengerter KR et al: Changing arteriosclerotic disease patterns and management strategies in lower-limb-threatening ischemia. Ann Surg 212:402, 1990
11. Wengerter KR, Veith FJ, Gupta SK et al: Prospective randomized multicenter comparison of in situ and reversed vein infrapopliteal bypasses. J Vasc Surg 13:189, 1991
12. Veith FJ, Gupta SK, Ascer E et al: Six-year prospective multicenter randomized comparison of autologous saphenous vein and expanded polytetrafluoroethylene grafts in infrainguinal arterial reconstructions. J Vasc Surg 3:104, 1986
13. Flinn WR, Rohrer MJ, Yao JST et al: Improved long-term patency of infragenicular PTFE grafts. J Vasc Surg 7:685, 1988
14. Patel KR, Semel L, Clauss RH: Extended reconstruction rate for limb salvage with intraoperative prereconstruction angiography. J Vasc Surg 7:531, 1988

15. Klamer TW, Lambert GE, Richardson JD et al: Utility of inframalleolar arterial bypass grafting. J Vasc Surg 11:164, 1990
16. Andros G, Harris RW, Salles-Cunha SX et al: Bypass grafts to the ankle and foot. J Vasc Surg 7:785, 1988
17. Bunt TJ: The role of a defined protocol for cardiac risk assessment in decreasing perioperative myocardial infarction in vascular surgery. J Vasc Surg 15:626, 1992
18. Cossman DV, Ellison JE, Wagner WH et al: Comparison of contrast arteriography to arterial mapping with color-flow duplex imaging in the lower extremities. J Vasc Surg 10:522, 1989
19. Moneta GL, Yeager RA, Antonovic R et al: Accuracy of lower extremity arterial duplex mapping. J Vasc Surg 15:275, 1992
20. Owen RS, Carpenter JP, Baum RA et al: Magnetic resonance imaging of angiographically occult runoff vessels in peripheral arterial occlusive disease. N Engl J Med 326:1577, 1992
21. Kozak BE, Bedell JE, Rosch J: Small vessel leg angiography for distal vessel bypass grafts. J Vasc Surg 8:711, 1988
22. Veith FJ, Gupta SK, Samson RH et al: Progress in limb salvage by reconstructive arterial surgery combined with new or improved adjunctive procedures. Ann Surg 194:386, 1981
23. Ascer E, Calligaro K, Veith FJ, Wengerter K: Graft angioplasty: use of the stenotic lesion as an inflow or outflow site in lower extremity arterial bypasses. J Vasc Surg 11:576, 1990
24. Ascer E, Veith FJ, Gupta SK et al: Short vein grafts: a superior option for arterial reconstructions to poor or compromised outflow tracts? J Vasc Surg 7:370, 1988
25. Veith FJ, Gupta SK, Samson RH et al: Superficial femoral and popliteal arteries as inflow sites for distal bypasses. Surgery 90:980, 1981
26. Sidaway AN, Menzoian JO, Cantelmo NL, LoGerfo FW: Effect of inflow and outflow sites on the results of tibioperoneal vein grafts. Am J Surg 152:211, 1986
27. Leather RP, Shah DM, Chang BB, Kaufman JL: Resurrection of the in-situ saphenous vein bypass 1000 cases later. Ann Surg 208:435, 1988
28. Rosenbloom MS, Walsh JJ, Schuler JJ et al: Long-term results of ingenicular bypasses with autogenous vein originating from the distal superficial femoral and popliteal arteries. J Vasc Surg 7:691, 1988
29. Marks J, King TA, Baele H et al: Popliteal-to-distal bypass for limb-threatening ischemia. J Vasc Surg 15:755, 1992
30. Schuler JJ, Flanigan DP, Williams LR et al: Early experience with popliteal to infrapopliteal bypass for limb salvage. Arch Surg 118:472, 1983
31. Cantelmo NL, Snow JR, Menzoian JO et al: Successful vein bypass in patients with an ischemic limb a palpable popliteal pulse. Arch Surg 121:217, 1986
32. Nunez AA, Veith FJ, Collier P et al: Direct approaches to the distal portions of the deep femoral artery for limb salvage bypasses. J Vasc Surg 8:576, 1988
33. Veith FJ, Ascer E, Gupta SK et al: Tibiotibial vein bypass grafts: a new operation for limb salvage. J Vasc Surg 2:552, 1985
34. Ascer E, Kirwin J, Mohan C, Gennaro M: The preferential use of the external iliac artery as an inflow source for redo femoro-popliteal and infrapopliteal bypass operations. J Vasc Surg 18:234, 1993
35. Imparato AM, Kim GE, Madayag M, Haveson S: Angiographic criteria for successful tibial arterial reconstructions. Surgery 74:830, 1973
36. Shah DM, Darling III RC, Chang BB et al: Is long bypass from groin to ankle a durable procedure? An analysis of a ten-year experience. J Vasc Surg 15:402, 1992
37. Corson JD, Brewster DC, LaSalle AJ, Darling RC: Comparative analysis of vein and prosthetic bypass grafts to the isolated popliteal artery. Surgery 91:448, 1982
38. Kram HR, Gupta SK, Veith FJ et al: Late results of two hundred seventeen femoropopliteal bypasses to isolated popliteal artery segments. J Vasc Surg 14:386, 1991
39. Wengerter KR, Yang PM, Veith FJ et al: A twelve year experience with popliteal-to-distal artery bypass: the significance and management of proximal disease. J Vasc Surg 15:143, 1992
40. Dalsing MC, White JV, Yao JST et al: Infrapopliteal bypass for established gangrene of the forefoot or toes. J Vasc Surg 2:669, 1985
41. Veterans Administration Cooperative Study Group 141: Comparative evaluation of prosthetic, reversed, and in situ vein bypass grafts in distal popliteal and tibial-peroneal revascularization. Arch Surg 123:434, 1988
42. Buchbinder D, Pasch AR, Rollins DL et al: Results of arterial reconstruction of the foot. Arch Surg 121:673, 1986
43. Taylor LM, Edwards JM, Porter JM: Present status of reversed vein bypass grafting: five year results of a modern series. J Vasc Surg 11:193, 1990
44. Mills JL, Taylor SM: Results of infrainguinal revascularization with reversed vein conduits: a modern control series. Ann Vasc Surg 5:156, 1991
45. Carney WI, Balko A, Barrett MS: In situ femoropopliteal and infrapopliteal bypass. Arch Surg 120:812, 1985
46. Bergamini TM, Towne JB, Bandyk DF et al: Experience with in situ saphenous vein bypasses during 1981 to 1989: determinant factors of long-term patency. J Vasc Surg 13:137, 1991
47. Imparato AM, Bracco A, Kim GE, Zeff R: Intimal and neointimal fibrous proliferation causing failure of arterial reconstructions. Surgery 72:1007, 1972
48. LoGerfo FW, Soncrant T, Teel T, Dewey CF: Boundary layer separation in models of side to end arterial anastomoses. Arch Surg 114:1369, 1979
49. Walden R, L'Italien G, Megerman J, Abbott WM: Matched elastic properties and successful arterial grafting. Arch Surg 115:1166, 1980
50. Abbott WM, Cambria RP: Control of physical characteristics (elasticity and compliance) of vascular grafts. p.

189. In Stanley JC (ed): Biologic and Synthetic Vascular Prostheses. Grune & Stratton, Orlando, 1982

51. Cambria RP, Megerman J, Abbott WM: Endothelial preservation in reversed and in situ autogenous vein grafts. Ann Surg 202:50, 1985

52. Bush HL, Graber JN, Jakubowski JA et al: Favorable balance of prostacyclin and thromboxane A$_2$ improves early patency of human in situ vein grafts. J Vasc Surg 1:149, 1984

53. Ad Hoc Committee on Reporting Standards, SVS/ISCVS: Suggested standards for reports dealing with lower extremity ischemia. J Vasc Surg 4:80, 1986

54. Hobson RW, Lynch TG, Jamil Z et al: Results of revascularization and amputation in severe lower extremity ischemia: a five-year clinical experience. J Vasc Surg 2:174, 1985

55. Rutherford RB, Jones DN, Bergentz SE et al: Factors affecting the patency of infrainguinal bypass. J Vasc Surg 8:236, 1988

56. Berkowitz HD, Greenstein SM: Improved patency in reversed femoral-infrapopliteal autogenous vein grafts by early detection and treatment of the failing graft. J Vasc Surg 5:755, 1987

57. Rafferty TD, Avellone JC, Farrell CJ et al: A metropolitan experience with infrainguinal revascularization. J Vasc Surg 6:365, 1987

58. Hall KV: The great saphenous vein used in situ as an arterial shunt after extirpation of the vein valves—a preliminary report. Surgery 51:492, 1962

59. Leather RP, Powers SR, Karmody AM: A reappraisal of the in-situ saphenous vein arterial bypass: its use in limb salvage. Surgery 86:453, 1979

60. Fogle MA, Whittemore AD, Couch NP, Mannick JA: A comparison of in situ and reversed saphenous vein grafts for infrainguinal reconstruction. J Vasc Surg 5:46, 1987

61. Bandyk DF, Kaebnick HW, Stewart GW, Towne JB: Durability of the in situ saphenous vein arterial bypass: a comparison of primary and secondary patency. J Vasc Surg 5:256, 1987

62. Mannick JA, Whittemore AD, Donaldson MC: Clinical and anatomic considerations for surgery in tibial disease and the results of surgery. Circulation, suppl. 83:I-81

63. Donaldson MC, Mannick JA, Whittemore AD: Causes of primary graft failure after in situ saphenous vein bypass grafting. J Vasc Surg 15:113, 1992

64. Graham JW, Lusby RJ: Infrapopliteal bypass grafting: use of upper limb vein alone and in autogenous composite grafts. Surgery 91:646, 1982

65. Harris RW, Andros G, Dulawa LB et al: Successful long-term limb salvage using cephalic vein bypass grafts. Ann Surg 200:785, 1984

66. Andros G, Harris RW, Salles-Cunha SX et al: Arm veins for arterial revascularization of the leg: arteriographic and clinical observations. J Vasc Surg 4:416, 1986

67. Balshi JD, Cantelmo NL, Menzoian JO, LoGerfo FW: The use of arm veins for infrainguinal bypass in end-stage peripheral vascular disease. Arch Surg 124:1078, 1989

68. Weaver FA, Barlow CR, Edwards WH et al: The lesser saphenous vein: autogenous tissue for lower extremity revascularization. J Vasc Surg 5:687, 1987

69. Chang BB, Paty PSK, Shah DM, Leather RP: The lesser saphenous vein: an underappreciated source of autogenous vein. J Vasc Surg 15:152, 1992

70. Yeager RA, Hobson II RW, Lynch TG et al: Analysis of factors influencing patency of polytetrafluoroethylene prostheses for limb salvage. J Surg Res 32:499, 1982

71. Christenson JT, Broome A, Norgren L, Eklof B: Revascularization of popliteal and below-knee arteries with polytetrafluoroethylene. Surgery 97:141, 1985

72. Bergan JJ, Veith FJ, Bernhard VM et al: Randomization of autogenous vein and polytetrafluoroethylene grafts in femoro-distal reconstruction. Surgery 92:921, 1982

73. Whittemore AD, Kent C, Donaldson MC et al: What is the proper role of polytetrafluoroethylene grafts in infrainguinal reconstruction? J Vasc Surg 10:299, 1989

74. Londrey GL, Ramsey DE, Hodgson KJ et al: Infrapopliteal bypass for severe ischemia: comparison of autogenous vein, composite, and prosthetic grafts. J Vasc Surg 13:631, 1991

75. Ascer E, Veith FJ, Gupta SK et al: Six year experience with expanded polytetrafluoroethylene arterial grafts for limb salvage. J Cardiovasc Surg (Torino) 5:468, 1985

76. Ascer E, Collier P, Gupta SK, Veith FJ: Reoperation for polytetrafluoroethylene bypass failure: the importance of distal outflow site and operative technique in determining outcome. J Vasc Surg 5:298, 1987

77. Klimach O, Charlesworth D: Femorotibial bypass for limb salvage using human umbilical vein. Br J Surg 70:1, 1983

78. Nevelsteen A, D'Hallewin MA, Deleersnijder J et al: The human umbilical vein graft in below-knee femoropopliteal and femorotibial surgery: an eight year experience. Ann Vasc Surg 1:328, 1986

79. Dardik H, Miller N, Dardik A et al: A decade of experience with the glutaraldehyde-tanned human umbilical cord vein graft for revascularization of the lower limb. J Vasc Surg 7:336, 1988

80. Hasson JE, Newton D, Waltman AC et al: Mural degeneration in the glutaraldehyde-tanned umbilical vein graft: incidence and implications. J Vasc Surg 4:243, 1986

81. Feinberg RL, Winter RP, Wheeler JR et al: The use of composite grafts in femorocrural bypasses performed for limb salvage: a review of 108 consecutive cases and comparison with 57 in situ saphenous vein bypasses. J Vasc Surg 12:257, 1990

82. Snyder SO, Gregory RT, Wheeler JR, Gayle RG: Composite grafts utilizing polytetrafluoroethylene–autogenous tissue for lower extremity arterial reconstructions. Surgery 90:881, 1981

83. Britton JP, Leveson SH: Distal arterial bypass by composite grafting. Br J Surg 74:249, 1987

84. Tyrrell MR, Grigg MJ, Wolfe JN: Is arterial reconstruction to the ankle worthwhile in the absence of autologous vein? Eur J Vasc Surg 3:429, 1989

85. Wheeler JR, Gregory RT, Snyder SO, Gayle RG: Goretex autogenous vein composite grafts for tibial reconstruction. J Vasc Surg 6:914, 1984

86. Sitman JV, Imbembo AL, Ricotta JJ et al: Dimethylsulfoxide treated, cryopreserved venous allografts in the arterial and venous systems. Surgery 95:154, 1984

87. Fujitani RM, Bassiouny HS, Gewertz BL et al: Cryopreserved saphenous vein allogenic homografts: an alternative conduit in lower extremity arterial reconstruction in infected fields. J Vasc Surg 15:519, 1992

88. Magometschnigg H, Kadletz M, Vodrazka M et al: Prospective clinical study with in vitro endothelial cell lining of expanded polytetrafluoroethylene grafts in crural repeat reconstruction. J Vasc Surg 15:527, 1992

89. Ortenwall P, Wadenvik H, Risberg B: Reduced platelet deposition on seeded versus unseeded segments of expanded polytetrafluoroethylene grafts: clinical observations after 6-month follow-up. J Vasc Surg 10:374, 1989

90. Herring MB, Compton RS, LeGrand DR et al: Endothelial seeding of polytetrafluoroethylene popliteal bypasses. J Vasc Surg 6:114, 1987

91. Ortenwall P, Wadenvik H, Kutti J, Risberg B: Reduction in deposition of indium 111-labelled platelets after autologous endothelial cell seeding of Dacron aortic bifurcation grafts in humans: a preliminary report. J Vasc Surg 6:17, 1987

92. Herring M, Baughman S, Glover J: Endothelium develops on seeded human arterial prosthesis: a brief clinical note. J Vasc Surg 2:727, 1985

93. Green RM, Roedersheimer R, DeWeese JA: Effects of aspirin and dipyridamole on expanded polytetrafluoroethylene graft patency. Surgery 92:1016, 1982

94. Kretschmer G, Wenzl E, Wagner O et al. Influence of anticoagulant treatment in preventing graft occlusion following saphenous vein bypass for femoropopliteal occlusive disease. Br J Surg 73:689, 1986

95. Clyne CAC, Archer TJ, Atuhaire LK et al: Random control trial of a short course of aspirin and dipyridamole (Persantin) for femorodistal grafts. Br J Surg 74:246, 1987

96. Kretschmer G, Wenzl E, Piza F et al: The influence of anticoagulant treatment on the probability of function in femoropopliteal vein bypass surgery: analysis of a clinical series (1970 to 1985) and interim evaluation of a controlled trial. Surgery 103:453, 1987

97. Kretschmer G, Herbst F, Prager M et al: A decade of oral anticoagulant treatment to maintain autologous vein grafts for femoropopliteal atherosclerosis. Arch Surg 127:1112, 1992

98. McCollum C, Alexander C, Kenchington G et al: Antiplatelet drugs in femoropopliteal vein bypasses: a multicenter trial. J Vasc Surg 13:150, 1991

99. Kohler TR, Kaufman JL, Kacoyanis G et al: Effect of aspirin and dipyridamole on the patency of lower extremity bypass grafts. Surgery 96:462, 1984

100. Ibahim IM, Sussman B, Dardik I et al: Adjunctive arteriovenous fistula with tibial and peroneal reconstruction for limb salvage. Am J Surg 140:246, 1980

101. Dardik H, Berry SM, Dardik A et al: Infrapopliteal prosthetic graft patency by use of the distal adjunctive arteriovenous fistula. J Vasc Surg 13:685, 1991

102. Harris PL, Campbell H: Adjuvant distal arteriovenous shunt with femorotibial bypass for critical ischemia. Br J Surg 70:377, 1983

103. Hinshaw DB, Schmidt CA, Hinshaw LB, Simpson JB: Arteriovenous fistula in arterial reconstruction of the ischemic limb. Arch Surg 118:589, 1983

104. Sommoggy S, Maurer PC, Dorrler et al: Femorodistal PTFE bypasses combined with distal arteriovenous fistula: a chance in critical limb ischemia. p. 98. In Veith FJ (ed): Current Critical Problems in Vascular Surgery. Vol. 2. Quality Medical Publishing, St. Louis, 1990

105. Snyder SO, Wheeler JR, Gregory RT, Gayle RG: Failure of arteriovenous fistulas at distal tibial bypass anastomotic sites. J Cardiovasc Surg (Torino) 26:137, 1985

106. Paty PSK, Shah DM, Saifi J et al: Remote distal arteriovenous fistula to improve infrapopliteal bypass patency. J Vasc Surg 1:171, 1990

107. Buchbinder D, Singh JK, Karmody AM et al: Comparison of patency rate and structural changes of in situ and reversed vein arterial bypass. J Surg Res 30:213, 1981

108. LoGerfo FW: Discussion of Leine AW, Bandyk DF, Bonier PH, Towne JB: Lessons learned in adopting the in situ saphenous vein bypass. J Vasc Surg 2:145, 1985

31

Surgical Management of Chronic Upper Extremity Ischemia

Thomas M. Bergamini

The management of patients with chronic upper extremity ischemia can be disconcerting even to the most experienced and skillful clinicians. The low prevalence of ischemia, as compared with that in the lower extremity, coupled with diverse etiologies for the occlusive process, can challenge diagnostic and therapeutic acumen.[1] Patients with significant arterial stenosis or short-segment occlusion may be asymptomatic because of well developed collaterals. Other patients may experience exertional arm pain but usually not to the same extent as those with a comparable level of ischemia in the legs. Patients with symptomatic chronic upper extremity ischemia tend to present with one of three clinical manifestations: arm claudication, digital ulceration or gangrene, or Raynaud's phenomena (episodic digital ischemia/pain). However, the differential diagnosis for these presenting symptoms and signs may be quite extensive in the individual patient. The astute clinician relies on patient history and level of arterial occlusion (based upon the physical examination, noninvasive vascular laboratory tests, and arteriography) to assign an etiology for the ischemia and formulate a treatment plan.

The medical history is most helpful in differentiating between the diverse etiologies of chronic upper extremity ischemia and thus identifying those patients with lesions amenable to surgical intervention. Hand and digit ischemia resulting from a systemic vasculitis, a hematologic disorder, or a connective tissue disease usually cannot be improved or corrected by surgical intervention owing to the distal nature of the lesions, but most patients can be managed effectively nonoperatively. Such patients will typically relate a prior history of an underlying systemic disease. McNamara et al.[2] reported that the diagnosis of scleroderma, systemic lupus erythematosus, or uremia preceded the resultant hand ischemia in a majority of cases. Patients with upper extremity ischemia due to a surgically correctable lesion will also frequently have a history suggestive of the etiology. For example, chronic upper extremity ischemia due to atherosclerosis, Takayasu's arteritis, trauma, or atheroembolism will have identifiable atherosclerotic risk factors, an obvious inflammatory stage of arteritis, remote arterial injury, or cardiac abnormality (aneurysm and/or arrhythmia), respectively. Careful questioning of patients is paramount in working through the differential diagnosis of chronic upper extremity ischemia.

The etiology of chronic upper extremity ischemia also correlates with the level of occlusive disease. Three levels of arterial involvement based on size and location that are useful for clinical diagnosis, are large (innominate and subclavian), medium (axillary and brachial), and small (radial, ulnar, and digital) arteries. In each arterial level a limited number of disease processes can be implicated for the occlusive lesion. Arteriosclerosis obliterans remains the primary disease involving the large arteries; trauma and atheroembolism are more common causes of lesions in the medium-sized arteries; for small distal arteries, vasculitis or hematologic and connective tissue disorders should be considered the most likely etiology for segmental or end-artery occlusions. By using a methodical evaluation process that includes physical examination (inspection, pulse palpation), nonivasive vascular laboratory testing, and arteriography, the level and morphology of upper extremity arterial occlusive lesions can be defined and this information used to determine the efficacy of surgical intervention and the type of procedure to be followed.

Table 31-1   History and Etiology of Chronic Upper Extremity Ischemia According to Anatomic Location

Representative History	Etiology
Large Arteries (Innominate/Subclavian)	
Elderly man with left arm claudication	Atherosclerotic disease
Woman <50 years old with left arm fatigue, inflammatory stage	Takayasu's disease
Middle-aged woman with bilateral arm claudication with arm elevation	Thoracic outlet syndrome
Medium-Sized Arteries (Axillary/Brachial)	
Arm or hand ischemia following transarterial catheterization	Trauma
Arm or hand ischemia in patient with atrial fibrillation	Macroembolism
Arm claudication >10 years following radiotherapy	Irradiation
Woman >50 years old with arm claudication, visual disturbances, and inflammatory stage	Giant cell arteritis
Small Arteries (Radial/Ulnar/Digital)	
Unilateral hand ischemia with history of repetitive trauma	Trauma (occupational disorder)
Hand ischemia with symptoms of thoracic outlet syndrome or palpable aneurysm	Microembolism
Hand ischemia with history of thrombosis	Hypercoagulable state
Man <50 years old, smoker, with hand ischemia	Buerger's disease

As with most vascular disorders, surgical intervention for upper extremity ischemia depends largely on the severity of ischemia, with underlying etiology and anatomic level of involvement being important predictors of outcome. Arterial bypass or repair is appropriate for patients with disabling arm claudication *or* digital ischemia (ulceration, tip gangrene) when the etiologic process is amenable to a surgical approach (Table 31-1). Clinically validated procedures for chronic upper extremity ischemia include direct arterial reconstruction/bypass, first thoracic rib resection, sympathectomy, or endovascular intervention by percutaneous transluminal balloon angioplasty (PTA). The patient population requiring upper extremity arterial surgery differs from that with critical lower limb ischemia. Surgical intervention for arterial occlusive disease of the upper extremity is performed in patients who are nearly a decade younger than those undergoing lower extremity arterial bypass.[3] As such, the longevity of patients undergoing upper extremity revascularization is greater; the 5-year survival rate is 80 percent compared with 50 percent for patients who have had lower extremity arterial bypass. This observation underscores the importance of proper patient selection for the type of revascularization procedure in order to maximize long-term patency.

This chapter reviews those chronic occlusive diseases of the upper extremity arterial tree that are amenable to direct surgical intervention. The etiologies of upper extremity ischemia are correlated with anatomic location, and key features of patients' history and examination, vascular laboratory testing, and arteriography are discussed. Finally, the results of surgical intervention for chronic upper extremity ischemia are presented relative to the etiology and anatomic level of disease.

DIFFERENTIAL DIAGNOSIS OF CHRONIC ISCHEMIA RELATIVE TO ANATOMIC INVOLVEMENT

Large Arteries (Innominate/Subclavian)

Atherosclerosis

Atherosclerosis is the most frequent cause of chronic arterial occlusive disease of the innominate and subclavian arteries.[4] Atherosclerotic stenoses tend to develop at the origin of the great vessels from the aortic arch and are focal, extending only for a short distance. The left subclavian artery is affected three to four times more frequently than the right. The majority of patients with hemodynamically significant atherosclerosis of aortic arch branches (pulse deficit in the upper extremity) are asymptomatic and require no treatment or intensive surveillance. Approximately 12 percent of patients who have a greater than 30 percent stenosis or occlusion of the subclavian or innominate arteries as demonstrated by angiography will require intervention.[5] Surgical repair is indicated for patients with disabling arm claudication, Raynaud's syndrome, or digital ulceration or gangrene. Atherosclerosis of the brachycephalic vessels may also be the site for embolization to more distal arteries of the upper extremities and thus may warrant direct surgical repair or bypass. An anomalous right subclavian artery, originating from the aortic arch distal to the left subclavian artery, has also been reported as a source of upper extremity ischemia due to occlusive disease or atheroembolism.[6]

Takayasu's Disease

Like atherosclerosis, nonspecific aortoarteritis (Takayasu's disease) involves the left subclavian artery more frequently than the right. Takayasu's disease can be distinguished from atherosclerotic disease by the age and sex of the patient and presenting clinical signs. This autoimmune disease occurs predominantly in women under the age of 50 years, in contrast to atherosclerosis, which is more common in elderly men. Half of patients with Takayasu's disease will relate a history of an acute inflammatory stage associated with a low-grade temperature, tachycardia, pain adjacent to the inflamed arteries, and easy fatiguability.[7] There may be a 5- to 20-year interval between the acute inflammatory stage(s) and the presentation with symptomatic arterial occlusive disease. Patients with chronic upper extremity symptoms due to Takayasu's disease merit surgical intervention only when symptoms are severe or limb-threatening because of the complexity of the repairs.

Thoracic Outlet Syndrome

Patients with chronic upper extremity ischemia due to thoracic outlet syndrome classically have symptoms that are exacerbated with arm elevation or exercise. Subclavian artery lesions (aneurysm, stenosis, or occlusion) produced by an anatomic thoracic outlet abnormality occurs in only 1 percent of cases.[8] These patients may present with diminished pulses and arm claudication, intermittent hand and digital ischemia, or Raynaud symptoms. Subclavian artery complications due to thoracic outlet syndrome are most common in patients with a anomalous cervical rib.[9] The ischemia produced by such lesions is typically distal in location (in the fingers or hand) and embolic in nature. Thoracic outlet syndrome has been reported following

shoulder or clavicle trauma and rarely, secondary to a tumor of the first rib.[10]

Medium-Sized Arteries (Axillary/Brachial)

Stenotic lesions or short segmental occlusions, not recognized after arterial trauma, are the most common manifestation of chronic ischemia produced by disease of the medium-sized arteries. Patients most commonly present several months following cardiac catheterization or a diagnostic arteriographic procedure, performed via the axillary or brachial artery approach, with the symptoms of arm claudication or fatigue with exercise. In a series reported by Gross et al.,[11] approximately one-half (47 percent) of patients treated for chronic upper extremity ischemia had iatrogenic injury of the axillary or brachial artery due to transarterial catheterization as the cause. The mean time interval between the invasive arterial procedure and operative treatment was 9 months.

Upper extremity ischemia can also result from compression and/or injury of the brachial artery by blunt trauma. This is most commonly observed in the acute situation following a supracondylar fracture of the humerus.[12] While rare, there have been reports of chronic upper extremity ischemia due to external arterial compression from humeral fracture or to congenital anomalies of the supracondylar process producing entrapment of the brachial artery.[13]

Macroembolism

Macroembolism of the axillary and brachial arteries can be subtle cause of chronic arterial insufficiency if not recognized and treated promptly. While the heart is the most common source of arterial embolism to the upper extremity, true or false aneurysms of the subclavian or axillary artery or poststenotic subclavian artery dilatation due to thoracic outlet syndrome can also harbor mural thrombi and be sources for distal embolism.[14] An infrequent source of upper extremity atheroembolism is the stump of an occluded axillofemoral graft.[15,16]

Radiation Injury

Irradiation-induced arterial occlusive disease resulting in chronic upper extremity ischemia is rare.[17] Patients present with arm claudication, digital ischemia, or Raynaud's symptoms, usually at least 10 years following radiotherapy for malignancy (breast cancer, melanoma, or lymphoma). The occurrence of arterial injury due to radiotherapy is dependent upon the radiation dose and prolonged patient survival after treatment of the primary cancer. At 5 to 10 years following irradiation, lesions such as fibrotic stenosis, periarterial fibrosis, mural thrombus and embolization can develop. After 20 years atherosclerosis may develop in the irradiated arterial segments.

Giant Cell Arteritis

Giant cell arteritis is a rare cause of upper extremity ischemia. Presenting symptoms and signs might include arm claudication, hand ischemia, or Raynaud's symptoms combined with the absence of upper extremity pulses. Giant cell arteritis can be differentiated from Takayasu's disease by the age of the patient, the constitutional symptoms of the acute inflammatory stage, and the response to steroid administration. In contrast to Takayasu's disease, giant cell arteritis usually occurs in older women (more than 50 years of age) and is associated with transient or permanent loss of vision due to an ischemic optic neuritis, with the absence of abdominal symptoms, and with dramatic improvement in symptoms with corticosteroid therapy.[1] The clinical diagnosis of giant cell arteritis can be substantiated by a temporal artery biopsy, but laboratory evidence supporting the diagnosis includes an elevated erythrocyte sedimentation rate and the presence of alkaline phosphatase, immunoglobulins, α_3-globulin, fibrinogen, C-reactive protein, and α_1-antitrypsin. Giant cell arteritis rarely involves the coronary, visceral, and cerebrovascular arteries, producing ischemia in these arterial circulations (e.g., myocardial infarction, stroke, or bowel ischemia).[18]

Small Arteries (Radial/Ulnar/Digital)

When chronic upper extremity ischemia is the result of distal small artery occlusion, the differential diagnosis includes innumerable systemic, hematologic, environmental, immunologic, and connective tissue disorders, conditions that are best managed without surgical intervention.[19] The clinician must be aware the clinical presentation of patients with these disease processes may be similar to that of patients with embolization from a more proximal, surgically correctable lesion. Overall, approximately two-thirds of patients with Raynaud's syndrome will eventually be diagnosed as having an associated systemic disease, the most common being a connective tissue disorder such as scleroderma. These diseases produce fixed occlusive lesions of the palmar and digital arteries, with occlusion proximal to the wrist a very infrequent occurrence. The ma-

jority of patients with such diseases have intermittent vasospasm of the hands and fingers, the condition characterizing Raynaud's syndrome. Digital ulceration is almost always accompanied by extensive palmar or digital artery obstruction.[19] It is of note that primary vasospastic Raynaud's syndrome (cold sensitivity) never produces digital ischemic ulcerations. The fact that certain etiologies of digital ulceration secondary to small artery disease are amenable to a surgical approach emphasizes the importance of establishing the correct diagnosis.[2] For example, in the select group of patients with chronic occlusive disease of the radial, ulnar, and/or digital arteries, ischemia due to trauma, microembolization from a proximal source, a hypercoagulable state, or Buerger's disease[20] can be improved with a surgical approach (Table 31-1).

Trauma

Direct trauma to the radial, ulnar, or palmar arteries can produce hand ischemia that is potentially surgically correctable. Occupations that involve repetitive blunt trauma to the hand (i.e., from a pneumatic drill or hammer) can damage the artery wall and result in stenosis, thrombosis, or aneurysm formation.[21,22] The ulnar artery is most commonly involved in such occupational injuries because of its anatomic location in the hypothenar eminence, a site of repetitive blunt trauma and vibration injury. This process has been termed the *hypothenar hammer syndrome,* and similar injury can occur in the thenar space involving the radial artery.[23] Ulnar artery thrombosis has also been reported following athletic activities such as catching a baseball or frisbee. Occlusion of the radial artery, in particular, is common following direct penetrating or blunt trauma or from transarterial catheters for arterial pressure monitoring or blood gas analysis. Patients with an incomplete palmar arch are at an increased risk of developing chronic hand ischemia due to injury of the radial or ulnar artery.[21]

Microembolisms

Microembolism to the radial, ulnar, or digital arteries can also produce chronic hand and/or digit ischemia. Possible embolic sources include the heart, a subclavian artery aneurysm, poststenotic subclavian artery dilatation due to thoracic outlet syndrome, and emoblization from an ulnar or radial artery aneurysm.[24] Patients with these latter lesions present with a tender, pulsatile mass in the thenar or hypothenar space, and digital ischemia is localized to only several digits (i.e., the fourth and fifth fingers) with embolization from an ulnar artery source.

Hypercoagulable States

Hypercoagulable states constitute an unusual cause of upper extremity ischemia and are usually the result of a spontaneous arterial thrombosis. Towne et al.[25] reported five patients with upper extremity ischemia due to an abnormality of the fibrinolytic system, specifically either a low level of plasminogen or an abnormal immunoreactive plasminogen. All these patients had presented with critical hand ischemia due to thrombosis of the brachial, radial, or ulnar artery. Four of them developed chronic ischemia due to persistent thrombosis of the radial, ulnar, or digital arteries despite attempted thrombectomy. Delayed recognition of the hypercoagulable state was the most important factor leading to the chronic ischemic condition.

Buerger's Disease

Thromboangiitis obliterans (Buerger's disease) is an inflammatory occlusive disease of the medium and small arteries of the upper extremity.[20,26,27] Patients are usually smokers who present at a young age (under 50 years) with chronic ischemic symptoms, such as arm claudication, Raynaud's syndrome, or digital ulceration or gangrene. The diagnostic criteria include a smoking history, onset before 50 years of age, infrapopliteal arterial occlusive disease, absence of atherosclerotic risk factors except smoking, and either infrabrachial arterial occlusive disease or superficial thrombophlebitis. The disease usually initially involves the peripheral arteries and progresses proximally. Abstinence from smoking and tobacco products is the only way to slow progression of the disease. The frequency of digital ulcer recurrence in patients with Buerger's disease is significantly higher for those who continue to smoke (48 percent) than for those who stop smoking (9.9 percent).[20] Although many patients require digital amputation, Buerger's disease of the upper extremity is associated with a low rate of major amputation (less than 2 percent). This outcome is in contrast to Buerger's disease of the lower extremity, for which below- or above-knee amputation is commonplace.[20,27]

EVALUATION OF CHRONIC UPPER EXTREMITY ISCHEMIA

Patients with chronic upper extremity ischemia typically demonstrate decreased or absent pulses and may have cutaneous signs of digital ischemia. Physical examination should include palpation for cervical ribs and clavicular abnormalities, in addition to careful pulse palpation and blood pressure measurements at several levels. Auscultation for bruits in the supraclavicular and subclavicular areas should be performed with and without arm abduction.[28] Most patients describe an exacerbation of symptoms in response to cold or emotional stimuli. Attacks of both vasospastic and obstructive Raynaud's syndrome can involve pallor of the affected part on exposure to cold, followed by cyanosis and rubor on rewarming, with a full recovery in 15 to 45 minutes. A tricolor response in the digits (white to blue to red) is not essential for diagnosis. Noninvasive hemodynamic testing followed by arteriography in patients identified as having obstructive lesions should be performed when evaluating chronic upper extremity ischemia. This diagnostic process will accurately determine the level and morphology of the occlusive disease.

Serologic laboratory tests are useful in the differential diagnosis, especially for diagnosing connective tissue diseases, such as systemic lupus erythematosus or scleroderma, that can cause chronic upper extremity ischemia. Takayasu's disease and giant cell arteritis are commonly associated with an elevated sedimentation rate. Laboratory testing is also essential for the diagnosis of hypercoagulable states, such as an abnormal plasminogen. Patients with Buerger's disease have been reported to have a distinctive pattern of HLA-A and HLA-B antigens.[26]

The noninvasive vascular laboratory provides an array of tests for the assessment of the patient with chronic upper extremity ischemia (Fig. 31-1). In general, the type of testing performed should be guided by patient history and physical findings. Routine testing should include measurement of segmental pressures (brachial, radial/ulnar, and digital) combined with pulse waveform analysis (Doppler and plethysmographic) in *both* upper extremities. In general, the difference in systolic blood pressure measurements between arms exceeds 20 mmHg in the presence of significant occlusive disease. Patients with normal brachial artery pressures but symptoms suggestive of proximal arterial disease should also undergo pressure measurements with Adson's maneuvers or arm abduction to evaluate whether a thoracic outlet (compression) syndrome is present. Patients with normal pulses and pressures to the level of the wrist should undergo digital photoplethysmography to obtain digital waveforms and pressures. The documentation of abnormal digital pressures and waveforms is diagnostic of fixed obstructive disease of the distal radial, ulnar, or digital arteries (obstructive Raynaud's syndrome). Patients with normal studies should undergo a cold tolerance test to confirm vasospastic Raynaud's syndrome.[29]

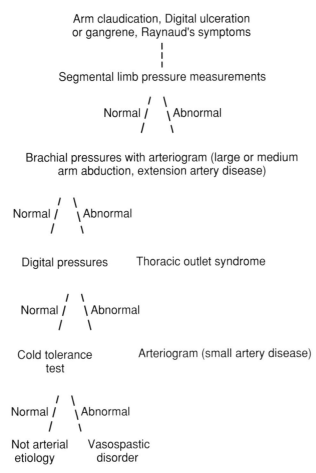

Figure 31-1 Algorithm for diagnostic evaluation.

Upper extremity arteriography should be the final step in the evaluation process for chronic upper extremity ischemia. Imaging should be performed from the aortic arch to the digital arteries[30] (Fig. 31-2). Normal anatomic variations of the upper extremity arteries must be considered when evaluating the arteriograms (Table 31-2). A femoral artery approach with selective catheterization of the subclavian and brachial arteries is the preferred angiographic method. Patients with symptoms of hand ischemia should have arteriography of both upper extremities with administration of intra-arterial vasodilators (papaverine or priscoline), since symmetric anatomic abnormalities may be present. Arteriographic findings, coupled with the history and the results of physical, laboratory, and noninvasive vascular examination should permit accurate diagnosis.

Each disease etiology has characteristic arteriographic findings. Atherosclerosis typically produces focal stenotic, irregular lesions at the origin of the aortic arch vessels. Patients with Takayasu's disease have long, diffuse stenotic segments, which gradually merge into normal-appearing distal artery, and also have an abundant collateral network associated with the arterial occlusions.[31] The thoracic outlet syndrome may be associated with a focal segmental stenosis of the subclavian artery as it crosses the first thoracic or anomalous cervical rib, often with a segment of poststenotic dilatation. With arm adduction, occlusion of the subclavian artery may be demonstrated. Atheroemboli to the brachial or a more distal artery can be recognized by an abrupt artery occlusion, and with recent embolization an intraluminal filling defect may be visualized. Unlike acute embolization, in chronic embolization collaterals can develop around the occlusion. Radiation-induced injury to the subclavian and axillary arteries is characterized by occlusive or stenotic lesions limited to the field of irradiation, with proximal and distal arterial anatomy appearing normal. Giant cell arteritis of the axillary or brachial arteries has unique characteristics, including long, smooth, tapered narrowing of arterial segments with interspersed areas of normal-caliber arteries. There is an absence of ulceration or plaque suggestive of atherosclerosis. Buerger's disease is characterized by abundant collaterals (described as spider leg configurations) associated with radial, ulnar, or digital artery stenosis or occlusion and by the absence of atherosclerotic changes in the proximal large arteries.[27] In the small and medium-sized arteries affected by Buerger's disease there is a smooth taper to an occluded segment, interspersed between segments with recanalized distal arteries, giving a corkscrew appearance. Arteriography of the palmar arch and digital arteries is very important in mapping any occlusive lesions at this level. Collagen vascular and systemic diseases are frequently associated with digital artery stenosis or occlusions. Patients with vasospastic Raynaud's syndrome demonstrate no arterial stenosis or occlusions on angiography.

SURGICAL INTERVENTION FOR CHRONIC UPPER EXTREMITY ISCHEMIA

Large Arteries (Innominate/Subclavian)

Surgical intervention for symptomatic atherosclerotic disease of the aortic arch and brachycephalic arteries is largely determined by the disease pattern. Patients with disease limited to a single vessel (e.g., subclavian or innominate) are optimally treated with an extrathoracic reconstructive procedure.[5,32] Crawford et al.[32] reported that 25 percent of the patients in

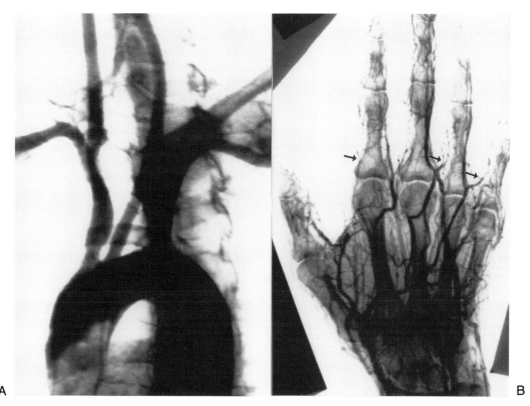

A
B

Figure 31-2 Aortic arch and upper extremity arteriogram of a patient with Raynaud's syndrome, digital ischemia, and a history of scleroderma reveals no significant disease of the aortic arch (**A**). The arteriogram of the hand (**B**) shows severe digital artery occlusive disease *(arrows)* due to the connective tissue disease. The patient was successfully treated by a nonsurgical approach.

Table 31-2 Frequency of Normal Anatomic Variations of Upper Extremity Arteries

Subclavian Artery	
Anomalous origin from the aortic arch	2%
Axillary/brachial/radial/ulnar arteries	
High origin of radial artery	14%
From axillary artery	12%
From brachial artery	2%
High origin of ulnar artery	3%
Palmar Arch	
Complete palmar arch	80%
Ulnar and radial artery origin	36%
Ulnar artery origin only	37%
Other	7%
Incomplete palmar arch	20%
Radial and ulnar artery origin	3%
Ulnar artery origin only	13%
Other	4%

(Data from Erlandson et al.[30] and Yao et al.[31])

their operative experience required bypass of more than one of the great vessels. In diffuse arch disease an adequate inflow vessel for an extrathoracic procedure may not be present, and treatment must be via a direct transthoracic approach. The first reconstructive procedure reported for atherosclerotic aortic arch disease involved multiple aortic arch vessels a prosthetic bifurcated graft being implanted in the ascending thoracic aorta and anastomosed to the innominate and right common carotid arteries.[33]

Extrathoracic reconstruction is, in general, preferred treatment because of equivalent graft patency, relief of symptoms, and a lower morbidity as compared with direct, transthoracic endarterectomy or bypass. A number of extrathoracic revascularization procedures have been described, including carotid-subclavian, carotid-carotid, subclavian-subclavian, axilloaxillary, and femoroaxillary bypass. Transposition of the subclavian artery to the adjacent common carotid artery is another option for patients with proximal subclavian occlusive disease. Carotid-subclavian bypass is the most frequently performed procedure for orificial arch vessel disease and the preferred procedure for patients with isolated subclavian artery occlusion or stenosis. The mortality rate associated with this procedure is approximately 1 to 2 percent.[34,35] Stroke occurs with an incidence of approximately 1 percent in patients with concomitant atherosclerotic disease involving carotid artery bifurcation.[32,34] Less common complications of carotid-subclavian bypass include phrenic nerve injury, thoracic duct disruption, and injury to sympathetic chain resulting in Horner's syndrome.

The low (approximately 1 to 2 percent) but disastrous morbidity of infection involving extrathoracic bypass grafts has prompted some surgeons to use only autogenous tissue. An autogenous tissue bypass is possible either by using the saphenous vein as a conduit for the carotid-subclavian bypass or by transposition of the subclavian artery to the adjacent common carotid artery. The transposition procedure is more technically demanding and requires a disease-free common carotid artery for inflow. For these reasons this procedure is not preferred by most surgeons, but long-term patency rates are equivalent to those of the carotid-subclavian bypass.[5] The preferred conduit (saphenous vein versus prosthetic graft) for a carotid-subclavian bypass is controversial.[35,36] Gerety et al.[36] reported no failures when carotid-subclavian bypasses were constructed by using a Dacron graft, but 5 of the 12 carotid-subclavian bypasses performed with saphenous vein thrombosed within the first year. Further confirmation of the inferior patency of saphenous veins is required since this result is at variance with other reports and may be related to technical factors such as vein quality and diameter.

Alternative extrathoracic surgical approaches to bypass of a left subclavian artery occlusion or stenosis include subclavian-subclavian, axilloaxillary, and femoroaxillary bypass. All are associated with a perioperative mortality rate of less than 5 percent. Long-term graft patency rates of subclavian-subclavian (95 percent) and axilloaxillary (76 to 100 percent) are equivalent to those reported for carotid-subclavian bypass. The femoroaxillary bypass had a lower long-term patency in the few cases reported.[34] The primary advantage of the alternative extrathoracic bypass procedures over carotid-subclavian bypass is a reduced risk of phrenic nerve or thoracic duct injury. However, injury to the brachial plexus can still occur and has been reported in as many as 10 percent of patients following axilloaxillary bypasses.[34] In addition, these bypasses have an increased risk of graft infection (4.1 percent) as compared with carotid-subclavian bypasses. The anatomic location of the bypass graft can also complicate management of patients who in the future may require median sternotomy for coronary artery bypass grafting

or tracheotomy. For the above reasons the alternative extrathoracic bypasses are not preferred over carotid-subclavian bypass, but they should be considered in selected high-risk patients in whom a carotid-subclavian bypass cannot be performed because of combined left common carotid and left subclavian artery occlusive disease or innominate artery occlusive disease.

Patients with symptomatic innominate artery stenosis or occlusion or with combined left common carotid and subclavian artery occlusion are not candidates for carotid-subclavian bypass because of inadequate inflow to both the carotid and subclavian arteries on the same side of the neck. Poor-risk patients with this unilateral, multifocal disease distribution are best treated with subclavian-subclavian, axilloaxillary, or carotid-carotid bypass graft (Fig. 31-3). In good-risk patients, however, the preferred treatment of innominate artery lesions or combined left common carotid and left subclavian artery lesions is a transthoracic arterial reconstructive procedure. Acceptable surgical approaches include endarterectomy or bypass grafting of the aortic arch vessels.[5,32] Innominate artery endarterectomy is reserved for patients who have disease limited to the distal innominate artery, which permits innominate artery clamping for proximal control and thus avoids potential injury to the aortic arch. Innominate artery endarterectomy and patch graft angioplasty was reported in eight cases by Crawford et al.[32] and in five cases by Zelenock et al.[5] with a low (< 5 percent) mortality and stroke rate and uniform long-term patency.

Patients who have occlusive lesions that involve the origins of the great vessels and the aortic arch are best treated with a transthoracic bypass procedure. In general, an 8- or 10-mm diameter knitted Dacron graft from the ascending aorta is anastomosed to one of the recipient vessels. A second tube graft is then placed end-to-side with respect to the first tube graft in the neck and anastomosed to other recipient outflow arteries. The use of this technique, as opposed to a prefabricated bifurcation graft, avoids tracheal compression and vein compression from the dual limbs exiting the mediastinum above the sternal notch.[32] The transthoracic procedures for aortic arch reconstruction have a less than 5 percent mortality and stroke rate.[5,32,34,35] The long-term patency rates, with a mean follow-up of 7.5 years, are higher than 80 percent,[32] and approximately 95 percent of patients experience relief of upper extremity symptoms. Recurrence of symptoms is typically due to new atherosclerotic lesions of the brachycephalic vessels rather than to graft occlusion.[5,32]

Patients with complex aortic arch lesions often have associated atherosclerotic lesions involving the carotid bifurcation or the vertebral or coronary arteries that

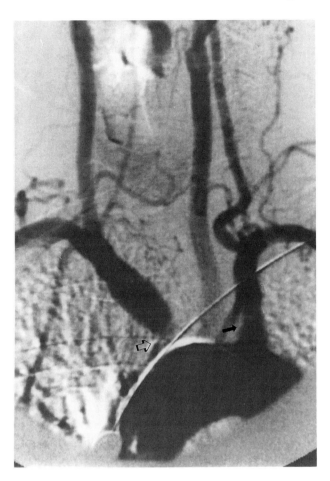

Figure 31-3 The arch aortogram of a high-risk patient with chronic right upper extremity ischemia and recurrent transient ischemic attacks of the right cerebral hemisphere demonstrated a 90 percent stenosis of the innominate artery *(open arrow)* and a 30 percent stenosis of the left subclavian artery *(closed arrow)*. The right carotid bifurcation and left common carotid artery had no significant disease. Possible surgical options include extrathoracic carotid-carotid bypass graft or a transthoracic aortic arch-to-carotid bypass. Occlusive disease of the proximal left subclavian artery precludes an extrathoracic subclavian or axillary artery bypass. Innominate artery endarterectomy is not indicated because the disease involves the proximal artery.

merit surgical treatment (Fig. 31-4). Performance of carotid endarterectomy or coronary artery bypass simultaneously with an extrathoracic or transthoracic aortic arch reconstruction causes no increase in the mortality and morbidity rates.[5,32] Crawford et al.[32] have reported long-term results of 37 patients who underwent simultaneous surgical treatment of aortic arch lesions and carotid or coronary artery disease with only one death. Chronic upper extremity ischemia due to macroembolism or microembolism from an aortic

arch vessel lesion is best treated with bypass graft and ligation of the vessel proximal to the distal graft anastomosis. Isolated left subclavian artery lesions that cause atheroemboli are best treated by carotid-subclavian bypass, with ligation of the subclavian artery proximal to the left vertebral artery. Lesions of the innominate artery that cause embolization can be treated with extrathoracic or transthoracic bypass grafts, with ligation of the proximal artery to prevent further potential for embolization. Innominate artery endarterectomy can also be effective in removing the embolic source when the disease involves only the distal artery.[32,37] Treatment of distal embolization from a true or false aneurysm of the subclavian artery or an aberrant right subclavian artery entails resection or bypass of the diseased artery.[38] Depending on the size and location of the subclavian artery aneurysm, the surgical approach may require a median sternotomy, left thoracotomy, or supraclavicular or subclavicular incision (Fig. 31-5). Aneurysms of branches of the major upper extremity arteries can be treated by ligation.[14] Treatment of an aberrant right subclavian artery can be by transposition of the right subclavian artery to the right common carotid artery via an extrathoracic procedure.

Surgical treatment of patients in the acute inflammatory stage of Takayasu's disease should be avoided. Patients with symptomatic chronic upper extremity ischemia, especially those with associated hypertension, beyond the acute inflammatory stage are best treated with surgical bypass grafting. The surgical approach may require an intrathoracic or extrathoracic approach, but a distal end-to-end arterial anastomosis is always the preferred method.[7] Patients with lesions isolated to a single subclavian or proximal common carotid artery can be treated with a carotid-subclavian bypass, and those with multiple aortic arch vessels diseased by nonspecific aortoarteritis are best treated by transthoracic bypass grafting. Endarterectomy should practically never be used for treatment of Takayasu's disease. Extrathoracic and transthoracic vascular reconstructions of aortic arch lesions due to Takayasu's disease are performed with less than 5 percent morbidity and mortality and a greater than 80 percent long-term patency and with excellent relief of symptoms.[5,32]

Patients with thoracic outlet syndrome as the etiology of chronic ischemic symptoms of the upper extremity are usually best treated with first and/or cervical rib resection. If there is evidence of intraluminal thrombus or peripheral embolism, repair of the arterial dilatation or aneurysm by resection and reconstruction should be performed concomitantly, with first rib resection and excision of fibrous ligaments or cervical rib, if present. Surgical reconstruction may require placement of an interposition graft, and in such cases auto-

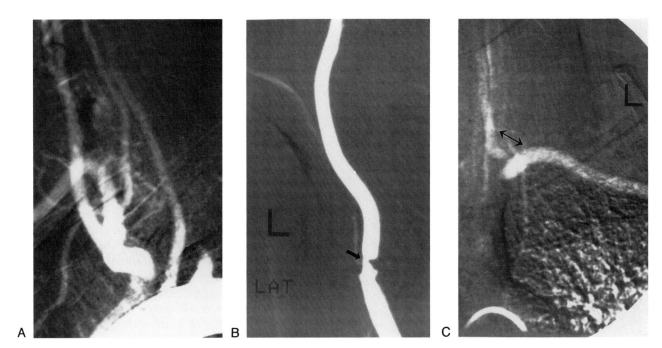

Figure 31-4 Arteriogram of a patient with **(A)** left arm claudication and dizziness due to proximal left subclavian artery occlusion *(open arrow)*, **(B)** 80 percent stenosis of the left internal carotid artery with an occluded external carotid artery *(closed arrow)*, and **(C)** retrograde flow in the left vertebral artery with delayed imaging of the left subclavian artery *(double-headed arrow)*. The patient was successfully treated with left carotid endarterectomy and carotid-subclavian bypass by using a segment of greater saphenous vein, which was opened longitudinally for a short distance at the carotid anastomosis for patch closure following endarterectomy.

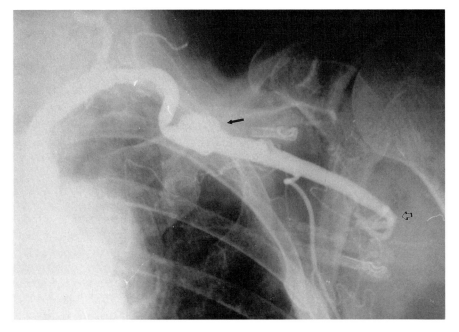

Figure 31-5 Arteriogram of a patient with a several-day history of left upper extremity ischemia, demonstrating subclavian artery aneurysm *(closed arrow)* and occlusion of the axillary artery due to embolization *(open arrow)*. The false aneurysm of the subclavian artery developed as a result of an unrecognized arterial injury following an automobile accident several years before. The patient was successfully treated with aneurysm resection via a subclavicular approach, (expanded polytetrafluoroethylene) interposition bypass graft, and embolectomy of the axillary artery.

genous saphenous vein is preferred over prosthetic material.[39] Patients with the thoracic outlet syndrome who have mild poststenotic dilatation (to less than twice the normal artery diameter) of the subclavian artery *and* no intraluminal thrombus or history of embolization can be effectively treated by first rib and/or cervical rib resection alone.[9] This surgical approach is based upon the fact that progression of subclavian artery disease is halted by correction of thoracic outflow abnormality.

Medium-Sized Arteries (Axillary/Brachial)

The surgical approach to lesions of the axillary and brachial arteries usually requires bypass grafting of the occluded arterial segments. The delayed recognition of arterial thrombosis following transarterial catheter injury, direct penetrating or blunt trauma, or macroembolism typically prohibits direct arterial repair or thromboembolectomy, making bypass grafting the preferred method of revascularization.[11,40] As in the case of chronic lower extremity ischemia, autogenous saphenous vein is the conduit of choice for upper extremity bypass grafting of axillary and brachial artery occlusive lesions. The graft may originate from the carotid, subclavian, axillary, or proximal brachial artery above the stenotic or occluded arterial segment. Bypasses to the brachial, radial, ulnar, and interosseous arteries have been successfully performed. Bypass grafts or cephalic or basilic vein using either reversed or in situ techniques have been reported.[11,34,40,41]

Upper extremity bypass grafting has a low (1 percent) mortality rate and good long-term patency. Gross et al,[11] reported no deaths for 27 axillary and brachial artery bypasses, but 3 of the 27 vein bypasses (11 percent) thrombosed in the early postoperative period, and late graft failures were observed. In a series of 33 bypass grafts for hand and forearm ischemia, McCarthy et al.[40] reported 2- and 3-year cumulative patency rates of 73 and 67 percent, respectively. Late patency was found to correlate with the level of the distal anastomoses, which was similar to the outcome following lower extremity bypass grafting. The 2-year patency rate for grafts to the brachial artery was 83 percent, compared with a 53 percent patency rate for grafts anastomosed to forearm arteries. Major upper extremity amputation was rarely required even after failure of the bypass graft.[11,40] In the one-quarter of patients who developed chronic upper extremity ischemia as a result of arterial trauma,[42] surgical intervention was associated with relief of symptoms and acceptable early and late graft patency.

Other uncommon causes of upper extremity ischemia that should be managed surgically include embolization from the occluded portion of an axillofemoral graft and brachial artery entrapment or compression following a supracondylar fracture of the humerus. The former problem should be treated by disconnection of the thrombosed axillofemoral graft and patch reconstruction of the subclavian or axillary artery.[15,16] Bony compression of the brachial artery after humerus fracture is best treated by removing the impinging bone, callous, or tendon.[12,13] The brachial artery entrapment syndrome that is due to a congenital anomaly of the supracondylar process is successfully treated by division of the fascial bands and resection of the supracondylar process.

Radiation-induced axillary and brachial artery stenotic or occlusive lesions are best treated with vein bypass grafts.[12,17] The arterial wall abnormalities are usually limited to the field of irradiation, which permits bypass from normal proximal arteries to the brachial, radial, or ulnar arteries that are outside the irradiation field. An autologous graft with vein harvested outside the field of irradiation is the conduit of choice. The greater saphenous vein is most commonly used. Tunneling of the bypass graft outside the field of irradiation, which avoids skin ulcerations or wound healing problems in the irradiated tissue, is optimal.

For patients with giant cell arteritis, surgery has a very limited role. The most effective treatment is steroid administration. Surgical intervention with bypass procedures is questionably indicated for those patients who have persistence of severe ischemia even after adequate steroid therapy. Successful upper extremity bypass grafts for giant cell arteritis have been reported, but in the majority of patients results have been extremely disappointing.[18,26] In patients with giant cell arteritis, surgical intervention is usually in the form of a temporal artery biopsy for diagnostic purposes.

Small Arteries (Radial/Ulnar/Digital)

Surgical intervention has a very limited role, if any, for patients with chronic upper extremity ischemia due to distal (small artery) occlusion. Cervical sympathectomy in patients with Raynaud's syndrome and digital ulceration has resulted in documented short-term benefit, with the least symptomatic patients perceiving the most benefit. However, recurrence of Raynaud's symptoms or of digital ulcerations is common. Similarly, attempts at arterial reconstruction for hand ischemia due to collagen vascular digital occlusive disease have given dismal results.[19,43] Overall, the response of the Raynaud's symptoms or digital ulcers to surgical intervention has not differed significantly from the response to medical management by local hand care and use of pharmacologic agents. The majority of patients can be effectively managed with a regimen of meticulous skin care and the avoidance of vasospasm (Table 31-3). Digital ulcers frequently heal with the use of topical antibiotics and dressing changes. Nifedipine (30 to 60 mg/day), the current drug of choice, can improve the Raynaud's symptoms in 50 to 60 percent of patients. Occasionally, sympatholytic agents, such as a combination of guanethidine (10 mg/day) and prazosin (1 to 2 mg/day), are needed for symptomatic relief. Surgical intervention for Raynaud's syndrome should be limited to those patients with a proximal source as the etiology.

Chronic upper extremity ischemia due to the delayed recognition of trauma or microembolism to the radial, ulnar, or digital arteries and ulnar artery thrombosis or aneurysm can be successfully treated with vein bypass of the injured artery or removal of the embolus source. For example, thrombosis of the ulnar artery due to repetitive trauma is best treated by vein bypass with proximal and distal arterial anastomoses to normal, nontraumatized artery.[23,44] Similarly, digital embolization from an ulnar artery aneurysm should be treated by aneurysm resection and interposition vein grafting of the ulnar artery. Clark et al.[24] have reported uniform graft patency and digital amputation rates with average 7-year follow-up following surgical intervention for this condition. A key predictor to the success of these distal revascularizations was the presence of a patent palmar arch for arterial runoff as documented by arteriography. Advances in microvascular surgical techniques can yield excellent early and long-term results of treatment of hand ischemia at the radial, ulnar, or digital anatomic level for specific indications and etiologies.

The surgical approach to patients with chronic upper extremity ischemia resulting from arterial thrombosis due to a hypercoagulable state is extremely challenging because of the extensive thrombosis that can develop in the upper extremity arterial tree. Patients with a viable upper extremity and no symptoms of critical limb ischemia are best treated with long-term oral anticoagulants to prevent recurrent arterial thrombosis.[25] Thrombolytic therapy or direct surgical thrombectomy should be attempted in patients with limb- or digit-threatening ischemia.

Surgical intervention also has a limited role in patients with thromboangiitis obliterans (Buerger's disease). Bypass grafting has been associated with an early failure rate of 50 percent or greater due to poor outflow.[20] The treatment of digital ulcerations of the upper extremity with thoracic or cervical sympathectomy is also of questionable benefit. Ohta et al.[20] reported 66 thoracic sympathectomies in 58 patients with 15 ulcer recurrences (26 percent) as compared with the total group, in which 148 (45 percent) of 328 patients had ulceration on more than one occasion. However, the number of patients in each group who continued to smoke after treatment was not given. In addition, the amputation rate in this series was only 1.7 percent. Mills et al.[27] reported a series of patients with upper extremity ischemia due to Buerger's disease among whom no sympathectomies were performed and no major upper extremity amputations were required. The most effective treatment of patients with chronic upper extremity ischemia due to Buerger's disease is smoking cessation and local skin care.

SUMMARY

In summary, surgical intervention for chronic upper extremity ischemia depends on the severity of presenting symptoms, its etiology, and the anatomic level of the arterial disease. A thorough history, physical examination, noninvasive vascular evaluation, and arteriography are essential to establish the proper diagnosis and formulate a treatment plan. Direct surgical repair or bypass of large or medium artery lesions is associated with a low morbidity and mortality and excellent long-term patency and limb salvage rates. The role of surgery is much more limited in the treatment of ischemia produced by arteritis, collagen vascular disease, connective tissue disorders, and other nonatherosclerotic arteriopathies. Endovascular techniques, such as balloon angioplasty or stenting, intra-arterial thrombolysis, or other forms of intra-arterial pharmacotherapy have a definite role in patients with chronic upper extremity ischemia, particularly in the treatment of acute exacerbations.

Table 31-3 Principles of the Nonsurgical Approach to Patients With Vasospastic and Occlusive Disorders of the Digital Arteries

Stop smoking
Avoid cold temperatures
Meticulous care of hands
Topical moisturizing agents
Topical antibiotics to ulcers
Calcium channel blocker (nifedipine)
Sympatholytic agent (guanethidine, prazosin)

REFERENCES

1. Machleder HI: Vascular Disorders of the Upper Extremity. 2nd Ed. Futura Publishing, New York, 1989
2. McNamara MF, Takaki HS, YAO JST et al: A systematic approach to severe hand ischemia. Surgery 83:1, 1978
3. Harris RW, Andros G, Dulawa LB et al: Large-vessel arterial occlusive disease in symptomatic upper extremity. Arch Surg 119:1277, 1984
4. Pearce WH, Yao JST: Upper extremity ischemia: overview. Semin Vasc Surg 3:207, 1990
5. Zelenock GB, Cronenwett JL, Graham LM et al: Brachycephalic arterial occlusions and stenosis. Arch Surg 120:370, 1985
6. Akers DL, Fowl RJ, Plettner J et al: Complications of anomalous origin of the right subclavian artery: case report and review of the literature. Ann Vasc Surg 5:385, 1991
7. Pokrovsky AV: Nonspecific aortoarteritis. p. 217. In Rutherford RB (ed): Vascular Surgery. 3rd Ed. WB Saunders, Philadelphia, 1989
8. Machleder HI: Thoracic outlet disorders: thoracic outlet compression syndrome and axillary vein thrombosis. p. 687. In Wilson SE, Veith FJ, Hobson RW (eds): Vascular Surgery. Principles and Practice. McGraw-Hill, New York, 1987
9. Scher LA, Veith FJ, Samson RH et al: Vascular complications of thoracic outlet syndrome J Vasc Surg 3:565, 1986
10. Melliere D, Yahia NEB, Etienne G et al: Thoracic outlet syndrome caused by tumor of the first rib. J Vasc Surg 14:235, 1991
11. Gross WS, Flanigan DP, Kraft RO et al: Chronic upper extremity arterial insufficiency. Etiology, manifestations, and operative management. Arch Surg 113:419, 1978
12. Holleman JH Jr, Hardy JD, Williamson JW et al: Arterial surgery for arm ischemia. A survey of 136 patients. Ann Surg 191:727, 1980
13. Talha H, Enon B, Chavalier JM et al: Brachial artery entrapment: compression by the supracondylar process. Ann Vasc Surg 1:479, 1986
14. Nijhuis HHAM, Muller-Wiefel H: Occlusion of the brachial artery by thrombus dislodged from a traumatic aneurysm of the anterior humeral circumflex artery. J Vasc Surg 13:408, 1991
15. Khalil IM, Hoballah JJ: Late upper extremity embolic complications of occluded axillofemoral grafts. Ann Vasc Surg 5:375, 1991
16. Bandyk DF, Thiele BL, Radke HM: Upper extremity emboli secondary to axillofemoral bypass grafts. Arch Surg 116:393, 1981
17. Kretschmer G, Niederle B, Polterauer P et al: Irradiation-induced changes in the subclavian and axillary arteries after radiotherapy for carcinoma of the breast. Surgery 99:658, 1986
18. Rivers SP, Baur GM, Inahara T et al: Arm ischemia secondary to giant cell arteritis. Am J Surg 143:554, 1982
19. Rivers SP, Porter JM: Raynaud's syndrome, upper extremity vasospastic disorders, and small artery occlusive disease. p. 696. In Wilson SE, Veith FJ, Hobson RW (eds): Vascular Surgery: Principles and Practice. McGraw-Hill, New York, 1987
20. Ohta T, Shionoya S: Fate of the ischemic limb in Buerger's disease. Br J Surg 75:259, 1988
21. Yao JST: Arterial surgery of upper extremity. p. 853. In Haimovici H (ed): Vascular Surgery. Principles and Techniques. 3rd Ed. Appleton & Lange, East Norwalk, CT, 1989
22. McGee GS, Pearce WH, McCarthy WJ et al: Hand ischemia. Semin Vasc Surg 3:242, 1990
23. Koman JA, Urbaniak JR: Ulnar artery insufficiency: a guide to treatment. J Hand Surg 6:16, 1981
24. Clark ET, Mass DP, Bassiouny HS et al: True aneurysmal disease in the hand and upper extremity. Ann Vasc Surg 5:276, 1991
25. Towne JB, Hussey CV, Bandyk DF: Abnormalities of the fibrinolytic system as a cause of upper extremity ischemia: a preliminary report. J Vasc Surg 7:661, 1988
26. Shionoya S: Buerger's disease (thromboangiitis obliterans). p. 207. In Rutherford RB (ed): Vascular Surgery. 3rd Ed. WB Saunders, Philadelphia, 1989
27. Mills JL, Taylor LM, Porter JM: Buerger's disease in the modern era. Am J Surg 154:123, 1987
28. Machleder HI: Vascular disease of the upper extremity and the thoracic outlet syndrome. P. 683. In Moore WS (ed): Vascular Surgery, A Comprehensive Review. 2nd Ed. Grune & Stratton, Orlando, 1986
29. Sumner DS: Noninvasive assessment of upper extremity and hand ischemia. J Vasc Surg 3:560, 1986
30. Erlandson EE, Forrest ME, Shields et al: Discriminant arteriographic criteria in the management of forearm and hand ischemia. Surgery 90:1025, 1981
31. Yao JST, Bergan JJ, Nieman HL: Arteriography for upper extremity and digital ischemia. In Nieman HL, Yao JST (eds): Angiography of Vascular Disease. Churchill Livingstone, New York, 1985
32. Crawford ES, Stowe CL, Powers RW Jr: Occlusion of the innominate, common carotid, and subclavian arteries: long-term results of surgical treatment. Surgery 94:781, 1983
33. DeBakey ME, Morris GC Jr, Jordan GL Jr et al: Segmental thrombo-obliterative disease of branches of aortic arch. JAMA 166:988, 1958
34. Whitehouse WM Jr, Zelenock GB, Wakefield TW et al: Arterial bypass grafts for upper extremity ischemia. J Vasc Surg 3:569, 1986
35. Provan JL: Arteriosclerotic occlusive arterial disease of brachycephalic and arch vessels p. 822. In Rutherford RB (ed): Vascular Surgery. 3rd Ed. WB Saunders, Philadelphia, 1989
36. Gerety RL, Andrus CH, May AG et al: Surgical treatment of occlusive subclavian artery disease. Circulation 64:228, 1981
37. Carlson RE, Ehrenfeld WK, Stoney RJ et al: Innominate artery endarterectomy. A 16-year experience. Arch Surg 112:1389, 1977

38. Roland CF, Cherry KJ Jr: Symptomatic atherosclerotic stenotic disease of an aberrant right subclavian artery. Ann Vasc Surg 5:196, 1991

39. Kieffer E, Ruotolo C: Arterial complications of thoracic outlet compression. p. 875. In Rutherford RB (ed): Vascular Surgery. 3rd Ed. WB Saunders, Philadelphia, 1989

40. McCarthy WJ, Flynn WR, Yao JST et al: Result of bypass grafting for upper limb ischemia. J Vasc Surg 3:741, 1986

41. Guzman-Stein G, Shubert W, Najarian DW et al: Composite in situ vein bypass for upper extremity revascularization. Plast Reconstr Surg 83:533, 1989

42. Braga PEG, Salgado AA, Zorn WGW et al: Course of the post-catheterization pulseless arm. J Cardiovasc Surg 25:236, 1984

43. Porter JM, Bardana EM, Baur GM et al: The clinical significance of Raynaud's syndrome. Surgery 80:756, 1976

44. Silcott GR, Polich VA: Palmar arch arterial reconstruction for the salvage of ischemic fingers. Am J Surg 142:219, 1981

32

Thrombolysis and Angioplasty in Upper Extremity Arterial Disease

Joseph Bonn

Michael C. Soulen

And with thy bloody and invisible hand,
Cancel and tear to pieces that great bond
Which keeps me pale!

William Shakespeare
Macbeth

Occlusive vascular disease of the upper extremity poses a particularly compelling clinical problem, since it occurs infrequently relative to lower extremity occlusive disease, reflects a somewhat different spectrum of etiologies, and has the potentially serious effect on lifestyle associated with functional compromise of the hand. The infrequency with which upper extremity arterial diseases are encountered and the broad range of underlying conditions that may contribute to their significance have resulted in a dearth of large-scale studies, either of the predisposing disorders or of the role of percutaneous vascular interventions such as thrombolysis and angioplasty in their management. The impact on a patient's quality of life caused by the loss of a fully functional arm and the unique sensory and motor functions of the hand, as compared with the loss of

ambulation sustained in lower extremity vascular disease, also sets these clinical entities apart.

Upper extremity occlusive arterial disorders can be divided into two large groups: those occurring commonly, such as atherosclerosis, thromboembolism (a manifestation of a host of underlying diseases), thoracic outlet syndrome, and trauma (both blunt and penetrating); and those occurring less commonly, such as aortoarteritis (Takayasu's arteritis), fibromuscular dysplasia, radiation arteritis, ergotism, and tumors, as well as the category of medium-small artery diseases occupied by thromboangiitis obliterans (Buerger's), Raynaud's disease, autoimmune/collagen vascular disorders, and chronic occupational trauma. The interventional vascular techniques of thrombolysis and angioplasty play significant but substantially different roles in the management of these disorders. Their relationship to well established surgical treatments is an evolving one and is the subject of continuing debate as improvements develop in percutaneous methods and as long-term data on their applications accumulate. This chapter focuses separately on each of these interventional modalities and the upper extremity occlusive arterial disorders that it treats; it reviews issues of patient evaluation and patient selection, outlines technique, and discusses published results.

THROMBOLYSIS

Thrombolysis, as one of several options in the treatment of peripheral occlusive arterial disease, has increasingly gained favor both as a primary treatment modality and as an adjunct to surgical treatments such as thromboembolectomy and bypass. The less invasive approach of regional thrombolysis and the ability of lytic agents to recanalize even the smallest peripheral vessels not only make it possible to restore flow in vessels too small to be thromboembolectomized but in so doing may reveal the underlying causative disorders and thereby lead to definitive treatment, while avoiding the potential deleterious effects of the balloon thromboembolectomy catheter on the arterial wall. Thrombolysis in the upper extremity carries with it a unique set of conditions; the wide-ranging list of possible underlying disorders, the proximity of catheters and thrombus to the cerebral vessel origins, the tendency of upper extremity arteries to vasospasm, and the limited tolerance for expansion in the fascial compartments of the forearm distinguish lytic therapy in the upper extremity from its counterpart in the lower extremity.

Etiologies

Upper extremity arterial occlusive disease can be concisely organized into three categories: embolic, traumatic, and manifestation of an underlying arterial disease.[1] Emboli to the upper extremity are much less common than to the lower extremity: one study of over 2000 cases of systemic emboli found them to involve the upper extremity in only 15 percent, whereas a smaller review of 25 extremity embolic cases found only 3 (12 percent) to involve the upper extremity.[2,3] Patients with upper extremity emboli characteristically present with acute onset of ischemic symptoms. Frequently no previous history of significant arm ischemia can be elicited. Often, however, there is a history of embolic episodes elsewhere, such as strokes, and a history of underlying heart disease, especially arrhythmias, previous myocardial infarction, or left ventricular aneurysm. Accurate diagnosis is critical in these patients since they may be at increased risk for future embolic episodes, they may require long-term anticoagulation, and any remaining thrombus at the source may eliminate them from consideration for thrombolysis.

Emboli to the upper extremity most commonly originate in the heart. Other sources include atheromata in the thoracic aortic arch, subclavian and axillary artery atherosclerotic lesions, and very rarely, paradoxical sources. Cardiac emboli are most commonly associated with atrial fibrillation; recent myocardial infarction, left ventricular mural thrombus, valvular disease, and bacterial endocarditis are less frequent associations.[1] Noncardiac emboli can originate in primary atherosclerotic lesions, post-traumatic subclavian-axillary pseudoaneurysms, aneurysms related to thoracic outlet syndrome, or the exposed thrombus at the axillary artery origin of a thrombosed axillofemoral bypass graft.[4-9]

When emboli travel to the upper extremity, they enter the brachiocephalic or subclavian artery and lodge at a point at which there is an abrupt change in caliber of the brachial artery at the trifurcation into the radial, ulnar, and interosseous arteries. Consequently, approximately 65 percent of emboli are found in the brachial artery, with 30 percent in the axillary artery and 5 percent in the subclavian artery. The source of the embolic material will influence the composition of the embolus; a cardiac embolus is a mixture of acute and organized chronic thrombus, and a noncardiac embolus is either thrombus (acute, chronic, or mixed) or a combination of atherosclerotic plaque and thrombus. This has important implications for treatment, since those emboli composed of organized thrombus and plaque are less likely to resolve with thrombolysis alone.

The traumatic causes of upper extremity thrombosis include penetrating trauma such as gunshot wounds and stabbings, intra-arterial injections of drugs (both self-administered and iatrogenic), and blunt trauma such as fractures and dislocations in all their permutations. An additional form of blunt trauma to be considered is chronic occupational trauma; in this case the unprotected segment of the ulnar artery impinges on the hook of the hamate, which leads to the hypothenar hammer syndrome. This repetitive blunt trauma results in aneurysm formation or ulnar artery thrombosis, with the aneurysm occasionally serving as a source of digital emboli.[10,11] The most common traumatic cause of upper extremity arterial thromboembolic disease, however, is iatrogenic, related to axillary and brachial artery catheterization for cardiac and peripheral angiography and to radial and brachial artery catheterization for pressure and oxygen monitoring.

Upper extremity arterial thromboembolism caused by an underlying or intrinsic vascular disorder covers a wide range of conditions, including failed surgical bypass grafts; atherosclerosis; connective tissue disorders such as scleroderma, giant cell arteritis, lupus, and

Takayasu's arteritis; an assortment of coagulation disorders; radiation vasculitis; drug toxicity (especially ergot alkaloids); and Buerger's disease.[12-18] While experience with lower extremity graft and atherosclerotic occlusions can often be translated to the upper extremity, optimal treatment mandates understanding and treating the underlying disorder as well as lysing the thombotic occlusion.

Scleroderma presents with a multifactorial propensity for vascular thrombosis; these factors include endothelial cell injury and coagulation alterations such as changes in plasminogen activators and plasminogen activator inhibitors. These changes occur in other rheumatic diseases as well, although without the severity usually seen in scleroderma.[12] Takayasu's arteritis is characterized by inflammatory changes in the media and adventitia, resulting in connective tissue proliferation and intimal thickening. The aorta and its proximal large branches and the pulmonary arteries are most commonly affected, and in the upper extremity one can find both long-segment stenoses and occlusions.[19]

Coagulation disorders, especially hypercoagulability, may account for a large number of unexplained thrombotic episodes. They are better understood when classified into primary and secondary hypercoagulable disorders.[13] Primary clinical conditions are those characterized by a clearly defined hemostasis abnormality, usually a congenital, fixed defect in the coagulation or fibrinolytic systems. These include antithrombin III deficiency; lupus anticoagulant; protein C and S deficiencies; and disorders of the fibrinolytic system, such as hypoplasminogenemia, abnormal plasminogen, plasminogen activator deficiency, factor XII deficiency, and dysfibrinogenemia. One of the most important of these primary disorders is antithrombin III deficiency, which may present as heparin resistance, thereby requiring an increased heparin dosage and occasionally fresh frozen plasma to prevent thrombosis during interventions. Another is lupus anticoagulant; patients with this disorder may benefit from preintervention treatment with steroids or antiplatelet agents, as well as from prolonged postintervention anticoagulation with heparin and warfarin. Patients with disorders of the fibrinolytic system such as diminished or abnormal plasminogen may be less likely to be helped by thrombolysis. They must be identified early in their care; suspicion should be raised by any patient with thrombosis of unusual location or extent beyond that expected from the injury or underlying disease, as well as an unusual number of previous arterial or venous thromboses.[14] These patients must undergo long-term anticoagulation with heparin and warfarin to preclude further thrombosis from the injury induced by the intervention.

Secondary hypercoagulability disorders can be classified by the origin of the abnormality, either as disorders of coagulation and fibrinolysis related to abnormal blood vessels and flow or as disorders of platelets.[13] Coagulation and fibrinolysis disorders include Trousseau's syndrome (the hypercoagulability associated with malignancy), pregnancy, oral contraceptive use, and the nephrotic syndrome. Blood vessel and flow abnormalities include venous stasis, presence of thrombus-inducing synthetic materials such as grafts, homocystinuria, hyperviscosity of blood, and thrombocytopenic thrombotic purpura. Platelet abnormalities include myeloproliferative disorders, paroxysmal nocturnal hemoglobinuria, hyperlipidemia, diabetes mellitus, and heparin-induced thrombocytopenia. The last is of particular importance since heparin administration to these patients not only results in thrombocytopenia but also can lead to thrombosis from a heparin-dependent antiplatelet antibody that accelerates platelet aggregation. Warfarin administration for 3 to 6 months is the effective alternative to heparin in these patients, but if thrombolysis is contemplated, the technique must consequently be adjusted.

Another underlying disorder that may manifest itself in upper extremity thrombosis is radiation-induced vasculitis, which is of particular concern in patients treated in the area of the subclavian and axillary arteries for breast cancer or lymphoma. A detailed history and knowledge of the treatment port is essential in evaluating these patients. Their presentation may vary with the length of time since irradiation: the first group may become symptomatic within 5 years, with simple mural thrombus at the exposed artery (occasionally embolizing to the digital arteries); the second group presents with fibrotic occlusion of the irradiated artery within 10 years of exposure; and the third group presents with more chronic changes (several decades after irradiation) from periarterial fibrosis and accelerated atherosclerosis.[15] Also to be considered are the combined effects in some patients of radiation-induced arterial injury and coexistent hypercoagulability, since these patients' risk of forming thrombus in the narrowed, fibrotic, and atherosclerotic artery is significantly increased.[16]

Arterial injury or spasm from drug toxicity usually results from complications of ergot alkaloids administered for migraine headaches, but in many locales it may also be induced by the intra-arterial injection of psychotropic drugs such as cocaine or heroin. Beyond their use in treating migraines, ergot alkaloids may be encountered as oxytocics for control of postpartum hemorrhage, as pressors to control postural hypotension, and in combination with heparin to reduce the incidence of deep venous thrombosis in high-risk patients. Arterial spasm from any medication may be reduced by oral calcium channel blockers such as nifedipine, intra-arterially administered nitroglycerin or tolazoline, and concomitant thrombolysis for any spasm-associated thrombosis.[17]

Buerger's disease, also known as thromboangiitis obliterans, may present with multiple segmental occlusions and high-grade stenoses of small peripheral arteries in the extremities, usually in patients with a history of heavy smoking and usually at a younger age than in the average patient with atherosclerosis. Distal arteries are affected more than larger proximal arteries, and thrombolysis is particularly indicated when these smaller vessels cannot be reached by embolectomy techniques. Treatment of the underlying small-vessel stenoses by small-balloon angioplasty after successful thrombolysis may preclude the need for high-risk distal surgical bypass.[18]

Patient Evaluation

The diversity of clinical conditions, both primary and secondary, that may result in upper extremity arterial thrombosis underscores the importance of a complete history and physical examination before considering more sophisticated evaluation. On the basis of this clinical information, decisions are made regarding imaging studies such as Doppler, echocardiography, magnetic resonance imaging (MRI), and angiography, in addition to the basic and sophisticated hematologic testing needed to establish the patient's coagulation status.

A systematic approach to the patient's history categorizes the ischemia by severity, vascular level, and extent. Determination of the timing and acuity of onset, as well as the existence of previous episodes or of associated vascular symptoms in the lower extremities or in the heart, will assist in the classification of the current episode. This in turn will direct the focus of the diagnostic workup and the subsequent therapy. The past medical history and review of systems should include investigations into trauma, cardiac disease, coagulation disorders, connective tissue disease, irradiation, previous vascular surgery, smoking, occupation, medications, and drug use. Potential contraindications to thrombolysis discovered at this point in the workup may include a history of recent myocardial infarction, stroke, bleeding episode, or surgery; a history of cardiac arrhythmia, valvular disease, or known cardiac thrombus; or a history of a hypercoagulable condition.

Physical examination of the upper extremity should focus on the extent of arterial insufficiency manifested by the loss of pulses and the degree and level of pallor and coolness, as well as on the severity of sensory and motor neurologic deficits. Palpation of bilateral axillary, brachial, radial, and ulnar pulses should be followed by an Allen's test to assess the relative degree of radial and ulnar artery inflow to the hand. A baseline neurologic examination is important if thrombolysis is to be initiated, for better evaluation of the patient at increased risk of cerebral thromboembolism owing to prolonged catheter placement across the great vessel origins or to cardiac thrombus fragmentation by circulating lytic agent.

Laboratory testing in the acute phase of diagnosis and treatment is devoted to evaluating simple parameters of the coagulation status such as prothrombin time (PT), activated partial thromboplastin time (aPTT), and platelet count. More specific indicators of coagulation disorders may take too long to obtain to influence the course of acute therapy, but their processing should begin as early as possible so that indications for longer-term therapy, such as anticoagulation with warfarin, can be determined. This is especially true if the pattern and extent of thrombosis or the history of repeated episodes raises the suspicion of a coexistent hypercoagulable state. Additional values such as serum creatinine and blood urea nitrogen may be helpful in assessing the patient's renal function and hydration status and in evaluating the relative risk of contrast medium exposure prior to the multiple arteriograms used to monitor thrombolysis. Baseline hemoglobin and hematocrit valves aid in the later evaluation of any hemorrhagic complications.

A Doppler study, utilizing both waveform analysis and imaging, may be helpful in assessing the location and extent of arterial disease and may assist in planning an intervention. In particular, vascular ultrasound imaging is helpful in detecting arterial aneurysms and pseudoaneurysms that may be obscured during arteriography by mural thrombus; it would be specifically indicated in a patient with a history of trauma or thoracic outlet syndrome.

Transthoracic echocardiography (TTE) is indicated when the emerging clinical picture points to an embolic etiology with the heart as a likely source, or when coexistent cardiac disease (arrhythmia, recent infarction, or valvular disease) raises the likelihood of cardiac thrombus being present and possibly increasing the risk of thrombolysis. A more invasive version, transesophageal echocardiography (TEE), has been shown to be more sensitive than TTE in detecting potential cardiac sources of emboli, such as left atrial appendage thrombus, left atrial thrombus, left ventricular apical thrombus, atrial septal defect (paradoxical emboli), and atrial septal aneurysm.[20] In one study a potential cardiac source of cerebral emboli was detected in 57 percent of patients by TEE, while TTE found such a source in only 15 percent of the study group. Of particular interest in this same study was the ability of TEE to detect a potential cardiac source in 39 percent of patients without clinical cardiac disease, while TTE found such sources in only 19 percent of the same group.[21] TEE was also shown in two other studies to detect atherosclerotic plaque protruding into the thoracic aortic arch. These unexpected findings in this relatively new technology raise the question of whether TEE should be performed prior to any upper extremity thrombolysis since it is more sensitive in detecting potential sources of emboli that may contraindicate this treatment.[5,6]

Arteriography remains the study of greatest yield in upper extremity arterial thrombosis, providing detailed information about the level and extent of the occlusion, the presence of collateral vessels, the size and condition of patent arteries, and often an impression as to whether the inciting insult was embolic or a result of in situ thrombosis.[7] Embolic disease, both the acute form and that resulting from chronic, repetitive embolization, often presents with discrete peripheral intraluminal filling defects, with poorly developed collateralization as compared with that seen with slowly progressive atherosclerosis.

Femoral access is most commonly used, as it carries the lowest risk of complications and is the route most familiar to angiographers; however, in rare circumstances such as severe aortoiliac disease the contralateral brachial or axillary approach may be safer to use for the diagnostic portion of the study. It is of utmost importance to begin with a thoracic aortogram to assess the aortic arch and the origin of the great vessels, especially the condition of the brachiocephalic and subclavian arteries. For investigation beyond these origins, the subclavian artery distal to the vertebral artery is selectively catheterized.

From this position, the arterial anatomy of the entire arm and hand is documented, with cut-film or digital technique depending on personal preference, the quality of the digital system, and contrast load considerations. The arm is placed in anatomic position or abducted at the shoulder to elicit changes from thoracic outlet syndrome. Particular attention must be paid to the presence of arterial anomalies, especially proximal origin of the radial artery, which is found in approximately 15 percent of cadaver studies, most commonly in the midbrachial position but occasionally in the high brachial or axillary artery. Other rare anomalies include proximal origin of the ulnar artery and the presence of superficial and accessory brachial arteries. Injections distal to anomalous origins can be mistakenly

interpreted as total occlusions of the anomalous branch.

Technical adjustments specific to the diagnostic evaluation of these occlusive cases include the frequent use of heparin-bonded catheters (Premier Biomedical, Woodlands, TX), both to decrease the risk of pericatheter thrombus formation in slow-flowing vessels and to decrease the risk of such thrombi embolizing to the cerebral vessels if the same catheter is used for thrombolysis and must rest across the origins of these vessels for a prolonged time. Arteriospasm can be reduced and visualization of collaterals and small digital arteries can be improved with gentle warming of the upper extremity and with aggressive vasodilatation, including pretreatment with calcium channel blockade (nifedipine, 10 mg sublingual) or with intra-arterial boluses of nitroglycerin (100-μg boluses, with attention to the systemic pressure) or tolazoline (15 to 25-mg boluses). Low-osmolar or nonionic contrast medium, especially in the dilute concentrations used in digital subtraction angiography, may be less painful to inject and may also reduce the incidence of significant arteriospasm. Magnification techniques, optimally requiring smaller focal spot tubes, considerably improve visualization of the most peripheral digital arteries, which is especially important in diagnosing small emboli and underlying small vessel disease.

Patient Selection

Determining the indications and contraindications of thrombolytic therapy in upper extremity arterial occlusive disease is in many ways similar to that in lower extremity disease. The decision hinges on a full knowledge of the patient's medical condition and of the etiology of the occlusion, as well as an awareness of the technical feasibility of the procedure and the pros and cons of alternative treatments. One must weigh the benefits of this less invasive therapy against its potential risks and the risks of conservative and surgical therapy.

One overview of patient selection proposes that thrombolysis is indicated in patients in whom the occlusion can be demonstrated, who are able to tolerate the potentially prolonged period of lysis, and who have no other contraindications.[22] The most important sign of a patient's ability to tolerate the pace of lytic therapy, which is slower than surgical thromboembolectomy, is the absence of significant sensory or motor neurologic deficits in the ischemic extremity (i.e., the absence of irreversible limb ischemia). Other absolute contraindications listed in Sullivan et al.'s report and in other reviews include stroke or transient ischemic attack within the last 6 months; major abdominal, thoracic or neurologic (including ophthalmologic) surgery within the last 2 months; recent gastrointestinal bleeding; severe impairment of liver function; and TTE evidence of left atrial or ventricular thrombus. Other authors propose as well that patients with recent penetrating trauma or vascular surgery in the ischemic limb may possess a relative contraindication, since they would incur a greater risk of hemorrhagic complications at the trauma or surgical site, and that patients with significant renal insufficiency may be at high risk for contrast-induced renal failure from the large, repetitive doses of contrast agent often required for the procedure.[23-28]

In patients with rapidly worsening sensory and motor deficits, the risk of irreversible ischemia developing during the several hours needed for thrombolysis is of great concern. Those patients who have already experienced prolonged and severe ischemia are also at greater risk for developing complications associated with revascularization of the extremity, including compartment syndromes (usually in the less forgiving forearm) caused by rhabdomyolysis or by thrombolysis-induced hemorrhage into the compartment. This potentially devastating syndrome is manifested primarily by pain (especially with passive stretching), swelling and tenderness, and loss of two-point discrimination. Recognition of a compartment syndrome, including determining forearm intracompartmental tissue pressures and acting on those greater than 30 mmHg by promptly decompressing the compartment with a fasciotomy, is vital to preserving limb function[29-32] (Fig. 32-1).

In the patient without any signs of irreversible ischemia, the suspected age of the thrombus (as estimated from the clinical history), while usually a general prognostic indicator for success, should not be a major factor in the selection criteria for thrombolysis. All patients without severe ischemic symptoms or other contraindications should undergo a trial of thrombolysis, which should include an attempt to recanalize the occlusion with conventional guidewire and catheter techniques, or if this fails, a less selective regional thrombolysis followed by a second, delayed attempt at guidewire and catheter recanalization.[22,33]

Technique

The primary goal of thrombolysis technique is to distribute the best lytic agent throughout the thrombus in the safest manner in order to produce the most effective combination of enzyme and substrate with the lowest risk of systemic complications. In addition, at the completion of thrombolysis one should be ready to

treat the uncovered cause or the underlying disease, with cooperative consultation of the vascular surgeon and the internist and with all available interventional, surgical, or medical techniques.

Experience in lower extremity regional thrombolysis has led most clinicians to choose urokinase (Abbokinase, from Abbott Laboratories, North Chicago, IL) as the lytic agent of choice for several reasons, including a very low incidence of induced allergic reactions, a low risk of systemic complications, and a rapid action. In addition, it has been shown in one study to achieve a greater therapeutic success rate and to be more cost-effective than streptokinase, while two other separate comparisons with streptokinase demonstrated urokinase to be successful more often and to cause significantly fewer major and minor hemorrhagic complications.[34-36] A comparison between recombinant tissue-type plasminogen activator and urokinase in a different study resulted in no significant difference in 30-day clinical success between the two agents, although there was a suggestion, not statistically significant, of fewer hemorrhagic complications in patients treated with urokinase.[26]

Initiation of thrombolysis may include systemic anticoagulation with heparin: a bolus of 3000 to 5000 units is followed by an infusion of between 800 and 1000 units per hour, depending on the patient's weight, to maintain the aPTT at approximately 1.5 to 2.0 times the control value for the duration of the procedure and often 12 to 24 hours beyond completion of thrombolysis, with checks of the aPTT every 6 hours to confirm the adequacy of the anticoagulation. Owing to their lack of sensitivity or specificity in predicting hemorrhagic complications, fibrinogen and fibrin split products are not followed routinely during thrombolysis.

The initial catheter approach for upper extremity thrombolysis commonly relies on the same femoral access and catheter used for the diagnostic portion of the procedure. The most optimal delivery of the lytic agent is directly into the thrombus and usually begins with crossing the occlusion by conventional guidewire and catheter technique; this can be performed with the original diagnostic catheter and a choice among several soft-tipped and torqueable 0.035- to 0.038-inch guidewires. The end-hole diagnostic catheter, once across the occlusion and confirmed to be in the distal lumen, is then withdrawn across the thrombus while a high-dose (usually 250,000 units) of urokinase is actively diffused throughout ("laced" into) the occlusion. This catheter is then positioned in the most proximal portion of the thrombus, whereupon the continuous infusion is begun. Follow-up arteriograms may be performed on a timed schedule or in response to changing clinical parameters. Our preference has been for a high-dose regi-

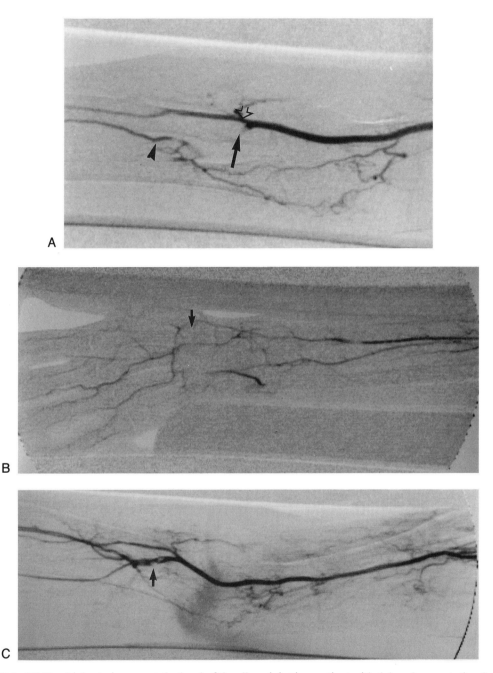

Figure 32-1 **(A)** Brachial arteriogram at the level of the elbow joint in a patient with delayed presentation 2 days after acute onset of upper extremity ischemia. Abrupt occlusion of the brachial artery *(closed arrow)* is demonstrated with continued patency of the radial artery due to its proximal origin *(open arrow)*. Collaterals reconstitute the interosseous artery *(arrowhead)*. **(B)** Runoff to the wrist and hand at presentation demonstrates the paucity of flow to the arch *(arrow)* and metacarpal branches through the attenuated radial and interosseous arteries. **(C)** Following high-dose thrombolysis with urokinase, the ulnar artery and interosseous artery are fully patent proximally, with a small residual thrombus demonstrated in the ulnar artery *(arrow)*. Delayed revascularization, however, resulted in a forearm compartment syndrome, requiring prompt treatment. Radial and ulnar pulses were full and recovery was uneventful after the forearm fasciotomies.

men for the first 2 hours after lacing, followed by tapered doses over subsequent 2-hour intervals as angiographic or clinical progress is demonstrated (Fig. 32-2).

Alternative techniques are to use one of several new multilumen or multiple-side-hole infusion catheters or to use perforated injectable guidewires, which track over smaller (0.018- to 0.035-inch) wires.[37,38] These new devices have the advantage of being able to lace the thrombus without having to be withdrawn by injecting lytic agent simultaneously through multiple ports positioned to span the length of the thrombus. Again, without moving the catheter or wire and without risking loss of access across the occlusion, the continuous infusion is begun; instead of percolating down the thrombus from the top, as with an end-hole catheter, the lytic agent spreads relatively evenly throughout the full volume of clot.

Another advantage of these multiport systems is that they can be passed coaxially through the end-hole diagnostic catheter, allowing the thrombolysis infusion to be split into both the end-hole catheter and the central coaxial catheter or injectable wire. This divided dose of lytic agent is designed to lyse the majority of the thrombus with the coaxial multiport catheter, which is embedded within the thrombus, its multiple ports spanning the length of the clot, while lysing the most proximal part of the thrombus column with the end-hole diagnostic catheter.

Protocols emphasizing higher doses and mechanical means of increasing the surface area of thrombus exposed to the lytic agent (pulsed-spray techniques, rotational catheters) have recently been introduced with the intention of improving efficacy, decreasing treatment time, lowering complication rates, lowering cost of care, and improving patient comfort.[24,39-43] At this time more clinical experience is needed to better understand the role these techniques might play in the future.

An alternative approach to upper extremity thrombolysis is to obtain the diagnostic study from the conventional femoral artery access but then to perform the therapeutic portion of the procedure with a separate antegrade brachial artery approach. A recent report describes the use of this technique to treat four patients with extensive hand and forearm thromboembolic disease in order to avoid prolonged catheterization across the origins of the great vessels to the head.[44] The procedure is limited to patients with thrombus distal to the antegrade brachial puncture site and entails the increased risk of brachial artery puncture, arteriospasm or nerve injury. A potential advantage, however, is that the more direct, antegrade approach may allow access into more distal vessels and thrombus in some patients,

thus allowing lacing and direct perfusion of clot in the palmar arches while reducing the risk of thromboembolic complications from the femoral access catheter in the aortic arch and subclavian artery. On the other hand, a further potential disadvantage is that complications at the brachial artery access site, such as severe spasm and thrombosis, may require surgical repair, since thrombolysis across the fresh brachial artery puncture site would involve a high risk of hemorrhagic complications.

Results

The vascular literature is replete with large series concentrating primarily on lower extremity thrombolysis but in which small numbers of patients with upper extremity ischemia have been included. Four studies, however, have focused solely on patients with upper extremity arterial occlusive disease, with promising results in the majority of cases.

One such study, published in 1984 with an updated review in 1985, describes the treatment with low-dose arterial streptokinase of nine patients with acute thrombosis and one patient with "chronic" disease (a 3-month history after placement of a radial artery blood-gas monitoring catheter).[45,46] Three of the patients with acute thrombosis had self-injected drugs; three occlusions were suspected to be embolic from the heart despite negative echocardiograms, including one in a patient with idiopathic thrombocytopenic purpura; two patients had in situ thrombosis; and in one patient a traumatic etiology, possibly thoracic outlet syndrome, was suspected. The proximal level of one occlusion occurred at the level of the brachial artery, extending into both radial and ulnar arteries, while all the other cases involved occlusions distal to the brachial artery trifurcation. After thrombolysis the nine patients with acute cases had excellent resolution of their symptoms, with one requiring fingertip amputations (instead of amputation of the majority of the hand). The patient with a chronic occlusion, however, showed no significant improvement and underwent surgical repair identical to that initially planned. No major complications were encountered.

Another study, published in 1990, reported on the treatment of eight patients, one with streptokinase and seven with high-dose regional urokinase.[33] Three patients with cardiac arrhythmias were suspected to have embolic occlusions; two patients had thrombosed surgical grafts; one patient had a combination of lupus erythematosus and atherosclerosis; one had a combination of thoracic outlet syndrome and polycythemia vera; and one had sustained injury to the brachial ar-

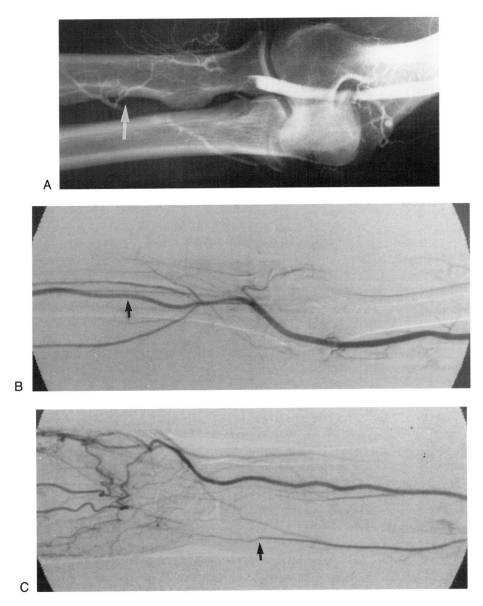

Figure 32-2 **(A)** Brachial arteriogram in a patient with acute upper extremity ischemia, demonstrating thrombo-embolic occlusion of the distal brachial artery with reconstitution by collaterals of the proximal radial artery *(arrow).* **(B)** Following high-dose thrombolysis with urokinase, the distal brachial artery, the dominant radial artery *(arrow),* the ulnar artery, and the displaced interosseous artery are recanalized and normal. Note the smaller caliber and angled origin of the latter two arteries, which might inhibit adequate balloon catheter embolectomy. **(C)** Following thrombolysis, the patent large radial artery fills the palmar arch and metarcarpal branches. The ulnar artery remains occluded distally *(arrow),* with collaterals to the ulnar aspect of the hand and a discontinuous arch. Several hours later the distal ulnar artery was found clinically to have recanalized.

tery during a cutdown for cardiac catheterization. The proximal level of occlusion was at the axillary artery in one patient, the subclavian artery in two, the brachial artery or graft in four, and distal to the brachial in one patient. Only one thrombus was laced, the other patients received high-dose urokinase infusions for 2 to 3 hours followed by lower doses for a mean infusion time of 23 hours, ranging from 0.5 to 72 hours. Five patients had full restoration of all pulses; in the other three a single wrist pulse was restored. Three patients required adjunctive percutaneous transluminal angioplasty of underlying stenoses. Complications included one groin hematoma, which was treated with surgical evacuation, and one irreversible occlusion of distal forearm artery by clot migration during lysis without other clinical sequelae.

A 1991 report described the treatment of 11 patients, of whom 6 were suspected to have cardiac thromboembolism, 1 had an underlying atherosclerotic stenosis, and 1 had a suspected embolus from a subclavian artery ulcerated plaque.[47] Regional high-dose urokinase using the modified McNamara protocol and a coaxial catheter system was successful in eight patients and failed in three; the failures occurred in a patient with an atherosclerotic lesion, in one with hypothenar hammer syndrome and organized ulnar artery thrombus, and one with atheroemboli in the palmar and digital arteries. No major complications were encountered, and the patients who failed lysis underwent successful surgery identical to that previously planned.

Another 1991 report described the treatment of six patients with high-dose regional urokinase, including initial lacing of the thrombus.[44] Two patients were suspected to have cardiac source emboli, one patient had severe atherosclerosis, one suffered blunt trauma, one had occlusion secondary to medication and local surgery, and one had no known cause. The average duration of thrombolysis was 16.2 hours, with a range of 10 to 26 hours. Four of the six patients underwent thrombolysis from an antegrade brachial artery puncture after the diagnostic study had been completed from a conventional femoral artery approach. Five patients recovered completely; one patient with severe digital ischemia and motor impairment before treatment had only mild improvement but underwent a less extensive limb salvage surgical procedure. A transient cerebrovascular accident, which resolved completely and was presumed to be due to pericatheter thrombus in the aortic arch, occurred in one of the two patients in whom thrombolysis was performed from the femoral access. In addition, one thrombotic occlusion of the femoral access site was lysed through the same sheath without significant sequelae.

A summary of these four reports reveals that of the 35 patients treated, 29 (83 percent), had complete resolution of their symptoms; however, 3 of these 29 patients required adjunctive percutaneous transluminal angioplasty of stenoses revealed after thrombolysis of their occlusions. Of the remaining 6 patients whose symptoms did not resolve with thrombolysis, 2 underwent less extensive surgery and 4 underwent the same surgery as would have been performed had thrombolysis not been attempted. The four major complications included only two that significantly altered the patient's care (a groin hematoma requiring surgical evacuation and a thrombosis of the femoral artery access site, which was successfully lysed from the same sheath), and two that did not substantially affect care (an asymptomatic occluded forearm artery and a transient stroke, which resolved completely).

Summary

The wider range of upper extremity thrombotic etiologies, the increased complexity of patient evaluation and selection, the greater potential for serious complications, and the relative lack of bypass grafts distinguishes thrombolysis in the upper extremity from its analogue in the lower extremity. Limited clinical series have demonstrated the value of thrombolysis in a diverse group of vascular disorders, both as a primary treatment modality and as an adjunct to percutaneous transluminal angioplasty and surgical therapy. As in many other percutaneous interventional techniques, early experience suggests that upper extremity arterial thrombolysis is associated with few serious complications when it fails, and tends to do so in a mode that leaves the patient no worse than if it had never been attempted.

ANGIOPLASTY

Percutaneous transluminal angioplasty, another option in the spectrum of treatments for upper extremity occlusive disease, plays a significant role mainly in the treatment of proximal and focal arterial stenoses. Atherosclerotic stenoses, the most common cause of upper extremity occlusive symptoms (discussed in detail below), are often amenable to percutaneous treatment. Other common causes of upper extremity ischemia are thoracic outlet syndrome and trauma. These disorders are frequently an indication for diagnostic arteriography but rarely are appropriately treated by the interventional radiologist. Thoracic outlet syndrome is caused by a primary musculoskeletal abnormality resulting in focal arterial compression. Since surgical treatment is required to decompress the thoracic outlet, any secondary vascular lesions can be corrected at the same time. Conversely, percutaneous dilatation of subclavian artery stenoses caused by thoracic outlet syndrome is unlikely to succeed if the inciting musculoskeletal abnormality is not repaired. Angiography is useful to document the extent of traumatic occlusion of arm vessels due to blunt or penetrating injury or brachial catheterization, but repair of these injuries is best done surgically.

Among the less common occlusive disorders, aortoarteritis (Takayasu's arteritis) and fibromuscular disease frequently are amenable to percutaneous angioplasty. Angioplasty has been used to treat radiation strictures, but experience is very limited.[48] Other rare causes of upper extremity occlusive disease include tumors, ergotism, and medium- to small-artery diseases such as arteriosclerosis obliterans, thromboangiitis obliterans, chronic occupational trauma, Raynaud's disease, and autoimmune collagen vascular diseases. Ergotism tends to respond to withdrawal of the ergot alkaloid, supplemented as needed by intra-arterial infusions of vasodilators and thrombolytic agents, while mechanical stenoses responsive to balloon dilatation are usually not present.[49,17] Similarly, narrowing of the subclavian, axillary, and brachial arteries caused by giant cell arteritis responds to steroid therapy, and transcatheter intervention is not necessary.[50] The medium- to small-artery disorders typically affect the vessels of the forearm, hand, and digits in diffuse patterns and generally are not amenable to transcatheter dilatation.

Results in Specific Diseases

Atherosclerosis

Atherosclerotic disease of the innominate and subclavian arteries causes symptoms far less frequently than atherosclerosis in the carotid or lower extremity vessels, thanks to the generous collateral network present around the shoulder. Angiographic surveys of over 8000 patients with symptoms of cerebrovascular insufficiency found significant subclavian, innominate, or vertebral artery stenoses in only about 15 percent of cases, with only 2 to 3 percent demonstrating steal physiology.[51,52] Among patients with anatomic lesions, only 5 percent have symptoms requiring intervention.[53] Concurrent carotid artery disease is present in up to one-third of patients, and correction of the carotid disease alone is often enough to relieve neurologic symptoms.[53]

Atherosclerotic lesions are usually ostial or located at vessel branch points, and symptomatic lesions are three to four times more common on the left side than on the right.[53] Symptoms are most often those of vertebrobasilar insufficiency (subclavian steal), with somewhat less than half of patients presenting with arm ischemia or a combination of central nervous system and arm symptoms. Angina in patients who have had internal mammary artery to coronary artery bypass (coronary-subclavian steal) has also been reported.[54-59] Tinnitus is a rare symptom of subclavian stenosis.[60] Indications for intervention are embolization, rest pain or gangrene of the upper extremity, debilitating central nervous system symptoms or arm claudication, and angina.

Surgical therapy is well established, extrathoracic by-

pass being the preferred operation currently.[51-53,61-64] Carotid-subclavian bypass or subclavian reimplantation into the common carotid artery are most often performed, although some surgeons advocate axilloaxillary bypass.[52] Operative morbidity and mortality for these procedures are in the 0 to 5 percent range, with neurologic morbidity approximately 1 percent. Clinical success rates are around 85 percent, and long-term graft patencies are 85 to 95 percent. Patients with diffuse disease of the brachiocephalic vessels who lack a good donor artery for extra-anatomic bypass require an intrathoracic approach for endarterectomy or bypass from the aorta. Morbidity and mortality from intrathoracic procedures are significantly higher (5 to 20 percent).

Patients with focal stenosis or occlusion of the subclavian artery are excellent candidates for percutaneous transluminal angioplasty (Fig. 32-3). Close to 1000 cases have been reported, with an average technical success rate of 93 percent.[65-78] Restenosis rates average 8.5 percent, with most recurrent lesions amenable to repeat angioplasty. The few studies that document long-term outcome suggest an 80 to 95 percent patency at 3 to 4 years, although as more experience accumulates, this prediction may become less optimistic.

In addition to being an effective procedure, subclavian angioplasty has proved to be gratifyingly safe. Early concerns about a hypothetical risk of vertebral embolization have been abolished by experimental and clinical experience. The reversed flow in the vertebral artery in patients with steal physiology persists for 2 to 20 minutes after angioplasty and appears to protect the brain from embolic particles.[74,79] Use of vasodilators or reactive hyperemia in the arm has been advocated to increase flow into the arm, further directing particles away from the cerebral circulation.[59,74] Some authors heparinize patients before performing subclavian angioplasty, while others do not consider this necessary.[68,80,81] Balloons can be inflated across the origin of the vertebral artery with impunity.[77] Among 398 patients undergoing subclavian angioplasty, complications were reported in 19 (4.8 percent). Nine (2.3 percent) of these were at the puncture site, and five (1.3 percent) were embolic events to the arm (three cases of transient digital ischemia and two brachial emboli requiring surgery). There was one stroke and one transient ischemic attack in the contralateral carotid distribution, the former following a postangioplasty arch injection and the latter following angioplasty of the contralateral internal carotid artery performed at the same time as the subclavian angioplasty.[82,83] One death within 30 days was reported, attributed to causes unrelated to the angioplasty.[79] We could find no reports in the English language literature of an embolic event to

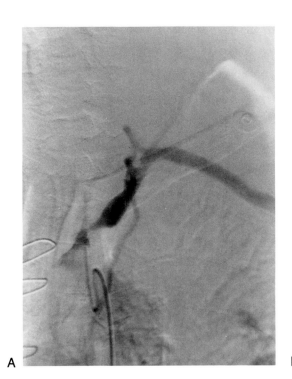
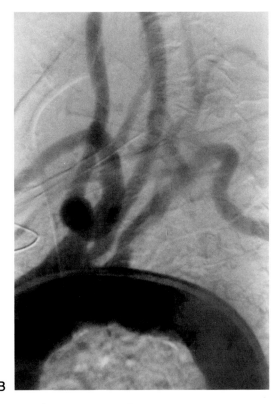

Figure 32-3 (A) Selective left subclavian artery injection in a patient with subclavian steal syndrome demonstrates a high-grade stenosis near the origin of the subclavian artery. Note the lack of antegrade flow in the left vertebral artery. A later film from the same injection (not shown) confirmed steal physiology. **(B)** Arch injection following left subclavian artery angioplasty. There is a mild residual stenosis. Antegrade flow in the vertebral artery has been restored.

the posterior circulation in a patient undergoing subclavian or innominate artery angioplasty. This remarkable safety record, combined with an efficacy similar to that of surgical therapy, makes percutaneous angioplasty the treatment of choice for short subclavian and innominate artery stenoses and occlusions in patients with ischemia of the posterior circulation or arm.

Coronary-subclavian steal has been recognized with increasing frequency as the use of the internal mammary artery as a bypass conduit has become popular. Several cases have been treated successfully by carotid-subclavian bypass.[55,56] Five patients have been treated successfully with percutaneous angioplasty, without complication[57-59,66] (Fig. 32-4). The 1 percent risk of embolization to the arm is of greater concern in these patients because of the possibility of compromising the internal mammary-coronary graft and causing myocardial ischemia or infarction. Maneuvers to increase blood flow to the arm distal to the origin of the internal mammary artery (vasodilators, reactive hyperemia) are recommended when dilating these patients.[59] Use of

the brachial or axillary approach is discouraged to avoid compromising the internal mammary artery origin and to preserve maximal flow down the arm.

Aortoarteritis

Nonspecific aortoarteritis (Takayasu's arteritis, pulseless disease) afflicts approximately 1 in 1000 persons in the United States and 6 in 1000 worldwide.[84] The mechanism of this disease has not been completely elucidated. It starts as a nonspecific inflammatory illness in the first two decades of life, which progresses to form fibrotic stenoses of the aorta and its major branches.[85] Symptoms of end-organ vascular insufficiency appear 5 to 10 years after the initial acute illness, which is often unremembered. In 90 percent of victims the disease appears present before the age of 30 years, and 75 percent of patients are female. Mortality rates at 10 years ranging from 11 to 73 percent have been reported if the vascular lesions are not corrected. The most common causes of death are stroke, heart failure, myocardial infarction, and renal failure.

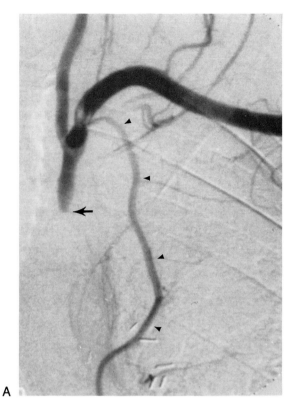

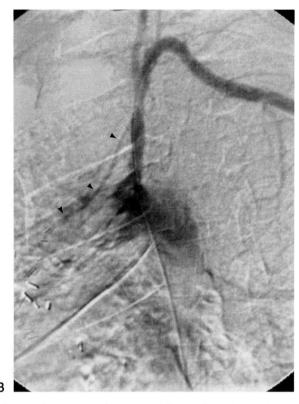

A   B

Figure 32-4 **(A)** Selective left subclavian arteriogram performed from a brachial approach in a patient with a left internal mammary artery (LIMA) to coronary artery graft who developed angina while exercising his left arm. The subclavian artery is occluded proximally *(arrow)*. The LIMA-coronary graft is patent *(arrowheads)*. An arch injection (not shown) confirmed steal physiology. **(B)** Arteriogram following subclavian artery angioplasty performed from a femoral approach demonstrates restoration of antegrade flow in the vertebral artery and continued patency of the LIMA graft *(arrowheads)*. (From Soulen and Sullivan,[59] with permission.)

The most common sites of vascular involvement are the aortic arch and its branches (75 percent of cases), of which the left subclavian artery is most often affected (55 percent), followed by the right subclavian (38 percent), left common carotid (30 percent), and right common carotid (15 percent).[86] Characteristically, lesions are multiple and symmetric. Neurologic symptoms are present in 80 percent of patients with disease involving the brachiocephalic arteries; 30 percent have had a stroke[85]; 80 percent have asymmetric blood pressure measurements in the arms; and 67 percent have a diminished or absent upper extremity pulse. Carotid and clavicular bruits are frequently present.

Angiographically, the typical subclavian lesion is a smoothly tapered stenosis, beginning within a few centimeters of the arch and extending to the origin of the vertebral artery.[85] Involvement of the vertebral artery is not common (15 percent of cases).[86] Distal branches are spared. Usually the aorta or other major branches are involved. The radiologic differential diagnosis includes atherosclerosis and fibromuscular dysplasia.

Atherosclerosis typically occurs after age 40, is more common in men, and favors vessel origins and bifurcations in the neck. At times the appearance of atherosclerosis may be indistinguishable from that of aortoarteritis. Fibromuscular dysplasia is quite rare in the subclavian artery, has a typical beaded appearance, and does not affect the aorta angiographically.

Surgical therapy for aortoarteritis of the subclavian artery depends upon the length of the vessel involved. If the ipsilateral carotid artery is normal, subclavian reimplantation into the carotid artery or carotid-subclavian bypass is the preferred operation. If the carotid artery is diseased, it is replaced and the subclavian artery is implanted into the carotid graft or is revascularized via another graft from the carotid graft or the aorta. We did not find success rates and mortality figures specific to subclavian artery repair, but in general surgical repair of aortoarteritis lesions seems to entail a higher mortality rate (4 to 27 percent) and lower graft patency rate than have been given for equivalent atherosclerotic lesions.[85]

Percutaneous transluminal angioplasty for treatment of aortoarteritis was first reported by Martin et al. in 1980.[87] One renal artery occlusion was recanalized and a subclavian artery stenosis was balloon-dilated, with patency at 4 and 12 months, respectively. Since then, over 70 angioplasties in more than 50 patients have been reported, including lesions in the aorta and the brachiocephalic, renal, visceral, and coronary arteries.[86-92] The overall success rate is approximately 88 percent, with an 18 percent restenosis rate. Almost all restenoses were redilated successfully. A delayed response to the primary dilatation occurs occasionally.[86,93] Among these reports are a total of 11 attempted dilatations of innominate or subclavian arteries,[86-88,90,92] of which 10 (91 percent), were technically successful, including 1 that restenosed and was successfully redilated at 15 months. As with other forms of arterial occlusive disease, angioplasty is indicated for patients with symptomatic focal stenoses or occlusions, while diffuse disease is better treated surgically. Park et al.[86] advocate excluding patients with serologic evidence of active disease (elevated erythrocyte sedimentation rate or C-reactive protein), although the effect of disease activity on the outcome of angioplasty is unknown. Dong et al.[89] reported 86 percent clinical success 6 months after renal angioplasty, even though 45 percent of the patients has an elevated erythrocyte sedimentation rate. On the other hand, patency of surgical bypass grafts drops from 88 percent in patients with chronic lesions to 53 percent in patients operated on during the active phase of disease. The role of adjunct medical therapy (steroids, nonsteroidal anti-inflammatory drugs, cyclophosphamide, and cyclosporine) remains to be elucidated.

Fibromuscular Dysplasia

The fibromuscular dysplasias (FMDs) are uncommon causes of symptoms of vascular insufficiency in the upper extremity. Although the renal and cerebral arteries are the usual sites affected by these diseases, the subclavian artery is the next most common site (9 percent of cases), and FMD has also been reported in the axillary and brachial arteries.[94-97] Patients with cerebral FMD are more likely to have associated subclavian disease (17 percent) than those with renal artery disease (3 percent).[94] Symptoms and signs of upper extremity FMD include claudication, subclavian steal, Raynaud's phenomenon, coldness, pallor, decreased or absent pulses, bruit, decreased blood pressure in the affected limb, distal embolization, muscle atrophy, and decreased limb length. Bilateral FMD of the subclavian artery can cause relative upper extremity hypotension, which masks underlying renovascular hypertension.[94]

Radiographically and pathologically, FMD in the upper extremities is almost always the medial fibroplasia subtype, with the characteristic "string of beads" appearance on angiograms.[97]

No one institution has a large experience with treatment of these lesions. Surgical dilatation or bypass, percutaneous transluminal angioplasty, and sympathectomy have all been reported in individual cases of FMD involving either the upper or lower extremity, with good results.[95-98]

Summary

A decade of experience involving close to 1000 procedures has established percutaneous transluminal angioplasty as a safe and effective treatment for innominate and subclavian artery stenoses and occlusions. The lower cost and morbidity of angioplasty combined with a clinical efficacy similar to that of surgery over the first few years after treatment make angioplasty the procedure of choice for these lesions. How the long-term patency of subclavian angioplasty compares with that of surgical bypass remains to be tested in a controlled fashion. As with most interventional procedures, early or late failure of angioplasty does not preclude subsequent surgery, which makes angioplasty an even more attractive first-line therapy.

REFERENCES

1. Ricotta JJ, Scudder PA, McAndrew JA et al: Management of acute ischemia of the upper extremity. Am J Surg 145:661, 1983
2. Jarrett F, Dacumos GC, Crummy AB et al: Late appearance of arterial emboli: diagnosis and management. Surgery 86:898, 1979
3. Champion HR, Gill W: Arterial embolus to the upper limb. Br J Surg 60(7):37, 1973
4. Sachatello CR, Ernst CB, Griffen WO Jr: The acutely ischemic upper extremity: selective management. Surgery 76:1002, 1974
5. Karalis DG, Chandrasekaran K, Victor MF et al: Recognition and embolic potential of intraaortic atherosclerotic debris. J Am Coll Cardiol 17:73, 1991
6. Tunick PA, Culliford AT, Lamparello PJ, Kronzon I: Atheromatosis of the aortic arch as an occult source of multiple systemic emboli. Ann Intern Med 114:391, 1991
7. Maiman MH, Bookstein JJ, Bernstein EF: Digital ischemia: angiographic differentiation of embolism from primary arterial disease. AJR 137:1183, 1981
8. Sullivan KL, Minken SL, White RI Jr: Treatment of a case of thromboembolism resulting from thoracic outlet syndrome with intra-arterial urokinase infusion. J Vasc Surg 7:568, 1988

9. Bandyk DF, Thiele BL, Radke HM: Upper-extremity emboli secondary to axillofemoral graft thrombosis. Arch Surg 116:393, 1981

10. Vayssairat M, Debure C, Cormier JM et al: Hypothenar hammer syndrome: seventeen cases with long-term follow-up. J Vasc Surg 5:838, 1987

11. Spencer-Green G, Morgan GJ, Brown L, Fitzgerald O: Hypothenar hammer syndrome: an occupational cause of Raynaud's phenomenon. J Rheumatol 14:1048, 1987

12. Fritzler MJ, Hart DA: Prolonged improvement of Raynaud's phenomenon and scleroderma after recombinant tissue plasminogen activator therapy. Arthritis Rheum 33:274, 1990

13. Perler BA: Review of hypercoagulability syndromes: what the interventionalist needs to know. J Vasc Intervent Radiol 2:183, 1991

14. Towne JB, Hussey CV, Bandyk DF: Abnormalities of the fibrinolytic system as a cause of upper extremity ischemia: a preliminary report. J Vasc Surg 7:661, 1988

15. Butler MJ, Lane RHS, Webster JHH: Irradiation injury to large arteries. Br J Surg 67:341, 1980

16. Bressler EL, Vogelzang RL, Atlas SW, Neiman HL: Radiation injury to the axillary artery presenting as distal thromboembolism. AJR 143:1079, 1984

17. Seifert KB, Blackshear WM Jr, Cruse CW et al: Bilateral upper extremity ischemia after administration of dihydroergotamine-heparin for prophylaxis of deep venous thrombosis. J Vasc Surg 8:410, 1988

18. Lang EV, Bookstein JJ: Accelerated thrombolysis and angioplasty for hand ischemia in Buerger's disease. Cardiovasc Intervent Radiol 12:95, 1989

19. Yamato M, Lecky JW, Hiramatsu K, Kohda E: Takayasu arteritis: radiographic and angiographic findings in 59 patients. Radiology 161:329, 1986

20. Kronzon I, Tunick PA, Freedberg RS et al: Transesophageal echocardiography is superior to transthoracic echocardiography in the diagnosis of sinus venosus atrial septal defect. J Am Coll Cardiol 17:537, 1991

21. Pearson AC, Labovitz AJ, Tatineni S, Gomez CR: Superiority of transesophageal echocardiography in detecting cardiac source of embolism in patients with cerebral ischemia of uncertain etiology. J Am Coll Cardiol 17:66, 1991

22. Sullivan KL, Gardiner GA Jr, Kandarpa K et al: Efficacy of thrombolysis in infrainguinal bypass grafts. Circulation, suppl. I, 83(2):I-99, 1991

23. Hirshberg A, Schneiderman J, Garniek A et al: Errors and pitfalls in intraarterial thrombolytic therapy. J Vasc Surg 10:612, 1989

24. Sullivan KL, Gardiner GA Jr, Shapiro MJ et al: Acceleration of thrombolysis with a high-dose transthrombus bolus technique. Radiology 173:805, 1989

25. McNamara TO, Fischer JR: Thrombolysis of peripheral arterial and graft occlusions: improved results using high-dose urokinase. AJR 144:769, 1985

26. Meyerovitz MF, Goldhaber SZ, Reagan K et al: Recombinant tissue-type plasminogen activator versus urokinase in peripheral arterial and graft occlusions: a randomized trial. Radiology 175:75, 1990

27. Hess H, Mietaschk A, Bruckl R: Peripheral arterial occlusions: a 6-year experience with local low-dose thrombolytic therapy. Radiology 163:753, 1987

28. Eisenbud DE, Brener BJ, Shoenfeld R et al: Treatment of acute vascular occlusions with intra-arterial urokinase. Am J Surg 160:160, 1990

29. Matsen FA III, Winquist RA, Krugmire RB: Diagnosis and management of compartmental syndromes. J Bone Joint Surg 62:286, 1980

30. Halpern AA, Nagel DA: Compartment syndromes of the forearm: early recognition using tissue pressure measurements. J Hand Surg 4:258, 1979

31. Gelberman RH, Garfin SR, Hergenroeder PT et al: Compartment syndromes of the forearm: diagnosis and treatment. Clin Orthop 161:252, 1981

32. Gelberman RH, Zakaib GS, Mubarak SJ et al: Decompression of forearm compartment syndromes. Clin Orthop 134:225, 1978

33. Widlus DM, Venbrux AC, Benenati JF et al: Fibrinolytic therapy for upper-extremity arterial occlusions. Radiology 175:393, 1990

34. Van Breda A, Graor RA, Katzen BT et al: Relative cost-effectiveness of urokinase versus streptokinase in the treatment of peripheral vascular disease. J Vasc Intervent Radiol 2:77, 1991

35. Belkin M, Belkin B, Bucknam CA et al: Intra-arterial fibrinolytic therapy. Arch Surg 121:769, 1986

36. Van Breda A, Katzen BT, Deutsch AS: Urokinase versus streptokinase in local thrombolysis. Radiology 165:109, 1987

37. Hicks ME, Picus D, Darcy MD, Kleinhoffer MA: Multilevel infusion catheter for use with thrombolytic agents. J Vasc Intervent Radiol 2:73, 1991

38. Mewissen MW, Minor PL, Beyer GA, Lipchik EO: Symptomatic native arterial occlusions: early experience with "over-the-wire" thrombolysis. J Vasc Intervent Radiol 1:43, 1990

39. McNamara T: Technique and results of "higher-dose" infusion. Cardiovasc Intervent Radiol 11:S48, 1988

40. Bildsoe MC, Moradian GP, Hunter DW et al: Mechanical clot dissolution: new concept. Radiology 171:231, 1989

41. Bookstein JJ, Fellmeth B, Roberts A et al: Pulsed-spray pharmacomechanical thrombolysis: preliminary clinical results. AJR 152:1097, 1989

42. Schmitz-Rode T, Gunther RW, Muller-Leisse C: US-assisted aspiration thrombectomy: in vitro investigations. Radiology 178:677, 1991

43. Schmitz-Rode T, Gunther RW: Percutaneous mechanical thrombolysis: a comparative study of various rotational catheter systems. Invest Radiol 26:557, 1991

44. Lamblase RE, Paolella LP, Haas RA, Dorfman GS: Extensive thromboembolic disease of the hand and forearm: treatment with thrombolytic therapy. J Vasc Intervent Radiol 2:201, 1991

45. Tisnado J, Bartol DT, Cho SR et al: Low-dose fibrinolytic therapy in hand ischemia. Radiology 150:375, 1984

46. Tisnado J, Cho SR, Beachley MC, Vines FS: Low-dose

fibrinolytic therapy in hand ischemia. Semin Intervent Radiol 2:367, 1985

47. Marx MV: Thrombolytic therapy for arterial occlusions of the upper extremities. p. 272. In Kadir S (ed): Current Practice of Interventional Radiology. 1st Ed. BC Decker, Philadelphia, 1991

48. Piedbois P, Becquemin JP, Blanc I et al: Arterial occlusive disease after radiotherapy: a report of fourteen cases. Radiother Oncol 17:133, 1990

49. Kramer RA, Hecker SP, Lewis BI: Ergotism: report of a case studied angiographically. Radiology 84:308, 1965

50. Joyce JW: The giant cell arteritides: diagnosis and the role of surgery. J Vasc Surg 3:827, 1986

51. Edwards WH, Mulherin JL Jr: The surgical approach to significant stenosis of vertebral and subclavian arteries. Surgery 87:20, 1980

52. Weiner RI, Deterling RA, Sentissi J, O'Donnell TF: Subclavian artery insufficiency. Arch Surg 122:876, 1987

53. Provan JL: Arteriosclerotic occlusive disease of the brachiocephalic and arch vessels. p. 822. In Rutherford RB (ed): Vascular Surgery. 3rd Ed. WB Saunders, Philadelphia, 1989

54. Granke K, Van Meter CH Jr, White CJ et al: Myocardial ischemia caused by postoperative malfunction of a patent internal mammary coronary graft. J Vasc Surg 11:659, 1990

55. Marshall WG, Miller EC, Kouchoukos NT: The coronary-subclavian steal syndrome: report of a case and recommendations for prevention and management. Ann Thorac Surg 46:93, 1988

56. Olson CO, Dunton RF, Maggs PR, Lahey SJ: Review of coronary-subclavian steal following internal mammary artery-coronary artery bypass surgery. Ann Thorac Surg 46:675, 1988

57. Meranze SG, McLean GK, Burke DR: Balloon dilation of a subclavian artery stenosis proximal to an internal mammary-coronary artery bypass graft. J Intervent Radiol 1:83, 1986

58. Ishii K, Hirota Y, Kita Y et al: Coronary-subclavian steal corrected with percutaneous transluminal angioplasty. J Cardiovasc Surg 32:275, 1991

59. Soulen MC, Sullivan KL: Subclavian artery angioplasty proximal to a left internal mammary-coronary artery bypass graft. Cardiovasc Intervent Radiol 14:355, 1991

60. Donald JJ, Raphael MJ: Case report: pulsatile tinnitus relieved by angioplasty. Clin Radiol 43:132, 1991

61. Beebe HG, Stark R, Johnson ML et al: Choices of operation for subclavian-vertebral disease. Am J Surg 139:616, 1980

62. Resnicoff SA, DeWeese JA, Rob CG: Surgical treatment of the subclavian steal syndrome. Circulation 41–42 (suppl. II):147, 1970

63. Deriu GP, Ballotta E: The surgical treatment of atherosclerotic occlusion of the innominate and subclavian arteries. J Cardiovasc Surg 22:532, 1981

64. Perler BA, Williams GM: Carotid-subclavian bypass: a decade of experience. J Vasc Surg 12:716, 1990

65. Dorros G, Lewin RF, Jamnadas P, Mathiak LM: Peripheral transluminal angioplasty of the subclavian and innominate arteries utilizing the brachial approach: acute outcome and follow-up. Cathet Cardiovasc Diagn 19:71, 1990

66. Levitt RG, Wholey MH, Jarmolowski CR: Subclavian artery angioplasty for treatment of upper extremity claudication, subclavian and coronary artery steal syndromes. J Vasc Intervent Radiol 2:48, 1991

67. Hüttl K, Simonffy A, Papp ZS: The role of PTA in the management of patients suffering lesions on the brachiocephalic arteries (BCA). J Vasc Intervent Radiol 2:49, 1991

68. Hebrang A, Maskovic J, Tomac B: Percutaneous transluminal angioplasty of the subclavian arteries: long-term results in 52 patients. AJR 156:1091, 1991

69. Nicholson AA, Kennan NM, Sheridan WG, Ruttley MS: Percutaneous transluminal angioplasty of the subclavian artery. Ann R Coll Surg 73:46, 1991

70. Gershony G, Basta L, Hagan AD: Correction of subclavian artery stenosis by percutaneous angioplasty. Cathet Cardiovasc Diagn 21:165, 1990

71. McNamara TO, Gardner K: Long-term results of brachiocephalic artery percutaneous transluminal angioplasty, abstracted. Radiology 177(P):262, 1990

72. Théron J, Courtheoux P, Alachkar F: Angioplasty of supraaortic arteries, abstracted. Program Abstracts, Cardiovascular and Interventional Radiology Society of Europe, Brussels, May 1990

73. Insall RL, Lambert D, Chamberlain J et al: Percutaneous transluminal angioplasty of the innominate, subclavian and axillary arteries. Eur J Vasc Surg 4:591, 1990

74. Becker GJ, Katzen BT, Dake MD: Noncoronary angioplasty. Radiology 170:921, 1989

75. Farina C, Mingoli A, Schultz RD et al: Percutaneous transluminal angioplasty versus surgery for subclavian artery occlusive disease. Am J Surg 158:511, 1989

76. Cook AM, Dyet JF: Six cases of subclavian stenosis treated by percutaneous angioplasty. Clin Radiol 40:352, 1989

77. Vitek JJ: Subclavian artery angioplasty and the origin of the vertebral artery. Radiology 170:407, 1989

78. Jaschke W, Menges HW, Ockert D et al: PTA of the subclavian and innominate artery: short- and long-term results. Ann Radiol (Paris) 32:29, 1989

79. Ringlestein EB, Zeumer H: Delayed reversal of vertebral artery blood flow following percutaneous transluminal angioplasty for subclavian steal syndrome. Neuroradiology 26:189, 1984

80. Vitek JJ, Keller FS, Duvall ER et al: Brachiocephalic artery dilation by percutaneous transluminal angioplasty. Radiology 158:779, 1986

81. Théron J: Angioplasty of supra-aortic arteries. Semin Intervent Radiol 4:331, 1987

82. Burke DR, Gordon RL, Mishkin JD et al: Percutaneous transluminal angioplasty of subclavian arteries. Radiology 164:699, 1987

83. Kachel R, Endert G, Basche S et al: Percutaneous trans-

luminal angioplasty (dilatation) of carotid, vertebral, and innominate stenoses. Cardiovasc Intervent Radiol 10:142, 1987
84. Jejeda C, Correa P: Non-syphilitic aortitis. Arch Pathol 87:177, 1969
85. Pokrovsky AV: Nonspecific aortoarteritis. p. 217. In Rutherford RB (ed): Vascular Surgery. 3rd Ed. WB Saunders, Philadelphia, 1989
86. Park JH, Han MC, Kim SH et al: Takayasu arteritis: angiographic findings and results of angioplasty. AJR 153:1069, 1989
87. Martin EC, Diamond NG, Casarella WJ: Percutaneous transluminal angioplasty in nonatherosclerotic disease. Radiology 135:27, 1980
88. Kumar S, Mandalam KR, Rao S et al: Percutaneous transluminal angioplasty in nonspecific aortoarteritis (Takayasu's disease): experience in 16 cases. Cardiovasc Intervent Radiol 12:321, 1989
89. Dong Z, Li S, Lu X: Percutaneous transluminal angioplasty for renovascular hypertension in arteritis: experience in China. Radiology 162:477, 1987
90. Hodgins GW, Dutton JW: Transluminal dilatation for Takayasu's arteritis. Can J Surg 27:355, 1984

91. Yagura M, Sano I, Akioka H et al: Usefulness of percutaneous transluminal angioplasty for aortitis syndrome. Arch Intern Med 144:1465, 1984
92. Staller BJ, Maleki M: Percutaneous transluminal angioplasty for innominate artery stenosis and total occlusion of subclavian artery in Takayasu's-type arteritis. Cathet Cardiovasc Diagn 16:91, 1989
93. Srur MF, Sos TA, Saddekni S et al: Intimal fibromuscular dysplasia and Takayasu arteritis: delayed response to percutaneous transluminal renal angioplasty. Radiology 157:657, 1985
94. Lüscher TF, Keller HM, Imhof HG et al: Fibromuscular hyperplasia: extension of the disease and therapeutic outcome. Nephron suppl. 1, 44:109, 1986
95. Iwai T, Konno S, Hiejima K et al: Fibromuscular dysplasia in the extremities. J Cardiovasc Surg 26:496, 1985
96. Drury JK, Pollock JG: Subclavian arteriopathy in the young patient. Br J Surg 68:617, 1981
97. Janevski BJ: Angiography of the Upper Extremity. Martinus Nijhoff, Boston, 1982
98. McCready RA, Pairolero PC, Hollier LH et al: Fibromuscular dysplasia of the right subclavian artery. Arch Surg 117:1243, 1982

Section VII

Arterial Aneurysms

Arterial aneurysms are a common clinical problem. Since they affect primarily the elderly, their incidence continues to rise as the general population ages. Technologies such as ultrasound and computed axial tomography have already increased incidental recognition of many small aneurysms. With current stresses on health care costs, appropriate management of all of these newly recognized aneurysms is a crucial issue in vascular diseases today.

The appropriate care of the aneurysm patient requires a diversified team of health care specialists. Basic scientists are rapidly discovering the molecular and genetic pathogenesis of aneurysms. They hope to provide clinical tests to screen high-risk patients who may eventually develop aneurysms. Epidemiologists are defining the natural history of aneurysms more accurately. On another front, the clinical approach depends on the integrated efforts of internists, radiologists, and surgeons. Expert cardiovascular anesthesia and postoperative care can now deliver the marginally healthy patient to a safe recovery. In this section, we have called upon several of these experts to comment on the current understanding and management of the most common types of arterial aneurysms.

Concepts rather than extraneous details are emphasized. A few case examples are used to illustrate clinical application of basic science. Numerous illustrations reinforce the key concepts. Likewise, selected references provide more details for those seeking further discussion.

Concepts of aneurysm pathogenesis have changed remarkably in the past 10 years. Simple atherosclerotic weakening of the arterial wall is no longer in vogue. Clinical features imply systemic connective tissue dis-order in many patients. Familial tendencies for aneurysms have been documented repeatedly. Specific genetic defects of collagen and an imbalance of proteolytic and antiproteolytic activity are being identified. Clinical laboratory tests for aneurysm predilection are on the horizon.

Traditional understanding of the natural history of aneurysms has also been challenged in the past five years. The limitations of previous autopsy and selected referral-practice studies have been realized. For example, several population-based studies of abdominal aortic aneurysms have arrived at strikingly similar conclusion: small aortic aneurysms do not cause much trouble, large aneurysms do. Unfortunately, most ruptured aneurysms are not only large but also previously unknown to the patient. Consequently, screening programs for abdominal aortic aneurysms are currently a hotly debated topic. Likewise, the natural history of small visceral and peripheral aneurysms need better definition.

Clinically, aneurysms present with a fascinating diversity of symptoms and signs. For example, a ruptured aneurysm can masquerade as acute congestive heart failure (aortocaval fistula). Claudication may be the presenting symptom for a thrombosed femoral aneurysm. Leg swelling from acute deep venous thrombosis may underly a large popliteal artery aneurysm compressing the popliteal vein. These are only a few examples of the unusual presentations of aneurysms.

In addition, aneurysms usually travel in the company of other medical conditions. The most common companion is coronary artery disease followed closely by chronic obstructive pulmonary disease. Two other serious associates with aneurysm disease can be chronic renal insufficiency and cirrhosis with portal hypertension. These medical threats, however, rarely elude a good history and physical examination. Most of these medical conditions can be improved before aneurysm operation. A variety of perioperative measures can be undertaken to minimize their adverse impact.

One of the greatest advances in modern aneurysm management has been accurate imaging of aneurysms. Ultrasound remains a cost-efficient and safe workhorse for identifying and measuring aneurysms. Computed tomography (CT) has overcome the difficulties of imaging thoracic and upper abdominal aneurysms. It has also enhanced recognition of other abdominal pathology that may co-exist with or mimic an aneurysm. CT has also assisted in the discovery of complications of aneurysm repair such as late development of new aneurysms or chronic graft infection. The value of arteriography, whether routine or selective, in mapping arterial occlusive disease associated with aneurysms cannot be overemphasized.

Until recently, treatment of aneurysms seemed straightforward. The adage was simply "find them and fix them." Repair was basically by an interposition graft (abdominal aortic aneurysm) or aneurysm liga-

tion with a bypass graft (popliteal aneurysms). The recent introduction of stent-graft combinations passed by retrograde transfemoral cutdown to repair abdominal aortic aneurysms adds another therapeutic option. Other alternatives are bound to appear.

Regardless of how an aneurysm is treated, every community must be prepared to treat symptomatic aneurysm patients or transport them to specialized surgical centers. Rapid transport of the symptomatic aneurysm patient is essential in saving lives and limbs. Helicopter pilots and nurses are examples of new members of the integrated health care team who are improving aneurysm results.

Finally, repair of a patient's aneurysm does not permanently assure good health. Coronary artery disease remains a continual threat. New aneurysms at other anatomic sites are always a possibility. Graft complications can present at any time during the patient's remaining life. All of these possibilities lead to one irrefutable recommendation: aneurysm patients must be observed closely throughout their lifetime. Once identified, the aneurysm patient must never be lost to follow-up.

33

Pathophysiology of Arterial Aneurysm Development

Jon R. Cohen
John W. Hallett, Jr.

Current understanding of the pathogenesis of aneurysms is based primarily on clinical and basic investigations of abdominal aortic aneurysms (AAAs). Whether the pathophysiology of AAAs is applicable to other anatomic sites is unclear; however, AAAs represent our best present model to study aneurysm pathophysiology.

AAAs occur below the renal arteries in 95 percent of cases and are usually associated with aortic atherosclerosis. The association of aortic aneurysms with infrarenal aortic atherosclerosis led to the theory that AAAs are random variants of atherosclerosis that occur at a weakened site in the arterial wall (Fig. 33-1). AAAs were thought to enlarge according to Laplace's law as a result of weakening in the aortic wall until eventual rupture. However, more recent clinical observations, genetic studies, and biochemical analysis indicate that aneurysms develop as a result of an alteration in systemic connective tissue metabolism.

CLINICAL OBSERVATIONS

Patients with abdominal aortic aneurysms frequently develop coronary artery disease. However, they rarely develop significant lower extremity arterial disease, and it is unusual for them to have claudication. In fact, instead of distal occlusive disease patients with aortic aneurysms frequently have other peripheral aneurysms, whereas in contrast, patients with aortoiliac occlusive disease frequently have distal occlusive disease but rarely have peripheral arterial aneurysms. In one large study of patients with aortic aneurysms,[1] approximately 5 percent had associated peripheral aneurysms, and multiple aneurysms occurred in over 80 percent of patients who had at least one peripheral aneurysm. Of patients with a common femoral artery aneurysm, 90 percent have an aortoiliac aneurysm and 60 percent have another femoral artery aneurysm. In patients with popliteal artery aneurysms, approximately 80 percent have second aneurysms; 65 percent have an aortic aneurysm, and 50 percent have bilateral popliteal artery aneurysms. Many patients with aneurysms have associated generalized arteriomegaly, and the diameters of blood vessels distal to the aneurysms are 40 to 50 percent larger than in patients with aortic occlusive disease.[2]

Another circumstance suggesting that a connective tissue defect occurs in patients with aneurysms is the more frequent coexistence of inguinal herniation in patients with AAAs as compared with patients with aortic occlusive disease. Patients with aneurysms have

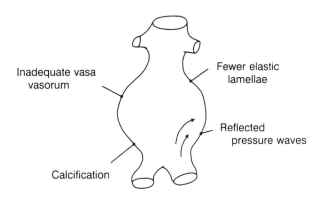

Figure 33-1 Factors that may predispose to aneurysm formation in the infrarenal abdominal aorta, especially when atherosclerosis is present.

more severe herniation, including more direct hernias, bilateral hernias, recurrent hernias, and early onset.[3] These observations suggest that connective tissue abnormalities of both the abdominal wall and the aortic wall result in hernia and aneurysms in the same patient. Tortuous carotid arteries have been found to be associated with aneurysms in up to 44 percent of cases but are found in only 10 percent of patients with routine carotid atherosclerosis.[4] Weakness in the arterial wall has been suggested as the cause of the tortuous carotid artery and the AAA in the same patient.

GENETIC REPORTS

Nine different reports of patients with familial aneurysms suggest that aneurysmal disease is transmitted genetically. Most recently a report of an infant with an aneurysm of the thoracoabdominal aorta and markedly elevated blood elastase activity was reported from Japan. This is the first report of a congenital aortic aneurysm linked directly to an increase in circulating proteolytic activity.[5]

In a recent study of first-degree relatives of patients with AAAs, the percentage of families with at least one affected first-degree relative was 15.4 percent. In 21 percent of the multiplex families, parent to offspring transmission of the AAA was noted. The relative risk of developing an AAA in this study was 3.97 for fathers, 4.03 for mothers, 9.92 for brothers, and 22.93 for sisters.[6] In a study of 14 families, the aortic aneurysm patient in each family had at least one blood relative with an aortic aneurysm and in two families the patient had two affected blood relatives.[7] After adjustment for age and sex in one study, there is an estimated 11.6

percent increase in aortic aneurysm risk among patients having an affected first-degree relative.[8] The genetic mechanisms of inheritance of AAAs has been studied in 50 families with 71 different affected individuals. The mechanism of inheritance has been suggested to be both X-linked and autosomal dominant, the X-linked variance being the most common type.[9] In one very interesting report, three brothers, the only siblings of one family, all underwent emergency surgery for ruptured aneurysms within a 12-month period.[10]

Several analyses of chromosome patterns in patients with aortic aneurysms have been reported. In one study a genetic variation in chromosome 16, which is responsible for the haptoglobin phenotype, was found to be associated with aneurysms.[11] The frequency of the haptoglobin α_1 allele was increased in aortic aneurysms as compared with controls. Interestingly, haptoglobin that contains the α_1 chain accelerates elastin degradation by elastase. In addition, a rare polymorphism of the cholesterol ester transfer protein locus was also more frequent in aneurysm patients. In another genetic study the α_1-antitrypsin phenotype associated with decreased circulating antiprotease activity (MZ phenotype) was found to occur more often in aneurysm patients.[12]

To date, seven studies have screened 1443 first-degree relatives of patients with aortic aneurysms. On combining the results of these seven studies, it is found that approximately 16 percent of the relatives of patients with aortic aneurysms have an aortic aneurysm (Table 33-1).

Table 33-1　Genetic Studies of Families with Abdominal Aortic Aneurysms

Study	No. of AAA Patients	First-Degree Relatives With AAA	
		No.	%
Johansen[8]	250	48	19%
Norrgard[7]	87	16	18%
Cole[13]	305	34	11%
Collin[14]	108	13	12%
Darling[15]	542	82	15%
Powell[11]	60	20	33%
Webster[6]	91	14	15%
Totals	1443	227	16%

Abbreviation: AAA, abdominal aortic aneurysm.

BIOCHEMICAL STUDIES

Elastin Metabolism

Many reports have documented increased proteolytic activity both in the aorta and in the circulating leukocytes in patients with AAAs as compared with patients with aortic occlusive disease and control subjects. These reports all suggest that an abnormally increased amount of elastase in the aortic wall is the significant factor in the development of aortic aneurysms.

Many factors have a direct effect on elastase and proteolytic activity; antiprotease activity (α_1-antitrypsin) and smoking are among those with major effects on circulating proteolytic activity. The relationship between elastase (the major proteolytic enzyme for elastin) and α_1-antitrypsin (the major elastase inhibitor) in the aortic wall is related directly to the different types of infrarenal aortic disease. Aortic elastase is significantly higher in patients with aortic aneurysms, multiple aneurysms, and ruptured aneurysms than in patients with aortic occlusive disease[17] (Fig. 33-2), and the inhibitor of elastase, α_1-antitrypsin, is significantly lower in patients with multiple aneurysms and ruptured aneurysms.[17] Furthermore, in a study of the breakdown of elastin into its by-product L-valylproline, patients with AAAs were found to have significantly higher elastin urine metabolites than patients with aortic occlusive disease and controls.[18]

Furthermore, in AAA patients the elastin content of the aortic wall is significantly less than in patients with aortic occlusive disease (Fig. 33-2). This decrease in elastin content is inversely correlated with the increase in elastase in the aortic wall.[19] Chemical studies of aneurysmal aortas confirm a significant deficiency of iron hematoxylin-reactive elastin, with a significant destruction of the elastin, as compared with patients with aortic occlusive disease.[20]

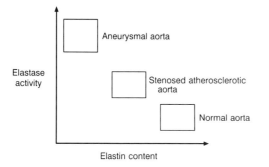

Figure 33-2 Elastin content and elastase activity in human aortic media. (Modified from Powell and Greenhalgh,[24] with permission.)

Many different types of elastase exist, including neutrophil and smooth muscle cell elastase. Neutrophils are chemotactic to the elastin fragments generated in the breakdown of elastin in aneurysmal tissue.[21] Smooth muscle cells also proliferate and secrete elastase in response to atherosclerosis. The increased delivery of proteolytic enzymes from both the neutrophils and smooth muscle cells in the aortic wall results in histologically disrupted elastic tissue as compared with occlusive disease patients and controls. There is also the possibility that a yet unknown metalloprotease in the aortic wall is responsible for the increased breakdown of elastin. Some data suggests that tissue inhibitor of metalloprotease is significantly lower in patients with AAAs than in control subjects.

Clinical observations from a population-based screening study suggest that increases in proteolytic activity have a significant effect on aneurysm development.[23] In this study male patients 74 years of age or older were screened for AAAs. Multiple risk factors were analyzed, but only three appeared significant, namely, history of smoking, angina, and impaired pulmonary elasticity [i.e., chronic obstructive pulmonary disease (COPD)]. Peripheral arterial occlusive disease, hypertension, and hyperlipidemia were not found to be suggestive. COPD results from increased pulmonary proteolytic activity and decreased antielastase activity. Smoking causes an increase in circulating proteolytic activity. The history of smoking and impaired pulmonary elasticity suggest that increased proteolytic activity may be a significant factor for the development of AAA and COPD in the same patient.

Collagen Metabolism

Abnormal collagen metabolism has been suggested as a cause for AAA development. Lower amounts of type III collagen have been found in some patients with familial aneurysms and abnormality of type III collagen has been suggested as a genetic factor in certain familial clusterings of aneurysm patients.[24] In one animal model of poststenotic dilatation, a twofold increase in collagenase activity as compared with controls occurred in the area of dilatation, with no change in elastase activity. This study suggested that collagenolysis may be induced by local flow and pressure changes and that aneurysms develop in response to altered hemodynamics.[25] In one study of the biosynthesis of type III collagen in aneurysm patients from cultured skin fibroblast, several patients with familial aneurysms had one normal allele and one allele coded for a structural mutation in type III collagen, which resulted in an imperfect triple helical collagen molecule.[26] However, a more recent study of collagen types in aneurysm patients and familial aneurysms found no type III collagen deficiency in either group.[27]

In studies of the mechanical properties of canine arteries before and after exposure to collagenase and elastase, all arteries exposed to elastase and mechanical forces developed aneurysms, which suggests that elastin provided the longitudinal retractive force. Furthermore, these studies indicated that the failure of elastin and not collagen was most likely responsible for the arteriomegaly and aneurysms seen with age and hypertension in humans.[28,29] Similar mechanical properties have been demonstrated in human iliac arteries treated with elastase and collagenase in the laboratory (Fig. 33-3). These studies also imply that the critical factor that precipitates rupture is collagenase activity.

Atherosclerosis and the Development of Aneurysms

Aneurysm development may be a result of atherosclerotic plaque regression in focal areas within the aorta. In a primate regression model of experimental atherosclerosis, aneurysms occurred in animals undergoing dietary cholesterol lowering. These studies suggest that aneurysm formation may occur at sites where atherosclerotic plaques atrophy, leaving the aortic wall too thin to resist the increasing wall tension that leads to aneurysmal development.[30]

Ruptured Aneurysms

Several clinical studies, genetic studies, and biochemical studies all suggest that aneurysm rupture may also occur as a result of increased proteolysis, with elastin and collagen breakdown (Fig. 33-4). One clinical report suggests that aneurysm rupture is hastened by other operative procedures as a result of increased circulating serum proteolytic activity.[31] An animal model has suggested that laparotomy alone upsets the dynamic equilibrium between synthesis and lysis of systemic connective tissue, resulting in increased aortic elastase activity after any type of abdominal procedure.[32]

Like the screening study of patients with asymptomatic AAAs, a regression analysis of aortic aneurysm rupture indicates that three variables may be important in aneurysm rupture; these include diastolic hypertension, initial aneurysm size, and the degree of obstructive pulmonary disease.[33] Since the mechanism for severe emphysema in COPD is probably an imbalance between elastase and antiprotease in the lung, it is possible that the association between COPD and aortic aneurysm rupture in the same patient is due to the fact that both entities occur by the same mechanism of increased systemic proteolysis.

Genetically, female members of families with aneurysms are strongly correlated with rupture of aortic aneurysms. The term *black widow syndrome* has been suggested to describe the fatal trait associated with female relatives of patients with aortic aneurysms.[15] Although aneurysms are more prevalent in men than in women, a family with a history of women with aneurysms increases rupture risk of the children, especially if the male spouse also has a family history of aneurysms.

UNIFIED HYPOTHESIS

These genetic studies, biochemical studies, and clinical observations provide the basis for a comprehensive hypothesis for the pathogenesis of aortic aneurysm de-

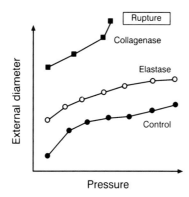

Figure 33-3 Effect of elastase and collagenase on both dilatation and rupture of human internal iliac arteries under increasing luminal pressure in the experimental laboratory. (Modified from Dobrin,[29] with permission.)

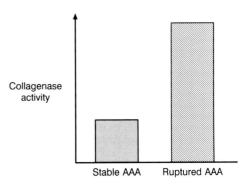

Figure 33-4 Collagenase activity in aortic media from stable and ruptured aortic aneurysms. (Adapted from Powell and Greenhalgh,[24] with permission.)

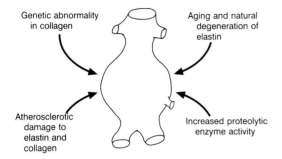

Figure 33-5 Genetic abnormality in collagen / Aging and natural degeneration of elastin / Atherosclerotic damage to elastin and collagen / Increased proteolytic enzyme activity

Figure 33-5 Multifactorial development of arterial aneurysms.

velopment (Fig. 33-5). Aneurysms probably are not merely random variants of atherosclerosis but rather develop in a logical stepwise progression, as listed below:

1. Aneurysm patients have a genetically determined increase in elastase, specifically an increase in both neutrophil and smooth muscle elastase. Some patients may also have defective collagen.
2. Serum proteolytic activity is in part determined by the genes for elastase production and is modified by other genes such as the α_1-antitrypsin phenotype, the haptoglobin phenotype, and environmental factors such as cigarette smoke.
3. During development of aortic atherosclerosis, which commonly occurs below the renal arteries in humans, elastin fragments and elastin peptides are exposed to the circulation. During the repair process, neutrophils are chemotactic to these aortic elastin fragments. The atherosclerotic fragments also act as stimulators of local smooth muscle proteolytic production. In aneurysm patients, as opposed to patients with aortic occlusive disease, increased amounts of proteolytic enzymes are delivered by elastase-laden neutrophils and smooth muscle cells in response to the atherosclerosis.
4. During the atherosclerotic process of arterial wall breakdown and repair, the increased delivery of proteolytic enzymes in aneurysm patients results in a chronic increase in aortic elastin breakdown, weakening of the aortic wall, and aneurysmal dilatation. Increased levels of collagenase may constitute the final factor that lowers the collagenous tensile strength sufficiently to cause rupture.
5. The many possible combinations of genetic and environmental factors that can occur from patient to patient is probably responsible for the large diversity of phenotypes seen clinically, such as patients with isolated aneurysms, multiple aneurysms, or massive arteriomegaly. This hypothesis suggests that aneurysms are indeed a variant of atherosclerosis, which is modified toward arterial dilatation and rupture both by increased proteolytic enzyme activity and by progressive deterioration of elastin and collagen.

CONCLUSION

At some future time we should have clinical laboratory tests that can identify patients who will develop aneurysms. The familial, and consequently genetic, predisposition to aneurysms is clear, but the exact genetic defect is unclear — in fact, there may be a variety of genetic defects, some of which may relate to collagen formation as implicated recently by a mutation in the gene for type III procollagen found in a family with aneurysms.[34] Other patients may have a genetic excess of proteolytic enzymes that break down elastin or collagen, while still others may have a deficiency of antiproteolytic enzymes that would normally prevent connective tissue destruction. Eventually, many of these genetic factors will be specifically identified and, it is to be hoped, will result in clinical tests that can screen patients at high risk for aneurysm disease so that any aneurysms found can be treated before complications arise.

REFERENCES

1. Dent TL, Lindenauer SM, Ernst, Fry WJ: Multiple arteriosclerotic arterial aneurysms. Arch Surg 105:338, 1972
2. Tilson MD, Dang C: Generalized arteriomegaly. Arch Surg 116:1030, 1981
3. Cannon DJ, Casteel L, Read RC: Abdominal aortic aneurysm, Leriche's syndrome, inguinal herniation and smoking. Arch Surg 119:387, 1984
4. Mukherjee D, Mayberry JC, Inahara T, Greig JD: The relationship of the abdominal aortic aneurysm to the tortuous internal carotid artery. Arch Surg 124:955, 1989
5. Tsuji A: An infant with aneurysm of the thoracoabdominal aorta and blood elastase activity. Pediatr Cardiol 11:179, 1990
6. Webster MW, St. Jean PL, Steed DL et al: Abdominal aortic aneurysm: results of a family study. J Vasc Surg 13:366, 1991
7. Norrgard O, Rais O, Angquist KA: Familial occurrence of abdominal aortic aneurysms. Surgery 95:650, 1984
8. Johansen K, Koepsell T: Familial tendency for abdominal aortic aneurysms. JAMA 256:1934, 1986
9. Tilson MD, Seashore MR: Fifty families with abdominal aortic aneurysms in two or more first-order relatives. Am J Surg 147:551, 1984
10. Clifton MA: Familial abdominal aortic aneurysms. Br J Surg 64:765, 1977
11. Powell JT, Bashir A, Dawson S et al: Genetic variation on chromosome 16 is associated with abdominal aortic aneurysm. Clin Sci 78:13, 1990
12. Cohen JR, Sarfati I, Ratner L, Tilson D: Alpha-1-antitrypsin phenotypes in patients with abdominal aortic aneurysms. J Surg Res 49:319, 1990

13. Cole CW, Barber GG, Bouchard A et al: Abdominal aortic aneurysm: consequences of a positive family history. Can J Surg 32:117, 1988

14. Collin J, Walton J: Is abdominal aortic aneurysm familial? Br Med J 299:493, 1989

15. Darling RC III, Brewster DC, Darling RC et al: Are familial abdominal aortic aneurysms different? J Vasc Surg 10:39, 1989

16. Powell JT, Greenhalgh RM: Multifactorial inheritance of abdominal aortic aneurysm. Eur J Vasc Surg 1:29, 1987

17. Cohen JR, Mandell C, Chang J, Wise L: Elastin metabolism of the infrarenal aorta. J Vasc Surg 7:210, 1988

18. Cohen JR, Dietzek A, Stein T, Wise L: Urinary L-valyl-proline in patients with aortic aneurysms. Surg Gynecol Obstet 168:507, 1989

19. Campa JS, Greenhalgh RM, Powell JT: Elastin degradation in abdominal aortic aneurysms. Atherosclerosis 65:13, 1987

20. Tilson MD: Histochemistry of aortic elastin in patients with nonspecific abdominal aortic aneurysmal disease. Arch Surg 123:503, 1988

21. Cohen JR, Keegan L, Sarfati I et al: Neutrophil chemotaxis and neutrophil elastase in the aortic wall in patients with abdominal aortic aneurysms. J Invest Surg 4:423, 1991

22. Brophy CM, Marks WH, Reilly JM, Tilson MD: Decreased tissue inhibitor of metalloproteinases (TIMP) in abdominal aortic aneurysm tissue: a preliminary report. J Surg Res 50:653, 1991

23. Bengtsson H, Bergqvist D, Ekberg O, Janzon L: A population-based screening of abdominal aortic aneurysms (AAA). Vasc Outlook 2(10):3, 1990

24. Powell JT, Greenhalgh RM: Cellular, enzymatic, and genetic factors in the pathogenesis of abdominal aortic aneurysms. J Vasc Surg 9:297, 1989

25. Zarins CK, Runyon-Hass A, Zatina MA et al: Increased collagenase activity in early aneurysmal dilatation. J Vasc Surg 3:328, 1986

26. Deak SB, Ricotta JJ, Deak ST et al: Abnormal type III collagen synthesis in patients with abdominal aortic aneurysms. Clin Res 37:33, 1989

27. Rizzo RJ, McCarthy WJ, Dixit SN et al: Collagen types and matrix protein content in human abdominal aortic aneurysms. J Vasc Surg 10:365, 1989

28. Dobrin PB, Schwartz TH, Baker WH: Mechanisms of arterial and aneurysmal tortuosity. Surgery 104:569, 1988

29. Dobrin PB: Pathophysiology and pathogenesis of aortic aneurysms: current concepts. Surg Clin North Am 69:687, 1989

30. Zarins CK, Xu C, Glagov S: Aneurysmal enlargement of the aorta during regression of experimental atherosclerosis. J Vasc Surg 12:246, 1990

31. Swanson RJ, Littooy FN, Hunt KT, Stoney RJ: Laparotomy as a precipitating factor in the rupture of intra-abdominal aneurysms. Arch Surg 115:299, 1980

32. Cohen JR, Schroder W, Mandell C, Wise L: Activation of rabbit elastase by non-aortic intra-abdominal surgery. Ann Vasc Surg 2:133, 1988

33. Cronenwett JL, Murphy TF, Zelenock GB et al: Actuarial analysis of variables associated with rupture of small abdominal aortic aneurysms. Surgery 98:472, 1985

34. Kontusaari S, Tromp G, Kuivaniemi H et al: A mutation in the gene for type III procollagen (COL3A1) in a family with aortic aneurysms. J Clin Invest 86:1465, 1990

34

Natural History of Aneurysms

David J. Ballard
John W. Hallett, Jr.

The primary question of interest with respect to the natural history of aneurysms, regardless of the location, is a probability of aneurysm rupture. While there have been several population-based studies of the natural history of abdominal aortic aneurysms (AAAs), only limited information is available regarding the natural history of aneurysms of the visceral, renal, and peripheral arteries. Because AAAs represent the most frequently encountered aneurysm management problem and because of the available scientific evidence regarding their natural history, this chapter focuses on the natural history of AAAs, although the limited published evidence regarding peripheral, thoracic, and thoracoabdominal aneurysms is also discussed.

ABDOMINAL AORTIC ANEURYSMS

Range of Complications

As indicated in Table 34-1, the potential specific clinical complications of AAAs are numerous. Because the major emphasis in clinical practice and in clinical investigation has been on the outcome of AAA rupture, the other complications of AAA listed in Table 34-1 have not been evaluated in a time-based probabilistic context.

Risk of Rupture

There have been several published population-based cohort studies of the risk of aneurysm rupture. The first and largest such cohort study[1] examined the risk of rupture among 176 residents of Rochester, Minnesota, in whom an unruptured AAA was documented on initial ultrasound evaluation. The cumulative incidence of AAA rupture in relation to initial maximal transverse diameter from these data is shown in Figure 34-1. By 8 years of follow-up, the cumulative incidence of rupture was 25 percent among patients with AAAs initially 5.0 cm or greater, 5 percent among patients with AAA initially 3.5 to 4.9 cm, and zero among patients with AAAs smaller than 3.5 cm. In a Cox model analysis of these data, a 1-cm larger initial diameter was associated with an increase of approximately 50 percent in the risk of rupture (adjusted hazard ratio, 1.55; 95 percent confidence interval, 1.04 to 2.32).

Several other community cohort studies have subsequently been published and have yielded very similar evidence of rupture risk. For example, Johansson et al.[2] reported that 3 of 42 patients studied in a community in Sweden who had an initial AAA diameter of less than 5.0 cm eventually experienced aneurysm rupture (mean follow-up, 5 years, 4 months). Although the study by Johansson et al. did not specifically provide

Table 34-1 Potential Specific Clinical
Complications of Abdominal Aortic Aneurysm

Rupture
Thrombosis
Disseminated intravascular coagulation
Embolism
Infection involving the aneurysm
Ureteral obstruction
Gastrointestinal obstruction
Bile duct compression
Symptomatic venous compression
Renal artery compression
Inflammatory aneurysm

Kaplan-Meier estimates of the cumulative incidence of rupture, the risk of rupture can be estimated from their published data to be approximately 7 percent at 5 years for patients in the less than 5.0 cm group. The 5-year risk of rupture for AAAs of at least 5.0 cm was approximately 40 percent. In another study from Sweden, Glimaker et al.[3] found that the cumulative incidence of rupture for AAAs smaller than 5.0 cm was 2.5 percent at 7 years among 110 residents of Uppsala. In these data, the risk of rupture at 3 years was 28 percent among 77 patients with an initial AAA diameter greater than 5.0 cm. The concept that the risk of rupture for AAAs smaller than 5.0 cm is substantially lower than for aneurysms at least 5.0 cm in diameter was further supported by a study of 208 patients who underwent more than one ultrasound or computed tomography (CT) scan at Ottawa Civic Hospital. In these data the 6-year cumulative incidence of rupture was 1 percent among patients with aneurysms smaller than

4 cm, 2 percent among patients with aneurysms 4.0 to 4.9 cm in diameter, and 20 percent among patients with aneurysms at least 5.0 cm in diameter.[4]

These population-based cohort studies, which have all been published since 1989, provide a substantially lower estimate of the risk of rupture for smaller AAAs than was reported in previous referral practice case series. Such series may systematically overestimate the risk of AAA rupture because of initial patient referral based on unusual AAA growth as documented in community care and also because of "lost follow-up" bias (i.e., inclusion of only individuals who returned to the referral center for additional AAA evaluation in the inception cohorts for the referral case series). For example, among 67 patients with AAAs smaller than 6.0 cm at the University of Michigan, Cronenwett et al. reported an annual rupture risk of 6 percent.[5] However, only 6 of the 12 cases included in this referral center case series actually involved documented rupture (the additional 6 patients had "acute expansion"). Thus, the actual annual rupture risk in this referral case series may have been closer to 3 percent. Several referral case series of larger aneurysms reported a clinically important risk of rupture for larger AAAs,[6,7] but none of these studies provided AAA size measurement by ultrasound or CT.

An autopsy-based study of AAA rupture had important influence on the clinical management of AAA in the 1970s and 1980s. Because of the important role of autopsy studies in surgical thinking, the limitations of these studies with respect to assessment of AAA rupture risk among living individuals must be addressed, and the data from these studies must be briefly reviewed. Although there are no national data regarding the percentage of individuals with AAA who undergo autopsy, the percentage of autopsy for all deaths during the past several decades in the United States has been reported to be approximately 10 percent.[8] Sudden death is one of several factors associated with the probability of undergoing autopsy. Because of the low overall probability of autopsy and the association of AAA rupture with sudden death, there is substantial potential for overestimating the prevalence of rupture at death among all deceased individuals with AAA when autopsy studies are the basis for such estimates. Given these circumstances, it is not surprising to find that in a region with the highest autopsy rate in the United States,[8] Sommerville et al. found that only 1 of 117 AAAs smaller than 4.5 cm (0.9 percent) was ruptured at autopsy at Mayo Clinic,[9] whereas Darling et al.[10] found a higher prevalence of rupture in a region with a lower autopsy rate (9.5 percent for AAAs below 4.0 cm, 23.4 percent for AAAs of 4.1–5.0 cm diameter). Furthermore, measurement of AAA at death may under-

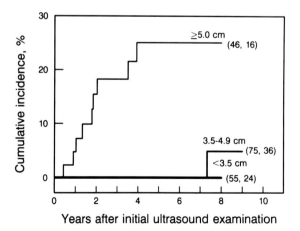

Figure 34-1 Cumulative incidence of rupture of AAAs according to the diameter of the aneurysm at the initial ultrasound examination (the numbers of patients under follow-up at 0 and 5 years are indicated in parentheses). (From Nevitt et al.,[1] with permission.)

estimate by approximately 0.5 cm the AAA size under in vivo aortic pressure.[1] Therefore, although autopsy studies have demonstrated that it is possible for a small AAA to rupture, these data cannot be used to evaluate the probability of rupture over a given period among living individuals with AAAs of a specific size.[9,10]

Risk Factors for Rupture

No population-based studies have documented risk factors other than AAA size for AAA rupture. In Cronenwett et al.'s analysis,[5] three factors were associated with rupture or acute expansion: diastolic blood pressure, initial AAA anterior and posterior diameter, and degree of obstructive pulmonary disease.

Expansion Rate

Valid information pertaining to the rate of expansion of AAA is important in AAA management because of the interrelationships of expansion rate, AAA size, and AAA rupture risk. Although AAAs clearly exist in three-dimensional space, most of the clinical research to date and the standard approach in clinical practice have focused on the maximal transverse diameter of the AAA as measured by ultrasound or CT.[11] For AAAs smaller than 5.0 cm, two population-based cohort studies have generated essentially similar results concerning the rate of size change. In a study of 27 residents of the Oxford Regional Health Authority, in whom AAA was detected through the Oxford screening program, Collin et al.[12] reported a median rate of size change of 0.22 cm/year. Among 91 residents of Rochester, Minnesota with AAAs smaller than 5.0 cm documented by ultrasound, Nevitt et al.[1] reported a median rate of size change of 0.21 cm/year. Among 103 residents of Rochester, Minnesota, 21 percent of individuals who underwent at least two or more ultrasound examinations had a AAA rate of size change of more than 0.4 cm/year (Fig. 34-2). Similar findings with re-

spect to AAA expansion rate have been published by Glimaker et al.[3] and by Guirguis and Barber.[4]

Survival

Several studies of survival among individuals with AAA, including the population-based study from Olmsted County, Minnesota, indicate that the majority of such persons will die from cardiovascular disease, rather than from aneurysm rupture.[13] In line with this observation, as compared with the general population, patients with AAAs have reduced survival, primarily owing to their increased cardiovascular disease mortality.[13,14]

Quality of Life and Functional Status

There is extremely limited information in the medical literature addressing the impact of the condition of AAA or of the diagnostic label of AAA on quality of life and functional status. Although several case studies have described patients without clinical evidence of AAA rupture who reported fear of or anxiety regarding the possibility of rupture, the frequency with which patients with unruptured AAA are afflicted with this potential impairment in their functional status or self-perceived quality of life is not described in the published literature. The impact of the diagnosis of AAA on quality of life and functional status and the role of elective surgical resection of AAA on quality of life and functional status are being explicitly addressed in three randomized trials of elective AAA surgery.[15-17]

Implications of AAA Natural History Data on Recommendations for AAA Screening

Several studies indicate that in the majority of individuals in the general population who have experienced AAA rupture, the aneurysm was not clinically recognized prior to rupture.[1] This observation has led, in part, to AAA screening recommendations.[18] Given the size distribution of AAAs, most of those that would be detected through aneurysm screening would be small.[19] As previously indicated, randomized trials are underway[15-17] that will provide more definitive evidence regarding the impact of elective surgery on the duration and quality of life of individuals with AAA. After these randomized trials have provided high-quality scientific evidence regarding the efficacy of elective aneurysm surgery, and when additional information regarding risk factors for AAA is available, it

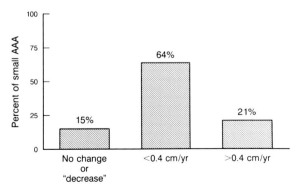

Figure 34-2 Expansion rates for small AAAs. (From Nevitt et al.,[1] with permission.)

will be possible to evaluate the potential effectiveness and cost-effectiveness of AAA screening programs.

FEMOROPOPLITEAL ANEURYSMS

Most of the natural history data on femoropopliteal aneurysms is based upon past retrospective reviews of patients who presented with symptomatic aneurysms or with large aneurysms that were easily detected on physical examination.[20-23] Population-based information from serial ultrasound examinations of a large series of patients is currently not available. Consequently, the current understanding of the outcome for femoral and popliteal aneurysms emphasizes their propensity for thrombosis, embolization, and limb-threatening ischemia. The size of the aneurysm does not appear to be as important as its configuration, tortuosity, and thrombus content, features that tend to result in sudden thrombosis and severe ischemia. In general, 30 to 50 percent of femoral or popliteal aneurysms present with severe lower limb ischemia. Without revascularization approximately 20 to 30 percent of such patients would eventually need an amputation.

THORACIC AND THORACOABDOMINAL ANEURYSMS

Data on the natural history of thoracic aortic aneurysms and thoracoabdominal aneurysms is also limited. One population-based study of thoracic aneurysms revealed a dismal 5-year patient survival of less than 20 percent. Approximately 75 percent of patients with identified thoracic aneurysms suffered rupture, usually within 2 years.[24] It must be emphasized that this study was based upon diagnosis by chest x-ray and autopsy and did not include recognition of many smaller thoracic aneurysms that can now be identified by CT scanning. Most of the aneurysms of this study would have been relatively large. With the advent of chest CT scanning, more accurate data for various aneurysm sizes should be available in the near future.

Likewise, our current knowledge of the natural course of thoracoabdominal aneurysms has been based primarily on one study.[25] This study included patients who were not thought to be fit for thoracoabdominal aneurysm repair or who refused such repair. At 5 years only one of four of these patients was still alive. Rupture was a common cause of death. Aside from this study, no studies of thoracoabdominal aneurysm prognosis based on serial CT scans are currently available.

Such information would be useful, since it would provide some estimate of rupture risk based upon aneurysm size.

REFERENCES

1. Nevitt MP, Ballard DJ, Hallett JW Jr: Prognosis of abdominal aortic aneurysms: a population-based study. N Engl J Med 321:1009, 1989
2. Johansson G, Nydahl S, Olofsson P, Swedenborg J: Survival in patients with abdominal aortic aneurysms: comparison between operative and nonoperative management. Eur J Vasc Surg 4:497, 1990
3. Glimaker H, Holmberg L, Elvin A et al: Natural history of patients with abdominal aortic aneurysm. Eur J Vasc Surg 5:125, 1991
4. Guirguis EM, Barber CG: The natural history of abdominal aortic aneurysms. Am J Surg 162:481, 1991
5. Cronenwett JL, Murphy TF, Zetenock GB et al: Actuarial analysis of variables associated with rupture of small abdominal aortic aneurysms. Surgery 98:472, 1985
6. Estes JE Jr: Abdominal aortic aneurysm: a study of one hundred and two cases. Circulation 2:258, 1950
7. Szilagyi DE, Elliott JP, Smith RF: Clinical fate of the patient with asymptomatic abdominal aortic aneurysm and unfit for surgical treatment. Arch Surg 104:600, 1972
8. Nemetz PN, Ludwig J, Kurland LT: Assessing the autopsy. Am J Pathol 128:362, 1987
9. Sommerville RL, Allen EV, Edwards JE: Bland and infected arteriosclerotic abdominal aortic aneurysms: a clinicopathologic study. Medicine (Baltimore) 38:207, 1959
10. Darling RC, Messina CR, Brewster DC, Ottinger LW: Autopsy study of unoperated abdominal aortic aneurysms: the case for early resection. Circulation 56:II-161, 1977
11. Cronenwett JL, Sargent SK, Wall WH et al: Variables that affect the expansion rate and outcome of small abdominal aortic aneurysms. J Vasc Surg 11:260, 1990
12. Collin J, Araujo L, Walton J: How fast do very small abdominal aortic aneurysms grow? Eur J Vasc Surg 3:15, 1989
13. Roger VL, Ballard DJ, Hallett JW Jr et al: Influence of coronary artery disease on morbidity and mortality following abdominal aortic aneurysmectomy: a population-based study, 1971–87. J Am Coll Cardiol 14:1245, 1989
14. Gersh BJ, Rihal CS, Rooke TW, Ballard DJ: Evaluation and management of patients with both peripheral vascular and coronary artery disease. J Am Coll Cardiol 18:203, 1991
15. Cole CW: Highlights of an international workshop on abdominal aortic aneurysms. Can Med Assoc J 141:393, 1989
16. Greenhalgh RM: When should the small asymptomatic aneurysm be operated upon? p. 457. In Greenhalgh RM,

Mannick JA (eds): The Cause and Management of Aneurysms. WB Saunders, London, 1990

17. Lederle FA: Management of small abdominal aortic aneurysms. Ann Intern Med 113:731, 1990
18. Oboler SK, LaForce FM: The periodic physical examination in asymptomatic adults. Ann Intern Med 110:214, 1989
19. Collin J, Araujo L, Walton J, Lindsell D: Oxford screening programme for abdominal aortic aneurysm in men aged 65 to 74 years. Lancet 2:613, 1988
20. Gifford RW, Hines EA, Janes JM: An analysis and follow-up study of one hundred popliteal aneurysms. Surgery 33:284, 1953

21. Cutler BS, Darling RC: Surgical management of arteriosclerotic femoral aneurysms. Surgery 74:764, 1973
22. Szilagyi DE, Schwartz RL, Reddy DJ: Popliteal arterial aneurysms. Arch Surg 116:724, 1981
23. Schellack J, Smith RB, Perdue GD: Nonoperative management of selected popliteal aneurysms. Arch Surg 122:372, 1987
24. Bickerstaff LK, Pairolero PC, Hollier LH et al: Thoracic aortic aneurysms: a population-based study. Surgery 92:1103, 1982
25. Crawford ES, DeNatale RW: Thoracoabdominal aortic aneurysm: observations regarding the natural course of the disease. J Vasc Surg 3:578, 1986

the adjacent femoral or popliteal veins or groin pain and femoral neuropathy from dissection of the hematoma into the femoral canal.

EROSION INTO ADJACENT STRUCTURES

Rarely, aneurysms erode or rupture into adjacent anatomic structures. Aneurysms that involve the innominate artery or the ascending or descending thoracic aorta can erode or rupture into the tracheobronchial tree, the pleural space, or the esophagus. Such patients present with a spectrum of symptoms that range from intermittent blood expectoration or melena to profuse bleeding with massive hemoptysis, hematemesis, hematochezia, and cardiovascular collapse. A chest x-ray or CT scan in this circumstance will show a mediastinal mass, aortic enlargement, or pleural effusion.

Abdominal aortic and iliac artery aneurysms can erode into the small or large intestine, the ureters, the inferior vena cava and iliac veins, or the left renal vein, the last of which is often retroaortic in location.

Primary aortoenteric or ilioenteric fistulae are very rare.[9,10] Abdominal aortic and iliac aneurysms that erode into the intestine are often associated with infection of the aneurysm. The most frequent location of the fistula is between the infrarenal abdominal aorta and the third or fourth portion of the duodenum, but communications can be formed between the aorta and iliac arteries and all regions of the abdominal intestinal tract.[9] Classically, these patients present with abdominal pain in association with a pulsatile abdominal mass and evidence of recent hemorrhage from the gastrointestinal tract. Fewer than one-half of patients with a primary aortoenteric fistula present with all three of these findings.[9,11] The intestinal bleeding is often slow and insidious at the onset, the so-called herald bleed.[10] Rarely is the initial clinical presentation that of severe hemorrhagic shock. Diagnosis requires a very high index of suspicion; despite treatment, the mortality remains high.

An aortocaval or iliocaval fistula can be caused by aneurysms involving the aortoiliac segments (Fig. 35-2). In my group's experience, approximately 8 of 10 major abdominal arteriovenous fistulae occur from spontaneous rupture of the aneurysm into an adjacent major vein. Rupture of an abdominal aortic aneurysm into the inferior vena cava is most frequent, while the second most common type of fistula results from rupture of an iliac aneurysm into the iliac vein. However, rupture of these aneurysms into the inferior vena cava or common iliac vein is unusual, occurring in less than

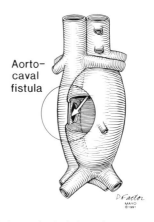

Figure 35-2 Schematic draining of an aortocaval fistula secondary to erosion or rupture of an abdominal aortic aneurysm into the inferior vena cava. (By permission of Mayo Foundation.)

1 percent of elective operations for abdominal aortic aneurysms and in less than 5 percent of all cases of ruptured aneurysms.[12]

Clinical presentation depends on the proximity of the fistula to the heart, as well as on the size of the fistula and the amount of shunted blood that passes from the arterial system into the venous system. Physiologically, these patients exhibit an increase in total blood volume and reductions in arterial pressure, peripheral resistance, and renal clearance, all of which are reversed by repair of the fistula.[13] Patients with more centrally located arteriovenous fistulas, such as between the abdominal aorta and inferior vena cava or between the iliac artery and iliac vein, can present with a constellation of symptoms and signs. With sudden, acute rupture of an aneurysm into a major vein, the signs and symptoms may be those of florid congestive heart failure, manifested by sudden cardiac decompensation, pulmonary edema, hypotension, tachycardia, and oliguria. With a more chronic, smaller erosion of the aneurysm into major veins, patients may present with compensated cardiac failure, symptoms of which include dyspnea on exertion, paroxysmal nocturnal dyspnea, or orthopnea. Examination in either case reveals distension of the jugular veins, bilateral pulmonary rales, and an S_3 heart sound. Additionally, patients may complain of abdominal, back, or flank pain and may develop lower limb swelling.[13,14] With a fistula between the aorta and left renal vein, patients complain of flank pain radiating into the groin, and they may have macroscopic or microscopic hematuria, which mimics the clinical presentation of patients with renal or ureteral stone disease. The key to diagnosis of an aortocaval or iliocaval fistula is the presence of a palpable, pulsatile abdominal mass in conjunction with an audible, continuous machinery-type abdominal bruit.

COMPRESSION OF ADJACENT STRUCTURES

Not only do aneurysms cause symptoms from rupture or from erosion into other structures, but they also cause symptoms simply by becoming enlarged and thereby encroaching on surrounding structures. Aneurysms involving the ascending aorta, transverse aortic arch, descending thoracic aortic, and brachiocephalic vessels can cause symptoms from compression of the tracheobronchial tree or esophagus, or impingement on the recurrent laryngeal nerve. These patients present with dyspnea on exertion, wheezing, stridor, and hoarseness. Compression of the esophagus, particularly in the case of an aberrant right subclavian artery aneurysm, can give rise to dysphagia, often termed *dysphagia lusoria*. A plain chest x-ray will often show a mediastinal mass and/or enlargement of the thoracic aorta, and bronchoscopy or endoscopy will show evidence of extrinsic compression of the trachea, bronchus, or esophagus.

Abdominal aortic and iliac aneurysms that compress major adjacent venous structures such as the inferior vena cava and iliac vein can present with unilateral or bilateral leg swelling. Rarely, aortic and iliac aneurysms compress the small bowel, mimicking the clinical presentation of patients with partial small bowel obstruction; the ureters, causing hydronephrosis and symptoms of ureteral obstruction; and even the bile ducts, resulting in painless jaundice.[15] Radiologic studies such as CT, ultrasound, excretory urography, and upper gastrointestinal contrast studies will help to confirm the etiology. Rarely, these studies show that the patient's symptoms may be due to a chronic contained rupture of an aneurysm, with compression of adjacent structures by the hematoma or false aneurysm. There may also be evidence of periaortitis or inflammation around the aneurysm.

Expansion of femoral and popliteal artery aneurysms can compress the femoral and popliteal veins, causing leg swelling and deep venous thrombosis (Fig. 35-3). Additionally, enlargement of femoral artery aneurysms can impinge upon the femoral nerve, resulting in femoral neuralgia. In this case the patient has dysesthesia along the anterior and medial aspect of the thigh and may develop muscle weakness involving the hip flexors and knee extensors.

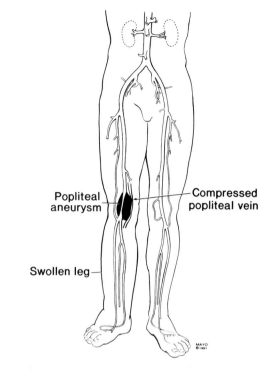

Figure 35-3 Schematic representation of a popliteal artery aneurysm that is compressing the adjacent popliteal vein causing a swollen leg. (By permission of Mayo Foundation.)

ARTERIAL ISCHEMIA

Aneurysms cause arterial ischemia from thrombosis or by distal embolization. While this is an uncommon mode of presentation for aneurysms of the aorta, it is a frequent presentation for symptomatic aneurysms of the femoral, popliteal, and brachiocephalic vessels (Fig. 35-4). Arterial ischemia caused by aneurysms in these locations can be either acute or chronic.

Acute arterial ischemia results from thrombosis of the aneurysm or macroembolization of thrombus or aneurysmal debris into large distal vessels. These patients present with pain, pallor, and pulselessness of the affected extremity. Typically, these symptoms occur at one arterial segment below the level of the thrombosis. The patient may have paresthesias and paralysis of the extremity, depending on the length of ischemia and the status of the collateral circulation. With acute aortic occlusion, as with thrombosis of an abdominal aortic aneurysm, both legs are ischemic. Examination reveals pale, cool, mottled skin, empty superficial veins, and absent arterial Doppler signals. With more profound degrees of ischemia there is often loss of motor function, loss of sensation to pinprick or light touch, and

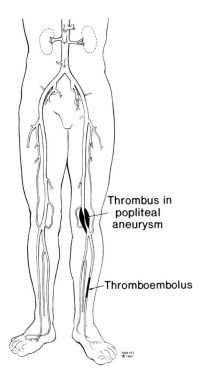

Figure 35-4 Aneurysms may be the source of distal thromboemboli. This is a common presentation of symptomatic peripheral artery aneurysms. (By permission of Mayo Foundation.)

muscle tenderness. Laboratory studies may confirm evidence of muscle injury with elevation of the serum creatinine kinase and aspartate serum transaminase levels and in some cases myoglobulinuria.

Acute arterial ischemia caused by aneurysms should be differentiated from that caused by cardiac emboli or in situ thrombosis of an atherosclerotic vessel. Careful history and physical examination are key elements in making this differentiation and should include a detailed examination of the heart (the supraclavicular and infraclavicular spaces), the neck (subclavian and axillary aneurysms), the abdomen (aortic aneurysms), and the legs (femoropopliteal aneurysms). Patients with cardiac emboli often have evidence of atrial or ventricular arrhythmias and a history of embolic events and may not have any previous symptoms or signs of peripheral arterial occlusive disease. The contralateral extremity often has normal pulses, with no evidence of aneurysmal enlargement of the vessels. In contrast, patients with in situ thrombosis of an atherosclerotic artery may give a history of limb claudication or previous vascular operations, will have an abnormal pulse examination in the contralateral extremity, and can have *trophic changes* of the skin and nail beds.

Important historical features in patients with acute thrombosis of an aneurysm include a family history of aneurysmal disease, previous aneurysm repair in another location, or radiologic documentation of aneurysms in other locations. Because of the high degree of bilaterality in patients with peripheral artery aneurysms ($\geq$ 50 percent),[7,8,16] careful evaluation and examination of the contralateral extremity is a necessity. The presence of a pulsatile mass in a similar anatomic region in the contralateral extremity is an important clue to diagnosis. In many cases the distal pulses in the contralateral extremity are intact. One other subtle clinical finding of interest occurs in patients with popliteal aneurysm thrombosis. The skin about the knee can be warm and slightly erythematous because of the increased blood flow through the collateral vessels. Thus, careful and detailed preoperative examination of the patient with acute arterial ischemia will often determine the etiology, which aids in planning appropriate intervention, whether arteriography or immediate operation.

Aneurysms also cause chronic ischemia, manifested as claudication, rest pain, or ischemic ulceration, which occur as a result of associated occlusive disease in the arterial segments above or below the aneurysm, or from chronic microembolization that has occluded the distal outflow vessels. Distal microembolization is perhaps the most significant and threatening problem in many of these patients.

In the brachiocephalic region, aneurysms of the innominate, subclavian, or carotid arteries can present with transient ischemic attacks or strokes because of embolization through the carotid or vertebrobasilar circulations. In the carotid circulation, emboli cause ipsilateral amaurosis fugax or transient monocular blindness, contralateral monoparesis or hemiparesis, contralateral sensory deficits, or speech disturbances. With vertebrobasilar embolization, patients present with diplopia or blurred vision, dysphasia, syncope, or bilateral motor or sensory deficits. Neurologic symptoms or signs are present in approximately 30 percent of patients with surgically treated brachiocephalic aneurysms.[6] Additionally, microembolization from aneurysms involving the innominate or subclavian arteries, the axillary artery, or even the ulnar artery (hypothenar hammer syndrome) can cause cyanosis of the fingers of the ipsilateral extremity, small punctate digital infarcts, splinter hemorrhages beneath the nail beds, or a very fine petechial rash.

At least one-half of patients with popliteal aneurysms present with symptoms of acute or chronic ischemia.[8] Similarly, 40 to 50 percent of those with femoral artery aneurysms present with limb-threatening problems.[7] Because acute or chronic limb ischemia frequently complicates femoral or popliteal artery aneurysms, identification and treatment of asymptomatic peripheral aneurysms are critical to minimizing limb loss.

INFECTED ANEURYSM

Aneurysms may be associated with infection or inflammation. Infection of an aneurysm occurs by several mechanisms.[17] First, septic emboli can lodge within the arterial wall and result in mycotic aneurysms. In the past this was most frequently associated with endocarditis (Fig. 35-5). The primary pathogens are Group D streptococci species.[17,18] Second, through hematogenous spread, *Staphylococcus* and *Salmonella* bacteria may produce a local arteritis that eventually causes aneurysmal degeneration of the vessel. *Salmonella* spp. are the most frequent cause of infection of aneurysms by this mechanism. Third, pre-existing aneurysms, most commonly atherosclerotic in origin, can become seeded by bloodborne bacteria. Gram-positive cocci, including *Staphylococcus epidermidis, Staphy-*

lococcus aureus, and streptococcal species, are the most frequent pathogens, but gram-negative bacilli and anaerobic bacteria are being isolated more commonly than in the past.[19,20] It is likely that infection of pre-existing aneurysms occurs because the local milieu, which includes a degenerated intima and atherosclerotic debris, allows for bacterial growth. This may account for the 15 to 20 percent positive culture rate of aneurysmal debris reported by others.[21-23] Primary infection of blood vessels or pre-existing aneurysms can also occur from local spread of adjacent infections or abscesses, although this is an infrequent occurrence.

The fourth major mechanism involves secondary infection from repeated trauma to an artery. Intravenous drug use with contaminated needles is a common cause of infected pseudoaneurysms of the brachial, femoral, and carotid arteries. Iatrogenic trauma from invasive catheterization procedures represents another increasingly common source of arterial pseudoaneurysms, which then become secondarily infected. Finally, in the era of cancer chemotherapy, immunocompromised patients represent a special subgroup susceptible to development of infected aneurysms. Fungal and mycobacterial organisms are often the etiologic agents. For example, infected abdominal aortic and femoral aneurysms have been reported following intravesical instillation of bacille Calmette-Guérin (BCG) vaccine for the treatment of bladder cancers.[24,25]

Patients with primary infected aneurysms are at high risk of death or limb loss, which ranges from approximately 5 percent for the treatment of localized infected false aneurysms of the femoral artery to over 70 to 90 percent for infected aortic aneurysms caused by gram-negative organisms or *Salmonella* spp.[17,20,26] These patients may present with very nonspecific, generalized constitutional symptoms or with catastrophic complications such as aneurysm rupture or profound sepsis.[27] Early diagnosis is crucial to avoid a disastrous outcome. The diagnosis of an infected aneurysm should be suspected in any patient with a known aneurysm or palpable pulsatile mass in the neck, arms, abdomen, or legs who presents with vague pain, intermittent low grade fevers or chills, generalized fatigue, weakness, or malaise.

Aneurysms may have surrounding inflammation without evidence of infection. These aneurysms have been termed *inflammatory aneurysms* and most frequently involve the abdominal aorta. This type of aneurysm represents approximately 4 to 5 percent of all abdominal aortic aneurysms.[28] The most common clinical presentation of inflammatory abdominal aortic aneurysms includes abdominal pain (60 percent of cases), weight loss (20 percent), and an elevation of the erythrocyte sedimentation rate (73 percent). Because of

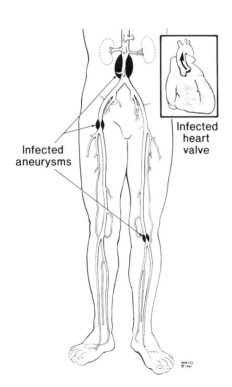

Figure 35-5 Infection of aneurysms can occur from a variety of mechanisms. As shown here, mycotic aneurysms due to septic emboli from infected heart valves can be present in the aorta, femoral arteries, or popliteal arteries. (By permission of Mayo Foundation.)

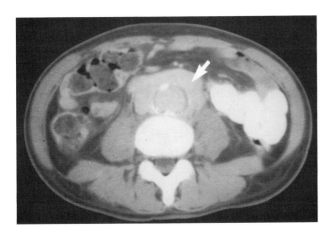

Figure 35-6 CT scan showing a contrast-enhanced rim surrounding a large inflammatory abdominal aortic aneurysm *(arrow).*

the associated inflammation of the retroperitoneal tissues, adjacent structures such as the duodenum (97 percent), the inferior vena cava (63 percent), left renal vein (51 percent), and ureter (23 percent) may be compressed and densely adherent to the aneurysm.[28] Nonetheless, very few patients present with symptoms referable to caval, left renal vein, intestinal, or ureteral obstruction. Since almost two-thirds of patients with this form of aortic aneurysm complain of back pain or abdominal pain, it is imperative that the clinician ascertain whether there is any evidence of leak or rupture of the aneurysm. CT is often performed as an initial diagnostic study and provides a tentative diagnosis of this type of aneurysm because of the presence of a contrast-enhanced rim about the anterior and lateral wall of the aneurysm (Fig. 35-6). Histologically, there is medial atrophy and degeneration, with marked thickening of the adventitial layer and infiltration by these layers by lymphocytes and plasma cells. Interestingly, once the aneurysm is repaired, the inflammatory process often resolves.

ASSOCIATED ANEURYSMS AND OCCLUSIVE DISEASE

The presence of an aneurysm in one region should be a clue that there may be aneurysms in other locations within the arterial system.[29] This is especially true with femoral or popliteal aneurysms, which occur bilaterally in approximately 50 to 70 percent of cases.[7,8,16] Additionally, brachiocephalic aneurysms are associated with aneurysms in other locations. In particular, almost 80 percent of patients with innominate aneurysms harbor additional aneurysms, usually in the tho-

racic or thoracoabdominal aorta or the aortoiliac segments and less frequently in the peripheral and visceral arteries. Association with other aneurysms is rare for patients with carotid aneurysms but occurs in almost one-third of those with subclavian aneurysms.[6] In contrast, patients with an abdominal aortic aneurysm have less than a 5 percent chance of harboring aneurysms in other locations, with one exception[29]; almost one-half of patients with *inflammatory* aortic aneurysms will have an aneurysm in another arterial segment, usually the iliac, femoral, popliteal, thoracic, or thoracoabdominal regions.[28]

Since many patients with aneurysmal disease have the same risk factors as those associated with arterial occlusive disease, these two entities may be present in the same patient (Fig. 35-7). This is not an uncommon relationship, especially with aortoiliac aneurysms, with as many as one-fourth of such patients having both aneurysmal and occlusive disease.[30-32] Because of this association, a careful history and thorough physical examination of all arterial segments are necessary. This will lessen the possibility of a patient developing unexpected complications from an undetected aneurysm in one region while being treated for symptomatic occlusive disease in another location.

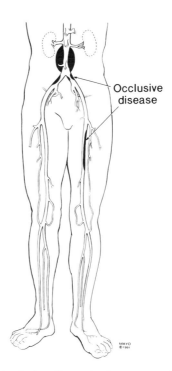

Figure 35-7 Occlusive disease in the common iliac and superficial femoral arteries in association with an abdominal aortic aneurysm. Aneurysms and atherosclerotic occlusive disease may coexist in the same patient. (By permission of Mayo Foundation.)

REFERENCES

1. Guirgins EM, Barbor GG: The natural history of abdominal aortic aneurysms. Am J Surg 162:481, 1991
2. Rutherford RB, Hollier LH (eds): Infrarenal aortic aneurysms. p. 909. In Vascular Surgery. 3rd Ed. WB Saunders, Philadelphia, 1989
3. Trastek VF, Pairolero PC, Joyce JW et al: Splenic artery aneurysms. Surgery 91:694, 1982
4. Erskine JM: Hepatic artery aneurysms. Vasc Surg 7:106, 1973
5. Graham LM, Stanley JL, Whitehouse WM Jr et al: Celiac artery aneurysms: historic (1945–1949) versus contemporary (1950–1984) differences in etiology and clinical importance. J Vasc Surg 5:757, 1985
6. Bower TC, Pairolero PC, Hallett JW Jr et al: Brachiocephalic aneurysms: the case for early recognition and repair. Ann Vasc Surg 5:125, 1991
7. Cutler BS, Darling RC: Surgical management of arterosclerotic femoral aneurysms. Surgery 74:764, 1973
8. Evans WE, Hayes JP: Atherosclerotic popliteal aneurysms. In Ernst CB, Stanley JC (eds): Current Therapy in Vascular Surgery. BC Decker, Philadelphia, 1987
9. Sweeney MS, Gadacz TR: Primary aortoduodenal fistula: manifestation, diagnosis, and treatment. Surgery 96:492, 1984
10. Steffes BC, O'Leary JP: Primary aortoduodenal fistula: a case report and review of the literature. Am Surg 46:121, 1980
11. Reckless JPD, McColl I, Taylor GW: Aorto-enteric fistulae: an uncommon complication of abdominal aortic aneurysms. Br J Surg 59:458, 1972
12. Baker PA, Scharzer LA, Ehrenhaft JL: Aortocaval fistula as a complication of abdominal aortic aneurysms. Surgery 72:933, 1972
13. Kazmier FJ, Harrison CE Jr: Acquired aortocaval fistulas. Am J Med 55:175, 1973
14. Reckless JPD, McColl I, Taylor GW: Aorto-caval fistulae: an uncommon complication of abdominal aortic aneurysms. Br J Surg 59:461, 1972
15. Bower TC, Cherry KJ, Pairolero PC: Unusual manifestations of abdominal aortic aneurysms. Surg Clin North Am 69:745, 1989
16. Anton GE, Hertzer NR, Beven EG et al: Surgical management of popliteal aneurysms: trends in presentation, treatment, and results from 1952–1984. J Vasc Surg 3:125, 1986
17. Wilson SE, Van Wagenen P, Panaro E Jr: Arterial infections. Curr Probl Surg 15:5, 1978
18. Brown SL, Busuttil RW, Baker JD et al: Bacteriologic and surgical determinants of survival in patients with mycotic aneurysms. J Vasc Surg 1:541, 1984
19. Bitseff EL, Edwards WH, Mulherin JL Jr et al: Infected abdominal aortic aneurysms. South Med J 80:309, 1987
20. Jarrett F, Darling RC, Mundth ED, et al: Experience with infected aneurysms of the abdominal aorta. Arch Surg 110:1281, 1975
21. Ilgenfritz FM, Jordan FT: Microbiological monitoring of aortic aneurysm wall and contents during aneurysmectomy. Arch Surg 123:506, 1988
22. Stonebridge PA, Mutirangura P et al: Bacteriology of aortic aneurysms. J R Coll Surg Edinb 35:42, 1990
23. Ernst CB, Campbell C Jr, Daugherty ME et al: Incidence and significance of intraoperative bacterial cultures during abdominal aneurysmectomy. Ann Surg 185:626, 1977
24. Bornet P, Pujade B, Lacaine F et al: Tuberculous aneurysm of the femoral artery: a complication of bacille Calmette-Guérin vaccine immunotherapy. J Vasc Surg 10:688, 1989
25. Woods JM, Schellack J, Stewart MT et al: Mycotic abdominal aortic aneurysm induced by immunotherapy with bacille Calmette-Guérin vaccine for malignancy. J Vasc Surg 7:808, 1988
26. Mendelowitz DS, Ramstedt R, Yao JST et al: Abdominal aortic salmonellosis. Surgery 85:514, 1979
27. Mundth ED, Darling RC, Alvarado RF et al: Surgical management of mycotic aneurysms and the complications of infection in vascular reconstructive surgery. Am J Surg 117:460, 1969
28. Pennell RC, Hollier LH, Lie JT et al: Inflammatory abdominal aortic aneurysms: a thirty year review. J Vasc Surg 2:859, 1985
29. Dent TL, Lindenau SM, Ernst CB, Fry WJ: Multiple atherosclerotic arterial aneurysms. Arch Surg 105:338, 1972
30. Johnston KW, Sobie TK: Multicenter prospective study of nonruptured abdominal aortic aneurysms. I: Population and operative management. J Vasc Surg 7:69, 1988
31. Nuno IN, Collins GM, Bardin JA et al: Should aortography be used routinely in the elective management of abdominal aortic aneurysms? Am J Surg 144:53, 1982
32. Bell DD, Gaspar RM: Routine aortography before abdominal aortic aneurysmectomy: a prospective study. Am J Surg 144:191, 1982

36

Preoperative Evaluation of Aneurysms

John W. Joyce

Arterial aneurysms are the most treatable of all potential cardiovascular catastrophes. Consequently, the evaluation of ancillary medical and surgical conditions is the foundation of sound counsel for the aneurysm patient who faces a major corrective operation. This chapter is directed to the clinical evaluation of aneurysmal disease and preoperative assessment of such patients.

Appreciation of three general characteristics of aneurysms allows a sound, logical approach. First, most aneurysms enlarge at a rate governed by the etiology of the lesion. Degenerative or dysplastic processes such as atherosclerosis, fibromuscular dysplasia, congenital defects of elastin and collagen, and syphilis engender growth measured over years. In contrast, when trauma, infection, or inflammation is causative, enlargement may be noted over days, weeks, or months. Second, because aneurysms tend to be multiple (Fig. 36-1), the discovery of one aneurysm must start the search for others; 3 percent of patients with abdominal aortic aneurysms (AAAs) and 10 to 12 percent of patients with thoracic aortic aneurysms have another aneurysm elsewhere.[1-3] Of patients with iliac, femoral, or popliteal artery aneurysms, 40 to 80 percent have a contralateral limb or proximal aneurysm at the time of diagnosis.[1,4,5] The third aspect of aneurysms to be emphasized is their diversified presentation and behavior at different anatomic sites, as detailed in Chapter 35.

DETECTION

The foundation for diagnoses of aneurysmal disease remains a competent historical and physical examination of the patient. Imaging by several techniques serves to confirm and quantitate the diagnosis, define complications, and in some cases screen for occult lesions.

History

The history may disclose prior aneurysmal disease, the presence of a pulsatile mass noted by the patient, or symptoms caused by the aneurysm or its complications. Risk factors predisposing to aneurysm formation must be sought specifically; they include hypertension, family history, cigarette smoking, and the presence of other predisposing diseases. Among predisposing conditions are atherosclerosis in the peripheral, cardiac, or carotid system; prior trauma; certain arteritides, including polyarteritis nodosa, Takayasu's and temporal arteritis, relapsing polychondritis, rheumatoid spondylitis, the Behçet syndrome, and Kawasaki disease; and hereditary disorders of connective tissue, specifically the Marfan and Ehlers-Danlos syndromes and occasionally mucopolysaccharidosis. While assessment of the arterial system is an intrinsic component of a general examination, it becomes critically important when

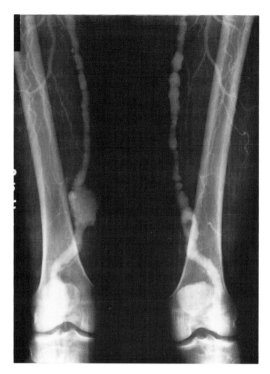

Figure 36-1 This 64-year-old man presented for advice regarding a 4.5-cm abdominal aortic aneurysm. These bilateral popliteal aneurysms were first appreciated by two-handed compression of the adductor muscle mass. Note the presence of arteriomegaly.

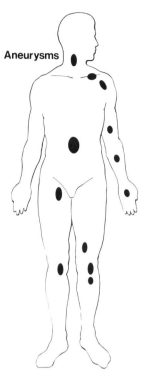

Figure 36-2 Sites of aneurysms palpable on physical examination. Most common are those of the abdominal aorta and the popliteal and femoral arteries. Infrequent sites of aneurysms are shown at the figure's left side at carotid, subclavian, axillary, and arm locations. Note the three areas where a popliteal aneurysm may be found.

clinical factors elevate suspicion of aneurysmal disease. Certain aneurysms will remain occult to history and examination when the lesion is small and the patient large. Specifically, aneurysms of the thoracic and thoracoabdominal aorta and of the iliac and visceral arteries are usually not detectable on physical examination but are recognized by imaging, surgery, or other investigations of associated symptoms.

Examination

Establishment of presence or absence of pulses, bruits, and aneurysms is the essential goal of the arterial examination. The skin, ocular fundus, and body habitus may provide additional information. Arteries always included are the radial, ulnar, subclavian, carotid, abdominal aorta, femoral, posterior tibial, and dorsalis pedis. The most common sites of aneurysm formation, in order of frequency, are the abdominal aorta and the popliteal and common femoral arteries, each accessible to palpation (Fig. 36-2). While upward of 80 percent of operated AAAs were detected by palpation in early reports, recent surveys suggest that the sensitivity of examination is in the 50 to 60 percent

range.[6-8] Most popliteal and femoral aneurysms are detectable by careful examination.[4,5]

Arterial size and pulsatility vary with the stature and conditioning of the patient. For a given patient, all pulses should correlate in magnitude, with the exception of the ulnar and dorsalis pedis, which may be less prominent. When a patient has one pulse that is slightly larger or more forceful than others, ectasia is suspected. An arbitrary definition of an aneurysm is a focal enlargement one and one-half times as large as the usual diameter of the artery. Tortuosity of the right common carotid, abdominal aorta, or wrist arteries can mimic an aneurysm. While careful palpation sometimes clarifies this question, ultrasound or arteriographic studies are generally required to settle it.

Diagnosis of an aneurysm is made with confidence when a palpable, often visible pulsation is transmitted to the fingers on either side of an enlarged vessel. Seroma surrounding an arterial graft is an exception to this rule; the tense fluid can transmit pulsations from a normal underlying prosthesis. A mass that pulsates on only part of its surface represents a mass plus a transmitted pulse (Fig. 36-3). Lesions adjacent to the abdominal aorta that can produce this phenomenon include horseshoe kidney, mesenteric and pancreatic cysts, and retroperitoneal tumors. Primary arterial tumors such as hemangioendotheliomas may also pulsate, but their firm, often irregular surface usually distinguishes them from true aneurysms.

I advocate the following techniques for examination of aneurysmal disease: (1) both patient and examiner should be in a relaxed position; (2) the examiner should use the surface area of two or more fingers on each side of the lesion; (3) the examiner should begin with light pressure, increasing it gradually as necessary; and (4) thumb contact should be avoided, as the examiner's own pulse may be transmitted.

For examination of the abdominal aorta, the patient should be supine on a firm surface, with arms at the side, and *knees flexed* to obtain maximum relaxation. The examination is initiated with eight fingers spread over the epigastrium; a diffuse pulsation is often seen or felt, even in obese patients. Subsequently, three or four fingers of each hand are slowly brought to press deeper on each side of the aorta until its pulsatility and dimensions are appreciated. Coaching the patient to relax and breathe, warning that modest discomfort may be felt, and penetrating to greater depth with each expiration enhance the difficult examination. AAAs may be noted below the xiphoid or at the umbilicus but more often

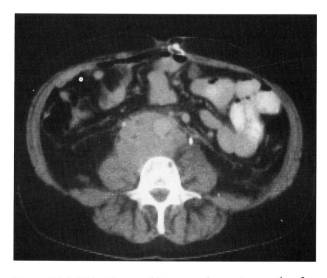

Figure 36-3 This 54-year-old man underwent operation for an abdominal aortic aneurysm. A dense, fibrotic mass was found, the abdomen was closed, and the patient was referred for definitive repair of what was thought to be an extensive inflammatory aneurysm. On examination, pulsatility was noted on only one surface, and a diagnosis of retroperitoneal mass with transmitted pulsation was made. At reoperation, biopsy confirmed an embryonal seminoma.

fill the epigastrium. Most are centered to the left of midline, but aortic tortuosity occasionally swings the mass more to the right. Extension of a pulsatile mass below the usual location of the umbilicus may represent overlap of a large aortic lesion but more often suggests extension into the iliac arteries. When the abdominal aorta is examined routinely, repetitive experience soon provides the examiner with confidence in differentiating a normal aorta from aneurysms as small as 3 or 4 cm in diameter in lean patients. Slight patient discomfort is common, but significant tenderness suggests a contained rupture, recent expansion, or an inflammatory aneurysm. I am unaware of rupture having occurred during examination of several thousand AAAs seen over four decades in my institution. (A solitary instance of rupture of an isolated iliac artery aneurysm occurred during digital examination of the rectum. The patient survived emergency repair.)

Aneurysms of limb arteries are detected readily by the technique described. Indeed, patients are often the first to note common femoral lesions while bathing. Popliteal artery aneurysms, second in frequency only to those of the abdominal aorta, are easily overlooked by both patient and physician, particularly when the latter accepts full pedal pulses as indirect evidence of popliteal integrity. The popliteal artery is best examined with the patient supine. The patient is encouraged to relax the knee into the cradle formed by two examining hands. Examination of the popliteal is incomplete unless three areas are assessed: most aneurysms are found at the joint crevice; an occasional lesion is found distal to the joint crevice, between the heads of the gastrocnemius muscle; and up to one-fourth of popliteal aneurysms occur in the portion of the popliteal artery arising at the adductor hiatus but proximal to the joint crevice and will be overlooked unless the adductor muscle mass is compressed between both hands of the examiner. This lesion is commonly associated with arteriomegaly and is usually bilateral (Fig. 36-1).

Aneurysms of the carotid, subclavian, and axillary systems are uncommon but accessible to palpation of the neck, supraclavicular space, and axilla—areas usually included in a general examination. Aneurysms in the muscular portion of the limbs or in the scalp, hands, and feet are random, self-apparent events and are usually the result of trauma, infected emboli, or occasionally, polyarteritis nodosa. An arteriovenous fistula may cause aneurysmal dilatation of the involved artery and vein and is accompanied by a continuous bruit.

Aneurysms of the visceral and iliac arteries and of the thoracic and thoracoabdominal aorta remain occult until quite large or symptomatic. Most visceral artery aneurysms are found incidentally to imaging or exploratory laparotomy or at the time symptoms appear.[9]

One-third or more of iliac aneurysms are extensions of aortic aneurysms. Isolated aneurysms of the common, external, or internal iliac artery are hidden in the pelvis and most often diagnosed secondary to imaging or rupture. Less than one-fifth are detected by abdominal examination or are suggested by pulsatility noted on rectal or pelvic examination.[10]

Asymptomatic thoracoabdominal aneurysms are diagnosed when imaging an associated thoracic aortic aneurysm or infrarenal AAA, from a retrocardiac shadow noted on chest roentgenograms, or during other imaging procedures. Most thoracic aortic aneurysms are discovered by chest roentgenograms. Larger lesions are noted during investigation of signs of mediastinal compression, such as cough, dysphagia, dysphonia, and hemoptysis, or during evaluation of aortic valve incompetence. Physical signs are late and include those of aortic valve incompetence, unilateral or bilateral jugular venous distension, and pulsatility in the upper intercostal interspaces or rarely, of the precordium.[2,3] Innominate artery aneurysms are rare and may present as pulsatility in the right supraclavicular space or as elevated right jugular venous distension. Most are detected as widening of the upper right mediastinum on a chest roentgenogram.[11]

Imaging

Chapter 37 on aneurysm imaging emphasizes the essential information that must be obtained after a good history and physical examination. Accurate measurements of aneurysm size and extent are critical to treatment decisions, especially in high-risk patients.[12,13]

Screening

Observations in the preceding chapters as well as the foregoing remarks define two sets of circumstances in which the clinician will use imaging to search for aneurysmal disease when the examination has not clearly established normalcy of the aorta and the iliac and popliteal arteries. The first set of circumstances comprises several clinical problems: (1) discovery of an aneurysm elsewhere; (2) unexplained acute occlusion of a distal artery; (3) microembolisms to the limbs, viscera, or kidney; (4) limb edema possibly caused by proximal aneurysm compression or fistula; and (5) a continuous bruit in the abdomen, chest, or limb.

Second, certain clinical settings establish a priority to monitor given patient populations for aneurysms. These populations include patients with heritable defects of connective tissue, the previously mentioned

vasculitides, trauma, syphilis, or tuberculosis. Knowledge of a familial tendency toward formation of abdominal aortic aneurysms has evolved, and both men and women with positive family history warrant surveillance as they age.[14-16]

A large number of people die without care or during emergency surgery from rupture of a previously undetected AAA. In view of the significant prevalence of hypertension, smoking, and associated occlusive disease of the coronary, limb, and carotid systems, reported among patients in all studies of the aneurysm, many screening studies have been performed with the goal of early detection and treatment. Most studies have used ultrasound because of its sensitivity, portability, and lower cost. The studies vary in format, controls, and populations, but the following selected observations are provocative.

The incidence of unknown AAA is about 5 to 10 percent in men aged 60 to 75 who have any manifestation of coronary disease, hypertension, or both.[7] The prevalence of an aneurysm is 15 percent in men aged 65 to 74 with intermittent claudication, in contrast to a 5 percent prevalence in those free of claudication. The prevalence of an aortic aneurysm in elderly Swedish men is at least 20 percent in those with angina and about 15 percent in those with prior myocardial infarction, as compared with prevalence rates of approximately 9 to 10 percent in those without these diagnoses.[18] Age increases the incidence of the aneurysm, which was noted as 83.2 per 100,000 patient-years at age 55 to 59 and 500 per 100,000 patient-years after age 80 in a controlled population study.[19] Both surgical and epidemiologic studies establish the aneurysm as more common in men. After age 65 the prevalence in women increases with age and becomes significant.[20,21]

Further definition of specific risks is needed, and cost/benefit ratios are debated. Nonetheless, the positive medical benefit of screening men over age 65 for the aneurysm has been detailed by Collin,[22] and he has calculated the cost per patient at only 11 percent that of an established breast screening program. Faced with a patient who has any risk factors for aneurysm, I screen periodically for AAA by examination and ultrasound.

PREOPERATIVE ASSESSMENT

The prototypical patient undergoing elective repair of an AAA is an elderly man (over 65 years of age), who is taking antihypertensive medication, who has smoked enough to have pulmonary damage, and (in at least 50 percent of cases) who has prior or current cardiac disease. He may also have renal impairment of varying severity and diabetes mellitus. He will be offered repair in the face of prior or current malignancy if the aneurysm is large or symptomatic and if the prognosis of the tumor is better than that of the aneurysm. An operative risk of 3 to 6 percent or less will be suggested, depending upon the details of the ancillary disease present.

The refinement of aneurysm surgery is such that medical problems (Fig. 36-4) far exceed surgical complications as the cause of operative mortality and morbidity. The remarkable success of surgical repair of potentially lethal aneurysms is dependent upon the recognition, quantitation, and perioperative management of the multiple significant deficits so often present.

Infection

The patient should be free of all systemic and focal bacterial infection prior to the elective repair of any aneurysm. This will minimize the uncommon but often devastating complication of subsequent prosthetic graft infection.

Hematologic

It is prudent to establish the integrity of the clotting mechanism from the patient and family history, platelet count, and both prothrombin and activated partial

thromboplastin times. This will identify congenital defects, defects that may be associated with occult hepatic disease, the occasional intravascular coagulopathy seen with symptomatic aneurysms, and possible platelet deficits induced by any of several drugs that the patient may have used recently. It is preferable that the patient be free of antiplatelet therapy for 10 to 14 days prior to the procedure to minimize the chance of perioperative bleeding.

A history of prior deep venous thromboembolic disease warrants consideration of anticoagulant prophylaxis during the recovery period.

Cardiac

Cardiac disease is the most common and threatening medical risk factor in aneurysm patients (Fig. 36-5). Significant hypertension and congestive heart failure are investigated, treated, and stabilized in the preoperative period. Potentially hazardous rhythm problems should be evaluated and managed with pharmacologic agents, pacing, or both as required. Critical aortic valve stenosis is to be appreciated and surgically corrected when present.

Myocardial infarction, and to a lesser extent acute cardiac failure and arrhythmias, are consistently identified as the major causes of death and morbidity following repair of atherosclerotic aneurysms.[23,24] This is to be expected, given the diffuse distribution of the atherosclerotic process. The incidence of clinically recognized markers of coronary disease in patients warranting repair of an AAA is consistently reported at 45 to 55 percent or higher.[23-25] Sensitive markers include infarction, congestive failure, angina, significant arrhythmia, reduced left ventricular function, abnormal resting electrocardiogram (ECG) and diabetes

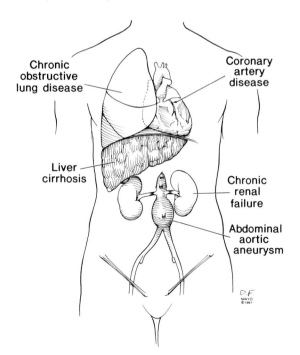

Figure 36-4 Common medical conditions that increase operative risk for aneurysm repair. (By permission of Mayo Foundation.)

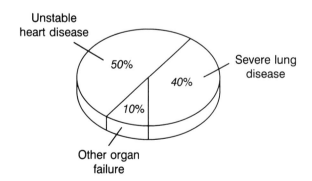

Figure 36-5 The most common medical problem increasing the risk of aortic aneurysm repair is unstable cardiac disease; this is followed closely by severe lung disease. Other organ failures are predominantly due to renal insufficiency. (From Hollier et al,[33] with permission.)

mellitus.[26] A significant additional incidence of occult coronary disease has been identified by various objective tests of the aneurysm population, whose activity level is often reduced by life-style, age, or impairment of the vascular, skeletal, or neurologic systems.[27–29] Noteworthy is the report of Hertzer and colleagues,[25] who performed coronary angiography on 1000 patients with significant aortic, peripheral, or carotid vascular disease. Among 263 patients with AAAs, aneurysms, 52 percent had clinical evidence of coronary disease. However, angiography revealed that only 6 percent had normal coronary arteries, 20 percent were judged to have severe correctable disease, and 5 percent had inoperable disease. Severe coronary disease was found in 15 percent without clinical evidence of the problem.[25]

Most patients undergoing aneurysm repair warrant some form of cardiac screening (Table 36-1). The only exception would be those with no clinically evident coronary disease and excellent exercise tolerance (e.g., walking 2 to 3 miles daily). Treadmill exercise testing has a sensitivity of only 65 percent and a significant incidence of both false positive and false negative results; also many patients are unfit to perform it. One study using exercise testing prior to vascular surgery reported no postoperative cardiac events in those achieving 75 percent or more of the maximum predicted heart rate, but a 26 percent incidence of perioperative infarction if this rate was not achieved and the ECG became abnormal.[30] Another report on ambulatory ECG monitoring of 176 patients undergoing vascular surgery included both asymptomatic patients and those with stable angina, prior infarction, or previous coronary artery bypass grafting (CABG). A positive test predicted postoperative ischemic events in 12 of 32 patients, and only one event occurred in 144 patients with a normal study. The test is relatively inexpensive but cannot be used when the baseline ECG is abnormal or the patient uses digoxin.[29] Abnormal exercise and dipyridamole thallium 201 distribution studies predict an approximate 24 percent risk of perioperative infarction and an 8 percent risk of cardiac death following vascular surgery.[28,31,32] Reduced left ventricular function and multiple ventricular wall deficits demonstrated by exercise MUGA[33] and exercise or dobutamine echocardiography are also predictive of significant coronary disease warranting angiographic definition.

I use treadmill testing when the patient's life-style suggests excellent exercise capacity. Thallium 201 redistribution studies are preferred when the patient is unable to exercise or has stable angina, prior infarction, or congestive heart failure. Coronary angiography is advised for those with unstable, class 3 or 4 angina and those with abnormal imaging studies.

CABG has significant benefit in those with left main or critical three-vessel occlusive disease and patients with left ventricular ejection fractions of less than 50 percent. It should precede vascular repair in these circumstances.

The role of percutaneous coronary angioplasty in reducing perioperative ischemic events is still being defined (Fig. 36-6). In a recent review of my own group's experience with 100 AAA patients needing preoperative coronary revascularization, the vast majority (86 percent) required CABG while only 14 percent were suitable for coronary balloon angioplasty (percutaneous transluminal coronary angioplasty [PTCA]) (Fig. 36-7). The advantage of PTCA, however, was earlier AAA repair (mean delay of 10 days) compared with 8 to 10 weeks for patients recovering from CABG. In the

Table 36-1 Recommendations for Preoperative Evaluation and Treatment of Coronary Artery and Valvular Heart Disease Prior to Aortic Aneurysm Repair

Class	Clinical Features	Recommendation
Class 1 (no clinically evident coronary artery disease)	No angina pectoris, no prior myocardial infarction, normal electrocardiogram, normal exercise and activity for age	Proceed with aneurysm repair under good cardiopulmonary monitoring
Class 2 (clinically evident coronary artery disease, stable)	Stable angina pectoris, prior myocardial infarction, abnormal electrocardiogram, sedate life-style with minimal physical activity	Noninvasive assessment of cardiac perfusion and ventricular function (see text); if significantly abnormal, coronary angiography and revascularization for critical disease
Class 3 (unstable coronary or valvular heart disease)	Progressive or unstable angina pectoris, myocardial infarction in previous 6 months, severely symptomatic valvular disease	Baseline noninvasive assessment of ventricular function; coronary and valvular angiography, with revascularization and/or valve repair before aneurysm repair

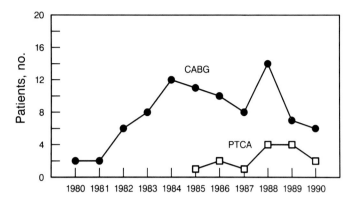

Figure 36-6 Relative utilization of coronary artery bypass grafting (CABG) and percutaneous transluminal coronary angioplasty (PTCA) to treat severe coronary atherosclerosis before elective repair of an AAA at the Mayo Clinic, 1980–1990. These 100 patients represent 4.1 percent of 2452 elective AAA repairs.

end all revascularized patients survived elective AAA repair, with only a 5 percent perioperative myocardial infarction rate. It should be emphasized that these 100 patients selected for coronary revascularization were a small (4.1 percent) subset of 2452 patients undergoing elective AAA repair over a 10-year period. The overall mortality for this entire cohort was only 2.9 percent. Consequently, most patients with coronary disease can safely undergo aneurysm repair with expert cardiovascular anesthesia, smooth surgical conduct, and intensive postoperative management.[34]

Renal

Renal insufficiency is identified in 4 to 17 percent of patients undergoing elective repair of an AAA.[24,35,36] This reflects predominantly the concomitant hypertension noted in 40 to 60 percent of patients undergoing the operation.[24,34,35,37] Significant renal artery stenosis has been documented by angiography in 13 to 22 percent of patients prior to surgery.[38,39] Simultaneous repair of the aneurysm and renal artery stenosis may be

elected when judged essential for management of hypertension; the operative mortality is 3 to 4 percent, an acceptable risk for the given clinical problems. Repair can be performed when creatinine values are in the 2 to 4 mg/dl range with minimal or no increase in mortality, and a modest incidence of postoperative azotemia, which is usually transient and rarely requires dialysis.[24,40,41] Creatinine values above 4 mg/dl do not preclude surgery; the need for dialysis becomes more likely but is not inevitable.[24,40,41] Patients with such values and those receiving chronic dialysis can be considered for surgery when the aneurysm is judged to be a significant threat and the need for long-term dialysis is acceptable to the patient.[41] Adequate preoperative hydration and intraoperative monitoring, fluid balance, and pharmacologic manipulations have established the current excellent level of operative safety for those with azotemia.

Renal imaging is desirable in selected patients prior to repair. Excretory urography or computed tomography (CT) scanning can detect clues of renal artery stenosis and occasional instances of ureteral obstruction, venous anomalies, or horseshoe kidney, each of which may alter surgical techniques or approach. When azotemia is significant, particularly in the diabetic patient, CT scanning can be performed without contrast agent. In some patients duplex ultrasound scanning will provide the needed information. Renal arteriography is indicated when renal artery stenosis is suspected and repair planned and when horseshoe kidney has been identified.

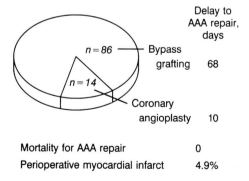

	Delay to AAA repair, days
Bypass grafting	68
Coronary angioplasty	10
Mortality for AAA repair	0
Perioperative myocardial infarct	4.9%

Figure 36-7 These data represent 100 patients who underwent preoperative coronary revascularization before elective repair of an AAA at the Mayo Clinic, 1980–1990.

Pulmonary

A history of prolonged cigarette smoking is reported in 45 to 85 percent of patients with AAA, which underscores the importance of tobacco abuse in the genesis of both atherosclerosis and aneurysms.[36,37] Clinically apparent obstructive lung disease is documented in 25 to 50 percent of patients undergoing aortic aneurysm repair. Respiratory insufficiency, however, is rarely responsible for postoperative death unless multisystem failure intervenes.[24,34,36,37,41] Spirometry and blood gas determinations are useful tests, as they predict the value of 2 to 3 days of preoperative pulmonary preparation with ventilatory exercise, bronchodilators, and in certain cases specific antibiotic therapy. Patients with a room air arterial oxygen pressure (PaO$_2$) of less than 50 mmHg and forced expiratory volumes less than 25 percent of predicted normal and those receiving home oxygen can tolerate repair.[34] While obstructive lung disease signals the need for preoperative preparation and increases postoperative ventilatory problems, repair of an AAA rarely needs to be denied because of respiratory status alone.

Carotid

Both patient and physician share the concern regarding possible perioperative stroke. Fortunately the overall incidence of central neurologic deficits with AAA repair ranges from 0.6 to 1.5 percent,[24,41,42] and the chance of fatal stroke is generally less than 1 percent on the basis of large operative series.[24,41-43] The incidence of perioperative stroke or transient ischemic attack has been reported as up to 3.1 percent when there is a prior history of such events.[24]

The presence of an asymptomatic bruit predicts a 2 to 10 percent chance of neurologic deficit with surgery. However, such events often do not correlate with extracranial occlusive disease but rather with hypotension, intracranial disease, and emboli from cardiac or aortic sources.[42,44] Abnormal ultrasound screening is associated with a stroke rate of 4 to 5 percent.[44,45]

It would seem logical to use duplex ultrasound screening or ocular pneumoplethysmography for those patients with a prior history of stroke or transient ischemic attack and those with bruits. The risk of death and stroke from carotid angiography and subsequent unilateral carotid endarterectomy is 1 to 2 percent, equaling or exceeding the risk of stroke and neurologic death from direct aneurysm repair. Proceeding with angiography and possible prophylactic carotid repair should be considered for those patients with significant bilateral stenoses on duplex scanning and those with recent transient ischemic attacks.

Asymptomatic carotid disease does not correlate well with the risk of perioperative stroke, but carotid stenosis documented by ultrasound is predictive of subsequent ischemic cerebral and cardiac events. These patients warrant surveillance.[42]

Arteriography

Arteriography is essential when planning repair of iliac and leg aneurysms (Table 36-2). It provides the knowledge of inflow, outflow, and the collateral internal iliac, profunda femoris, and geniculate arteries that is needed in planning the type and extent of procedure. Arch aortography, with multiple views, can be critical in planning repair of carotid, brachiocephalic, and high descending thoracic and thoracoabdominal aneurysms. Details of the comorbidity of the aorta and these vessels, as well as the relationship of the lesions to the arch, affect the type and extent of the procedure and the proper placement of clamps during surgery and define the need to support the cerebral circulation. Thoracoabdominal aneurysm repair requires preoperative definition of visceral and/or renal arteries when they are involved in the aneurysm.

Many surgeons use aortography prior to the repair of all AAAs. Advocates note that this defines the upper and lower limits of the lesion, recognizes significant renal, visceral, and runoff stenoses, and may reveal multiple renal arteries, small visceral aneurysms, and horseshoe kidney.[38,46,47] Others use aortography selectively, thus reducing the potential for contrast-induced nephropathy, embolization, and wound complications, as well as overall cost. They argue that the extent of the aneurysm and horseshoe kidney can usually be determined by examination or other forms of imaging and that many variables can be recognized and accommodated during operation. They reserve aortography for symptomatic visceral artery stenosis, suspected renal artery stenosis causing hypertension or azotemia, clinically significant ileofemoral stenosis, associated

Table 36-2 Recommendations for Arteriography Before Elective Aneurysm Repair

Type of Aneurysm	Arteriography
Carotid/brachicephalic	Routine
Thoracic/thoracoabdominal	Optional[a]
Abdominal	Selective
	Suspected renal or visceral stenosis
	Evident aortoiliac occlusive disease
	Horseshoe kidney
	Associated femoropopliteal aneurysms
Femoropopliteal	Routine

[a] If the thoracic or thoracoabdominal aneurysm involves major brachiocephalic or abdominal visceral arteries, arteriography is recommended.

ileofemoropopliteal aneurysmal disease, known horseshoe kidney, or prior colectomy.[48,49] Gaspar et al.[49] offer careful analysis supporting this as an effective approach, and this has long been the practice in my institution.[48]

REFERENCES

1. Dent TL, Lindenauer M, Ernst CB, Fry WJ: Multiple arteriosclerotic arterial aneurysms. Arch Surg 105:338, 1972
2. Pressler V, McNamara JJ: Aneurysms of the thoracic aorta: review of 260 cases. J Thorac Cardiovasc Surg 89:50, 1985
3. Joyce JW, Fairbairn JF II, Kincaid OW, Juergens JL: Aneurysms of the thoracic aorta: a clinical study with special reference to prognosis. Circulation 29:176, 1964
4. Wychulis AR, Spittell JA Jr, Wallace RB: Popliteal aneurysms. Surgery 68:942, 1970
5. Pappas GK, Janes JM, Bernatz PE et al: Femoral aneurysms: review of surgical management. JAMA 190:489, 1964
6. Demos NJ: Severe vascular impairment of the left half of the colon. Surg Gynecol Obstet 117:205, 1963
7. Lederle FA, Walker JM, Reinke DB: Selective screening for abdominal aortic aneurysms with physical examination and ultrasound. Arch Intern Med 148:1753, 1988
8. Littooy FN, Steffan G, Greisler HP et al: Use of sequential B-mode ultrasonography to manage abdominal aortic aneurysms. Arch Surg 124:419, 1989
9. Stanley JC, Thompson NW, Fry WJ: Splanchnic artery aneurysms. Arch Surg 101:689, 1970
10. McCready RA, Pairolero PC, Gilmore JC et al: Isolated iliac artery aneurysms. Surgery 93:688, 1983
11. Brewster DC, Moncure AC, Darling RC et al: Innominate artery lesions: problems encountered and lessons learned. J Vasc Surg 2:99, 1985
12. Bernstein EF, Chan EL: Abdominal aortic aneurysm in high-risk patients: outcome of selective management based on size and expansion rate. Ann Surg 200:255, 1984
13. Gomez MN, Choyke PL: Pre-operative evaluation of abdominal aortic aneurysms: ultrasound or computed tomography? J Cardiovasc Surg (Torino) 28:159, 1974
14. Darling RC III, Brewster DC, Darling RC et al: Are familial abdominal aortic aneurysms different? J Vasc Surg 10:39, 1989
15. Norrgard L, Rais O, Angquist KA: Familial occurrence of abdominal aortic aneurysms. Surgery 95:650, 1984
16. Johansen K, Koepsell T: Familial tendency for abdominal aortic aneurysms. JAMA 256:1934, 1986
17. Collin J, Araujo L, Waldton J, Lindsell D: Oxford screening program for abdominal aortic aneurysms in men aged 65 to 74 years. Lancet 2:613, 1988
18. Bergqvist D, Bengtsson J, Sternby NH: Associated atherosclerotic manifestations. p. 47. In Greenhalgh RM, Mannick JA (eds): The Cause and Management of Aneurysms. WB Saunders, London, 1990

19. Melton LJ, Bickerstaff LK, Hollier LH et al: Changing incidence of abdominal aortic aneurysms: a population-based study. Am J Epidemiol 120:379, 1984
20. Collin J: The epidemiology of abdominal aortic aneurysms. Br J Hosp Med 64(July):7, 1988
21. Office of Population, Censuses and Surveys: Mortality Statistics. England and Wales. Her Majesty's Stationery Office, London, 1984
22. Collin J: The value of screening for abdominal aortic aneurysm by ultrasound. p. 447. In Greenhalgh RM, Mannick JA (eds): The Cause and Management of Aneurysms. WB Saunders, London, 1990
23. Hertzer NR: Fatal myocardial infarction following abdominal aortic aneurysm resection: three hundred forty-three patients followed six to eleven years postoperatively. Ann Surg 192:667, 1980
24. Johnson KW, Scobie TK: Multicenter prospective study of nonruptured abdominal aortic aneurysms. 1. Population and operative management. J Vasc Surg 7:69, 1988
25. Hertzer NR, Beven EG, Young JR et al: Coronary artery disease in peripheral vascular patients: a classification of 1000 coronary angiograms and results of surgical management. Ann Surg 199:223, 1984
26. Cooperman M, Pflug B, Martin EW Jr et al: Cardiovascular risk factors in patients with peripheral vascular disease. Surgery 84:505, 1978
27. Pasternack PF, Imparato AM, Bear G et al: The value of radionuclide angiogram in the prediction of perioperative myocardial infarction in patients undergoing abdominal aortic aneurysm resection. J Vasc Surg 1:320, 1984
28. Boucher CA, Brewster DC, Darling KC et al: Determination of cardiac risk by dipyridamole-thallium imaging before peripheral vascular surgery. N Engl J Med 312:389, 1985
29. Raby KE, Goldman L, Creager MA et al: Correlation between perioperative ischemia and major cardiac events after peripheral vascular surgery. N Engl J Med 321:1296, 1989
30. Cutler BS, Wheeler HB, Paraskos JA, Cardullo PA: Applicability and interpretation of electrocardiographic stress testing in patients with peripheral vascular disease. Am J Surg 141:507, 1981
31. Cutler BS, Leppo JA: Dipyridamole thallium 201 scintigraphy to detect coronary artery disease before abdominal aortic surgery. J Vasc Surg 5:91, 1987
32. Eagle KA, Singer DE, Brewster DC et al: Dipyridamole-thallium scanning in patients undergoing vascular surgery. Optimizing preoperative evaluation of cardiac risk. JAMA 257:2185, 1987
33. Hollier LH, Reigel MM, Kazmier FJ et al: Conventional repair of abdominal aortic aneurysm in the high-risk patient: a plea for abandonment of nonresective treatment. J Vasc Surg 3:712, 1986
34. McCabe CJ, Coleman WS, Brewster DC: The advantage of early operation for abdominal aortic aneurysm. Arch Surg 116:1025, 1981
35. Young AE, Sandberg GW, Couch NP: The reduction of mortality of abdominal aortic aneurysm resection. Am J Surg 134:585, 1977

36. O'Donnell TF Jr, Darling RC, Linton RR: Is 80 years too old for aneurysmectomy? Arch Surg 111:11250, 1976

37. Gaspar MR: Role of arteriography in the evaluation of aortic aneurysms: the case against. p. 250. In Bergan JJ, Yao JST (eds): Aneurysms: diagnosis and treatment. Grune & Stratton, Orlando, 1982

38. Brewster DC, Retana A, Watman AC et al: Angiography and the management of aneurysms of the abdominal aorta: its value and safety. N Engl J Med 292:822, 1975

39. Stewart MT, Smith RB, Fulenwider JT et al: Concomitant renal revascularization in patients undergoing aortic surgery. J Vasc Surg 2:400, 1985

40. Cohen JR, Mannick JA, Couch NP et al: Abdominal aortic aneurysm repair in patients with perioperative renal failure. J Vasc Surg 3:867, 1986

41. Diehl JT, Cali RF, Hertzer NR, Beven EG: Complications of abdominal aortic aneurysm reconstruction: an analysis of perioperative risk factors in 557 patients. Ann Surg 197:49, 1983

42. Barnes RW, Liebman PR, Marszalck PB et al: The natural history of asymptomatic carotid disease in patients undergoing cardiovascular surgery. Surgery 90:1075, 1981

43. Crawford ES, Saleh SA, Babb JW et al: Infrarenal abdominal aortic aneurysm. Ann Surg 193:699, 1981

44. Treiman RL, Foran RF, Cohen JL et al: Carotid bruit: a follow-up report on its significance in patients undergoing an abdominal aortic operation. Arch Surg 114:1138, 1979

45. Turnipseed WD, Berkoff HA, Belzer FO: Postoperative stroke in cardiac and peripheral vascular disease. Ann Surg 192:365, 1980

46. Bauer GM, Porter JM, Eidelmiller LR et al: The role of arteriography in abdominal aortic aneurysm. Am J Surg 136:184, 1978

47. Couch NP, O'Mahoney J, McIrvine A et al: The place of abdominal aortography in abdominal aortic aneurysm resection. Arch Surg 118:1029, 1983

48. Bell DD, Gaspar MR: Routine aortography before abdominal aortic aneurysmectomy: prospective study. Am J Surg 144:191, 1982

49. Gaspar MR, Campbell JJ, Bell DD: Role of arteriography in assessment of abdominal aortic aneurysm. p. 251. In Ernst CB, Stanley JC (eds): Current Therapy in Vascular Surgery. 2nd Ed. BC Decker, Philadelphia, 1991

37

Imaging of Aneurysms

Anthony W. Stanson

ABDOMINAL AORTIC ANEURYSMS

A number of imaging modalities now exist by which aneurysms can be studied (see Ch. 14). The main diagnostic technique for confirming the *presence* of an aneurysm of the abdominal aorta is ultrasound. It is cost-effective, noninvasive, and technically simple to perform. Furthermore the equipment is portable, in contrast to computed tomography (CT), magnetic resonance imaging (MRI), and angiography. Extensive mapping of the main arterial segments from the low abdominal aorta to the popliteal arteries can be performed, except for the deep iliac artery segments, which are usually obscured by bowel gas.

Clinical management of aneurysms is dependent upon their size (Fig. 37-1). In the initial evaluation and subsequent follow-up of a patient with a known aneurysm, accurate measurement of diameter and interval change in diameter is vital to the course of treatment. But how accurate can measurements from the various imaging modalities be? Overall the reproducibility of aneurysm diameter measurement is within 3 to 5 mm.[1] High-quality CT or MRI scanning with critical assessment of measurement site may allow the best accuracy, with about 3 mm of variance.[2]

To accurately measure an aneurysm requires finding the largest diameter. This may not be a simple task because some aneurysms have irregular contours as well as areas of eccentric expansion. Additionally, it is important to find the pathway of the longitudinal axis of the artery, since a measurement perpendicular to this axis gives the true diameter (Fig. 37-2). Almost

never is this axis a straight line (even in a normal aorta) because of lordosis of the lumbar spine and the lateral drift of the aorta from the left side in the upper abdomen to near the midline in the midabdomen. Indeed, perhaps no arterial segment is oriented in a straight line to any given plane. Of course when there is aortic tortuosity, the pathway of the longitudinal axis is even more erratic. Each imaging modality presents its own problem in establishing the measurement plane relative to the long axis of the aneurysm. A simple CT scan experiment using a water-filled plastic cylinder, which illustrates the effect of object angulation upon the image, is given in Figure 37-3. The principles also apply to images obtained by ultrasound and MRI.

IMAGING TECHNIQUES

There are five diagnostic imaging studies available to determine aneurysm size. They are, in ascending order of cost, plain film of abdomen (anteroposterior [AP] and lateral views), ultrasound, CT scanning, MRI, and angiography (arteriography). Consideration must be given to the measurement accuracy of each of these examinations.

Plain Radiographic Films

Plain films of the abdomen (AP and lateral views of the lumbar spine) were the standard diagnostic study before development of ultrasound and CT scanning.

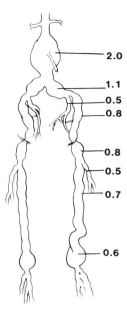

Figure 37-1 Maximum normal diameter (cm) of adult arteries.

This is an inexpensive method, but unfortunately most aneurysms are not sufficiently calcified to be adequately evaluated. In addition, those that have enough calcium may be difficult to measure accurately because of film magnification factors. However, for purposes of a follow-up examination, plain films usually can be compared accurately, especially if the aneurysm is stable. Of course, the relationships between the patient and the film and the x-ray tube and the film must be the same from the first examination to the next to keep magnification factors constant. There is little demand today for plain film evaluation of aneurysmal disease. Its role has been largely preempted by ultrasound.[1]

Ultrasound

Ultrasound is an ideal diagnostic tool to evaluate aneurysms of the abdominal aorta (Fig. 37-4), as well as those of the femoral and popliteal arteries.[1] The examination is not as expensive as CT, MRI, or angiography. Although ultrasound costs more than twice as much as plain films, its diagnostic impact makes ultrasound cost-effective in comparison. Ultrasound has the advantage of yielding nonmagnified images, which are obtained noninvasively in a short time and do not depend upon the presence of calcification. Measurements are relatively easy to obtain, but care must be taken to ensure that the transducer beam is truly perpendicular to the longitudinal axis of the aneurysm. Unfortunately, the central axis through the abdominal aorta is neither constant nor predictable. Failure to recognize the plane that is perpendicular to the long axis results in an oblique measurement, which is falsely large. An additional problem with ultrasound measurement is the difficulty in establishing the exact echogenic interface of the front and back walls of the aorta. Dense calcific deposits cast shadows that somewhat obscure borders. The interface of adjacent tissues and imprecise electronic gain settings on the machine can also obscure the precise border of an aneurysm. In most patients measurement accuracy is within a 3 to 5-mm variance for abdominal aortic aneurysm.

Computed Tomography

A third choice for an imaging modality is CT scanning. With this technique also, no inherent magnification is recorded on the images. Spatial resolution is better than 1 mm with current machines. Measure-

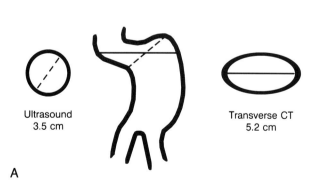

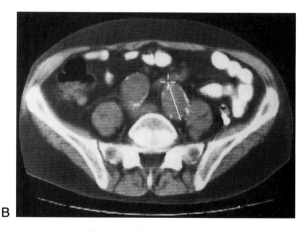

Figure 37-2 (A) Variation in aneurysm size measured by ultrasound and CT scan. **(B)** Incorrect measurement axis through an oblique path of the left iliac artery aneurysm. Adjacent CT scan sections cephalad and caudad show that the iliac artery is coursing dorsally, following the sacral curve. The short axis would be the correct direction in which to measure for the diameter of this aneurysm.

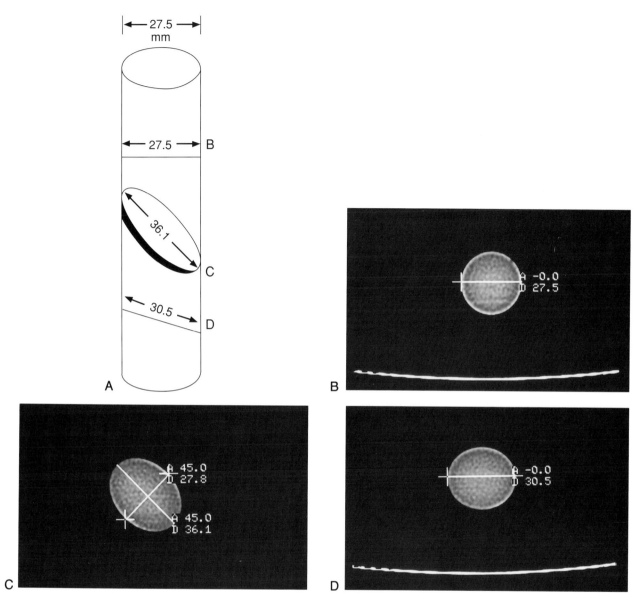

Figure 37-3 Measurements of the diameter of a phantom made of water in a plastic cylinder and scanned by CT **(A)**. The cylinder is in the long axis of the scanner, and the CT section is a true cross section and is measured at a CT angle of zero degrees for a diameter of 27.5 mm **(B)**. The cylinder is sharply angulated in two planes. The short axis diameter is 27.8 mm, which is the true diameter of the cylinder and is found at a 45-degree angle; the long axis measurement is 36.1 mm **(C)**. The cylinder is angulated laterally a few degrees, and the diameter now measures 30.5 mm along the horizontal axis (CT angle of zero degrees), which is falsely large **(D)**.

ments can be made in any direction of the cross-sectional images, but the two dimensions that are traditionally used are the AP and lateral diameters. However, these dimensions may not necessarily establish the true size of an aneurysm unless the long axis happens to be perpendicular to the plane of the CT cross-sectional image. It is therefore important to consider whether the CT image is an oblique section

through the aneurysm, in which case the shortest diameter gives the more accurate measurement, with the greatest diameter representing a falsely large measurement. If the aneurysm is truly oval in configuration, however, the short axis measurement would be falsely small (Fig. 37-5). By studying the adjacent image levels and noting the shape and drift of the aorta, an accurate size assessment of the aorta can be made. This ap-

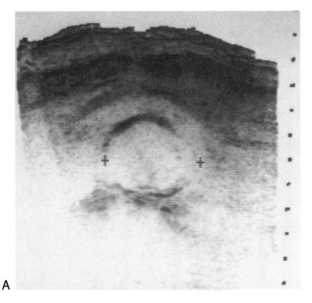
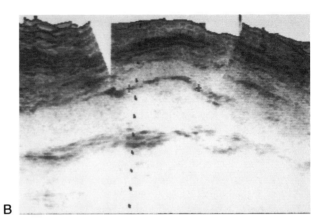

Figure 37-4 Periaortitis (inflammatory aneurysm) of the infrarenal abdominal aorta associated with a small aneurysm. This ultrasound examination of cross-sectional (**A**) and longitudinal (**B**) views shows the characteristic hypoechoic band (+) of tissue anterior and lateral to the aorta.

proach to the analysis of aneurysm diameter will usually resolve differences between ultrasound and CT measurements.

Another factor to be considered by clinicians when measuring aneurysms from CT films is the measurement scale. This is a centimeter reference printed on the side and/or top of the image, and its scale changes as the size of the field of view, also printed on the film, is changed. When looking at the images on film, one must use this reference scale. Although this seems obvious, it is easy to omit this detail when comparing two or more

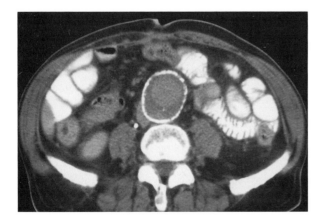

Figure 37-5 CT scan of abdomen. Aneurysm of the low abdominal aorta is oval in shape. The largest diameter is a measurement taken at an angle of about 15 degrees and is the true diameter.

CT studies. The temptation to use a caliper on one scan and to transfer it to the same image on the printout from another examination will lead to inaccuracy unless the size of the field of view is the same for both. Sometimes different CT machines may have been used for sequential examinations, and even if the same field-of-view size is chosen, the printed image may not be identical. By independently comparing measurement scales, one can avoid such errors.

In summary, the accuracy of measuring abdominal aortic aneurysms, which should be within a 3- to 5-mm range by any method, is probably a little better than this with CT; however, careful attention must be given to a variety of technical and geometric issues.

Extended CT Imaging Information

Beyond establishing the presence and size of an aneurysm, imaging modalities provide a window to other anatomic conditions in the adjacent region as well as within the aneurysm. The impact of the development of CT to display morphology of disease has been immeasurable. Diseases of the aorta are good examples. The younger physician can only imagine what it was like to have practiced medicine without CT scanning.

Very specific information about the aorta can be obtained from the CT scan.[3,4] Sometimes intraluminal thrombus is present and produces peculiar calcific deposits that are not to be confused with atheromatous intimal calcification (Fig. 37-5), since such confusion would falsely lead to the diagnosis of an aortic dissection.[5,6] Patency of the aortic lumen is established when intravenous contrast material is used (Fig. 37-6). The thickness of the aortic wall can be assessed, especially in cases of periaortitis, also called inflammatory aneurysm[7] (Fig. 37-7). It is often possible to identify the ureters, which may become entrapped in the inflammation of the aortic adventitia. Identification of symptomatic inflammatory aneurysm is important, not only in order to protect the ureters at operation but also to avoid the mistaken diagnosis of a leaking aneurysm. In addition, periaortitis can be part of the spectrum of retroperitoneal fibrosis; the periaortic thickening can occur without any true aneurysm of the aorta.

CT provides valuable information about the structures around an aneurysm and consequently can assist in patient evaluation or in surgical planning[2-4,8] (Fig. 37-8). The retroperitoneum can be thoroughly evaluated for hemorrhage, adenopathy, and renal disease or pancreatic disease in patients with sudden onset of back pain (Figs. 37-9 to 37-13). CT scanning also provides information about the location of an aneurysm relative to the visceral arteries. Ideally, the CT scan sections should be relatively thin (5 or 6 mm) and should be contiguous in order to permit identification and correlation of adjacent small structures. If metallic surgical clips have been deposited in the operative bed, the CT scan will record these as tissue-obscuring artifacts that preclude a diagnostic image. The celiac, superior mesenteric, and main renal arteries can be identified in most cases (Fig. 37-14). However, accessory renal arteries may be missed. This is also true for the multiple arteries of a horseshoe kidney, some of which arise from the iliac arteries. Major venous structures, such as

a retroaortic left renal vein (Fig. 37-15) or persistent left inferior vena cava, can also be assessed. The iliac arteries are usually well seen by CT scanning, including the main trunk of the internal iliac arteries, which may be aneurysmal in arteriomegaly. (Ultrasound is often not able to investigate the pelvic arteries adequately because of overlying bowel gas.)

After aortic graft surgery, CT is an excellent diagnostic modality for follow-up studies or for diagnosing complications such as anastomotic aneurysms, infection, and expansion of the graft fabric. It offers highly specific information, which usually exceeds that of angiography and ultrasound, especially in the retroperitoneum. CT scan often delineates complicated anatomy, which helps with preoperative planning.[3,4,9]

The fabric of the graft can usually be seen on scans performed before administration of intravenous contrast material (Figs. 37-16 and 37-17). Detectability of graft fabric is dependent upon the fabric type; the ability to see the fabric allows specific assessment of the postoperative bed.[10] Perigraft fluid can be identified and followed in its natural course of resorption over a few weeks. If it persists or reappears, infection must be excluded. Fluid collections around the operative bed can be evaluated and aspirated or drained as indicated by CT guidance. Such intervention is not advocated until there is a pressing clinical need. If the duodenum crosses graft fabric without intervening fat, graft erosion of the duodenum may be present or may subsequently develop. By identifying the cephalad and caudad limits of an arterial graft, aneurysms at the anastomosis and those of the graft fabric (Fig. 37-18) or of the adjacent native vessel can be distinguished.

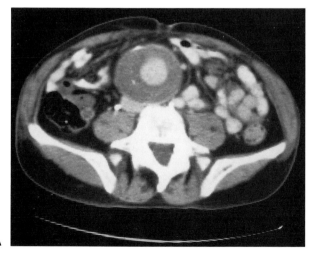

A

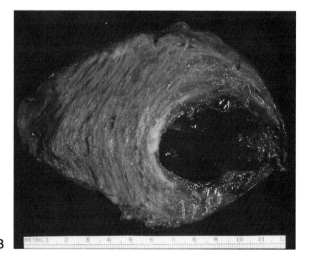

B

Figure 37-6 (A) CT scan with intravenous contrast material shows a relatively small lumen within a large infrarenal abdominal aortic aneurysm. Note the small calcific deposit within the thrombus at 8 o'clock from the lumen. **(B)** Thrombus (T) from large aneurysm with small lumen (L).

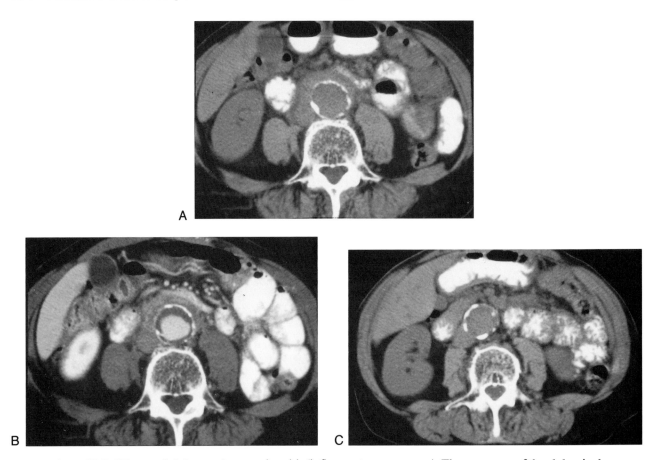

Figure 37-7 CT scan of abdomen shows periaortitis (inflammatory aneurysm). The aneurysm of the abdominal aorta is small. The rind of tissue is primarily anterior **(A)**; it enhances with intravenous contrast material **(B)**. Two years later the inflammatory mass has cleared **(C).**

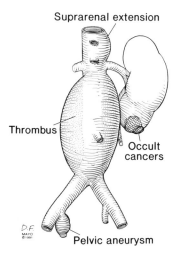

Figure 37-8 CT scanning can reveal findings that are sometimes difficult to visualize by ultrasound (e.g., suprarenal aneurysm, occult tumors, and pelvic aneurysms.) (By permission of Mayo Foundation.)

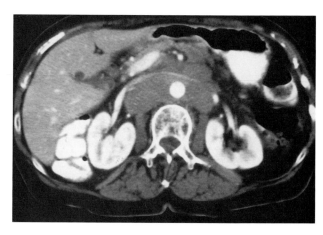

Figure 37-9 CT scan of abdomen shows lymphoma presenting as acute back pain and as a palpable, pulsatile abdominal mass simulating aortic aneurysm. Note the adenopathy around a normal aorta.

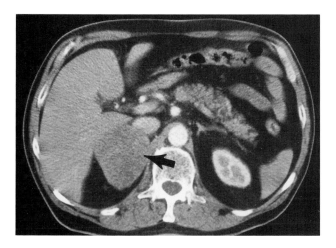

Figure 37-10 CT examination shows a large mass in the right adrenal gland *(arrow)*. This was found to be a pheochromocytoma, which presented as acute abdominal and back pain. Aortic dissection or rupture of an aortic aneurysm was considered in the clinical evaluation. Obesity precluded adequate abdominal palpation of the aorta.

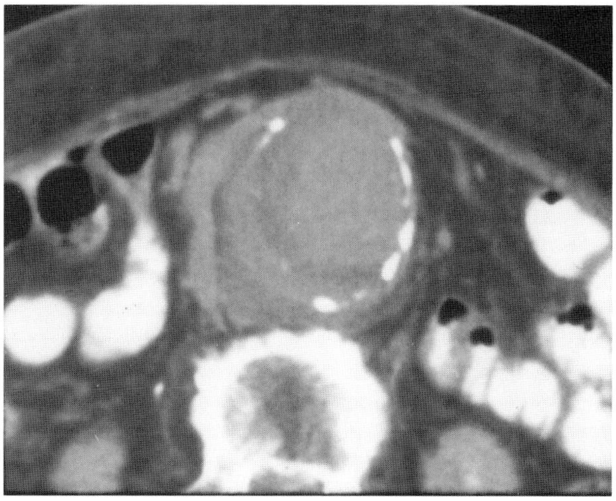

Figure 37-12 CT scan of abdomen, showing contained rupture of an abdominal aortic aneurysm. Note that at 7 to 8 o'clock, posterior to the aorta, there is extraluminal fluid obliterating the normal expected fat pad between the aorta and the vertebral body.

Magnetic Resonance Imaging

Magnetic resonance imaging, in cross section, is similar to CT scanning, but it also offers the capacity for additional views in coronal and sagittal planes. However, spatial resolution for the abdominal aorta is not quite as good as with CT scanning, and the procedure costs more and takes longer to perform. In the approaching era of managed health care, MRI may not be an ideal modality for evaluating or following abdominal aortic aneurysms.

Many of the regional imaging features of CT scanning are seen also with MRI. Certain pulse sequences and vascular imaging programs provide a good display

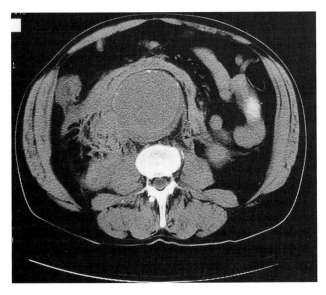

Figure 37-11 Rupture of a large abdominal aortic aneurysm. The CT scan shows the perforation at the 8 o'clock position with adjacent hematoma in the retroperitoneal space.

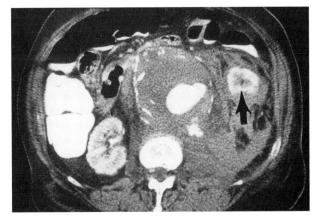

Figure 37-13 CT scan of abdomen, showing rupture of a large abdominal aortic aneurysm. Note the extravasation of contrast material at the 5 o'clock position of the aorta in addition to the large quantity of blood in the retroperitoneum, which displaces the left kidney (arrow) anteriorly.

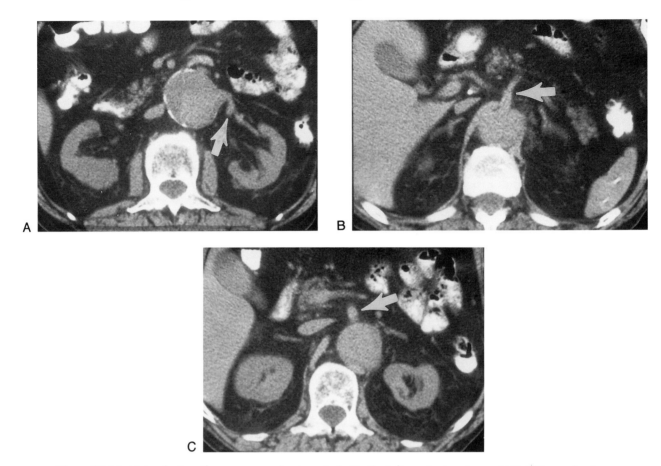

Figure 37-14 Abdominal aortic aneurysm extends cephalad to the left renal artery *(arrow)* **(A).** CT examination allows identification of the celiac artery *(arrow)* **(B)** and the superior mesenteric artery *(arrow)* **(C).** The aorta is ectatic at these levels.

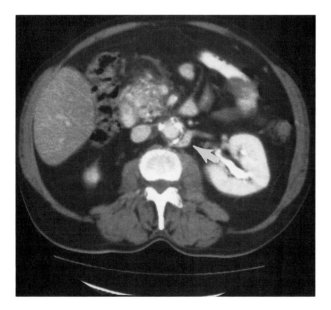

Figure 37-15 CT scan of abdomen. Example of retroaortic left renal vein *(arrow).* There is severe calcific, atheromatous disease of the aorta and the origins of the renal arteries.

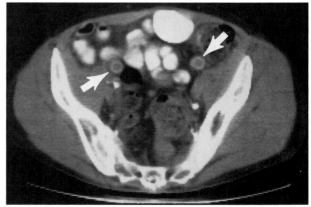

Figure 37-16 CT scan of the pelvis without contrast enhancement shows arterial graft fabric of the limbs as opaque rings *(arrows)* on this scan.

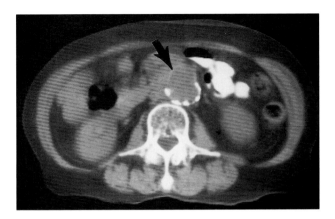

Figure 37-17 Aortic graft fabric *(arrow)* is identified at the proximal (end-to-side) anastomosis on this CT scan.

of the visceral vessels,[2] and moreover, the retroperitoneal structures are well seen. MRI does not involve x-ray exposure, and intravenous contrast material would rarely be necessary. These features must be weighed against a higher cost and limited access to the equipment.

Arteriography

Historically, angiography was the imaging modality of choice for aortic disease. It allows a global view of the visceral arteries and the proximal aorta as well as the iliac arteries distally.[11,12] However, this is an invasive procedure of great expense. A major pitfall with arteriography is inability to determine aneurysm size accurately. Often thrombus on the aneurysm wall is not appreciated unless calcium is detected in the intima to demarcate the outer border. This is true in the abdominal region as well as in the femoropopliteal arteries. Also, the problem of image magnification is present here, just as with plain films. Correction for this, whenever possible, is cumbersome and time-consuming and requires a biplane series.

However, in spite of the imaging capability of ultrasound, CT scanning, and MRI, aortography still has its place for the study of aneurysms.[11,12] For example, assessment of the patency of the visceral arteries may be important to properly plan a surgical correction. The presence and location of multiple renal arteries can be determined. In cases of arteriomegaly it is desirable to have a map of the pelvic and leg arteries because often additional sites of aneurysms may be present.

CLINICAL APPLICATIONS

Arteriomegaly

Arteriomegaly is characterized by a diffuse pattern of arterial ectasia extending from the low abdominal aorta to the popliteal arteries. The degree of arterial dilatation varies considerably from patient to patient. The incidence in our practice is about 2 percent among patients who come for femoral arteriography.[13] Men are far more frequently affected than women. Approximately one-fourth of these patients have more significant dilatation, resulting in aneurysms at multiple sites, which can become quite large, especially in the popliteal segment. The finding of popliteal aneurysms is an important clue, which almost always indicates that arteriomegaly is present and other sites of aneurysms must be sought. In most cases the aneurysms are found between the abdominal aorta and the popliteal segments, but visceral and brachiocephalic arteries may also be affected.

Attempts have been made to classify arteriomegaly by location of the aneurysms—above, below, or both above and below the inguinal ligament.[13] This may be useful for surgical consideration. It is interesting to note that the external iliac artery is almost always spared and is thus a suitable site for placing the anastomosis for an aortoiliac graft.

It is important that an imaging study encompass a large anatomic zone because of the diffuse nature of aneurysm sites (Fig. 37-19). Angiography is well suited for arteriomegaly. Ultrasound is also excellent for the femoral and popliteal arteries as well as the low abdominal aorta. However, because there is a high incidence of emboli to the lower leg arteries, angiography is frequently required to evaluate the distal arteries available for bypass grafting. Because of the diffuse ectasia and multiple aneurysms, the arterial flow is very slow, which makes the angiogram difficult to complete. In an effort to overcome this tourniquets are sometimes used on the legs to augment flow by reactive hyperemia. It is important that they not be applied to a site at which an aneurysm could become compressed and produce iatrogenic embolism. Below-knee sites are satisfactory for tourniquet placement because aneurysms rarely involve tibial arteries.

Suspected Rupture

The patient who presents with acute back pain is frequently thought to have a ruptured abdominal aor-

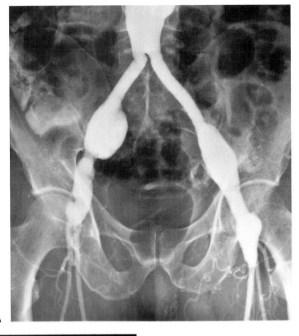

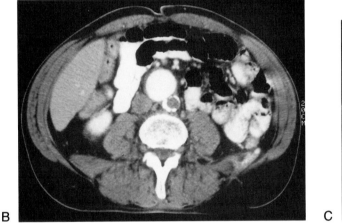
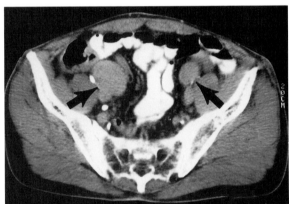

Figure 37-18 Abdominal aortogram shows aneurysms at multiple sites along the course of the aortobifemoral graft **(A)**. The proximal anastomosis by CT scan is end-to-side, and there is marked expansion of the fabric diameter **(B)**. Both iliac limbs **(C)** are also expanded, but here the fabric had split open anteriorly and the lumen was contained by reactive fibrous tissue.

tic aneurysm. Once the physical examination has been completed to exclude other causes of pain, a CT scan may offer the best means of arriving at a diagnosis. Aortic rupture is usually easily detected by CT[9,14–16] (Figs. 37-11 to 37-13). At times the images are exceptionally dramatic because of retroperitoneal hemorrhage. Impending aortic rupture can also be detected by CT as the lack of a sharp border to an aneurysm. A contained rupture has smooth boundaries but obliter-

ates adjacent fat tissue planes, especially those posteriorly adjacent to the vertebral bodies (Figs. 37-12 and 37-20). Both these conditions may also be identified by the presence of aneurysm contents beyond a calcified intimal border. On occasion a patient thought to have a symptomatic aortic aneurysm is found by the CT scan to have some other disease process such as retroperitoneal lymphadenopathy or lymphoma or dissection of the aorta (Figs. 37-9 and 37-21).

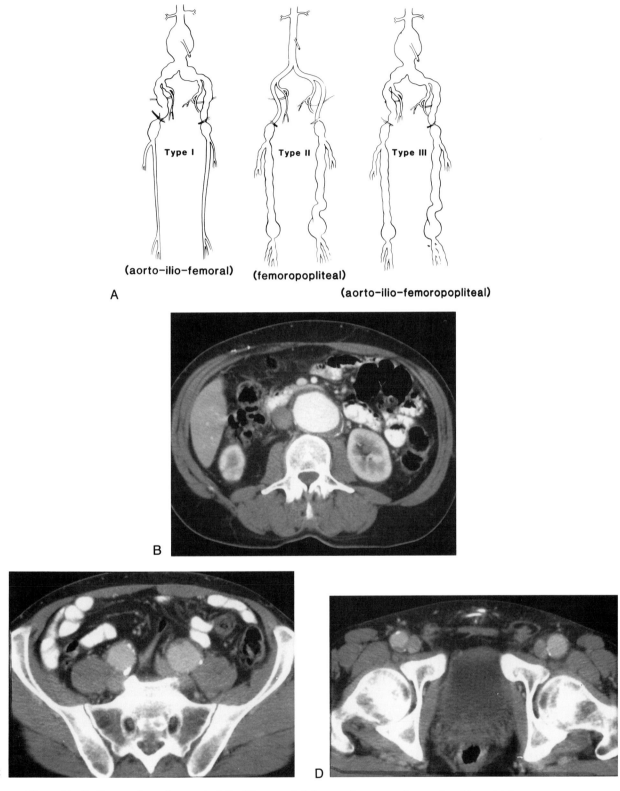

Figure 37-19 Types of arteriomegaly **(A)**. CT scan of abdomen shows arteriomegaly with multiple aneurysms: **(B)** abdominal aorta, **(C)** common iliac arteries, and **(D)** common femoral arteries.

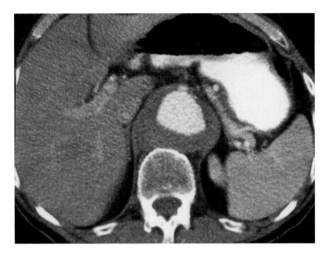

Figure 37-20 CT scan of abdomen, showing false aneurysm of the aorta at the thoracolumbar junction. This was secondary to a penetrating atheromatous ulcer of the posterior wall. There is no calcification of the intima in this region, and therefore it is difficult to predict the nature of this lesion. However, at the 8 o'clock position soft tissue or fluid density encroaches upon the fat plane between the posterior aorta and the vertebral body. This indicates a false aneurysm, not a simple aneurysm.

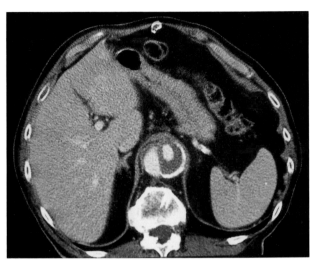

Figure 37-21 CT scan of abdomen shows aortic dissection at the thoracolumbar junction, forming a small aneurysm in its total size.

AORTIC ATHEROSCLEROTIC ULCERS

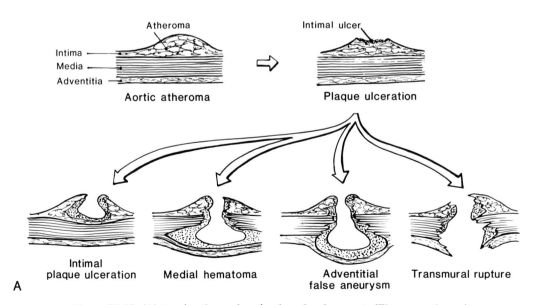

Figure 37-22 **(A)** Aortic atherosclerotic ulcer development. *(Figure continues.)*

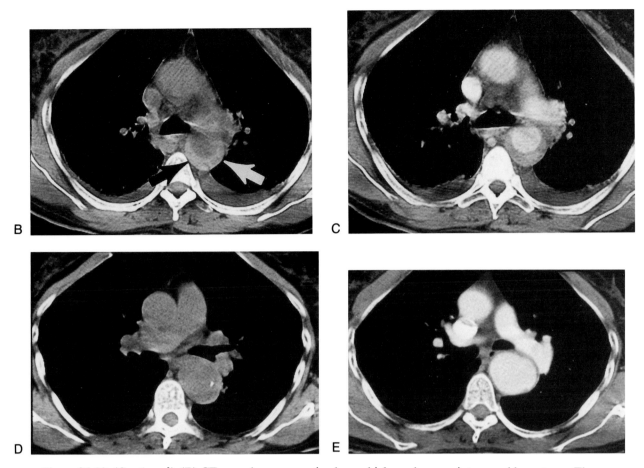

Figure 37-22 *(Continued).* **(B)** CT scan shows an aortic ulcer, which produces an intramural hematoma. The acute hematoma is identified on the nonenhanced scan as a high-density crescent *(arrow)* in the posterior wall of the descending thoracic aorta. **(C)** After injection of intravenous contrast material, the high-density hematoma loses its specific appearance. **(D)** Scan made 3 weeks later shows that the hematoma no longer has its high-density appearance. This is the natural maturation of a hematoma as shown by CT scan. **(E)** Eventually the aortic ulcer-hematoma complex matures to an eccentric aneurysm of the descending thoracic aorta. The hematoma has resorbed, and the new lumen is aneurysmal. In Fig. D, the calcification in the descending thoracic aorta at the 4 o'clock position is atheromatous disease of the intima. At this phase and on this single scan, the significance of the calcium deposit is nonspecific.

Aneurysm Following Dissection

Occasionally an aortic dissection results in aneurysm formation. This occurs when distal reentry sites allow continued pulsatile pressure upon the false lumen. A CT scan is well suited to follow increases in aortic diameter throughout the length of the aorta. Over time, false lumina may partially thrombose, and the wall of the false lumen may show deposits of calcium, causing confusion as to which is the true lumen.

Penetrating Atheromatous Ulcer

In addition to the "classic" type of aortic dissection, there is another type of dissection, that presents with similar clinical symptoms. The initial imaging studies, however, reveal an intramural hematoma rather than a false lumen.[17] This hematoma is the result of an atheromatous ulcer that penetrates into the media, causing a hemorrhage that becomes circumferential and does not distort the true lumen (Fig. 37-22). The outer diameter of the aorta becomes expanded by a few millimeters and in some cases up to about 1 cm. The site of origin of the atheromatous ulcer is almost always in the descending thoracic segment, usually in the middle and distal thirds. The vertical length of the hematoma is variable, but it often extends cephalad to the isthmus and caudad to the upper abdominal level.

The best imaging modality for this lesion is a CT scan. A series should be obtained before and after injection of intravenous contrast material. The initial scans will show the hematoma as a high-density crescent in the aortic wall.[18] This high density persists for about 2 weeks, after which the hematoma becomes isodense with the lumen of the aorta (Fig. 37-22). The intramural thickness stays the same in the acute phase unless further dissection occurs, an event usually recognized by recurrent pain.

Another value of the noncontrast scan is that the position of intimal atheromatous calcification can be seen (Fig. 37-22). This is a very important diagnostic feature when examining all arteries by CT. Intimal calcification should be in close approximation to the outer border of the aorta. Whenever it is displaced from the outer wall, there is disease in the wall, which may take the form of the false lumen of classic dissection, the hematoma of penetrating atheromatous ulcer, false aneurysm, or periaortitis.

In the initial report of a series of penetrating atheromatous ulcers, surgical intervention was recommended. In contrast, a subsequent report indicated that some patients who are treated medically survive without rupture.[19] Follow-up of these patients by CT scans shows an interesting development in the aorta — the hematoma reabsorbs and the lumen expands (Fig. 37-22). Usually, the outer diameter remains the same in the region of the ulcer, but in some cases an eccentric aneurysm can be the result (Fig. 37-22). At other areas along the length of the hematoma, some expansion of the lumen as well as some contraction of the outer diameter can occur.

False Aneurysm

False aneurysm of the aorta is not common. The etiology is usually focal disruption of an atheromatous ulcer or, less commonly, infection or giant cell arteritis (Figs. 37-23 and 37-24). Usually these are found in the descending thoracic and upper abdominal segments. The lesion is often detected by a chest x-ray and then evaluated by CT or sometimes by angiography. The CT findings are usually suggestive of something other than the more frequently seen degenerative aneurysm. Often intimal calcification is displaced from the outer

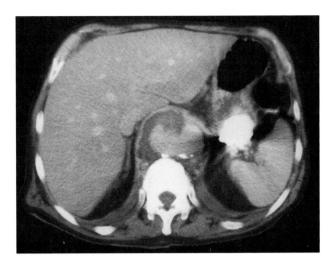

Figure 37-23 Infected false aneurysm of the aorta at the thoracolumbar junction. Contrast-enhanced CT scan shows an irregular, expanded lumen. Note the absence of fat at the angles between the posterior wall of the aorta at 5 o'clock and 7 o'clock and the spine.

wall. Also, the borders are eccentric, and local tissue planes of periaortic fat are obliterated (Figs. 37-23 and 37-24).

Pulsatile Abdominal Mass

The physical examination of a patient with a pulsatile abdominal mass should usually lead to the correct diagnosis of aneurysm, and assessment by ultrasound should be sufficient. On occasion no aneurysm is found, or if one is found it is too small to account for the

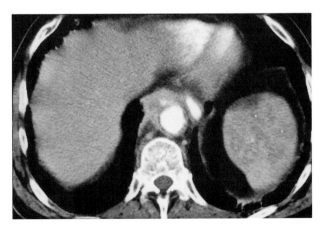

Figure 37-24 CT scan of abdomen, showing infected false aneurysm of the aorta at the thoracolumbar junction. Note the small collection of contrast material at the 10 o'clock position within the compartment of hematoma and abscess.

palpable mass. A CT scan can be helpful to exclude a tumor in the mesentery or retroperitoneum[14] (Fig. 37-9). Rarely, nothing is found by CT scan except a lordotic spine with the aorta somewhat closer to the anterior abdominal wall than expected. Even more rarely, a hematoma in the rectus abdominis muscle can simulate a pulsatile mass in a thin patient.

REFERENCES

1. Maloney JD, Pairolero PC, Smith BF et al: Ultrasound evaluation of abdominal aortic aneurysms. Circulation 56:II-80, 1977
2. Pavone P, Di Cesare E, Di Renzi P et al: Abdominal aortic aneurysm evaluation: comparison of US, CT, MRI, and angiography. Magn Reson Imaging 8:199, 1990
3. Todd GJ, Nowygrod R, Benvenisty A et al: The accuracy of CT scanning in the diagnosis of abdominal and thoracoabdominal aortic aneurysms. J Vasc Surg 13:302, 1991
4. Vowden P, Wilkinson D, Ausobsky JR, Kester RC: A comparison of three imaging techniques in the assessment of an abdominal aortic aneurysm. J Cardiovasc Surg 30:891, 1989
5. Machida K, Tasala A: CT patterns of mural thrombus in aortic aneurysms. J Comput Assist Tomogr 4:840, 1980
6. Torres WE, Maurer DE, Steinberg HV et al: CT of aortic aneurysms: the distinction between mural and thrombus calcification. AJR 150:1317, 1988
7. Pennell RC, Hollier LH, Lie JT et al: Inflammatory abdominal aortic aneurysms: a thirty-year review. J Vasc Surg 2:859, 1985
8. Papanicolau N, Wittenberg J, Ferrucci JT et al: Preoperative evaluation of abdominal aortic aneurysms by computed tomography. AJR 146:711, 1986
9. Johnson WC, Gale ME, Gerzof SG et al: The role of computed tomography in symptomatic aortic aneurysms. Surg Gynecol Obstet 162:49, 1986
10. Brown OW, Stanson AW, Pairolero PC, Hollier LH: Computerized tomography following abdominal aortic surgery. Surgery 91:716, 1982
11. Brewster DC, Retana A, Waltman AC, Darling RC: Angiography in the management of aneurysms of the abdominal aorta: its value and safety. N Engl J Med 292:822, 1975
12. Couch NP, O'Mahony J, McIrvine A et al: The place of abdominal aortography in abdominal aortic aneurysm resection. Arch Surg 118:1029, 1983
13. Hollier LH, Stanson AW, Gloviczki P et al: Arteriomegaly: classification and morbid implications of diffuse aneurysmal disease. Surgery 93:700, 1983
14. Kvilekval KH, Best IM, Mason RA et al: The value of computed tomography in the management of symptomatic abdominal aortic aneurysms. J Vasc Surg 12:28, 1990
15. Sterpetti AV, Blair EA, Schultz RD et al: Sealed rupture of abdominal aortic aneurysm. J Vasc Surg 11:430, 1990
16. Clayton MJ, Walsh JW, Brewer WH: Contained rupture of abdominal aortic aneurysms: sonographic and CT diagnosis. AJR 138:154, 1982
17. Stanson AW, Kazmier FJ, Hollier LH et al: Penetrating atherosclerotic ulcers of the thoracic aorta: natural history and clinicopathologic correlations. Ann Vasc Surg 1:15, 1986
18. Welch TJ, Stanson AW, Sheedy PF et al: Radiographic evaluation of penetrating aortic atherosclerotic ulcer. Radiographics 10:675, 1990
19. Hussain S, Glover JL, Bree R, Bendick PJ: Penetrating atherosclerotic ulcers of the thoracic aorta. J Vasc Surg 9:71, 1989

38

Management of Aneurysms

John W. Hallett, Jr.

Synthetic or autogenous grafting remains the treatment of choice for most arterial aneurysms (Figs. 38-1 and 38-2). The era of simply ligating, wiring, or "tailoring" (aneurysmorrhaphy) aneurysms is long past.[1] Recent percutaneous interventional techniques, however, have demonstrated possible future alternatives to standard surgical correction. For example, Parodi et al.[2] have recently treated several abdominal aortic aneurysms (AAAs) by transfemoral passage of collapsed synthetic grafts into the aorta with graft placement by expandable intraluminal stents (Fig. 38-3). Although investigational, these new interventional approaches may eventually change aneurysm management for selected patients. Likewise, no definitive medical therapy exists for aneurysms, although antihypertensives, especially beta blockers, may retard expansion and reduce rupture risk.[3] These medications may become more important in treating the increasing number of clinically recognized small aneurysms. For now, grafting is the safest and most durable approach to an aneurysm. Consequently, this chapter emphasizes the key concepts of surgical management.

PATIENT SELECTION

Nearly all patients with arterial aneurysms can successfully undergo surgical repair. The number of aneurysm patients in the United States exceeds hundreds of thousands.[4] Worldwide, several million aneurysms exist, and recognition is increasing steadily with greater use of ultrasound and computed tomography (CT).

Limited surgical resources prevent repairing all of them, so certain criteria must be used to select those patients who are most likely to benefit from surgical repair. Patient selection can be discussed conveniently in four broad categories: (1) aneurysm symptoms and signs; (2) aneurysm size, configuration, and content; (3) patient health; and (4) surgical expertise.

Aneurysm Symptoms and Signs

As soon as an aneurysm becomes symptomatic, its natural history changes dramatically. For example, 30 percent of painful abdominal aortic aneurysms rupture within 30 days and 80 percent within 1 year.[5] Likewise, 20 to 30 percent of patients with thrombosed popliteal aneurysms suffer limb loss if surgical revascularization is not undertaken.[6] Other symptoms or signs that necessitate surgical intervention include septicemia from infected aneurysms; lower-extremity venous obstruction from large popliteal aneurysms; incapacitating claudication from thrombosed aneurysms; peripheral thromboembolism from a proximal aneurysm; and congestive heart failure from an aortocaval fistula. Regardless of aneurysm size, such symptoms mandate urgent repair.

Aneurysm Size, Configuration, and Content

Since arterial diameter is the key determinant of rupture risk, aneurysm size is the most important factor influencing patient selection for elective repair of

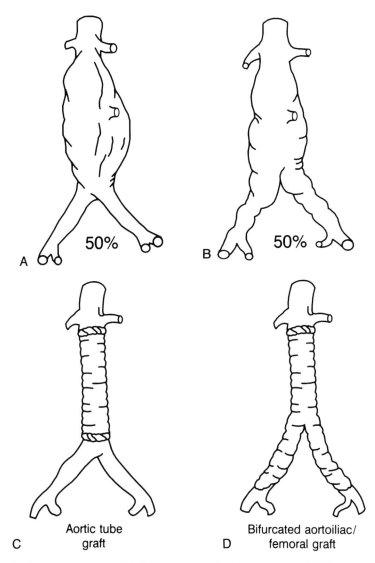

Figure 38-1 Abdominal aortic aneurysms **(A & B)** are treated with Dacron or PTFE (polytetrafluoroethylene) aortic tube **(C)** or bifurcated grafts **(D)**. (By permission of Mayo Foundation.)

asymptomatic aneurysms. Physicians, however, must be cautious in setting "legal limits" for operation. The variability of aneurysm measurement has already been mentioned. Consequently, size zones of relative rupture risk (e.g., for AAA, 3.0 to 4.9 cm, 5.0 to 6.9 cm, and >7 cm) are more appropriate than any specific size. Generally, any AAA larger than 5 cm in a good-risk patient should be repaired.[7] In a very poor-risk patient, it may be more appropriate to wait until the AAA expands toward the 6 to 7 cm range or until medical risks are minimized.[8,9]

Although many small aneurysms can be safely followed, some should be considered for repair. For example, an otherwise healthy 62-year-old patient with a 4.0 to 5.0 cm AAA may choose elective repair over continued observation. Small aneurysms may also require correction for (1) associated aortic or renal occlusive disease, (2) rapid expansion, (3) difficulty in serial follow-up, (4) extreme patient anxiety about the aneurysm, or (5) a strong family history of rupture. Several studies consistently report that about one-third of small AAAs aneurysms are repaired eventually, while the remainder can be followed safely with a low risk of rupture.[10–12]

With other types of aneurysms, size is not as important as content or configuration. Femoral artery aneurysms tend to develop thrombus, leading to occlusion[13] (Fig. 38-4). Ultrasound can not only measure femoral aneurysm size but can also reveal associated stenosis and thrombosis, all of which are indications for repair.

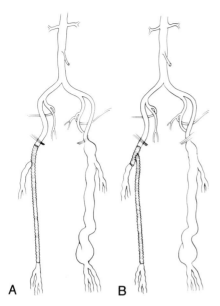

Figure 38-2 Either synthetic **(A)** or autogenous **(B)** vein grafts are used to correct femoropopliteal aneurysms. (By permission of Mayo Foundation.)

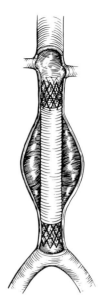

Figure 38-3 Selected abdominal aortic aneurysms have been treated by a graft-stent combination placed by retrograde passage from a femoral artery cutdown. (From Parodi et al.,[2] with permission.)

The configuration of popliteal aneurysms, which includes tortuosity and kinking across the knee joint, predisposes to thrombosis and embolization (Fig. 38-5). Ultrasound can usually map a tortuous or kinked aneurysm and reveal any thrombotic content. Consequently, arterial configuration and content are generally more important than size for lower extremity aneurysms.[14,15-18] For example, a small, tortuous popliteal aneurysm with intraluminal thrombus and decreased peripheral pulses resulting from chronic arterial occlusive disease or past thromboembolism needs repair before occlusion threatens limb viability.

Patient Health

Although aneurysm symptoms and size are the most important factors influencing surgical intervention, patient health must receive equal attention. Operative

mortality for otherwise healthy patients is low (2 to 3 percent) while poor-risk patients (Table 38-1) may face a mortality of at least 8 to 10 percent[19-21] (Table 38-2). High-risk medical conditions include (1) severe coronary and valvular heart disease[21,22]; (2) decompensated chronic obstructive pulmonary disease[23]; (3) chronic renal failure[24]; (4) hepatic cirrhosis with portal hypertension; and (5) chronic hematologic disorders associated with bleeding dysfunction (Table 38-1 and Fig. 38-6). Although these risk factors cannot be eliminated, they can often be alleviated before operation. The best example is coronary revascularization for unstable angina pectoris before AAA repair.[25] About 5 percent of AAA patients will have unstable coronary or valvular heart disease that needs preoperative correction.[26] The subsequent AAA operative mortality of these patients is low and similar to that of patients without evident heart disease.[25,26]

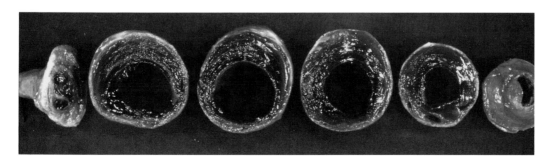

Figure 38-4 These cross sections of a large femoral aneurysm display considerable intraluminal thrombus.

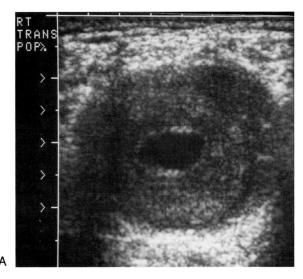
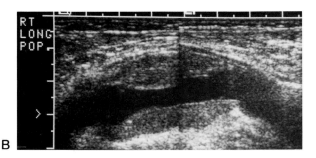

Figure 38-5 Duplex ultrasound scan demonstrates a large popliteal aneurysm with thrombus. **(A)** Transverse section; **(B)** longitudinal view.

Surgeon's Expertise and Hospital Size

Recent studies confirm that the surgeon's experience is also an important predictor of elective mortality.[27] For example, low-volume surgeons who perform one to five AAA operations per year) have an average elective aneurysm mortality rate of 9 percent as compared with high-volume surgeons (> 25 AAA procedures per

year), with a 4 percent mortality rate. To a lesser extent, the hospital's volume of such operations is important. Low-volume hospitals (one to five AAA operations per year) have an average elective operative mortality rate of 12 percent as compared with high-volume hospitals (more than 40 AAA operations per year), where the elective operative mortality rate is 5 percent. Specialized surgical centers achieve the lowest operative mortalities for both good (2 to 3 percent) and poor-risk (5 to 10 percent) aneurysm patients.[28]

Exclusion for Aneurysm Repair

Only an occasional patient is not a candidate for repair of a symptomatic, ruptured, or large aneurysm. This group would include patients with terminal ma-

Table 38-1 Criteria for High Risk

Age	>85 years
Renal	Serum creatinine ≥ 3 mg/dl
Pulmonary	Receiving oxygen at home PO_2 <50 mmHg FEF_{25-75} <25% of predicted value
Hepatic	Biopsy-proven cirrhosis with ascites
Abdominal	Retroperitoneal fibrosis
Cardiac	Class 3–4 angina Resting LVEF <30% Recent CHF (30 days) Complex ventricular ectopy Large LV aneurysm Severe valvular disease Recurrent CHF or angina after CABG Severe CAD by angiography (unreconstructed)

Abbreviations: FEF_{25-75}, mean forced expiratory flow in midportion of expiratory curve; LVEF, left ventricular ejection fraction; CHF, congestive heart failure; LV, left ventricular; CABG, coronary artery bypass grafting; CAD, coronary artery disease.
(From Hollier et al.,[28] with permission.)

Table 38-2 Comparative Mortality of 458 Consecutive AAA Repairs at the Mayo Clinic

	No. of Patients	No. of Deaths	Mortality Rate (%)
High risk	106	6	5.7
Non-high risk	294	5	1.7
Exclusions			
Rupture	26	6	23.1
AAA + renal	32	1	3.1

Abbreviations: AAA, abdominal aortic aneurysmectomy; renal, renovascular procedure.
(From Hollier et al.,[28] with permission.)

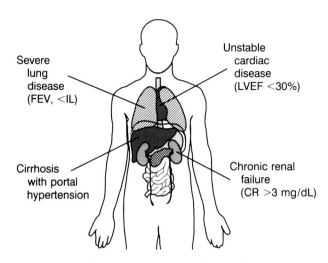

Figure 38-6 Clinical factors that significantly increase operative mortality for repair of an aortic aneurysm.

lignancies, end-stage multiorgan failure, or living wills refusing any surgery.

SURGICAL PROCEDURE

Principles

Direct in situ arterial grafting is the treatment of choice for most aneurysms. Prior to direct grafting, ligation of aneurysms was practiced with some success, since collateral blood flow could prevent limb loss in many patients. This practice evolved toward aneurysmorrhaphy (partial excision of the aneurysm sac and reclosure of the artery to a smaller diameter),[1] an approach that maintained direct arterial flow but obviously left a portion of the aneurysmal artery intact. The next surgical advance came with the classic 1952 report of Charles DuBost and associates of Paris.[29] Their resection of an abdominal aortic aneurysm, with reestablishment of arterial continuity by a preserved human arterial graft, seemed to solve two problems, elimination of the aneurysm and preservation of arterial flow. To the dismay of surgeons and patients, the arterial homografts tended to degenerate into aneurysms themselves. The introduction of Dacron and PTFE (polytetrafluoroethylene) prostheses solved this problem and alleviated the final dilemma of aortic aneurysm treatment, namely, providing an adequate supply of grafts for thousands of aneurysm repairs each year.

The only important exception to direct in situ graft repair is encountered when there is local infection of the aneurysm and surrounding tissues.[30-32] This situation requires resection of the infected aneurysm, closure of the proximal and distal arteries, drainage of any abscess, and extra-anatomic bypass grafting. However, a few aneurysm infections are confined to the arterial wall and thrombus, are not associated with infection of adjacent tissues, and are not surrounded by an abscess. In these selected cases success can be achieved by complete resection of the aneurysm *without opening* it; direct in situ grafting, with coverage by clean, fresh tissue; and administration of systemic antibiotics.[33,34]

Although direct in situ aortic grafting is clearly the procedure of choice for an AAA, aneurysm ligation and extra-anatomic bypass have been advocated by some surgeons for high-risk patients.[35] The perceived benefit has been less morbidity and mortality. The data do not appear, however, to support this perception for most patients.[36,37] In fact, a ligated aneurysm under pressure from residual lumbar arteries can still rupture. Aneurysm ligation may be appropriate for a rare patient, but most specialized surgical centers have argued for its abandonment in favor of standard aneurysm repair by an experienced anesthesia and surgical team.[28,36,37] Whether the extraperitoneal approach to the AAA has an advantage over the standard midline abdominal incision in such patients is still debated.[38]

Technical Difficulties

Certain anatomic features increase the technical difficulty of aneurysm repair.[19,20] Good preoperative imaging will detect most of them and allow their safe handling without complicating mistakes in aneurysm exposure and repair. The more common anatomic challenges are as follows:

1. *Extensive thoracoabdominal aneurysm.* An aneurysm extending along a major section of the aorta predisposes to spinal cord ischemia and paraplegia as well as to intestinal and renal artery problems.[39-44] Those that extend from the high thoracic to low abdominal aorta (Crawford type II) (Fig. 38-7 and Table 38-3) place the patient at greatest risk of postoperative paraplegia (29 percent).[39] Such aneurysms may involve numerous lumbar arteries, including the critical radicular artery of Adamkiewicz between T8 and L2. Likewise, these aneurysms involve the origin of the renal and intestinal arteries. The Crawford graft inclusion (Fig. 38-8) technique has simplified and shortened renal and visceral artery reconstruction and ischemia times.[39,40] Renal failure requiring hemodialysis, however, still affects about 10 percent of such patients.[39] Finally, the most common postoperative problem is prolonged respiratory insufficiency, which occurs in 25 to 30 percent of patients.[39,42] Mortality rises dramatically (to 40 percent) for patients who require tracheotomy.[44]

2. *Inflammatory aneurysms.* Classically inflammatory aneurysms involve the abdominal aorta[45-47] (Fig. 38-9).

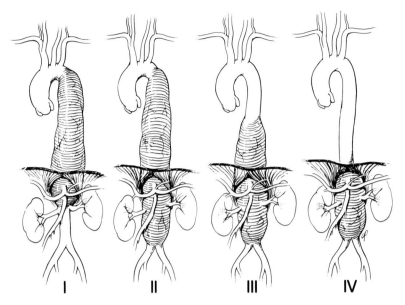

Figure 38-7 Anatomic classification of thoracoabdominal aneurysms. (From Crawford,[39] with permission.)

They probably represent an excessive autoimmune type of inflammatory response to atherosclerosis and typically are *not* infected with bacteria or other organisms. They present technical danger to the surgeon because of adhesion or incorporation of the adjacent duodenum, left renal vein, and ureters. Injury to these neighboring structures is minimized by working around them rather than dissecting them out of the aneurysm wall.

3. *Horseshoe kidneys.* These structures may present two technical challenges[48-50] (Fig. 38-10). First, their presence on top of the aortic aneurysm requires some mobilization of the renal isthmus to allow clamping and grafting. Second, they may have multiple renal arteries that require reimplantation into the graft.
4. *Internal iliac artery aneurysms.* These aneurysms may present problems with controlled back-bleeding and pel-

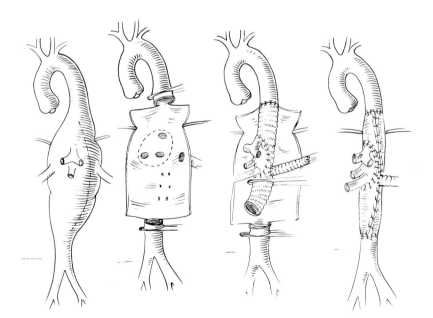

Figure 38-8 Crawford graft inclusion technique for thoracoabdominal aneurysm repair. (From Pairolero and Bernatz,[1] with permission.)

Table 38-3 Results of Surgical Treatment of
Thoracoabdominal Aortic Aneurysms

Extent	No. of Patients	Deaths (%)	Paraplegia (%)	Hemodialysis (%)
I	270	23 (9)	38 (14)	20 (7)
II	353	36 (10)	102 (29)	34 (10)
III	285	25 (9)	16 (6)	28 (10)
IV	285	19 (7)	10 (4)	24 (8)
Total	1193	103 (9%)	166 (14%)	106 (9%)

(From Crawford,[39] with permission.)

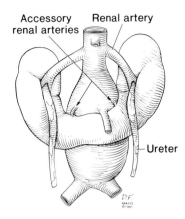

Figure 38-10 Horseshoe kidneys complicate about one in 200 abdominal aortic aneurysms. They may have multiple renal arteries. (By permission of Mayo Foundation.)

vic ischemia if both internal iliac arteries are ligated.[51] Generally, maintaining flow into one internal iliac artery will prevent pelvic and colonic ischemia.

5. *Venous anomalies.* Venous anomalies of the left renal vein (Fig. 38-11) and vena cava (Fig. 38-12) can complicate exposure and clamping of the proximal aortic neck of the aneurysm. Generally, a retroaortic left renal vein is slightly lower than a normally anterior left renal vein and can be inadvertently injured during mobilization and clamping of the aorta.

6. *Diffuse femoropopliteal arteriomegaly.* This condition (Fig. 38-13) is challenging because limb salvage depends on maintaining adequate profunda femoris and popliteal-to-tibial arterial flow despite extensive aneurysms and sometimes limited autogenous vein for multiple bypasses.[52] Such patients may require numerous, staged operations over their lifetimes.

Graft Materials

Three basic materials or tissues are used to repair most aneurysms; namely, Dacron, PTFE, and autogenous vein. Long-term follow-up has confirmed the durability of Dacron in the aortoileofemoral and vein in the femoropopliteal region.[16,18,53–55) The choice of graft material depends on aneurysm location (Fig. 38-14). Large arteries such as the aorta the iliac and common femoral arteries are replaced with Dacron or PTFE. Softer woven, coated, or knitted Dacron or PTFE grafts are currently popular for the aorta since these products have low porosity and do not leak much blood. Although PTFE grafts are available for aortic reconstruction, this material is used primarily for femoropopliteal aneurysm repairs. If saphenous vein is available, it is preferable to PTFE for repair of popliteal aneurysms that cross the knee joint.

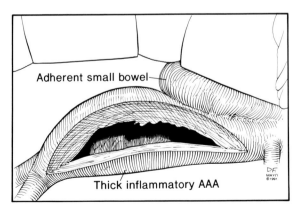

Figure 38-9 Inflammatory abdominal aortic aneurysms usually adhere to the duodenum. (By permission of Mayo Foundation.)

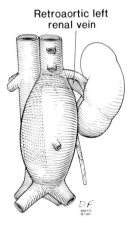

Figure 38-11 About 3 to 5 percent of patients have a retroaortic left renal vein, which passes behind the aneurysm neck and can be injured during aortic clamping. (By permission of Mayo Foundation.)

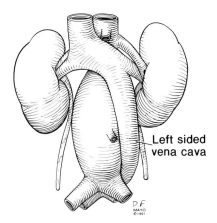

Figure 38-12 A left-sided vena cava can make exposure of the aneurysm neck more difficult than usual. (By permission of Mayo Foundation.)

Anesthetic Management

Many facets of anesthetic management lead to a good outcome in aneurysm surgery. All of them cannot be mentioned here, but a few central concepts deserve emphasis. In essence, good anesthetic management prevents serious ischemia of certain key organs, namely, the heart, kidneys, and spinal cord (thoracoabdominal aneurysms).

1. *Cardiac protection.* The first requirement is good monitoring; an arterial line and continuous electrocardiogram (ECG) are essential. Although not mandatory, a Swan-Ganz pulmonary artery catheter should be used in pa-

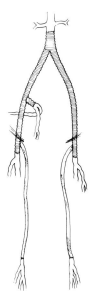

Figure 38-13 Diffuse arteriomegaly of aortoiliac and femoropopliteal arteries may require multiple grafts. (By permission of Mayo Foundation.)

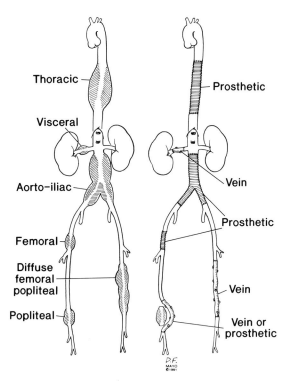

Figure 38-14 Choice of graft material for various anatomic locations. (By permission of Mayo Foundation.)

tients with serious coronary artery or valvular heart disease and poor ventricular function. Intraoperative transesophageal two-dimensional echocardiography has also been helpful in patients in whom actual visualization of cardiac valves and wall motion is needed. The use of this monitoring mode in high-risk aneurysm patients with bad hearts is likely to increase. The second essential for cardiac protection is maximizing cardiac output,[56] which requires optimizing intravascular fluid balance before and after aortic cross-clamping. Next, reducing afterload resistance during aortic clamping usually requires nitroprusside. Finally, intravenous nitroglycerin may play a role in alleviating myocardial ischemia.
2. *Renal protection.* Protection of the kidneys depends mainly on adequate intravenous hydration, monitored by urine output and cardiac filling (e.g., wedge pressure, 8–12 mmHg). Low-dose dopamine (2 to 3 μg/kg/min) is another useful adjunct to promote renal vasodilatation and flow. Urinary output is also enhanced by 12.5 g of intravenous mannitol before aortic clamping.
3. *Prevention of spinal cord ischemia.* This remains the key challenge of thoracoabdominal aneurysm repair. Unfortunately, no single measure prevents paraplegia, although several factors appear beneficial.[57,58] Every effort must be made to limit the extent of lumbar artery ligation. When possible, lumbar arteries should be included in proximal, distal, and large patch anastomoses. Catheter drainage of spinal fluid (Fig. 38-15) for abnormally high (>15 to 20 mmHg) spinal fluid pressure may alleviate spinal cord

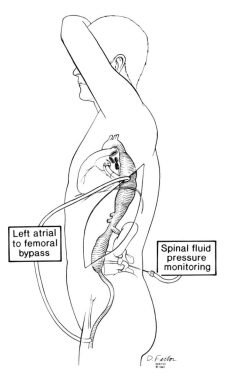

Figure 38-15 Two adjunctive measures to protect spinal cord perfusion are spinal fluid pressure monitoring with drainage and left atrial-to-femoral bypass. (By permission of Mayo Foundation.)

compartment syndrome. Use of shunts or left atrial-to-femoral bypass pumps may enhance distal spinal cord perfusion and alleviate cardiac afterload, but their benefit has not been clearly proved by any study. Although experimental, administration of free-radical scavengers may play a role.[57]

4. *Body core temperature maintenance.* Temperature maintenance also needs attention[59] because hypothermia (body temperature below 33°C) causes significant capillary leak syndrome, coagulopathy, and life-threatening ventricular arrhythmias (Fig. 38-16). A warm (70 to 75°F) ambient operating room temperature during induction and preparation is especially helpful. Warm intravenous fluids also help. Recently, the Bair Hugger warming tent (Fig. 38-17) for the thorax and head has added a valuable adjunct to keeping the patient warm.

Blood Transfusion

Repair of most aortic and some peripheral arterial aneurysms requires blood transfusion. In fact, 95 percent of aortic aneurysm patients receive at least 2 to 3 units of bank blood during operation. Intraoperative red cell salvage by rapid autotransfusion devices has significantly reduced the need for any homologous blood[60,61] (Fig. 38-18). At least 70 percent of routine AAA repairs can now be completed with *only* the patient's reinfused packed red blood cells (Fig. 38-19). Rapid autotransfusers wash, process, and pack a unit (225 ml) of red cells in 5 minutes. During an uncomplicated AAA repair, 2 to 3 units of blood are returned. The chance that additional bank blood will be needed is increased by (1) complex aortic operations or reoperations; (2) pre-existing anemia (hemoglobin less than 11 g); and (3) multiple passes of aspirated blood through the autotransfusers (red cell trauma and hemolysis). Since most aneurysms need urgent repair, multiple red cell deposits by the patient over several weeks are usually not possible.

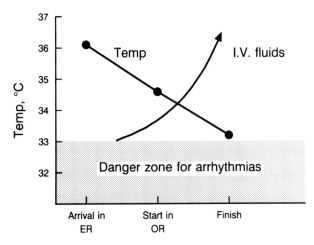

Figure 38-16 Hypothermia during aneurysm surgery causes (1) a capillary leak syndrome requiring increased fluid replacement, (2) coagulopathy due to platelet dysfunction, and (3) ventricular arrhythmias.

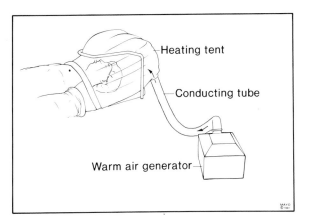

Figure 38-17 A forced air heating tent over the upper body and head can maintain core temperature during major aneurysm operations (Bair Hugger warming tent). (By permission of Mayo Foundation.)

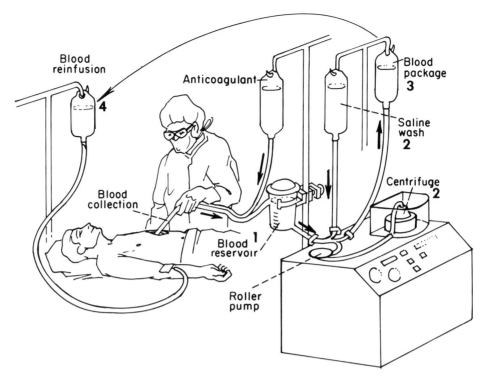

Figure 38-18 Rapid autotransfusion devices pack washed red blood cells (hematocrit, 50 to 55, volume, 225 ml) for return in 5 minutes. (From Hallett,[61] with permission.)

Intraoperative Monitoring of Peripheral Perfusion

Along with intra-abdominal bleeding, graft thrombosis or peripheral thromboembolism is one of the most common early complications of any aneurysm repair.[18,19] A thrombotic complication affects 3 to 5 percent of patients.[18,19,54,55] Use of intraoperative heparin may lessen the risk but does not eliminate it. In nearly every case, thrombosis or embolism occurs in the operating room and can be detected and frequently corrected there.

Several methods of intraoperative monitoring can detect the thrombosis and embolism; these include (1) pedal pulse examination, (2) Doppler signal analysis at the ankle and foot, (3) calf plethysmographic pulse

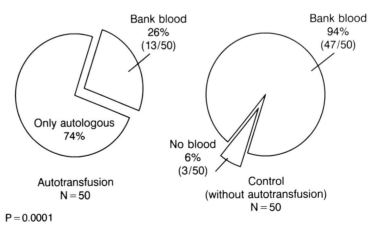

Figure 38-19 Intraoperative blood usage. Rapid autologous cell salvage and return reduce significantly the need for any bank blood during aortic surgery. (From Hallett,[61] with permission.)

waveforms, and (4) electromagnetic measurement of graft flows. In addition, an operative arteriogram or duplex ultrasound analysis can assess femoropopliteal grafts and runoff. In a recent prospective study using a combination of pulses, Doppler signals, and calf pulse volume recordings, my colleagues and I detected intra-operative thrombotic problems in 2 percent of AAA repairs and successfully corrected all of them before leaving the operating room. Thus, the key concept is that intraoperative monitoring of peripheral perfusion decreases the risk of the patient returning to the operating room with a postoperative thrombotic complication.

SPECIAL PROBLEMS

Ruptured Aneurysms

Ruptured AAA is a common surgical emergency of the aged.[62-64] This trend is likely to continue since at least one-half of patients presenting with a ruptured AAA did not know of their aneurysm.[65] They obviously never had a chance for elective repair.

In marked contrast to elective AAA surgical mortalities of 2 to 5 percent, approximately 50 percent of patients arriving at a hospital with a ruptured AAA will die.[66-70] This dismal outlook has not changed much in 20 years. The most critical factors predicting death from rupture remain profound shock, pre-existing cardiorespiratory disease, and technical complications.[65-68] Ruptured aneurysms need an expeditious trip to the operating room and expert control of the proximal aorta. Several factors are essential in the successful management of ruptured aneurysms (Fig. 38-20).

1. *Rapid transport.* Patients with suspected AAA rupture should be transported rapidly by helicopter or ambulance to a major hospital, where a surgical team should be waiting for initial assessment and resuscitation. An operating room should be ready as soon as the patient arrives.
2. *Accurate diagnosis.* If the diagnosis of ruptured AAA is in question and the patient is hemodynamically stable, an abdominal CT scan or ultrasound evaluation should be considered (Fig. 38-21). An ECG should be obtained to rule out acute myocardial infarction. A toxic drug screen should be made for any elderly, psychotic patient who is receiving psychotropic agents and has acute circulatory collapse.
3. *Immediate operation.* A patient who has a known AAA and a clinical presentation consistent with acute rupture should be taken *directly* to the operating room without delay in the emergency area.
4. *Temperature control.* Cold kills! Patients with a ruptured AAA and shock become hypothermic quickly. Those

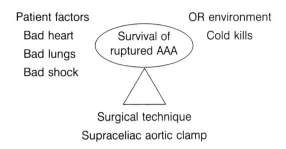

Figure 38-20 Survival of a patient with a ruptured aortic aneurysm depends on patient factors, operating room environment, and surgical skill.

with a body temperature below 33°C develop a capillary leak syndrome necessitating massive fluid resuscitation, manifest a diffuse coagulopathy, and frequently slip suddenly into life-threatening cardiac arrhythmias (Fig. 38-16). The two most useful means of preventing hypothermia are (1) to warm the operating room to 70 to 75°F *before* the patient enters the operating room and (2) to use the Bair Hugger warming tent over the upper thorax and head (Fig. 38-17).

5. *Autotransfusion.* Use of rapid cell savers should be routine in addition to banked blood products.
6. *Intravenous antibiotics.* These must not be forgotten.
7. *Low-dose intravenous dopamine.* Dopamine at a dose of 2 to 3 μg/kg/min has a vasodilatory effect for both renal and mesenteric circulations and may alleviate acute renal failure and bowel ischemia.
8. *Swan-Ganz pulmonary artery catheter.* Use of this catheter facilitates fluid and cardiac management.
9. *Supraceliac aortic clamping at the diaphragm.* Such clamping should be used liberally when large perirenal hematomas are present[71] (Fig. 38-22).

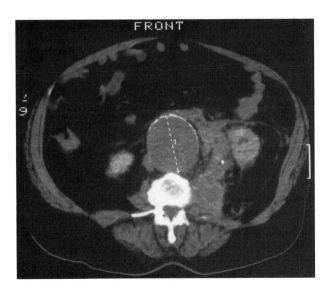

Figure 38-21 CT scan showing large abdominal aortic aneurysm with a left-sided rupture and hematoma.

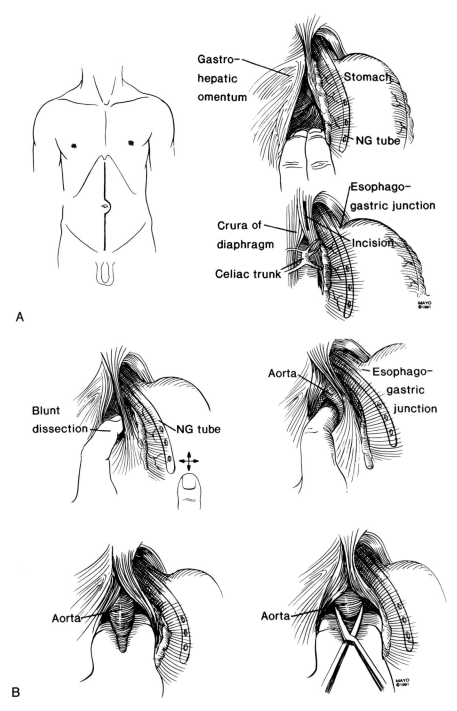

Figure 38-22 Supraceliac aortic clamping is useful for large abdominal aortic aneurysms and huge retroperitoneal hematomas that obscure the proximal aneurysm neck at the renal level. (Modified from Veith et al.,[71] and by permission of Mayo Foundation.)

10. *Systemic heparin.* Generally, large doses (5000 units or more) are unnecessary, although distal low-dose heparin irrigation or a small systemic dose (2500 to 3000 units) may minimize lower limb thrombotic complications.
11. A *low-porosity (woven or collagen-coated knit) straight tube graft.* This should be used whenever possible.
12. *Bowel viability.* If questionable, this can be checked by an intravenous fluoroscein (two ampules) examination.
13. *Good peripheral perfusion.* This should be ensured by palpable pulses or by good Doppler signals or calf plethysmographic pulse volume recordings before the patient leaves the operating room.
14. *Assisted ventilation.* This should be continued until excessive body edema recedes.
15. *Flexible sigmoidoscopy.* This test should be performed for any suspicion of colonic ischemia (e.g., early profuse diarrhea and systemic toxicity).

Long-term outcome for survivors is excellent and not significantly different from that for survivors of elective repair.[72] These patients should be checked periodically (every 2 to 5 years) for any graft-related complications or other aneurysms, and any of their siblings and children older than 50 years should be checked for AAAs because of the increasing awareness of the familial tendency of aortic aneurysms.[73]

Associated Operations with Aneurysm Repair

Occasionally, another surgical problem coexists with an aneurysm. Two common examples are gallstones and inguinal hernias. Should such problems be corrected at the same time that the aneurysm is repaired? The answer is debatable.[74-82] In general the safest approach is to repair only the aneurysm and delay other elective abdominal operations until later. This approach minimizes the chance of graft contamination and subsequent infection. Additional operations performed together with AAA repair appear to increase morbidity and mortality.[73]

Exceptions to this rule do arise. One common problem is severe stenosis of both renal arteries, causing uncontrolled hypertension or renal insufficiency.[80] One or both renal artery lesions should be corrected concomitantly with the AAA repair. Likewise, severe occlusive disease of the celiac and superior mesenteric arteries may require bypass if the inferior mesenteric artery is ligated. Certainly a large inferior mesenteric artery, in the face of an occluded superior mesenteric artery needs reimplantation or bypass during infrarenal AAA repair.

Although asymptomatic gallstones or hernias can be left alone, select intra-abdominal pathology can be treated safely after AAA grafting and retroperitoneal closure. Examples include recently symptomatic gallstones,[75] renal cancer, and an occasional colon tumor.[77-79] Such colon tumors are usually bleeding cancers of the right colon, for which a right hemicolectomy can be performed safely after AAA repair and retroperitoneal closure. When a left colon tumor is present, a large aneurysm is usually repaired first and the colon tumor is resected a few weeks later when the patient is ready. Rarely, it is necessary to resect an obstructed colon cancer and perform a colostomy *after* resection of a large or symptomatic aneurysm.

A 1980 report warned that laparotomy alone increased the risk of rupture if an aortic aneurysm was not concomitantly corrected.[83] The aortic aneurysms in this study, however, were generally large (more than 7 cm). A subsequent study published in 1991, did not find such an increased rupture risk (mean diameter 5.6 cm, range 3.0 to 8.5 cm) at the time of surgery.[84] Nonetheless, our bias remains to repair large (more than 6 cm) aortic aneurysms at the time of surgery for other concomitant abdominal problems provided that gross contamination of the aortic graft can be avoided.

REFERENCES

1. Pairolero PC, Bernatz PE: Aneurysms. p. 1. In Goldsmith HS (ed): Practice of Surgery. Harper & Row, Philadelphia, 1983
2. Parodi JC, Palmaz JC, Barrone HD: Transfemoral intraluminal graft implantation for abdominal aortic aneurysm. Ann Vasc Surg 5:491, 1991
3. Leach SD, Toole AL, Stern H et al: Effect of β-adrenergic blockade on the growth rate of abdominal aortic aneurysms. Arch Surg 123:606, 1988
4. Hallett JW: Optimal sizes of abdominal aortic aneurysms for surgery in good-risk and poor risk patients. In Veith FJ (ed): Current Critical Problems in Vascular Surgery. Quality Medicals, St. Louis, 1991
5. Gliedman ML, Ayers WB, Vestal BL: Aneurysms of the abdominal aorta and its branches: a study of untreated patients. Ann Surg 146:207, 1957
6. Gifford RW, Hines EA, Janes JM: An analysis and follow-up study of one hundred popliteal aneurysms. Surgery 33:284, 1953
7. Nevitt MP, Ballard DJ, Hallett JW: Prognosis of abdominal aortic aneurysms. N Engl J Med 321:1009, 1989
8. Bernstein EF, Fisher JC, Varco RL: Is excision the optimum treatment for all abdominal aortic aneurysms? Surgery 61:83, 1967
9. Bernstein EF, Chan EL: Abdominal aortic aneurysm in high-risk patients. Ann Surg 200:255, 1984
10. Cronenwett JL, Sargent SK, Wall MH et al: Variables that affect the expansion rate and outcome of small abdominal aortic aneurysms. J Vasc Surg 11:260, 1990

11. Treiman RL, Hartunian SL, Cossman DV et al: Late results of small untreated abdominal aortic aneurysms. Ann Vasc Surg 5:359, 1991

12. Brown PM, Pattenden R, Gutelius JR: The natural history of small abdominal aortic aneurysm — the Kingston abdominal aortic aneurysm study. J Vasc Surg 15:21, 1992

13. Cutler BS, Darling RC: Surgical management of arteriosclerotic femoral aneurysms. Surgery 74:764, 1973

14. Szilagyi DE, Schwartz RL, Reddy DJ: Popliteal arterial aneurysms. Arch Surg 116:724, 1981

15. Reilly MK, Abbott WM, Darling RC: Aggressive surgical management of popliteal artery aneurysms. Am J Surg 145:498, 1983

16. Anton GE, Hertzer NR, Beven EG et al: Surgical management of popliteal aneurysms: trends in presentation, treatment, and results from 1952 to 1984. J Vasc Surg 3:125, 1986

17. Schellack J, Smith RB, Perdue GD: Nonoperative management of selected popliteal aneurysms. Arch Surg 122:372, 1987

18. Dawson I, van Bockel JH, Brand R, Terpstra JL: Popliteal artery aneurysms: long-term follow-up of aneurysmal disease and results of surgical treatment. J Vasc Surg 13:398, 1991

19. Johnston KW, Scobie TK: Multicenter prospective study of nonruptured abdominal aortic aneurysms. Part I. Population and operative management. J Vasc Surg 7:69, 1988

20. Johnston KW: Multicenter prospective study of nonruptured abdominal aortic aneurysm. Part II. Variables predicting morbidity and mortality. J Vasc Surg 9:437, 1989

21. Roger VL, Ballard DJ, Hallett JW et al: Influence of coronary artery disease on morbidity and mortality after abdominal aortic aneurysmectomy: a population-based study, 1971–1987. J Am Coll Cardiol 14:1245, 1989

22. Gersh BJ, Rihal CS, Rooke TW, Ballard DJ: Evaluation and management of patients with both peripheral vascular and coronary artery disease. J Am Coll Cardiol 18:203, 1991

23. Robison JG, Beckett WC, Mills JL et al: Aortic reconstruction in high-risk pulmonary patients. Ann Surg 210:112, 1989

24. Cohen JR, Mannick JA, Couch NP, Whittemore AD: Abdominal aortic aneurysm repair in patients with preoperative renal failure. J Vasc Surg 3:867, 1986

25. Hertzer NR, Young JR, Beven EG et al: Late results of coronary bypass in patients with infrarenal aortic aneurysms: the Cleveland Clinic study. Ann Surg 205:360, 1987

26. Golden MA, Whittemore AD, Donaldson MC, Mannick JA: Selective evaluation and management of coronary artery disease in patients undergoing repair of abdominal aortic aneurysms: a 16-year experience. Ann Surg 212:415, 1990

27. Veith FJ, Goldsmith J, Leather RP, Hannan EL: The need for quality assurance in vascular surgery. J Vasc Surg 13:523, 1991

28. Hollier LH, Reigel MM, Kazmier FJ et al: Conventional repair of abdominal aortic aneurysm in the high-risk patient: a plea for abandonment of nonresective treatment. J Vasc Surg 3:712, 1986

29. Dubost C, Allary M, Oeconomos N: Resection of an aneurysm of the abdominal aorta. Arch Surg 64:512, 1952

30. Jarrett F, Darling RC, Mundth ED, Austen WG: Experience with infected aneurysms of the abdominal aorta. Arch Surg 110:1281, 1975

31. Perry MO: Infected aortic aneurysm. J Vasc Surg 2:597, 1985

32. Brown SL, Busuttil RW, Baker JD et al: Bacteriologic and surgical determinants of survival in patients with mycotic aneurysms. J Vasc Surg 1:541, 1984

33. Walker WE, Cooley DA, Duncan JM et al: The management of aortoduodenal fistula by in situ replacement of the infected abdominal aortic graft. Ann Surg 205:727, 1985

34. Bandyk DF, Bergamini TM, Kinney EV et al: In situ replacement of vascular prostheses infected by bacterial biofilms. J Vasc Surg 13:575, 1991

35. Karmody AM, Leather RP, Goldman M: The current position of nonresective treatment for abdominal aortic aneurysm. Surgery 94:591, 1983

36. Lynch K, Kohler T, Johansen K: Nonresective therapy for aortic aneurysm: results of a survey. J Vasc Surg 4:469, 1986

37. Schwartz RA, Nichols WK, Silver D: Is thrombosis of the infrarenal abdominal aortic aneurysm an acceptable alternative? J Vasc Surg 3:448, 1986

38. Cambria RP, Brewster DC, Abbott WM et al: Transperitoneal versus retroperitoneal approach for aortic reconstruction: a randomized prospective study. J Vasc Surg 11:314, 1990

39. Crawford ES: Thoracoabdominal and proximal aortic replacement for extensive aortic aneurysmal disease. p. 351. In Greenhalgh RM, Mannick JA (eds): The Course and Management of Aneurysms. WB Saunders, London, 1990

40. Crawford ES, Crawford JL, Safi HJ et al: Thoracoabdominal aortic aneurysms: preoperative and intraoperative factors determining immediate and long-term results of operations in 605 patients. J Vasc Surg 3:389, 1986

41. Crawford ES, DeNatale RW: Thoracoabdominal aortic aneurysm: observations regarding the natural course of the disease. J Vasc Surg 3:578, 1986

42. Hollier LH, Symmonds JB, Pairolero PC et al: Thoracoabdominal aortic aneurysm repair: analysis of postoperative morbidity. Arch Surg 123:871, 1988

43. Cambria RP, Brewster DC, Moncure AC et al: Recent experience with thoracoabdominal aneurysm repair. Arch Surg 124:620, 1989

44. Svensson LG, Hess KR, Coselli JS et al: A prospective study of respiratory failure after high-risk surgery on the thoracoabdominal aorta. J Vasc Surg 14:271, 1991

45. Pennell RC, Hollier LH, Lie JT et al: Inflammatory abdominal aortic aneurysms: a thirty-year review. J Vasc Surg 2:859, 1985

46. Crawford JL, Stowe CL, Safi HJ et al: Inflammatory aneurysms of the aorta. J Vasc Surg 2:113, 1985
47. Lindblad B, Almgren B, Bergqvist D et al: Abdominal aortic aneurysm with perianeurysmal fibrosis: experience from 11 Swedish vascular centers. J Vasc Surg 13:231, 1991
48. Sidell PM, Pairolero PC, Payne WS et al: Horseshoe kidney associated with surgery of the abdominal aorta. Mayo Clin Proc 54:97, 1979
49. Bietz DS, Merendino KA: Abdominal aneurysm and horseshoe kidney: a review. Ann Surg 181:333, 1975
50. Connelly TL, McKinnon W, Smith RB, Perdue GD: Abdominal aortic surgery and horseshoe kidney: report of six cases and a review. Arch Surg 115:1459, 1980
51. Gloviczki P, Cross SA, Stanson AW et al: Ischemic injury to the spinal cord or lumbosacral plexus after aorto-iliac reconstruction. Am J Surg 162:131, 1991
52. Hollier LH, Stanson AW, Gloviczki P et al: Arteriomegaly: classification and morbid implications of diffuse aneurysmal disease. Surgery 93:700, 1983
53. Darling RC, Brewster DC: Elective treatment of abdominal aortic aneurysms. World J Surg 4:661, 1980
54. Crawford ES, Saleh SA, Babb JW: Infrarenal abdominal aortic aneurysm: factors influencing survival after operation performed over a 25-year period. Ann Surg 193:699, 1981
55. Olsen PS, Schroeder T, Agerskov K et al: Surgery for abdominal aortic aneurysm. J Cardiovasc Surg 32:636, 1991
56. Whittemore AD, Clowes AW, Hechtman HB, Mannick JA: Aortic aneurysm repair: reduced operative mortality associated with maintenance of optimal cardiac performance. Ann Surg 192:414, 1980
57. Svensson LG, Von Ritter CM, Groeneveld HT et al: Cross-clamping of the thoracic aorta. Ann Surg 204:38, 1986
58. Hollier LH: Protecting the brain and spinal cord. J Vasc Surg 5:524, 1987
59. Bourchier RG, Gloviczki P, Larson MV et al: The mechanisms and prevention of intravascular fluid loss after occlusion of the supraceliac aorta in dogs. J Vasc Surg 13:637, 1991
60. Hallett JW, Popovsky M, Ilstrup D: Minimizing blood transfusions during abdominal aortic surgery: recent advances in rapid autotransfusion. J Vasc Surg 5:601, 1987
61. Hallett JW: Minimizing the use of homologous blood products during repair of abdominal aortic aneurysms. Surg Clin North Am 69:817, 1989
62. Hoffman M, Avellone JC, Plecha FR et al: Operation for ruptured abdominal aortic aneurysms: a community-wide experience. Surgery 91:597, 1982
63. Johansen K, Kohler TR, Nicholls SC et al: Ruptured abdominal aortic aneurysm: the Harborview experience. J Vasc Surg 13:240, 1991
64. Crawford ES: Ruptured abdominal aortic aneurysm: an editorial. J Vasc Surg 13:348, 1991
65. Gloviczki P, Pairolero PC, Mucha P et al: Ruptured abdominal aortic aneurysms: repair should not be denied. J Vasc Surg 15:851, 1992
66. Wakefield TW, Whitehouse WM, Wu SC et al: Abdominal aortic aneurysm ruptured: statistical analysis of factors affecting outcome of surgical treatment. Surgery 91:586, 1982
67. Donaldson MC, Rosenberg JM, Bucknam CA: Factors affecting survival after ruptured abdominal aortic aneurysm. J Vasc Surg 2:564, 1985
68. Ouriel K, Geary K, Green RM et al: Factors determining survival after ruptured aortic aneurysm: the hospital, the surgeon, and the patient. J Vasc Surg 11:493, 1990
69. Mannick JA, Whittemore AD: Management of ruptured or symptomatic abdominal aortic aneurysms. Surg Clin North Am 68:377, 1988
70. Sullivan CA, Rohrer MJ, Cutler BS: Clinical management of the symptomatic but unruptured abdominal aortic aneurysm. J Vasc Surg 11:799, 1990
71. Veith FJ, Gupta S, Daly V: Technique for occluding the supraceliac aorta through the abdomen. Surg Gynecol Obstet 151:427, 1980
72. Rohrer MJ, Cutler BS, Brownell Wheeler H: Long-term survival and quality of life following ruptured abdominal aortic aneurysm. Arch Surg 123:1213, 1988
73. Johansen K, Koepsell T: Familial tendency for abdominal aortic aneurysms. JAMA 256:1934, 1986
74. Bickerstaff LK, Hollier LH, Van Peenen HJ et al: Abdominal aortic aneurysm repair combined with a second surgical procedure—morbidity and mortality. Surgery 95:487, 1984
75. Ouriel K, Ricotta JJ, Adams JT, Deweese JA: Management of cholelithiasis in patients with abdominal aortic aneurysm. Ann Surg 198:717, 1983
76. Fry RE, Fry WJ: Cholelithiasis and aortic reconstruction: the problem of simultaneous surgical therapy. J Vasc Surg 4:345, 1986
77. Nora JD, Pairolero PC, Nivatvongs S et al: Concomitant abdominal aortic aneurysm and colorectal carcinoma: priority of resection. J Vasc Surg 9:630, 1989
78. Velanovich V, Andersen CA: Concomitant abdominal aortic aneurysm and colorectal cancer: A decision analysis approach to a therapeutic dilemma. Ann Vasc Surg 5:449, 1991
79. Lobbato VJ, Rothenberg RE, LaRaja RD, Georgiou J: Coexistence of abdominal aortic aneurysm and carcinoma of the colon: a dilemma. J Vasc Surg 2:724, 1985
80. Hallett JW, Fowl R, O'Brien PC et al: Renovascular operations in patients with chronic renal insufficiency: do the benefits justify the risks? J Vasc Surg 5:622, 1987
81. Szilagyi ED, Elliott JP, Berguer R: Coincidental malignancy and abdominal aortic aneurysm. Arch Surg 95:402, 1967
82. Morgan RJ, Abbott WM: Safe management of patients with simultaneously occurring prostatism and abdominal aortic aneurysm. Am J Surg 143:319, 1982
83. Swanson RJ, Littooy FN, Hunt TK, Stoney RJ: Laparotomy as a precipitating factor in the rupture of intra-abdominal aneurysms. Arch Surg 115:299, 1980
84. Durham SJ, Steed DL, Moosa HH et al: Probability of rupture of an abdominal aortic aneurysm after an unrelated operative procedure: a prospective study. J Vasc Surg 13:248, 1991

39

Alternatives to Resective Therapy for Abdominal and Pelvic Aneurysms

B. Clay Parker

ABDOMINAL AORTIC ANEURYSMS

Indisputably, the treatment of choice for abdominal aortic aneurysms is direct surgical repair. As described in Chapters 33 to 38, the results of this therapy are generally excellent and, with careful attention to preoperative evaluation and postoperative care, can be accomplished with low morbidity and mortality, even in elderly patients and in patients with significant medical disease.[1-3] However, occasional patients are encountered with sizable or symptomatic abdominal aortic aneurysms, whom end-stage cardiac, pulmonary, or renal disease places at unacceptably high risk for standard surgical repair. Likewise, extensive prior abdominal operations, intra-abdominal adhesions, multiple stomata, intra-abdominal infection, and intra-abdominal neoplastic disease can occasionally present prohibitive technical hurdles to standard surgery. In this small subset of patients, nonresective therapy, combining induced aneurysm thrombosis and extra-anatomic (axillobifemoral) bypass grafting may be considered.[1,3-5] The predominant advantages of this modality are avoidance of aortic cross-clamping with the resultant rapid increase in cardiac afterload; less blood loss; shorter operating time[4,5]; and because the peritoneal

cavity is not entered, a more rapid return of bowel function.[5]

The earliest nonresective methods involved initial placement of an extra-anatomic bypass, followed by ligation of the abdominal aorta and iliac arteries proximal and distal to the aneurysm sac.[6,7] Alternatively, ligation of the iliac arteries alone was performed in some cases, with the expected result of thrombosis of the aortic aneurysm up to the first major branch vessels, generally the renal arteries. Subsequently, transcatheter occlusion techniques have been used as an adjunct in aneurysm thrombosis.[4-6,8,9]

Preliminary evaluation of the aneurysm prior to inducing thrombosis by ligation or transcatheter embolization requires angiography.[4,5,9] The predominant issues to be addressed by angiography include the possible presence of accessory renal arteries relative to the aneurysm, inferior mesenteric artery patency, hypogastric artery patency, and infrainguinal arterial runoff. Inferiorly located accessory renal arteries may be at risk in the course of induced aneurysm thrombosis, which could be potentially critical in patients with marginal renal reserve.[4,6,9] Inferior mesenteric artery patency is not found in most aneurysms over 6 cm in diameter. However, patency of this vessel may indicate that it is a significant source of perfusion of the lower gastrointestinal tract, as well as an important source of collateral perfusion to the superior mesenteric artery, the pelvic organs, and the lower extremities. In this setting, thrombosis of such an important arterial supply could be devastating.[4,9,10,11] Evaluation of the infrainguinal arterial runoff provides useful information prior to axillofemoral bypass grafting, since poor infragraft runoff serves to further compromise this graft's already limited long-term patency.[12]

Angiographic demonstration of hypogastric artery occlusion allows exclusion of the aneurysm by ligation of the external iliac arteries distally via groin incisions. If the hypogastric arteries are patent, ligation of the distal common iliac arteries via a retroperitoneal approach is required to exclude the aneurysm from direct arterial pressure.[4-6] When the common iliac arteries are aneurysmal, separate ligation of the proximal internal and external iliac arteries must be carried out. With distal ligation alone as the method to induce thrombosis of an abdominal aortic aneurysm, a 70 percent success rate has been reported.[5] In those aneurysms that remain nonthrombosed, transaxillary angiography should be performed to determine the location of the runoff vessel responsible for continued aortic patency. Transcatheter embolization can be undertaken in the same setting.[4-6,9] A variety of embolic agents, including coils, Gelfoam, thrombin, detachable balloons, autologous clot, and tissue adhesives have been described for use in occluding the responsible vessel and/or the aortic aneurysm itself to effect clotting.[4-6,9,13] An alternative approach, which further limits the amount of surgical trauma to the patient, is ligation of the distal external iliac arteries at the time of axillobifemoral grafting (regardless of the status of the hypogastric arteries), followed by transaxillary aortography, with selective embolization of the hypogastric arteries or aneurysm sac as needed to induce complete thrombosis of the aortic aneurysm.[13]

Reported complications of induced aneurysm thrombosis include infection, coagulopathy, and renal and/or intestinal ischemia.[1,14-16] Most of these complications are presented in the literature as case reports, which makes evaluation of a true complication rate difficult. A more bothersome aspect of nonresective therapy has been continued aneurysm expansion and rupture. In a review of six collective series reporting a total of 87 patients, Inahara et al.[14] found seven cases of post-treatment aortic aneurysm rupture (8 percent). A nationwide survey of vascular surgeons by Lynch et al.[17] revealed a 3.3 percent rupture rate in a collective series of 118 aneurysms treated by proximal and distal ligation and a 20 percent rupture rate in a collective series of 88 patients treated by distal ligation.

Thus, the potential complications and inferior results in preventing aneurysm rupture as compared with standard surgical treatment limit the utility of nonresective therapy, especially in view of the excellent safety and efficacy of arterial grafting for aneurysm management. Despite these drawbacks, nonresective therapy may be a reasonable treatment choice in the limited subset of patients with far advanced cardiac, pulmonary, and/or renal disease or in patients with anatomic prohibitions to standard surgical abdominal aortic aneurysm repair. Percutaneous arterial grafting is undergoing evaluation as an alternative, minimally invasive method of aneurysm treatment[18,19] and may replace aneurysm exclusion and in some cases, standard surgical grafting for treatment of aortic aneurysms.

HYPOGASTRIC ARTERY ANEURYSMS

Patients with hypogastric artery aneurysms may also benefit from transluminal occlusion techniques. Hypogastric artery aneurysms are quite rare as isolated lesions (0.4 percent of all arterial aneurysms),[20] although they may be seen more frequently in conjunction with aneurysms of the abdominal aorta and common iliac arteries. Symptoms of these true pelvic aneurysms are usually gastrointestinal, genitourinary, or neurologic in nature, owing to local mass effect.[21] The location of these aneurysms makes evaluation by physical examination difficult, although a pulsatile mass may be felt on careful rectal or vaginal examination in up to 55 percent of patients with such lesions.[22] Because of the inaccessability of these aneurysms to physical examination, the clinical presentation in one-third to one-half of cases is rupture.[22,23] These lesions are best detected by abdominal-pelvic computed tomographic (CT) scanning, with magnetic resonance imaging (MRI) and ultrasound playing supplementary roles.

The treatment of hypogastric aneurysms has historically been surgical, with mortality rates of 7 percent for elective and 42 percent for emergent operations.[24] A variety of surgical techniques have been described, including extirpation of the aneurysm by direct arterial reconstruction; endoaneurysmorrhaphy with oversewing of the back-bleeding outflow vessels and subsequent obliteration of the aneurysm cavity; proximal and distal ligation; and proximal ligation only.[21,25-28] Although the first three of these techniques offer the advantage of total exclusion of the aneurysm from arterial pressure, these procedures can be technically difficult or impossible, especially in cases of large aneu-

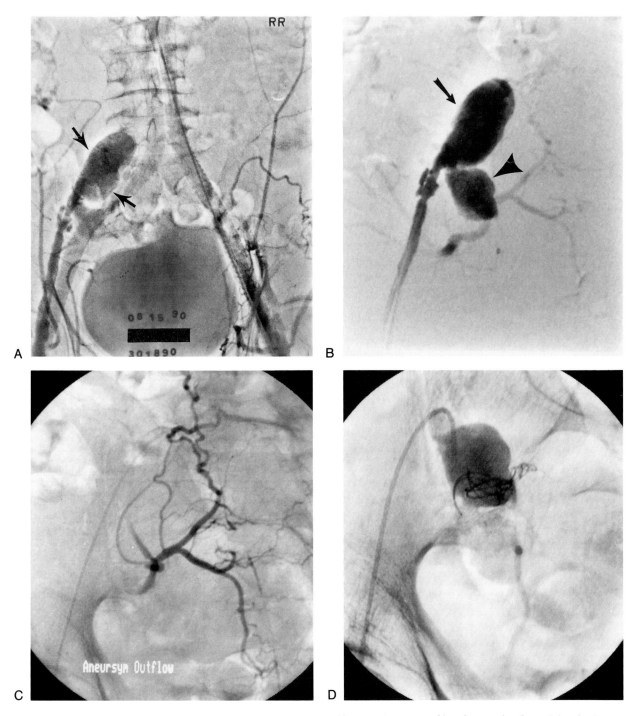

Figure 39-1 This 61-year-old man had undergone aortobifemoral bypass grafting for repair of an abdominal aortic aneurysm. Prior pelvic surgery and medical illness placed him at prohibitive risk for surgical repair. **(A)** Late film of a pelvic arteriogram demonstrates right common iliac and hypogastric aneurysm *(arrows)* (aortobifemoral graft placed previously for abdominal aortic aneurysm repair). **(B)** Selective right iliac arteriogram confirms the aneurysms of the common iliac artery *(arrow)* and hypogastric artery *(arrowhead)*. **(C)** Selective catheterization of the hypogastric aneurysm allows evaluation of aneurysm outflow via sacral branches. Occlusion at origin of outflow branch preserves integrity of these branches, prevents inadvertent distal embolization during aneurysm occlusion, and prevents retrograde filling of aneurysm after proximal embolization. **(D)** Hypogastric aneurysm filled with coils and autologous clot. *(Figure continues.)*

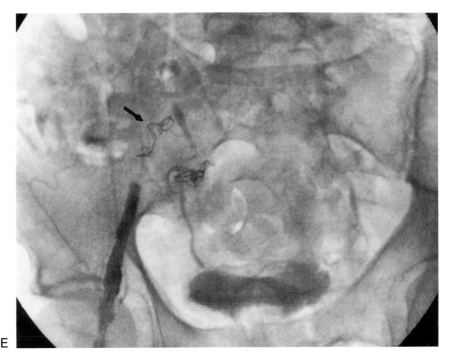

E

Figure 39-1 *(Continued)* **(E)** Final result after embolization of aneurysm inflow external iliac artery with coils *(arrow).* Total occlusion of aneurysm subsequently documented by CT.

rysms with adherence to local pelvic viscera and deep pelvic location.[21,26] Proximal ligation only is technically much easier to accomplish, though pelvic collateral vessels allow a mechanism for continued patency or recurrence of the aneurysm. Indeed, recurrent hypogastric aneurysms have been reported following proximal ligation only.[25,28] In a review of 28 cases treated in this manner, Brin and Busuttil reported five recurrences with one rupture.[25]

The technical difficulties of optimal surgical repair and the feasibility of superselective catheterization of the hypogastric branch vessels have prompted the use of transcatheter embolization as an alternative treatment modality.[29] We have treated three hypogastric artery aneurysms in this manner with aneurysm thrombosis successfully achieved in each instance (Figs. 39-1 and 39-2). Initial angiographic evaluation prior to hypogastric aneurysm embolization should include evaluation of concomitant aneurysmal disease of the abdominal aorta, common iliac arteries, and contralateral hypogastric artery, which may also require treatment. The patency of the inferior mesenteric and contralateral hypogastric arteries should also be evaluated, as these vessels may provide important collateral arterial supply to the pelvic viscera following hypogastric occlusion.[10,11]

Subsequently, the hypogastric artery aneurysm should be selectively catheterized, and via superselective angiographic methods, arterial outflow from the aneurysm should be demonstrated. Selection of these outflow vessels may be accomplished with a standard 5 French angiographic catheter, or may require coaxial placement of a 3 French tapered catheter system through a 5 French angiographic catheter that has been placed selectively in the aneurysm. With evaluation of the arterial outflow in this manner, it is feasible to occlude these outflow vessels selectively by using a combination of embolic materials, including embolic coils, Gelfoam, glue, and autologous clot. Thus, an effective "distal ligation" of the aneurysm can be accomplished. Subsequently, the aneurysm cavity itself can be filled with additional embolic material to the neck of the hypogastric artery, which results in complete aneurysm thrombosis and functional "proximal ligation." Significant series of hypogastric aneurysm embolization cases are not available for determination of success rates, complication rates, or recurrence rates. Nelson[30] found that 12 of 13 patients with unrepaired hypogastric aneurysms died. In light of this, we would recommend hypogastric aneurysm embolization as a treatment option in nonsurgical candidates.

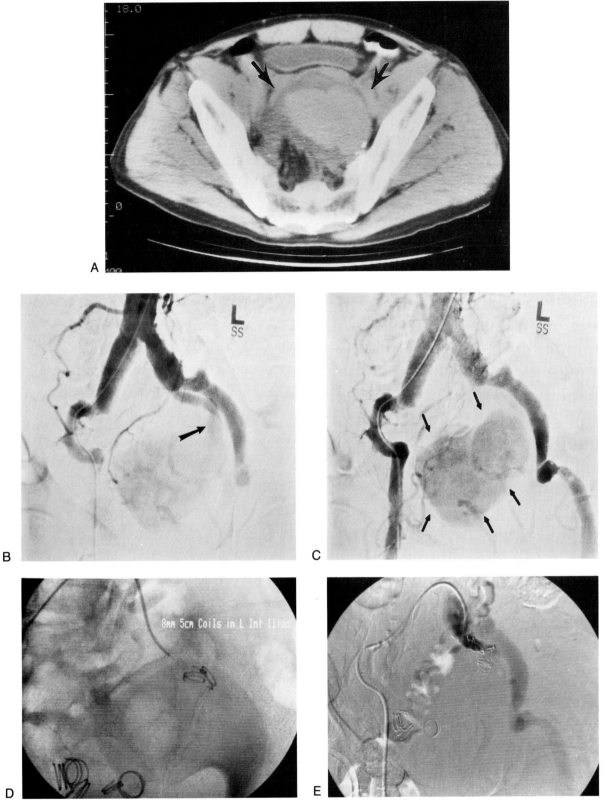

Figure 39-2 This 71-year-old man had a history of left leg pain. Severe underlying medical illness made him an unacceptable surgical candidate. **(A)** CT scan demonstrates large aneurysm *(arrows)* with minimal thrombosis. The site of origin is unclear. **(B)** Early film from pelvic angiogram demonstrates filling of aneurysm from left hypogastric artery *(arrow)*. **(C)** Later phase of pelvic angiogram better demonstrates aneurysm *(arrows)*. **(D)** Multiple coils placed during embolization. **(E)** Selective hypogastric angiogram after embolization documents complete occlusion. Reflux of contrast agent is seen in external iliac artery.

REFERENCES

1. Johnson K: Treatment options for aneurysms in high risk patients. Surg Clin North Am 69:765, 1989
2. Bernstein EF, Chan EL: Abdominal aortic aneurysm in high risk patients. Ann Surg 200:255, 1984
3. Kwaan JHM, Khan RS, Connally JE: Total exclusion technique for the management of abdominal aortic aneurysms. Am J Surg 146:93, 1983
4. Leather RP, Shah D, Goldman M et al: Nonresective treatment of abdominal aortic aneurysms. Arch Surg 114:1402, 1979
5. Karmody AM, Leather RP, Goldman M et al: The current position of nonresective treatment for abdominal aortic aneurysm. Surgery 94:591, 1983
6. Bergner R, Feldman AJ, Karmody AM: Intravascular thrombosis of abdominal aortic aneurysm in high risk patients. Vasc Diagn Ther 2:24, 1981
7. Blaisdell FW, Hall AD, Thomas AN: Ligation treatment of abdominal aortic aneurysms. Am J Surg 109:560, 1965
8. Carrasco H, Parry CE: Transcatheter embolization of abdominal aortic aneurysms. AJR 138:729, 1982
9. Goldman ML, Sarrafizadeh MS, Phillip PK et al: Bucrylate embolization of abdominal aortic aneurysms: an adjunct to nonresective therapy. AJR 135:1195, 1980
10. Iliopoulos JL, Howonitz PE, Pierce GE et al: The critical hypogastric circulation. Am J Surg 154:671, 1987
11. Iliopoulos JL, Hermreck AS, Thomas JH et al: Hemodynamics of the hypogastric arterial circulation. J Vasc Surg 9:637, 1989
12. Rutherford RB, Pott A, Pearce WH: Extra-anatomic bypass: a closer view. J Vasc Surg 6:437, 1987
13. Savarese RP, Rosenfeld JC, ReLaurentis DA: Alternatives in the treatment of abdominal aortic aneurysms. Am J Surg 142:226, 1981
14. Inahara T, Geary GL, Mukherjee D, Egan JM: The contrary position to the nonrestrictive treatment for abdominal aortic aneurysm. J Vasc Surg 2:42, 1985
15. Cho SI, Johnson WC, Birch HL et al: Lethal complications associated with nonrestrictive treatment of abdominal aortic aneurysms (sic). Arch Surg 117:1214, 1982
16. Schwartz RA, Nichols WK, Silva D: Is thrombosis of the infrarenal abdominal aortic aneurysm an acceptable alternative? J Vasc Surg 3:448, 1986
17. Lynch K, Kohler TR, Johansen K: Nonresective therapy for aortic aneurysm: results of a survey. J Vasc Surg 4:469, 1986
18. Mirch D, Wright KC, Wallace S et al: Percutaneously placed endovascular grafts for aortic aneurysms: feasibility study. Radiology 170:1033, 1989
19. Cragg AH, Lund G, Rysavy JA et al: Percutaneous arterial grafting. Radiology 150:45, 1984
20. Silver D, Anderson EE, Porter JM: Isolated hypogastric artery aneurysm. Arch Surg 95:308, 1967
21. Krupski WC, Bass A, Rosenberg GD et al: The elusive isolated hypogastric artery aneurysm: novel presentation. J Vasc Surg 10:557, 1989
22. Richardson JW, Greenfield LJ: Natural history and management of iliac aneurysms. J Vasc Surg 8:165, 1988
23. Markowitz AM, Norman JC: Aneurysms of the iliac artery. Ann Surg 154:777, 1961
24. Lowry SF, Kraft RO: Isolated aneurysms of the iliac artery. Arch Surg 113:1289, 1978
25. Brin BJ, Busuttil RW: Isolated hypogastric artery aneurysms. Arch Surg 117:1329, 1982
26. Matsuhara J, Nagasue M, Tsuchishima S et al: Bilateral ruptured isolated internal iliac artery aneurysms — report of a case and review of the literature. Jpn J Surg 19:760, 1989
27. Byrne JL, Zaman SN, Meade JW et al: Operative management of bilateral internal iliac artery aneurysms. J Cardiovasc Surg (Torino) 30:241, 1989
28. Golden RL, Bauman J, Johnstone M et al: Recurrent giant hypogastric artery aneurysm — a case report. Angiology 620, 1988
29. Perdue GD, Mittenthal MJ, Smith RB et al: Aneurysms of the internal iliac artery. Surgery 93:243, 1983
30. Nelson RP: Isolated internal iliac artery aneurysms and their urologic manifestations. J Urol 124:300, 1980

40

Long-Term Prognosis and Follow-Up of Aneurysm Patients

John W. Hallett, Jr.

The triumph of modern aneurysm surgery has been prolongation of life and limb for many patients. A single aneurysm operation, however, does not free the patient from the risk of future aneurysms or other cardiovascular events. These patients remain at lifelong risk of new aneurysms, graft complications, heart attacks, and strokes. Fortunately, regular checkups can detect some of these problems before they become serious. This chapter describes the nature and prevalence of these problems and, more importantly, emphasizes the value of long-term patient and graft surveillance.

PROLONGATION OF LIFE

Surgical correction of aortic aneurysms gained a firm and essentially unchallenged place in medicine during the late 1950s and 1960s. Szilagyi and colleagues[1] receive much of the credit for emphasizing the contribution of abdominal aortic aneurysmectomy to prolongation of life. They reported that 5-year survival following repair of an abdominal aortic aneurysm (AAA) was at least 50 percent, compared with only 15 to 20 percent for aneurysms not surgically treated. Rupture caused death in 35 percent of nonsurgical cases, most of which involved large aneurysms (>6 cm). This study also revealed that coronary or cerebral atherosclerosis presented the next most impor-

tant risk to life. More recent surgical series report 5-year survivals following AAA repair in the 70 to 80 percent range for patients without clinically evident coronary artery disease (CAD) and 50 to 60 percent for those with CAD[2-6] (Fig. 40-1). With thoracoabdominal aneurysm repair, 5-year survival was also good for patients with no heart disease (60 percent) but somewhat poorer for those with heart disease (50 percent).[7]

The main area of continuing controversy surrounds smaller (<5 cm) aortic aneurysms.[8] Some surgeons advocate repairing all of them in anticipation of eventual expansion, possible rupture, and declining patient health. Recent data, however, confirm a low rupture risk for small aneurysms[9-14]; rupture of an AAA less than 5 cm in diameter is a rare event. The most common cause of death for a patient with a small aneurysm is not rupture but myocardial infarction. These cardiac findings suggest that discovery of a small aneurysm should alert the physician to efforts to identify and treat any associated severe heart disease.

LIMB SALVAGE

The benefit of repairing femoral or popliteal aneurysms is saving limb function.[15-20] The vast majority of prophylactically operations for popliteal aneurysms will achieve excellent early (95 percent) and late (90

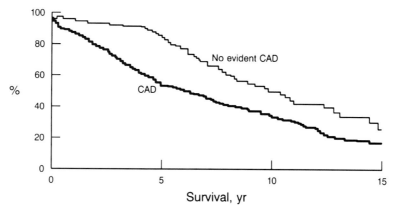

Figure 40-1 Survival after elective repair of infrarenal abdominal aortic aneurysms. (Modified from Crawford et al.,[2] with permission.)

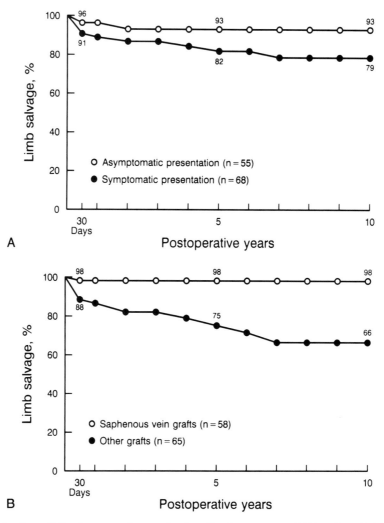

Figure 40-2 Limb salvage following operative repair of popliteal aneurysms. **(A)** Based on clinical symptoms. **(B)** Based on type of graft. (Adapted from Anton et al.,[19] with permission.)

percent at 10 years) limb salvage (Fig. 40-2). In contrast, repair of symptomatic popliteal aneurysms that has a slightly lower 10-year salvage rate (80 percent). Prognosis is especially poor for patients who present with prolonged acute ischemia and poor runoff. Graft patency is also better for those patients who undergo operation for asymptomatic popliteal aneurysms and those who receive vein grafts (Fig. 40-3).

MULTIPLE ANEURYSMS

The connective tissue disorder of aneurysmal disease makes multiple aneurysms possible in every patient[21,22] (Fig. 40-4). For example, at least 5 percent of patients with one aortic aneurysm will eventually develop a new one requiring another operation[23] (Figs. 40-5 and 40-6). Most of these new aneurysms are rec-

ognized relatively late (i.e., 5 to 15 years after the first repair).[24] They are more prevalent in patients with long-standing hypertension. In the lower extremities, bilaterality of popliteal aneurysms is well known (50 percent of cases).[15-20] The presence of an aortic aneurysm in a patient presenting with a popliteal aneurysm is also common (30 percent of cases).[15-20] All these findings support close long-term surveillance of aneurysm patients.

GRAFT COMPLICATIONS

Late graft complications (Figs. 40-7 and 40-8) are relatively uncommon but do affect 3 to 5 percent of patients.[2,11,23,25] These include anastomotic problems, graft infections or enteric erosions, fabric degeneration, and graft thrombosis. Anastomotic false aneurysms in

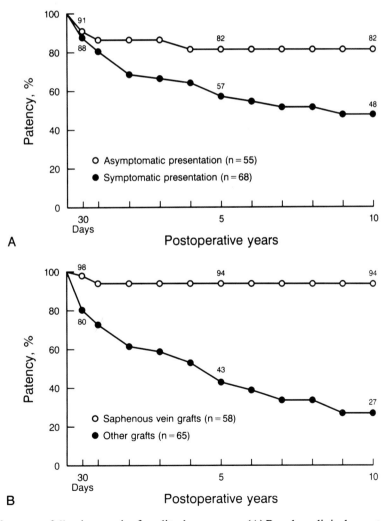

Figure 40-3 Graft patency following repair of popliteal aneurysms. **(A)** Based on clinical symptoms. **(B)** Based on type of graft. (Adapted from Anton et al.,[19] with permission.)

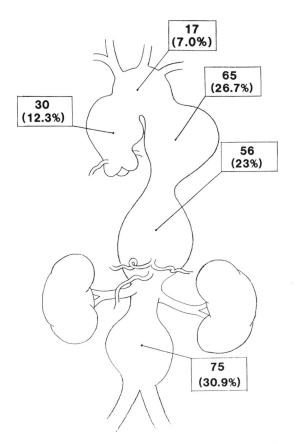

Figure 40-4 Location of aortic aneurysms in 102 patients with 243 multiple aortic aneurysms (From Gloviczki et al.,[21] with permission.)

the abdomen may remain silent until catastrophic rupture occurs. The best method of early detection is periodic ultrasound or computed tomography (CT) scanning of aortic grafts. Graft infections are rare (1 to 2 percent of cases) but may present insidiously with malaise, low-grade fevers, weight loss, and enlarging pseudoaneurysms. More dramatic presentations include gastrointestinal bleeding from a graft erosion into the gut or septicemia in a leg joint from mycotic emboli. Fabric degeneration with serious graft dilatation is infrequent but is seen occasionally with ultralightweight knitted grafts implanted in the early 1970s.[26] Finally, graft thrombosis is rare with abdominal aortic grafts for aneurysmal disease but is an important problem in aortofemoral bypass grafts (10 to 15 percent of cases in nonsmokers and 20 to 30 percent in smokers at 5 years).[27] Saphenous vein grafts for femoropopliteal aneurysms also achieve patency at 5 years (80 to 90 percent) as compared with synthetic grafts (40 to 50 percent) with good runoff and 20 to 30 percent with poor runoff).[19]

CARDIOVASCULAR EVENTS

New aneurysms and graft complications are not, however, the most common cause of late morbidity and mortality in aneurysm patients—cardiovascular events are more threatening by a large margin.[3,5,6] Population-based studies that included all aneurysm patients in a single community revealed alarming late results for those with clinically evident CAD.[6] By 8 years postaneurysmectomy, 60 percent had sustained a myocardial infarction or died of cardiac causes. Sur-

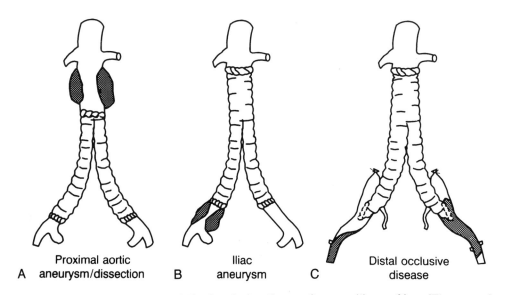

| A | Proximal aortic aneurysm/dissection | B | Iliac aneurysm | C | Distal occlusive disease |

Figure 40-5 (A–C) New aneurysms and distal occlusive disease after aortoiliac grafting. *(Figure continues.)*

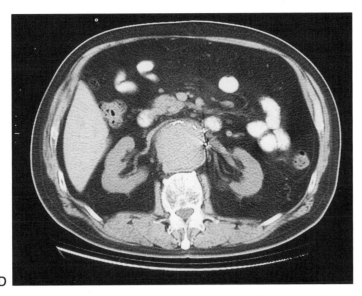

D

Figure 40-5 *(Continued.)* **(D)** New abdominal aortic aneurysm, recognized 6 years after an aortoiliac graft for an abdominal aortic aneurysm. (From Hallett and Calcagno,[24] with permission.)

vival was poor (30 to 40 percent) for those with CAD. In encouraging contrast to these dismal results are the results for patients with no evident CAD, who had a 70 percent survival at 5 years and a 60 percent survival at 8 years, with only a 15 percent risk of a cardiac event. Although less common than cardiac morbidity, cerebrovascular disease has been found to cause stroke in 5 percent of aneurysm patients at 5 years and in 10 percent by 10 years.[28] Hypertension appears to be a significant factor in both cardiac and cerebral events and in lowering late survival (Fig. 40-9).[2,23]

RECOMMENDATIONS

The life-long threat of new aneurysms and cardiovascular events emphasizes the need for long-term follow-up (Table 40-1). Prevention of complications begins with patient education—physicians must convince patients that periodic rechecks are worthwhile, should discuss control of blood pressure with them, and should not overlook the benefit of smoking cessation. Patients must be told to report new or unstable angina pectoris or dyspnea on exertion. They should be aware

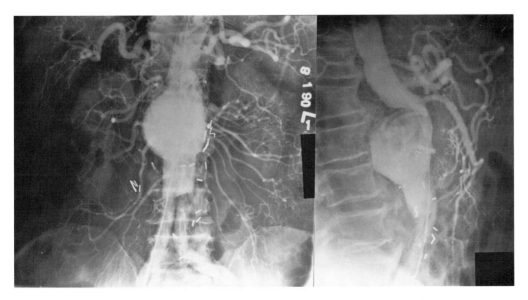

Figure 40-6 An aortogram showing the juxtarenal aortic aneurysm of Figure 40-5.

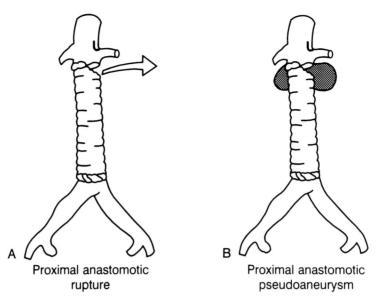

Figure 40-7 Late graft complications following aortic tube grafts for abdominal aortic aneurysm. Proximal anastomotic rupture **(A)** is often associated with an anastomotic pseudoaneurysm **(B)**.

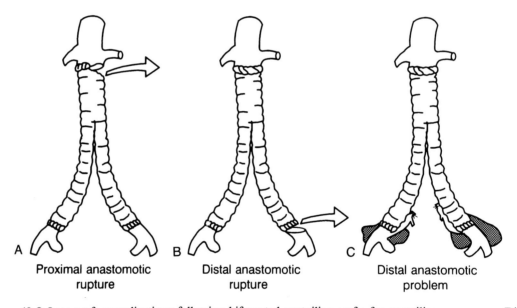

Figure 40-8 Late graft complications following bifurcated aortoiliac grafts for aortoiliac aneurysms. Distal anastomotic problems are just as prevalent as proximal anastomotic problems.

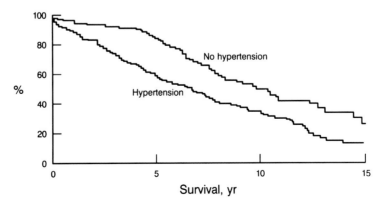

Figure 40-9 Effect of hypertension on survival after elective repair of infrarenal abdominal aortic aneurysms. (Modified from Crawford et al.,[2] with permission.)

Table 40-1 Recommended Follow-up of Aneurysm Patients

Type of Original Aneurysm	History/ Physical Examination[a]	Chest X-ray	Ultrasound[b]	CT Scan
Aortic/iliac	Yearly	q 1–2 years	q 1–2 years	For thoracoabdominal grafts or abnormal or inadequate ultrasound
Femoral	Yearly	q 1–2 years	Yearly	NA
Popliteal	Yearly	q 1–2 years	Yearly	NA

Abbreviations: CT, computed tomography; NA, not applicable in most patients.
[a] Any new or progressive cardiac or cerebrovascular symptoms deserve evaluation. Hypertension needs good control.
[b] Ultrasound of aortic graft, femoral, and popliteal arteries.

that prophylactic antibiotics are advisable for persons with synthetic grafts if they are receiving other surgical or dental care or if they develop any bacterial infections.

The frequency and content of periodic checkups are debatable.[29] A reasonable approach for *all* aneurysm patients is a yearly review of any cardiovascular symptoms along with a check of blood pressure, cervical bruits, and abdominal and peripheral pulses. Any new cardiac symptoms should prompt an electrocardiogram and some form of noninvasive cardiac testing. New cerebrovascular symptoms or cervical bruits should be investigated initially with ocular pneumoplethysmography or carotid duplex ultrasound scanning.

A more difficult question concerns the frequency of imaging an aneurysm graft. Each year or every 2 years, surveillance for new aneurysm or graft complications can be performed with a chest x-ray and an ultrasound study of the abdominal aorta and femoropopliteal arteries. Any questionable abnormalities of the abdominal aorta, suprarenal area, or thoracoabdominal segment should be evaluated with a CT scan.[30,31] The CT scan is also the best method to follow thoracoabdominal aneurysm grafts. Peripheral femoropopliteal grafts can be followed by ankle-brachial pressure indices or by duplex ultrasound.

FUTURE NEEDS

The need for long-term periodic checkups of the patient's cardiac status, graft function, and possible new aneurysms is clearly established. In contrast, the frequency and type (imaging) of surveillance are unresolved issues. The cost of follow-up is also not inconsequential. Consequently, future clinical trials need to

address the most cost-effective methods to maintain the patient's health and the graft's function.

REFERENCES

1. Szilagyi DE, Smith RF, DeRusso FJ et al: Contribution of abdominal aortic aneurysmectomy to prolongation of life. Ann Surg 164:678, 1966
2. Crawford ES, Saleh SA, Babb JW III et al: Infrarenal abdominal aortic aneurysm: factors influencing survival after operation performed over a 25-year period. Ann Surg 193:699, 1981
3. Hollier LH, Plate G, O'Brien PC et al: Late survival after abdominal aortic aneurysm repair: influence of coronary artery disease. J Vasc Surg 1:290, 1984
4. Reigel MM, Hollier LH, Kazmier FJ et al: Late survival in abdominal aortic aneurysm patients: the role of selective myocardial revascularization on the basis of clinical symptoms. J Vasc Surg 5:222, 1987
5. Hertzer NR: Fatal myocardial infarction following abdominal aortic aneurysm resection: 343 patients followed 6–11 years postoperatively. Ann Surg 192:667, 1980
6. Roger VL, Ballard DJ, Hallett JW Jr et al: Influence of coronary artery disease on morbidity and mortality after abdominal aortic aneurysmectomy: a population-based study, 1971–1987. J Am Coll Cardiol 14:1245, 1989
7. Crawford ES, Crawford JL, Safi HJ et al: Thoracoabdominal aortic aneurysms: preoperative and intraoperative factors determining immediate and long-term results of operations in 605 patients. J Vasc Surg 3:389, 1986
8. Hallett JW Jr: Optimal sizes of abdominal aortic aneurysms for surgery in good-risk and poor-risk patients. In Veith FJ (ed): Current Critical Problems in Vascular Surgery. Quality Medicals, St. Louis, 1991
9. Nevitt MP, Ballard DJ, Hallett JW Jr: Prognosis of abdominal aortic aneurysms. N Engl J Med 321:1009, 1989

10. Cronenwett JL, Sargent SK, Wall MH et al: Variables that affect the expansion rate and outcome of small abdominal aortic aneurysms. J Vasc Surg 11:260, 1990

11. Johansson G, Nydahl S, Olofsson P, Swedenborg J: Survival in patients with abdominal aortic aneurysms: comparison between operative and nonoperative management. Eur J Vasc Surg 4:497, 1990

12. Gillmaker H, Holmberg L, Elvin A et al: Natural history of patients with abdominal aortic aneurysm. Eur J Vasc Surg 5:125, 1990

13. Treiman RL, Hartunian SL, Cossman DV et al: Late results of small untreated abdominal aortic aneurysms. Ann Vasc Surg 5:359, 1991

14. Brown PM, Pattenden R, Gutelius JR: The natural history of small abdominal aortic aneurysm: the Kingston abdominal aortic aneurysm study. J Vasc Surg 15:21, 1992

15. Edmunds LH, Darling RC, Linton RR: Surgical management of popliteal aneurysms. Circulation 32:517, 1965

16. Vermilion BD, Kimmins SA, Pace WG, Evans WE: A review of one hundred forty-seven popliteal aneurysms with long-term follow-up. Surgery 90:1009, 1981

17. Reilly MK, Abbott WM, Darling RC: Aggressive surgical management of popliteal artery aneurysms. Am J Surg 145:498, 1983

18. Whitehouse WM, Wakefield TW, Graham LM et al: Limb-threatening potential of arteriosclerotic popliteal artery aneurysms. Surgery 93:694, 1983

19. Anton GE, Hertzer NR, Beven ED et al: Surgical management of popliteal aneurysms: trends in presentation, treatment, and results from 1952 to 1984. J Vasc Surg 3:125, 1986

20. Dawson I, van Bockel JH, Brand R, Terpstra JL: Popliteal artery aneurysms: long-term follow-up of aneurysmal disease and results of surgical treatment. J Vasc Surg 13:398, 1991

21. Gloviczki P, Pairolero P, Welch T et al: Multiple aortic aneurysms: the results of surgical management. J Vasc Surg 11:19, 1990

22. Crawford ES, Coselli JS, Svensson LG et al: Diffuse aneurysmal disease (chronic aortic dissection, Marfan, and mega aorta syndromes) and multiple aneurysm. Ann Surg 211:521, 1990

23. Plate G, Hollier LH, O'Brien P et al: Recurrent aneurysms and late vascular complications following repair of abdominal aortic aneurysms. Arch Surg 120:590, 1985

24. Hallett JW, Calcagno D: Long-term results of straight and bifurcated aortic grafts for abdominal aortic aneurysm repair: a population-based experience. p. 301. In Greenhalgh RM, Hollier LH (eds): The Maintenance of Arterial Reconstruction. WB Saunders, London, 1991

25. Calcagno D, Hallett JW, Ballard DJ et al: Late iliac artery aneurysms and occlusive disease following aortic tube grafts for abdominal aortic aneurysm repair: a 35-year experience in one community. Ann Surg 214:733, 1991

26. Nunn DB, Carter MM, Donohue MT, Hudgins PC: Postoperative dilation of knitted Dacron aortic bifurcation graft. J Vasc Surg 12:291, 1990

27. Krupski WC: The peripheral vascular consequences of smoking. Ann Vasc Surg 5:291, 1991

28. Plate G, Hollier LH, O'Brien PC et al: Late cerebrovascular accidents after repair of abdominal aortic aneurysms. Acta Chir Scand 154:25, 1988

29. Harris PL: Follow-up after reconstructive arterial surgery. Eur J Vasc Surg 5:369, 1991

30. Brown OW, Stanson AW, Pairolero PC, Hollier LH: Computerized tomography following abdominal aortic surgery. Surgery 91:716, 1982

31. Stanford W, Rooholamini SA, Galvin JR: Ultrafast computed tomography in the diagnosis of aortic aneurysms and dissections. J Thorac Imaging 5:32, 1990

Index

Page numbers followed by f indicate figures; those followed by t indicate tables.

A

Abdominal aorta
  aneurysms of. *See* Abdominal aortic
    aneurysms (AAA).
  duplex scanning of, in renovascular hyper-
    tension, 697
  examination of, 581
  traumatic injury of, angiography in, 218
Abdominal aortic aneurysms (AAA),
    565–568
  complications of, 565, 566t
  compression of adjacent structures by,
    574
  computed tomography of, 595f
  erosion of, 573
  imaging of, 589, 590f, 591f
  nonresective treatment of, 621–622
  pathophysiology of, 559–563, 560f
    atherosclerosis and, 562
    clinical observations and, 559–560
    collagen metabolism and, 561–562,
      562f
    elastin metabolism and, 561, 561f
    genetic factors in, 560, 560t
    ruptured aneurysms and, 562, 562f
    unified hypothesis of, 562–563, 563f
  quality of life and functional status and,
    567
  rupture of, 562, 562f, 615
    expansion rate and, 567, 567f
    risk of, 565–567, 566f
  screening for, 567–568

size of, 606
survival and, 567
Abdominal mass, pulsatile, imaging and,
    602–603
Ablative surgery, in chronic venous
    insufficiency, of lower extremity,
    987–988
Abnormal arteriovenous communications
    (AVC), 1107
Absolute alcohol, in arteriovenous malfor-
    mations, 1129
Acceleration index (AI), 186
Acceleration time (AT), 186
Acceleration time ratio (ATR), 186
Acidic fibroblast growth factor (aFGF), in
    intimal hyperplasia, 25
Activated clotting factors, thrombus forma-
    tion and, 124
Activated partial thromboplastin time (aPTT),
    monitoring of heparin therapy using,
    879
Acute extremity ischemia, 303
  embolization and thrombosis and. *See*
    Embolism, peripheral; Thrombosis,
    peripheral.
  fibrinolytic system and. *See* Fibrinolytic
    system.
  graft failure causing. *See* Graft failure.
  pathophysiology of, 305–309
  reperfusion syndrome and, 305–306,
    306f
  skeletal muscle ischemia-reperfusion
    injury and, 306–308, 308f

clinical modification of, 308–309
thrombolytic therapy for. *See* Percu-
    taneous intra-arterial thrombolysis
    (PIAT); Thrombolytic therapy.
traumatic, 303, 399–416. *See also specific*
    vessels.
  amputation and, 411
  arteriography in. *See* Arteriography, in
    traumatic injuries.
  in children, 416, 416t
  diagnosis of, 400–404
  drug abuse and, 411–412
  etiology of, 399
  fasciotomy in. *See* Fasciotomy.
  history in, 400–401
  iatrogenic injuries and. *See* Iatrogenic
    injuries.
  location of, 400, 400t
  management of, 404
  mechanism of, 400
  physical examination in, 401
  primary versus interposition grafts in,
    404–405, 405t
Acute renal failure (ARF), aortoiliac opera-
    tions and, 1154–1155
Acute tubular necrosis (ATN), acute
    rejection distinguished from,
    187–188
Adventitial cystic disease. *See* Cystic
    disease, adventitial.
Age. *See also* Children; Infants.
  deep venous thrombosis and, 120
  fibrinolysis and, 323

Chronic venous insufficiency (CVI), 941–948, 951–960
  ambulatory compression in, 952–958
    adjunctive devices and, 957–958
    Circ-Aid device and, 957, 957f
    elastic compression stockings and, 952–956, 953t
      Oregon protocol for treatment of venous ulceration and, 953, 954f, 955f, 955–956
    Unna boot and, 956, 957t
  anatomy and physiology of, 941–942, 942f
  complications of surgical treatment of, 1209–1212, 1210t–1212t
  continuous wave Doppler studies in, 945–946
  deep, surgical management of, 988–995
    cross-femoral venous bypass in, 992–993
    iliac vein decompression in, 993–994
    inferior vena caval reconstruction in, 994
    saphenopopliteal bypass in, 993
    valvuloplasty in, 988, 989t, 990, 991–992
    vein segment transposition in, 990, 1210–1211
    vein valve transplantation in, 990–991
  descending phlebography in, 943–944, 944f
  diagnosis of, 952
  duplex scanning in, 946–947, 947f, 948f
  history in, 943
  of lower extremity, 983–995
    communicating vein, surgical management of, 987–988
    diagnosis of, 984, 985f, 986
    pathophysiology and clinical manifestations of, 983–984, 984t
    superficial, surgical management of, 986–987
    surgical management of, 986–995
  pathogenesis of, 951–952
  pharmacologic therapy in, 958–959
    anticoagulants and, 959
    fibrinolysis-enhancing agents and, 958
    pentoxifylline and, 959
    phlebotropic agents and, 958–959
    prostaglandins and, 959
  physical examination in, 943
  plethysmography in, 944–945, 945f
  post-thrombotic, 1211
  pressure measurements in, 945
  roentgenographic studies in, 943
  sclerotherapy in, 960

surgical management of, deep venous insufficiency and. *See* Chronic venous insufficiency (CVI), deep, surgical management of.
  topical preparations in, 959–960
  treatment of, complications of, 1209–1212, 1210t–1212t
  of upper extremity, 973–981
    axillosubclavian obstruction in absence of trauma of thrombosis and, 975
    diagnosis of, 975–976
    iatrogenic trauma to axillosubclavian veins and, 975
    indications for surgical treatment of, 976f, 976–977, 977t
    operative procedures for, 977–979, 979f, 979t, 980f, 981
    spontaneous axillosubclavian venous thrombosis and, 974f, 974–975
Circ-Aid device, in chronic venous insufficiency, 957, 957f
Circle of Willis, in subclavian steal syndromes, 78
Claudication. *See also* Intermittent claudication.
  in aortoiliac disease, treatment of, 471
  hemodynamics in, exercise testing and, 149, 149f
  neurogenic, 424
  surgical management of, 494
  vasculogenic, 424
Clavicular resection, in chronic venous insufficiency of upper extremity, 978
Claviculectomy, medial, in chronic venous insufficiency of upper extremity, 978
Clot extraction, emergency, in acute lower limb ischemia, 359
Coagulation, thrombus formation and, 124–125
Coagulopathies. *See also* Hypercoagulable states.
  endovascular intervention and, 1227
  minimizing, 1152
  pulmonary angiography and, 925
  upper extremity arterial disease and, 541
Coarctation
  of the aorta, adult, 268
  atherosclerotic, angiography in, 209, 209f
Cockett's veins, 131
Coils, steel, for transcatheter embolization, 827–828, 828f
Colestipol, plaque growth and, 9
Colic artery
  left, 796
  middle, 771, 771f, 772f

right, 771, 771f
Collagen
  in arterial wall, 63–64
  metabolism of, abdominal aortic aneurysms and, 561–562, 562f
Collateral circulation
  arterial, in subclavian steal syndromes, 78
  carotid angiography and, 274–275
  hemodynamics and, 68–69, 69f, 70f
  intestinal, 796
  splanchnic artery operations and, 1193, 1193f
Colon. *See also headings beginning with* terms Bowel *and* Intestinal.
  vascular anatomy of, 770–771, 771f, 772f, 773
Color Doppler, in deep venous thrombosis, 869, 871f, 874, Plate 60–1
Color-flow imaging
  in aortoiliac and lower extremity arterial disease, 180, 181, 183
  in peripheral arterial disease, 428–429
  physics of, 170–171, Plate 12–2, Plate 12–3
  of portal vein, 758
  in renal artery disease, 184
  in visceral vascular disorders, 752–753
Common carotid artery, balloon injury of, in rat, 18
Common femoral artery
  arteriovenous graft placement in, 1056, 1057f
  as inflow for infrapopliteal bypass grafting, 512
Communicating veins, 941–942, 942f
  chronic insufficiency of, 984
    surgical management of, 986–987
  incompetent, 984, 1209
    surgical management of, 987–988
  of lower extremity, 131
Compartment syndromes
  fasciotomy in. *See* Fasciotomy.
  percutaneous intra-arterial thrombolysis and, 369–370
  tissue pressures measurement in, 409
Compliance mismatch, graft patency and, 92f–94f, 92–93
Compression sclerotherapy (CST)
  complications of, 1208f, 1208–1209
  in varicose veins, 1205, 1208
Compression stockings, in chronic venous insufficiency, 952–956, 953t
  of lower extremity, 986
  Oregon protocol for treatment of venous ulceration and, 953, 954f, 955f, 955–956